Medical
Biochemistry

THIRD EDITION

John W Baynes PhD

Carolina Distinguished Professor Emeritus
Department of Chemistry and Biochemistry
Graduate Science Research Center
University of South Carolina
Columbia, South Carolina
USA

Marek H Dominiczak MD FRCPath FRCP(Glas)

Professor in the Medical Faculty
University of Glasgow

Consultant Biochemist
NHS Greater Glasgow and Clyde
Gartnavel General Hospital
Glasgow
UK

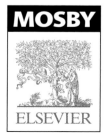

MOSBY an imprint of Elsevier Limited

MOSBY
ELSEVIER

First published 1999
Second Edition 2005
Third Edition 2009
   Reprinted 2009

ISBN: 978-0-323-05371-6

British Library Cataloguing in Publication Data
A catalogue record for this book is available from the British Library

Library of Congress Cataloging in Publication Data
A catalog record for this book is available from the Library of Congress

Notice
Medical knowledge is constantly changing. Standard safety precautions must be followed, but as new research and clinical experience broaden our knowledge, changes in treatment and drug therapy may become necessary or appropriate. Readers are advised to check the most current product information provided by the manufacturer of each drug to be administered to verify the recommended dose, the method and duration of administration, and contraindications. It is the responsibility of the practitioner, relying on experience and knowledge of the patient, to determine dosages and the best treatment for each individual patient. Neither the Publisher nor the author assume any liability for any injury and/or damage to persons or property arising from this publication.

The Publisher

Printed in China
Last digit is the print number: 9 8 7 6 5 4 3 2

Contents

Preface

We are delighted to present the third edition of *Medical Biochemistry*. It has been rewarding to see the previous editions of the text adopted at an increasing number of universities across the world. In the third edition, our aim remains the same: to provide a biochemical foundation for the study of clinical medicine – with maximum practical relevance. The ultimate goal is to help shape a scientifically informed clinician.

The third edition has again been substantially updated. Chapters on lipids, biochemical endocrinology and glucose homoeostasis have been rewritten, and the ones on regulation of gene expression and recombinant DNA technology have been updated to include recent developments in these rapidly evolving fields. We also recruited several new authors to provide a new perspective on the coverage of some complex topics such as protein and nucleotide biosynthesis, and DNA and RNA. We have added a new chapter on systems biochemistry, the-omics: genomics, proteomics and metabolomics, to complement existing chapters on biotechnology and gene expression. All chapters have been revised with emphasis on clarity of presentation. We were also keen to remove redundant or outdated matter. Literature references have been updated throughout, and there are now many more references to relevant websites. In this edition, we have removed the Question Bank (Self Assessment), because these resources, and much more, are available at the Elsevier website: www.student consult.com, to which the reader is referred.

We have included many new cross-references: these take the reader to related subjects and clinical cases in different chapters of the book. This way the Clinical, Diagnostic or Advanced Knowledge boxes complement text in several different chapters. Remember, however, that using these cross-references is optional: each chapter is also a self-contained story.

In this edition the reader will see more emphasis on signaling systems and cascades of regulatory reactions. We have focused on these complex pathways because regulation of signal transduction provides enormous potential for development of novel therapies. A word of warning: the reader will soon notice that terminology in the gene expression and signaling fields is often difficult for the nonspecialist (as well as the specialist!). Many names of genes and transcription factors are enigmatic, at best. The ones we have included here are not to be memorized but to provide a coherent picture and a fact-based model for other systems in regulatory biology.

The strength of the book is that it marries (we hope happily) aspects of 'conventional' biochemistry with a substantial amount of molecular biology. Our judgment on how much of each to include was driven by pragmatism: the relevance of a given subject to today's practice of medicine.

The text touches upon several interdisciplinary interfaces, the most important being the one between biochemistry and molecular biology. There are others: the chapters on water and electrolyte metabolism and on acid-base balance in traditional teaching belong to physiology. We believe, however, that they are essential for the understanding of biochemistry in medicine. We have also included a substantial amount of 'diagnostic' (clinical) biochemistry, which illuminates interpretation of tests commonly used in clinical practice. This not only makes the book more valuable for a medical student but extends its usefulness to those with either a medical or science background who intend to pursue a career in laboratory medicine.

Our hope is that *Medical Biochemistry* offers the reader a broad perspective on biochemistry and on its future potential. If it manages this, it is because our contributors represent a very broad range of expertise – they include investigators involved in cutting-edge basic research as well as experienced clinicians who spend most of their time on the wards and in the outpatient clinics. Therefore, we believe, one classic criticism of a medical biochemistry textbook does not apply here: this is not a book where clinicians theorize about science, or scientists about clinical practice, it is an integrated work that genuinely combines research and practice.

We hope it makes an enjoyable read. We look forward to hearing your comments and suggestions.

List of Contributors

Gary A Bannon PhD
Director
Section on Protein Analytics
Regulatory Division
Monsanto
St Louis, MO, USA

John W Baynes PhD
Carolina Distinguished Professor Emeritus
Department of Chemistry and Biochemistry
Graduate Science Research Center
University of South Carolina
Columbia, SC, USA

Robert Best PhD
Professor
Division of Medical Genetics
School of Medicine
University of South Carolina
Columbia, SC, USA

Franklyn F Bolander Jr MD PhD
Associate Professor in Biological Sciences
Department of Biological Sciences
University of South Carolina
Columbia, SC, USA

Iain Broom MBChB MIBiol FRCPath FRCP
Professor of Clinical Biochemistry; Consultant in Clinical
Biochemistry and Metabolic Medicine
The Robert Gordon University
School of Life Sciences
Aberdeen, UK

James A Carson PhD
Associate Professor
Department of Exercise Science
University of Southern Carolina
Columbia, SC, USA

Wayne M Carver PhD
Associate Professor
Department of Cell and Developmental Biology and
Anatomy
University of South Carolina
School of Medicine
Columbia, SC, USA

Marek H Dominiczak MD FRCPath FRCP(Glas)
Professor in the Medical Faculty
University of Glasgow;
Consultant Biochemist
cNHS Greater Glasgow and Clyde
Gartnavel General Hospital
Glasgow, UK

Alan D Elbein PhD
Professor and Chair
Department of Biochemistry and Molecular Biology
University of Arkansas for Medical Sciences
Little Rock, AR, USA

Alex Farrell FRCPath (deceased)
Formerly Consultant Immunologist; Head of
Department of Clinical Immunology, Immunopathology,
Histocompatibility and Immunogenetics
Western Infirmary
Glasgow, UK

William D Fraser BSc MD MRCP FRCPath
Professor of Clinical Biochemistry
Department of Clinical Chemistry
Royal Liverpool University Hospital
Liverpool, UK

Junichi Fujii PhD
Professor
Department of Biomolecular Function
Graduate School of Medical Science
Yamagata University
Yamagata, Japan

Peter J Galloway DCH FRCP (Edin) FRCPath
Consultant Chemical Pathologist
NHS Greater Glasgow and Clyde
Yorkhill Hospital for Sick Children
Glasgow, UK

Helen S Goodridge BSc PhD
Research Scientist
Immunobiology Research Institute
Cedars-Sinai Medical Center
Los Angeles, CA, USA

J Alastair Gracie BSc PhD
Senior University Teacher
Division of Immunology, Infection and Inflammation
Glasgow Biomedical Research Centre
University of Glasgow
Glasgow, UK

Alehandro Gugliucci MD PhD
Professor of Biochemistry
Touro University
Vallejo, CA, USA

Margaret M Harnett BSc PhD
Professor of Immune Signalling
Division of Immunology, Infection and Inflammation
Glasgow Biomedical Research Centre
University of Glasgow
Glasgow, UK

Simon Heales PhD FRCPath
Consultant Clinical Scientist
Department of Clinical Biochemistry
National Hospital for Neurology and Neurosurgery
London, UK

George M Helmkamp Jr PhD
Professor of Biochemistry
Department of Biochemistry and Molecular Biology
University of Kansas School of Medicine
Kansas City, KS, USA

D Margaret Hunt BA PhD
Associate Professor
Department of Pathology and Microbiology
University of South Carolina School of Medicine
Columbia, SC, USA

Andrew Jamieson MBChB(Hons) PhD FRCP(Glas)
Consultant Physician
Department of Medicine
Hairmyres Hospital
East Kilbride, UK

Alan F Jones DPhil FRCP FRCPath
Consultant Physician and Chemical Pathologist
Department of Clinical Biochemistry and Immunology
Birmingham Heartlands and Solihull NHS Trust
Birmingham, UK

Gur Prasad Kaushal PhD
Professor of Medicine
Department of Medicine, Division of Nephrology
University of Arkansas for Medical Sciences
Little Rock, AR, USA

W Stephen Kistler PhD
Professor of Biochemistry
Department of Chemistry
University of South Carolina
Columbia, SC, USA

Walter Kolch MD DR MED HAB
Professor of Molecular Cell Biology
Beatson Institute for Cancer Research
Glasgow, UK

Utkarsh V Kulkarni MBBS MD MRCP DipRCPath
Senior Research Fellow
Centre for Obesity Research and Epidemiology
The Robert Gordon University
Aberdeen, UK

Gordon Lowe MD FRCP
Professor of Vascular Medicine
Division of Cardiovascular Medical Sciences
University of Glasgow
Royal Infirmary
Glasgow, UK

Masatomo Maeda PhD
Professor of Pharmaceutical Sciences
Laboratory of Biochemistry and Molecular Biology
Graduate School of Pharmaceutical Sciences
Osaka University
Osaka, Japan

Jeffrey R Patton PhD
Associate Professor
Department of Pathology, Microbiology and
Immunology
School of Medicine
University of South Carolina
Columbia, SC, USA

Andrew Pitt BSc DPhil
Director
Sir Henry Wellcome Functional Genomics Facility;
Senior Lecturer
Department of Integrative and Systems Biology
University of Glasgow
Glasgow, UK

Allen B Rawitch PhD
Professor of Biochemistry and Molecular Biology
Office of Academic Affairs
University of Kansas Medical Center
Kansas City, KS, USA

Peter F Semple MD FRCP
Senior Lecturer; Consultant Physician
Department of Medicine and Therapeutics
University of Glasgow
Western Infirmary
Glasgow, UK

Robert K Semple PhD MRCP
Wellcome Trust Clinician Scientist Fellow
Department of Clinical Biochemistry
Cambridge University
Cambridge, UK

L William Stillway PhD
Professor of Biochemistry and Molecular Biology
Department of Biochemistry and Molecular Biology
Medical University of Southern Carolina
Charleston, SC, USA

Mirosława Szczepaùska-Konkel PhD
Professor of Clinical Biochemistry
Laboratory of Cellular and Molecular Nephrology
Polish Academy of Sciences Medical Research Centre
Medical School of Gdansk
Gdansk, Poland

Naoyuki Taniguchi MD PhD
Professor
Department of Biochemistry
Osaka University Medical School
Osaka, Japan

Yee Ping Teoh MBDS MRCP DipRCPath
Consultant Chemical Pathologist
Department of Medical Biochemistry
Wrexham Maelor Hospital
Wrexham, UK

Edward J Thompson PhD MD DSc FRCPath FRCP
Professor of Neurochemistry
Department of Neuroimmunology
Institute of Neurology
National Hospital for Nervous Diseases
London, UK

Robert Thornburg PhD
Professor of Biochemistry
Department of Biochemistry, Biophysics and Molecular
Biology
Iowa State University
Ames, IA, USA

A Michael Wallace BSc MSc PhD FRCPath
Professor, University of Strathclyde
Consultant Clinical Scientist
Department of Clinical Biochemistry
Royal Infirmary
Glasgow, UK

Dedication

John Baynes
To all the co-authors, who have contributed their expertise
and guidance to Medical Biochemistry

Marek Dominiczak
To my teachers, H Gemmel Morgan and Stefan Angielski
To Anna, my parents and Peter Jacob
To my students and trainees
To those who will shape the future of biochemistry

Acknowledgments

We thank the contributors to this edition for their effort and expertise and for coping with the many editors' requests. We welcome new contributors to this edition: Wayne Carver, Alistair Gracie, Alejandro Gugliucci, Walter Kolch, Utkarsh Kulkarni, Jeffrey Patton, and Yee Ping Teoh. We again thank Peter Semple for scrutinizing the clinical boxes and Peter Galloway for reviewing and contributing many pediatric cases for the second edition. We were greatly saddened by the untimely death of Alex Farrell who wrote the original chapter on the immune system.

We thank our students for their comments, which they share with us in the teaching laboratories and at lectures and tutorials, and for reviews, suggestions and criticisms posted on the web. We are also indebted to many doctors and nurses whom we met on ward rounds, and particularly to the members of the Nutrition Team in Glasgow where multidisciplinary discussions channel expertise from different fields into patient care.

We thank the team at Elsevier – Alex Stibbe, Kate Dimock, Nani Clansey and Kerrie-Anne McKinlay – for expertly guiding this edition from the idea, through writing and proofs, to publication. We are grateful to the artists for their continuing efforts in preparing the illustrations and to the proofreaders, Anne Powell and Punella Theakes, for their thoroughness. As before, we greatly appreciate the invaluable secretarial assistance of Ms. Jacky Gardiner in Glasgow.

Abbreviations

A	adenine	bw	body weight
ACE	angiotensin-converting enzyme	C	cytosine
acetyl-CoA	acetyl-coenzyme A	CA	carbonic anhydrase
ACh	acetylcholine	CAD	caspase-dependent endonuclease
ACTase	aspartate carbamoyl transferase	CAIR	carboxyaminoimidazole ribonucleotide
ACTH	adrenocorticotropic hormone		
ADC	AIDS-dementia complex	cAMP	cyclic AMP
ADH	alcohol dehydrogenase	CAT	catalase
ADH	antidiuretic hormone (also known as AVP)	CD	cluster designation: classification system for cell surface molecules
ADP	adenosine diphosphate	CDGS	carbohydrate-deficient glycoprotein syndromes
AFP	α-fetoprotein		
AGE	advanced glycoxidation (glycation) end-product	CDK	cyclin-dependent kinase
		CDKI	cyclin-dependent kinase inhibitor
AHF	antihemophilic factor	CDP	cytidine diphosphate
AICAR	5-aminoimidazole-4-carboxamide ribonucleotide	CFTR	cystic fibrosis transmembrane conductance regulator
AIDS	acquired immunodeficiency syndrome	cGMP	cyclic GMP
		CITP	carboxy terminal procollagan extension peptide
AIR	5-aminoimidazole ribonucleotide		
ALDH	aldehyde dehydrogenase	CML	chronic myeloid leukemia
ALP	alkaline phosphatase	CMP	cytidine monophosphate
ALT	alanine aminotransferase	CNS	central nervous system
AML	acute myeloblastic leukemia	COAD	chronic obstructive airways disease (synonym: COPD)
AMP	adenosine monophosphate		
APC	adenomatous polyposis coli (gene)	COMT	catecholamine-O-methyl transferase
APO-1	'death domain'-receptor Fas	COPD	chronic obstructive pulmonary disease (synonym: COAD)
apoA, B etc	apolipoprotein A, B etc		
APRT	adenosine phosphoribosyl transferase	CoQ_{10}	coenzyme Q_{10} (ubiquinone)
		COX-1	cyclooxygenase-1
APTT	activated partial thromboplastin time	CPK	creatine phosphokinase
		CPS I, II	carbamoyl phosphate synthetase I, II
ARDS	acute respiratory distress syndrome		
AST	aspartate aminotransferase	CPT I, II	carnitine palmitoyl transferase I, II
ATF	activation transcription factor	CREB	cAMP-responsive element-binding protein
ATM	ataxia telangiectasia-mutated gene		
ATP	adenosine triphosphate	CRGP	calcitonin-related gene peptide
AVP	arginine-vasopressin (same as antidiuretic hormone)	CRH	corticotropin-releasing hormone
		CRP	C-reactive protein
AZT	3′-azido-3′-deoxythymidine	CSF	cerebrospinal fluid
2,3-BPG	2,3-bisphosphoglycerate	CT	calcitonin
Bcl-2	B cell lymphoma protein 2	CTP	cytidine triphosphate
bp	base pair	CVS	chorionic villous sampling
BUN	blood urea nitrogen equivalent of (but not the same as) blood urea	DAG	diacylglycerol
		DCC	'delete in colon carcinoma' gene

DEAE	diethylaminoethyl		Fru-6-P	fructose-6-phosphate
DGGE	denaturing-gradient gel electrophoresis		FSF	fibrin-stabilizing factor
DHAP	dihydroxyacetone phosphate		FSH	follicle-stimulating hormone
DIC	disseminated intravascular coagulation		G	guanine
			G3PDH	glyceraldehyde-3-phosphate dehydrogenase
DIPF	diisopropylphosphofluoride		GABA	γ-amino butyric acid
DNA	deoxyribonucleic acid		GAG	glycosaminoglycan
DNP	2,4-dinitrophenol		Gal	galactose
Dol-P	dolichol phosphate		Gal-1-P	galactose-1-phosphate
Dol-PP-GlcNAc	dolichol pyrophosphate-acetylglucosamine		GalNAc	N-acetylgalactosamine
			GalNH$_2$	galactosamine
DOPA	dihydroxyphenylalanine		GAP	guanosine–triphosphatase activating protein
DPPC	dipalmitoylphosphatidylcholine			
EBV	Epstein–Barr virus		GAR	glycinamide ribonucleotide
ECF	extracellular fluid		GDH	glutamate dehydrogenase
ECM	extracellular matrix		GDP	guanosine diphosphate
EDRF	endothelium-derived relaxing factor (NO)		GDP-D-Man	guanosine diphosphate-D-mannose
EDTA	ethylenediaminetetraacetic acid		GDP-L-Fuc	guanosine diphosphate-L-fucose
EF-1,2	elongation factor-1, -2		GDP-Man	guanosine diphosphate-mannose
EF2	eukaryotic elongation factor		GFAP	glial fibrillary acid protein
EGF	epidermal growth factor		γGT	γ-glutamyl transferase
eIF-3	eukaryotic cell initiation factor(-3)		GH	growth hormone
ELK	transcription factor		GHRH	growth hormone-releasing hormone
ER	endoplasmic reticulum			
ERK	extracellular-regulated kinase		GIP	glucose-dependent insulinotropic peptide
ESR	erythrocyte sedimentation rate			
F-ATPase	coupling factor-type ATPase		GIT	gastrointestinal tract
FACIT	fibril-associated collagen with interrupted triple helices		GK	glucokinase
			Glc	glucose
FAD	flavin adenine dinucleotide		Glc-1-P	glucose-1-phosphate
FADD	a 'death domain' accessory protein		Glc-6-P	glucose-6-phosphate
FADH$_2$	reduced flavin adenine dinucleotide		Glc-6-Pase	glucose-6-phosphatase
			GlcN-6-P	glucosamine-6-phosphate
FAICAR	5-formylaminoimidazole-4-carboxamide ribonucleotide		GlcNAc	N-acetylglucosamine
			GlcNAc-1P	N-acetylglucosamine-1-phosphate
FAP	familial adenomatous polyposis		GlcNAc-6-P	N-acetylglucosamine-6-phosphate
Fas	apoptosis signaling molecule: a 'death domain' accessory protein (CD95)		GlcNH$_2$	glucosamine
			GlcUA	D-glucuronic acid
			GLP-1	glucagon-like peptide-1
FBPase	fructose bisphosphatase		GLUT	glucose transporter (GLUT-1 to GLUT-5)
FCγR	group of immunoglobulin receptors			
			GM1	monosialoganglioside 1
FDP	fibrin degradation product		GMP	guanosine monophosphate
FGAR	formylglycinamide ribonucleotide		GnRH	gonadotropin-releasing hormone
FGF	fibroblast growth factor		GP1b-IXa (etc.)	glycoprotein receptor 1b-IXa (etc.)
FHH	familial hypocalciuric hypercalcemia		GPx	Glutathione peroxidase
			GRE	glucocorticoid response element
FMN	flavin mononucleotide		GSH	reduced glutathione
FMNH$_2$	reduced flavin mononucleotide		GSSG	oxidized glutathione
FRAXA	fragile X syndrome		GTP	guanosine triphosphate
Fru-1,6-BP	fructose-1,6 bisphosphate		GTPase	guanosine triphosphatase
Fru-2,6-BP	fructose-2,6 bisphosphate		5-HIAA	5-hydroxyindoleacetic acid
Fru-2,6-BPase	fructose-2,6 bisphosphatase		5-HT	5-hydroxytryptamine

Hb	hemoglobin	JNK	Jun N-terminal kinase
HCM	hypercalcemia associated with malignancy	K	equilibrium constant
		kb	kilobase
Hct	hematocrit	kbp	kilobase pair(s)
HDL	high-density lipoprotein	KCCT	kaolin-cephalin clotting time
HGF-R	hepatocyte growth factor receptor	KIP2	cell cycle regulatory molecule
		K_m	Michaelis constant
HGPRT	hypoxanthine-guanine phospho-ribosyl transferase	LACI	lipoprotein-associated coagulation inhibitor
HIV	human immunodeficiency virus	LCAT	lecithin: cholesterol acyltransferase
HLA	human leukocyte antigen (system)	LDH	lactate dehydrogenase
		LDL	low-density lipoprotein
HLH	helix-loop-helix (motif)	LH	luteinizing hormone
HMG	hydroxymethylglutaryl	LPL	lipoprotein lipase
HMWK	high-molecular-weight kininogen	LPS	lipopolysaccharide
		LRP-LDL	LDL-receptor-related protein
HNPCC	hereditary nonpolyposis colorectal cancer	M-CSF-R	macrophage colony-stimulating factor receptor
hnRNA	heteronuclear ribonucleic acid	Malonyl-CoA	malonyl-coenzyme A
HPLC	high-pressure liquid chromatography	Man	mannose
		Man-1-P	mannose-1-phosphate
HPT	hyperparathyroidism	Man-6-P	mannose-6-phosphate
HRT	hormone replacement therapy	MAO	monoamine oxidase
HTGL	hepatic triglyceride lipase	MAPK	mitogen-activated protein kinase (a superfamily of signal-transducing kinases)
HTH	helix-turn-helix (motif)		
ICAM-1	intracellular cell adhesion molecule-1		
		Mb	myoglobin
ICF	intracellular fluid	MCHC	mean corpuscular hemoglobin concentration
IDDM	Type 1 diabetes mellitus (term now substituted by Type 1 diabetes mellitus)		
		MCP-1	monocyte chemoattractant protein-1
IDL	intermediate-density lipoprotein	MCV	mean corpuscular volume
		MDR	multidrug resistance
IdUA	L-iduronic acid	MEK	mitogen-activated protein kinase kinase
IFN-γ	interferon-γ		
Ig	immunoglobulin	MEK	protein kinase belonging to the MAPK superfamily
IGF	insulin growth factor		
IGF-I	insulin-like growth factor-I	MEN IIA	multiple endocrine neoplasia type IIA
IL	interleukin (IL-1–IL-29)		
IMP	inosine monophosphate	met-tRNA	methionyl-tRNA
Inr	initiator (nucleotide sequence of a gene)	MGUS	monoclonal gammopathy of uncertain significance
IP_1 I-1-P_1, I-4-P_1 (etc.)	inositol monophosphate	MHC	major histocompatibility complex
IP_2, I-1, 3-P_2, I-1, 4-P_2	inositol bisphosphate		
IP_3, I-1,4, 5-P_3	inositol trisphosphate	mRNA	messenger ribonucleic acid
IP_4, I-1,3,4, 5-P_4	inositol tetraphosphate	MPO	myeloperoxidase
IRE	iron response element	MRP	multidrug resistance-associated protein
IRF-BP	IRE-binding protein		
IRMA	immunoradiometric assay	MS	mass spectrometry
ITAM	immunoreceptor tyrosine activation motif	MSH	melanocyte-stimulating hormone
ITIM	immunoreceptor tyrosine inhibition motif	MSUD	maple syrup urine disease
		MyoD	muscle cell-specific transporter factor
JAK	Janus kinase		

Na$^+$/K$^+$-ATPase	sodium-potassium ATPase
NABQI	N-acetyl benzoquinoneimine
NAC	N-acetylcysteine
NAD$^+$	nicotinamide adenine dinucleotide (oxidized)
NADH	nicotinamide adenine dinucleotide (reduced)
NADP$^+$	nicotinamide adenine dinucleotide phosphate (oxidized)
NADPH	nicotinamide adenine dinucleotide phosphate (reduced)
NANA	N-acetyl neuraminic acid (sialic acid)
NF	nuclear factor
NF-II	type II neurofibromatosis
NGF	nerve growth factor
NIDDM	noninsulin-dependent diabetes mellitus
NMDA	N-methyl-D-aspartate
NPY	neuropeptide Y
NSAID	nonsteroidal antiinflammatory drug
nt	nucleotide (as measure of size/length of a nucleic acid)
1,25(OH)$_2$D$_3$	1,25-dihydroxy vitamin D$_3$
OGTT	oral glucose tolerance test
8-oxo-Gua	8-oxo-2'-deoxyguanosine
OxS	oxidative stress
P-ATPase	phosphorylation-type ATPase
3-PG	3-phosphoglycerate
p38RK	p38-reactivating kinase
Pa	Pascal
PA	phosphatidic acid
PAF	platelet-activating factor
PAGE	polyacrylamide gel electrophoresis
PAI-1	plasminogen activator inhibitor type 1
PAPS	phosphoadenosine phosphosulfate
PC	phosphatidyl choline
PC	pyruvate carboxylase
PCP	phencyclidine
PCR	polymerase chain reaction
PDE	phosphodiesterase
PDGF	platelet-derived growth factor
PDH	pyruvate dehydrogenase
PDK	phosphatidylinositol trisphosphate-dependent kinase
PE	phosphatidyl ethanolamine
PEP	phosphoenolpyruvic acid
PEPCK	phosphoenolpyruvate carboxykinase
PF3	platelet factor 3
PFK-1 (-2)	phosphofructokinase-1 (-2)
PGG$_2$	prostaglandin G$_2$ (etc.)
PGK	phosphoglycerate kinase
PGM	phosphoglucomutase
PHHI	persistent hyperinsulinemic hypoglycemia of infancy
PHP	pseudohypoparathyroidism
Pi	inorganic phosphate
PI-3-K	phosphoinositide-3-kinase
PICP	amino terminal procollagen extension peptide
PIP$_2$/PIP$_3$	phosphatidylinositol bisphosphate/trisphosphate
PK	pyruvate kinase
PKA/PKC	protein kinase A/C
PKU	phenylketonuria
PL	phospholipase A etc
PLA/PLC	phospholipase A/C
PMA	phorbol myristic acetate
PNS	peripheral nervous system
PPi	inorganic pyrophosphate
PRL	prolactin
PrP	prion protein
PRPP	5-phosphoribosyl-α-pyrophosphate
PS	phosphatidyl serine
PTA	plasma thromboplastin antecedent
PTH	parathyroid hormone
PTHrP	parathyroid hormone-related protein
PTK	protein tyrosine kinase
PTPase	phosphotyrosine phosphatase
Py	pyrimidine base (in a nucleotide sequence)
R	receptor (with qualifier, not alone)
RAIDD	a 'death domain' accessory protein
Rb	retinoblastoma protein
RBC	red blood cell
RDS	respiratory distress syndrome
RER	rough endoplasmic reticulum
RFLP	restriction fragment length polymorphism
RIP	a 'death domain' accessory protein
RKK	p38RK homolog of MEK
RNA	ribonucleic acid
RNAPol II	RNA polymerase II
RNR	ribonucleotide reductase
RNS	reactive nitrogen species

ROS	reactive oxygen species	TBG	thyroid-binding globulin
S	Svedberg unit	TCA	tricarboxylic acid cycle
SACAIR	5-aminoimidazole-4-(N-succinylocarboxamide) ribonucleotide	TF	transcription factor (with qualifier)
SAM	S-adenosyl methionine	TFPI	tissue factor pathway inhibitor
SAP1	transcription factor	TG	triacylglycerol (triglyceride)
SAPK	stress-activated protein kinase	TGF(-β)	transforming growth factor(-β)
SCIDS	severe combined immunodeficiency syndrome	T_{max}	renal transport maximum
scuPA	single-chain urinary-type plasminogen activator	TNF	tumor necrosis factor
		TNF-R	tumor necrosis factor receptor
SD	standard deviation	tPA	tissue-type plasminogen activator
SDS	sodium dodecyl sulfate	TRADD	a 'death domain' accessory protein
SDS-PAGE	sodium dodecyl sulfate-polyacryl-amide gel electrophoresis	TRAFS	a 'death domain' accessory protein
SGLT	Na^+-coupled glucose symporter	TRH	thyrotropin-releasing hormone
SEK	SAPK homolog of MEK	TSH	thyroid-stimulating hormone (thyrotropin)
SER	smooth endoplasmic reticulum		
ser-P	serine phosphate	TTP	thymidine triphosphate
SH	(figs only) steroid hormone	TXA_2	thromboxane A_2
SH2	Src-homology region-2	U	uridine
SIADH	syndrome of inappropriate antidiuretic hormone secretion	UCP	uncoupling protein
		UDP	uridine diphosphate
snRNA	small nuclear RNA	UDP-Gal	UDP-galactose
SOD	superoxide dismutase	UDP-GalNAc	UDP-N-acetylgalactosamine
SPCA	serum prothrombin conversion accelerator	UDP-Glc	UDP-glucose
		UDP-GlcNAc	UDP-N-acetylglucosamine
Src	a protein tyrosine kinase	UDP-GlcUA	UDP glucuronic acid
SRE	steroid response element	UMP	uridine monophosphate
SRP	signal recognition particle	uPA	urinary-type plasminogen activator
SSCP	single-strand conformational polymorphism		
SSRI	selective serotonin reuptake inhibitor	UV	ultraviolet
		VCAM-1	vascular cell adhesion molecule-1
STAT	signal transducer and activator of transcription	VDCC	voltage-dependent calcium channel
SUR	sulfonylurea receptor	VIP	vasoactive intestinal peptide
T	thymine	VLDL	very low-density lipoprotein
T tubule	transverse tubule	vWF	von Willebrand factor
T_3	tri-iodothyronine	WAF1	cell cycle regulator
T_4	thyroxine	X-SCID	X-linked severe combined immunodeficiency
TAG	triacylglycerol (triglyceride)	XMP	xanthine monophosphate
TAP	transporters associated with antigen presentation	XO	xanthine oxidase
		ZP3	zona pellucida 3 glycoprotein
TB	tuberculosis		

1. Introduction

J W Baynes and M H Dominiczak

BIOCHEMISTRY AND CLINICAL MEDICINE

Overview

Medical biochemistry covers aspects of biochemistry relevant to medicine and explains how the body works as a chemical system. It explains how it malfunctions in disease and tells how therapies are designed to restore body function. It provides a foundation for understanding the action of new drugs, such as antidepressants, drugs used to treat diabetes, hypertension and heart failure, and those that lower blood lipids. It helps to understand clinical applications of recombinant proteins and viral vectors. Medical biochemistry also contributes to understanding how lifestyle, and particularly diet, influence our performance, as well as how the organism ages. It describes how cellular signaling and communications systems are involved in response to endogenous and environmental stresses, and the action of new drugs which act through them. It also addresses the enormous progress made in recent years in understanding human genetics and provides a framework for appreciating the emerging fields of nutrigenomics and pharmacogenomics, that will hopefully create a basis for treatments customized to an individual's genetic make-up.

Focus

The human organism is, on the one hand, a tightly controlled, integrated metabolic system and on the other, a system that is open and communicates with its environment. Despite these two seemingly contradictory characteristics, the body manages to maintain its internal environment for decades. We regularly top up our fuel (consume food) and water, and take up oxygen from inspired air to use for oxidative metabolism (respiration is in fact a controlled, low-temperature combustion reaction). We then use the energy generated from metabolism to perform work and to maintain body temperature. We get rid of (exhale or excrete) carbon dioxide, water and nitrogenous waste. The amount and quality of food we consume have significant impact on our health – both malnutrition and obesity are currently major public health issues worldwide. One of the most important reasons to study biochemistry is to understand the interplay of nutrition, metabolism and genetics in health and disease.

ENTIRE BIOCHEMISTRY ON TWO PAGES

Editors say that any text can be shortened, no matter how important the details. Below we have attempted to condense our book to less than two pages. This gives a very general overview but also creates a useful mental framework for further study. The highlighted terms take you through the contents of the following chapters.

The major structural components of the body are proteins, carbohydrates and lipids

Proteins are building blocks and catalysts; as structural units, they form the architectural framework of our tissues; as enzymes, together with helper molecules known as **coenzymes** and **cofactors**, they catalyze and control biochemical reactions.

Carbohydrates and **lipids** are used primarily as energy sources. Their storage forms in the body are glycogen and triglycerides, Carbohydrates are also present as glycoconjugates with proteins and lipids, and lipids form the backbone of biological membranes.

Chemical variables, such as **pH, oxygen tension, inorganic ion and buffer concentrations,** define the homeostatic environment in which metabolism takes place. Small changes in this environment, for example, less than a tenth of a pH unit, can be life-threatening. All therapies, including emergency interventions, aim to maintain its stability.

Blood is the medium for exchange of gases, fuels, metabolites and information between tissues. Blood plasma is an accessible 'window' on metabolism and serves as a source of clinical information for the diagnosis and management of disease. The **blood coagulation system** and the **immune system** defend against disturbances in this environment.

Biological membranes compartmentalize metabolic pathways. They play a fundamental role in **ion and metabolite transport,** and also in **transducing signals** from one cell to another. Most of the body's energy is consumed to maintain ion and metabolite gradients across biological membranes; nerve and muscle function, and the red blood cell are critically dependent on membrane potentials, which are used for nerve transmission, muscle contraction and maintenance of cell shape.

Energy released from nutrients is distributed throughout the cell in the form of adenosine triphosphate

The recovery and utilization of energy in biological systems occur through **oxidative phosphorylation** which takes place in the **mitochondria**. This process involves oxygen consumption, or **respiration**, by which we capture the energy of fuels, produce a hydrogen ion gradient and convert this energy to **adenosine triphosphate (ATP)**. Biochemists call ATP the 'common currency of metabolism' for exchange of metabolic energy. It transduces energy from fuel metabolism for use in work, transport and biosyntheses.

Central pathways of carbohydrate and lipid metabolism are access routes to other processes

Sugars and fats are our primary sources of energy but our nutritional requirements also include amino acids or **proteins** and micronutrients – **vitamins and trace elements**.

Glucose is metabolized through **glycolysis**, a universal anaerobic pathway for energy production. Glycolysis transforms glucose into pyruvate, setting the stage for oxidative metabolism in the mitochondria. It also produces metabolites that are the starting points for synthesis of **amino acids**, **proteins**, **lipids** and **nucleic acids**. Glycolytic enzymes are regulated by several mechanisms: small-molecule effectors, reversible and irreversible chemical modification of key enzymes, and by control of gene expression.

The maintenance of a normal concentration of blood glucose is essential for our survival and is linked to the metabolism of **glycogen**, the short-term storage form of glucose. Glucose homeostasis is regulated by hormones (primarily insulin and glucagon and also epinephrine) that coordinate metabolic activities among cells and organs.

Oxygen is essential for survival but can also be toxic

During aerobic metabolism, pyruvate is transformed into **acetyl coenzyme A (acetyl-CoA)**, which is the common intermediate in the metabolism of carbohydrates, lipids and amino acids. Acetyl-CoA enters the central metabolic engine of the cell, the **tricarboxylic acid cycle (TCA cycle)** in the mitochondrion. Acetyl-CoA is oxidized to **carbon dioxide** and reduces the important coenzymes **nicotinamide adenine dinucleotide (NAD^+)** and **flavin adenine dinucleotide (FAD)**. Reduction of these nucleotides captures the energy from fuel oxidation, and they are in turn the substrates for the final pathway: **oxidative phosphorylation**. They become oxidized by molecular oxygen through a chain of **electron transport** reactions, providing the energy for **synthesis of ATP**.

While oxygen is essential for aerobic metabolism, it can also cause oxidative stress and widespread tissue damage during inflammation. To protect us from the more damaging effects of oxygen, we are endowed with powerful **antioxidant defenses**.

Eating and fasting shift body metabolism between the anabolic and catabolic states

Life can be divided into a continuous cycle of eating and not eating. The main pathways of carbohydrate and lipid metabolism are partially reversible and their direction changes in response to food intake. The direction of metabolism is constantly shifting during the feed–fast cycle. In the fed state, the active pathways are **glycolysis**, **glycogen synthesis**, **lipogenesis** and **protein synthesis**, rejuvenating tissues and storing the excess of metabolic fuel. In the fasting state, the direction of metabolism is reversed: glycogen and lipid stores are degraded through **glycogenolysis** and **lipolysis**. Protein is converted into glucose by the pathway of **gluconeogenesis**, and other biosynthetic processes are slowed down. Derangements of fuel metabolism, which often develop with age, lead to **diabetes** and **dyslipidemias** and are major contributors to **atherosclerosis**.

Tissues perform specialized functions

These functions include muscle contraction, nerve conduction, immune surveillance, hormonal signaling, maintenance of pH and electrolyte balance, detoxification of foreign substances and bone formation. Specialized microstructures, such as **glycoconjugates** (glycoproteins, glycolipids and proteoglycans), play a crucial role in tissue organization, cell–cell interactions and in the structure and function of the extracellular matrix.

Genome and cellular signaling underlie it all

The genome provides the mechanism of conservation and transfer of genetic information, the regulation of the expression of constituent genes and the control of protein synthesis. Protein synthesis is controlled by information encoded in **deoxyribonucleic acid (DNA)** and transcribed into **ribonucleic acid (RNA)**, which is then translated into peptides that fold into **functional protein molecules**. The spectrum of expressed proteins and the control of their temporal expression during development, adaptation and aging are responsible for our protein make-up.

Applications of **recombinant DNA** and polymerase chain reaction (PCR) technology have revolutionized the work of clinical laboratories during the last decade. The recent ability to scan the entire genome and the potential of **proteomics** create an opportunity to gain new insights into the dynamics of gene-driven protein synthesis. Finally, **cell growth, cellular signaling** and **repair mechanisms** are important for survival, and the time-dependent decline in these systems leads to **aging** and development of diseases such as **cancer**.

We have summarized it all in Figure 1.1, which looks not unlike the plan of the London Underground (see Further Reading). Don't be intimidated by the many as yet unfamiliar terms and refer back to this figure as you study different chapters to see how your understanding of biochemistry increases.

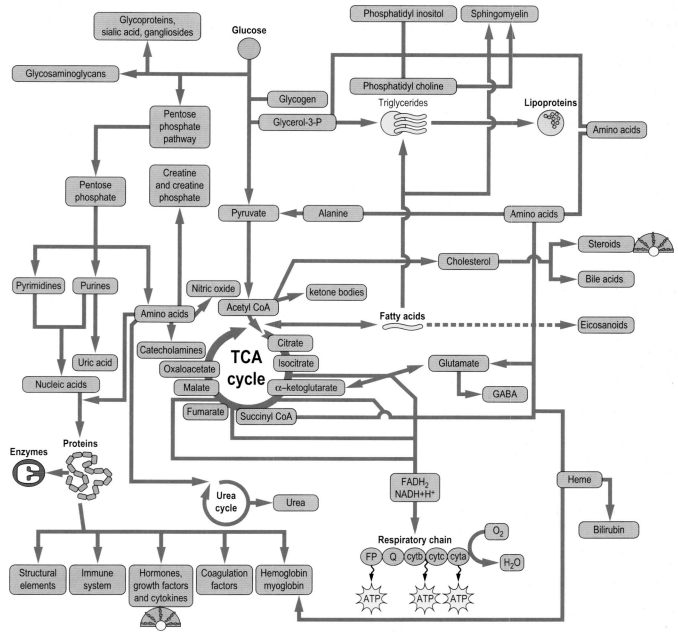

Fig 1.1 **Biochemistry: all in one.** Interrelationships between biochemical pathways. This figure has been designed to give you a bird's-eye view of the field. It may help to structure your study or revision. Refer back to it as you study this book and see how you gain perspective on biochemistry. GABA, γ-aminobutyrate; glycerol-3-P, glycerol-3-phosphate; CoA, coenzyme A; TCA, tricarboxylic acid cycle; cyt, cytochrome; FP, flavoprotein; Q, coenzyme Q_{10}; ATP, adenosine 5′-triphosphate.

THE FINAL WORD

In today's medical education, students direct their learning to acquire knowledge that should be a framework for career-long study. Studying medicine piecemeal by narrow specialties is less valuable than integrated learning, which allows you to place acquired knowledge in a wider context. This book attempts to do just that for biochemistry. We encourage the student to think all the time about clinical issues and relate gained knowledge to everyday clinical situations.

As you consult this book, keep in mind that it is not designed to be a review text or resource for preparation for multiple choice exams. These resources are provided separately on our website. This text is an integrated, clinically oriented presentation of aspects of biochemistry relevant to medicine: a resource for your clinical career. It is shorter than many of the heavy tomes in our discipline and is focused not on the accumulation of factual knowledge but on the development of ideas and relationships that we hope you will retain in your recall memory, and which will be helpful to you in clinical practice, long after you leave the lecture hall.

Most of all, *Medical Biochemistry* was written because we believe that understanding biochemistry helps in the practice of clinical medicine. Therefore, in the text we link basic science to situations which a physician encounters at the bedside, in the doctor's office and when dealing with the clinical laboratory. Our clinical cases have been scrutinized by clinicians and laboratorians who deal with real patients every day to make sure that they reflect practical problems that you will face in your career as a physician. We hope that the concepts learned here will help you then – and benefit your patients.

Further reading

Cooke M, Irby DM, Sullivan W, Ludmerer KM. American medical education 100 years after the Flexner report. *N Engl J Med* 2006; **355**: 1339–1344.

Dominiczak MH. Teaching and training laboratory professionals for the 21st century. *Clin Chem Lab Med* 1998; **36**: 133–136.

Jolly B, Rees L (eds). *Medical education in the millennium*. Oxford: Oxford University Press, 1998.1–268.

Ludmerer KM. Learner-centered medical education. *N Engl J Med* 2004; **351**: 1163–1164.

2. Amino Acids and Proteins

N Taniguchi

LEARNING OBJECTIVES

After reading this chapter you should be able to:

- Classify the amino acids based on their chemical structure and charge.
- Explain the meaning of the terms pK_a and pI as they apply to amino acids and proteins.
- Describe the elements of the primary, secondary, tertiary, and quaternary structure of proteins.
- Describe the principles of ion exchange and gel filtration chromatography, and electrophoresis and isoelectric focusing, and describe their application in protein isolation and characterization.
- Explain the principle of MALDI-TOF and electrospray mass spectrometry and their application to proteomics.

INTRODUCTION

Proteins are the primary structural and functional polymers in living systems. They have a broad range of activities, including catalysis of metabolic reactions and transport of vitamins, minerals, oxygen, and fuels. Some proteins make up the structure of tissues, while others function in nerve transmission, muscle contraction and cell motility, and still others in blood clotting and immunologic defenses, and as hormones and regulatory molecules. Proteins are synthesized as a sequence of amino acids linked together in a linear polyamide (polypeptide) structure, but they assume complex three-dimensional shapes in performing their function. There are about 300 amino acids present in various animal, plant and microbial systems, but only 20 amino acids are coded by DNA to appear in proteins. Many proteins also contain modified amino acids and accessory components, termed prosthetic groups. A range of chemical techniques is used to isolate and characterize proteins by a variety of criteria, including mass, charge and three-dimensional structure. Proteomics is an emerging field which studies the full range of expression of proteins in a cell or organism, and changes in protein expression in response to growth, hormones, stress, and aging.

AMINO ACIDS

Stereochemistry: configuration at the α-carbon, D- and L-isomers

Each amino acid has a central carbon, called the α-carbon, to which four different groups are attached (Fig. 2.1):

- a basic amino group ($-NH_2$)
- an acidic carboxyl group ($-COOH$)
- a hydrogen atom ($-H$)
- a distinctive side chain ($-R$).

One of the 20 amino acids, proline, is not an α-amino acid but an α-imino acid (see below). Except for glycine, all amino acids contain at least one asymmetric carbon atom (the α-carbon atom), giving two isomers that are optically active, i.e. they can rotate plane-polarized light. These isomers, referred to as stereoisomers or enantiomers, are said to be chiral, a word derived from the Greek word for hand. Such isomers are nonsuperimposable mirror images and are analogous to left and right hands, as shown in Figure 2.2. The two amino acid configurations are called D (for dextro or right) and L (for levo or left). All amino acids in proteins are of the L-configuration, because proteins are biosynthesized by enzymes that insert only L-amino acids into the peptide chains.

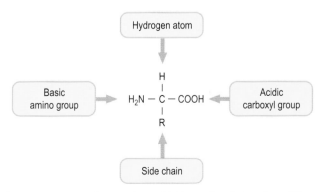

Fig. 2.1 **Structure of an amino acid.** Except for glycine, four different groups are attached to the α-carbon of an amino acid. Table 2.1 lists the structures of the R groups.

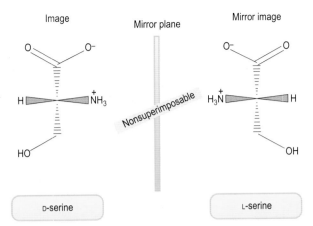

Fig. 2.2 **Enantiomers.** The mirror-image pair of amino acids. Each amino acid represents nonsuperimposable mirror images. The mirror-image stereo-isomers are called enantiomers. Only the L-enantiomers are found in proteins.

Classification of amino acids based on chemical structure

The properties of each amino acid are dependent on its side chain (—R); the side chains are the functional groups that are the major determinants of the structure and function of proteins, as well as the electrical charge of the molecule. Knowledge of the properties of these side chains is important for understanding methods of analysis, purification, and identification of proteins. Amino acids with charged, polar or hydrophilic side chains are usually exposed on the surface of proteins. The nonpolar hydrophobic residues are usually buried in the hydrophobic interior or core of a protein and are out of contact with water. The 20 amino acids in proteins encoded by DNA are listed in Table 2.1 and are classified according to their side chain functional groups.

Aliphatic amino acids

Alanine, valine, leucine, and isoleucine, referred to as aliphatic amino acids, have saturated hydrocarbons as side chains. Glycine, which has only a hydrogen side chain, is also included in this group. Alanine has a relatively simple structure, a side chain methyl group, while leucine and isoleucine have *sec*- and *iso*-butyl groups. All of these amino acids are hydrophobic in nature.

Aromatic amino acids

Phenylalanine, tyrosine, and tryptophan have aromatic side chains. The nonpolar aliphatic and aromatic amino acids are normally buried in the protein core and are involved in hydrophobic interactions with one another. Tyrosine has a

The 20 α-amino acids specified by the genetic code

Amino acids	Structure of R moiety
Aliphatic amino acids	
glycine (Gly, **G**)	—H
alanine (Ala, **A**)	—CH₃
valine (Val, **V**)	
leucine (Leu, **L**)	
isoleucine (Ile, **I**)	
Sulfur-containing amino acids	
cysteine (Cys, **C**)	
methionine (Met, **M**)	
Aromatic amino acids	
phenylalanine (Phe, **F**)	
tyrosine (Tyr, **Y**)	
tryptophan (Trp, **W**)	
Imino acid	
proline (Pro, **P**)	(Whole structure)
Neutral amino acids	
serine (Ser, **S**)	
threonine (Thr, **T**)	
asparagine (Asn, **N**)	
glutamine (Gln, **Q**)	
Acidic amino acids	
aspartic acid (Asp, **D**)	
glutamic acid (Glu, **E**)	
Basic amino acids	
histidine (His, **H**)	
lysine (Lys, **K**)	
arginine (Arg, **R**)	

Table 2.1 **The 20 amino acids found in proteins.** The three-letter and single-letter abbreviations in common use are given in parentheses.

weakly acidic hydroxyl group and may be located on the surface of proteins. Reversible phosphorylation of the hydroxyl group of tyrosine in some enzymes is important in the regulation of metabolic pathways. The aromatic amino acids are responsible for the ultraviolet absorption of most proteins, which have absorption maxima ~280 nm. Tryptophan has a greater absorption in this region than the other two aromatic amino acids. The molar absorption coefficient of a protein is useful in determining the concentration of a protein in solution, based on spectrophotometry. Typical absorption spectra of aromatic amino acids and a protein are shown in Figure 2.3.

 ## NONPROTEIN AMINO ACIDS

Some amino acids occur in free or combined states, but not in proteins. Measurement of abnormal amino acids in urine (aminoaciduria) is useful for clinical diagnosis (see Chapter 19). In plasma, free amino acids are usually found in the order of 10–100 μmol/L, including many that are not found in protein. Citrulline, for example, is an important metabolite of L-arginine and a product of nitric oxide synthase, an enzyme that produces nitric oxide, an important vasoactive signaling molecule. Urinary amino acid concentration is usually expressed as μmol/g creatinine. Creatinine is an amino acid derived from muscle and is excreted in relatively constant amounts per unit body mass per day. Thus, the creatinine concentration in urine, normally about 1 mg/mL, can be used to correct for urine dilution. The most abundant amino acid in urine is glycine, which is present as 400–2000 μg/g creatinine.

Neutral polar amino acids

Neutral polar amino acids contain hydroxyl or amide side chain groups. Serine and threonine contain hydroxyl groups. These amino acids are sometimes found at the active sites of catalytic proteins, enzymes (Chapter 6). Reversible phosphorylation of peripheral serine and threonine residues of enzymes is also involved in regulation of energy metabolism and fuel storage in the body (Chapter 13). Asparagine and glutamine have amide-bearing side chains. These are polar but uncharged under physiological conditions. Serine, threonine and asparagine are the primary sites of linkage of sugars to proteins, forming glycoproteins (Chapter 26).

Acidic amino acids

Aspartic and glutamic acids contain carboxylic acids on their side chains and are ionized at pH 7.0 and, as a result, carry negative charges on their β- and γ-carboxyl groups, respectively. In the ionized state, these amino acids are referred to as aspartate and glutamate, respectively.

Basic amino acids

The side chains of lysine and arginine are fully protonated at neutral pH and, therefore, positively charged. Lysine contains a primary amino group (NH_2) attached to the terminal ε-carbon of the side chain. The ε-amino group of lysine has a $pK_a \approx 11$. Arginine is the most basic amino acid ($pK_a \approx 13$)

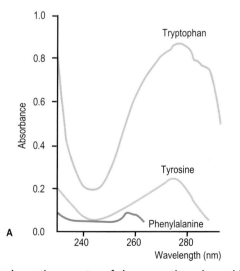
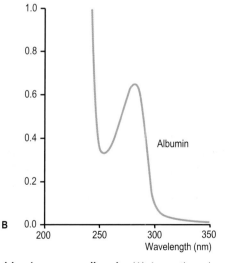

Fig. 2.3 **Ultraviolet absorption spectra of the aromatic amino acids and bovine serum albumin.** (A) Aromatic amino acids such as tryptophan, tyrosine, and phenylalanine have absorbance maxima at ~280 nm. Each purified protein has a distinct molecular absorption coefficient at around 280 nm, depending on its content of aromatic amino acids. (B) A bovine serum albumin solution (1 mg dissolved in 1 ml of water) has an absorbance of 0.67 at 280 nm using a 1 cm cuvette. The absorption coefficient of proteins is often expressed as $E_{1\%}$ (10 mg/mL solution). For albumin, $E_{1\% 280nm} = 6.7$. Although proteins vary in their Trp, Tyr, and Phe content, measurements of absorbance at 280 nm are useful for estimating protein concentration in solutions.

and its guanidine group exists as a protonated guanidinium ion at pH 7.0.

Histidine ($pK_a \approx 6$) has an imidazole ring as the side chain and functions as a general acid–base catalyst in many enzymes. The protonated form of imidazole is called an imidazolium ion.

Sulfur-containing amino acids

Cysteine and its oxidized form, cystine, are sulfur-containing amino acids characterized by low polarity. Cysteine plays an important role in stabilization of protein structure, since it can participate in formation of a disulfide bond with other cysteine residues to form cystine residues, crosslinking protein chains and stabilizing protein structure. Two regions of a single polypeptide chain, remote from each other in the sequence, may be covalently linked through a disulfide bond (intrachain disulfide bond). Disulfide bonds are also formed between two polypeptide chains (interchain disulfide bond), forming covalent protein dimers. These bonds can be reduced by enzymes or by reducing agents such as 2-mercaptoethanol or dithiothreitol, to form cysteine residues. Methionine is the third sulfur-containing amino acid and contains a nonpolar methyl thioether group in its side chain.

Proline, a cyclic imino acid

Proline is different from other amino acids in that its side chain pyrrolidine ring includes both the α-amino group and the α-carbon. This imino acid forces a 'bend' in a polypeptide chain, sometimes causing abrupt changes in the direction of the chain.

Classification of amino acids based on the polarity of the amino acid side chains

Table 2.2 depicts the functional groups of amino acids and their polarity (hydrophilicity). Polar side chains can be involved in hydrogen bonding to water and to other polar groups and are usually located on the surface of the protein. Hydrophobic side chains contribute to protein folding by hydrophobic interactions and are located primarily in the core of the protein or on surfaces involved in interactions with other proteins.

Ionization state of an amino acid

Amino acids are amphoteric molecules – they have both basic and acidic groups. Monoamino and monocarboxylic acids are ionized in different ways in solution, depending on the solution's pH. At pH 7, the 'zwitterion' $^+H_3N-CH_2-COO^-$ is the dominant species of glycine in solution, and the overall molecule is therefore electrically neutral. On titration to acidic pH, the α-amino group is protonated and positively charged, yielding the cation $^+H_3N-CH_2-COOH$, while titration with alkali yields the anionic $H_2N-CH_2-COO^-$ species.

$$^+H_3N-CH_2-COOH \overset{H^+}{\rightleftarrows} {}^+H_3N-CH_2-COO^- \overset{OH^-}{\rightleftarrows}$$
$$H_2N-CH_2-COO^-$$

pK_a values for the α-amino and α-carboxyl groups and side chains of acidic and basic amino acids are shown in

Summary of the functional groups of amino acids and their polarity			
Amino acids	**Functional group**	**Hydrophilic (polar) or hydrophobic (apolar)**	**Examples**
acidic	carboxyl, —COOH	polar	Asp, Glu
basic	amine, —NH$_2$	polar	Lys
	imidazole	polar	His
	guanidino	polar	Arg
neutral	glycine, —H	nonpolar	Gly
	amides, —CONH$_2$	polar	Asn, Gln
	hydroxyl, —OH	polar	Ser, Thr,
	sulfhydryl, —SH	nonpolar	Cys
aliphatic	hydrocarbon	nonpolar	Ala, Val, Leu, Ile, Met, Pro
aromatic	C-rings	nonpolar	Phe, Trp, Tyr

Table 2.2 **Summary of the functional groups of amino acids and their polarity.**

Table 2.3. The overall charge on a protein depends on the contribution from basic (positive charge) and acidic (negative charge) amino acids, but the actual charge on the protein varies with the pH of the solution. To understand how the side chains affect the charge on proteins, it is worth recalling the Henderson–Hasselbalch equation.

Henderson-Hasselbalch equation and pK_a

The general dissociation of a weak acid, such as a carboxylic acid, is given by the equation:

$$HA \rightleftharpoons H^+ + A^- \tag{1}$$

where HA is the protonated form (conjugate acid or associated form) and A^- is the unprotonated form (conjugate base, or dissociated form).

The dissociation constant (K_a) of a weak acid is defined as the equilibrium constant for the dissociation reaction (1) of the acid:

$$K_a = \frac{[HA][A^-]}{[HA]} \tag{2}$$

The hydrogen ion concentration $[H^+]$ of a solution of a weak acid can then be calculated as follows. Equation (2) can be rearranged to give:

$$[H^+] = K_a \times \frac{[HA]}{[A^-]} \tag{3}$$

Equation (3) can be expressed in terms of a negative logarithm:

$$-\log[H^+] = -\log K_a - \log\frac{[HA]}{[A^-]} \tag{4}$$

pK values and ionized groups in proteins			
Group	Acid (protonated form) (conjugate acid)	H$^+$ + Base (unprotonated form) (conjugate base)	pK_a
terminal carboxyl residue (α-carboxyl)	—COOH (carboxylic acid)	—COO$^-$ + H$^+$ (carboxylate)	3.0–5.5
aspartic acid (β-carboxyl)	—COOH	—COO$^-$ + H$^+$	3.9
glutamic acid (γ-carboxyl)	—COOH	—COO$^-$ + H$^+$	4.3
histidine (imidazole)	(imidazolium)	(imidazole)	6.0
terminal amino (α-amino)	—NH$_3$$^+$ (ammonium)	—NH$_2$ + H$^+$ (amine)	8.0
cysteine (sulfhydryl)	—SH (thiol)	—S$^-$ + H$^+$ (thiolate)	8.3
tyrosine (phenolic hydroxyl)	(phenol)	(phenolate)	10.1
lysine (ε-amino)	—NH$_3$$^+$	—NH$_2$ + H$^+$	10.5
arginine (guanidino)	(guanidinium)	(guanidino)	12.5

Table 2.3 **Typical pK_a values for ionizable groups in proteins.** Actual pK_a values may vary by as much at three pH units, depending on temperature, buffer, ligand binding, and especially neighboring functional groups in the protein.

Since pH is the negative logarithm of $[H^+]$, i.e. $-\log[H^+]$, and pK_a equals the negative logarithm of the dissociation constant for a weak acid, i.e. $-\log K_a$, the Henderson–Hasselbalch equation (5) can be developed and used for analysis of acid–base equilibrium systems:

$$pH = pK_a + \log\frac{[A^-]}{[HA]} \qquad (5)$$

For a weak base, such as an amine, the dissociation reaction can be written as:

$$RNH_3^+ \rightleftharpoons H^+ + RNH_2 \qquad (6)$$

and the Henderson–Hasselbalch equation becomes:

$$pH = pK_a + \log\frac{[RNH_2]}{[RNH_3^+]} \qquad (7)$$

From equations (5) and (7), it is apparent that the extent of protonation of acidic and basic functional groups, and therefore the net charge, will vary with the pK_a of the functional group and the pH of the solution. For alanine, which has two functional groups with $pK_a = 2.4$ and 9.8, respectively (Fig. 2.4), the net charge varies with pH, from $+1$ to -1. At a point intermediate between pK_{a1} and pK_{a2}, alanine has a net zero charge. This pH is called its isoelectric point, pI (see Fig. 2.4).

BUFFERS

Buffers are solutions that minimize a change in $[H^+]$, i.e. pH, on addition of acid or base. A buffer solution, containing a weak acid or weak base and a counter-ion, has maximal buffering capacity at its pK_a, i.e. when the acidic and basic forms are present at equal concentrations. The acidic, protonated form reacts with added base, and the basic unprotonated form neutralizes added acid, as shown below for an amino compound:

$$RNH_3^+ + OH^- \rightleftharpoons RNH_2 + H_2O$$
$$RNH_2 + H^+ \rightleftharpoons RNH_3^+$$

An alanine solution (see Fig. 2.4) has maximal buffering capacity at pH 2.4 and 9.8, i.e. at the pK_a of the carboxyl and amino groups, respectively. When dissolved in water, alanine exists as a dipolar ion, or zwitterion, in which the carboxyl group is unprotonated ($-COO^-$) and the amino group is protonated ($-NH_3^+$). The pH of the solution is 6.1 and the pI halfway between the pK_a of the amino and carboxyl groups. The titration curve of alanine by NaOH (see Fig. 2.4) illustrates that alanine has minimal buffering capacity at its pI, and maximal buffering capacity at a pH equal to the pK_{a1} or pK_{a2}.

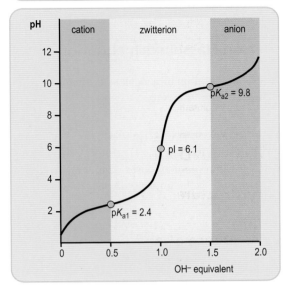

Fig. 2.4 **Titration of amino acid.** The curve shows the number of equivalents of NaOH consumed by alanine while titrating the solution from pH 0 to pH 12. Alanine contains two ionizable groups: an α-carboxyl group and an α-amino group. As NaOH is added, these two groups are titrated. The pK_a of the α-COOH group is 2.4, whereas that of the α-NH$_3^+$ group is 9.8. At very low pH, the predominant ion species of alanine is the fully protonated form:

$$^+H_3N-\overset{\overset{\textstyle CH_3}{|}}{C}H-COOH$$

At the mid-point in the first stage of the titration (pH 2.4), equimolar concentrations of proton donor and proton acceptor species are present, providing good buffering power.

$$^+H_3N-\overset{\overset{\textstyle CH_3}{|}}{C}H-COOH \quad H_2N-\overset{\overset{\textstyle CH_3}{|}}{C}H-COO^-$$

The second stage of the titration corresponds to the removal of a proton from the $-NH_3^+$ group of alanine. The pH at the mid-point of this stage is 9.8, equal to the pK_a for the $-NH_3^+$ group. The titration is complete at a pH of about 12, at which point the predominant form of alanine is:

$$H_2N-\overset{\overset{\textstyle CH_3}{|}}{C}H-COO^-$$

The pH at which a molecule has no net charge is known as its isoelectric point, pI. For alanine, it is calculated as:

$$pI = \left[\frac{pK_{a1} + pK_{a2}}{2}\right] = \left[\frac{2.4 + 9.8}{2}\right] = \frac{12.2}{2} = 6.1$$

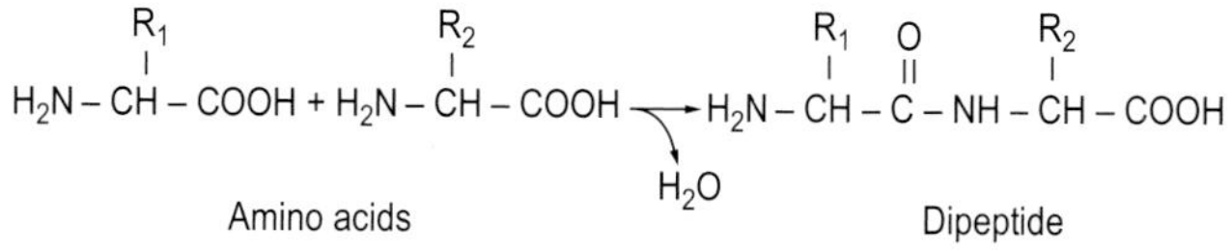

Fig. 2.5 Structure of a peptide bond.

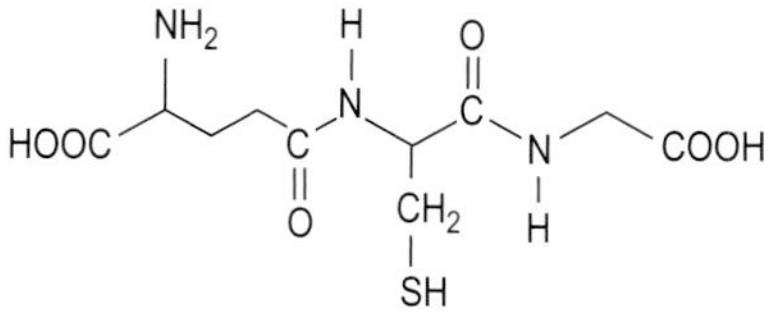

Fig. 2.6 Structure of glutathione.

PEPTIDES AND PROTEINS

Primary structure of proteins

The primary structure of the protein is the linear sequence of amino acids

In proteins, the carboxyl group of one amino acid is linked to the amino group of the next amino acid, forming an amide (peptide) bond; water is eliminated during the reaction (Fig. 2.5). The amino acid units in a peptide chain are referred to as amino acid residues. A peptide chain consisting of three amino acid residues is called a tripeptide, e.g. glutathione in Fig. 2.6. By convention, the amino terminus (N-terminus) is taken as the first residue, and the sequence of amino acids is written from left to right. When writing the peptide sequence, one uses either the three-letter or the one-letter abbreviations of amino acids, such as Asp-Arg-Val-Tyr-Ile-His-Pro-Phe-His-Leu or D-R-V-Y-I-H-P-F-H-L (see Table 2.1). This peptide is angiotensin, a peptide hormone that affects blood pressure. The amino acid residue having a free amino group at one end of the peptide, Asp, is called the N-terminal amino acid (amino terminus), whereas the residue having a free carboxyl group at the other end, Leu, is called the C-terminal amino acid (carboxyl terminus). Proteins contain between 50 and 2000 amino acid residues. The mean molecular mass of an amino acid residue is about 110 dalton units (Da). Therefore the molecular mass of most proteins is between 5500 and 220000Da. Human carbonic anhydrase I, an enzyme that plays a major role in acid–base balance in blood (Chapter 24), is a protein with a molecular mass of 29000Da (29kDa).

The charge and polarity characteristics of a peptide chain

The amino acid composition of a peptide chain has a profound effect on its physical and chemical properties. Proteins rich in aliphatic or aromatic amino groups are relatively insoluble in water and are likely to be found in cell membranes. Proteins rich in polar amino acids are more water soluble. Amides are neutral compounds so that the amide backbone of a protein, including the α-amino and α-carboxyl groups from which it is formed, does not contribute to the charge of the protein. Instead, the charge on the protein is dependent on the side chain functional groups of amino acids. Amino acids with side chain acidic (Glu, Asp) or basic (Lys, His, Arg) groups will confer charge and buffering capacity to a protein. The balance between acidic and basic side chains in a protein determines its isoelectric point (pI) and net charge in solution. Proteins rich in lysine and arginine are basic in solution and have a positive charge at neutral pH, while acidic proteins, rich in aspartate and glutamate, are acidic and have a negative charge. Because of their side chain functional groups, all proteins become more positively charged at acidic pH and more negatively charged at basic pH. Proteins are an important part of the buffering capacity of blood cells and biological fluids.

GLUTATHIONE

Glutathione (GSH) is a tripeptide with the sequence L-γ-glutamyl-L-cysteinyl-glycine (Fig. 2.6). If the thiol group of the cysteine is oxidized, the disulfide GSSG is formed. GSH is the major peptide present in the cell. In the liver, the concentration of GSH is ~5mmol/L. GSH plays a major role in the maintenance of cysteine residues in proteins in their reduced (sulfhydryl) forms and in antioxidant defenses (Chapter 37). The enzyme γ-glutamyl transpeptidase is involved in the metabolism of glutathione and is a plasma biomarker for some liver diseases, including hepatocellular carcinoma and alcoholic liver disease.

Secondary structure is determined by hydrogen bonding interactions of carbonyl and amide residues in the peptide backbone

The secondary structure of a protein refers to the local structure of the polypeptide chain. This structure is determined by hydrogen bond interactions between the carbonyl oxygen group of one peptide bond and the amide hydrogen of another nearby peptide bond. There are two types of secondary structure: the α-helix and the β-pleated sheet.

The α-helix

The α-helix is a rod-like structure with the peptide chain tightly coiled and the side chains of amino acid residues

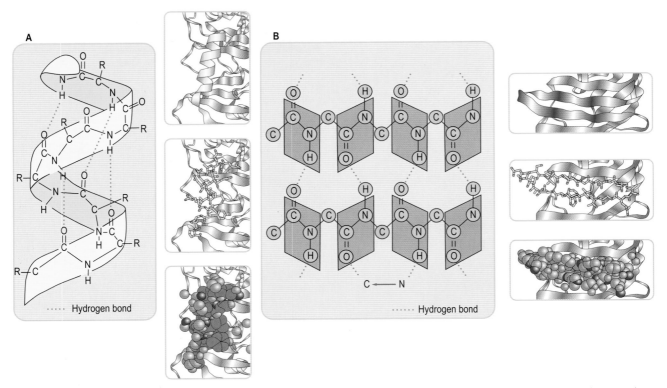

Fig. 2.7 **Protein secondary structural motifs.** (A) An α-helical secondary structure. Hydrogen bonds between 'backbone' amide NH and C═O groups stabilize the α-helix. Hydrogen atoms of OH, NH or SH group (hydrogen donors) interact with free electrons of the acceptor atoms such as O, N or S. Even though the bonding energy is lower than that of covalent bonds, they play a pivotal role in the stabilization of protein molecules. R, side chain of amino acids which extend outward from the helix. Ribbon, stick and space-filling models are shown. (B) The parallel β-sheet secondary structure. In the β-conformation, the backbone of the polypeptide chain is extended into a zigzag structure. When the zigzag polypeptide chains are arranged side by side, they form a structure resembling a series of pleats. Ribbon, stick and space-filling models are also shown.

extending outward from the axis of the spiral. Each amide carbonyl group is hydrogen bonded to the amide hydrogen of a peptide bond that is four residues away along the same chain. There are on average 3.6 amino acid residues per turn of the helix, and the helix winds in a right-handed (clockwise) manner in almost all natural proteins (Fig. 2.7A).

The β-pleated sheet

If the H-bonds are formed between peptide bonds in different chains, the chains become arrayed parallel or antiparallel to one another in what is commonly called a β-pleated sheet. The β-pleated sheet is an extended structure as opposed to the coiled α-helix. It is pleated because the carbon—carbon (C—C) bonds are tetrahedral and cannot exist in a planar configuration. If the polypeptide chain runs in the same direction, it forms a parallel β-sheet (Fig. 2.7B), but in the opposite direction, it forms an antiparallel structure. The β-turn or β-bend refers to the segment in which the polypeptide abruptly reverses direction. Glycine (Gly) and proline (Pro) residues often occur in β-turns on the surface of globular proteins.

COLLAGEN

Human genetic defects involving collagen illustrate the close relationship between amino acid sequence and three-dimensional structure. Collagens are the most abundant protein family in the mammalian body, representing about a third of body proteins. Collagens are a major component of connective tissue such as cartilage, tendons, the organic matrix of bones, and the cornea of the eye.

Comment. Collagen contains 35% Gly, 11% Ala, and 21% Pro plus Hyp (hydroxyproline). The amino acid sequence in collagen is generally a repeating tripeptide unit, Gly-Xaa-Pro or Gly-Xaa-Hyp, where Xaa can be any amino acid; Hyp = hydroxyproline. This repeating sequence adopts a left-handed helical structure with three residues per turn. Three of these helices wrap around one another with a right-handed twist. The resulting three-stranded molecule is referred to as tropocollagen. Tropocollagen molecules self-assemble into collagen fibrils and are packed together to form collagen fibers. There are metabolic and genetic disorders which result from collagen abnormalities. Scurvy, osteogenesis imperfecta (Chapter 28) and Ehlers–Danlos syndrome result from defects in collagen synthesis and/or crosslinking.

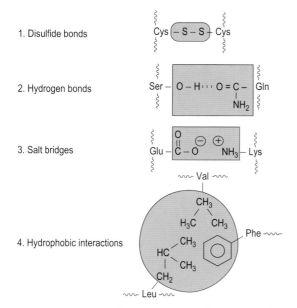

1. Disulfide bonds

2. Hydrogen bonds

3. Salt bridges

4. Hydrophobic interactions

Fig. 2.8 **Elements of tertiary structure of proteins.** Examples of amino acid side chain interactions contributing to tertiary structure.

Tertiary structure results from folding of the peptide chain

The three-dimensional, folded and biologically active conformation of a protein is referred to as its tertiary structure. This structure reflects the overall shape of the molecule. The tertiary structure of proteins is determined by X-ray crystallography and nuclear magnetic resonance spectroscopy. The folded conformation of proteins that contain more than 200 residues consists of several smaller folded units termed domains.

The three-dimensional tertiary structure of a protein is stabilized by interactions between side chain functional groups: covalent disulfide bonds, hydrogen bonds, salt bridges, and hydrophobic interactions (Fig. 2.8). The side chains of tryptophan and arginine serve as hydrogen donors, whereas asparagine, glutamine, serine, and threonine can serve as both hydrogen donors and acceptors. Lysine, aspartic acid, glutamic acid, tyrosine, and histidine also can serve as both donors and acceptors in the formation of ion pairs (salt bridges). Two opposite-charged amino acids, such as glutamate with a γ-carboxyl group and lysine with an ε-amino group, may form a salt bridge, primarily on the surface of proteins (see Fig. 2.8).

Compounds such as urea and guanidine hydrochloride frequently cause denaturation or loss of secondary and tertiary structure when present at high concentrations such as, for example, 8 mol/L urea. These reagents are called denaturants or chaotropic agents.

LENS DISLOCATION IN HOMOCYSTEINURIA (INCIDENCE: 1 IN 350 000)

The most common ocular manifestation of homocystinuria (Chapter 19) is lens dislocation occurring around age 10 years. Fibrillin, found in the fibers that support the lens, is rich in cysteine residues. Disulfide bonds between these residues are required for the crosslinking and stabilization of protein and lens structure. Homocysteine, a homolog of cysteine, can disrupt these bonds by homocysteine-dependent disulfide exchange.

Another equally rare sulfur amino acid disorder – sulfite oxidase deficiency – is also associated with lens dislocation by a similar mechanism (usually presenting at birth with early refractory convulsions). Marfan's syndrome, also associated with lens dislocation, is associated with mutations in the fibrillin gene (Chapter 28).

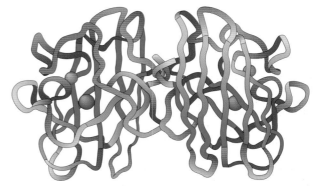

Fig. 2.9 **Three-dimensional structure of a dimeric protein.** Quaternary structure of Cu,Zn-superoxide dismutase from spinach. Cu,Zn-superoxide dismutase has a dimeric structure, with a monomer molecular mass of 16 000 Da. Each subunit consists of eight antiparallel β-sheets called a β-barrel structure, in analogy with geometric motifs found on native American and Greek weaving and pottery. Courtesy of Dr Y Kitagawa.

Quaternary structure is formed by interactions between peptide chains

Quaternary structure refers to a complex or an assembly of two or more separate peptide chains that are held together by noncovalent or, in some cases, covalent interactions. In general, most proteins larger than 50 kDa consist of more than one chain and are referred to as dimeric, trimeric or multimeric proteins. Many multisubunit proteins are composed of different kinds of functional subunits, such as the regulatory and catalytic subunits. Hemoglobin is a tetrameric protein (Chapter 5), and beef heart mitochondrial ATPase has 10 protomers (Chapter 9). The smallest unit is referred to as a monomer or subunit. Figure 2.9 indicates the structure of

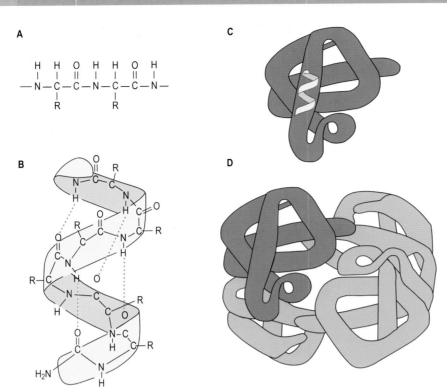

A

B

C

D

Fig. 2.10 **Primary, secondary, tertiary, and quaternary structures.** (A) The primary structure is composed of a linear sequence of amino acid residues of proteins. (B) The secondary structure indicates the local spatial arrangement of polypeptide backbone yielding an extended α-helical or β-pleated sheet structure as depicted by the ribbon. Hydrogen bonds between the 'backbone' amide —NH— and —CO— groups stabilize the helix. (C) The tertiary structure illustrates the three-dimensional conformation of a subunit of the protein while the quaternary structure (D) indicates the assembly of multiple polypeptide chains into an intact, tetrameric protein.

the dimeric protein Cu,Zn-superoxide dismutase. Figure 2.10 is an overview of the primary, secondary, tertiary, and quaternary structures of a tetrameric protein.

PURIFICATION AND CHARACTERIZATION OF PROTEINS

Protein purification procedures take advantage of separations based on charge, size, binding properties, and solubility. The complete characterization of the protein requires an understanding of its amino acid composition, its complete primary, secondary and tertiary structure and, for multimeric proteins, its quaternary structure.

In order to characterize a protein, it is first necessary to purify the protein by separating it from other components in complex biological mixtures. The source of the proteins is commonly blood or tissues, or microbial cells such as bacteria and yeast. First, the cells or tissues are disrupted by grinding or homogenization in buffered isotonic solutions, commonly at physiologic pH and at 4°C to minimize protein denaturation during purification. The 'crude extract' containing organelles such as nuclei, mitochondria, lysosomes, microsomes, and cytosolic fractions can then be fractionated by high-speed centrifugation or ultracentrifugation. Proteins that are tightly bound to the other biomolecules or membranes may be solubilized using organic solvent or detergent.

 ## POSTTRANSLATIONAL MODIFICATIONS OF PROTEINS

Most proteins undergo some form of enzymatic modification after the synthesis of the peptide chain. The 'posttranslational' modifications are performed by processing enzymes in the endoplasmic reticulum, Golgi apparatus, secretory granules, and extracellular space. The modifications include proteolytic cleavage, glycosylation, lipation and phosphorylation. Mass spectrometry (below) is a powerful tool for detecting such modifications, based on differences in molecular mass (see Chapter 33).

Salting out (ammonium sulfate fractionation)

The solubility of a protein is dependent on the concentration of dissolved salts, and the solubility may be increased by the addition of salt at a low concentration (salting in) or decreased by high salt concentration (salting out). When ammonium sulfate, one of the most soluble salts, is added to a solution of a protein, some proteins precipitate at a given salt concentration while others do not. Human serum immunoglobulins are precipitable by 33–40% saturated $(NH_4)_2SO_4$, while albumin remains soluble. Saturated ammonium sulfate is about 4.1 mol/L. Most proteins will precipitate from an 80% saturated $(NH_4)_2SO_4$ solution.

Separation on the basis of size

Dialysis and ultrafiltration

Small molecules, such as salts, can be removed from protein solutions by dialysis or ultrafiltration. Dialysis is performed by adding the protein–salt solution to a semipermeable membrane tube (commonly a nitrocellulose or collodion membrane). When the tube is immersed in a dilute buffer solution, small molecules will pass through and large protein molecules will be retained in the tube, depending on the pore size of the dialysis membrane. This procedure is particularly useful for removal of $(NH_4)_2SO_4$ or other salts during protein purification, since the salts will interfere with the purification of proteins by ion exchange chromatography (below). Figure 2.11 illustrates the dialysis of proteins.

Ultrafiltration has largely replaced dialysis for purification of proteins. This technique uses pressure to force a solution through a semipermeable membrane of defined, homogeneous pore size. By selecting the proper molecular weight cut-off value (pore size) for the filter, the membranes will allow solvent and lower molecular weight solutes to permeate the membrane, forming the filtrate, while retaining higher molecular weight proteins in the retentate solution. Ultrafiltration can be used to concentrate protein solutions or to accomplish dialysis by continuous replacement of buffer in the retentate compartment.

Gel filtration (molecular sieving)

Gel filtration, or gel permeation, chromatography uses a column of insoluble but highly hydrated polymers such as dextrans, agarose or polyacrylamide. Gel filtration chromatography depends on the differential migration of dissolved solutes through gels that have pores of defined sizes. This technique is frequently used for protein purification and for desalting protein solutions. Figure 2.12 describes the principle of gel filtration. There are commercially available gels

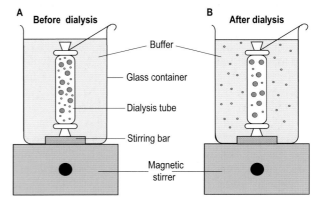

Fig. 2.11 **Dialysis of proteins.** Protein and low-molecular-mass compounds are separated by dialysis on the basis of size. (A) A protein solution with salts is placed in a dialysis tube in a beaker and dialyzed with stirring against an appropriate buffer. (B) The protein is retained in the dialysis tube, whereas salts will exchange through the membrane. By use of a large volume of external buffer, with occasional buffer replacement, the protein will eventually be exchanged into the external buffer solution.

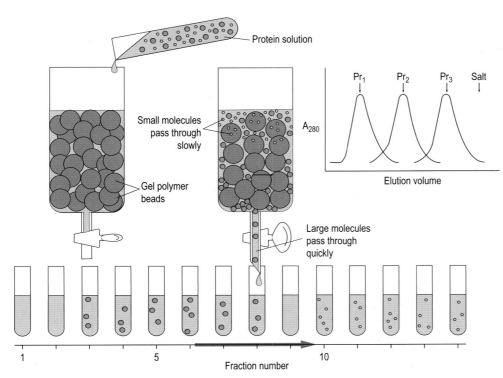

Fig. 2.12 **Fractionation of proteins by size: gel filtration chromatography of proteins.** Proteins with different molecular sizes are separated by gel filtration based on their relative size. The smaller the protein, the more readily it exchanges into polymer beads, whereas larger proteins may be completely excluded. Larger molecules flow more rapidly through this column, leading to fractionation on the basis of molecular size. The chromatogram on the right shows a theoretical fractionation of three proteins, Pr_1–Pr_3, of decreasing molecular weight.

made from carbohydrate polymer beads designated as dextran (Sephadex series), polyacrylamide (Bio-Gel P series), and agarose (Sepharose series), respectively. The gels vary in pore size and one can choose the gel filtration materials according to the molecular weight fractionation range desired.

Separation on the basis of charge: ion exchange chromatography

When a charged ion or molecule with one or more positive charges exchanges with another positively charged component bound to a negatively charged immobilized phase, the process is called cation exchange. The inverse process is called anion exchange. The cation exchanger, carboxymethyl-cellulose $(O-CH_2-COO^-)$, and anion exchanger, diethyl-aminoethyl (DEAE) cellulose $(-O-C_2H_4-NH^+[C_2H_5]_2)$, are frequently used for the purification of proteins. Consider purifying a protein mixture containing albumin and immunoglobulin. At pH 7.5, albumin, with a pI of 4.8, is negatively charged; immunoglobulin with a pI ~8 is positively charged. If the mixture is applied to a DEAE column at pH 7, the albumin sticks to the positive-charged DEAE column whereas the immunoglobulin passes through the column. Figure 2.13 illustrates the principle of ion exchange chromatography. As with gel permeation chromatography, proteins can be separated from one another, based on small differences in their pI. Adsorbed proteins are commonly eluted with a gradient formed from two or more solutions with different pH and/or salt concentrations. In this way, proteins are gradually eluted from the column and are well resolved based on their pI.

Affinity chromatography

Affinity chromatography is a convenient and specific method for purification of proteins. A porous chromatography column matrix is derivatized with a ligand that interacts with, or binds to, a specific protein in a complex mixture. The protein of interest will be selectively and specifically bound to the ligand while the others wash through the column. The bound protein can then be eluted by a high salt concentration, mild denaturation or by a soluble form of the ligand or ligand analogs (Chapter 6).

Determination of purity and molecular weight of proteins by sodium dodecyl sulfate-polyacrylamide gel electrophoresis (SDS-PAGE)

Electrophoresis can be used for the separation of a wide variety of charged molecules, including amino acids, polypeptides, proteins, and DNA. When a current is applied to molecules in dilute buffers, those with a net negative charge at the selected pH migrate toward the anode and those with a net positive charge toward the cathode. A porous support, such as paper, cellulose acetate or polymeric gel, is commonly used to minimize diffusion and convection.

Like chromatography, electrophoresis may be used for preparative fractionation of proteins at physiologic pH. Different soluble proteins will move at different rates in the electrical field, depending on their charge to mass ratio. A denaturing detergent, sodium dodecyl sulfate (SDS), is commonly used in a polyacrylamide gel electrophoresis (PAGE) system to

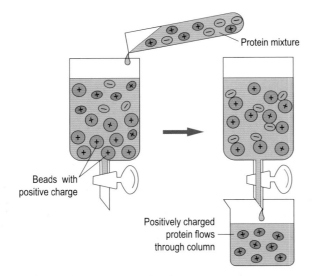

Beads with positive charge

Protein mixture

Positively charged protein flows through column

Fig. 2.13 **Fractionation of proteins by charge: ion exchange chromatography.** Mixtures of proteins can be separated by ion exchange chromatography according to their net charges. Beads that have positive-charge groups attached are called anion exchangers, whereas those having negative-charge groups are cation exchangers. This figure depicts an anion exchange column. Negatively charged protein binds to positively charged beads, and positively charged protein flows through the column.

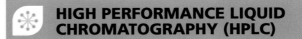

HIGH PERFORMANCE LIQUID CHROMATOGRAPHY (HPLC)

HPLC is a powerful chromatographic technique for high-resolution separation of proteins, peptides, and amino acids. The principle of the separation may be based on the charge, size or hydrophobicity of proteins. The narrow columns are packed with a noncompressible matrix of fine silica beads coated with a thin layer of a stationary phase. A protein mixture is applied to the column, and then the components are eluted by either isocratic or gradient chromatography. The eluates are monitored by ultraviolet absorption, refractive index or fluorescence. This technique gives high-resolution separation.

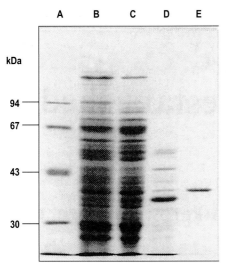

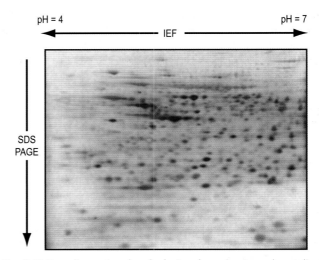

Fig. 2.14 **SDS-PAGE.** Sodium dodecyl sulfate-polyacrylamide gel electrophoresis is used to separate proteins on the basis of their molecular weights. Larger molecules are retarded in the gel matrix, whereas the smaller ones move more rapidly. Lane A contains standard proteins with known molecular masses (indicated in kDa on the left). Lanes B, C, D and E show results of SDS-PAGE analysis of a protein at various stages in purification: B = total protein isolate; C = ammonium sulfate precipitate; D = fraction from gel permeation chromatography; E = purified protein from ion exchange chromatography.

Fig. 2.15 **Two-dimensional gel electrophoresis.** A crude rat liver extract was first subjected to isoelectric focusing (IEF) in cylindrical gel within the pH range 4–7. The gel was then laid horizontally on a second slab gel and separated by SDS-PAGE according to molecular mass. The gel was then stained with Coomassie Blue.

separate and resolve protein subunits according to molecular weight. The protein preparation is usually treated with both SDS and a thiol reagent, such as β-mercaptoethanol, to reduce disulfide bonds. Because the binding of SDS is proportional to the length of the peptide chain, each protein molecule has the same mass-to-charge ratio and the relative mobility of the protein is proportional to the molecular mass of the polypeptide chain. Varying the state of crosslinking of the polyacrylamide gel provides selectivity for proteins of different molecular weights. A purified protein preparation can be readily analyzed for homogeneity on SDS-PAGE by staining with sensitive and specific dyes, such as Coomassie Blue, or with a silver staining technique, as shown in Figure 2.14.

Isoelectric focusing (IEF)

Isoelectric focusing (IEF) is used to separate proteins on the basis of their pI by conducting electrophoresis in a microchannel or gel containing a pH gradient. A protein applied to the system will be either positively or negatively charged, depending on its amino acid composition and the ambient pH. Upon application of a current, the protein will move towards either the anode or cathode until it encounters that part of the system which corresponds to its pI, where the protein has no charge and will cease to migrate. IEF is used in conjunction with SDS-PAGE for two-dimensional gel electrophoresis (Fig. 2.15). This technique is particularly useful for the fractionation of complex mixtures of proteins for proteomic analysis (see above).

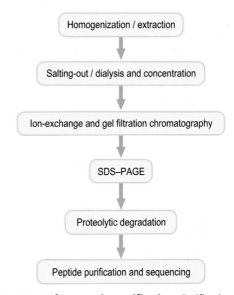

Fig. 2.16 **Strategy for protein purification.** Purification of a protein involves a sequence of steps in which contaminating proteins are removed, based on difference in size, charge and hydrophobicity. Purification is monitored by SDS-PAGE (see Fig. 2.14). The primary sequence of the protein is determined by automated Edman degradation of peptides (see Fig. 2.18). The three-dimensional structure of the protein may be determined by X-ray crystallography.

ANALYSIS OF PROTEIN STRUCTURE

The typical steps in the purification of a protein are summarized in Figure 2.16. Once purified, for the determination of its amino acid composition, a protein is subjected to hydrolysis, commonly in 6 mol/L HCl at 110°C in a sealed and evacuated tube for 24–48 h. Under these conditions, tryptophan,

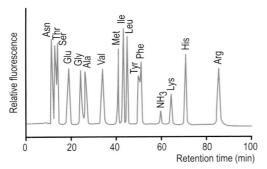

Fig. 2.17 **Typical chromatogram from an amino acid analysis by cation exchange chromatography.** A protein hydrolysate is applied to the cation exchange column in a dilute buffer at acidic pH (~3.0), at which all amino acids are positively charged. The amino acids are then eluted by a gradient of increasing pH and salt concentrations. The most anionic (acidic) amino acids elute first, followed by the neutral and basic amino acids. Amino acids are derived by post-column reaction with a fluorogenic compound, such as o-phthalaldehyde.

cysteine and most of the cystine are destroyed, and glutamine and asparagine are quantitatively deaminated to give glutamate and aspartate, respectively. Recovery of serine and threonine is incomplete and decreases with increasing time of hydrolysis. Alternative hydrolysis procedures may be used for measurement of tryptophan, while cysteine and cystine may be converted to an acid-stable cysteic acid prior to hydrolysis. Following hydrolysis, the free amino acids are separated on an automated amino acid analyzer using an ion exchange column or, following pre-column derivatization with colored or fluorescent reagents, by reversed-phase high-performance liquid chromatography (HPLC). The free amino acids fractionated by ion exchange chromatography are detected by reaction with a chromogenic or fluorogenic reagent, such as ninhydrin or dansyl chloride, Edman's reagent (see below) or o-phthalaldehyde. These techniques allow the measurement of as little as 1 pmol of each amino acid. A typical elution pattern of amino acids in a purified protein is shown in Figure 2.17.

Determination of the primary structure of proteins

Information on the primary sequence of a protein is essential for understanding its functional properties, the identification of the family to which the protein belongs, as well as characterization of mutant proteins that cause disease. A protein may be cleaved first by digestion by specific endoproteases, such as trypsin (Chapter 6), V8 protease or lysyl endopeptidase, to obtain peptide fragments. Trypsin cleaves peptide bonds on the C-terminal side of arginine and lysine residues, provided the next residue is not proline. Lysyl endopeptidase is also frequently used to cleave at the C-terminal side of lysine. Cleavage by chemical reagents such as cyanogen bromide is also useful. Cyanogen bromide cleaves on the C-terminal side of methionine residues.

THE PROTEOME

A proteome is defined as the full complement of proteins produced by a particular genome; changes in cellular and tissue proteomes occur in response to hormonal signaling during development, and environmental stresses. Proteomics is defined as the qualitative and quantitative comparison of proteomes under different conditions. In one approach to analyze the proteome of a cell, proteins are extracted and subjected to two-dimensional polyacrylamide gel electrophoresis (2D-PAGE). Individual protein spots are identified by staining, then extracted and digested with proteases. Small peptides from such a gel are sequenced by mass spectrometry, permitting the identification of the protein. A typical analysis of a rat liver extract is shown in Fig. 2.15. In 2D-differential gel electrophoresis (DIGE), two proteomes may be compared by labeling their proteins with different fluorescent dyes, e.g. red and green. The labeled proteins are mixed, then fractionated by 2D-PAGE. Proteins present in both proteomes will appear as yellow spots, while unique proteins will be red or green, respectively (see Chapter 36).

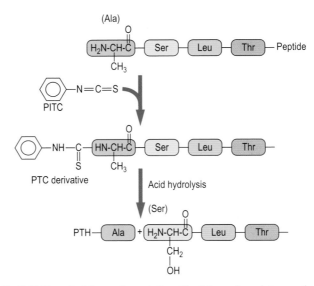

Fig. 2.18 **Steps in Edman degradation.** The Edman degradation method sequentially removes one residue at a time from the amino end of a peptide. Phenyl isothiocyanate (PITC) converts the N-terminal amino group of the immobilized peptide to a phenylthiocarbamyl derivative (PTC amino acid) in alkaline solution. Acid treatment removes the first amino acid as the phenylthiohydantoin (PTH) derivative, which is identified by HPLC.

Before cleavage, proteins with cysteine and cystine residues are reduced by 2-mercaptoethanol and then treated with iodoacetate to form carboxymethylcysteine residues. This avoids spontaneous formation of inter- or intramolecular disulfides during analyses.

The cleaved peptides are then subjected to reverse-phase HPLC to purify the peptide fragments, and then sequenced on an automated protein sequencer, using the Edman degradation technique (Fig. 2.18). The sequence of overlapping

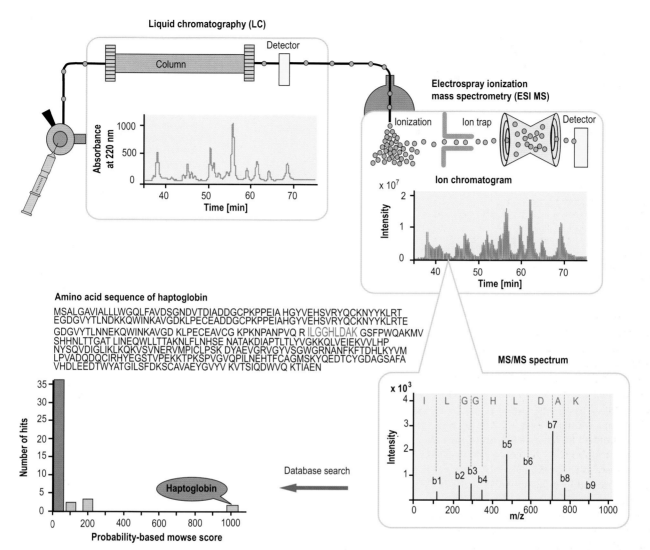

Fig. 2.19 **Identification of proteins by HPLC electrospray ionization-liquid chromatography mass spectrometry (HPLC-ESI-MS/MS).** The protein is digested with trypsin and the tryptic peptides are fractionated on a reversed-phase HPLC system, using a gradient of increasing concentration of organic solvent in water. The quality of peptide fractionation is monitored by ultraviolet detection, measuring the absorbance of the peptide bond (~220 nm). The peptides (in solution) are injected directly into the mass spectrometer. The ESI interface has a high vacuum liquid inlet system in which the majority of solvent is rapidly evaporated and a voltage is applied to ionize the peptides. The peptide ions are enriched in an 'ion trap', then extracted according to their molecular mass (m/z = mass/charge ratio). They are then fragmented by collision with gas molecules and the fragments are further analyzed in a second mass spectrometer module, a process known as tandem mass spectrometry (MS/MS). Because peptide bonds fragment in a characteristic manner, to the left and right of the α carbon, fragments are obtained which differ in molecular weight according to the amino acid sequence of the peptide. The b-ions shown here represent the series of fragment obtained on cleavage at the amino terminus. A complementary series of y-ions is obtained on fragmentation from the carboxyl end. The mass of the peptides and fragment ion patterns are analyzed to obtain the sequence of amino acids, which is then compared to a protein database (see websites at end of chapter). In the example shown, the peptide is identified as ILGGHLDAK, which is found in the haptoglobin molecule. More than a single peptide is commonly used for unambiguous identification of a protein.

peptides is then used to obtain the primary structure of the protein. Mass spectrometry is more commonly used today to obtain both the molecular mass and sequence of polypeptides simultaneously (see below). Both techniques can be applied directly to proteins or peptides recovered from SDS-PAGE or two-dimensional electrophoresis (IEF plus SDS-PAGE). Once the partial amino acid sequence is obtained, one can determine the nucleotide sequence of the DNA that encodes this

polypeptide segment. After chemically synthesizing this DNA, it can be used to identify and isolate the gene containing its nucleotide sequence (Chapter 34).

Protein sequencing and identification can also be done by electrospray ionization liquid chromatography tandem mass spectrometry (HPLC-ESI-MS/MS) (Fig. 2.19). This technique is sufficiently sensitive that proteins isolated by 2D-PAGE (see Fig. 2.15), typically less than 1 μg of protein per spot, can be

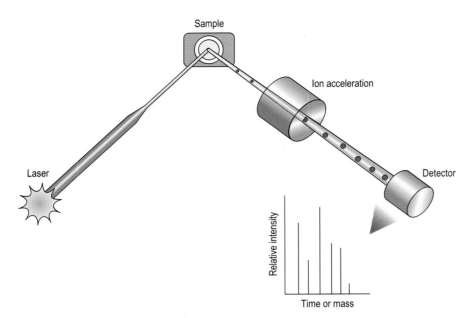

Sample

Ion acceleration

Laser

Detector

Relative intensity

Time or mass

Fig. 2.20 **Matrix-assisted laser desorption ionization-time of flight mass spectrometry (MALDI-TOF MS).** Proteins or peptides are mixed with a matrix material and dried on a sample plate; the matrix is designed to absorb light at a specific laser wavelength, generating heat. The protein or peptides are ionized and desorbed by a pulse of laser irradiation, and the ionized particles are accelerated in a voltage gradient at a rate that is dependent on their mass-to-charge (m/z) ratio. Each ion reaches the detector after a time (TOF) that is directly related to its molecular mass. These ions may then be fragmented to obtain amino acid sequence formation.

 ## PROTEIN FOLDING AND FOLDING DISEASE

For proteins to function properly, they must fold into the correct shape. Proteins have evolved so that one fold is more favorable than all others – the native state. Numerous proteins assist other proteins in the folding process. These proteins, termed chaperones, include 'heat shock' proteins, HSP 60 and HSP 70, and protein disulfide isomerase. A protein folding disease is a disease that is associated with abnormal conformation of a protein. This occurs in chronic, age-related diseases, such as Alzheimer's disease, amyotrophic lateral sclerosis, and Parkinson's disease.

digested with trypsin in situ, then extracted from the gel and identified, based on their amino acid sequence. This technique, as well as a complementary technique called matrix-assisted laser desorption ionization-time of flight (MALDI-TOF) MS/MS (Fig. 2.20), can be applied for determination of the molecular weight of intact proteins, as well as for sequence analysis of peptides, leading to unambiguous identification of a protein.

Determination of the three-dimensional structure of proteins

X-ray crystallography and NMR spectroscopy are usually used for determination of the three-dimensional structure of proteins. X-ray crystallography depends on the diffraction of X-rays by the electrons of the atoms constituting the molecule. However, since the X-ray diffraction caused by an

 ## CREUTZFELDT–JAKOB DISEASE

A 56-year-old male cattle rancher presented with epileptic cramp and dementia and was diagnosed as having Creutzfeldt–Jakob disease, a human prion disease. The prion diseases, also known as transmissible spongiform encephalopathies, are neurodegenerative diseases that affect both humans and animals. This disease in sheep and goats is designated as scrapie, and in cows as spongiform encephalopathy (mad cow disease). The diseases are characterized by the accumulation of an abnormal isoform of a host-encoded protein, prion protein-cellular form (PrPC), in affected brains.

Comment. Prions appear to be composed only of PrPSc (scrapie form) molecules, which are abnormal conformers of the normal, host-encoded protein. PrPC has a high α-helical content and is devoid of β-pleated sheets, whereas PrPSc has a high β-pleated sheet content. The conversion of PrPC into PrPSc involves a profound conformational change. The progression of infectious prion diseases appears to involve an interaction between PrPC and PrPSc, which induces a conformational change of the α-helix-rich PrPC to the β-pleated sheet-rich conformer of PrPSc. PrPSc-derived prion disease may be genetic or infectious. The amino acid sequences of different mammalian PrPCs are similar, and the conformation of the protein is virtually the same in all mammalian species.

individual molecule is immeasurably weak, the protein must exist in the form of a well-ordered crystal, in which each molecule has the same conformation in a specific position and orientation on a three-dimensional lattice. Based on diffraction of a collimated beam of electrons, the distribution of the electron density, and thus the location of atoms, in the crystal can be calculated to determine the structure of the protein. For protein crystallization, the most frequently used method is the hanging drop method which involves the use of a simple apparatus that permits a small portion of a protein solution (typically $10\,\mu l$ droplet containing $0.5–1\,mg/$ protein) to evaporate gradually to reach the saturating point at which the protein begins to crystallize. NMR spectroscopy is usually used for structural analysis of small organic compounds, but high-field NMR is also useful for determination of the structure of a protein in solution and complements information obtained by X-ray crystallography.

Summary

There are thousands of different proteins in cells, and each protein has a different structure and function. The higher order structure of a protein is the product of its primary, secondary, tertiary, and quaternary structure. Purification and characterization of proteins are essential for elucidating their structure and function. By taking advantage of differences in their size, solubility, charge and ligand binding properties, proteins can be purified to homogeneity using various chromatographic and electrophoretic techniques. The molecular mass and purity of a protein, and its subunit composition, can be determined by SDS-PAGE. The primary structure can be determined by hydrolysis of a protein and automated Edman degradation. Deciphering the primary and three-dimensional structures of a protein by X-ray analysis or NMR spectroscopy leads to an understanding of structure–function relationships in proteins. Mass spectrometry has become a powerful technique for elucidating protein structure, chemical modification, function and homology.

ACTIVE LEARNING

1. Mass spectrometry analysis of blood, urine and tissues is now being applied for clinical diagnosis. Discuss the merits of this technique with respect to specificity, sensitivity, through-put and breadth of analysis, including proteomic analysis for diagnostic purposes.
2. Review the importance of protein misfolding and deposition in tissues in age-related chronic diseases.

Further reading

Dominguez DC, Lopes R, Torres ML. Proteomics: clinical applications. *Clin Lab Sci* 2007; **20**: 245–248.

Frydman J. Folding of newly translated proteins *in vivo*: the chaperones. *Annu Rev Biochem* 2001; **70**: 603–647.

Imai J, Yashiroda H, Maruya M, Yahara I, Tanaka K. Proteasomes and molecular chaperones: cellular machinery responsible for folding and destruction of unfolded proteins. *Cell Cycle* 2003; **2**: 585–590.

Kovacs GG, Budka H. Prion diseases: from protein to cell pathology. *Am J Pathol* 2008; **172**: 555–565.

Marouga R, David S, Hawkins E. The development of the DIGE system: 2D fluorescence difference gel analysis technology. *Anal Bioanal Chem* 2005; **382**: 669–678.

Matt P, Fu Z, Ru Q, Van Eyk JE. Biomarker discovery: proteome fractionation and separation in biological samples. *J Physiol Genomics* 2008; **14**: 12–17.

Shkundina, IS, Ter-Avanesyan, MD. Prions. *Biochemistry* (Moscow) 2007; **72**:1519-1536.

Valentine JS, Hart PJ. Misfolded CuZnSOD and amyotrophic lateral sclerosis. *Proc Natl Acad Sci USA* 2003; **100**: 3617–3622.

Walsh CT. *Posttranslational modification of proteins: expanding nature's inventory*, 3rd edn. Colorado: Roberts & Co., 2007.

Websites

Amino acids: www.owlnet.rice.edu/~bios301/Bios301/lecture/301_4_2006.pdf

Protein structure (graphics, videos, general): www3.interscience.wiley.com:8100/legacy/college/boyer/0471661791/structure/jmol_intro/sec_str.htm

Molecular visualization: http://molvis.sdsc.edu/index.htm

Collagen: www.messiah.edu/departments/chemistry/molscilab/Jmol/collagen/chapter1.htm

Protein databanks: www.pdb.org and http://us.expasy.org

3. Carbohydrates and Lipids

J W Baynes

LEARNING OBJECTIVES

After reading this chapter you should be able to:

- Describe the structure and nomenclature of carbohydrates.
- Identify the major carbohydrates in the human body and in our diet.
- Distinguish between reducing and nonreducing sugars.
- Describe various types of glycosidic bonds in oligosaccharides and polysaccharides.
- Identify the major classes of lipids in the human body and in our diet.
- Describe the types of bonds in lipids and their sensitivity to saponification.
- Explain the general role of triglycerides, phospholipids and glycolipids in the body.
- Outline the general features of the fluid mosaic model of the structure of biologic membranes.

INTRODUCTION

This chapter describes the structure of carbohydrates and lipids found in the diet and in tissues. These two classes of compounds differ significantly in physical and chemical properties. Carbohydrates are hydrophilic; the smaller carbohydrates, such as milk sugar and table sugar, are soluble in aqueous solution, while polymers such as starch or cellulose form colloidal dispersions or are insoluble. Lipids vary in size, but rarely exceed 2 kDa in molecular mass; they are insoluble in water but soluble in organic solvents. In contrast to proteins, carbohydrates and lipids are major sources of energy and are stored in the body in the form of energy reserves – glycogen and triglycerides (fat). Both carbohydrates and lipids may be bound to proteins and have important structural and regulatory functions, which are elaborated in later chapters. This chapter ends with a description of the fluid mosaic model of biological membranes, illustrating how protein, carbohydrates and lipids are integrated into the structure of biological membranes that surround the cell and intracellular compartments.

CARBOHYDRATES

Nomenclature and structure of simple sugars

The classic definition of a carbohydrate is a polyhydroxy aldehyde or ketone. The simplest carbohydrates, having two hydroxyl groups, are glyceraldehyde and dihydroxyacetone (Fig. 3.1). These three-carbon sugars are trioses; the suffix 'ose' designates a sugar. Glyceraldehyde is an aldose, and dihydroxyacetone a ketose sugar. Prefixes and examples of longer chain sugars are shown in Table 3.1.

Numbering of the carbons begins from the end containing the aldehyde or ketone functional group. Sugars are classified into the D or L family, based on the configuration around the highest numbered asymmetric center (Fig. 3.2). In contrast to the L-amino acids, nearly all sugars found in the body have the D configuration.

An aldohexose, such as glucose, contains four asymmetric centers, so that there are 16 (2^4) possible stereoisomers, depending on whether each of the four carbons has the D or L configuration (see Fig. 3.2). Eight of these aldohexoses are D-sugars. Only three of these are found in significant amounts in the body: glucose (blood sugar), mannose and galactose (see Fig. 3.2). Similarly, there are four possible epimeric D-ketohexoses; fructose (fruit sugar) (see Fig. 3.2) is the only ketohexose present at significant concentration in our diet or in the body.

Because of their asymmetric centers, sugars are optically active compounds. The rotation of plane polarized light may be dextrorotatory ($+$) or levorotatory ($-$). This designation

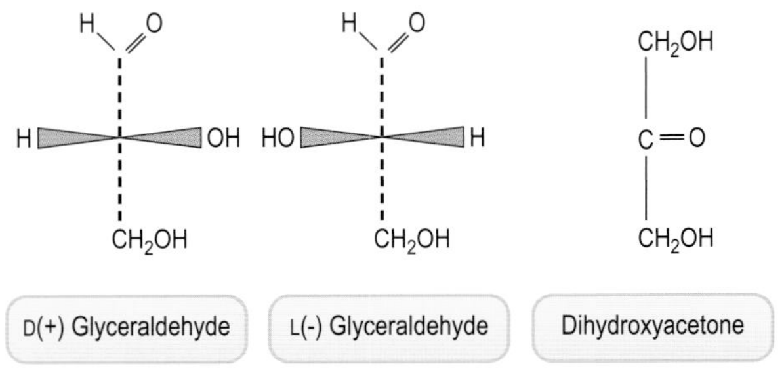

D(+) Glyceraldehyde   L(-) Glyceraldehyde   Dihydroxyacetone

Fig. 3.1 **Structures of the trioses.** D- and L-glyceraldehyde (aldoses) and dihydroxyacetone (a ketose).

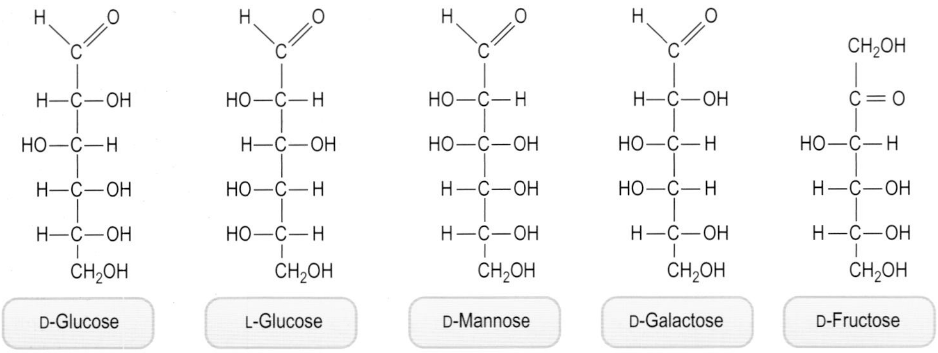

Fig. 3.2 **Structures of hexoses: D- and L-glucose, D-mannose, D-galactose and D-fructose.** The D and L designations are based on the configuration at the highest numbered asymmetric center, C-5 in the case of hexoses. Note that L-glucose is the mirror image of D-glucose, i.e. the geometry at all of the asymmetric centers is reversed. Mannose is the C-2 epimer, and galactose the C-4 epimer of glucose. These linear projections of carbohydrate structures are known as Fischer projections.

Classification of carbohydrates by length of the carbon chain

Number of carbons	Name	Examples in human biology
Three	triose	glyceraldehyde, dihydroxyacetone
Four	tetrose	erythrose
Five	pentose	ribose, ribulose*, xylose, xylulose*, deoxyribose
Six	hexose	glucose, mannose, galactose, fucose, fructose
Seven	heptose	sedoheptulose*
Eight	octose	none
Nine	nonose	neuraminic (sialic) acid

*The syllable 'ul' indicates that a sugar is ketose; the formal name for fructose would be 'gluculose'. As with fructose, the keto group is located at C-2 of the sugar, and the remaining carbons have the same geometry as the parent sugar.

Table 3.1 **Classification of carbohydrates by length of the carbon chain.**

is also commonly included in the name of the sugar; thus D(+)-glucose or D(−)-fructose indicates that the D form of glucose is dextrorotatory, while the D form of fructose is levorotatory.

Cyclization of sugars

The linear sugar structures shown in Figure 3.2 imply that aldose sugars have a chemically reactive, easily oxidizable, electrophilic, aldehyde residue; aldehydes such as formaldehyde or glutaraldehyde react rapidly with amino groups in protein to form Schiff base (imine) adducts and crosslinks during fixation of tissues. However, glucose is relatively resistant to oxidation and does not react rapidly with protein. As shown in Figure 3.3, glucose exists largely in nonreactive, inert, cyclic hemiacetal conformations, >99.99% in aqueous solution at pH 7.4 and 37°C. Of all the D-sugars in the world, D-glucose exists to the greatest extent in these cyclic conformations, making it the least oxidizable and least reactive with protein. It has been proposed that the relative chemical inertness of glucose is the reason for its evolutionary selection as blood sugar.

When glucose cyclizes to a hemiacetal, it may form a furanose or pyranose ring structure, named after the 5- and 6-carbon cyclic ethers, furan and pyran (see Fig. 3.3). Note that the cyclization reaction creates a new asymmetric center at C-1; the -OH group at C-1 may assume either the D or L configuration. C-1 is known as the anomeric carbon. The preferred conformation for glucose is the β-anomer (~65%) in which the hydroxyl group on C-1 is oriented equatorial to the ring. The β-anomer is the most stable form of glucose because all of the hydroxyl groups, which are bulkier than hydrogen, are oriented equatorially, in the plane of the ring. The α- and β-anomers of glucose can be isolated in pure form by selective crystallization from aqueous and organic solvents. They have different optical rotations, but equilibrate with one another over a period of hours in aqueous solution to form the equilibrium mixture of 65:35 β:α anomer. These differences in structure may seem unimportant, but in fact some metabolic pathways use one anomer but not the other, and vice versa. Similarly, while the fructopyranose conformations are the primary forms of fructose in aqueous solution, most of fructose metabolism proceeds from the furanose form.

In addition to the basic sugar structures discussed above, a number of other common sugar structures are presented in Figure 3.4. These sugars, deoxysugars, aminosugars and sugar acids are found primarily in oligosaccharide or polymeric structures in the body, e.g. ribose in RNA and deoxyribose in DNA, or they may be attached to proteins or lipids to form glycoconjugates (glycoproteins or glycolipids, respectively). Glucose is the only sugar found to a significant extent as a free sugar (blood sugar) in the body.

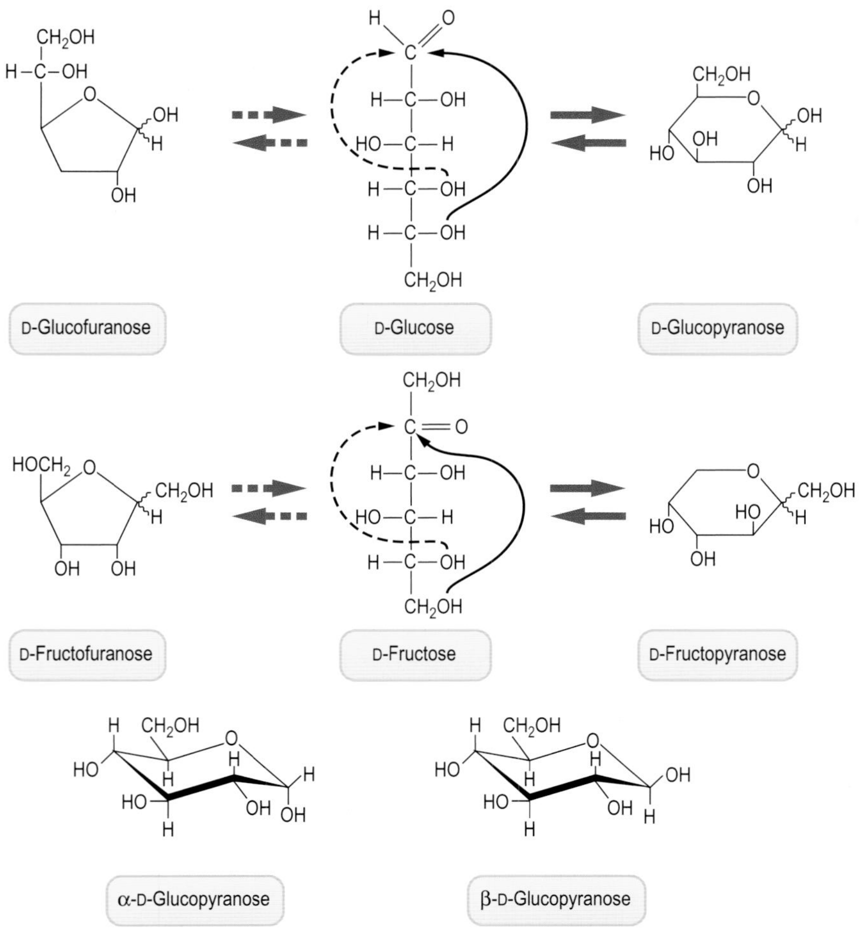

Fig. 3.3 **Linear and cyclic representations of glucose and fructose.** (Top) There are four cyclic forms of glucose, in equilibrium with the linear form: α- and β-glucopyranose and α- and β-glucofuranose. The pyranose forms account for over 99% of total glucose in solution. These cyclic conformations are known as Haworth projections; by convention, groups to the right in Fischer projections are shown above the ring, and groups to the left, below the ring. The squiggly bonds to H and OH from *C*-1, the anomeric carbon, indicate indeterminate geometry and represent either the α or the β anomer. (Middle) The linear and cyclic forms of fructose. The ratio of pyranose:furanose forms of fructose in aqueous solution is ~3:1. The ratio shifts as a function of temperature, pH, salt concentration and other factors. (Bottom) Stereochemical representations of the chair forms of α- and β-glucopyranose. The preferred structure in solution, β-glucopyranose, has all of the hydroxyl groups, including the anomeric hydroxyl group, in equatorial positions around the ring, minimizing steric interactions.

Disaccharides, oligosaccharides and polysaccharides

Carbohydrates are commonly coupled to one another by glycosidic bonds to form disaccharides, trisaccharides, oligosaccharides and polysaccharides. Saccharides composed of a single sugar are termed homoglycans, while saccharides with complex composition are termed heteroglycans. The name of the more complex structures includes not only the name of the component sugars, but also the ring conformation of the sugars, the anomeric configuration of the linkage between sugars, the site of attachment of one sugar to another, and the nature of the atom involved in the linkage, usually an oxygen or *O*-glycosidic bond, sometimes a nitrogen or *N*-glycosidic bond. Figure 3.5 shows the structure of several common disaccharides in our diet: lactose (milk sugar), sucrose (table sugar), maltose and isomaltose, which are products of digestion of starch, cellobiose, which is obtained on hydrolysis of cellulose, and hyaluronic acid.

THE INFORMATION CONTENT OF COMPLEX GLYCANS

Sugars are attached to each other in glycosidic linkages between hemiacetal carbon of one sugar and a hydroxyl group of another sugar. Two glucose residues can be linked in many different linkages (i.e. α1,2; α1,3; α1,4; α1,6; β1,2; β1,3; β1,4; β1,6; α,α1,1; α, β1,1; β,β1,1) to give 11 different disaccharides, each with different chemical and biologic properties. Two different sugars, such as glucose and galactose, can be linked either glucose → galactose or galactose → glucose and these two disaccharides can have a total of 20 different isomers. In contrast, two identical amino acids, such as two alanines, can only form one dipeptide, alanyl-alanine. And two different amino acids, i.e. alanine and glycine, can only form two dipeptides, alanyl-glycine and glycyl-alanine. As a result, sugars have the potential to provide a great deal of chemical information. As outlined in Chapters 26 and 27, carbohydrates bound to proteins and lipids in cell membranes can serve as recognition signals for both cell–cell and cell–pathogen interactions.

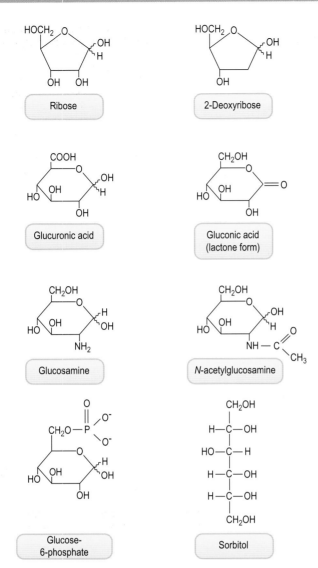

Fig. 3.4 **Examples of various types of sugars found in human tissues.** Ribose, the pentose sugar in ribonucleic acid (RNA); 2-deoxyribose, the deoxypentose in DNA; glucuronic acid, an acidic sugar formed by oxidation of *C*-6 of glucose; gluconic acid, an acidic sugar formed by oxidation of *C*-1 of glucose, shown in the δ-lactone form; glucosamine, an amino sugar; *N*-acetylglucosamine, an acetylated amino sugar. Glucose-6-phosphate, a phosphate ester of glucose, an intermediate in glucose metabolism; sorbitol, a polyol formed on reduction of glucose.

Differences in linkage make a big difference in biochemistry and nutrition. Thus, amylose, a component of starch, is an α-1→4-linked linear glucan, while cellulose is a β-1→4-linked linear glucan. These two polysaccharides differ only in the anomeric linkage between glucose subunits, but they are very different molecules. Starch is soluble in water, cellulose is insoluble; starch is pasty, cellulose is fibrous; starch is digestible, while cellulose is indigestible by humans; starch is a food, rich in calories, while cellulose is roughage.

REDUCING SUGAR ASSAY FOR BLOOD GLUCOSE

The original assays for blood glucose measured the reducing activity of blood. These assays work because glucose, at 5 mM concentration, is the major reducing substance in blood. The Fehling and Benedict assays use alkaline cupric salt solutions. With heating, the glucose decomposes oxidatively, yielding a complex mixture of organic acids and aldehydes. Oxidation of the sugar reduces cupric ion (blue-green color) to cuprous ion (orange-red color) in solution. The color yield produced is directly proportional to the glucose content of the sample. Reducing sugar assays do not distinguish glucose from other reducing sugars, such as fructose or galactose. In diseases of fructose and galactose metabolism, such as hereditary fructose intolerance of galactosemia (Chapter 29), these assays could yield positive results, creating the false impression of diabetes.

LIPIDS

Lipids are localized primarily to three compartments in the body: plasma, adipose tissue and biological membranes. This introduction will focus on the structure of fatty acids (the simplest form of lipids, found primarily in plasma), triglycerides (the storage form of lipids, found primarily in adipose tissue), and phospholipid (the major class of membrane lipids in all cells). Steroids, such as cholesterol, and (glyco)sphingolipids will be mentioned in the context of biological membranes, but these lipids and others, such as the eicosanoids, will be addressed in detail in later chapters.

Fatty acids

Fatty acids exist in free form and as components of more complex lipids. As summarized in Table 3.2, they are long, straight chain alkanoic acids, most commonly with 16 or 18 carbons. They may be saturated or unsaturated, the latter containing 1–5 double bonds, all in *cis* geometry. The double bonds are not conjugated, but separated by methylene groups.

Fatty acids with a single double bond are described as monounsaturated, while those with two or more double bonds are described as polyunsaturated fatty acids. The polyunsaturated fatty acids are commonly classified into two groups, ω-3 and ω-6 fatty acids, depending on whether the first double bond appears three or six carbons from the terminal methyl group. The melting point of fatty acids, as well as that of more complex lipids, increases with the chain length of the fatty acid, but decreases with the number of double bonds. The *cis*-double bonds place a kink in the linear structure of the fatty acid chain, interfering with close packing,

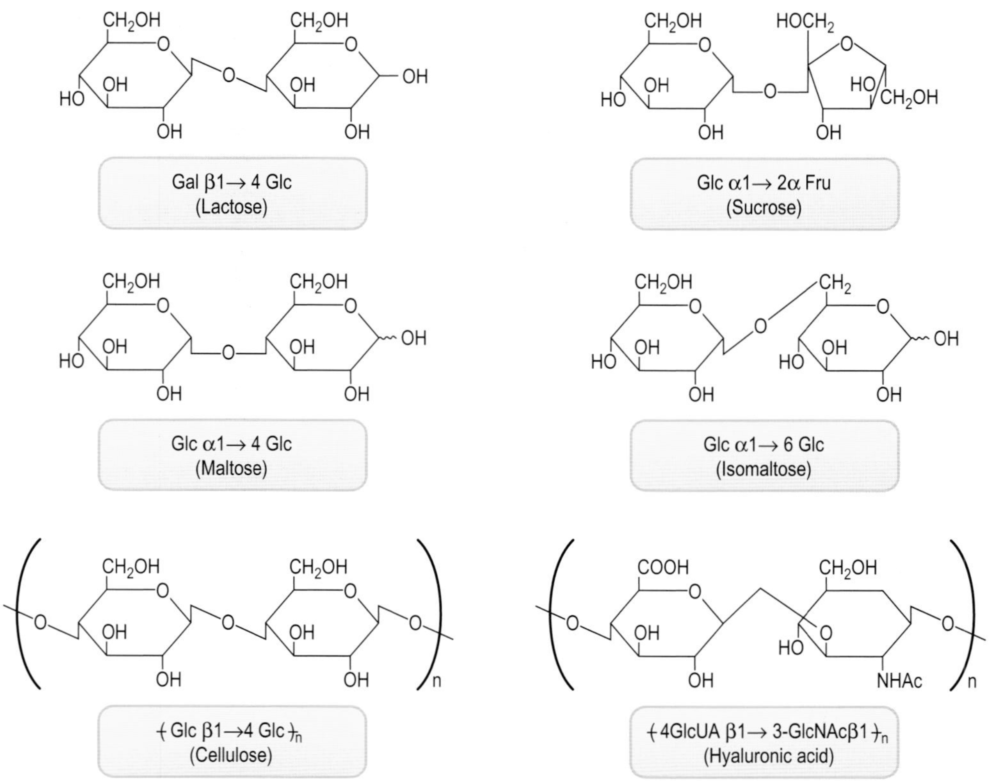

Fig. 3.5 **Structures of common disaccharides and polysaccharides.** Lactose (milk sugar); sucrose (table sugar); maltose and isomaltose, disaccharides formed on degradation of starch; and repeating disaccharide units of cellulose (from wood) and hyaluronic acid (from vertebral disks). Fru, fructose; Gal, galactose; Glc, glucose; GlcNAc, *N*-acetylglucosamine; GlcUA, glucuronic acid.

Naturally occurring fatty acids					
Carbon atoms		**Chemical formula**	**Systematic name**	**Common name**	**Melting point (°C)**
Saturated fatty acids					
12	12:0	$CH_3(CH_2)_{10}COOH$	*n*-dodecanoic	lauric	44
14	14:0	$CH_3(CH_2)_{12}COOH$	*n*-tetradecanoic	myristic	54
16	16:0	$CH_3(CH_2)_{14}COOH$	*n*-hexadecanoic	palmitic	63
18	18:0	$CH_3(CH_2)_{16}COOH$	*n*-octadecanoic	stearic	70
20	20:0	$CH_3(CH_2)_{18}COOH$	*n*-eicosanoic	arachidic	77
Unsaturated fatty acids					
16	16:1; ω-6, Δ^9	$CH_3(CH_2)_5CH{=}CH(CH_2)_7COOH$		palmitoleic	-0.5
18	18:1; ω-9, Δ^9	$CH_3(CH_2)_7CH{=}CH(CH_2)_7COOH$		oleic	13
18	18:2; ω-6, $\Delta^{9,12}$	$CH_3(CH_2)_4CH{=}CHCH_2CH{=}CH(CH_2)_7COOH$		linoleic	-5
18	18:3; ω-3, $\Delta^{9,12,15}$	$CH_3CH_2CH{=}CHCH_2CH{=}CHCH_2CH{=}CH(CH_2)_7COOH$		linolenic	-11
20	20:4; ω-6, $\Delta^{5,8,11,14}$	$CH_3(CH_2)_4CH{=}CHCH_2CH{=}CHCH_2CH{=}CHCH_2CH{=}CH(CH_2)_7COOH$		arachidonic	-50

Table 3.2 **Structure and melting point of naturally occurring fatty acids.** For unsaturated fatty acids, the 'ω' designation indicates the location of the first double bond from the methyl end of the molecule; the Δ superscripts indicate the location of the double bonds from the carboxyl end of the molecule. Unsaturated fatty acids account for about two-thirds of all fatty acids in the body; oleate and palmitate account for about one half and one quarter of total fatty acids in the body.

BUTTER OR MARGARINE?

There is continuing debate among nutritionists about the health benefits of butter versus margarine in foods.

Comments. Butter is rich in both cholesterol and triglycerides containing saturated fatty acids, which are dietary risk factors for atherosclerosis. Margarine contains no cholesterol and is richer in unsaturated fatty acids. However, the unsaturated fatty acids in margarine are mostly the unnatural *trans*-fatty acids formed during the partial hydrogenation of vegetable oils. *Trans*-fatty acids affect plasma lipids in the same fashion as saturated fatty acids, suggesting that there are comparable risks associated with the consumption of butter or margarine. The resolution of this issue is complicated by the fact that various forms of margarine, for example soft-spread and hard-block types, vary significantly in their content of *trans*-fatty acids. Partially hydrogenated oils are more stable than the natural oils during heating; when used for deep-frying, they need to be changed less frequently. Despite the additional expense, the food and food-service industries have gradually shifted to the use of natural oils, rich in unsaturated fatty acids and without *trans*-fatty acids, for cooking and baking.

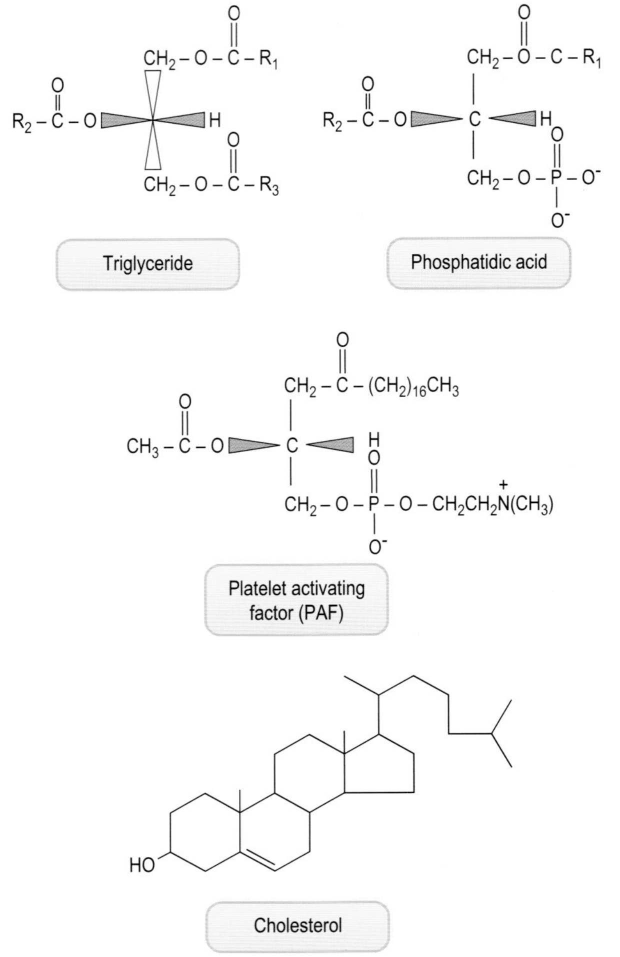

Fig. 3.6 **Structure of four lipids with significantly different biological functions.** Triglycerides are storage fats. Phosphatidic acid is a metabolic precursor of both triglycerides and phospholipids (see Fig. 3.7). Cholesterol is less polar than phospholipids; the hydroxyl group tends to be on the membrane surface, while the polycyclic system intercalates between the fatty acid chains of phospholipids. Platelet-activating factor, a mediator of inflammation, is an unusual phospholipid, with a lipid alcohol rather than an esterified lipid at the *sn*-1 position, an acetyl group at *sn*-2, and phosphorylcholine esterified at the *sn*-3 position.

therefore requiring a lower temperature for freezing, i.e. they have a lower melting point.

Triacylglycerols (triglycerides)

Fatty acids in plant and animal tissues are commonly esterified to glycerol, forming a triacylglycerol (triglyceride) (Fig. 3.6), either oils (liquid) or fats (solid). In humans, triglycerides are stored in solid form (fat) in adipose tissue. They are degraded to glycerol and fatty acids in response to hormonal signals, then released into plasma for metabolism in other tissues, primarily muscle and liver. The ester bond of triglycerides and other glycerolipids is also readily hydrolyzed ex vivo by a strong base, such as NaOH, forming glycerol and free fatty acids. This process is known as saponification; one of the products, the sodium salt of the fatty acid, is soap.

Glycerol itself is does not have a chiral carbon, but the numbering is standardized using the stereochemical numbering (*sn*) system, which places the hydroxyl group of C-2 on the left; thus all glycerolipids are derived from L-glycerol (see Fig. 3.6). Triglycerides isolated from natural sources are not pure compounds, but mixtures of molecules with different fatty acid composition, e.g. 1-palmitoyl, 2-oleyl, 3-linoleoyl-L-glycerol, where the distribution and type of fatty acids vary from molecule to molecule.

Phospholipids

Phospholipids are polar lipids derived from phosphatidic acid (1,2-diacyl-glycerol-3-phosphate) (see Fig. 3.6). Like triglycerides, the glycerophospholipids contain a spectrum of fatty acids at the *sn*-1 and *sn*-2 position, but the *sn*-3 position is occupied by phosphate esterified to an amino compound. The phosphate acts as a bridging diester, linking the diacylglyceride to a polar, nitrogenous compound, most frequently choline, ethanolamine or serine (Fig. 3.7). Phosphatidylcholine (lecithin), for example, usually contains palmitic acid or stearic acid at its *sn*-1 position and an 18-carbon, unsaturated fatty acid (e.g. oleic, linoleic or linolenic) at its *sn*-2 position. Phosphatidylethanolamine

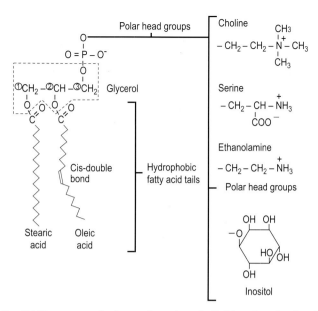

Fig. 3.7 **Structure of the major phospholipids of animal cell membranes.** Phosphatidylcholine, phosphatidylserine, phosphatidylethanolamine and phosphatidylinositol (see also Chapter 27).

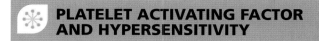

PLATELET ACTIVATING FACTOR AND HYPERSENSITIVITY

Platelet activating factor (PAF; see Fig. 3.6.) contains an acetyl group at carbon-2 of glycerol and a saturated 18-carbon alkyl ether group linked to the hydroxyl group at carbon-1, rather than the usual long-chain fatty acids of phosphatidylcholine. It is a major mediator of hypersensitivity reactions, acute inflammatory reactions, and anaphylactic shock, and affects the permeability properties of membranes, increasing platelet aggregation and causing cardiovascular and pulmonary changes, including edema and hypotension. In allergic persons, cells involved in the immune response become coated with immunoglobulin E (IgE) molecules that are specific for a particular antigen or allergen, such as pollen or insect venom. When these individuals are reexposed to that antigen, antigen–IgE complexes form on the surface of the inflammatory cells and activate the synthesis and release of PAF.

(cephalin) usually has a longer chain polyunsaturated fatty acid at the *sn*-2 position, such as arachidonic acid. These complex lipids contribute charge to the membrane: phosphatidylcholine and phosphatidylethanolamine are zwitterionic at physiologic pH and have no net charge, while phosphatidylserine and phosphatidylinositol are anionic. A number of other phospholipid structures with special functions will be introduced in later chapters.

When dispersed in aqueous solution, phospholipids spontaneously form lamellar structures and, under suitable conditions, they organize into extended bilayer structures – not only lamellar structures but also closed vesicular structures termed liposomes. The liposome is a model for the structure of a biological membrane, a bilayer of polar lipids with the polar faces exposed to the aqueous environment and the fatty acid side chains buried in the oily, hydrophobic interior of the membrane. The liposomal surface membrane, like its component phospholipids, is a pliant, mobile and flexible structure at body temperature.

Biological membranes also contain another important amphipathic lipid, cholesterol, a flat, rigid hydrophobic molecule with a polar hydroxyl group (see Fig. 3.6). Cholesterol is found in all biomembranes and acts as a modulator of membrane fluidity. At lower temperatures it interferes with fatty acid chain associations and increases fluidity, and at higher temperatures it tends to limit disorder and decrease fluidity. Thus, cholesterol-phospholipid mixtures have properties intermediate between the gel and liquid crystalline states of the pure phospholipids; they form stable but supple membrane structures.

STRUCTURE OF BIOMEMBRANES

Eukaryotic cells have a plasma membrane, as well as a number of intracellular membranes that define compartments with specialized functions; differences in both membrane protein and lipid composition distinguish these organelles (Table 3.3). In addition to the major phospholipids described in Figure 3.7, other important membrane lipids include cardiolipin, sphingolipids (sphingomyelin and glycolipids), and cholesterol, which are described in detail in later chapters. Cardiolipin (diphosphatidyl glycerol) is a significant component of the mitochondrial inner membrane, while sphingomyelin, phosphatidylserine and cholesterol are enriched in the plasma membrane (see Table 3.3). Some lipids are distributed asymmetrically in the membrane, e.g. phosphatidylserine and phosphatidylethanolamine are enriched on the inside, and phosphatidylcholine and sphingomyelin on the outside, of the red blood cell membrane. The protein to lipid ratio also differs among various biomembranes, ranging from about 80% (dry weight) lipid in the myelin sheath that insulates nerve cells, to about 20% lipid in the inner mitochondrial membrane. Lipids affect the structure of the membrane, the activity of membrane enzymes and transport systems, and membrane function in processes such as cellular recognition and signal transduction. Exposure of phosphatidylserine in the outer leaflet of the erythrocyte plasma membrane increases the cell's adherence to the vascular wall and is a signal for macrophage recognition and phagocytosis. Both of these recognition processes probably contribute to the natural process of red cell turnover in the spleen.

Phospholipid composition of organelle membranes from rat liver						
	Mitochondria	Microsomes	Lysosomes	Plasma membrane	Nuclear membrane	Golgi membrane
Cardiolipin	18	1	1	1	4	1
Phosphatidylethanolamine	35	22	14	23	13	20
Phosphatidylcholine	40	58	40	39	55	50
Phosphatidylinositol	5	10	5	8	10	12
Phosphatidylserine	1	2	2	9	3	6
Phosphatidic acid	–	1	1	1	2	<1
Sphingomyelin	1	1	20	16	3	8
Phospholipids (mg/mg protein)	0.18	0.37	0.16	0.67	0.50	0.83
Cholesterol (mg/mg protein)	<0.01	0.01	0.04	0.13	0.04	0.08

Table 3.3 **Phospholipid composition of organelle membranes from rat liver**. This table shows the phospholipid composition (%) of various organelle membranes together with weight ratios of phospholipids and cholesterol to protein.

The fluid mosaic model

The generally accepted model of biomembrane structure is the fluid mosaic model proposed by Singer & Nicolson in 1972. This model represents the membrane as a fluid-like phospholipid bilayer into which other lipids and proteins are embedded (Fig. 3.8). As in liposomes, the polar head groups of the phospholipids are exposed on the external surfaces of the membrane, with the fatty acyl chains oriented to the inside of the membrane. Whereas membrane lipids and proteins easily move on the membrane surface (lateral diffusion), 'flip-flop' movement of lipids between the outer and inner bilayer leaflets rarely occurs without the aid of the membrane enzyme flippase.

Membrane proteins are classified as integral (intrinsic) or peripheral (extrinsic) membrane proteins. The former are embedded deeply in the lipid bilayer and some of them traverse the membrane several times (transmembrane proteins) and have both internal and external polypeptide segments that participate in regulatory processes. In contrast, peripheral membrane proteins are bound to membrane lipids and/or integral membrane proteins (see Fig. 3.8); they can be removed from the membrane by mild chaotropic agents, such as urea, or mild detergent treatment without destroying the integrity of the membrane. In contrast, transmembrane proteins can be removed from the membrane only by treatments that dissolve membrane lipids and destroy the integrity of the membrane. Most of the transmembrane segments of integral membrane proteins form α-helices. They are composed

primarily of amino acid residues with nonpolar side chains – about 20 amino acid residues forming six to seven α-helical turns are enough to traverse a membrane of 5 nm (50 Å) thickness. The transmembrane domains interact with one another and with the hydrophobic tails of the lipid molecules, often forming complex structures, such as channels involved in ion transport processes (see Fig. 3.8 and Chapter 8).

Although this model is basically correct, there is growing evidence that many membrane proteins have limited mobility and are anchored in place by attachment to cytoskeletal proteins. Membrane substructures, described as lipid rafts, also demarcate regions of membranes with specialized composition and function. Specific phospholipids are also enriched in regions of the membrane involved in endocytosis and junctions with adjacent cells.

A major role of membranes is to maintain the structural integrity and barrier function of cells and organelles. However, membranes are not rigid or impermeable; they are fluid, and their components often move around in a directed fashion under the control of intracellular motors. The fluidity is essential for membrane function and cell viability; when bacteria are transferred to lower temperature, they respond by increasing the content of unsaturated fatty acids in membrane phospholipids, thereby maintaining membrane fluidity at low temperature. The membrane also mediates the transfer of information and molecules between the outside and inside of the cell, including cellular recognition, signal transduction processes and metabolite and ion

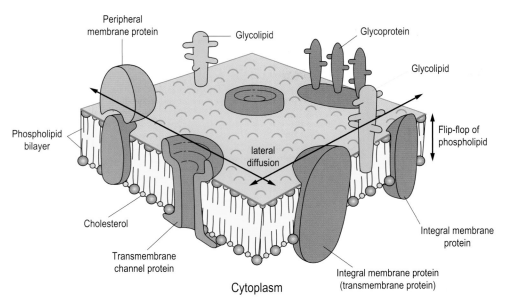

Peripheral membrane protein
Glycolipid
Glycoprotein
Glycolipid
Phospholipid bilayer
lateral diffusion
Flip-flop of phospholipid
Cholesterol
Transmembrane channel protein
Integral membrane protein
Integral membrane protein (transmembrane protein)
Cytoplasm

Fig. 3.8 **Fluid mosaic model of the plasma membrane.** In this model, proteins are embedded in a fluid phospholipid bilayer; some are on one surface (peripheral) and others span the membrane (transmembrane). Carbohydrates, covalently bound to some proteins and lipids, are not found on all subcellular membranes, e.g. mitochondrial membranes. On the plasma membrane, they are located almost exclusively on the outer surface of the cell (see also Chapter 8).

 ## MEMBRANE PATCHES

Although the fluid mosaic model is basically correct, it is recognized that there are membrane regions with unique protein and lipid compositions. Caveolae, 50–100 nm plasma membrane invaginations, and lipid rafts are plasma membrane patches (microdomains) important for signal transduction and endocytosis. These patches are enriched in cholesterol and sphingolipids, and the interaction of the long saturated fatty acid tails of sphingolipids with cholesterol results in the stabilization of the fluid environment. The patches are detergent insoluble and show high buoyant density on sucrose density gradient centrifugation. Pathogens such as viruses, parasites, bacteria and even bacterial toxins may enter into the host cells through binding to specific components of caveolae. Classic examples of patches enriched in a particular protein are the purple membrane of *Halobacterium halobium* containing bacteriorodopsin, and gap junctions containing connexin. Bacteriorodopsin is a light driven-proton pump which generates a H^+-concentration gradient across the bacterial membrane, providing energy for nutrient uptake for bacterial growth. Gap junctions between uterine muscle cells increase significantly during the late stages of pregnancy. They provide high-capacity channels between cells and permit coordinated contraction of the uterus during labor.

transport; fluidity is essential for these functions. Overall, cell membranes, which are often viewed by microscopy as static, are well-organized, flexible and responsive structures. In fact, the microscope picture is like a high-speed stop-action photo of a sporting event; it may look peaceful and still but there's a lot of action going on.

 ## MEMBRANE PERTURBATION BY AMPHIPATHIC COMPOUNDS

Amphipathic compounds have distinct polar and nonpolar moieties. They include many anesthetics and tranquilizers. The pharmacologic activities of these compounds are dependent on their ability to interact with membranes and perturb membrane structure. A number of antibiotics and natural products, such as bile salts and fatty acids, are also amphipathic. While effective at therapeutic concentrations, some of these drugs exhibit detergent-like action at moderate to high concentrations and disrupt the bilayer structure, resulting in membrane leakage.

 ## MEMBRANE ANCHORING PROTEINS

Lateral movements of some membrane proteins are restricted by their tethering to macromolecular assemblies inside (cytoskeleton) and/or outside (extracellular matrix) the cell and, in some cases, to membrane proteins of adjacent cells, e.g. in tight junctions between epithelial cells. Lateral diffusion of erythrocyte integral membrane proteins, band 3 (an anion transporter) and glycophorin, is limited by indirect interaction with spectrin, a cytoskeletal protein, through ankyrin and band 4.1 protein, respectively. Such interactions are so strong that they limit lateral diffusion of band 3. Genetic defects of spectrin cause hereditary spherocytosis and elliptocytosis, diseases characterized by altered red cell morphology. Ankyrin mutation affects the localization of plasma membrane proteins in cardiac muscle, causing cardiac arrhythmia, a risk factor for sudden cardiac death.

ACTIVE LEARNING

1. Compare the caloric value of starch and cellulose. Explain the difference.
2. Explain why disaccharides such as lactose, maltose and isomaltose are reducing sugars, but sucrose is not.
3. What does the iodine number of a lipid indicate about its structure?
4. Review the industrial process for making soaps.
5. Review the history of models for biologic membranes. What are the limitations of the original Singer–Nicolson model?

Summary

Following the previous chapter on amino acids and proteins, this chapter provides a broader foundation for further studies in bio-chemistry, by introducing the basic structural features and physical and chemical properties of two major building blocks – carbohydrates and lipids. Knowledge of the structure of carbo-hydrates is essential for the chapters on intermediary metabolism and on the biosynthesis and function of glycoproteins, glycolipids and proteoglycans. Understanding the function of lipids in the structure of biological membranes lays a foundation for under-standing function of membranes in transport, signal transduction and electrochemical processes involved in energy production, nerve transmission and muscle contraction.

Further reading

Samad A, Sultana Y, Aqil M. Liposomal drug delivery systems: an update. *Curr Drug Deliv* 2007;**4**:297–305.

Sengupta P, Baird B, Holowka D. Lipid rafts, fluid/fluid phase separation, and their relevance to plasma membrane structure and function. *Semin Cell Dev Biol* 2007;**18**:583–590.

Singer SJ. Some early history of membrane molecular biology. *Annu Rev Physiol* 2004;**66**:1–27.

van Deurs B, Roepstorff K, Hommelgaard AM, Sandvig K. Caveolae: anchored, multifunctional platforms in the lipid ocean. *Trends Cell Biol* 2003;**13**:92–100.

Vereb G, Szöllosi J, Matkó J et al. Dynamic, yet structured: the cell membrane three decades after the Singer–Nicolson model. *Proc Natl Acad Sci USA* 2003;**100**:8053–8058.

Zhang YM, Rock CO. Membrane lipid homeostasis in bacteria. *Nat Rev Microbiol* 2008;**6**:222–233.

Websites

Sugar structure: http://bama.ua.edu/~lsbusenlehner/Chapter7a.pdf
Sugar chemistry: www.cem.msu.edu/~reusch/VirtualText/carbhyd.htm
Phospholipids: www.cyberlipid.org/phlip/phli01.htm
Membrane phospholipids: http://cellbio.utmb.edu/cellbio/membrane_intro.htm
History of membrane models: www1.umn.edu/ships/9-2/membrane.htm
Singer–Nicolson drawings: http://cnx.org/content/m15255/latest/
Soaps and saponification: www.kitchendoctor.com/articles/soap.html

4. Blood: Cells and Plasma Proteins

W D Fraser

LEARNING OBJECTIVES

After reading this chapter you should be able to:

- Describe the major components of blood.
- Explain the difference between plasma and serum.
- Define the roles of plasma proteins and their broad classification.
- Identify diseases associated with deficiency of specific proteins.
- Discuss the structure and function of the immunoglobulins.
- Appreciate the pathologic significance of monoclonal gammopathy.
- Define the acute phase response and the change it induces in the concentrations of circulating plasma proteins.

INTRODUCTION

Blood functions as a transport and distribution system for the body, delivering essential nutrients to tissues and at the same time removing waste products. It is composed of an aqueous solution containing molecules of varying sizes and a number of cellular elements. Some of the components of blood perform important roles in the body's defense against external insult and in the repair of damaged tissues.

Importantly for a clinician, plasma is also a 'window' on metabolism. Because it is easy to obtain, many diagnostic laboratory tests in biochemistry, hematology and immunology are performed on plasma samples.

The most commonly used tests are listed in the Appendix together with their reference values.

PLASMA AND SERUM

Plasma is the natural environment of blood cells but most chemical measurements are done in serum

The formed elements of blood are suspended in an aqueous solution that is termed plasma. Plasma is the supernatant obtained by centrifuging a blood sample that has been treated with an anticoagulant to prevent clotting of red cells. Serum is the supernatant obtained if a blood sample is allowed to clot (usually requires 30–45 minutes) and then centrifuged. In laboratory practice, the most common anticoagulants are lithium heparinate and ethylenediamine tetraacetic acid (EDTA). Heparinate prevents clotting by binding to thrombin. EDTA and citrate bind Ca^{2+} and Mg^{2+}, thus interfering with the action of calcium/magnesium-dependent enzymes (prothrombin-converting complex, thromboplastin and thrombin) involved in the clotting cascade. When blood is collected for transfusion, citrate is used as an anticoagulant. During clotting, fibrinogen is converted to fibrin as a result of proteolytic cleavage by thrombin, and so a major difference between plasma and serum is the absence of fibrinogen in serum.

FORMED ELEMENTS OF BLOOD

There are three major cellular components circulating in the bloodstream.

Erythrocytes

Erythrocytes are not complete cells, as they do not possess nuclei and intracellular organelles. They are cellular remnants, containing specific proteins and ions, which can be present in high concentrations. Erythrocytes are the end-product of erythropoiesis in the bone marrow, which is under the control of erythropoietin produced by the kidney (Fig. 4.1). Hemoglobin is synthesized in the erythrocyte precursor cells (erythroblasts and reticulocytes) under a tight control dictated by the concentration of heme, the synthesis of which involves the chelation of reduced ferrous iron (Fe^{2+}) by four nitrogen atoms in the center of a porphyrin ring (see Chapter 29). The main functions of erythrocytes are the transport of oxygen and the removal of carbon dioxide and hydrogen ion; as they lack cellular organelles, they are not capable of protein synthesis and repair. As a result, erythrocytes have a finite life span of 60–120 days before being trapped and broken down in the spleen.

Leukocytes

Leukocytes are cells, the main function of which is to protect the body from infection (see Chapter 38).

Most leukocytes are produced in the bone marrow, some are produced in the thymus, and others mature within several tissues (Fig. 4.2) (see Chapter 38). Leukocytes can control their own synthesis by secreting into the blood signal peptides that subsequently act on the bone marrow stem cells. In order to

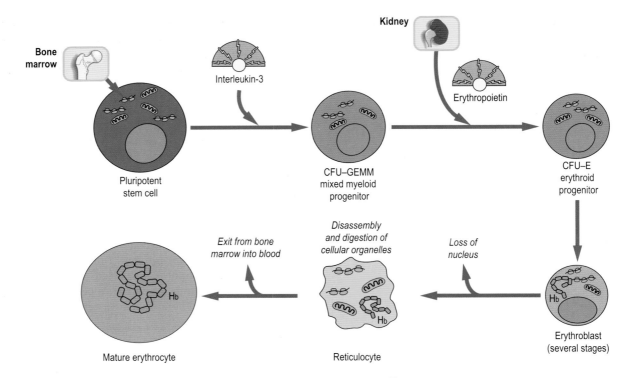

Fig. 4.1 **Simplified scheme of the formation of erythrocytes.** In an average day, 10^{11} erythrocytes are formed. Hemoglobin is synthesized in the erythrocyte and reticulocyte before the loss of ribosomes and mitochondria. CFU, colony-forming unit; GEMM, granulocyte, erythroid, monocyte, megakaryocyte; CFU-E, colony-forming unit erythroid.

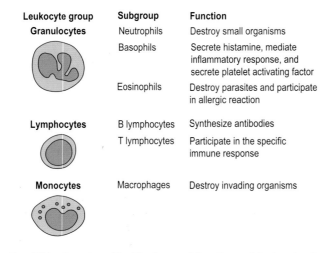

Leukocyte group	Subgroup	Function
Granulocytes	Neutrophils	Destroy small organisms
	Basophils	Secrete histamine, mediate inflammatory response, and secrete platelet activating factor
	Eosinophils	Destroy parasites and participate in allergic reaction
Lymphocytes	B lymphocytes	Synthesize antibodies
	T lymphocytes	Participate in the specific immune response
Monocytes	Macrophages	Destroy invading organisms

Fig. 4.2 **Leukocytes.** Classification and functions of leukocytes (see also Chapter 38).

function correctly, leukocytes have the ability to migrate out of the bloodstream into surrounding tissues.

Thrombocytes (platelets)

Thrombocytes (platelets) are not true cells, but are membrane-bound fragments derived from megakaryocytes residing in the bone marrow. They have a key role in the process of blood clotting (see Chapter 7).

PLASMA PROTEINS

Plasma proteins can be broadly classified into two groups: those, including albumin, that are synthesized by the liver,

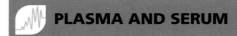

PLASMA AND SERUM

The role of the clinical laboratory

The clinical laboratory performs a large number of biochemical analyses on body fluids, which can give answers to specific clinical questions about an individual patient. Such analyses are usually requested to aid in the diagnosis or treatment of specific conditions. The majority of specimens received by the laboratory are blood and urine samples. Whereas some measurements are performed on whole blood, serum or plasma are preferred for most analyses of molecules and ions. In general, the time devoted to the analysis of each sample is relatively short, but the entire process from a request for analysis to receipt of a result involves many steps and can take several hours. Throughout the process, constant checking and quality assurance are performed to ensure that the produced results are analytically and clinically valid. An outline of the laboratory workflow is shown in Figure 4.3.

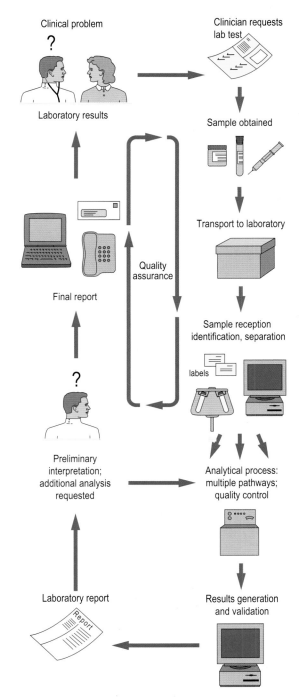

Fig. 4.3 **The function of the clinical laboratory.** Flow diagram indicating the steps involved in the generation of results from the clinical laboratory.

and the immunoglobulins, which are produced by plasma cells of the bone marrow, usually as part of the immune response.

A number of plasma proteins have the ability to bind certain ligands with a high affinity and specificity. These proteins can then act as a reservoir for the ligand and help control its distribution and availability by transporting it to tissues throughout the body. Binding to a protein can also render a toxic substance less harmful to the tissues. Major binding proteins and their ligands are shown in Table 4.1.

Transport proteins and their ligands	
Proteins	**Ligands**
Cation binding	
Albumin	Divalent and trivalent cations, e.g. Cu^{2+}, Fe^{3+}
Ceruloplasmin	Cu^{2+}
Transferrin	Fe^{3+}
Hormone binding	
Thyroid-binding globulin (TBG)	Thyroxine (T_4), tri-iodothyronine (T_3)
Cortisol-binding globulin (CBG)	Cortisol
Sex hormone-binding globulin (SHBG)	Androgens (testosterone), estrogens (estradiol)
Hemoglobin/protoporphyrin binding	
Albumin	Heme, bilirubin, biliverdin
Haptoglobin	Hemoglobin dimers
Fatty acid binding	
Albumin	Nonesterified fatty acids, steroids

Table 4.1 **Transport proteins and their ligands.** Almost all plasma proteins bind ligands, and this is a major function of many proteins. Albumin can bind many molecules weakly and nonspecifically, but other proteins bind tightly to specific molecules – for example, transferrin is specific for ferric iron (Fe^{3+}).

NEPHROTIC SYNDROME

A 44-year-old woman was admitted to hospital because of weakness, anorexia, recurrent infections, bilateral leg edema, and breathlessness. Her plasma albumin concentration was 19 g/L (normal range 36–52 g/L) and her urinary protein excretion 10 g/24 h (normal value <0.15 g/24 h). There was microscopic hematuria. Renal biopsy confirmed the diagnosis as membranoproliferative glomerulonephritis.

Comment. This woman had the classic triad of the nephrotic syndrome: hypoalbuminemia, proteinuria, and edema. The nephritis has resulted in damage to the glomerular basement membrane, with resultant leak of albumin. Continued loss of albumin exceeds the synthetic capacity of the liver, and results in hypoalbuminemia; consequently, the capillary osmotic pressure is significantly reduced. This leads to both peripheral (leg) edema and pulmonary edema (breathlessness). With increasing glomerular damage, proteins of larger molecular mass, such as immunoglobulins and complement (Chapter 38), are lost.

Albumin

Albumin, in addition to its functions as a protein reserve in nutritional depletion and as an osmotic regulator, is a major transport protein

Albumin, the predominant plasma protein having no known enzymatic or hormonal activity, accounts for approximately 50% of the protein found in human plasma, and is present normally at a concentration of 35–45 g/L. It is easy to isolate and has been extensively studied. With a molecular weight of about 66 kDa, albumin is one of the smallest plasma proteins and, given its highly polar nature, dissolves easily in water. At pH 7.4, it is an anion with 20 negative charges per molecule; this gives it a vast capacity for nonselective binding of many ligands. The presence of large amounts of albumin in the body (4–5 g/kg body weight), with at least 38% being present intravascularly, also helps to explain the critical role it has in exerting colloid osmotic pressure.

The rate of synthesis of albumin (14–15 g daily) is dependent on nutritional status, especially on the extent of amino acid deficiencies. The half-life of albumin is about 20 days, and degradation appears to occur by pinocytosis in all tissues. Importantly, although the albumin level reflects the nutritional status in the longer term, in hospitalized patients short-term changes in plasma albumin concentration are usually due to overhydration (see Chapter 23).

Albumin is the primary plasma protein responsible for the transport of hydrophobic fatty acids, bilirubin, and drugs

Albumin demonstrates a unique ability to solubilize, in aqueous phase, a range of substances that include the long-chain fatty acids, sterols, and several synthetic compounds. The transport of long-chain fatty acids underpins much of the body's distribution of energy-rich substrates. Through binding, consequently solubilizing and ultimately transporting fatty acids such as stearic acid, oleic acid and palmitic acid, albumin enables the transport of these hydrophobic molecules in the predominantly hydrophilic milieu of the plasma. Associative studies have demonstrated the presence of numerous fatty acid binding sites on the albumin molecule, with variable affinities. The highest affinity sites are believed to lie in the globular segments within specialized clefts of the albumin molecule (Fig. 4.4).

In addition to binding fatty acids, albumin has an important role in binding unconjugated bilirubin, thereby rendering it not only water soluble and transportable from the reticuloendothelial system to the liver, but also temporarily nontoxic. In the presence of excessively high concentrations of unconjugated bilirubin, the binding capacity of albumin

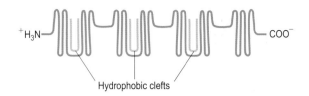

Fig. 4.4 **Molecular model of human albumin.** The hydrophobic clefts are globular segments of albumin that bind fatty acids with high affinity.

is exceeded and in children this can contribute to the development of kernicterus (see Chapter 29).

The presence of sites within the albumin molecule that are capable of binding a variety of drugs, including salicylates, barbiturates, sulfonamides, penicillin and warfarin, is of great pharmacologic relevance. Chiefly, such interactions are weak and the ligands become easily displaced by competitors for the binding site. Given such binding, not only does albumin play a part in drug solubilization but it may also determine the proportion of free, and thus pharmacologically active, drug available in the plasma.

Somewhat surprisingly, albumin is not essential for human survival and rare congenital defects have been described where there is hypoalbuminemia or complete absence of albumin (analbuminemia).

Proteins that transport metal ions

The ability of proteins to bind and transport metal ions is of major importance

Iron is an essential element for many metabolic processes and is an important component of the heme proteins, myoglobin, hemoglobin, and cytochromes. Within the plasma, iron is transported bound to transferrin as ferric ions (Fe^{3+}) and is released from the protein into tissues after it has bound to specific cell receptors and the resulting complex has been internalized. The iron is then deposited in storage sites as ferritin or hemosiderin, or is used in synthesis of heme proteins. The binding of ferric ions to transferrin protects against the toxic effects of these ions. In inflammatory reactions, the iron-transferrin complex is degraded by the reticuloendothelial system without a corresponding increase in the synthesis of either of its components; this results in low plasma concentrations of transferrin and iron.

■ Ferritin is the major iron storage protein found in almost all cells of the body. It acts as the reserve of iron in the

✳ HEMOLYSIS AND FREE HEMOGLOBIN

Handling of free hemoglobin

When erythrocytes are prematurely hemolyzed, they release hemoglobin into the plasma, where it dissociates into dimers that bind to haptoglobin. The hemoglobin–haptoglobin complex is metabolized more rapidly than haptoglobin alone, in the cells of the liver and reticuloendothelial system, producing an iron–globulin complex and bilirubin. This prevents the loss of iron in the urine. When excessive hemolysis occurs, the plasma haptoglobin concentration can become very low. If hemoglobin breaks down into heme and globin, the free heme is bound by hemopexin; unlike haptoglobin, which is an acute phase protein, hemopexin is not affected by acute phase response. The heme–hemopexin complex is taken up by liver cells, where iron binds to ferritin. A third complex, called methemalbumin, can form between oxidized heme and albumin. These mechanisms have evolved to allow the body not only to scavenge iron and prevent major losses, but also to complex the free heme, which is toxic to many tissues.

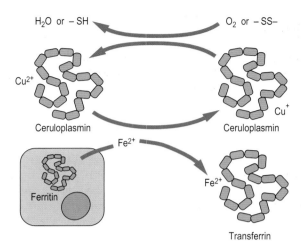

Fig. 4.5 **Plasma ferroxidase activity of ceruloplasmin.** Oxidation of Fe^{2+} by ceruloplasmin permits the binding and transport of iron by plasma transferrin. The cuprous ion (Cu^{2+}) bound to ceruloplasmin is regenerated by reaction with oxygen or with oxidized thiol groups.

liver and bone marrow. The concentration of ferritin in plasma is proportional to the amount of stored iron, therefore measurement of plasma ferritin is one of the best indicators of iron deficiency.

- Hemosiderin is a derivative of ferritin and is found in the liver, spleen, and bone marrow. It is insoluble in aqueous solutions, and forms aggregates that slowly release iron when deficiency occurs.
- Ceruloplasmin is the major transport protein for copper, an essential trace element. Ceruloplasmin helps export copper from the liver to peripheral tissues, and is essential for the regulation of the oxidation reduction reactions, transport, and utilization of iron (Fig. 4.5). Increased concentrations of ceruloplasmin occur in active liver disease and in tissue damage.

Low concentrations of ceruloplasmin and total copper are observed in Wilson's disease, the autosomal recessive disorder of copper transport. The genetic defect is on chromosome 13 resulting in a mutation in copper-transporting P-type adenosine triphosphatase (ATP7B) which is responsible for transport of copper into ceruloplasmin and elimination of copper through bile. Mutation of ATP7B results in the accumulation of copper in the liver, brain and kidney. These mutations are readily identified by haplotype and mutational analysis and so genetic screening of patients and their families for Wilson's disease is possible (see also Chapter 11).

⌖ WILSON'S DISEASE

A 14-year-old girl was admitted as an emergency. She was jaundiced with abdominal pain and had an enlarged, tender liver with drowsiness and asterixis (flapping tremor) due to acute liver failure. Previous history revealed behavior disturbance, difficulty with movement in the recent past, and truancy from school. Her ceruloplasmin concentration was 50 mmol/L (normal range 200–450 mmol/L (20–45 mg/dL)), serum copper was 8 mmol/L (normal range 10–22 μmol/L (65–144 μg/dL)), urinary excretion of copper was 2.2 mmol/24 h (normal range 2–3.9 μmol/24 h (13–25 μg/dL)), and a liver biopsy established the diagnosis of Wilson's disease.

Comment. This case highlights the importance of measurement of ceruloplasmin. In Wilson's disease, a deficiency of ceruloplasmin results in low plasma concentrations of copper. The metabolic defect is in the excretion of copper in bile and its reabsorption in the kidney; copper is deposited in liver, brain, and kidney. Liver symptoms are present in patients of younger age, and cirrhosis and neuropsychiatric problems are manifest in those who are older. Detection of low plasma concentrations of ceruloplasmin and copper, increased urinary excretion of copper, and markedly increased concentrations of copper in the liver confirm the diagnosis.

Immunoglobulins

Immunoglobulins are proteins produced in response to foreign substances (antigens; see also Chapter 38)

The immune system may be conceptualized as two independent entities, served by separate lymphoid cells: thymically derived T lymphocytes oversee immunoregulation and cell-based immune function, and B lymphocytes that synthesize and secrete antibodies (immunoglobulins). These antibodies are proteins, produced by the immune system, which have a defined specificity for a foreign particle (immunogen) that stimulated their synthesis. Not all foreign substances entering the body can elicit this response, however; those that do are called immunogens, whereas any agent that can be bound by an antibody is termed an antigen.

The immunoglobulins are a uniquely diverse group of molecules, recognizing and reacting with a wide range of specific antigenic structures (epitopes) and giving rise to a series of effects that result in the eventual elimination of the presenting antigen. Some immunoglobulins have additional effector functions; for example, IgG is involved in complement activation.

Structure of immunoglobulins

Immunoglobulins share a common Y-shaped structure of two heavy and two light chains

The immunoglobulin is a Y-shaped molecule containing two identical units termed heavy (H) chains and two identical, but smaller, units termed light (L) chains. Several H chains exist, and the nature of the H chain determines the class of immunoglobulin: IgG, IgA, IgM, IgD and IgE are characterized by γ, α, μ, δ and ε heavy chains, respectively. L chains are of only two types, κ and λ, and both types may be found in any one class of immunoglobulin, although obviously not within the same molecule. Each polypeptide chain within the immunoglobulin is characterized by a series of globular regions, which have considerable sequence homology and, in evolutionary terms, are probably derived from protogene duplication.

The N-terminal domains of both H and L chains contain a region of variable amino acid sequence (the V region); together, these regions determine antigenic specificity. Both H and L chains are required for full antibody activity, as the physically apposed V regions in the L and H chains form a functional pocket into which the epitope fits; this is termed the antibody recognition (Fab_2) region. The domain immediately adjacent to the V region is much less variable, in both H and L chains. The remainder of the H chain consists of a further constant region (Fc region) consisting of a hinge region and two additional domains. This constant region is responsible for immunoglobulin functions other than epitope recognition, such as complement activation (Chapter 38). This basic structure of immunoglobulins is depicted in Figure 4.6. When antigen binds to the immunoglobulin, conformational changes are transmitted through the hinge region of the antibody, to the Fc region, which is then said to have become activated.

The immunoglobulin G molecule

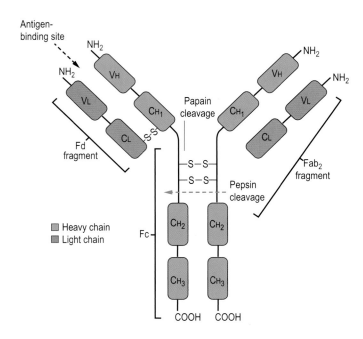

Pentameric IgM

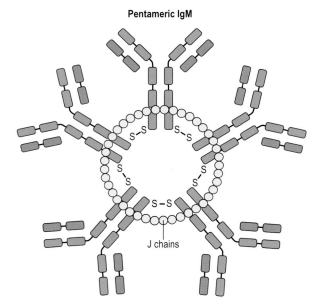

Fig. 4.6 **The structure of immunoglobulins.** Diagrammatic representation of the basic structure of a monomeric immunoglobulin and that of pentameric immunoglobulin (IgM). V, variable region; C, constant region; H, heavy chain; L, light chain; J chain, joining chain; Fab_2, fragment generated by pepsin cleavage of the molecule; Fc, Fd, fragments generated by papain proteolysis.

Major immunoglobulins

IgG is the most common immunoglobulin that protects tissue spaces and freely crosses the placenta

IgG, with an overall molecular mass of 160 kDa, consists of the basic 2H2L immunoglobulin subunit joined by a variable number of disulfide bonds. The γ H chains have several antigenic and structural differences, allowing classification of IgG into a number of subclasses according to the type of H chain present; however, functional differences between the subclasses are minor.

IgG circulates in high concentrations in the plasma, accounting for 75% of immunoglobulin present in adults, and has a half-life of 22 days. It is present in all extracelluar fluids, and appears to eliminate small, soluble antigenic proteins through aggregation and enhanced phagocytosis by the reticuloendothelial system. From weeks 18–20 of pregnancy, IgG is actively transported across the placenta and provides humoral immunity for the fetus and neonate before maturation of the immune system.

IgA is found widely in secretions and presents an antiseptic barrier, which protects mucosal surfaces

IgA has an H chain similar to the γ chain of IgG, and α chains possess an extra 18 amino acids at its C-terminus. The extra peptide sequence enables the binding of a 'joining' or J chain. This short (129-residue) acidic glycopeptide, synthesized by plasma cells, allows dimerization of secretory IgA. IgA is often found in noncovalent association with the so-called secretory component, a highly glycosylated 71 kDa polypeptide, synthesized by mucosal cells and capable of protecting IgA against proteolytic digestion.

IgA represents 7–15% of plasma immunoglobulins and has a half-life of 6 days. It is found, in particular in the dimerized form, in parotid, bronchial, and intestinal secretions. It is a major component of colostrum (the first milk from the mother's breasts after the birth of a child). IgA appears to function as the primary immunologic barrier against pathogenic invasion of mucous membranes. It can promote phagocytosis, cause eosinophilic degranulation, and activate complement via the so-called alternative pathway.

IgM is confined to the intravascular space and helps eliminate circulating antigens and microorganisms

Immunoglobulins belonging to this final major class are polyvalent, with a high molecular mass. IgM has a basic form similar to that of IgA, having the extra H chain domain that allows for J chain binding, and is thus capable of polymerization. IgM normally circulates as a pentamer, with a molecular mass of 971 kDa, linked by disulfide bonds and the J chain (see Fig. 4.6).

IgM accounts for 5–10% of plasma immunoglobulins and has a half-life of 5 days. With its polymeric nature and

MULTIPLE MYELOMA

A 65-year-old man presented with a sudden onset of low back pain. Radiography revealed a crush fracture of the second lumbar vertebra, and discrete and so-called 'punched out' lesions in the skull. Serum electrophoresis demonstrated the presence of a monoclonal immunoglobulin. This proved to be an IgG immunoglobulin and, on electrophoresis, excess free κ chains (Bence-Jones protein) were found in the patient's urine.

Comment. Multiple myeloma affects men and women with equal incidence and presents mostly after the age of 50 years. The clinical features are due to both the malignant proliferation of monoclonal plasma cells and the synthesis and secretion of antibody by these cells. Bone lesions affect the skull, vertebrae, ribs, and pelvis. There may be generalized osteoporosis and pathologic fractures. In up to 20% of cases, no plasma protein is detected, although Bence-Jones proteins are present in urine. Such cases are commonly associated with suppression of production of other immunoglobulins (immunoparesis). The presence of excess light chains may cause renal failure as a result of the deposition of Bence-Jones proteins in the renal tubules or amyloidosis. Other common findings in myelomatosis include anemia and hypercalcemia.

high molecular mass, most IgM is found confined to the intravascular space, although lesser amounts may be found in secretions, usually in association with secretory component. It is the first antibody to be synthesized after an antigenic challenge.

Minor immunoglobulins

IgD is the surface receptor for antigen in B lymphocytes

IgD differs from the standard immunoglobulin structure chiefly by its high carbohydrate content of numerous oligosaccharide units, resulting in an increased molecular mass of 190 kDa. δ chains are characterized by having only a single interconnecting disulfide bridge, and an elongated hinge region that is particularly susceptible to proteolysis.

Accounting for less than 0.5% of circulating plasma immunoglobulin mass, IgD has a role that remains elusive although, as a surface component of the mature B cell, it probably has some role in response to antigens. Rare cases of isolated IgD deficiency seem to be associated with no obvious pathology.

IgE is present only in trace amounts and acts to bind antigen and promote a release of vasoactive amines from mast cells

Similar to IgM in its unit structure, IgE has ε heavy chains that consist of five, rather than four, domains, but J chain binding and polymers do not occur. The extended H chain helps to explain the high molecular mass of IgE which is approximately 200 kDa.

IgE has a high affinity for binding sites on mast cells and basophils. Antigenic binding at the Fab$_2$ region induces crosslinking of the high-affinity receptor, granulation of the cell, and release of vasoactive amines. By this mechanism, IgE plays a major part in allergy/atopy and mediates antiparasitic immunity.

Monoclonal immunoglobulins

Monoclonal immunoglobulins are the product of a single B cell, and arise from benign or malignant transformations of B cells

Monoclonal immunoglobulins result from the proliferation of a single B cell clone, which thus produces identical antibodies. Usually, these are structurally normal molecules but sometimes they may be in some way fragmented or truncated. The absolute physical identity of the monoclonal immunoglobulins leads to a single band in gel electrophoresis, revealed by protein staining as a single, dense band in the γ region (the paraprotein band) (Fig. 4.7).

Monoclonal immunoglobulins are associated with diverse malignant pathologies such as myeloma and Waldenström's macroglobulinemia, and also with more benign transformations that are usually termed monoclonal gammopathies of uncertain significance (MGUS).

THE ACUTE PHASE RESPONSE AND C-REACTIVE PROTEIN

The acute phase response is a nonspecific response to tissue injury or infection; it affects several organs and tissues

During the acute phase response, there is a characteristic marked increase in the synthesis of some proteins (predominantly in the liver), along with a decrease in the plasma concentration of some others (Fig. 4.8). An increase in the synthesis of proteins such as proteinase inhibitors (α_1-antitrypsin), coagulation proteins (fibrinogen, prothrombin), complement proteins, and C-reactive protein is of obvious clinical benefit. The synthesis of albumin, transthyretin (prealbumin), and transferrin decreases during the acute phase response, and they are thus termed the 'negative acute phase reactants'.

C-reactive protein (CRP) is a major component of the acute phase response and a marker of bacterial infection. It is synthesized in the liver and is constructed of five polypeptide subunits, having a molecular weight of around 130 kDa. It is present in only minute quantities (<1 mg/L in normal serum)

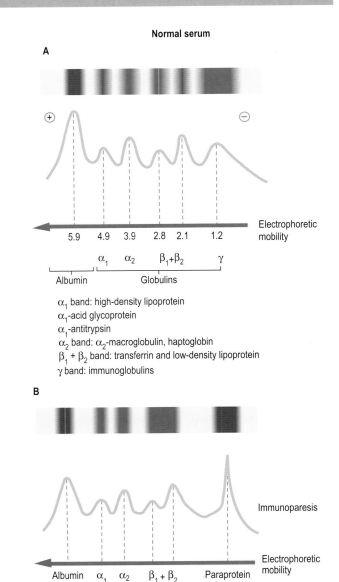

Normal serum

A

α_1 band: high-density lipoprotein
α_1-acid glycoprotein
α_1-antitrypsin
α_2 band: α_2-macroglobulin, haptoglobin
$\beta_1 + \beta_2$ band: transferrin and low-density lipoprotein
γ band: immunoglobulins

B

Fig. 4.7 **Comparison of gel electrophoretic appearance of normal serum and that containing monoclonal immunoglobulins.** The scanning pattern peaks (solid line) represent the relative concentrations of the separated proteins. (A) Normal serum. (B) Monoclonal gammopathy: a strongly stained band is present in the γ-globulin region on electrophoresis, and there is an associated reduction of staining in the remainder of the γ-region (immunoparesis).

and is believed to mediate binding of foreign polysaccharides, phospholipids, and complex polyanions, and also activating complement via the classic pathway (see Chapter 38). Measurement of CRP concentration in plasma is an essential test in diagnosis and monitoring of infection and sepsis.

In addition, using an assay for CRP, which is approximately 100 times more sensitive than the conventional CRP

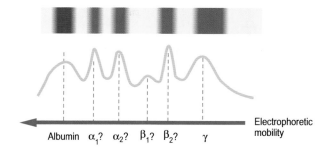

 Fig. 4.8 **Acute phase response.** Gel electrophoretic pattern observed in serum during the acute phase response. Albumin is decreased, the sum of α_1- and α_2-globulins is increased, β_1-globulins are decreased, β_2-globulins are increased and there is a mild increase in γ-globulins.

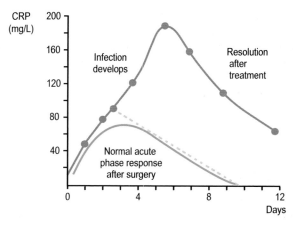

Fig. 4.9 **C-reactive protein (CRP) and the postoperative acute phase reaction.** The concentration of CRP increases as part of the acute phase response to surgical trauma, and a further increase may be observed if recovery is complicated by infection. (The dotted line represents response to uncomplicated surgery.)

ACUTE PHASE RESPONSE

A 45-year-old woman suffered severe lower limb injuries in a road traffic accident. After her admission to hospital, biochemical profiling revealed slightly decreased concentrations of total serum protein (58 g/L; normal 60–80 g/L) and serum albumin (38 g/L; normal 36–52 g/L). Serum electrophoresis revealed an increase in the α_1 and α_2 protein fractions. Four days after her operation, the patient's condition deteriorated and she developed an increased temperature, sweating, and confusion. An acute infection was diagnosed and treatment with appropriate antibiotics was commenced. CRP concentrations peaked 5 days after the operation (Fig. 4.9).

Comment. Increased concentrations of α_1 and α_2 proteins (which include α_1-antitrypsin, α_1-acid glycoprotein, and haptoglobin), together with a decrease in serum albumin concentration, suggest an acute phase response. This response is also associated with an increase in CRP, the erythrocyte sedimentation rate (ESR), and increased plasma viscosity. A therapeutic response to treatment of infection can be assessed by a decrease in plasma CRP concentration.

measurement method, one may detect minimal fluctuations in the concentration of this protein. Very small increases in CRP concentration seem to reflect a state of chronic low-grade inflammation which is associated, for instance, with an increased risk of cardiovascular disease (see Chapter 18). Other inflammatory conditions such as inflammatory bowel disorders, type 2 diabetes and the metabolic syndrome (see Chapter 21), and also abdominal aortic aneurysm and premature rupture of membranes during pregnancy, have been associated with these minute increases in serum CRP concentration.

Summary

- The formed elements of blood are erythrocytes, leukocytes and platelets. They are suspended in an aqueous solution (plasma) and have several specialized functions such as transport of oxygen, destruction of external agents, and clotting of blood. Plasma which is allowed to clot yields serum. Most biochemical tests are done on serum. To obtain plasma, blood must be taken into a test tube containing an anticoagulant.

- Plasma contains many proteins broadly classified into albumin and globulins (predominantly immunoglobulins). Albumin functions as a major transport protein for several ligands – trace metals, hormones, bilirubin, and free fatty acids.

- Other proteins are more specialized: they bind specific ligands, e.g. ceruloplasmin binds Cu^{2+} and thyroid-binding globulin (TBG) binds thyroid hormones.

- Immunoglobulins are unique molecules that participate in the defense against antigens that may enter or attempt to enter the body. They have a common structure and five classes of immunoglobulin exist with different protective functions.

- Changes in the concentration of plasma proteins give important clinical information. A characteristic pattern with decreased albumin, transthyretin and transferrin and increased α_1-antitrypsin, fibrinogen and C-reactive protein indicates the acute phase response.

- Serum and urine protein electrophoresis is an important way of identifying the presence of monoclonal immunoglobulins.

ACTIVE LEARNING

1. Compare and contrast plasma and serum and discuss the different types of blood samples taken for laboratory tests.
2. Discuss the transport role of serum albumin.
3. Describe the core structure of immunoglobulins and different roles played in immunity by different classes of immunoglobulins.
4. How does the acute phase reaction affect the results of blood tests?
5. Characterize Wilson's disease.
6. How is hemoglobin handled if erythrocytes become disrupted?

Further reading

Anderson KC, Shaughnessy JD, Barlogie B, Harousseau JL, Roodman GD. Multiple myeloma. *Hematology*. American Society of Hematology Education Program Book 2002;214-240. (Full text available at *www.asheducationbook.org*)

El-Youssef M. Wilson's disease. *Mayo Clin Proc* 2003;**78**:1126–1136.

Hayashi T, Hideshima T, Anderson KC. Novel therapies for multiple myeloma. *Br J Haematol* 2003;**120**:10–17.

Lewis SM, Bain B, Bates I (eds). *Practical haematology*, 9th edn. London: Churchill Livingstone, 2001.

Pepys MB, Hirschfield GM. C-reactive protein: a critical update. *J Clin Invest* 2003; **111**:1805–1812. (full text available at *www.jci.org*)

Jialal I, Devaraj S. Venugopal SK. C-reactive protein: risk marker or mediator in atherothrombosis. *Hypertension* 2004;**44**:6–11.

Zimmermann MA, Selzman CH, Cothren C. Diagnostic implications of C-reactive protein. *Arch Surg* 2003;**138**:220–224.

5. Oxygen Transport

G M Helmkamp

LEARNING OBJECTIVES

After reading this chapter you should be able to:

- Describe the mechanism of oxygen binding to myoglobin and hemoglobin.
- Describe conformational differences between deoxygenated and oxygenated hemoglobins.
- Define the concept of cooperativity in oxygen binding to hemoglobin.
- Describe the Bohr effect and its role in modulating the binding of oxygen to hemoglobin.
- Explain how 2,3-bisphosphoglycerate interacts with hemoglobin and influences oxygen binding.
- Summarize the processes by which carbon dioxide is transported from peripheral tissues to the lungs.
- Describe the major classifications of hemoglobinopathies.
- Describe the molecular basis of sickle cell disease.

INTRODUCTION

With the evolution of metazoan organisms $\sim 0.5 \times 10^9$ years ago, life became dependent on an oxygen (O_2)-based recovery of energy from chemical bonds. Vertebrates are aerobic organisms with a closed circulatory system and a mechanism for extraction of O_2 from air (or water) and release of carbon dioxide (CO_2) in waste products. Inspired O_2 leads to an efficient utilization of metabolic fuels, such as glucose and fatty acids; expired CO_2 is a major product of cellular metabolism. This utilization of O_2 as a metabolic substrate is accompanied by the generation of free radical species that are capable of damaging virtually all biological macromolecules. Organisms protect themselves from radical damage in several ways: sequestering O_2, limiting their production, and detoxifying them. Heme proteins, interestingly, participate in these protective mechanisms. The major heme proteins in mammals are myoglobin (Mb) and hemoglobin (Hb). Mb is found primarily in skeletal and striated muscle and serves to store O_2 in the cytoplasm and deliver it on demand to the mitochondrion. Hb is restricted to erythrocytes where it facilitates the transport of O_2 and CO_2 between the lungs and peripheral tissues. This chapter presents the molecular features of Mb and Hb, the biochemical and physiologic relationships between the structures of Mb and Hb and their interaction with O_2 and other small molecules, and the pathologic aspects of selected Hb mutations.

Properties of oxygen

The introduction of O_2 into the Earth's anaerobic biosphere occurred $\sim 2.5 \times 10^9$ years ago and led to its current level in air of 21%. In mixtures of gases, each component makes a specific contribution, known as its partial pressure (Dalton's Law), that is directly proportional to its concentration. It is also customary to use the partial pressure of a gas as a measure of its concentration in physiologic fluids. For atmospheric O_2 at a barometric pressure (sea level) of 760 mmHg or torr (101.3 kPascal or kPa; 1 atmosphere absolute or ATA), the partial pressure of oxygen, pO_2, is 150–160 mmHg. The amount of O_2 in solution is, in turn, directly proportional to its partial pressure. Thus, in arterial blood (37°C, pH 7.4) the pO_2 is ~ 100 mmHg, which produces a concentration of dissolved O_2 of 0.13 mmol/L. This level of dissolved O_2, however, is inadequate to support efficient aerobic metabolism.

Rather, the major fraction of O_2 transported in blood and stored in muscle is complexed with the iron (ferrous, Fe^{2+}) proteins Hb and Mb, respectively. Hb is a tetrameric protein with four O_2-binding sites (heme groups). In arterial blood with a Hb concentration of 150 g/L (2.3 mmol/L) and O_2 saturation of 97.4%, the contribution of protein-bound O_2 is about 8.7 mmol/L. This concentration represents a dramatic 67-fold increase over physically dissolved O_2. The total oxygen-carrying capacity of arterial blood, in dissolved and protein-bound forms, is ~ 8.8 mmol/L – almost 200 ml of dissolved oxygen per liter of blood.

CHARACTERISTICS OF MAMMALIAN GLOBIN PROTEINS

Globins constitute an ancient family of soluble metalloproteins whose structure and functions have been characterized in microorganisms, plants, invertebrates, and vertebrates. Present-day globins, with their spectacular diversity of function, most likely evolved from a single ancestral globin. While the extent of amino acid identity among invertebrate and

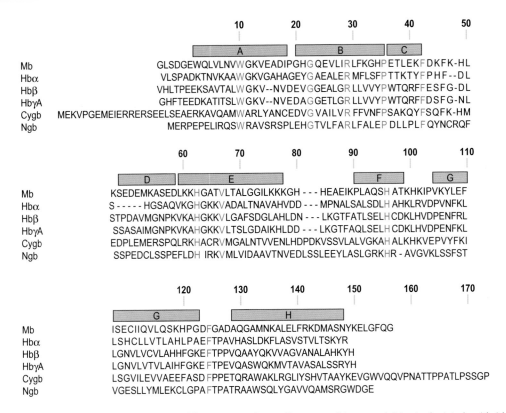

Fig. 5.1 **Human globin amino acid sequences are highly conserved.** An alignment of human globins is depicted, with identical amino acid residues in orange. The two residues in green, PheCD1 (F) and HisF8 (H), are absolutely conserved in all metazoan globins. Helical segments in myoglobin are identified by the blue bars. Mb, myoglobin; Hbα, α-globin; Hbβ, β-globin; HbγA, γA-globin; Cygb, cytoglobin; Ngb, neuroglobin.

vertebrate globins varies widely and can often appear random, two features are noteworthy: the invariant residues PheCD1 and HisF8 and characteristic patterns of hydrophobic residues in helical segments (Fig. 5.1). Human Mb consists of a single globin polypeptide (153 amino acid residues, 17053 Da). Human Hb is a tetrameric assembly of two α-globin polypeptides (141 residues, 15868 Da) and two β-globin polypeptides (146 residues, 15126 Da). A single heme prosthetic group is noncovalently associated with each globin apoprotein.

The secondary structure of mammalian globins is dominated by a high proportion of α-helix, with over 75% of the amino acids associated with eight helical segments. These α-helices are organized into a tightly packed, nearly spherical, tertiary structure, designated the globin fold (Fig. 5.2). So universal is this overall tertiary structure among all globins that the conventional nomenclature for globin residues follows that defined initially for sperm whale Mb, namely helices A, B, C, etc., starting at the N-terminus, separated by corners AB, BC, etc., with residues numbered within each helix and corner. For example, residue A14, an amino acid that participates in electrostatic stabilization between helix A and the GH corner, corresponds to Lys[15] in insect Hb, Lys[16] in Mb and α-globin, and Lys[17] in β-globin (arrow, lower center, Fig. 5.2).

Polar amino acids are located almost exclusively on the exterior surface of globin polypeptides and contribute to the remarkably high solubility of these proteins (e.g. 370 g/L

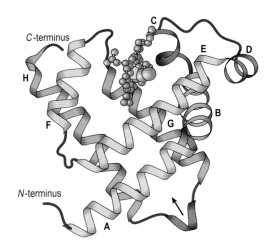

Fig. 5.2 **Myoglobin is a compact globular protein.** In this drawing of mammalian Mb only the globin polypeptide backbone is shown, with emphasis on the high proportion of secondary structure (exclusively α-helix). The two-layer, three-over-three arrangement of α-helices is highlighted by the light and dark shades of red. The heme group is illustrated as a 'ball-and-stick' structure.

(5.7 mmol/L) Hb in the erythrocyte). Amino acids that are both polar and hydrophobic, such as threonine, tyrosine and tryptophan, are oriented with their polar functions toward the protein's exterior. Hydrophobic residues are buried within

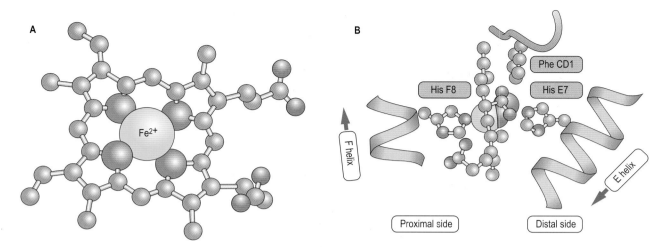

Fig. 5.3 **Heme is a complex of porphyrin and iron.** (A) In this view the carbon framework of protoporphyrin IX, a conjugated tetrapyrrole ring, is shown in gray; O_2 molecules are red. Iron (yellow sphere) prefers six ligands in an octahedral coordination geometry; pyrrole nitrogen atoms (blue spheres) provide four of these. PheCD1 makes critical hydrophobic and electrostatic stacking interactions with the porphyrin ring. (B) In the oxygenated globin structure, the planar heme is positioned between the proximal and distal histidines (HisF8 and HisE7, respectively); only HisF8 has an imidazole nitrogen (blue sphere) close enough to bond with iron. The α-helices that contain these histidines are shown in pink. In deoxygenated globins, the sixth position remains vacant, leaving a pentacoordinated iron. In the oxygenated state, O_2 occupies the sixth position. Both porphyrin propionate moieties participate in hydrogen and electrostatic bonding interactions with globin side chains and solvent.

the interior, where they stabilize the folding of the polypeptide and form a pocket that accommodates the heme prosthetic group. Notable exceptions to this general distribution of amino acid residues in globins are the two histidines that play indispensable roles deep within the heme pocket (Fig. 5.3). The side chains of these histidines are oriented perpendicular to and on either side of the heme prosthetic group. One of the side chain imidazole nitrogens of the invariant proximal histidine (HisF8) is close enough to bond directly to the pentacoordinate Fe^{2+} atom. On the opposite side of the heme plane the distal histidine (HisE7), which is too far from the heme iron for direct bonding, functions critically to stabilize bound O_2 by hydrogen bonding.

Structure of the heme prosthetic group

Heme, the O_2-binding moiety common to Mb and Hb, is a porphyrin molecule to which an iron atom (Fe^{2+}) is coordinated (see Fig. 5.3). The Fe-porphyrin prosthetic group is planar and hydrophobic, with the exception of two propionate groups which are exposed to solvent. Heme becomes an integral component of the globin holoprotein during polypeptide synthesis; it is heme that gives globins, as well as blood and muscle, their characteristic purple-red color – purple in the deoxygenated state, red in the oxygenated state.

Globins increase the aqueous solubility of the otherwise poorly soluble, hydrophobic heme prosthetic group. Once sequestered inside a hydrophobic pocket created by the folded globin polypeptide, heme is in a protective environment that minimizes the spontaneous oxidation of Fe^{2+} to Fe^{3+} (rusting) in the presence of O_2. Such an environment is also essential for globins to bind and release O_2. Should the iron atom become oxidized to the ferric state, heme can no longer interact reversibly with O_2, compromising its function in O_2 storage and transport.

Myoglobin: an oxygen storage protein

Located in the cytosol of skeletal, cardiac and some smooth muscle cells, Mb binds O_2 that has been released by Hb in the tissue capillaries and subsequently diffused into tissues. This stored O_2 is readily available to organelles, particularly the mitochondrion, that carry out oxidative metabolism. With its single ligand-binding site, the reversible reaction of Mb with O_2:

$$Mb + O_2 \rightleftharpoons Mb \cdot O_2$$

may be described by the following equations:

$$K_a = [Mb \cdot O_2]/[Mb][O_2]$$

$$Y = [Mb \cdot O_2]/\{[Mb \cdot O_2] + [Mb]\}$$

where K_a is an affinity or equilibrium constant and Y is the fractional O_2 saturation. Combining these two equations, expressing the concentration of O_2 in terms of its partial

HYPERBARIC O₂ THERAPY FOR ACUTE CARBON MONOXIDE POISONING

A 22-year-old pregnant woman, carrying a fetus of 31 weeks gestational age, was transported to the maternity clinic of a hospital for suspected CO poisoning. The patient was experiencing headache, nausea, and visual abnormalities. She stated that her workplace had been undergoing repairs to the heating and ventilation systems during the past 2 weeks, and on the day of her hospital visit the fire department had evacuated the building after detecting a high level of CO (200 ppm), compared to a typical urban street level of 10 ppm. Vital signs were blood pressure of 116/68 mmHg, pulse rate of 100, and respiratory rate of 24. Noteworthy in the patient's evaluation was a carboxy-Hb (Hb:CO) component of 15% of total Hb at time of admission (normal = 3%, but may exceed 10% in heavy smokers). Fetal monitoring indicated a fetal heart rate of 135, with occasional, moderate irregularities. Uterine contractions were occurring every 3–5 min. The patient was treated in the hospital's hyperbaric O₂ chamber: 30 min at 2.5 ATA, then 60 min at 2.0 ATA. She also received magnesium sulfate intravenously to resolve the premature contractions. The patient was discharged 2 days later. She delivered a healthy female infant at

38 weeks of gestational age who, on examination at birth and at 6 weeks of age, exhibited no apparent sequelae to her in utero exposure to CO or 100% O₂.

Comment. Carbon monoxide is a normal product of heme catabolism and has a range of physiologic activities in vascular, neuronal and immunologic systems. Like O₂, CO also binds to heme prosthetic groups. Because the affinity of globin-bound heme for CO is about 250 times that for O₂, prolonged exposure of hemoglobin to exogenous CO would be virtually irreversible ($t_{1/2}$ for reversal in blood ~4–8 h) and lead to highly toxic levels of carboxy-Hb. Hyperbaric O₂ is the treatment of choice for severe or complicated CO poisoning. The administration of 100% O₂ at 2–3 ATA creates arterial and tissue pO₂ values of 2000 mmHg and 400 mmHg respectively (~20 times normal). The immediate result is a reduction in the $t_{1/2}$ of carboxy-Hb to less than 30 min. Hyperbaric O₂ is also used in the treatment of decompression sickness, arterial gas embolism, radiation-induced or ischemic tissue injury, and severe hemorrhage (compare box on p. 523).

pressure pO₂, and substituting the term P_{50} for $1/K_a$ yields the equation for the O₂ saturation curve of Mb:

$$Y = pO_2/\{pO_2 + P_{50}\}$$

By definition, the constant P_{50} is the value of pO₂ at which $Y = 0.5$ or half the ligand sites are occupied (saturated by O₂). In a plot of Y versus pO₂, the equation for ligand binding by Mb describes a hyperbola (Fig. 5.4) with a P_{50} of 4 mmHg. The low value of P_{50} reflects a high affinity for O₂. In the capillary beds of muscle tissues, pO₂ values are in the range of 20–40 mmHg. Predictably, working muscles exhibit lower pO₂ values than muscles at rest. With its high affinity for O₂, myocyte Mb readily becomes saturated with O₂ that has entered from the blood. As O₂ is consumed during aerobic metabolism, O₂ dissociates through mass action from Mb and diffuses into mitochondria, the power plants of the muscle cell.

Hemoglobin: an oxygen transport protein

Hb is the principal O₂-transporting protein in human blood; it is localized exclusively in erythrocytes. Adult Hb (HbA) is a tetrahedral array of two identical α-globin and two identical β-globin subunits, a geometry that predicts several types of subunit–subunit interactions in the quaternary structure (Fig. 5.5). Importantly, within the Hb tetrahedron each subunit is in contact with the other three. Experimental analysis of the quaternary structure indicates multiple noncovalent interactions (hydrogen and electrostatic bonds) between each pair of dissimilar subunits, i.e. at the α–β interfaces. In contrast,

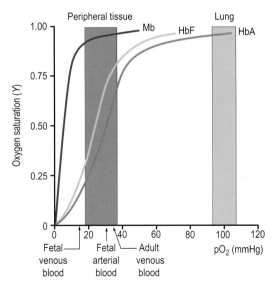

Fig. 5.4 **Oxygen saturation curves of myoglobin and hemoglobin.** Mb and Hb have different O₂ saturation curves. The fractional saturation (Y) of O₂-binding sites is plotted against the concentration of O₂ (pO₂ (mmHg)). Curves are shown for Mb, fetal Hb (HbF), and adult Hb (HbA). Also indicated, by arrows and shading, are the normal levels of O₂ measured in various adult and fetal blood samples.

there are fewer and predominantly hydrophobic interactions between identical subunits, at the α_1–α_2 or β_1–β_2 interfaces. The actual number and nature of contacts differ in the presence or absence of O₂ and allosteric effectors. Strong associations within each αβ heterodimer and at the interface between

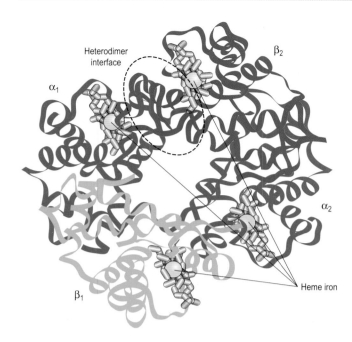

Fig. 5.5 **Hemoglobin is a tetramer of four globin subunits.** Hb is a tetrahedral complex of two identical α-globins (α₁ and α₂, greens) and two identical β-globins (β₁ and β₂, reds). With this geometry each globin subunit contacts the other three subunits, creating the interfaces and interactions that define cooperativity. One of the heterodimer interfaces is outlined in a dashed oval.

the two heterodimers (see Fig. 5.5) are now recognized as major factors determining O_2 binding and release. Thus, Hb is more appropriately considered a dimer of heterodimers, $(\alpha\beta)_2$, rather than an $\alpha_2\beta_2$ tetramer. Although a solution of HbA is theoretically a dynamic mixture of heterodimers and tetramers, under physiological conditions (high Hb and neutral pH) the equilibria greatly favor the tetramer: >99% for oxygenated Hb, >99.9% for deoxygenated Hb.

Interactions of hemoglobin with oxygen

As a gas delivery vehicle, Hb must be able to bind O_2 efficiently as it enters the lung alveoli during respiration and to release O_2 to the extracellular environment with similar efficiency as erythrocytes circulate through tissue capillaries. This remarkable duality of function is achieved by cooperative interactions among globin subunits. When deoxygenated Hb becomes oxygenated, significant structural changes extend throughout the protein molecule. In the heme pocket, as a consequence of O_2 coordination to iron and a new orientation of atoms in the heme structure, the proximal histidine and helix F to which it belongs shift their positions (see Fig. 5.3). This subtle conformational change triggers major structural realignments elsewhere within that globin subunit. In turn, these tertiary structural changes are transmitted, even amplified, in the overall quaternary structure such that a 12–15° rotation and a 0.10nm displacement of the

$\alpha_1\beta_1$ dimer relative to the $\alpha_2\beta_2$ dimer take place. Because of the inherent asymmetry of the $\alpha_2\beta_2$ tetramer, these combined motions result in quite dramatic changes within and, more importantly, between the $\alpha\beta$ heterodimers. Because of structural changes in hemoglobin as a result of binding of oxygen and other effectors, the binding affinity for subsequent molecules of oxygen may be increased (positive cooperativity) or decreased (negative cooperativity).

Hb can bind up to four molecules of O_2. With its multiple ligand-binding sites and structural changes in response to binding, the oxygen affinity and the fractional saturation of Hb are more complex functions than those of Mb. Consequently, the equation for the fractional O_2 saturation curve must be modified to:

$$Y = pO_2{}^n/\{pO_2{}^n + P_{50}{}^n\}$$

where n is the Hill coefficient. In a plot of Y versus pO_2 when $n > 1$, the equation for ligand binding describes a sigmoid (S-shaped) curve (see Fig. 5.4). The Hill coefficient, determined experimentally, is a measure of cooperativity among ligand-binding sites, i.e. the extent to which the binding of O_2 with one subunit influences the affinity of O_2 with other subunits. For fully cooperative binding, n is equal to the number of sites, an indication that binding at one site maximally enhances binding at other sites in the same molecule. The normal Hill coefficient for adult Hb ($n \sim 2.7$) reflects strongly cooperative ligand binding. Hb has a considerably lower affinity for O_2, reflected in a P_{50} of 27 ± 2 mmHg, compared to myoglobin ($P_{50} = 4$ mmHg). In the absence of cooperativity, even with multiple sites, the Hill coefficient would be 1, i.e. binding of one molecule of O_2 would not influence the binding of other molecules. Decreased or absent cooperativity is observed for Hb mutants that have lost functional subunit–subunit contacts (Table 5.1). The steepest slope of the saturation curve for Hb lies in a range of pO_2 that is found in most tissues (see Fig. 5.4). Thus, relatively small changes in pO_2 will result in considerably larger changes in the interaction of Hb with O_2. Accordingly, slight shifts of the curve in either direction will also dramatically influence O_2 affinity.

The mechanism underlying the cooperativity in oxygen binding by hemoglobin involves a shift between two conformational states of the hemoglobin molecule which differ in oxygen affinity. These two quaternary conformations are known as the T (tense) and R (relaxed) states, respectively. In the T state, interactions between the heterodimers are stronger; in the R state, these noncovalent bonds are, in summation, weaker. O_2 affinity is lower for the T state and higher for the R state. The transition between these structures is accompanied by the dissolution of existing noncovalent bonds and formation of new ones at the heterodimer interfaces (Fig. 5.6). Contact between the two $\alpha\beta$ heterodimers (see Fig. 5.5) is stabilized by a mixture of hydrogen and electrostatic bonds. Approximately 30 amino acids participate in the noncovalent interactions that characterize the deoxygenated and oxygenated Hb conformations.

Classification and examples of hemoglobinopathies

Classification	Common name	Mutation	Frequency	Biochemical changes	Clinical consequences
abnormal solubility	HbC	$Glu^{6(\beta)} \rightarrow Lys$	common	cellular crystallization of oxygenated protein; increased fragility	mild hemolytic anemia; splenomegaly (enlarged spleen)
decreased O_2 affinity	Hb Titusville	$Asp^{94(\alpha)} \rightarrow Asn$	very rare	heterodimer interface altered to stabilize T state; decreased cooperativity	mild cyanosis (blue-purple skin coloration from deoxygenated blood)
increased O_2 affinity	Hb Helsinki	$Lys^{82(\beta)} \rightarrow Met$	very rare	reduced binding of 2,3-BPG in T state	mild polycythemia (increased erythrocyte count)
ferric heme (methemoglobin)	HbM Boston	$His^{58(\alpha)} \rightarrow Tyr$	occasional	altered heme pocket (mutation of distal His)	cyanosis of skin and mucous membranes; decreased Bohr effect
unstable protein	Hb Gun Hill	$\Delta\beta91–95$	very rare	misfolding caused by loss of Leu in heme pocket and shorter helix	formation of Heinz bodies (inclusions of denatured Hb); jaundice (yellow coloration of integument and sclera); pigmented urine
abnormal synthesis	Hb Constant Spring	$ter^{142(\alpha)} \rightarrow Gln$	very rare	loss of termination codon; decreased mRNA stability	α-thalassemia (hemolytic anemia, splenomegaly and jaundice)

Table 5.1 **Classification and examples of hemoglobinopathies.** Hemoglobinopathies are usually classified according to the most prominent change to the protein's structure, function or regulation. Initial identification of a mutation often involves electrophoretic or chromatographic analysis, as shown in Fig 5.9 for HbSC, a double heterozygous genotype associated with a sickle cell disease-like phenotype. Δ = deletion mutant.

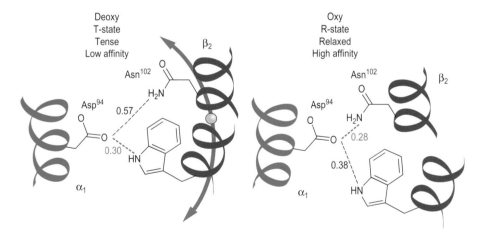

Fig. 5.6 **Noncovalent bonds differ in deoxygenated and oxygenated hemoglobin.** In the middle of the interface between the two αβ heterodimers are the residues $Asp^{94(\alpha)}$ on the α_1-globin of one heterodimer and $Trp^{37(\beta)}$ and $Asn^{102(\beta)}$ on the β_2-globin of the other heterodimer (see dashed oval in Fig. 5.5). Each has side chain atoms capable of noncovalent interactions. (Left) In the deoxygenated T state the distance between the Asp and Trp residues favors a hydrogen bond, whereas the distance between Asp and Asn is too great. (Right) As a result of the conformational changes that accompany the transition to the oxygenated R state, the distance between Asp and Trp is now too large, but that between Asp and Asn is compatible with formation of a new hydrogen bond. Elsewhere along this interface, other bonds are created and broken. An identical alignment of residues and noncovalent interactions is found between the α_2- and β_1-globin monomers. Distances are shown in nm. Hydrogen bonds are commonly 0.27–0.31 nm in length.

Several models have been developed to describe the transition between the T and R states of Hb. At one extreme is a model in which each Hb subunit sequentially responds to O_2 binding with a conformational change, thereby permitting hybrid intermediates of the T and R states. At the opposite extreme is a model in which all four subunits switch concertedly; hybrid states are forbidden, and O_2 binding shifts the equilibrium between T and R states. The molecular structures of deoxygenated and partially and fully ligated Hb have been studied extensively by a broad range of thermodynamic and kinetic techniques. Yet, progress toward reconciling inconsistencies among classic and more recent models has been slow.

PULSE OXIMETRY

Pulse oximetry ('pulse-ox') is a noninvasive method of estimating the oxygen saturation of arterial Hb. Two physical principles are involved: first, the visible and infrared spectral characteristics of oxy- and deoxy-Hb are different; second, arterial blood flow has a pulsatile component that results from volume changes with each heart beat. Transmission or reflectance measurements are made in a translucent tissue site with reasonable blood flow, commonly a finger, toe or ear of adults and children, or a foot or hand of infants. The photodetector and microprocessor of the pulse oximeter permit a calculation of oxygen saturation (SpO$_2$ = saturation of peripheral oxygen) that typically correlates within 4–6% of the value found by arterial blood gas analysis. Pulse oximetry is used to monitor the cardiopulmonary status during local and general anesthesia, in intensive care and neonatal units, and during patient transport. Body movement, radiated ambient light, elevated bilirubin, artificial or painted fingernails can interfere with pulse oximetry. Conventional, two-wavelength instruments 'assume' that the optical measurements are associated with oxygenated and deoxygenated hemoglobins; they cannot discriminate among oxy-, carboxy- and met-Hb. Newer technologies, however, utilize six or eight wavelengths and permit multiple Hb species discrimination with an accuracy of ±2.0% and a precision of ±1.0%.

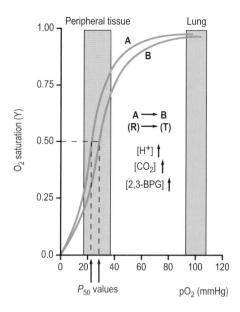

Fig. 5.7 **Allosteric effectors decrease the oxygen affinity of hemoglobin.** O$_2$ interaction with Hb is regulated by allosteric effectors. Under physiologic conditions HbA exhibits a highly cooperative O$_2$ saturation curve. With an increase in the erythrocyte concentration of any of three allosteric effectors, H$^+$, CO$_2$ or 2,3-bisphosphoglycerate (2,3-BPG), the curve shifts to the right (position B), indicating a decreased affinity for O$_2$ (increase in P_{50} value). Actions of the effectors that modulate O$_2$ affinity appear to be additive. Conversely, a decrease in any of the allosteric effectors shifts the curve to the left (position A). Increasing temperature will also shift the curve to the right. The sensitivity of O$_2$ saturation to H$^+$ is known as the Bohr effect. Normal ranges of O$_2$ measured in pulmonary and peripheral tissue capillaries are indicated by shaded areas.

ALLOSTERIC MODULATION OF THE OXYGEN AFFINITY OF HEMOGLOBIN

Allosteric proteins and effectors

Hb is one of the best studied examples of an allosteric protein, a protein that exhibits changes in ligand (or substrate) affinity under the influence of small molecules (see also Chapter 6 and Figure 6.11). These small molecules, called allosteric (meaning other place or site) effectors, bind to proteins at sites that are spatially distinct from the ligand-binding sites. Through long-range conformational effects, they alter the ligand or substrate binding affinity of the protein. Allosteric proteins are typically multisubunit proteins. The O$_2$ binding affinity of Hb is affected positively by O$_2$, as well as by a number of chemically diverse allosteric effectors, including H$^+$, CO$_2$, and 2,3-bisphosphoglycerate (2,3-BPG) (Fig. 5.7). When an allosteric effector affects its own binding to the protein (at other sites), the process is termed homotropic, e.g. the effect of binding of O$_2$ at one site on Hb enhances the affinity for binding of O$_2$ to other sites on Hb. When the allosteric effector is different from the ligand whose binding is altered, the process is termed heterotropic, e.g. the effect of H$^+$ on the P_{50} for oxygen binding to Hb. These interactions lead to horizontal shifts in the O$_2$ binding curves (see Fig. 5.7).

Bohr effect

The O$_2$ affinity of Hb is exquisitely sensitive to pH, a phenomenon known as the Bohr effect. The Bohr effect is most readily described as a right shift in the O$_2$ saturation curve with decreasing pH. Thus, an increased concentration of H$^+$ (decreased pH) favors an increased P_{50} (lower affinity) for O$_2$ binding to Hb, equivalent to an H$^+$-dependent shift of Hb from the R to the T state.

To understand the Bohr effect at the level of protein structure and to appreciate the role of H$^+$ as a heterotropic allosteric effector, it is important to recall that Hb is a highly charged molecule. The residues that participate in the Bohr effect include the *N*-terminal Val amino group of α-globin and the *C*-terminal His side chain of β-globin. The pK_a values of these weak acids differ sufficiently between the deoxygenated and oxygenated forms of Hb to cause the uptake of 1.2–2.4 protons by the deoxygenated, compared to oxygenated, tetramer.

Identification of specific amino acid residues of the α- and β-globins that participate in the Bohr effect is complicated by differential interactions of other charged solutes with deoxy- and oxy-Hb. Thus, a preferential binding of a given anion, i.e. Cl^- and/or organic phosphates, to deoxygenated Hb involves the alteration of the pKs of some cationic groups, thereby contributing to the overall observed Bohr effect. For example, there is compelling evidence showing that $Val^{1(\alpha)}$ is relevant to the Bohr effect only in the presence of Cl^-. The pK_a of this group shifts from 8.0 in deoxygenated Hb to 7.25 in ligated Hb in the presence of physiological Cl^- (~100 mmol/L). Further, the participation of the $Val^{1(\alpha)}$ groups in the chloride-dependent Bohr effect is strongly modulated by CO_2 because of the formation of CO_2 (carbamino) adducts of Hb (below).

As Hb binds O_2, protons dissociate from selected weak acid functions. Conversely, in acidic media, protonation of the conjugate bases inhibits O_2 binding. During their circulation between pulmonary alveoli and peripheral tissue capillaries, erythrocytes encounter markedly different conditions of pO_2 and pH. The high pO_2 in the lungs promotes ligand saturation and forces protons from the Hb molecule to stabilize the R state. In the capillary bed, particularly in metabolically active tissues, the pH is slightly lower, due to the production of acidic metabolites, such as lactate. Oxygenated Hb, upon entering this environment, will acquire some 'excess' protons and shift toward the T state, promoting release of O_2 for uptake by tissues for aerobic metabolism.

Effects of CO₂ and temperature

Closely related to the Bohr effect is the ability of CO_2 to alter the O_2 affinity of Hb. Like the negative allosteric effect of H^+, the increase in pCO_2 in venous capillaries decreases the affinity of Hb for O_2. Accordingly, a right shift in the ligand saturation curve occurs as pCO_2 increases. It should be emphasized that the allosteric effector is, in fact, CO_2, not HCO_3^-. CO_2 reacts reversibly with the unprotonated N-terminal amino groups of the globin polypeptides to form carbamino adducts:

$$Hb\!-\!NH_2 + CO_2 \rightleftharpoons Hb\!-\!NHCOO^- + H^+$$

This transient covalent chemical modification of Hb is not only a specialized example of allosteric control, resulting in a stabilization of deoxygenated Hb; it also represents one form of transport of CO_2 to the lungs for clearance from the body. Between 5% and 10% of the total CO_2 content of blood exists as carbamino adducts.

There is a strong physiologic correlation between pCO_2 and the O_2 affinity of Hb. CO_2 is a major product of mitochondrial oxidation and, like H^+, is particularly abundant in metabolically active tissues. Upon diffusing into blood, CO_2 can react with oxygenated Hb, shift the equilibrium toward the T state, and thereby promote the dissociation of bound O_2 (see Fig. 5.7). The vast majority of peripheral tissue CO_2, however, is hydrated in the presence of erythrocyte carbonic anhydrase to carbonic acid (H_2CO_3), a weak acid that dissociates partially to H^+ and HCO_3^-:

$$CO_2 + H_2O \rightleftharpoons H_2CO_3 \text{ enzyme-catalyzed reaction}$$
$$H_2CO_3 \rightleftharpoons H^+ + HCO_3^- \text{ spontaneous acid dissociation}$$

 ## ARTIFICIAL HEMOGLOBINS

The supply-and-demand curves of whole blood and packed red cell availability and utilization point to an impending crisis and the need to develop alternatives. Red cell substitutes are transfusion alternatives that are potentially useful during major surgical procedures and hemorrhagic shock emergencies. Three types of artificial O_2 carriers have been investigated: Hb-based oxygen carrier (HBOC), liposome-encapsulated Hb, and perfluorocarbon emulsion. HBOCs are hemoglobins derived from allogeneic, xenogeneic or recombinant sources that have been modified by polymerization, crosslinkage or conjugation. These modifications facilitate purification and sterilization, and minimize toxicity and immunogenicity. They are also necessary to stabilize the acellular Hb tetramers; otherwise the hemoglobin dissociates into dimers and monomers in plasma and is excreted in urine.

Several HBOCs have progressed through extensive clinical evaluation. One of these is HBOC-201, a glutaraldehyde-polymerized bovine Hb that has received approval for human use in South Africa for acute anemia secondary to surgical procedures.

A polymerized, pyridoxylated human Hb is in phase 3 trials in the United States, but concerns have been raised regarding product safety and protocol ethics. A conjugated HBOC, in which polyethylene glycol is attached to surface Lys residues on human Hb, has completed phase 2 investigation. The polymerized forms have O_2 affinity (P_{50}) in the range 16–38 mmHg and diminished cooperativity (n ~1.3–2.1); the conjugated Hb exhibits a very high O_2 affinity (5–6 mmHg), a Hill coefficient of 1.2, and a Bohr effect half that of native Hb.

Adverse effects are not uncommon with HBOCs. Increased vasoconstriction with subsequent hypertension occurs, a result of increased binding of nitric oxide (NO) by acellular Hb and altered stimulation of catecholamine release. Other problems include increased heme oxidation to met-Hb, elevated iron deposition in tissues, gastrointestinal distress, neurotoxicity, and interference with diagnostic measurements. Molecular engineering of human Hb, now underway in a number of laboratories, seeks to improve O_2 binding, allosteric properties, and side effects of HBOCs.

Interestingly, from both carbamino adduct formation and hydration/dissociation reactions involving CO_2, an additional pool of protons is generated, protons that become available to participate in the Bohr effect and facilitate O_2—CO_2 exchange. During its return to the lungs, blood transports two forms of CO_2: carbamino-Hb and the H_2CO_3/HCO_3^- acid–conjugate base pair. Blood and Hb are now exposed to a low pCO_2, and through mass action the carbamino adduct formation is reversed and binding of O_2 is again favored. Similarly, in the pulmonary capillaries, erythrocyte carbonic anhydrase converts H_2CO_3 to CO_2 and H_2O, which are expired into the atmosphere.

Working muscles not only produce the allosteric effectors H^+ and CO_2 as byproducts of aerobic metabolism, but they also liberate heat. Because the binding of O_2 to heme is an exothermic process, the O_2 affinity of Hb decreases with increasing temperature. Thus, the microenvironment of an exercising muscle profoundly favors a more efficient release of Hb-bound O_2 to the surrounding tissue.

Effect of 2,3-bisphosphoglycerate

2,3-Bisphosphoglycerate (2,3-BPG), an organic phosphate compound, is another important modulator of the O_2 affinity of Hb. 2,3-BPG is synthesized in human erythrocytes in a one-step shunt off the glycolytic pathway (Chapter 12). Like H^+ and CO_2, 2,3-BPG is an indispensable negative allosteric effector that, when bound to Hb, causes a marked increase in P_{50} (see Fig. 5.7). Were it not for the high erythrocyte concentration of 2,3-BPG (~4.1 mmol/L, nearly equal to that of Hb), the O_2 saturation curve of Hb would approach that of Mb!

At one end of the twofold symmetry axis within the quaternary structure of Hb there is a shallow cleft defined by cationic amino acids of the juxtaposed β-globin subunits (Fig. 5.8). A single molecule of 2,3-BPG binds to this site.

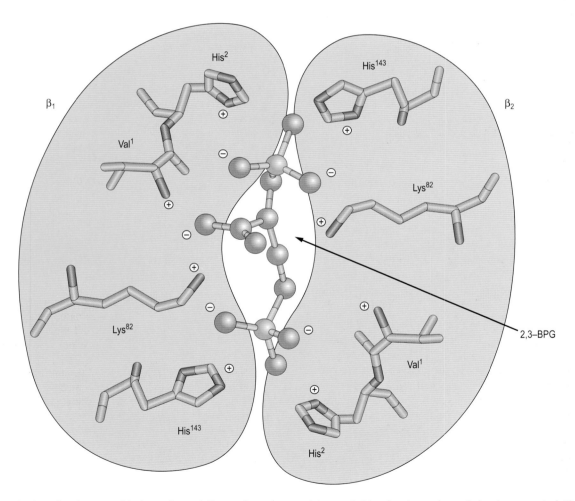

Fig. 5.8 **2,3-Bisphosphoglycerate binds preferentially to deoxygenated hemoglobin.** On the surface of the deoxygenated Hb tetramer where the two β-globins (purple) interact, there is a cleft formed by the *N*-terminal amino acid residue (Val[1(β)]) and the side chains of His[2(β)], Lys[82(β)], and His[143(β)] (stick models). This site consists of eight cationic groups, sufficient to bind with high affinity one molecule of 2,3-BPG (ball-and-stick model; phosphorus, orange), a molecule with five anionic groups at physiologic pH. This array of positive charges does not exist in oxygenated Hb. In fetal Hb (HbF) His[143(β)] is replaced by a Ser residue.

A critical consequence of the conformational differences between the T and R states is that deoxygenated Hb preferentially interacts with the negatively charged 2,3-BPG. Multiple electrostatic interactions stabilize the complex between the polyanionic effector and deoxygenated Hb. The cleft is too narrow in fully oxygenated Hb to accommodate 2,3-BPG.

The importance of 2,3-BPG as an allosteric effector is underscored by observations that its concentration in the erythrocyte changes in response to various physiologic and pathologic conditions. During chronic hypoxia (decreased pO_2) secondary to pulmonary disease, anemia or shock, the level of 2,3-BPG increases. Such compensatory increases have also been described in cigarette smokers and on adaptation to high altitudes. The net result is a greater stabilization of the deoxygenated, low-affinity T state and a further shift of the saturation curve to the right, thereby facilitating release of more O_2 to tissues. Under most circumstances, the rightward shift has an insignificant effect on the O_2 saturation of Hb in the lungs.

SELECTED TOPICS

Interaction of hemoglobin with nitric oxide

Nitric oxide (NO) is a gaseous free radical capable of oxidative modification (nitration, nitrosation, nitrosylation) of biological macromolecules. Yet this highly reactive molecule, also known as endothelium-derived relaxing factor (EDRF), is synthesized in endothelial cells and participates in normal vascular physiology, including vasodilation (smooth muscle), hemostasis (platelet), and adhesion molecule expression (endothelial cell) (see box on p. 76). Erythrocytes are the largest intravascular reservoir of bioactive NO, and Hb is indispensable for its formation, storage, and release. SNO-Hb is the product of S-nitrosylation of the $Cys^{93\beta}$ side chains of Hb. These Cys thiol groups can accept NO by transfer from intracellular S-nitrosoglutathione or from heme-bound NO (nitrosyl-Hb). NO is released by exchange from SNO-Hb to Cys side chains of anion exchanger 1, an erythrocyte membrane protein that can then deliver NO to the plasma. The formation and breakdown of SNO-Hb are sensitive to pO_2, deoxygenation/oxygenation status, and the T state/R state conformational transition; SNO-Hb also binds O_2 more tightly.

Another remarkable process within the erythrocyte is the allosterically regulated conversion of nitrite (NO_2^-) to NO, a reaction performed by deoxygenated Hb. This intrinsic 'nitrite reductase' activity takes advantage of the moderate NO_2^- concentration in the erythrocyte (up to 0.3 μmol/L). While the chemistry is complex, the reaction is thought to yield a labile intermediate nitrosyl-met(ferric)Hb that can readily transfer NO to $Cys^{93(\beta)}$ on oxygenated Hb.

ACUTE MOUNTAIN SICKNESS (TOO HIGH, TOO FAST)

Acute mountain sickness (AMS) develops in individuals who ascend rapidly to ambient conditions of hypobaric hypoxia. Symptoms include shortness of breath, rapid heart rate, headache, nausea, anorexia, and sleep disturbance. These can develop at altitudes of 2000 m (25% incidence) and higher to 4000 m or more (50% incidence). The most severe form is high-altitude cerebral edema (2% incidence), a potentially fatal condition characterized by ataxia and other neuromuscular and neurologic problems. At 4000 m the barometric pressure is 460 mmHg, leading to an ambient partial pressure of O_2 of 96 mmHg (sea level, 160). Physiologic calculations yield values of a tracheal pO_2 of 86 mmHg (sea level, 149), an alveolar pO_2 of 50 mmHg (sea level, 105), and an arterial pO_2 of 45 mmHg (sea level, 100). At this arterial partial pressure of O_2, Hb saturation is only 81% (see Fig. 5.4). Consequently, the O_2 carrying capacity of arterial blood decreases to ~160 mL/L (sea level, 198). Hypoxia can also lead to overperfusion of vascular beds, endothelial leakage, and edema. Humans adapt to high altitude (acclimatization) by several mechanisms. Hyperventilation is a critical short-term response that serves to decrease alveolar pCO_2 and, in turn, increase alveolar pO_2. Arterial pH is also increased during hyperventilation, leading to a higher affinity of Hb for O_2. A gradual increase in 2,3-BPG typically occurs in response to chronic hypoxia. Another important adaptive mechanism is polycythemia, an increase in erythrocyte concentration that results from erythropoietin stimulation of bone marrow cells. Within one week of acclimatization the Hb concentration can increase by as much as 20% to provide near-normal arterial O_2 content.

Neuroglobin and cytoglobin: minor mammalian hemoglobins

Two other globins have recently been identified in humans. Neuroglobin (Ngb) is expressed primarily in the central nervous system and some endocrine tissues; cytoglobin (Cygb) is ubiquitously expressed, primarily in cells of fibroblast origin. Tissue concentrations of both are <1 mmol/L. The Ngb polypeptide has 151 amino acid residues (16 933 Da), whereas Cybg contains 190 residues (21 405 Da), with 'extensions' of 20 amino acids at both the N- and C-termini (see Fig. 5.1). Both human proteins share only about 25% sequence identity with Mb and Hb. Yet all key elements of the globin fold are present: the three-over-three α-helix sandwich; proximal and distal His residues; and a hydrophobic, heme-containing pocket.

In contrast to Mb and Hb, Ngb and Cygb contain hexacoordinate hemes for both the Fe^{2+} and Fe^{3+} valency states. The distal HisE7, serving as the sixth ligand, must be displaced to permit binding of O_2. Yet the O_2 affinities of Ngb

A college student with severe muscle spasms in her arms, numbness in her extremities, some dizziness, and respiratory difficulty was brought to the student health center. The patient had been vigorously exercising in an attempt to relieve the stress of forthcoming examinations when she suddenly began to experience forced, rapid breathing. Suspecting hyperventilation, a health care worker began to reassure the student and helped her recover by getting her to breathe into a paper bag. After 20 minutes the spasms ceased, feeling returned to her fingers, and the lightheadedness resolved.

Comment. Alveolar hyperventilation is an abnormally rapid, deep, and prolonged breathing pattern that leads to respiratory alkalosis, i.e. a profound decrease in pCO_2 and an increase in blood pH that can be attributed to an increased loss of CO_2 from the body. With decreased $[CO_2]$ and $[H^+]$, two allosteric effectors of O_2 binding and release, the affinity of Hb for O_2 increases sufficiently to reduce the efficiency of delivery of O_2 to peripheral tissues, including the central nervous system. Another characteristic of alkalosis is a decreased level of ionized calcium in plasma, a situation that contributes to muscle spasms and cramps. In general, hyperventilation is triggered by hypoxemia, pulmonary and cardiac diseases, metabolic disorders, pharmacologic agents, and anxiety.

and Cygb are surprisingly high, with P_{50} values in the range 1–7.5 mmHg and 0.7–1.8 mmHg, respectively, compared to a $P_{50} \approx 27$ mmHg for Hb. Binding of O_2 to the dimeric Cygb is cooperative (Hill coefficient, 1.2–1.7) but independent of pH. On the other hand, monomeric Ngb exhibits a pH-dependent O_2 affinity. The functions of these minor globins remain elusive. Ngb appears to be comparable to Mb, mediating the delivery of O_2 to retina mitochondria. Cygb has been proposed to function as an enzyme cofactor, supplying O_2 for the hydroxylation of Pro and Lys side chains in some proteins.

Normal hemoglobin variants

Over 95% of the Hb found in adult humans is HbA, with the $\alpha_2\beta_2$ globin subunit composition. HbA_2 accounts for 2–3% of the total and has an $\alpha_2\delta_2$ polypeptide composition. HbA_2 is elevated in β-thalassemia, a disease characterized by a deficiency in β-globin biosynthesis. Functionally, these two adult hemoglobins are indistinguishable. Not surprisingly, mutations of the gene encoding δ-globin are without clinical consequence.

Another minor Hb is fetal Hb, HbF; its subunits are α-globin and γ-globin. While it accounts for no more than 1% of adult Hb, HbF predominates in the fetus during the second and third trimesters of gestation and in the neonate. Gene switching on chromosome 11 causes HbF to decrease shortly after birth. The most striking functional difference between HbF and HbA is its decreased sensitivity to 2,3-BPG. Comparison of the primary structures of the β- and γ- polypeptides reveals a replacement of $His^{143\beta}$ by Ser in γ-globin (see Fig. 5.1). Consequently, two of the cationic groups that participate in the binding of the anionic allosteric effector are no longer available (see Fig. 5.8). Predictably, the interaction of 2,3-BPG with HbF is weaker, resulting in an increased affinity for O_2 (P_{50} of 19 mmHg for HbF compared to 27 mmHg for HbA) and a greater stabilization of the oxygenated R state. The direct benefit of this structural and functional change in the HbF isoform is a more efficient transfer of O_2 from maternal HbA to fetal HbF (see Fig. 5.4). Separation of these and other Hb variants in the clinical laboratory is performed by electrophoretic and chromatographic analysis (Fig. 5.9).

Sickle cell disease, a common hemoglobinopathy

Sickle cell disease (SCD), an inherited disorder of Hb structure, is characterized by a tendency for erythrocytes to distort and limit blood flow in capillary beds. Clinically, an individual with SCD presents with intermittent episodes of hemolytic anemia, resulting from chronic lysis of red cells, and painful vasoocclusive crises. Common features also include impaired growth, increased susceptibility to infections, and multiple organ damage. In the African-American population, SCD affects 70–75 000 individuals, a frequency of ~0.2%. Heterozygous, mostly asymptomatic carriers number 8% in this same population. Sickle cell disease has a prevalence of 40% in some regions of equatorial Africa.

SCD is caused by an inherited, single point mutation in the gene encoding β-globin, leading to the expression of the Hb variant HbS. Indeed, HbS has been studied biochemically, biophysically, and genetically for over 50 years, making SCD the paradigm of a molecular disease. The mutation is $Glu^{6(\beta)} \rightarrow Val$: a surface-localized charged amino acid is replaced by a hydrophobic residue. Valine on the mutant β-globin subunit fits into a complementary pocket (sometimes called a 'sticky patch') formed on the β-globin subunit of a deoxygenated Hb molecule, a pocket that becomes exposed only upon the release of bound O_2 in tissue capillaries.

HbA remains a true solute at rather high concentrations, largely as a result of a polar exterior surface that is compatible and nonreactive with nearby Hb molecules. In contrast, HbS, when deoxygenated, is less soluble. It forms long, filamentous polymers that readily precipitate, distorting erythrocyte morphology to the characteristic sickle shape. In the homozygous individual with SCD (HbS/HbS), the complex process of nucleation and polymerization occurs rapidly, producing about 10% of circulating erythrocytes that are sickled. In the heterozygous individual (HbA/HbS, sickle

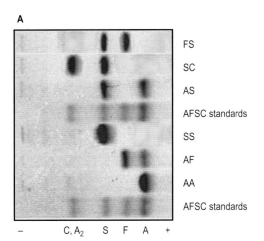

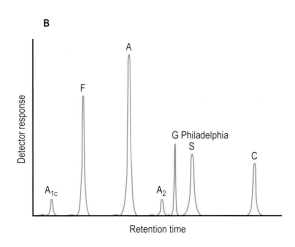

Fig. 5.9 **Normal and abnormal hemoglobins can be separated by electrophoretic and chromatographic methods.** (A) This panel shows cellulose acetate electrophoresis (pH 8.4) of blood samples obtained for neonatal screening. This rapid technique will tentatively identify HbS and HbC, two common mutant hemoglobins in the African-American population. Additional tests are required for a definitive diagnosis. FS, newborn with sickle cell disease; SC, double heterozygote child with sickle cell-like disease; AS, child with sickle cell trait; AF, normal neonate. (B) This trace illustrates high-pressure liquid chromatography (HPLC) with a cation-exchanger solid phase, a technique capable of separating and quantifying more than 40 hemoglobins. HPLC may also be used to measure HbA_{1c}, a glycated protein that provides information on the progression and treatment of diabetes mellitus. Also shown is the elution profile of Hb G Philadelphia ($Asn^{68(\alpha)} \rightarrow Lys$), a common but benign variant that co-migrates with HbS on electrophoresis.

 ## ACQUIRED METHEMOGLOBINEMIA

In a rural region of the state, a 4-month-old infant was seen at the local emergency room for episodes of seizures, breathing difficulty, and vomiting. The infant's skin and mucous membranes were bluish, indicating cyanosis. Analysis of arterial blood revealed a chocolate brown color, a normal pO_2, an O_2 saturation of 60%, and a met-Hb (ferric-heme) level of 35%. The tentative cause of the acute toxic methemoglobinemia was found to be well water contaminated by a nitrate/nitrite concentration of 34mg/L. The infant was treated successfully by intravenous administration of methylene blue (1–2 mg/kg) that serves to accelerate indirectly the enzymatic reduction of met-Hb to normal (ferrous) Hb by NADPH met-Hb reductase, which is normally a minor pathway for conversion of met-Hb to Hb.

Comment. Met-Hb is formed when the ferrous iron of heme is oxidized to ferric iron; it is produced spontaneously at a low rate and more rapidly in the presence of certain drugs, nitrites, and aniline dyes. In genetic forms of methemoglobinemia, mutation of either the proximal or distal His to Tyr makes the heme iron more susceptible to oxidation (see Table 5.1). The extent of oxidation in Hb tetramers can range from one heme group to all four. Erythrocytes contain an NADH-cytochrome b_5 reductase, or NADH diaphorase, that is responsible for the majority of met-Hb reduction. Infants are particularly vulnerable to methemoglobinemia because their level of NADH-cytochrome b_5 reductase is half that of adults. Moreover, their higher level of HbF is more sensitive to oxidants compared to HbA.

 ## HEMOGLOBIN A_{1c} – A MIRROR OF DIABETES MELLITUS MANAGEMENT

Adult blood contains a number of chemically modified Hb subfractions. One of these is HbA_{1c}, a glycated Hb that is normally present at levels of 4–6% of the HbA fraction. Glycated Hb is formed in vivo by the nonenzymatic attachment of D-glucose to primary amino groups of globin polypeptides. A relatively fast and reversible initial reaction produces a labile aldimine (Schiff base), which slowly rearranges to a stable ketoamine (Amadori product). The modification specific to HbA_{1c} occurs at the N-terminal residue of the two β-globin polypeptides. The level of HbA_{1c} increases with mean blood glucose concentration over the previous 3–6 weeks; it can rise to 14% or more in some patients with high blood glucose. Measurements of HbA_{1c} are used routinely to monitor glycemic control in the treatment of diabetes mellitus, with a target goal for most patients of <7% HbA_{1c}. Quantitative methods include HPLC, mass spectrometry, and immunoturbidimetric assays. See Chapter 21 for further discussion.

cell trait), the kinetics of sickling are decreased by at least a factor of 1000, thereby accounting for the asymptomatic nature of this genotype. In dilute solution, HbS has interactions with O_2 (P_{50} value, Hill coefficient) that are similar to those for HbA. However, the Bohr effect on concentrated

HbS is more pronounced, leading to greater release of O_2 in the capillaries and increased propensity for sickling.

Sickled erythrocytes exhibit less deformability. They no longer move freely through the microvasculature and often block blood flow, especially in the spleen and joints. Moreover, these cells lose water, become fragile, and have a considerably shorter life span, leading to hemolysis and anemia. Except during extreme physical exertion, the heterozygous individual appears normal. For reasons that remain to be elucidated, heterozygosity is associated with an increased resistance to malaria, specifically growth of the infectious agent *Plasmodium falciparum* in the erythrocyte. This observation represents an example of a selective advantage that the HbA/HbS heterozygote exhibits over either the HbA/HbA normal or the HbS/HbS homozygote and probably offers an explanation for the persistence of HbS in the gene pool.

Other hemoglobinopathies

More than 900 mutations in the genes encoding the α- and β-globin polypeptides have been documented. As with most mutational events, the majority of these lead to few, if any, clinical problems. There are, however, several hundred mutations that give rise to abnormal Hb and pathologic phenotypes. Hb mutants or hemoglobinopathies are usually named after the location (hospital, city or geographical region) in which the abnormal protein was first identified. They are classified according to the type of structural change and altered function and the resulting clinical characteristics (see Tables 5.1, 5.2). While many of these mutants have predictable phenotypes, others are surprisingly pleiotropic in their impact on multiple properties of the Hb molecule. With few exceptions, Hb variants are inherited as autosomal recessive traits. Occasionally, double heterozygotes are identified, e.g. HbSC (Fig. 5.9).

ANALGESIC TREATMENT OF SICKLE CELL VASOOCCLUSIVE CRISES

Acute vasoocclusive crises are the most common problem reported by individuals with SCD; they are also the most frequent reason for emergency room treatment and hospital admission. Episodes of vasoocclusive pain are unpredictable and are often excruciating and incapacitating. The origin of this progressive pain involves altered rheologic and hematologic properties of erythrocytes attributable to HbS polymerization and aggregation. Microvascular dysfunction is precipitated by an inflammatory response, indicated by elevation of plasma acute phase proteins. Ultimately, impaired vasomotor responses in arterioles and adhesive interactions between sickled erythrocytes and endothelial cells in postcapillary venules restrict blood flow to tissues throughout the body.

Epidemiologic data indicate that ~5% of patients with SCD can expect to experience 3–10 episodes of severe pain annually. Typically, the pain crisis resolves within 5–7 days, but a severe crisis may cause pain that persists for weeks. To provide relief to the patient, nonnarcotic, narcotic, and adjuvant analgesics are used alone or in combination. The severity and duration of the pain dictate the most appropriate analgesic regimen. Parenterally administered opioids (morphine, hydromorphone, meperidine) are frequently used for treatment of severe pain in vasoocclusive crises. Several recent studies suggest additional options for the patient and physician: continuous intravenous infusion of a nonsteroidal antiinflammatory drug (ketorolac) and continuous epidural administration of local anesthetic (lidocaine) and opioid analgesic (fentanyl) effectively decreased pain that was unresponsive to conventional measures. In addition to analgesia, oxygen therapy and fluid management are also initiated.

SEPARATION OF HEMOGLOBIN VARIANTS AND MUTANTS; DIAGNOSIS OF HEMOGLOBINOPATHIES

The mobility of a protein during electrophoresis or chromatography is determined by its charge and interaction with the matrix. Three commonly used techniques provide sufficient resolution to separate Hb variants differing in a single charge from HbA: electrophoresis, isoelectric focusing, and ion exchange chromatography. Electrophoretic and chromatographic separations of Hb are illustrated in Figure 5.9. The volume of hemolysate required (<100 µL) makes these techniques suitable for neonatal and adult blood samples. Quantification is performed by scanning densitometry or absorption spectrometry. Indications of abnormalities in screening tests are followed by complete blood count (Table 5.2), additional protein analysis, and DNA analysis to identify specific mutations to the globin genes.

COMPLETE BLOOD COUNT

A complete blood count (CBC) provides information on blood cell populations and their characteristics. Data are obtained from whole blood samples by automated hematology analysis. Some instruments also provide leukocyte differentials, reticulocyte count, and red cell morphology. A typical printout of the results for one individual and the reference range is shown in Table 5.2.

Complete blood count (CBC)		
Parameter	**Patient**	**Reference value (SI units)***
white blood cell count, WBC	6.82×10^9/L	$4.0–11.0 \times 10^9$/L
red cell count, RBC	4.78×10^{12}/L	$4.0–5.2 \times 10^{12}$/L (F); $4.5–5.9 \times 10^{12}$/L (M)
hemoglobin, HGB	6.1 mmol/L	7.4–9.9 mmol/L (F); 8.4–10.9 mmol/L (M)
hematocrit, HCT	33.4%	41–46% (F); 37–49% (M)
mean corpuscular volume, MCV	71.9 fL	80–96 fL
mean corpuscular hemoglobin, MCH	21.3 pg/cell	26–34 pg/cell
mean corpuscular hemoglobin concentration, MCHC	296 g/L	320–360 g/L
red cell distribution width, RDW	17.7%	11.5–14.5%
platelet count, PLT	274×10^9/L	$150–350 \times 10^9$/L
mean platelet volume, MPV	8.6 fL	6.4–11.0 fL

*F, female; M, male; fL, 10^{-15} L; pg, 10^{-12} g. To convert mmol Hb/L to g Hb/dL, multiply by 0.01611. See also reference values in the Appendix.

Table 5.2 **Complete blood count (CBC).** Automated laboratory evaluation of blood provides invaluable information for the diagnosis and monitoring of health problems. The complete blood count, performed on a sample of whole blood, includes counts of red cells (erythrocytes), white cells (leukocytes), and platelets and quantitative indices of the red cells (MCV, MCH, MCHC, and RDW). The results describe the hematopoietic status of the bone marrow and the presence of anemia and its possible cause. Data presented are characteristic of an individual with iron deficiency anemia: low HGB, low MCV (microcytosis), and low MCH (hypochromia). See also reference values in the Appendix.

Summary

This chapter describes two important proteins that reversibly interact with O_2: myoglobin (Mb), a tissue oxygen storage molecule, and hemoglobin (Hb), a blood oxygen transport molecule. Both use an ancient heme-containing polypeptide domain motif to sequester O_2 and increase its solubility. These proteins must function efficiently in rather different biochemical environments to sustain aerobic metabolism. As a tetramer of globins, Hb is one of the best characterized examples of cooperativity in ligand interactions. With its wide variety of effector molecules, Hb is also a prototype of an allosteric protein. Conformational changes in both the tertiary and quaternary structures characterize the transition between deoxygenated and oxygenated states. Mutations to globin genes lead to a spectrum of structural and functional variants, among which are fetal Hb and sickle cell disease.

ACTIVE LEARNING

1. Discuss why some genetic mutations to α-globin or β-globin result in a pathologic phenotype while the majority remain silent or benign. Describe the mutations that are the most difficult to detect.
2. Speculate on the mechanisms by which an adult with sickle cell disease would benefit from a fetal hemoglobin (HbF) level of 20%.
3. Many hemoglobin-based oxygen carriers (HBOCs) have a decreased sensitivity to pH and an increased susceptibility to oxidation. Discuss the consequences of a reduced Bohr effect to oxygen delivery to the periphery, tissue acid–base balance, and CO_2 transport to the lungs.
4. Summarize the observations of experimental animals in which the gene encoding myoglobin has been ablated ('knocked out').

Further reading

Allen BW, Piantadosi CA. How do red blood cells cause hypoxic vasodilation? The SNO-hemoglobin paradigm. *Am J Physiol Heart Circ Physiol* 2006;**291**: H1507–H1512.

Clarke C. Acute mountain sickness: medical problems associated with acute and subacute exposure to hypobaric hypoxia. *Postgrad Med J* 2006;**82**:748–753.

Frenette PS, Atweh GF. Sickle cell disease: old discoveries, new concepts, and future promise. *J Clin Invest* 2007;**117**:850–858.

Jahr JS, Walker V, Manoochehri K. Blood substitutes as pharmacotherapies in clinical practice. *Curr Opin Anesthesiol* 2007;**20**:325–330.

Juurlink DN, Buckley NA, Stanbrook MB, Isbister GK, Bennett M, McGuigan MA. Hyperbaric oxygen for carbon monoxide poisoning. *Cochrane Database of Systematic Reviews* 2005;(1):Issue 1.

Ou CN, Rognerud CL. Diagnosis of hemoglobinopathies: electrophoresis vs. HPLC. *Clin Chim Acta* 2001;**313**:187–194.

Pesce A, Bolognesi M, Bocedi A et al. Neuroglobin and cytoglobin. Fresh blood for the vertebrate globin family. *EMBO Reports* 2002;**3**:1146–1151.

Schnog JB, Duits AJ, Muskiet FAJ et al. Sickle cell disease: a general review. *Neth J Med* 2004;**62**:364–374.

Wu L, Wang R. Carbon monoxide: endogenous production, physiological functions, and pharmacological applications. *Pharmacol Rev* 2005;**57**:585–630.

Websites

A database of human hemoglobin variants and thalassemia (links to sites describing human hemoglobinopathies and thalassemias): http://globin.cse.psu.edu/globin/hbvar/

The Red Cell and Anemia (detailed five-part presentation by pathologist E Uthman):

- Blood cells and the CBC: http://web2.airmail.net/uthman/blood_cells.html
- Anemia: Pathophysiologic Consequences, Classification, and Clinical Investigation: http://web2.airmail.net/uthman/anemia/anemia.html
- Nutritional Anemias and Anemia of Chronic Disease: http://web2.airmail.net/uthman/nutritional_anemia/nutritional_anemia.html
- Hemolytic Anemias: http://web2.airmail.net/uthman/hemolytic_anemia/hemolytic_anemia.html
- Hemoglobinopathies and Thalassemias: http://web2.airmail.net/uthman/hemoglobinopathy/hemoglobinopathy.html

Sickle Cell Information Center (comprehensive site for both patients and professionals): www.scinfo.org/

Animations:

- Interactive examination (Jmol format) of hemoglobin and heme structures, binding of oxygen, and impact of sickle cell disease mutation. Molecular Visualization Resources, University of Massachusetts: http://www.umass.edu.molvis/tutorials/hemoglobin
- In-depth tutorial probe (Jmol format) of myoglobin and hemoglobin structures and ligand binding. © Interactive Concepts in Biochemistry, Science Technologies, John Wiley & Sons Publishers: http://www3.interscience.wiley.com:8100/legacy/college/boyer/0471661791/structure/HbMb/hbmb.htm

6. Catalytic Proteins – Enzymes

J Fujii

LEARNING OBJECTIVES

After reading this chapter you should be able to:

- Describe the characteristics of enzymatic reactions from the viewpoint of free energy, equilibrium and kinetics.
- Discuss the structure and composition of enzymes, including the role of cofactors, and conditions that affect enzymatic reactions.
- Describe enzyme kinetics based on the Michaelis–Menten equation and the significance of the Michaelis constant (K_m).
- Describe the elements of enzyme structure that explain their substrate specificity and catalytic activity.
- Describe regulatory mechanisms affecting enzymatic reactions, including regulation by allosteric effectors and covalent modification.
- Differentiate among the major types of enzyme inhibition from the viewpoint of enzyme kinetics.
- Discuss the therapeutic use of enzyme inhibitors and the diagnostic utility of clinical enzyme assays.

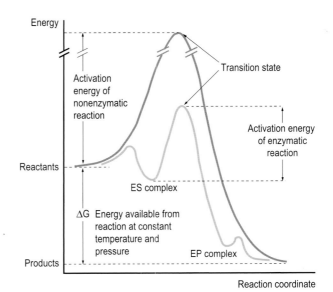

Fig. 6.1 **Reaction profile for enzymatic and nonenzymatic reactions.** The basic principles of an enzyme-catalyzed reaction are the same as any chemical reaction. When a chemical reaction proceeds, the substrate must gain activation energy to reach a point called the transition state of the reaction, at which the energy level is maximum. Since the transition state of the enzyme-catalyzed reaction has a lower energy than that of the uncatalyzed reaction, the reaction can proceed faster. ES complex, enzyme–substrate complex; EP complex, enzyme–product complex.

INTRODUCTION

Almost all biological functions are supported by chemical reactions catalyzed by biological catalysts, called enzymes. Efficient metabolism is controlled by orderly, sequential, and branching metabolic pathways. Enzymes accelerate chemical reactions under physiologic conditions, at 37°C and neutral pH. However, an enzyme cannot alter the equilibrium for a reaction; it can only accelerate the reaction rate, by decreasing the activation energy of the reaction (Fig. 6.1). Regulation of enzymatic activities allows metabolism to adapt to rapidly changing conditions. Nearly all enzymes are proteins, although some ribonucleic acid molecules, termed ribozymes, also have catalytic activity (Chapter 32). Based on analysis of the human genome, it is estimated that about a quarter of human genes encode for enzymes that catalyze metabolic reactions.

ENZYMATIC REACTIONS

Factors affecting enzymatic reactions

Effect of temperature

In the case of an inorganic catalyst, the reaction rate increases with the temperature of the system, and high temperature may be used to accelerate a reaction. In contrast, enzymes normally function as catalysts at constant (ambient or body) temperature. In in vitro assays, however, enzyme activity increases with temperature, but then declines at higher temperature. Thus, enzymes display a temperature optimum in vitro. This happens because enzymes, like all proteins, denature at high temperature and lose activity.

Effect of pH

Every enzyme has a pH optimum because ionizable amino acids, such as histidine, glutamate, and cysteine, participate in the catalytic reactions. Cytosolic enzymes have pH optima in the pH 7–8 range. Pepsin, which is secreted by gastric cells and functions in gastric juice, has a pH optimum of 1.5–2.0; trypsin and chymotrypsin have alkaline pH optima, consistent with their digestive activity in alkaline pancreatic juice; lysosomal enzymes typically have acidic pH optima. The pH sensitivity of enzymes results from the effect of pH on the ionic charge of amino acid side chains of enzymes. Various solutes, including substrates, products, metal ions and regulatory molecules, also affect the rate of enzymatic reactions.

Definition of enzyme activity

For the purposes of standardization, the activity of an enzyme is measured under defined conditions (temperature, pH, buffer, substrate and coenzyme concentration). The rate or velocity (v) of an enzymatic reaction under these conditions is defined as the rate of conversion of substrate to product per unit of time. A unit of enzyme is a measure of the amount of enzyme. The commonly used international unit (IU) for an enzyme is the amount of enzyme that catalyzes conversion of one micromole of substrate to product per min (1 IU = 1 μmol/min). The *katal* is an international unit for the amount of enzyme that catalyzes conversion of 1 mole of substrate into 1 mole of product per second (1 kat = 1 mol/s). Because the katal is generally a very small number, the much larger international unit is more commonly used as the standard unit of activity.

The specific activity of an enzyme, a measure of activity per amount of protein, is expressed as μmol/min/mg of protein or IU/mg of protein. The specific activity of enzymes varies greatly among tissues, depending on the metabolic function of the tissue. The enzymes for cholesterol synthesis, for example, have a higher specific activity (IU/mg tissue) in liver than in muscle, consistent with the role of liver in biosynthesis of cholesterol. The specific activity of an enzyme is useful for estimating its purity – the higher the specific activity of an enzyme, the higher its purity or homogeneity.

Reaction specificity and substrate specificity are determined by the structure of the active site

Most enzymes are highly specific for both the type of reaction catalyzed and the nature of the substrate(s). Reaction specificity, i.e. the reaction that the enzyme catalyzes, is determined chemically by the amino acid residues in the catalytic center of the enzyme. In general, the active site of the enzyme is composed of the substrate binding site and the catalytic site. Substrate specificity is determined by the size, structure, charges, polarity, and hydrophobicity of the substrate binding site. This is because the substrate must bind in the active site as the first step in the reaction, setting the stage for catalysis. Highly specific enzymes such as catalase and urease, which degrade H_2O_2 and urea respectively, catalyze only one specific chemical reaction, but some enzymes have broader substrate specificity. The serine proteases are a typical example of such a group of enzymes. These are a family of closely related enzymes, such as the pancreatic enzymes, chymotrypsin, trypsin, and elastase, which contain a reactive serine residue in the catalytic site. They catalyze the hydrolysis of peptide bonds on the carboxyl side of a limited range of amino acids in protein. Although they have similar structures and catalytic mechanisms, their substrate specificities are quite different because of structural features of the substrate binding site (Fig. 6.2).

Isozymes are enzymes that catalyze the same reaction, but differ in their primary structure and/or subunit composition. Levels of some tissue-specific enzymes and isozymes are measured in serum for diagnostic purposes (Fig. 6.3 and Table 6.1).

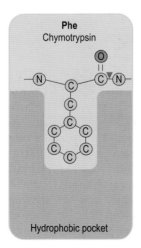
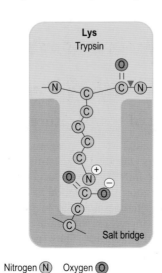
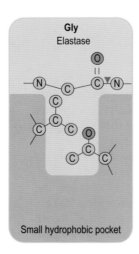

Fig. 6.2 **Characteristics of the substrate-binding sites in the serine proteases chymotrypsin, trypsin, and elastase.** In chymotrypsin a hydrophobic pocket binds aromatic amino acid residues such as phenylalanine (Phe). In trypsin, the negative charge of the aspartate residue in the substrate binding site promotes cleavage to the carboxyl side of positively charged lysine (Lys) and arginine (Arg) residues. In elastase, side chains of valine and threonine block the substrate binding site and permit binding of amino acids with small or no side chains, such as glycine (Gly).

Cleavage site → Carbon Ⓒ Nitrogen Ⓝ Oxygen Ⓞ

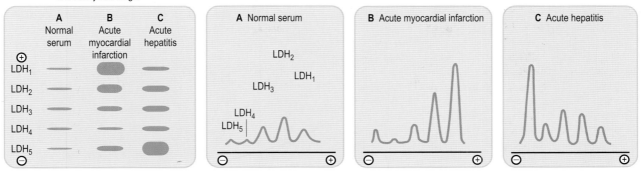

Electrophoretic analysis of LDH isozymes on gel

Fig. 6.3 **Densitometric patterns of the LDH isozymes in serum of patients diagnosed with myocardial infarction or acute hepatitis.** Isozymes, differing slightly in charge, are separated by electrophoresis on cellulose acetate, visualized using a chromogenic substrate, and quantified by densitometry. Total serum LDH activity is also increased in these patients. Since hemolysis releases LDH from red blood cells and affects diagnosis, blood samples should be treated with care. The LDH measurements for the diagnosis of myocardial infarction have now been superseded by assay of plasma troponin levels.

Some enzymes used for clinical diagnosis of disease

Enzyme	Tissue source(s)	Diagnostic use
AST	heart, skeletal muscle, liver, brain	liver disease
ALT	liver	liver disease, e.g hepatitis (ALT > AST)
amylase	pancreas, salivary gland	acute pancreatitis, biliary obstruction
CK	skeletal muscle, heart, brain	muscular dystrophy, myocardial infarction
GGT	liver	hepatitis, cirrhosis
LDH	heart, liver erythrocytes	lymphoma, hepatitis
lipase	pancreas	acute pancreatitis, biliary obstruction
alkaline phosphatase	osteoblast	bone disease, bone tumors
acid phosphatase	prostate	prostate cancer

AST, aspartate aminotransferase; ALT, alanine aminotransferase; CK, creatine phosphokinase; GGT, γ glutamyl transferase; LDH, lactate dehydrogenase.

Table 6.1 **Some enzymes used for clinical diagnosis of disease.**

Nomenclature of enzymes

A systematic classification is required to organize the different enzymes that catalyze the many thousands of reactions that take place in our body. All enzymes are assigned

Enzyme classification

Class	Reaction	Enzymes
1. Oxidoreductases	$A_{red} + B_{ox} \rightarrow A_{ox} + B_{red}$	dehydrogenases, peroxidases
2. Transferases	$A—B + C \rightarrow A + B—C$	hexokinase, transaminases
3. Hydrolases	$A—B + H_2O \rightarrow$ $A—H + B—OH$	alkaline phosphatase, trypsin
4. Lyases (synthases)	$A(XH)—B \rightarrow$ $A—X + B—H$	carbonic anhydrase, dehydratases
5. Isomerases	$A \rightleftharpoons ISO—A$	triose phosphate isomerase, phosphoglucomutase
6. Ligases (synthetases)	$A + B + ATP \rightarrow$ $A—B + ADP + Pi$	pyruvate carboxylase, DNA ligases

Table 6.2 **Enzyme classification.** Major classes of enzymes.

a four-digit enzyme classification (EC) number. The first digit indicates membership of one of the six major classes of enzymes shown in Table 6.2. The next two digits indicate substrate subclasses and sub-subclasses; the fourth digit indicates the serial number of the specific enzyme. The transfer of reducing equivalents from one redox system to another is catalyzed by the oxidoreductases (Class 1). The transfer of other functional groups from one substrate to another is catalyzed by the transferases (Class 2). The hydrolases (Class 3) catalyze group transfer, but the acceptor molecule is exclusively a water molecule. Reactions involving the addition or removal of H_2O, NH_3, or CO_2 are catalyzed by lyases (Class 4), also called synthases. Isomerases (Class 5) catalyze

TISSUE SPECIFICITY OF LACTATE DEHYDROGENASE ISOZYMES

A 56-year-old female was admitted to an intensive care unit. The patient had suffered from a slight fever for 1 week, and had some chest pain, and difficulty breathing for the past 24 h. No abnormality was found on chest X-ray or by electrocardiography. However, a blood test showed white blood cells 12 100/mm^3 (normal: 4000–9000/mm^3), red blood cells 240 × 10^4/mm^3, hemoglobin 8.6 g/dL, lactate dehydrogenase (LDH) 1400 IU/L (normal: 200–400 IU/L). Levels of other enzymes were normal. Based on the blood tests, the LDH isozyme profile and other data, the patient was eventually diagnosed with malignant lymphoma.

Comment. LDH is a tetrameric enzyme, composed of two different 35 kDa subunits. The heart contains mainly the H type, and skeletal muscle and the liver the M type subunit, which are encoded by different genes. Five types of tetrameric isozymes can be formed from these subunits: H$_4$ (LDH$_1$), H$_3$M$_1$ (LDH$_2$), H$_2$M$_2$ (LDH$_3$), H$_1$M$_3$ (LDH$_4$), and M$_4$ (LDH$_5$). Since isozyme distributions differ among tissues, it is possible to diagnose tissue damage by assaying total LDH activity and then by isozyme profiling (Fig. 6.3).

 ### PROPORTION OF ENZYME GENES IN WHOLE HUMAN GENOME

About a quarter of genes encode enzymes. Names of enzyme groups with number and proportion (percentage in parenthesis) in a total of 26 383 human genes were as follows: transferase, 610 (2.0); synthase and synthetase, 313 (1.0); oxidoreductase, 656 (2.1); lyase, 117 (0.4); ligase, 56 (0.2); isomerase, 163 (0.5); hydrolase, 1227 (4.0); kinase, 868 (2.8); nucleic acid enzyme, 2308 (7.5). Original data (Venter *et al.* *Science* 2001;**291**:1335) are quoted here, and so classification does not exactly match the nomenclature in Table 6.2.

 ### ISOZYMES

Isozyme profiles are often performed in the clinical laboratory for diagnostic purposes (see Fig. 6.3). The definition of isozymes is often operational, i.e. based on simple and reproducible assay methods that sometimes do not require precise analysis of enzyme structure. The term isozyme is commonly used to refer to: (1) genetic variants of an enzyme; (2) genetically independent proteins with little homology; (3) heteropolymers of two or more noncovalently bound polypeptide chains; (4) unrelated enzymes that catalyze similar reactions, e.g. enzymes conjugated with different prosthetic groups or requiring different coenzymes or cofactors; (5) different forms of a single polypeptide chain, e.g. varying in carbohydrate composition, deamination of amino acids, or proteolytic modification.

isomerization reactions by rearranging atoms within a molecule, and thus do not affect the atomic composition of the substrate. Ligases, also called synthetases (Class 6), use ATP to catalyze energy-dependent synthetic reactions. In general, enzymes are cited by their common name, such as bovine pancreatic ribonuclease, but EC designations are essential for some purposes, e.g. for access information in protein data banks (Chapter 2) and for research on structure–function relationships.

Roles of coenzymes

Helper molecules referred to as coenzymes play an essential part in enzyme-catalyzed reactions. Enzymes with covalently or noncovalently bound coenzymes are referred to as holoenzymes. A holoenzyme without a coenzyme is termed an apoenzyme. Coenzymes are divided into two categories. Soluble coenzymes bind reversibly to the protein moiety of the enzyme. They are often modified during the enzymatic reaction, then dissociate from the enzyme and are recycled by another enzyme; oxidoreductases, discussed in Chapter 9, have coenzymes that may be oxidized by one enzyme, then reduced and recycled by another. Coenzymes, such as coenzyme A, assist in the transport of intermediates from one enzyme to another during a sequence of reactions. Most coenzymes are vitamin derivatives. Derivatives of the B vitamins, niacin and riboflavin, act as coenzymes for

oxidoreductase reactions. The structure and function of coenzymes will be described in later chapters. Prosthetic groups are tightly bound, often covalently linked, to an enzyme and remain associated with the enzyme during the entire catalytic cycle. Some enzymes require inorganic (metal) ions, frequently termed cofactors, for their activity, e.g. blood-clotting enzymes that require Ca^{2+} and oxidoreductases, which use iron, copper, and manganese.

ENZYME KINETICS

The Michaelis–Menten equation: a simple model of an enzymatic reaction

Enzyme reactions are multistep in nature and comprise several partial reactions. In 1913, long before the structure of proteins was known, Michaelis and Menten developed a simple model for examining the kinetics of enzyme-catalyzed reactions (Fig. 6.4). The Michaelis–Menten model assumes that the substrate S binds to the enzyme E, forming an essential

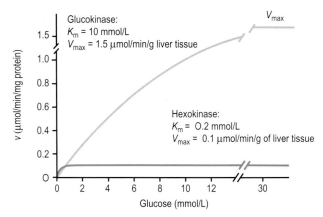

Fig. 6.4 **Properties of glucokinase and hexokinase.** Glucokinase and hexokinase catalyze the same reaction, phosphorylation of glucose to glucose 6-phosphate (Glc-6-P). They exhibit different kinetic properties and have different tissue distributions and physiologic functions.

intermediate, the enzyme-substrate complex (ES), which then undergoes reaction on the enzyme surface and decomposes to E+ product (P). The model assumes that E, S, and ES are all in rapid equilibrium with one another, so that a steady-state concentration of ES is rapidly achieved, and that decomposition of the ES complex to E + P is the rate-limiting step in catalysis.

The catalytic constant, k_{cat}, also known as the turnover number, is a rate constant which describes how quickly an enzyme can catalyze a reaction. The k_{cat} is defined as the number of substrate molecules that can be converted per enzyme molecule per unit time. The proportion of ES, in relation to the total number of enzyme molecules $[E]_t$, i.e. the ratio $[ES]/[E]_t$, limits the velocity of an enzyme (v) so that:

$$v = k_{cat}[ES]$$

Since E, S, and ES are all in chemical equilibrium, the enzyme achieves maximal velocity, V_{max}, at very high (saturating) substrate concentrations [S], when $[ES] \approx [E]_t$. Thus:

$$V_{max} = k_{cat}[E]_t$$

For the dissociation of the ES complex, the law of mass action yields:

$$K_d = \frac{[E][S]}{[ES]}$$

Given that:

$$[E]_t = [E] + [ES]$$

it can be shown that:

$$\frac{[ES]}{[E]_t} = \frac{[S]}{(K_m + [S])}, \text{ where } K_m = K_d$$

Consequently, v is given by:

$$v = \frac{(k_{cat}[E]_t[S])}{(k_m + [S])}$$

Since $k_{cat}[E]_t$ corresponds to the maximum velocity, V_{max}, that is attained at high (saturating) substrate concentrations, we obtain the Michaelis–Menten equation:

$$v = \frac{(V_{max}[S])}{(K_m + [S])}$$

Analysis of the above equations indicates that the Michaelis constant, K_m, is expressed in units of concentration and corresponds to the substrate concentration at which v is 50% of the maximum velocity, i.e. $[ES] = \frac{1}{2}[E]_t$ and $v = V_{max}/2$.

The Michaelis–Menten model is based on the assumptions that:

- E, S, and ES are in rapid equilibrium
- there are no forms of the enzyme present other than E and ES
- the conversion of ES into E + P is a rate-limiting, irreversible step. While all enzyme catalyzed reactions are theoretically reversible, initial velocities are normally measured, i.e. when product concentration, and therefore the reverse reaction, is negligible.

ISOZYMES: GLUCOKINASE AND HEXOKINASE

Hexokinase catalyzes the first step in glucose metabolism in all cells, namely the phosphorylation reaction of glucose by adenosine triphosphate (ATP) to form glucose 6-phosphate (Glc-6-P):

glucose + ATP → glucose 6-phosphate + ADP

This enzyme has a low K_m for glucose (0.2 mmol/L) and is inhibited allosterically by its product, Glc-6-P. Since normal glucose levels in blood are about 5 mmol/L and intracellular levels are 0.2–2 mmol/L, hexokinase efficiently catalyzes this reaction (50–90% of V_{max}) under normal conditions, e.g. in muscle.

Hepatocytes, which store glucose as glycogen, and pancreatic β-cells, which regulate glucose consumption in tissues and its storage in liver by secreting insulin, contain an isozyme called glucokinase. Glucokinase catalyzes the same reaction as hexokinase, but has a higher K_m for glucose (10 mmol/L) and is not inhibited by the product, Glc-6-P. Since glucokinase has a much higher K_m than hexokinase, glucokinase phosphorylates glucose with increasing efficiency as blood glucose levels increase following a meal (see Fig. 6.4). One of the physiologic roles of glucokinase in the liver is to provide Glc-6-P for the synthesis of glycogen, a storage form of glucose. In the pancreatic β-cell, glucokinase functions as the glucose sensor, determining the threshold for insulin secretion. Mice lacking glucokinase in the pancreatic β-cell die within 3 days of birth of profound hyperglycemia, because of failure to secrete insulin (see also Chapter 21).

Similar types of kinetic models have been developed for describing the kinetics of multisubstrate, multiproduct enzymes.

Use of the Lineweaver–Burk and Eadie–Hofstee plots for estimating K_m and V_{max}

In a plot of reaction rate versus substrate concentration, the rate of the reaction approaches the maximum velocity (V_{max}) asymptotically (Fig. 6.5A), so that it is difficult to obtain accurate values for V_{max} and, as a result, K_m (substrate concentration required for half-maximal activity), by simple extrapolation. To solve this problem, several linear transformations of the Michaelis–Menten equation have been developed.

Lineweaver–Burk plot

The Lineweaver–Burk, or double reciprocal, plot is obtained by taking the reciprocal of the steady-state Michaelis–Menten equation (Fig. 6.5B). By rearranging the equation, we obtain:

$$\frac{1}{v} = \left(\frac{1}{V_{max}}\right) + \left\{\left(\frac{k_m}{V_{max}}\right)\left(\frac{1}{[S]}\right)\right\}$$

This equation yields a straight line ($y = mx + b$), with $y = 1/v$, $x = 1/[S]$, m = slope, b = y intercept. Therefore, a graph of $1/v$ versus $1/[S]$ (Fig. 6.5B) has a slope of K_m/V_{max}, a $1/v$ intercept of $1/V_{max}$ and a $1/[S]$ intercept of $-1/K_m$. Although the Lineweaver–Burk plot is widely used for kinetic analysis of enzyme reactions, because reciprocals of the data are calculated, a small experimental error, especially at low substrate concentration, can result in a large error in the graphically determined values of K_m and V_{max}. An additional disadvantage is that important data obtained at high substrate concentrations are concentrated into a narrow region near the $1/v$ axis.

Eadie–Hofstee plot

A second, widely used linear form of the Michaelis–Menten equation is the Eadie–Hofstee plot (Fig. 6.5C). This is described by the equation:

$$v = V_{max} - \left(K_m \times \frac{v}{[S]}\right)$$

In this case, a plot of v versus $v/[S]$ has a y axis (v-intercept) of V_{max}, an x axis ($v/[S]$) intercept of V_{max}/K_m and a slope of $-K_m$. The Eadie–Hofstee plot does not compress the data at high substrate concentrations.

MECHANISM OF ENZYME ACTION

Enzymes vary significantly in their mechanism of action. In some cases catalysis is carried out on the bound substrate, without a stable covalent interaction between enzyme and

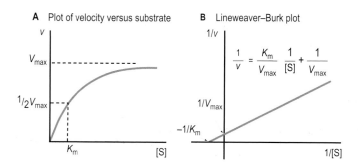

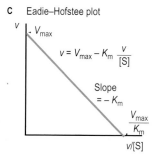

Fig. 6.5 **Enzyme kinetics plot.** Kinetic representations of the properties of enzymes. (A) Michaelis–Menten plot of velocity (v) versus substrate concentration ([S]). (B) Lineweaver–Burk plot. (C) Eadie–Hofstee plot.

substrate. In other cases, a covalent intermediate is formed on, and then released from, the enzyme and, in others, all the action takes place on a coenzyme which forms a covalent bond with substrate. The mechanisms of action of many enzymes are discussed in later chapters in this text.

The serine proteases, introduced in Figure 6.2, are representative of enzymes that form a covalent intermediate with their substrates. These enzymes cleave peptide bonds in proteins and, as in all enzymatic reactions, functional groups on amino acid side chains participate in the enzyme-catalyzed reaction. In the serine protease family, an active site serine residue catalyzes cleavage of the peptide bond. The functional group on serine, a primary alcohol, is not among the more reactive functional groups in organic chemistry. To enhance its activity in serine proteases, this serine residue is part of a 'catalytic triad', in the case of chymotrypsin: Asp^{102}, His^{57} and Ser^{195} (Fig. 6.6).

Concerted hydrogen bonding interactions between these amino acids increase the nucleophilicity of the serine residue, so that it can attack the carbonyl carbon atom of the peptide bond in the substrate. Chymotrypsin is specific for cleavage on the carboxyl side of peptide bonds containing aromatic amino acids, such as phenylalanine. The mechanism of the enzymatic reaction is outlined in Figure 6.7, showing the formation and cleavage of an enzyme bound intermediate.

Trypsin and elastase, two other digestive enzymes with different amino acid specificities, are similar to chymotrypsin in many respects. About 40% of the amino acid sequences of these three enzymes are identical, and their three-dimensional structures are very similar. All three enzymes contain the aspartate-histidine-serine catalytic triad, and are inactivated by reaction of fluorophosphates with the active serine residue. The nerve gas, diisopropylfluorophosphate, forms a sterically hindered, very slowly hydrolyzed serine-diisopropylphospate ester.

ENZYME INHIBITION

Enzymes may be inhibited in different ways

Among numerous substances affecting metabolic processes, enzyme inhibitors are particularly important. Many drugs, either naturally occurring or synthetic, act as enzyme inhibitors. Metabolites of these compounds may also inhibit enzyme activity. Most enzyme inhibitors act reversibly, but there are also irreversible inhibitors that permanently modify the target enzyme. Using the Lineweaver–Burk plots, it is possible to distinguish three forms of reversible inhibition: competitive, uncompetitive, and noncompetitive inhibition.

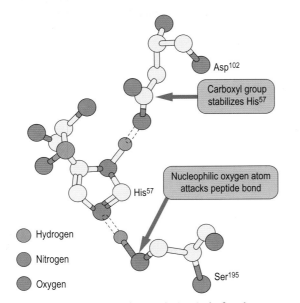

Fig. 6.6 **A schematic model of a catalytic triad of serine protease.**

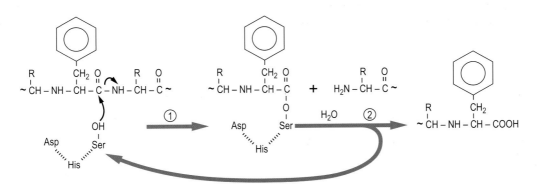

Fig. 6.7 **Mechanism of action of chymotrypsin.** The active site serine residue attacks the carbonyl group of the peptide bond on the carboxyl side of a phenylalanine residue. The carboxy-terminal peptide is released and the amino-terminal peptide remains an enzyme-bound intermediate – the amino-terminal peptide linked with its carboxy-terminal phenylalanine esterified to the active site serine residue. The ester bond is hydrolyzed in the second step of the reaction to release the amino-terminal peptide and regenerate active enzyme.

Competitive inhibitors cause an apparent increase in K_m, without changing V_{max}

An enzyme can be inhibited competitively by substances that are similar in chemical structure to the substrate. These compounds bind in the active site and compete with substrate for the active site of the enzyme; they cause an apparent increase in K_m, but no change in V_{max} (Fig. 6.8). The inhibition is not the result of an effect on enzyme activity, but on substrate access to the active site. The reaction scheme for competitive inhibition is:

$$E\begin{matrix}+S\rightleftharpoons ES\rightarrow E+P\\+\\{}^+I\rightleftharpoons EI\end{matrix}$$

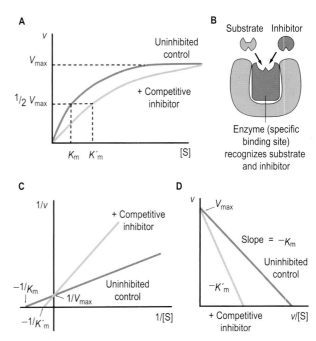

Fig. 6.8 **Competitive enzyme inhibition.** (A) Plot of velocity versus substrate concentration. (B) Mechanism of competitive inhibition. (C) Lineweaver–Burk plot in the presence of a competitive inhibitor. (D) Eadie–Hofstee plot in the presence of a competitive inhibitor. K'_m is the apparent K_m in presence of inhibitor.

 TREATMENT OF HYPERTENSION WITH AN INHIBITOR OF ANGIOTENSIN-CONVERTING ENZYME (ACE)

A 50-year-old man was admitted to hospital suffering from general fatigue, a stiff shoulder, and headache. The patient was 1.8 m tall and weighed 84 kg. His blood pressure was 196/98 mmHg (normal below 140/90 mmHg; optimal below 120/80 mmHg) and his pulse was 74. He was diagnosed as hypertensive. The patient was given captopril, an angiotensin-converting enzyme (ACE) inhibitor. After 5 days' treatment, his blood pressure returned to near-normal levels.

Comment. Renin in the kidney converts angiotensinogen into angiotensin I, which is then proteolytically cleaved to angiotensin II by ACE. Angiotensin II increases renal fluid and electrolyte retention, contributing to hypertension. Inhibition of ACE activity is therefore an important target for hypertension treatment. Captopril inhibits ACE competitively, decreasing blood pressure. (See also Chapter 23.)

 METHANOL POISONING CAN BE TREATED BY ETHANOL ADMINISTRATION

A 46-year-old male presented to the emergency room 7 h after consuming a large quantity of bootleg alcohol. He could not see clearly and complained of abdominal and back pain. Laboratory results indicated severe metabolic acidosis, a serum osmolality of 465 mmol/kg (reference range 285–295 mmol/kg), and serum methanol level of 4.93 g/L (156 mmol/L!). By aggressive treatment, including an ethanol drip, bicarbonate, and hemodialysis, he survived and regained his eyesight.

Comment. Methanol poisoning is uncommon but extremely hazardous. Ethylene glycol poisoning is more common and exhibits similar clinical characteristics. The most important initial symptom of methanol poisoning is visual disturbance. Laboratory evidence of methanol poisoning includes severe metabolic acidosis and increased plasma solute (methanol) concentration. Methanol is slowly metabolized to formaldehyde, which is then rapidly metabolized to formate by alcohol dehydrogenase. Formate accumulates during methanol intoxication and is responsible for the metabolic acidosis in the early stage of intoxication. In later stages, lactate may also accumulate as a result of formate inhibition of respiration. Ethanol is metabolized by alcohol dehydrogenase, which binds ethanol with much higher affinity than either methanol or ethylene glycol. Ethanol is therefore a useful agent to inhibit competitively the metabolism of methanol and ethylene glycol to toxic metabolites. The unmetabolized methanol and ethylene glycol are gradually excreted in urine. Early treatment with ethanol, together with alkali to combat acidosis and hemodialysis to remove methanol and its toxic metabolites, yields a good prognosis.

The inhibition constant (K_i) is the dissociation constant of the enzyme–inhibitor complex (EI) and the lower the K_i, the more efficient the inhibition of enzyme activity. Regardless of the K_i, however, the rate of the enzyme-catalyzed reaction in the presence of a competitive inhibitor can be increased by increasing the substrate concentration, since substrate, at higher concentration, competes more effectively with the inhibitor.

Both K_m and V_{max} decrease in uncompetitive inhibition

An uncompetitive inhibitor binds only to the enzyme–substrate complex and not to the free enzyme. The equation below shows the reaction scheme for uncompetitive inhibition. In this case, the K_i is the dissociation constant for the enzyme–substrate–inhibitor complex (ESI).

$$E + S \rightleftharpoons ES \underset{\searrow E+P}{\overset{+I \rightleftharpoons ESI}{}}$$

The inhibitor causes a decrease in V_{max} because a fraction of the enzyme–substrate complex is diverted by the inhibitor to the inactive ESI complex. Binding of the inhibitor and the increase in the ESI complex may also affect the dissociation of substrate, causing an apparent decrease in K_m, i.e. an apparent increase in substrate affinity.

V_{max} decreases in noncompetitive inhibition

A noncompetitive inhibitor can bind either to the free enzyme or to the enzyme–substrate complex. Thus, noncompetitive inhibition is more complex than other types of inhibition. The equation below shows the reaction scheme observed for noncompetitive inhibition.

$$
\begin{array}{ccc}
E & + S \rightleftharpoons ES & \rightarrow E + P \\
+ & & + \\
I & & I \\
\updownarrow & & \updownarrow \\
EI & & ESI
\end{array}
$$

Many drugs and poisons irreversibly inhibit enzymes

Prostaglandins are key inflammatory mediators. Their synthesis is initiated by cyclooxygenase-mediated oxidation and cyclization of arachidonate under inflammatory conditions (Chapter 40). Compounds that suppress cyclooxygenase have antiinflammatory activity. Aspirin (acetylsalicylic acid), one of the most popular drugs, inhibits cyclooxygenase activity by acetylating Ser[530], which blocks access of arachidonate to the active site of the enzyme. Other nonsteroidal antiinflammatory drugs (NSAIDs), such as indomethacin, inhibit

ENZYME INHIBITION: TRANSITION STATE INHIBITION AND SUICIDE SUBSTRATE

Enzymes catalyze reactions by inducing the transition state of the reaction. It should therefore be possible to construct molecules that bind very tightly to the enzyme by mimicking the transition state of the substrate. Transition states themselves cannot be isolated, because they are not a stable arrangement of atoms, and some bonds are only partially formed or broken. But for some enzymes, analogs can be synthesized that are stable, but still have some of the structural features of the transition state.

Penicillin (Fig. 6.9) is a good example of a transition state analog. It inhibits the transpeptidase that crosslinks bacterial cell wall peptidoglycan strands, the last step in cell wall synthesis in bacteria. It has a strained four-membered lactam ring that mimics the transition state of the normal substrate. When penicillin binds to the active site of the enzyme, its lactam ring opens, forming a covalent bond with a serine residue at the active site. Penicillin is a potent irreversible inhibitor of bacterial cell wall synthesis, making the bacterium osmotically fragile and unable to survive in the body.

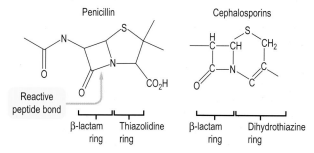

Fig. 6.9 **Structure of penicillin showing the reactive peptide bond in the β-lactam ring and core structure of cephalosporins.** Penicillins contain β-lactam ring in conjunction with thiazolidine ring. Cephalosporins are another class of compounds containing the β-lactam ring fused to a six-membered dihydrothiazine ring. Because of their effectiveness and lack of toxicity, β-lactam compounds are widely used antibiotics. Bacteria with β-lactamase, which breaks the β-lactam ring, are resistant to these antibiotics.

cyclooxygenase activity by reversibly blocking the arachidonate binding site.

Disulfiram (Antabuse®) is a drug used for the treatment of alcoholism. Alcohol is metabolized in two steps to acetic acid. The first enzyme, alcohol dehydrogenase, yields acetaldehyde, which is then converted into acetic acid by aldehyde dehydrogenase. The latter enzyme has an active site cysteine residue that is irreversibly modified by disulfiram, resulting in accumulation of alcohol and acetaldehyde in the blood. People who take disulfiram become sick because of the accumulation of acetaldehyde in blood and tissues, leading to alcohol avoidance.

Alkylating reagents, such as iodoacetamide (ICH_2CONH_2), irreversibly inhibit the catalytic activity of some enzymes by modifying essential cysteine residues. Heavy metals, such as mercury and lead salts, also inhibit enzymes with active site sulfhydryl residues. The mercury adducts are often reversible by thiol compounds. Eggs or egg-white are sometimes administered as an antidote for accidental ingestion of heavy metals; the egg white protein, ovalbumin, is rich in sulfhydryl groups, traps the free metal ions and prevents their absorption from the gastrointestinal tract.

In many cases, irreversible inhibitors are used to identify active-site residues involved in enzyme catalysis and to gain insight into the mechanism of enzyme action. By sequencing or mass spectrometric analysis of the modified peptide, it is possible to identify the specific amino acid residue modified by the inhibitor and involved in catalysis.

REGULATION OF ENZYME ACTIVITY

In multistep metabolic pathways, the slowest step limits the overall rate of the reaction. It is therefore most efficient to regulate the metabolic pathway by controlling key enzymes that are involved in this 'rate-limiting' step. Generally, five independent mechanisms are involved in the regulation of enzyme activity.

■ The expression of the enzyme protein from the corresponding gene changes in response to the cell's changing environment or metabolic demands.

■ Enzymes may be irreversibly activated or inactivated by proteolytic enzymes.

■ Enzymes may be reversibly activated or inactivated by covalent modification, such as phosphorylation.

■ Allosteric regulation modulates the activity of key enzymes through reversible binding of small molecules at sites distinct from the active site in a process that is relatively rapid and, hence, the first response of cells to changing conditions.

■ The degradation of enzymes by intracellular proteases in the lysosome or by proteasomes in the cytosol also determines the lifetimes of the enzymes and consequently enzyme activity over a much longer period of time.

Proteolytic activation of digestive enzymes

Some enzymes are stored in a specific organelle or compartment, such as exocytotic vesicles in cells, in inactive precursor forms termed proenzymes or zymogens. Several digestive enzymes are stored as inactive zymogens in the pancreas. The zymogens are secreted in pancreatic juice following a meal and are activated in the gastrointestinal tract; trypsinogen is converted into trypsin by the action of intestinal enteropeptidase. Enteropeptidase, located on the inner surface of the duodenum, hydrolyzes an *N*-terminal peptide from the inactive trypsinogen. Rearrangement of the tertiary structure yields

the proteolytically active form of trypsin. The active trypsin then digests other zymogens, such as procarboxypeptidase, proelastase and chymotrypsinogen, as well as other trypsinogen molecules (Chapter 10). Similar proteolytic cascades are observed during blood clotting and fibrinolysis (dissolution of clots) (Chapter 7).

Since the pancreas is an important organ for controlling blood glucose, the unregulated activation of these enzymes would cause inflammation and destruction of the pancreas (pancreatitis), possibly leading to destruction of β-cells and development of diabetes.

Allosteric regulation of rate-limiting enzymes in metabolic pathways

The substrate saturation curve for an 'isosteric' (single shape) enzyme is hyperbolic (see Fig. 6.5A). In contrast, allosteric enzymes show sigmoidal plots of reaction velocity versus substrate concentration [S] (Fig. 6.10). An allosteric effector molecule binds to the enzyme at a site that is distinct and physically separate from the substrate-binding site, and affects substrate binding (K_m) and/or k_{cat}. In some cases, the substrate may exert allosteric effects; this is referred to as a homotropic effect. If the allosteric effector is different from the substrate, it is referred to as a heterotropic effect. Homotropic effects are observed when the reaction of one substrate molecule with a multimeric enzyme affects the binding of a second substrate molecule at a different active site on the enzyme. The interaction between subunits makes the binding of substrate cooperative and results in a sigmoidal curve in the plot of *v* versus [S]. This effect is essentially identical with that described for the binding of O_2 to hemoglobin

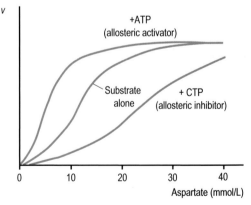

Fig. 6.10 **Allosteric regulation of ATCase.** Plot of velocity (*v*) versus substrate concentration in the presence of an allosteric activator or allosteric inhibitor. Aspartate transcarbamoylase (ATCase) is an example of an allosteric enzyme. Aspartate (substrate) homotropically regulates ATCase activity, providing sigmoidal kinetics. CTP, an endproduct, heterotropically inhibits, but ATP, a precursor, heterotropically activates ATCase. This enzyme is described in more detail in Chapter 30 (compare Fig. 5.7).

HEMOPHILIA IS CAUSED BY A DEFECT IN ZYMOGEN ACTIVATION

A child was admitted to hospital with muscle bleeding affecting the femoral nerve. Laboratory findings indicated a blood-clotting disorder, hemophilia A, resulting from deficiency of Factor VIII. Factor VIII was administered to the patient to restore blood-clotting activity.

Comment. Formation of a blood clot results from a cascade of zymogen-activation reactions. Over a dozen different proteins, known as blood-clotting factors, are involved. In the final step, the blood clot is formed by conversion of a soluble protein, fibrinogen (Factor I), into an insoluble, fibrous product, fibrin, which forms the matrix of the clot. This last step is catalyzed by the serine protease, thrombin (Factor IIa). Hemophilia is a disorder of blood clotting caused by a defect in one of the sequence of clotting factors. Hemophilia A, the major (85%) form of hemophilia, is caused by a defect of clotting Factor VIII (see Chapter 7).

NUCLEOSIDE ANALOGS ARE USED AS ANTIVIRAL AGENTS

Nucleoside analogs such as acyclovir and ganciclovir have been used for treatment of herpes simplex virus (HSV), varicella-zoster (VZV), and cytomegalovirus (CMV). They are prodrugs that are activated by phosphorylation and terminate viral DNA synthesis by inhibiting the viral DNA polymerase reaction. The thymidine kinase (TK), more properly a nucleoside kinase, of the viruses phosphorylate these compounds to their monophosphate form. Cellular kinases next add phosphates to form the active triphosphate compounds, which are competitive inhibitors of the viral DNA polymerase during DNA replication (Chapter 31). While viral TK has low substrate specificity and efficiently phosphorylates nucleoside analogs, cellular nucleoside kinases have high substrate specificity and barely phosphorylate the nucleoside analogs. Thus, virus-infected cells are prone to be arrested at a specific cell cycle stage, G_2-M checkpoint (Chapter 43), but uninfected cells are resistant to the nucleoside analogs.

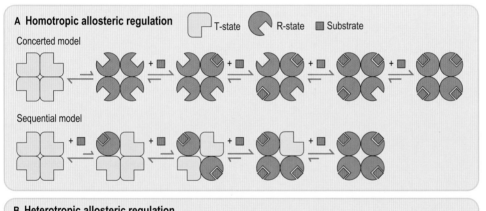

Fig. 6.11 **Schematic representation of allosteric regulation.** (A) In homotropic regulation, the substrate acts as an allosteric effector. Two models are presented. In the concerted model, all of the subunits convert from the T (tense; low affinity for substrate)- into the R (relaxed; high affinity for substrate)- state at the same time; in the sequential model, they change one by one, with each substrate-binding reaction. (B) In heterotropic regulation, the effector is distinct from the substrate, and binds at a structurally different site on the enzyme. Positive and negative effectors stabilize the enzyme in R- and T-state, respectively.

(Chapter 5), except that in the case of enzymes, substrate binding leads to an enzyme-catalyzed reaction.

Positive and negative cooperativity

Positive cooperativity indicates that the reaction of a substrate with one active site makes it easier for another substrate to react at another active site. Negative cooperativity means that the reaction of a substrate with one active site makes it more difficult for a substrate to react at the other active site. Since the affinity of the enzyme changes with substrate concentration, it cannot be described by simple Michaelis–Menten kinetics. Instead, it is characterized by the substrate concentration giving a half-maximal rate, $[S]_{0.5}$, and the Hill coefficient (H) (Chapter 5). The H-values are larger than 1 for enzymes with positive cooperativity and less than 1 for those with negative cooperativity. For most allosteric enzymes, intracellular substrate concentrations are poised near the $[S]_{0.5}$, so that the enzyme's activity responds to slight changes in substrate concentration.

The model most often invoked to rationalize allosteric behavior was established by Monod, Wyman and Changeaux, the so-called concerted model (Fig. 6.11). As with O_2 binding to Hb, in the absence of substrate, the enzyme has a low affinity for substrate and is in the T-state (tense state). The

INSECTICIDE POISONING

A 55-year-old man was spraying an insecticide containing organic fluorophosphates in a rice field. He suddenly developed a frontal headache, eye pain, and tightness in his chest, typical signs of overexposure to toxic organic fluorophosphates. He was taken to hospital and treated with an intravenous injection of 2 mg of atropine sulfate, and gradually recovered.

Comment. Organic fluorophosphates form covalent phosphoryl-enzyme complexes with both serine proteases and esterases, such as acetylcholinesterase, irreversibly inhibiting the enzymes. Acetylcholinesterase terminates the action of acetylcholine during neuromuscular activity (Chapter 42) by hydrolyzing the acetylcholine to acetate and choline. Inhibition of this enzyme prolongs the action of acetylcholine, leading to constant neuromuscular stimulation. Atropine does not affect the activity of acetylcholinesterase, but competitively blocks acetylcholine binding and muscle stimulation at the neuromuscular junction.

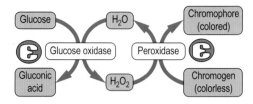

Fig. 6.12 **The glucose oxidase/peroxidase assay for blood glucose.** The color produced in this assay is directly proportional to blood glucose concentration.

enhancing assay sensitivity by ~50%. The H_2O_2 produced in the oxidase reaction is then used in a peroxidase reaction to oxidize a chromogen to yield a colored chromophore. The color yield is directly proportional to the glucose content of the sample. There are fluorometric versions of this assay for high sensitivity, and one commercial analyzer uses an oxygen electrode to measure the rate of decrease in oxygen concentration in the sample, which is also directly proportional to the glucose concentration.

Reagent strips and glucometers

People with diabetes normally monitor their blood glucose several times a day using reagent strips and glucose meters. The reagent strips are impregnated with a glucose oxidase-peroxidase (GOP) reagent. In the manual version of this assay, the extent of color change on a dipstick is related to glucose concentration – typically on a 1–4 scale. Modern glucometers use a small drop of blood (~1 μL) and amperometric electrodes to measure the current produced by the redox reaction catalyzed by glucose dehydrogenase (GDH), which oxidizes glucose to gluconic acid but reduces a coenzyme, rather than oxygen. These assays are commonly used where rapid or frequent measurements of blood glucose are required. When the GOP and GDH assays were compared at high altitude on a trek up Mount Kilimanjaro, the GOP assay, which depends on ambient oxygen, had a greater error. Both methods were less accurate at the low temperatures at high altitude.

other conformation of the enzyme is the R-state (relaxed state). Binding of allosteric effector molecules shifts the fraction of enzyme from one state to the other. While enzymes are shifted to the R-state by the binding of positive allosteric effector molecules, they are stabilized in the T-form by negative allosteric effector molecules. In this model, all the active sites in the R-state are the same and all have higher substrate affinity than in the T-state. Because the transition between the T- and R-states occurs at the same time for all subunits, this is called the concerted (two-state) model. An alternative model, the so-called sequential (multistate) model, was proposed by Koshland, Nèmethy and Filmer. It postulates that each subunit changes independently to a different conformation and that different subunits may have different affinities for substrate. It is now recognized that both models are applicable to different enzymes.

ENZYMATIC MEASUREMENT OF BLOOD GLUCOSE

The glucose-oxidase peroxidase assay

In the clinical laboratory today, plasma and urinary glucose are measured by automated enzymatic methods. The most common assay procedure uses a mixture of glucose oxidase and peroxidase (Fig. 6.12). Glucose oxidase is highly specific for glucose, but oxidizes only the β-anomer of the sugar, which represents ~64% of glucose in solution. The assay mixture is therefore supplemented with mutarotase, which rapidly catalyzes the interconversion of the anomers,

Kinetic assays

In the assay described in Figure 6.12 and plotted for several glucose concentrations in Figure 6.13A, the reaction is allowed to proceed to its endpoint, i.e. until all the glucose has been oxidized, then the color change is measured. The color yield is then plotted against a standard to determine blood glucose concentration (Fig. 6.13B). High-throughput kinetic analyzers estimate the glucose concentration in a sample by measuring the initial rate of the reaction. Analysis of the kinetic plots in Figure 6.13A, for example, indicates that both the endpoint and the rate of the glucose oxidase assay

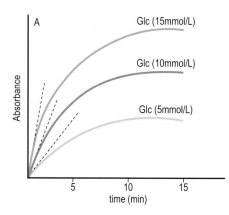

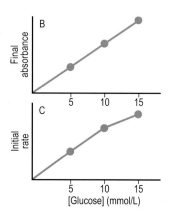

Fig. 6.13 **Glucose oxidase/peroxidase assays – endpoint versus kinetic assays.** (A) Graphical analysis of an endpoint assay. (B) The final (endpoint) absorbances are plotted as a function of glucose concentration, yielding a straight line. (C) Initial rates of reactions are estimated by multiple measurements early in the assay (dotted lines in frame A), and plotted versus glucose concentration. Nonlinear plots, when obtained, are analyzed by computer.

are dependent on glucose concentration. Thus, the analyzer can measure the change in absorbance (or some other parameter) during the early stages of the reaction and compare this rate to that of a standard solution to estimate the glucose concentration (Fig. 6.13C). These assays are performed on flow-injection or centrifugal analyzers to insure rapid mixing of reagents and sample. Kinetic analyzers are inherently faster than endpoint assays because they estimate glucose concentration before the assay reaches its endpoint. These assays work because glucose oxidase and glucose dehydrogenase have a high K_m for glucose. At the concentrations of glucose found in blood, the rate of the oxidase reaction is proportional to glucose concentration, i.e. in the first order region of the Michaelis–Menten equation where the substrate concentration is less than the K_m (see Fig. 6.5A).

Summary

Most metabolism is catalyzed by biological catalysts called enzymes. Their catalytic activities are apparent at body temperature, and they are strictly regulated by several mechanisms. Both covalent and noncovalent modifications are involved in this regulation and allow for efficient metabolic control. Enzyme activity can be inhibited (or activated) by synthetic compounds (drugs), exogenous compounds (toxins), and endogenous compounds (allosteric effectors). Kinetic analyses of enzymatic reaction are beneficial for evaluating the biological role of enzymes and for elucidating their reaction mechanisms. In addition, assays of enzymes in blood are useful for diagnosis of some diseases.

Further reading

Crusat M, de Jong M. Neuraminidase inhibitors and their role in avian and pandemic influenza. *Antivir Ther* 2007;**12**:593–602.

Lopez-Otin C, Matrisian LM. Emerging roles of proteases in tumour suppression. *Nat Rev Cancer* 2007;**7**:800–808.

Matchar DB, McCrory DC, Orlando LA et al. Systematic review: comparative effectiveness of angiotensin-converting enzyme inhibitors and angiotensin II receptor blockers for treating essential hypertension. *Ann Intern Med* 2008; **148**(1):16–29.

Nordlund P, Reichard P. Ribonucleotide reductases. *Annu Rev Biochem* 2006;**75**: 681–706.

Öberg D, Östenson C-G. Performance of glucose dehydrogenase-and glucose oxidase-based blood glucose meters at high altitude and low temperature. *Diabetes Care* 2005;**28**:1261.

Ryter SW, Alam J, Choi AM. Heme oxygenase-1/carbon monoxide: from basic science to therapeutic applications. *Physiol Rev* 2006;**86**:583–650.

Stancoven A, McGuire DK. Preventing macrovascular complications in type 2 diabetes mellitus: glucose control and beyond. *Am J Cardiol* 2007;**99**(11A): 5H–11H.

Witt H, Apte MV, Keim V, Wilson JS. Chronic pancreatitis: challenges and advances in pathogenesis, genetics, diagnosis, and therapy. *Gastroenterology* 2007;**132**: 1557–1573.

ACTIVE LEARNING

1. In a multistep sequence of enzymatic reactions, where is the most effective site for controlling the flux of substrate through the pathway? What effect will an inhibitor of a rate-limiting enzyme have on the concentration of substrates in a multistep pathway?
2. Most drugs are designed to inhibit specific enzymes in biologic systems. The drug Prozac has had a profound effect on the medical treatment of depression. Review the history of development of Prozac, illustrating the importance of specificity in the mechanism of drug action.
3. Discuss some examples of reversible and irreversible enzyme inhibitors used in medical practice.
4. Knock-out mice are mice that lack a specific gene. Discuss the impact of KO mice on the direction of drug development in the pharmaceutical industry.

Websites

Clinical Enzymology: www.labtestsonline.org/

International Federation of Clinical Chemistry and Laboratory Medicine: www. ifcc.org/

Enzymology news articles: www.newsrx.com/library/topics/Enzymology.html

Enzyme structures database: www.ebi.ac.uk/thornton-srv/databases/enzymes/

Chymotrypsin, mechanism of action: www.chembio.uoguelph.ca/educmat/ chm258/lecture12.pdf

Serine proteases: www.med.unibs.it/~marchesi/pps97/course/section12/ serprot1.html

Enzyme nomenclature: www.chem.qmul.ac.uk/iubmb/enzyme/

Enzyme classification: www.chem.qmul.ac.uk/iubmb/enzyme/rules.html

7. Hemostasis and Thrombosis

G Lowe

LEARNING OBJECTIVES

After reading this chapter you should be able to:

- Outline the sequential mechanisms involved in normal hemostasis.
- Summarize the processes through which the vessel wall regulates hemostasis and thrombosis.
- Describe the role of platelets in hemostasis and thrombosis.
- Outline pathways through which antiplatelet drugs act.
- Describe the pathways of blood coagulation, and how these are tested in the clinical hemostasis laboratory to identify coagulation disorders.
- Describe the physiologic inhibitors of blood coagulation.
- Outline pathways through which anticoagulant drugs act.
- Describe the main components of the fibrinolytic system.
- Describe how thrombolytic (fibrinolytic) drugs act.

INTRODUCTION

Circulation of the blood within the cardiovascular system is essential for transportation of gases, nutrients, minerals, metabolic products, and hormones between different organs. It is also essential that blood should not leak excessively from blood vessels when they are injured by the traumas of daily life. Animal evolution has therefore resulted in the development of an efficient but complex series of hemodynamic, cellular, and biochemical mechanisms that limit such blood loss by forming platelet-fibrin plugs at sites of vessel injury (hemostasis). Genetic disorders that result in loss of individual protein functions, and therefore in excessive bleeding (e.g. hemophilia), have played an important part in the identification of many of the biochemical mechanisms in hemostasis.

It is essential also that these hemostatic mechanisms are appropriately controlled by inhibitory mechanisms, otherwise an exaggerated platelet-fibrin plug may produce local occlusion of a major blood vessel (artery or vein) at its site of origin (thrombosis), or may break off and block a blood vessel downstream (embolism). Arterial thrombosis is the major cause of heart attacks, stroke, and nontraumatic limb amputations in developed countries. Venous thrombosis and embolism are also major causes of death and disability. Clinical use of antithrombotic drugs (antiplatelet, anticoagulant, and thrombolytic agents) is now widespread in developed countries, and requires an understanding of how they interfere with hemostatic mechanisms to exert their antithrombotic effects.

HEMOSTASIS

Hemostasis means 'the arrest of bleeding'

After tissue injury that ruptures smaller vessels (including everyday trauma, injections, surgical incisions, and tooth extractions), a series of interactions between the vessel wall and the circulating blood normally occurs, resulting in cessation of blood loss from injured vessels within a few minutes (hemostasis). Hemostasis results from effective sealing of the ruptured vessels by a hemostatic plug composed of blood platelets and fibrin. Fibrin is derived from circulating fibrinogen, whereas platelets are small cell fragments that circulate in the blood and have an important role in the initiation of hemostasis.

Hemostasis requires the effective, coordinated function of blood vessels, platelets, coagulation factors and the fibrinolytic system

Figure 7.1 provides an overview of hemostatic mechanisms and illustrates some of the interactions between blood vessels, platelets, and the coagulation system in hemostasis; each of these components of hemostasis also interacts with the fibrinolytic system. The initial response of small blood vessels to injury is arteriolar vasoconstriction, which temporarily reduces local blood flow. Flow reduction transiently reduces blood loss, and may also promote formation of the platelet-fibrin plug. Activation of blood platelets is followed by their adhesion to the vessel wall at the site of injury, and their subsequent aggregation to each other, building up an occlusive platelet mass that forms the initial (primary) hemostatic plug. This platelet plug is friable and, unless subsequently stabilized by fibrin, will be washed away by local blood pressure when vasoconstriction reverses.

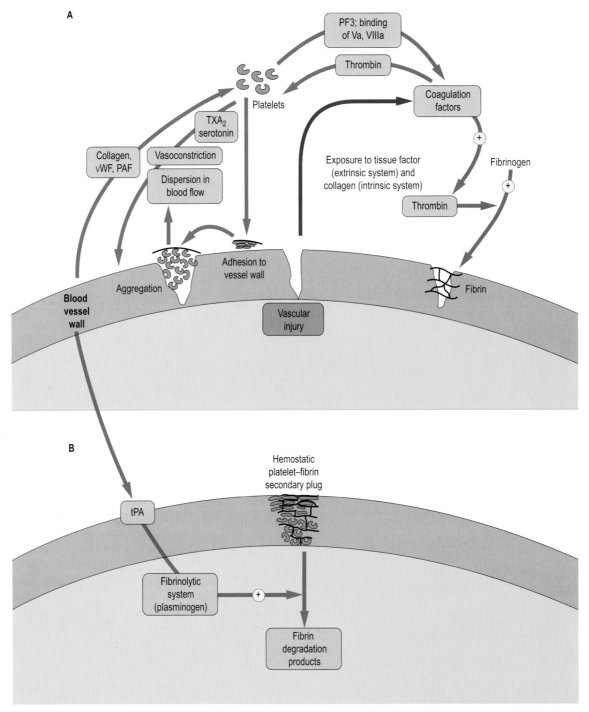

Fig. 7.1 **Overview of hemostatic mechanisms.** (A) Vascular injury sets in motion a series of events that culminate in formation of a primary plug of platelets. This can be dispersed by blood flowing through the vessel unless the plug is stabilized. (B) The primary plug is stabilized by a network of fibrin (formed from crosslinked fibrinogen). The secondary plug is stable and is degraded only when the fibrinolytic system has been activated. PAF, platelet activating factor; PF3, platelet factor 3; tPA, tissue-type plasminogen activator; TXA$_2$, thromboxane A$_2$; Va, activated coagulation factor V; VIIIa, activated coagulation factor VIII; vWF, von Willebrand factor.

Vascular injury also activates coagulation factors, which interact sequentially to form thrombin, which converts circulating soluble plasma fibrinogen to insoluble, crosslinked fibrin. This forms the subsequent (secondary) hemostatic plug, which is relatively resistant to dispersal by blood flow or fibrinolysis.

There are two pathways of the activation of coagulation factors: the extrinsic pathway which is initiated by the exposure of the flowing blood to tissue factor, released from subendothelial tissue; and the intrinsic pathway which has an important amplification role in generating thrombin and fibrin.

Causes of excessive bleeding		
	Congenital	Acquired
Vessel wall	disorders of collagen synthesis (Ehlers–Danlos syndrome)	vitamin C deficiency (scurvy) corticosteroid excess
Platelets	vWF deficiency (von Willebrand disease) platelet GPIb-IX deficiency (Bernard–Soulier syndrome) platelet GPIIb-IIIa deficiency (Glanzmann's thrombasthenia)	antiplatelet drugs (e.g. aspirin) defective formation of platelets excessive destruction of platelets
Coagulation	coagulation factor deficiencies (hemophilias): factor VIII factor IX factor XI fibrinogen etc.	vitamin K deficiency (factors II, VII, IX, X) oral anticoagulants (vitamin K antagonists, e.g. warfarin) liver disease disseminated intravascular coagulation (DIC)
Fibrinolysis	antiplasmin deficiency PAI-1 deficiency	fibrinolytic drugs (e.g. tPA, urokinase, streptokinase)

Table 7.1 **Congenital and acquired causes of excessive bleeding.** GPIb-IX, GPIIb-IIIa, glycoprotein receptors Ib-IX and IIb-IIIa; PAI-1, plasminogen activator inhibitor type 1

The lysis of fibrin is as important to health as its formation

Hemostasis is a continuous process throughout life, and would result in excessive fibrin formation and vascular occlusion if unchecked. Evolution has therefore produced a fibrinolytic system; this is activated by local fibrin formation, resulting in local generation of plasmin, an enzyme which digests fibrin plugs (in parallel with tissue repair processes), thus maintaining vascular patency. Digestion of fibrin results in generation of circulating fibrin degradation products (FDP). These are detectable in plasma of healthy individuals at low concentration, which illustrates that fibrin formation and lysis are continuing processes in health.

Excessive bleeding may result from defects in each of the components of hemostasis, which may be caused by disease (congenital or acquired) or by antithrombotic drugs (Table 7.1).

The vascular, platelet, coagulation and fibrinolytic components of hemostasis will now be discussed in turn.

THE VESSEL WALL

Vascular injury has a key role in initiating local formation of the platelet-fibrin plug and in its subsequent removal by the fibrinolytic system

All blood vessels are lined by a flat sheet of endothelial cells, which have important roles in the interchange of chemicals, cells, and microbes between the blood and the body tissues. Endothelial cells in the smallest blood vessels (capillaries) are supported by a thin layer of connective tissue, rich in collagen fibers, called the intima. In veins, a thin layer (the media) of contractile smooth muscle cells allows some venoconstriction: for example, superficial veins under the skin constrict in response to surface cooling. In arteries and arterioles, a well-developed muscle layer allows powerful vasoconstriction, including the vasoconstriction after local injury that forms part of the hemostatic response. Larger vessels also have a supportive connective tissue outer layer (the adventitia).

Normal endothelium has an antithrombotic surface

Intact normal endothelium does not initiate or support platelet adhesion or blood coagulation. Its surface is antithrombotic. This thrombo-resistance is partly due to endothelial production of two potent vasodilators and inhibitors of platelet function: prostacyclin (prostaglandin I_2, PG_{I2}) and nitric oxide, otherwise known as endothelium-derived relaxing factor (EDRF) (see box on p. 76).

The vasoconstriction that occurs after vascular injury is partly mediated by two platelet activation products: serotonin (5-hydroxytryptamine), and thromboxane A_2 (TXA_2), a product of platelet prostaglandin metabolism. In addition, after a vascular injury that disrupts the endothelial cell lining, flowing blood is exposed to subendothelial collagen, which activates the intrinsic pathway of blood coagulation. The endothelial cell damage also exposes flowing blood to subendothelial tissue factor, which activates the extrinsic pathway of blood coagulation (see Fig. 7.1).

PROSTACYCLIN AND NITRIC OXIDE

Exposure of flowing blood to collagen as a result of endothelial damage also stimulates platelet activation. Platelets bind to collagen via von Willebrand factor (vWF), which is released from the endothelial cells. vWF in turn binds both to collagen fibers and to platelets (via a platelet membrane glycoprotein receptor, GPIb-IX). Platelet-activating factor (PAF) from the vessel wall may also activate platelets in hemostasis (see Fig. 7.1; see also box on p. 29).

PROSTACYCLIN AND NITRIC OXIDE: BIOCHEMICAL MEDIATORS OF VASOCONSTRICTION AND VASODILATATION

The diameters of arteries and arterioles throughout the body continuously alter to regulate blood flow according to local and general metabolic and cardiovascular requirements. Control mechanisms include neurogenic (sympathetic/adrenergic; see Chapter 41) and myogenic pathways, and local biochemical mediators, including prostacyclin (PGI_2) and nitric oxide.

Prostacyclin is the major arachidonic acid metabolite formed by vascular cells. It is a potent vasodilator, and also a potent inhibitor of platelet aggregation. It has a short half-life in plasma (3 min).

Nitric oxide is also a potent vasodilator formed by vascular endothelial cells, also with a short half-life. It was initially termed endothelium-derived relaxing factor (EDRF). In common with that of prostacyclin, its generation by endothelial cells is enhanced by many compounds, and also by blood flow and shear stress. In the normal circulation, nitric oxide appears to have a key role in flow-mediated vasodilatation. It is synthesized by two distinct forms of endothelial nitric oxide synthase (eNOS): constitutive and inducible. Constitutive eNOS rapidly provides relatively small amounts of nitric oxide for short periods, related to vascular flow regulation. The beneficial effects of nitrate drugs in hypertension and angina may partly reflect their effects on this pathway (see Chapter 18). Inducible eNOS is stimulated by cytokines in inflammatory reactions, and releases large amounts of nitric oxide for long periods. Its suppression by glucocorticoids may partly account for their anti-inflammatory effects.

Both prostacyclin and nitric oxide appear to exert their vasodilator actions by diffusing locally from endothelial cells to vascular smooth muscle cells, where they stimulate guanylate cyclase, resulting in increased formation of cyclic guanosine 3′,5′-monophosphate (cGMP) and relaxation of vascular smooth muscle via alteration of the intracellular calcium concentration (see Chapter 40).

Thromboxane A$_2$ and aspirin

It has already been noted that PGI_2, the major arachidonic acid metabolite formed by vascular cells, is a potent vasodilator and inhibitor of platelet aggregation. In contrast, the major arachidonic acid metabolite formed by platelets is thromboxane A_2 (TXA_2), which is a potent vasoconstrictor and stimulates platelet aggregation. In common with prostacyclin, TXA_2 has a short half-life. In the late 1970s, Salvador Moncada and John Vane contrasted the effects of PGI_2 and TXA_2 on blood vessels and platelets, and hypothesized that a balance between these two compounds was important in the regulation of hemostasis and thrombosis.

Congenital deficiencies of cyclooxygenase or thromboxane synthase (the enzymes involved in TXA_2 synthesis) result in a mild bleeding tendency. Ingestion of even low doses of acetylsalicylic acid (aspirin) irreversibly acetylates cyclooxygenase and suppresses TXA_2 synthesis and platelet aggregation for several days, resulting in an antithrombotic effect and a mild bleeding tendency. Bleeding is especially likely from the stomach, as a result of the formation of stomach ulcers secondary to the inhibition of cytoprotective gastric mucosal prostaglandins by aspirin. Although in persons at high risk of arterial thrombosis (e.g. previous myocardial infarction or stroke) this bleeding tendency is outweighed by a reduction in risk of thrombosis, aspirin is contraindicated in individuals with a history of bleeding disorders, or existing stomach or duodenal ulcers.

Collagen has a key role in the structure and hemostatic function of small blood vessels

Because collagen has a key role in the structure and hemostatic function of small blood vessels, vascular causes of excessive bleeding include congenital or acquired deficiencies of collagen synthesis (see Table 7.1). Congenital disorders include the rare Ehlers–Danlos syndrome. Acquired disorders include the relatively common vitamin C deficiency, scurvy (see Chapter 11), and excessive exogenous or endogenous corticosteroids.

PLATELETS

Blood platelets form the initial hemostatic plug in small vessels, and the initial thrombus in arteries and veins.

Platelets are circulating, anuclear microcells of mean diameter 2–3 mm. They are fragments of bone marrow megakaryocytes, and circulate for about 10 days in the blood. The concentration of platelets in normal blood is $150 - 400 \times 10^9/L$ ($150 - 400 \times 10^3/mm^3$).

Platelet-related bleeding disorders

Congenital defects in platelet adhesion/aggregation can cause lifelong excessive bleeding

A simple screening test – measurement of the skin bleeding time (normal range, 2–10 minutes) – is sufficient to detect congenital defects of platelet adhesion/aggregation, in which the time is characteristically prolonged. The most common such defect is von Willebrand disease (see Table 7.1), a group of autosomal dominant disorders that result in low plasma concentrations of vWF multimers. These multimers are composed of subunits (molecular weight 250 kDa) that

PLATELET ACTIVATION EXPOSES GLYCOPROTEIN RECEPTORS

Platelets can be activated by several chemical agents, including adenosine diphosphate (ADP, released by platelets, erythrocytes, and endothelial cells), epinephrine, collagen, thrombin, and PAF; by immune complexes (generated during infections); and by high physical shear stresses (shear stress is the tangential force applied to the cells by the flow of blood). Most of the chemical agents appear to act by binding to specific receptors on the platelet surface membrane. After receptor stimulation, several pathways of platelet activation can be initiated, resulting in several phenomena:

■ **change in platelet shape** from a disk to a sphere with extended pseudopodia, which facilitates aggregation and coagulant activity
■ **release of several compounds involved in hemostasis** from intracellular granules, for example ADP, serotonin, TXA_2, and vWF
■ **aggregation**, via exposure of GPIb-IX membrane receptor and linking by vWF (under high shear conditions), and via exposure of another membrane glycoprotein receptor, GPIIa-IIIb, and linking by fibrinogen (under low shear conditions)
■ **adhesion to the vessel wall** via exposure of the GPIb-IX membrane receptor, through which vWF binds platelets to subendothelial collagen.

Finally, stimulation of the platelet membrane receptor triggers the activation of platelet membrane phospholipases, which hydrolyze membrane phospholipids, releasing arachidonic acid. Arachidonic acid is metabolized by cyclooxygenase and thromboxane synthase to TXA_2, a potent but labile (half-life 30 sec) mediator of platelet activation and vasoconstriction.

PLATELET MEMBRANE RECEPTORS AND THEIR LIGANDS vWF AND FIBRINOGEN

Platelets have a key role in hemostasis and thrombosis, through adhesion to the vessel wall and subsequent aggregation to form a platelet-rich hemostatic plug or thrombus. These processes involve exposure of specific membrane glycoprotein receptors after platelet activation by several compounds.

Platelet receptor GPIb-IX plays a key part in the adhesion of platelets to subendothelium. It binds vWF, which also interacts with specific subendothelial receptors, including those on subendothelial collagen. Congenital deficiencies of GPIb-IX (Bernard–Soulier syndrome) or, more commonly, of vWF result in a bleeding tendency. In contrast, high plasma concentrations of vWF are associated with increased risk of thrombosis. For patients at high risk of thrombosis, therapeutic strategies directed against vWF (for example, anti-vWF antibodies) are currently being developed, to reduce the thrombotic risk.

Another receptor, GPIIb-IIIa, has a key role in platelet aggregation. After platelet activation, hundreds of thousands of GPIIb-IIIa receptors can be exposed in a single platelet. These receptors interact with fibrinogen or vWF, which bind platelets together, forming a hemostatic or thrombotic plug. Congenital deficiency of GPIIb-IIIa (the rare Glanzmann's thrombasthenia) causes a severe bleeding disorder; in contrast, deficiencies of either fibrinogen or vWF cause a milder bleeding disorder, because these two ligands can substitute for each other. High plasma concentrations of fibrinogen are associated with increased risk of thrombosis, partly because of its platelet-binding activity. For patients at high risk of thrombosis, inhibitors of the GPIIb-IIIa receptor (such as antireceptor antibodies) are being developed and are proving to be clinically effective.

are released from endothelial cells (and platelet granules) and circulate in plasma at a concentration of 1 mg/dL. Not only does vWF have an important role in platelet hemostatic function but it also transports coagulation factor VIII (antihemophilic factor) in the circulation and delivers it to sites of vascular injury. Hence, plasma concentrations of factor VIII may also be low in von Willebrand disease. Treatment of this disease is to increase the low plasma vWF activity, usually by means of desmopressin (a synthetic analog of vasopressin (see Chapter 23) which releases vWF from endothelial cells into plasma). Sometimes this is done using concentrates of VWF.

Less common congenital bleeding disorders include GPIb-IX deficiency (Bernard–Soulier syndrome), GPIIb-IIIa deficiency (Glanzmann's thrombasthenia), and fibrinogen deficiency (because fibrinogen bridges GPIIb-IIIa receptors of adjacent platelets).

Acquired disorders of platelets include a low platelet count (thrombocytopenia), which may be the result of either defective formation of platelets by bone marrow megakaryocytes (as in marrow neoplasia or aplasia), or excessive destruction of platelets (e.g. by antiplatelet antibodies, or in splenomegaly or disseminated intravascular coagulation, DIC).

Antiplatelet drugs

Antiplatelet drugs are used in the prevention or treatment of arterial thrombosis; their sites of action are illustrated in Figure 7.2. As described above, aspirin inhibits cyclooxygenase and hence reduces the formation of TXA_2. Because it also has the effect of reducing the formation of PGI_2, which itself has antiplatelet activity, agents acting more specifically as thromboxane synthase inhibitors or thromboxane receptor antagonists have also been investigated as potential antiplatelet agents, but do not appear to be more effective than aspirin. Dipyridamole acts by reducing the availability of ADP,

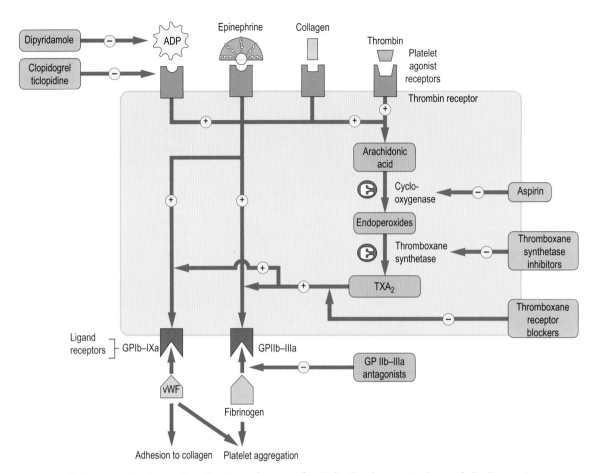

Fig. 7.2 **Pathways of platelet activation and mechanisms of action of antiplatelet drugs.** Stimulation of platelet agonist receptors results in exposure of platelet ligand receptors, partly through the platelet prostaglandin (cyclooxygenase) pathway. Ligand receptors bind vWF and fibrinogen in platelet adhesion/aggregation. vWF, von Willebrand factor; TXA_2, thromboxane A_2.

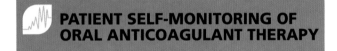

PATIENT SELF-MONITORING OF ORAL ANTICOAGULANT THERAPY

Oral anticoagulant therapy (e.g. with warfarin) is given long-term to patients at risk of thrombosis within the chambers of the heart (e.g. patients with atrial fibrillation or heart valve prostheses), which may embolize to the brain causing a stroke. Monitoring of the prothrombin time every few weeks is essential to minimize the risk not only of thromboembolism but also of excessive bleeding. Up to 1% of the adult population in developed countries now receive long-term oral anticoagulants, hence traditional monitoring by doctors and nurses (taking blood samples, sending them to the laboratory, getting results, and giving dosage instructions to patients) has become a huge workload. In recent years, portable prothrombin time measuring devices have been developed which selected patients can use for self-monitoring. A 'finger-stick' capillary sample is drawn into the machine, and the result displayed to the patient (similar to blood glucose self-monitoring by persons with diabetes). Computer algorithms have also been developed which track the patient's prothrombin time results and oral anticoagulant doses, and can recommend appropriate changes in dose.

and ticlopidine and clopidogrel inhibit the ADP receptor (see Fig. 7.2). These drugs have antithrombotic effects similar to those of aspirin, but cause less gastric bleeding because they do not interfere with synthesis of prostaglandins in the stomach. GPIIb-IIIa antagonists are used in acute coronary thrombosis. Each of these antiplatelet drugs adds to the antithrombotic efficacy of aspirin but also increases the risk of bleeding when used in combination.

COAGULATION

Blood coagulation factors interact to form the secondary, fibrin-rich, hemostatic plug in small vessels, and the secondary fibrin thrombus in arteries and veins.

Plasma coagulation factors are identified by Roman numerals: they are listed in Table 7.2, together with some of their properties. Tissue factor was formerly known as factor III, calcium ion as factor IV; factor VI does not exist. Congenital deficiencies of other coagulation factors (I–XIII) result in excessive bleeding, which illustrates their physiologic

Coagulation factors and their properties

Factor	Synonyms	Molecular weight (Da)	Plasma concentration (mg/dL)
I	Fibrinogen	340 000	200–400
II	Prothrombin	70 000	10
III	Tissue factor (thromboplastin)	44 000	0
IV	*Calcium ion	40	9–10
V	Proaccelerin, labile factor	330 000	1
VII	Serum prothrombin conversion accelerator (SPCA), stable factor	48 000	0.05
VIII	Antihemophilic factor (AHF)	330 000	0.01
(vWF)		(250 000)n	1
IX	Christmas factor	55 000	0.3
X	Stuart–Prower factor	59 000	1
XI	Plasma thromboplastin antecedent (PTA)	160 000	0.5
XII	Hageman factor	80 000	3
XIII	Fibrin-stabilizing factor (FSF)	320 000	1–2
Prekallikrein	Fletcher factor	85 000	5
High molecular weight kininogen (HMWK)	Fitzgerald, Flaujeac or Williams factor, contact activation cofactor	120 000	6

*To convert calcium ion to mmol/L multiply by 0.2495

Table 7.2 **Coagulation factors and some of their properties.** n indicates number of subunits.

importance in hemostasis. The exception is factor XII deficiency, which does not increase the bleeding tendency, despite prolonging blood clotting times in vitro; the same is true for its cofactors, prekallikrein or high-molecular-weight kininogen (HMWK). A possible explanation for this is given below.

Figure 7.3 illustrates the currently accepted scheme of blood coagulation. Since the early 1960s, this has been accepted as a 'waterfall' or 'cascade' sequence of interactive proenzyme to enzyme conversions, each enzyme activating the next proenzyme in the sequence(s). Activated factor enzymes are designated by the letter 'a', for example factor XIa. Traditionally, the scheme has been divided into three parts:

- the intrinsic pathway
- the extrinsic pathway
- the final common pathway.

These are described below. They are distinguished on the basis of the nature of the initiating factor and its corresponding test in the clinical hemostasis laboratory; hence, three tests of coagulation are performed in clinical laboratories on citrated, platelet-poor plasma:

- activated partial thromboplastin time (APTT)
- prothrombin time
- thrombin time.

Platelet-poor plasma is used in these tests because the platelet count influences clotting time results. To obtain the platelet-poor plasma, citrate anticoagulant is added to blood to sequester calcium ions reversibly, and the blood is centrifuged at 2000g for 15 minutes. The coagulation time tests are initiated by adding calcium and appropriate initiating agents.

The intrinsic pathway

The term 'intrinsic' implies that no extrinsic factor such as tissue factor or thrombin is added to the blood, other than a contact with nonendothelial 'surface'. The clinical test of this pathway is the activated partial thromboplastin time (APTT), also known as the kaolin-cephalin clotting time (KCCT) because kaolin (microparticulated clay) is added as a standard 'surface' and cephalin (brain phospholipid extract) as a substitute for platelet phospholipid. The normal range of the APTT is about 30–50 seconds; prolongations are observed in deficiencies of factors XII (or its cofactors, prekallikrein or HMWK), XI, IX (or its cofactor, factor VIII), X (or its cofactor, factor V), prothrombin (factor II) or fibrinogen (factor I) (see Table 7.1). The test is used to exclude the common congenital hemophilias (deficiencies of factors VIII, IX or XI; see Table 7.2), and to monitor heparin treatment (see box). Hemophilias caused by factor VIII or IX deficiency occur in about 1 in 10 000 males; inheritance is X-linked recessive, transmitted by carrier females. Treatment is usually with factor VIII or IX concentrates.

The extrinsic pathway

The term 'extrinsic' refers to the effect of tissue factor, which (after combining with coagulation factor VII) greatly

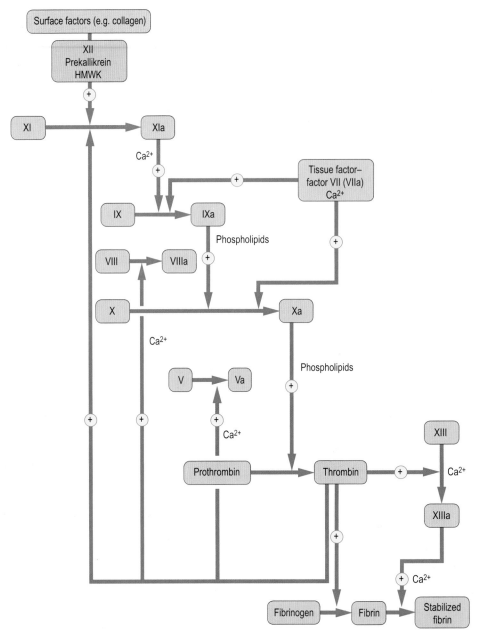

Fig. 7.3 **Blood coagulation: activation of coagulation factors.** After the initiation of blood coagulation, the coagulation factor proenzymes are activated sequentially: activated factor enzymes are designated by the letter 'a'. The purple box indicates contact factors that have no apparent function in in vivo hemostasis. Phospholipids are supplied in vivo by platelets. HMWK, high-molecular-weight kininogen.

accelerates coagulation, by activating both factor IX and factor X (see Fig. 7.3). Tissue factor is a polypeptide that is expressed in all cells other than endothelial cells. The clinical test of this pathway is the prothrombin time (PT), in which tissue factor is added to plasma. The normal range is about 10–15 seconds; prolongations are observed in deficiencies of factors VII, X, V, II or I. In clinical practice, the test is used to diagnose both the rare congenital defects of these factors and, much more commonly, acquired bleeding disorders, resulting from:

- **vitamin K deficiency** (e.g. malabsorption, obstructive jaundice; see Chapter 11) which reduces hepatic synthesis of factors II, VII, IX and X. Treatment is by injections of vitamin K
- **oral anticoagulants** (e.g. warfarin) which are vitamin K antagonists, reducing hepatic synthesis of these factors. Excessive bleeding in patients taking warfarin can be treated by stopping the drug, giving vitamin K or replacing factors II, VII, IX and X with fresh frozen plasma or concentrates

ANTITHROMBIN DEFICIENCY

A 40-year-old man was admitted from the emergency room of his local hospital because of acute pain and swelling of his left leg 10 days after recent major surgery. Ultrasound imaging of the leg confirmed occlusion of the left femoral vein by thrombus.

Comment. He was prescribed anticoagulant therapy with low molecular weight heparin at standard doses. The patient volunteered a strong family history of 'clots in the legs' at a young age. A thrombophilia screening test was performed, and showed a low plasma antithrombin level.

CLASSIC HEMOPHILIA: CONGENITAL FACTOR VIII DEFICIENCY

A 3-year-old boy was admitted from the emergency room of his local hospital because of extensive bruising after a fall down a few stairs. A routine coagulation screen test showed a greatly prolonged APTT of more than 150 sec (normal range, 30–50 sec). Assay of coagulation factor VIII showed a very low level; the vWF level was normal. His mother recollected a family history of excessive bleeding which had affected her brother and father.

Comment. Because of this typical history of an X-linked recessive bleeding disorder, a low coagulation factor VIII level, and a normal vWF level, a diagnosis of classic hemophilia (congenital factor VIII deficiency) was made. The family were referred to the local hemophilia center and counseled about the risks of further affected sons and carrier daughters. The child was treated with intravenous factor VIII concentrate for the presenting bleed, and for future bleeds, injuries or surgery.

■ **liver disease**, which reduces hepatic synthesis of these factors. For example, the prothrombin time is a prognostic marker of liver failure after acetaminophen (paracetamol) overdose (see Chapter 29). Treatment is by replacing factors II, VII, IX and X with fresh frozen plasma or concentrates.

The final common pathway

The third part of coagulation is tested clinically by the thrombin time, in which exogenous thrombin is added to plasma. The normal range of values is about 10–15 seconds; prolongations are observed in fibrinogen deficiency. This may be congenital or due to acquired consumption of fibrinogen in disseminated intravascular coagulation (DIC), or may occur after administration of fibrinolytic drugs (see below). Treatment is with fresh frozen plasma or fibrinogen concentrates.

Thrombin

Thrombin converts circulating fibrinogen to fibrin and activates factor XIII which crosslinks the fibrin, forming a clot. It is currently believed that activation of blood coagulation is usually initiated by vascular injury, causing exposure of flowing blood to tissue factor, which results in activation of factors VII and IX. Subsequently, activation of factors X and II (prothrombin) occurs preferentially at sites of vascular injury, and upon activated platelets, which provide procoagulant activity (platelet factor 3, PF3) as a result of exposure of negatively charged platelet surface membrane phospholipids, such as phosphatidylserine. This is accompanied by the exposure, on activated platelets, of high-affinity binding sites for several activated coagulation factors (especially factors Va and VIIIa), and provision of platelet phospholipid, which further catalyzes coagulation activation. As a result of these biochemical interactions (see Fig. 7.1 and Fig. 7.4), thrombin and fibrin formation are efficiently localized at sites of vascular injury.

Thrombin has a central role in hemostasis

Not only does thrombin convert circulating fibrinogen to fibrin at sites of vascular injury, producing the secondary, fibrin-rich hemostatic plug, it also activates factor XIII (transglutaminase), which crosslinks such fibrin, rendering it resistant to dispersion by local blood pressure or by fibrinolysis (see Figs 7.1 and 7.3). Furthermore, thrombin stimulates its own generation in a positive feedback cycle in two ways:

■ **it catalyzes activation of factor XI**: this may explain why congenital deficiencies of factor XII, prekallikrein or HMWK are not associated with excessive bleeding (see Fig. 7.4)
■ **it catalyzes activation of factors VIII and V.**

Thrombin also activates platelets (see Fig. 7.2).

Now that the central role of thrombin in hemostasis and thrombosis has been recognized, there is current interest in the development of direct antithrombins as antithrombotic drugs; these include examples such as hirudin (originally obtained from the medicinal leech, *Hirudo medicinalis*) and its synthetic derivatives.

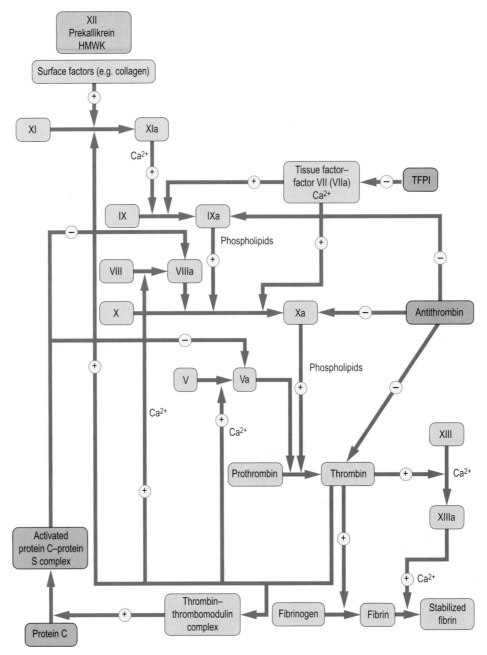

Fig. 7.4 **Sites of action of blood coagulation inhibitors.** Antithrombin, protein C and protein S, and tissue factor pathway inhibitor (TFPI).

Coagulation inhibitors are essential to prevent excessive thrombin formation and thrombosis

Three systems of coagulation inhibitors have been identified (see Fig. 7.4 and Table 7.3).

- **Antithrombin**: this is a protein synthesized in the liver. Its activity is catalyzed by the antithrombotic drug heparin, and by heparin-like endogenous glycosaminoglycans (GAGs) that are present on the surface of vascular endothelial cells. It inactivates not only thrombin, but also factors IXa and Xa (see Fig. 7.4). Congenital antithrombin deficiency results in increased

risk of venous thromboembolism. Heparin injections are given in the treatment of acute venous or arterial thrombosis; they are usually replaced by oral anticoagulants such as warfarin for longer-term anticoagulation.

- **Protein C and its cofactor, protein S**: these are vitamin K-dependent proteins, synthesized in the liver. When thrombin is generated, it binds to thrombomodulin (molecular weight 74 kDa), which is present on the surface of vascular endothelial cells. The thrombin–thrombomodulin complex activates protein C, which forms a complex with its cofactor, protein S. This complex selectively degrades factors Va and VIIIa by limited proteolysis (see Fig. 7.4).

Properties of coagulation inhibitors		
Inhibitor (synonym)	Molecular weight	Plasma concentration (mg/dL)
Antithrombin (antithrombin III)	65 000	18–30
Protein C	56 000	0.4
Protein S	69 000	2.5
Tissue factor pathway inhibitor, TFPI (lipoprotein-associated coagulation inhibitor, LACI)	32 000	0.1

Table 7.3 **Properties of coagulation inhibitors**.

Properties of the components of fibrinolytic system		
Component (synonym)	Molecular weight	Plasma concentration (mg/dL)
Plasminogen	92 000	0.2
Tissue-type plasminogen activator, tPA	65 000	5 (basal)
Urinary-type plasminogen activator type 1, uPA	54 000	20
Plasminogen activator inhibitor type 1, PAI-1	48 000	200
Antiplasmin (α_2 antiplasmin)	70 000	700

Table 7.4 **Properties of the components of fibrinolytic system**.

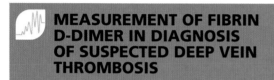

MEASUREMENT OF FIBRIN D-DIMER IN DIAGNOSIS OF SUSPECTED DEEP VEIN THROMBOSIS

Fibrin D-dimer (a degradation product of crosslinked fibrin and a marker of fibrin turnover) is normally present in blood at concentrations less than 0.25 g/L. In deep vein thrombosis of the leg (DVT), deposition of a large mass of crosslinked fibrin within the leg veins, followed by partial lysis by the body's fibrinolytic system, increases fibrin turnover and blood D-dimer levels are elevated. Many patients attend accident and emergency departments with a swollen and/or painful leg, which may be due to DVT. Rapid immunoassays for blood D-dimer can be performed in the emergency department, and are now widely used as a adjunct to clinical diagnosis. About one-third of patients with clinically suspected DVT have normal D-dimer levels, which in combination with a low clinical score usually excludes the diagnosis and may allow early discharge of such patients without the need for further investigation or treatment. In patients with raised D-dimer levels, heparin treatment is started and imaging of the leg performed (usually by ultrasound) to confirm the presence and extent of DVT.

Hence, this pathway forms a negative feedback upon thrombin generation. Congenital deficiencies of protein C or protein S result in increased risk of venous thromboembolism; a further cause of increased risk of venous thromboembolism is a mutation in coagulation factor V (factor V Leiden), which confers resistance to its inactivation by activated protein C. This mutation is common, occurring in about 3% of the population in Western countries.

Tissue factor pathway inhibitor (TFPI): this protein is synthesized in endothelium and the liver; it circulates bound to lipoproteins. It inhibits the tissue factor–VIIa complex (see Fig. 7.4), which may explain the severe

bleeding in hemophilia caused by deficiency in factor VIII or IX (failure to sustain thrombin and fibrin formation). Conversely, deficiency of TFPI does not appear to increase the risk of thrombosis.

FIBRINOLYSIS

The fibrinolytic system also limits excessive fibrin formation

The coagulation system acts to form fibrin; the fibrinolytic system acts to limit excessive formation of fibrin (both intra- and extravascular) through plasmin-mediated fibrinolysis. Circulating plasminogen binds to fibrin via lysine-binding sites; it is converted to active plasmin by plasminogen activators. Tissue-type plasminogen activator (tPA) is synthesized by endothelial cells; it normally circulates in plasma in low basal concentrations (5 ng/mL), but is released into plasma by stimuli that include venous occlusion, exercise, and epinephrine. Together with plasminogen, it binds strongly to fibrin, which stimulates its activity (the K_m for plasminogen decreases from 65 to 0.15 μmol/L in the presence of fibrin), thereby localizing plasmin activity to fibrin deposits. Excessive tPA activity in plasma is normally prevented by an excess of its major inhibitor, plasminogen activator inhibitor type 1 (PAI-1), which is synthesized by both endothelial cells and hepatocytes. Urinary-type plasminogen activator (uPA) circulates in plasma both as an active single-chain precursor form, uPA (scuPA, pro-urokinase) and as a more active two-chain form (tcuPA, urokinase). One activator of scuPA is surface-activated coagulation factor XII, which therefore links the coagulation and fibrinolytic systems. The major components of the fibrinolytic system are illustrated in Table 7.4 and Figure 7.5.

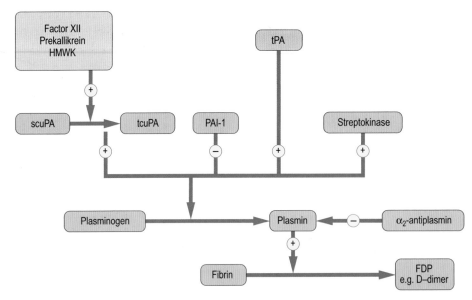

Fig. 7.5 **The fibrinolytic system.** Plasminogen can be activated to plasmin by uPA (urokinase), tPA or streptokinase. uPA and tPA are inhibited by plasminogen activator inhibitor type 1 (PAI-1). Plasmin is inhibited by antiplasmin. Plasmin degrades fibrin to fibrin degradation products (FDP). HMWK, high-molecular-weight kininogen; scuPA, prourokinase; tcuPA, urokinase; tPA, tissue-type plasminogen activator.

ANTITHROMBOTIC TREATMENT IN MYOCARDIAL INFARCTION

Occlusion of a coronary artery by thrombus causes death of that part of the heart muscle which is supplied by the artery (myocardial infarction). In acute myocardial infarction, the patient typically experiences severe, substantial chest pain.

Aspirin and heparin are also usually given in acute myocardial infarction and other acute coronary syndromes, to inhibit the platelet and fibrin components of the developing coronary artery thrombus.

Many patients with evolving acute myocardial infarction were candidates for thrombolytic treatment with a plasminogen activator drug, given intravenously. Prompt thrombolysis dissolved the coronary artery thrombus, reduced the size of the infarct, and reduced the risk of complications, including death and heart failure. However, in recent years direct removal of the thrombus (percutaneous coronary intervention) is given instead of thrombolytic therapy, because unlike thrombolytic therapy it does not increase the risk of bleeding for example into the brain.

Comment. Thrombolytic drugs are also used in some carefully selected patients with early evolving ischemic stroke; or in some patients with massive pulmonary embolism. Thrombolytic drugs include tissue-type and urinary-type plasminogen activators (tPA and uPA) (see Fig. 7.5), produced by recombinant gene technology, or their synthetic variants. All thrombolytic drugs can cause bleeding (see Table 7.1), as a result of lysis of hemostatic plugs in addition to the target thrombi.

Excessive formation of plasmin is normally prevented by:

- binding of 50% of plasminogen to histidine-rich glycoprotein (HRG)
- rapid inactivation of free plasmin by its major inhibitor, α_2-antiplasmin.

The physiologic importance of PAI-1 and α_2-antiplasmin is illustrated by the increased bleeding tendency that is associated with the rare cases of their congenital deficiencies (see Table 7.1); the excessive plasma plasmin activity which results from the deficiencies has the effect of lysing hemostatic plugs.

Summary

- Hemostasis constitutes a number of processes which guard the body against blood loss.
- Injury to the blood vessel wall sets in motion complex phenomena which involve blood platelets (activation, adhesion, aggregation) and a cascade of coagulation factors, classified into intrinsic, extrinsic and final common pathways.
- The integrity of these three systems may be tested by simple laboratory tests.
- Deficiencies of factors participating in the coagulation cascade, and/or disordered platelet function, result in bleeding disorders.
- Eventually, blood clots are degraded by the fibrinolytic system. The process of fibrinolysis prevents thrombotic phenomena and there is normally a balance between hemostasis and thrombosis.

ACTIVE LEARNING

Test your knowledge

1. When a patient presents with excessive bleeding from multiple sites, what laboratory tests should be done to identify the likely cause of their hemostatic defect?
2. When a patient presents with a painful swollen leg, possibly due to acute deep venous thrombosis (DVT), what laboratory tests can be performed to help the clinician to:
   - establish or exclude this diagnosis?
   - monitor anticoagulant treatment, after the diagnosis has been confirmed?
3. When a patient presents with acute coronary artery thrombosis (evolving to myocardial infarction), what antithrombotic drugs should be urgently considered to reduce the risk of complications?

- Aspirin and heparin are used in patients with acute myocardial infarction or other acute coronary syndromes.
- Aspirin (or other antiplatelet agents) are also used to reduce risk of recurrent myocardial infarction and stroke.
- Anticoagulant drugs (e.g. heparin then warfarin) are used in treatment of acute venous thrombosis or embolism.
- Anticoagulant drugs (e.g warfarin) are used long term to prevent thromboembolism from the heart (atrial fibrillation, heart valve prostheses).

Further reading

de Moerloose P (ed). State of the art 2007. *J Thromb Haemostas* 2007;**5(suppl 1)**: 1–331.

Mannucci PM, Levi M. Prevention and treatment of major blood loss. *N Engl J Med* 2007; **356**: 2301–2311.

Marsh N (ed). State of the art 2005. *J Thromb Haemostas* 2005;**3(8)**:1553–1904.

8. Membranes and Transport

M Maeda

LEARNING OBJECTIVES

After reading this chapter you should be able to:

- Describe the differences between passive and active carrier-mediated transport systems.
- Describe the basic features of membrane channels and pores.
- Give several specific examples of ion and substrate transport systems, including coupled transport systems.
- Describe several characteristic diseases resulting from defects in membrane transport.

INTRODUCTION

As discussed in Chapter 3, biomembranes are not rigid or impermeable, but highly mobile and dynamic structures. The plasma membrane is the gatekeeper of the cell. It controls not only the access of inorganic ions, vitamins and nutrients, but also the entry of drugs and the exit of waste products. Integral transmembrane proteins have important roles in transporting these molecules through the membrane and often maintain concentration gradients across the membranes. K^+, Na^+ and Ca^{2+} concentrations in the cytoplasm are maintained at ~140, 10, and 10^{-4} mmol/L (546, 23, and 0.0007 mg/dL), respectively, by transporter proteins, whereas those outside (in the blood) are ~5, 145, and 1–2 mmol/L (20, 333, and 7–14 mg/dL), respectively. The driving force for transport of ions and maintenance of ion gradients is directly or indirectly provided by ATP. The transport properties of membranes will be illustrated by several important examples.

TYPES OF TRANSPORT PROCESSES

Simple diffusion through the phospholipid bilayer

Small, nonpolar molecules (such as O_2, CO_2, N_2) and uncharged polar molecules (such as urea, ethanol, and small organic acids) move through membranes by simple diffusion without the aid of membrane proteins (Table 8.1 and Fig. 8.1A). The direction of net movement of these species is always 'downhill', along the concentration gradient, from high to low concentration to establish equilibrium.

Transport systems of biomembranes						
Type		Transport protein (example)	Energy coupling	Specificity	Saturability	Rate (molecules/ transport protein/s)
Passive transport or diffusion	simple diffusion	−	−	−	−	
	facilitated diffusion	+	−	+	+	
	transporter	(GLUT-1~5)				~10^2
	channel	(H_2O, Na^+, K^+, Ca^{2+}, Cl^-)				10^7–10^8
Active transport	primary	+	+	+	+	10^2–10^4
	secondary	+	+	+	+	10^0–10^{2*}
	symporter	(SGLT-1, 2, neutral amino acids)				
	antiporter	(Cl^-/HCO_3^-, Na^+/Ca^{2+}, Na^+/H^+)				
	uniporter	(Glutamate)				

Table 8.1 **Classification of transport systems of biomembranes.** Transport systems are classified according to the role of transport proteins and energy coupling. Typical substrates for various types of channels are shown in the parentheses. *The Cl^-/HCO_3^- antiporter seems to be an exception to secondary active transport systems, as its transport rate is high, at 10^5 molecules/transport protein/s.

A Transport and energy coupling

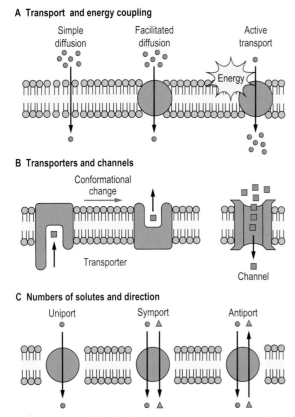

B Transporters and channels

C Numbers of solutes and direction

Fig. 8.1 **Various models of solute movement across membranes.**

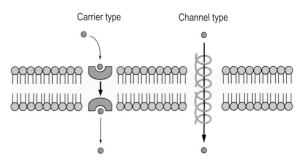

Fig. 8.2 **Mobile ion carriers and channel-forming ionophores.** Ionospheres permit net movement of ions only down their electrochemical gradients.

The hydrophobicity of the molecules is an important requirement for simple diffusion across the membrane, as the interior of the phospholipid bilayer is hydrophobic. The rate of transport of these molecules is, in fact, closely related to their partition coefficient between oil and water.

Although water molecules can be transported by simple diffusion, channel proteins (see below) are believed to control the movement of water across most membranes, especially in the kidney for concentration of the urine. Mutation in a water channel protein gene (aquaporin-2) causes diuresis in some patients with nephrogenic diabetes insipidus, a disease characterized by excessive urination but without the hyperglycemia characteristic of diabetes mellitus (see Chapter 23).

Transport mediated by membrane proteins

Transport of larger, polar molecules, such as amino acids or sugars, into a cell requires the involvement of membrane proteins known as transporters, also called porters, permeases, translocases or carrier proteins. The term 'carrier' is also applied to ionophores, which move passively across the membrane together with the bound ion (Fig. 8.2). Transporters are as specific as enzymes for their substrates, and work by

 MEMBRANE PERMEABILITY

Antibiotics that induce ion permeability

Peptide antibiotics act as ionophores and increase the permeability of membranes to specific ions; bactericidal effects of ionophores are attributed to disturbance of the ion transport systems of bacterial membranes. Ionophores permit net movement of ions only down their electrochemical gradients. There are two classes of ionophores: mobile ion carriers (or caged carriers) and channel formers (Fig. 8.2). Valinomycin is a typical example of a mobile ion carrier. It is a cyclic peptide with a lipophilic exterior and ionic interior. It dissolves in the membrane and diffuses between the inner and outer surfaces. K^+ binds in the central core of valinomycin, and the complex diffuses across the membrane, releasing the K^+ and gradually dissipating the K^+ gradient. The carrier type-ionophores, nigericin and monensin, exchange H^+ for Na^+ and K^+, respectively. Ionomycin and A23187 are Ca^{2+} ionophores.

The β-helical gramicidin A molecule, a linear peptide with 15 amino acid residues, forms a pore. The head-to-head dimer of gramicidin A makes a transmembrane channel that allows movement of monovalent cations (H^+, Na^+, and K^+).

Polyene antibiotics such as amphotericin B and nystatin exert their cytotoxic action by rendering the membrane of the target cell permeable to ions and small molecules. Formation of a sterol–polyene complex is essential for the cytotoxic function of these antibiotics, as they display a selective action against organisms in which the membranes contain sterols. Thus they are active against yeasts, a wide variety of fungi, and other eukaryotic cells but have no effect on bacteria. Because their affinity for ergosterol, a fungal membrane component, is higher than that for cholesterol, these antibiotics have been used for the treatment of topical infections of fungal origin.

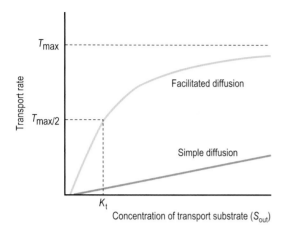

Fig. 8.3 **Comparison of the transport kinetics of facilitated diffusion and simple diffusion.** The rate of transport of substrate is plotted against the concentration of substrate in the extracellular medium. In common with enzyme catalysis, transporter-catalyzed uptake has a maximum transport rate, T_{max} (saturable). K_t is the concentration at which the rate of substrate uptake is half-maximal. For simple diffusion, the transport rate is slower and directly proportional to substrate concentration.

one of two mechanisms: facilitated diffusion or active transport. Facilitated diffusion catalyzes the movement of a substrate through a membrane down a concentration gradient and does not require energy. In contrast, active transport is a process in which substrates are transported uphill, against their concentration gradient. Active transport must be coupled to an energy-producing reaction (see Fig. 8.1A).

Saturability and specificity are important characteristics of membrane transport systems

The rate of facilitated diffusion is generally much greater than that of simple diffusion: transport proteins catalyze the transport process. In contrast to simple diffusion, in which the rate of transport is directly proportional to the substrate concentration, facilitated diffusion is a saturable process, having a maximum transport rate, T_{max} (Fig. 8.3). When the concentration of extracellular molecules (transport substrates) becomes very high, the T_{max} is achieved by saturation of the transporter proteins with substrate. The kinetics of facilitated diffusion for substrates can be described by the same equations that are used for enzyme catalysis (e.g. Michaelis–Menten and Lineweaver–Burk type equations) (see Chapter 6):

$$S_{out} + \text{transporter} \underset{}{\overset{K_t}{\rightleftharpoons}} (S \cdot \text{transporter complex}) \rightarrow S_{in}$$

where K_t is the dissociation constant of the substrate–transporter complex, and S_{out} is the concentration of transport substrate. Then the transport rate, t, can be calculated as:

$$t = \frac{T_{max}}{\left[1 + \dfrac{K_t}{S_{out}}\right]}$$

where the K_t is the concentration that gives the half-maximal transport rate. The K_t for a transporter is conceptually the same as the K_m for an enzyme.

The transport process is usually highly specific: each transporter transports only a single species of molecules or structurally related compounds. The red blood cell GLUT-1 transporter has a high affinity for D-glucose, but 10–20 times

CYSTINOSIS

An 18-month-old child presented with polyuria, failure to thrive and an episode of severe dehydration. Urine dipstick testing demonstrated glucosuria and proteinuria, with other biochemical analyses showing generalized aminoaciduria and phosphaturia.

Comment. This is a classic presentation of infantile cystinosis, resulting from accumulation of cystine in lysosomes because of a defect in the lysosomal transport protein, cystinosine. Cystine is poorly soluble, and crystalline precipitates form in cells throughout the body. In vitro experiments with cystine loading have shown that renal proximal tubular cells become ATP-depleted, resulting in impairment of ATP-dependent ion pumps with consequent electrolyte imbalances and metabolite losses. Treatment with cysteamine increases the transport of cystine from lysosomes, delaying the decline in renal function. Cysteamine is a weak base; it forms a mixed disulfide with cysteine, which is then secreted through a cationic amino acid transporter. If untreated, renal failure occurs by 6–12 years of age. Unfortunately, there is further accumulation of cystine in the central nervous system, despite therapy, with long-term neurologic damage.

HARTNUP DISEASE

A 3-year-old boy had been on holiday to Spain and developed pellagra-like skin changes on his face, neck, forearms and dorsal aspects of his hands and legs. His skin became scaly, rough and hyperpigmented. The child was brought to the GP complaining of headaches and weakness. Urinalysis demonstrated gross hyperaminoaciduria of neutral monoamino-monocarboxylic acids (i.e. alanine, serine, threonine, asparagine, glutamine, valine, leucine, isoleucine, phenylalanine, tyrosine, tryptophan, histidine and citrulline).

Comment. These neutral amino acids share a common transporter which is expressed only on the luminal border of epithelial cells in the renal tubules and intestinal epithelium. The pellagra-like dermatitis (see Chapter 11) and neurologic involvement resemble nutritional niacin deficiency. The reduced tryptophan intake results in reduced nicotinamide production. The disease is easily treated with oral nicotinamide and application of sun-blocking agents to exposed areas.

lower affinity for the related sugars, D-mannose and D-galactose. The enantiomer L-glucose is not transported; its K_t is more than 1000 times higher than that of the D-form.

Characteristics of glucose transporters (uniporters)

Glucose transporters are essential for facilitated diffusion of glucose into cells. The GLUT family of glucose transporters includes GLUT-1 to GLUT-5 (Table 8.2) and others. They are transmembrane proteins similar in size, all having about 500 amino acid residues and 12 transmembrane helices. GLUT-1, in red blood cells, has a K_m of ~2 mmol/L. The GLUT-1 transporter operates at about 40% of T_{max} under fasting conditions (glucose concentration of 5 mmol/L; 90 mg/dL); this level of activity is sufficient to meet the needs of the red cell (Chapter 12). In contrast, pancreatic islet β-cells express GLUT-2, with a K_m of more than 10 mmol/L (180 mg/dL). In response to the intake of food and the resulting increase in blood glucose concentration, GLUT-2 molecules respond by increasing the uptake of glucose into β-cells, stimulating insulin secretion (Chapter 21). Cells in insulin-sensitive tissues such as muscle and adipose have GLUT-4. Insulin stimulates translocation of GLUT-4 from intracellular vesicles to the plasma membrane, facilitating glucose uptake during meals.

Classification of glucose transporters			
Transporter	K_t for D-glucose transport (mM)	Substrate	Major sites of expression
Facilitated diffusion (uniporter) (passive transport)			
GLUT-1	1–2	glucose, galactose, mannose	erythrocyte, blood–tissue barriers
GLUT-2	15–20	glucose, fructose	liver, intestine, kidney, pancreatic β-cells, brain
GLUT-3	1.8*	glucose	ubiquitous
GLUT-4	5	glucose	skeletal and cardiac muscles, adipose tissues
GLUT-5	6–11**	fructose	intestine
Na⁺-coupled symporter (active transport)			
SGLT-1	0.35	glucose (2Na⁺/1 glucose), galactose	intestine, kidney
SGLT-2	1.6	glucose (1Na⁺/1 glucose)	kidney

Table 8.2 **Classification of glucose transporters.** K_m values are determined from the uptake of 2-deoxy-D-glucose (*), a nonmetabolizable analog of glucose, and fructose (**).

DEFECTIVE GLUCOSE TRANSPORT ACROSS THE BLOOD–BRAIN BARRIER AS A CAUSE OF SEIZURES AND DEVELOPMENTAL DELAY

A male infant at the age of 3 months suffered from recurrent seizures. His cerebrospinal fluid (CSF) glucose concentrations were low (0.9–1.9 mmol/L; 16–34 mg/dL), and the ratio of CSF to blood glucose ranged from 0.19 to 0.33; the normal value is 0.65. The potential causes of low CSF glucose concentrations, such as bacterial meningitis, subarachnoid hemorrhage, and hypoglycemia, were not present and high CSF lactate values would be found in all these conditions except hypoglycemia. In contrast, the CSF lactate concentrations were consistently low (0.3–0.4 mmol/L; 3–4 mg/dL) compared with the normal value (~2.2 mmol/L; ~20 mg/dL). These findings suggested a defect in transport of glucose from the blood to the brain.

Comment. Assuming that the activity of GLUT-1 glucose transporter in the erythrocyte reflects that of the brain microvessels, a transport assay was carried out using his erythrocytes. The T_{max} for uptake of glucose by the patient's erythrocytes was 60% of the mean normal value, suggesting a heterozygous defect. A ketogenic diet (a high-fat, low-protein, low-carbohydrate diet) was started, since the brain can use ketone bodies as oxidizable fuel sources, and the entry of ketone bodies into the brain is not dependent on the glucose transporter system. The patient stopped having seizures within 4 days after beginning the diet.

Transport by channels and pores

Channels are often pictured as tunnels across the membrane, in which binding sites for substrates (ions) are accessible from either side of the membrane at the same time (see Fig. 8.1B). Conformational changes are not required for the translocation of substrates entering from one side of the membrane to exit on the other side. However, voltage changes and ligand binding induce conformational changes in channel structure that have the effect of opening or closing the channels – processes known as voltage or ligand 'gating'. Movement of molecules through channels is fast in comparison with the rates achieved by transporters (see Table 8.1).

The terms 'channel' and 'pore' are sometimes used interchangeably. However, 'pore' is used most frequently to describe more open, somewhat nonselective structures that discriminate between substrates, e.g. peptides or proteins, on the basis of size. The term 'channel' is usually applied to more specific ion channels.

Three examples of pores important for cellular physiology

The gap junction between endothelial, muscle, and neuronal cells is a cluster of small pores, in which two cylinders of six connexin subunits in the plasma membranes join each other to form a pore about 1.2–2.0 nm (12–20 Å) in diameter. Molecules smaller than about 1 kDa can pass between cells through these gap junctions. Such cell–cell interchange is important for physiologic communication or coupling, for example in the concerted contraction of uterine muscle during labor and delivery. Mutations of the genes encoding connexin 26 and connexin 32 cause deafness and Charcot–Marie–Tooth disease, respectively.

Nuclear pores have a radius of about 9.0 nm (90 Å) through which larger proteins and nucleic acids enter and leave the nucleus.

A third class of pores is important for protein sorting. Mitochondrial proteins encoded by nuclear genes are transported to this organelle through pores in the outer mitochondrial membrane. Nascent polypeptide chains of secretory proteins and plasma membrane proteins also pass through pores in the endoplasmic reticulum membrane during biosynthesis of the peptide chain.

Active transport

ATP is a high-energy product of metabolism and is often described as the 'energy currency' of the cell (Chapter 9). The phosphoanhydride bond of ATP releases free energy when it is hydrolyzed to produce adenosine diphosphate (ADP) and inorganic phosphate. Such energy is used for synthesis of large and small cellular molecules, cell movement, and uphill transport of molecules against concentration gradients. Primary active transport systems use ATP directly to drive transport; secondary active transport uses an electrochemical gradient of Na^+ or H^+ ions, or a membrane potential produced by primary active transport processes. Sugars and amino acids are generally transported into cells by secondary active transport systems.

The most important primary active transport systems are ion pumps (ion transporting ATPases or pump ATPases)

The pump ATPases are classified into four groups (Table 8.3; see also Figs 23.3–23.5). Coupling factor ATPases

Various primary active transporters in eukaryotic cells				
Group	Member	Location	Substrate(s)	Functions
F-ATPase (coupling factor)	H^+-ATPase	mitochondrial inner membrane	H^+	ATP synthesis driven by electrochemical gradient of H^+
V-ATPase (vacuolar)	H^+-ATPase	cytoplasmic vesicles (lysosome, secretory granules), plasma membranes (ruffled border of osteoclast, kidney epithelial cell)	H^+	activation of lysosomal enzymes, accumulation of neurotransmitters, turnover of bone, acidification of urine
P-ATPase (phosphorylation)	Na^+/K^+-ATPase	plasma membranes (ubiquitous, but abundant in kidney and heart)	Na^+ and K^+	generation of electrochemical gradient of Na^+ and K^+
	H^+/K^+-ATPase	stomach (parietal cell in gastric gland)	H^+ and K^+	acidification of stomach lumen
	Ca^{2+}-ATPase	sarcoplasmic reticulum and endoplasmic reticulum	Ca^{2+}	Ca^{2+} sequestration into sarcoplasmic (endoplasmic) reticulum
	Ca^{2+}-ATPase	plasma membrane	Ca^{2+}	Ca^{2+} excretion to outside of the cell
	Cu^{2+}-ATPase	plasma membrane and cytoplasmic vesicles	Cu^{2+}	Cu^{2+} absorption from intestine and excretion from liver
ABC transporter (ATP binding cassette)	P-glycoprotein	plasma membrane	various drugs	excretion of harmful substances, multidrug resistance for anticancer drugs
	MRP	plasma membrane	glutathione conjugate	detoxification, multidrug resistance
	CFTR*	plasma membrane	Cl^-	cAMP-dependent chloride channel, regulation of other channels
	TAP	endoplasmic reticulum	peptide	presentation of peptides for immune response

*Some ABC transporters function as channels or channel regulators. MRP, multidrug resistance-associated protein; CFTR, cystic fibrosis transmembrane conductance regulator; TAP, transporter associated with antigen processing.

Table 8.3 **Primary active transporters in eukaryotic cells.** Various examples of primary active transporters (ATP-powered pump ATPases) are listed, together with their location.

MENKES AND WILSON'S DISEASES

X-linked Menkes disease is a lethal disorder that occurs in 1 in 100 000 newborn infants and is characterized by abnormal and hypopigmented hair, a characteristic facies, cerebral degeneration, connective tissue and vascular defects, and death by the age of 3 years. A copper-transporting P-ATPase that is expressed in all tissues except liver is defective in this disease (see Table 8.3). In patients with Menkes disease, copper enters the intestinal cells but is not transported further, resulting in severe copper deficiency. Subcutaneous administration of a copper histidine complex may be an effective treatment if started early.

The gene for Wilson's disease also encodes a copper-transporting P-ATPase and is 60% identical with that of the Menkes gene. It is expressed in liver, kidney, and placenta. Wilson's disease occurs in 1 in 35 000–100 000 newborns and is characterized by failure to incorporate copper into ceruloplasmin in the liver and failure to excrete copper from the liver into bile, resulting in toxic accumulation of copper in the liver and also in the kidney, brain, and cornea. Liver cirrhosis, progressive neurologic damage, or both, occur during childhood to early adulthood. Chelating agents such as penicillamine are used for treatment of patients with this disease. Oral zinc treatment may be useful for decreasing the absorption of dietary copper.

Comment. Copper is an essential trace metal and an integral component of many enzymes. However, it is toxic in excess, because it binds to proteins and nucleic acids, enhances the generation of free radicals, and catalyzes oxidation of lipids and proteins in membranes (Chapter 37).

(F-ATPases) in mitochondrial, chloroplast, and bacterial membranes hydrolyze ATP and transport hydrogen ions (H^+). As discussed in detail in the next chapter, the mitochondrial F-ATPase works in the backward direction, synthesizing ATP from ADP and phosphate as protons move down an electrochemical (concentration and charge) gradient generated across the inner mitochondrial membrane during oxidative metabolism. The product, ATP, is released into the mitochondrial matrix, but is needed for biosynthetic reactions in the cytoplasm. ATP is transported to the cytoplasm through an ATP-ADP translocase in the mitochondrial inner membrane. This translocase is an example of an antiport system (see Fig. 8.1C); it allows one molecule of ADP to enter only if one molecule of ATP exits simultaneously.

Cytoplasmic vesicles, such as lysosomes, endosomes, and secretory granules, are acidified by a V-type (vacuolar) H^+-ATPase in their membranes. Acidification by this V-ATPase is important for the activity of lysosomal enzymes that have acidic pH optima, and for the accumulation of drugs and neurotransmitters in secretory granules. The V-ATPase also acidifies the extracellular environments of osteoclasts and renal epithelial cells. Defects in the osteoclast plasma membrane V-ATPase result in osteopetrosis (increased bone density), while mutation of the ATPase in collecting ducts of the kidney causes renal tubular acidosis. F- and V-type ATPases are structurally similar, and seem to be derived from a common ancestor. The ATP-binding catalytic subunit and the subunit forming the H^+ pathway are conserved between these ATPases.

P-ATPases form phosphorylated intermediates that drive ion translocation: the 'P' refers to the phosphorylation. These transporters have an active-site aspartate residue that is reversibly phosphorylated by ATP during the transport process. The P-type Na^+/K^+-ATPase in various tissues and the Ca^{2+}-ATPase in the sarcoplasmic reticulum have important roles in maintaining cellular ion gradients.

Na^+/K^+-ATPases also create an electrochemical gradient of Na^+ that produces the driving force for uptake of nutrients from the intestine (below). The discharge of this electrochemical gradient is also fundamental to the process of nerve transmission (Chapter 40). Mutations of P-ATPase genes cause Brody cardiomyopathy (Ca^{2+}-ATPase), familial hemiplegic migraine type 2 (Na^+/K^+-ATPase), and Menkes and Wilson diseases (Cu^{2+}-ATPases).

The ATP-binding cassette (ABC) transporters comprise the fourth active transporter family. 'ABC' is the abbreviation for 'ATP-binding cassette', referring to an ATP-binding region in the transporter (see Table 8.3). P-glycoprotein

 ## ABC TRANSPORTER DISEASES

Human genome data suggest that there are about 50 genes for ABC transporters. An unusually wide range of diseases are caused by defects in ABC transporters, including Tangier disease, Stargardt disease, progressive intrahepatic cholestasis, Dubin-Johnson syndrome, pseudoxanthoma elasticum, familial persistent hyperinsulinemic hypoglycemia of infancy (PHHI), adrenoleukodystrophy, Zellweger syndrome, sitosterolemia and cystic fibrosis.

Cystic fibrosis (CF) is the most common potentially lethal autosomal recessive disease of Caucasian populations, affecting 1 in 2500 newborns. CF is usually manifested as exocrine pancreatic insufficiency, an increase in the concentration of chloride ions (Cl^-) in sweat, male infertility, and airway disease, which is the major cause of morbidity and mortality. The pancreatic and lung pathology results from the increased viscosity of secreted fluids (mucoviscoidosis). CF is caused by mutations in the gene CFTR (cystic fibrosis transmembrane conductance regulator) which encodes a Cl^- channel. ATP binding to CFTR is required for channel opening. The lack of this channel activity in epithelia of CF patients affects both ion and water secretion.

('P' = permeability) and MRP (multidrug resistance-associated protein), which have a physiological role in excretion of toxic metabolites and xenobiotics, contribute to resistance of cancer cells to chemotherapy. TAP transporters, a class of ABC transporters associated with antigen presentation, are required for initiating the immune response against foreign proteins; they mediate antigen peptide transport from the cytosol into endoplasmic reticulum. Some ABC transporters are present in peroxisomal membrane where they appear to be involved in the transport of peroxisomal enzymes necessary for oxidation of very long-chain fatty acids. Defects of ABC transporters are associated with a number of diseases (see box on p. 92).

Uniport, symport, and antiport are examples of secondary active transport

Transport processes may be classified into three general types: uniport (monoport), symport (cotransport) and antiport (countertransport) (see Fig. 8.1). Transport substrates move in the same direction during symport, and in opposite directions during antiport. Uniport of charged substrates may be electrophoretically driven by the membrane potential of the cell. The movement of one substrate uphill, against its concentration gradient, can be driven by antiport of another

substrate (usually a cation such as Na^+ or H^+) down a gradient. The proteins participating in these transport systems are termed uniporters, symporters, and antiporters, respectively (see Table 8.1). Some examples are presented below.

Examples of transport systems and their coupling

Ca^{2+} transport and mobilization in muscle

Striated muscle (skeletal and cardiac) is composed of bundles of muscle cells (Chapter 20). Each cell is packed with bundles of actin and myosin filaments (myofibrils) that produce contraction. During muscle contraction, nerves at the neuromuscular junction stimulate local depolarization of the membrane by opening voltage-dependent Na^+ channels. The depolarization spreads rapidly into invaginations of the plasma membrane called the transverse (T) tubules, which extend around the myofibrils (see Fig. 20.5).

Voltage-dependent Ca^{2+} channels (VDCC) located in the T tubules of skeletal muscle change their conformation in response to membrane depolarization, and directly activate a Ca^{2+}-release channel in the sarcoplasmic reticulum membrane, a network of flattened tubules that surrounds each myofibril in the muscle cell cytoplasm. The escape of Ca^{2+} from the lumen (interior compartment) of the sarcoplasmic reticulum increases the cytoplasmic concentration of Ca^{2+} (depolarization-induced Ca^{2+} release) about 100-fold, from 10^{-4} mmol/L (0.0007 mg/L) to about 10^{-2} mmol/L (0.07 mg/dL), triggering ATP hydrolysis by myosin, which initiates muscle contraction. A Ca^{2+}-ATPase in the sarcoplasmic reticulum then hydrolyzes ATP to transport Ca^{2+} back out of the cytoplasm into the lumen of the sarcoplasmic reticulum, decreasing the cytoplasmic Ca^{2+} and allowing the muscle to relax (Fig. 8.4, left).

In cardiac muscle, VDCCs permit the entry of a small amount of Ca^{2+}, which then stimulates Ca^{2+} release through the Ca^{2+} channel from the lumen of the sarcoplasmic reticulum (Ca^{2+}-induced Ca^{2+} release). Not only the sarcoplasmic reticulum Ca^{2+}-ATPase, but also an Na^+/Ca^{2+}-antiporter and a plasma membrane Ca^{2+}-ATPase are responsible for pumping out cytoplasmic Ca^{2+} from heart muscle (Fig. 8.4, right). The rapid restoration of ion gradients allows for rhythmic contraction of the heart.

Role of Na^+/K^+-ATPase in glucose uptake

The transport of blood glucose into cells is generally by facilitated diffusion, as the intracellular concentration of glucose is typically less than that of blood (see Table 8.2). In contrast, the transport of glucose from the intestine into blood involves both facilitated diffusion and active transport

ION GRADIENTS

Concentration gradient and electrochemical gradient of ions

The permeability of most nonelectrolytes through membranes can be analyzed by assuming that the rate-limiting step is the diffusion within the lipid bilayer. Their permeability across a phospholipid bilayer is experimentally shown to be a function of the partition coefficient into organic solvents. The relative rate of simple diffusion of a molecule across the membrane is therefore proportional to the concentration gradient across the bilayer and to the hydrophobicity of the molecule. For charged molecules and ions, transport across the membrane must be facilitated by a transporter or channel, and is driven by the electrochemical gradient, a combination of the concentration gradient (chemical potential) and the voltage gradient across the membrane (electric potential). These forces may act in the same direction or in opposite directions.

In the case of Na^+ ions, the concentration difference between outside (145 mM) and inside (12 mM) the cell is about a factor of 10, being maintained by the Na^+/K^+-ATPase. The Na^+/K^+ATPase is an electrogenic, pumping out three Na^+ and pumping in two K^+ ions, generating an inside-negative membrane potential. K^+ leaks out through K^+ channels, down its concentration gradient (140 mM to 5 mM), further increasing the electric potential. The concentration gradient of Na^+ ions and the electric potential (inside negative) power the import and export of other molecules with Na^+ against their concentration gradient by symporters and antiporters, respectively.

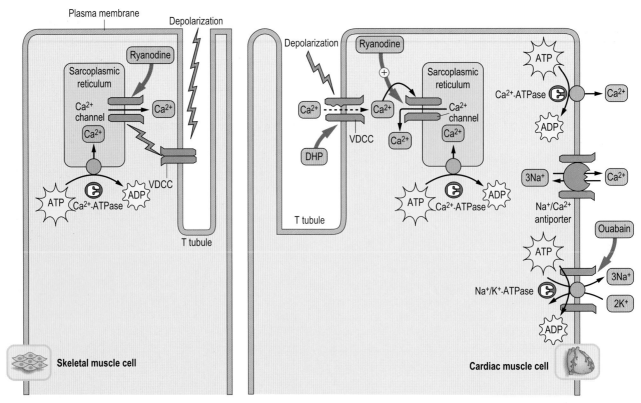

Fig. 8.4 **Ca²⁺ movement in muscle contraction cycle.** Roles of transporters in Ca^{2+} movements in skeletal (left) and cardiac (right) muscle cells during contraction. Thick arrows indicate the binding sites for inhibitors. In skeletal muscle, VDCCs directly activate release of Ca^{2+} from the sarcoplasmic reticulum. The increased cytoplasmic Ca^{2+} concentration triggers muscle contraction. A Ca^{2+}-ATPase in the sarcoplasmic reticulum pumps Ca^{2+} back into the lumen, decreasing the cytoplasmic Ca^{2+} concentration, and the muscle relaxes. In heart muscle, VDCCs allow entry of a small amount of Ca^{2+}, which induces release of Ca^{2+} from the lumen of sarcoplasmic reticulum. Two types of Ca^{2+}-ATPases and an Na^+/Ca^{2+}-antiporter are responsible for pumping cytoplasmic Ca^{2+} out of the muscle cell. The Na^+/Ca^{2+}-antiporter uses the sodium (Na^+) gradient produced by Na^+/K^+-ATPase to antiport Ca^{2+}. DHP, dihydropyridine, nifedipine, a calcium channel blocker used for treatment of hypertension.

processes (Fig. 8.5). Active transport is especially important for maximal recovery of sugars from the intestine when the intestinal concentration of glucose falls below that in the blood.

An Na^+-coupled glucose symporter SGLT1, driven by an Na^+ gradient formed by Na^+/K^+-ATPase, transports glucose into the intestinal epithelial cell, while GLUT-2 facilitates the downhill movement of glucose into the portal circulation (see Fig. 8.5). A similar pathway operates in the kidney.

The kidneys constitute an ultrafiltration system that filters small molecules from blood. However, glucose, amino acids, many ions, and other nutrients in the ultrafiltrate are almost completely reabsorbed in the proximal tubules, by symport processes. Glucose is reabsorbed primarily by sodium glucose transporter 2 (SGLT2; one-to-one Na^+:Glc stoichiometry) into renal proximal tubular epithelial cells. Much smaller amounts of glucose are recovered by SGLT1 in a later segment of the tubule, which couples transport of one molecule of glucose to two sodium ions. The concentration of Na^+ in the filtrate is 140 mmol/L (322 mg/dL), while that inside the epithelial cells is 30 mmol/L (69 mg/dL), so that Na^+ flows 'downhill' along its gradient, dragging glucose 'uphill' against its concentration gradient. As in intestinal epithelial cells, the low intracellular concentration of Na^+ is maintained by an Na^+/K^+-ATPase on

 MODULATION OF TRANSPORTER ACTIVITY IN DIABETES

The ATP-sensitive K^+ channel (K_{ATP}) participates in regulation of insulin secretion in pancreatic islet β-cells. When the blood concentration of glucose increases, glucose is transported into the β-cell through a glucose transporter (GLUT-2) and metabolized, resulting in an increase in cytoplasmic ATP concentration. The ATP binds to the regulatory subunit of the K^+ channel, K_{ATP}-β (called the sulfonylurea receptor, SUR1), causing structural change of a K_{ATP}-α subunit, which closes the K_{ATP} channel. This induces depolarization of the plasma membrane (decreased voltage gradient across the membrane) and activates voltage-dependent calcium (Ca^{2+}) channels (VDCCs). The entry of Ca^{2+} stimulates exocytosis of vesicles that contain insulin. The binding of sulfonylureas such as tolubutamide and glibenclamide to K_{ATP}-β on the outside of the plasma membrane is thought to mimic the regulatory effect of intracellular ATP. Sulfonylureas stimulate insulin secretion, which decreases blood glucose concentration in diabetes. Defective K_{ATP} channels, which are unable to transport K^+, induce low blood glucose concentration, a condition called persistent hyperinsulinemic hyperglycemia of infancy (PHHI), that occurs in 1 per 50 000 persons as a result of loss of K^+-channel function and continuous insulin secretion (see Chapter 21).

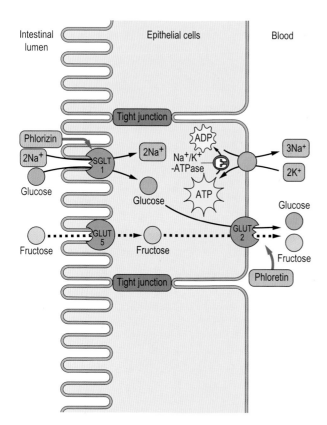

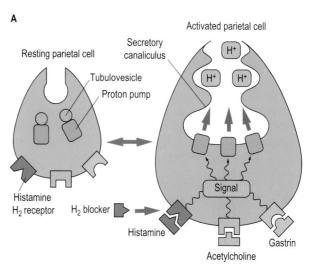

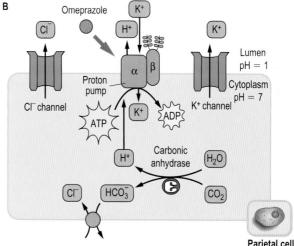

Fig. 8.5 **Glucose transport from intestinal lumen into the blood.** Glucose is pumped into the cell through the Na^+-coupled glucose symporter (SGLT1), and passes out of the cell by facilitated diffusion mediated by the GLUT-2 uniporter. The Na^+ gradient for glucose symport is maintained by the Na^+/K^+-ATPase, which keeps the intracellular concentration of Na^+ low. SGLT1 is inhibited by phlorizin and GLUT-2 by phloretin. Phloretin-insensitive GLUT-5 catalyzes the uptake of fructose by facilitated diffusion. The fructose is then exported through GLUT-2. A defect of SGLT1 causes glucose/galactose malabsorption. Adjacent cells are connected by impermeable tight junctions, which prevent solutes from crossing the epithelium.

✳ VARIOUS DRUGS INHIBIT TRANSPORTERS IN MUSCLE

Phenylalkylamine (verapamil), benzodiazepine (diltiazem), and dihydropyridine (DHP; nifedipine) are Ca^{2+}-channel blockers that inhibit VDCCs (see Fig. 8.4). Ryanodine inhibits the Ca^{2+}-release channel in the sarcoplasmic reticulum. These drugs are used as antihypertensive agents to inhibit the increase in cytoplasmic Ca^{2+} concentration and thus the force of muscle contraction. In contrast, cardiac glycosides such as ouabain and digoxin increase heart muscle contraction and are used for treatment of congestive heart failure. They act by inhibiting the Na^+/K^+-ATPase that generates the Na^+ concentration gradient used to drive export of Ca^{2+} by the Na^+/Ca^{2+} antiporter. Snake venoms such as α-bungarotoxin, and tetrodotoxin from the puffer fish inhibit voltage-dependent Na^+ channels. Lidocaine, an Na^+-channel blocker, is used as a local anesthetic and antiarrhythmic drug. Inhibition of Na^+ channels represses transmission of the depolarization signal.

Fig. 8.6 **Acid secretion from gastric parietal cells.** (A) Acid secretion is stimulated by extracellular signals and accompanied by morphologic changes in parietal cells, from resting (left) to activated (right). The proton pump (H^+/K^+-ATPase) moves to the secretory canaliculus (plasma membrane) from cytoplasmic tubulovesicles. H_2-blockers compete with histamine at the histamine H_2-receptor. (B) Ion balance in the parietal cell. The H^+ transported by the proton pump are supplied by carbonic anhydrase. Bicarbonate, the other product of this enzyme, is antiported with Cl^-, which is secreted through a Cl^- channel. The potassium ions imported by the proton pump are again excreted by a K^+ channel. The proton pump has catalytic α- and glycosylated β-subunits. The drug omeprazole covalently modifies cysteine residues located in the extracytoplasmic domain of the α-subunit and inhibits the proton pump. Thick arrows indicate the binding sites for inhibitors.

the opposite side of the tubular epithelial cell, which antiports three cytoplasmic sodium ions for two extracellular potassium ions, coupled with hydrolysis of a molecule of ATP.

Acidification of gastric juice by a proton pump in the stomach

The lumen of the stomach is highly acidic (pH ≈ 1) because of the presence of a proton pump (H^+/K^+-ATPase; P-ATPase in Table 8.3) that is specifically expressed in gastric parietal

INHIBITING THE GASTRIC PROTON PUMP AND ERADICATION OF *HELICOBACTER PYLORI*

Chronic strong acid secretion by the gastric proton pump injures the stomach and the duodenum, leading to gastric and duodenal ulcers. Proton pump inhibitors such as omeprazole are delivered to parietal cells from the circulation after oral administration. Omeprazole is a prodrug: it accumulates in the acidic compartment, as it is a weak base, and is converted to the active compound under the acidic conditions in the gastric lumen. The active form covalently modifies cysteine residues located in the extracytoplasmic domain of the proton pump. H_2-blockers (receptor antagonists) such as cimetidine and ranitidine indirectly inhibit acid secretion by competing with histamine for its receptor (see Fig. 8.6).

Comment. Infection of the stomach by *Helicobacter pylori* also causes ulcers and is associated with an increased risk of gastric adenocarcinoma. Recently, antibiotic treatment has been introduced to eradicate *H. pylori*. Interestingly, antibiotic treatment together with omeprazole is much more effective, possibly because of an increased stability of the antibiotic under the weakly acidic condition produced by proton pump inhibition.

cells. The gastric proton pump is localized in intracellular vesicles in the resting state. Stimuli such as histamine and gastrin induce fusion of the vesicles with the plasma membrane (Fig. 8.6A). The pump antiports two cytoplasmic protons and two extracellular potassium ions, coupled with hydrolysis of a molecule of ATP; thus it is called an H^+/K^+-ATPase. The counter-ion Cl^- is secreted through a Cl^- channel, producing hydrochloric acid (HCl) (gastric acid) in the lumen (Fig. 8.6B).

Summary

Most of the permeability properties of the membrane are determined by transport proteins, which are integral membrane proteins. Protein-mediated transport is a saturable process with high substrate specificity. Facilitated diffusion is catalyzed by transporters that permit the movement of ions and molecules down concentration gradients, whereas uphill or active transport requires energy. Primary active transport is catalyzed by pump ATPases that use energy produced by ATP hydrolysis. Secondary active transport uses electrochemical gradients of Na^+ and H^+, or membrane potential produced by primary active transport processes. Uniport, symport, and antiport are examples of secondary active transport.

ACTIVE LEARNING

1. Describe the similarities between the kinetics of enzyme action and transport processes. Compare the properties of various glucose transporters with those of hexokinase and glucokinase, both kinetically and in terms of physiologic function.
2. Identify a number of transport inhibitors used in clinical medicine, e.g. Ca^{2+}-channel blockers, laxatives and inhibitors of gastric acid secretion.
3. Investigate the process of glucose transport across the blood–brain barrier and explain the pathogenesis of hypoglycemic coma.
4. Study the role and specificity of ABC transporters in multidrug resistance to chemotherapeutic agents.

Numerous substrates such as ions, nutrients, small organic molecules including drugs and peptides, and proteins are transported by various transporters. All these transporters are indispensable for homeostasis. The expression of unique sets of transporters is important for specific cell functions such as muscle contraction, nutrient and ion absorption by intestinal epithelial cells, resorption of nutrients by kidney cells, and secretion of acid from gastric parietal cells.

Further reading

Camargo SM, Brockenhauer D, Kleta R. Aminoacidurias: clinical and molecular aspects. *Kidney Int* 2008;**73**:918–925.

Klein I, Sarkadi B, Varadi A. An inventory of the human ABC proteins. *Biochim Biophys Acta* 1999;**1461**:237–262.

Lage H. ABC-transporters: implications on drug resistance from microorganisms to human cancers. *Int J Antimicrob Agents* 2003;**22**:188–199.

Linton KJ. Structure and function of ABC transporters. *Physiology* 2007;**22**:122–130.

Wood IS, Trayhurn P. Glucose transporters (GLUT and SGLT): expanded families of sugar transport proteins. *Br J Nutr* 2003;**89**:3–9.

Websites

General reviews:
- http://fajerpc.magnet.fsu.edu/Education/2010/Lectures/12_Membrane_Transport.htm
- http://users.rcn.com/jkimball.ma.ultranet/BiologyPages/D/Diffusion.html#direct
- www.rpi.edu/dept/bcbp/molbiochem/MBWeb/mb1/part2/carriers.htm
Human ABC transporters : http://nutrigene.4t.com/humanabc.htm
P-ATPase: http://biobase.dk/%7Eaxe/Patbase.html
Animation:
- www.stolaf.edu/people/giannini/biological%20anamations.html
- www.wiley.com/legacy/college/boyer/0470003790/animations/membrane_transport/membrane_transport.htm
- www.phschool.com/science/biology_place/biocoach/biomembrane1/quiz.html

9. Bioenergetics and Oxidative Metabolism

L W Stillway

LEARNING OBJECTIVES

After reading this chapter you should be able to:

- Describe how thermodynamics is related to nutrition and obesity.
- Outline the mitochondrial electron transport system showing eight major electron carriers.
- Explain how ubiquinone, heme and the iron–sulfur complexes participate in electron transport.
- Define membrane potential and explain its role in ATP synthesis and thermogenesis.
- Explain the role of uncoupling proteins in thermogenesis.
- Describe the mechanism of ATP synthase.
- Describe the effects of inhibitors such as rotenone, antimycin A, carbon monoxide, cyanide and oligomycin on oxygen uptake by mitochondria.

INTRODUCTION

Oxidation of metabolic fuels is essential to life. In higher organisms, fuels such as carbohydrates and lipids are metabolized to carbon dioxide and water, generating a central metabolic currency, adenosine triphosphate (ATP). Most metabolic energy is produced by oxidation-reduction (redox) reactions in mitochondria. The regulation of energy metabolism is no small feat, because warm-blooded animals have such variable demands for energy from such processes as thermogenesis at low temperatures, stimulation of ATP synthesis during stress, degradation of excess food, efficient use of nutrients during starvation, and coupling of ATP synthesis with the rate of respiration during work and exercise. This chapter will provide an introduction to the concept of free energy, oxidative phosphorylation and the transduction of energy from fuels into useful work. The pathways and specific molecules through which electrons are transported to oxygen and the mechanism of generation of ATP will be described and related to the structure of the mitochondrion, the powerhouse of the cell and the major source of cellular ATP. Lastly, these biochemical processes will be applied to human health and disease.

OXIDATION AS A SOURCE OF ENERGY

Energy content of foods

Nutrition and disorders such as obesity, diabetes, and cancer all require an understanding of thermodynamics. Obesity, for example, is a disorder in which there is an imbalance between energy intake and expenditure. It is therefore important that the energy content of foods be known. The commonly accepted energy values for the four major food categories are shown in Table 9.1; alcohol is included because it is a significant dietary component for some people. These values are obtained by completely burning (oxidizing) samples of each food. Biologically, about 40% of food energy is conserved as ATP, and the remaining 60% is liberated as heat.

The basal metabolic rate (BMR)

The basal metabolic rate (BMR) is the total heat energy released from the body at rest

Virtually all of the reactions in the body are exothermic, and the sum of all reactions at rest is called the basal metabolic rate (BMR), which can be measured by two basic methods: direct calorimetry, where the total heat liberated by

The energy value of food		
Metabolic fuel	**Energy content**	
	kJ/g	kcal/g
fats	38	9
carbohydrates	17	4
proteins	17	4
alcohol	29	7

Table 9.1 **Energy content of the major classes of food.** Note that the thermodynamic term, kcal (energy required to increase the temperature of 1 kg (1 L) of water by 1°C), is equivalent to the common nutritional Calorie (capital C), i.e. 1 Cal = 1 kcal, 1 kcal = 4.2 kJ.

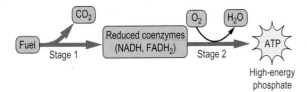

Fig. 9.1 **Stages of fuel oxidation.** NADH, reduced nicotinamide adenine dinucleotide; FADH$_2$, reduced flavin adenine dinucleotide.

an animal is measured over time, and indirect calorimetry, where the BMR is calculated from the quantity of oxygen consumed, which is directly related to the BMR. Adult men (70 kg) have a BMR of about 7500 kJ (1800 kcal) and women about 5400 kJ (1300 kcal) per day; the BMR may vary by a factor of two between individuals, depending on age, sex, body mass and composition. Heat production by mitochondria accounts for the largest portion of the BMR. Elevated thyroid hormones increase the BMR. The BMR is measured under controlled conditions: after an 8-hour sleep, in the reclining position, in the postabsorptive state, typically after a 12-hour fast.

Another measure often used is the RMR, or resting metabolic rate, which is virtually the same as the BMR but measured under less restrictive conditions. The RMR is a measure of minimum energy expenditure at rest; it is typically about 70% of total daily energy expenditure. Exercise scientists frequently use the term MET, Metabolically Equivalent Task, as a measure of energy expenditure at rest. Slow to vigorous walking is a 2–4 MET/h activity; vigorous running on a treadmill may consume more than 15 MET/h.

Stages of fuel oxidation

The oxidation of fuels can be divided into two general stages: production of reduced nucleotide coenzymes during the oxidation of fuels, and use of the free energy from oxidation of the reduced coenzymes to produce ATP (Fig. 9.1).

FREE ENERGY

The Gibbs' free energy (ΔG) of a reaction is the maximum amount of energy that can be obtained from a reaction at constant temperature and pressure. The units of free energy are kcal/mol (kJ/mol). It is not possible to measure the absolute free energy content of a substance directly, but when reactant A reacts to form product B, the free energy change in this reaction, ΔG, can be determined.

For the reaction A $\rightarrow$ B:

$$\Delta G = G_B - G_A$$

where G_A and G_B are the free energy of A and B, respectively. All reactions in biologic systems are considered to be reversible reactions, so that the free energy of the reverse reaction, B $\rightarrow$ A, is numerically equivalent, but opposite in sign to that of the forward reaction.

If there is a greater concentration of B than of A at equilibrium, the conversion A $\rightarrow$ B is favorable – that is, the reaction tends to move forward from a standard state in which A and B are present at equal concentrations. In this case, the reaction is said to be a spontaneous or exergonic reaction, and the free energy of this reaction is defined as negative: that is, $\Delta G < 0$, indicating that energy is liberated by the reaction. Conversely, if the concentration of A is greater than that of B at equilibrium, the forward reaction is termed unfavorable, nonspontaneous or endergonic, and the reaction has a positive free energy: that is, B tends to form A, rather than A to form B. In this case, energy input would be required to push the reaction A $\rightarrow$ B forward from its equilibrium position to the standard state in which A and B are present at equal concentrations. The total free energy available from a reaction depends on both its tendency to proceed forward from the standard state (ΔG) and the amount (moles) of reactant converted to product.

The free energy of metabolic reactions is related to their equilibrium constants

Thermodynamic measurements are based on standard-state conditions where reactant and product are present at 1 molar concentrations, the pressure of all gases is 1 atmosphere and the temperature is 25°C (298°K). Most commonly, the concentrations of reactants and products are then measured after equilibrium is attained. Standard free energies are represented by the symbol $\Delta G°$ and biological standard free energy change by $\Delta G°'$, with the accent symbol designating pH 7.0. The free energy available from a reaction may be calculated from its equilibrium constant by the Gibbs equation:

$$\Delta G°' = -RT \ln K'eq$$

where T is absolute temperature (°Kelvin), $\ln K'eq$ is the natural logarithm of the equilibrium constant for the reaction at pH 7, and R is the gas constant:

$$R = 8.3 \, J \, K^{-1} \, mol^{-1} \quad or \quad \sim 2 \, cal \, K^{-1} \, mol^{-1}$$

Several common metabolic intermediates that you will encounter in your studies are listed in Table 9.2, along with the equilibrium constants and free energies for their hydrolysis reactions. Those intermediates with free energy changes equal to or greater than that of ATP, the central energy transducer of the cell, are considered to be high-energy compounds, and generally have either anhydride or thioester bonds. The lower-energy compounds listed are all phosphate esters and, in comparison, do not yield as much free energy on hydrolysis.

Thermodynamics of hydrolysis reactions			
Metabolite	**K′eq**	**$\Delta G°'$**	
		$(kJ\,mol^{-1})$	**$(kcal\,mol^{-1})$**
phosphoenolpyruvate	1.2×10^{11}	-61.8	-14.8
phosphocreatine	9.6×10^{8}	-50.2	-12.0
1,3-bisphosphoglycerate	6.8×10^{8}	-49.3	-11.8
pyrophosphate	9.7×10^{5}	-33.4	-8.0
acetyl coenzyme A	4.1×10^{5}	-31.3	-7.5
ATP	2.9×10^{5}	-30.5	-7.3
glucose-1-phosphate	5.5×10^{3}	-20.9	-5.0
fructose-6-phosphate	7.0×10^{2}	-15.9	-3.8
glucose-6-phosphate	3.0×10^{2}	-13.8	-3.3

Table 9.2 **Thermodynamics of hydrolysis reactions.** Equilibrium constants and free energy of hydrolysis of various metabolic intermediates at pH 7 ($\Delta G°'$).

The hydrolysis reaction of glucose-6-phosphate (Glc-6-P) is written as:

$$Glc\text{-}6\text{-}P + H_2O \rightarrow Glucose + Pi$$

$$\Delta G°' = -13.8\,kJ/mol\,(-3.3\,kcal/mol)$$

This reaction has a negative free energy and occurs spontaneously. The reverse reaction, synthesis of Glc-6-P from glucose and phosphate, would require input of energy.

CONSERVATION OF ENERGY BY COUPLING WITH ADENOSINE TRIPHOSPHATE

Living systems must transfer energy from one molecule to another without losing all of it as heat. Some of the energy must be conserved in a chemical form in order to drive nonspontaneous biosynthetic reactions. In fact, nearly half of the energy obtained from the oxidation of metabolic fuels is channeled into the synthesis of ATP, a universal energy transducer in living systems. ATP is often referred to as the common currency of metabolic energy, because it is used to drive so many energy-requiring reactions. ATP consists of the purine base adenine, the five-carbon sugar ribose, and α, β, and γ phosphate groups (Fig. 9.2). The two anhydride linkages are said to be high-energy bonds, because their hydrolysis yields a large negative change in free energy. When ATP is used for metabolic work, these high-energy linkages are broken and ATP is converted to ADP or to AMP.

ATP is commonly used to drive biosynthetic reactions

The free energy of a high-energy bond, such as the phosphate anhydride bonds in ATP, can be used to drive or push forward reactions that would otherwise be unfavorable. In fact, nearly all biosynthetic pathways are thermodynamically unfavorable, but are made favorable by coupling various reactions with hydrolysis of high-energy compounds. For example, the first step in the metabolism of glucose is the synthesis of Glc-6-P. As shown in Table 9.2, this is not a favorable reaction: the hydrolysis ($\Delta G°' = -13.8\,kJ/mol$ or $-3.3\,kcal/mol$), rather than synthesis ($\Delta G°' = +13.8\,kJ/mol$ or $+3.3\,kcal/mol$), of Glc-6-P is the favored reaction. However, as shown below, the synthesis of Glc-6-P (reaction I) can be energetically coupled to the hydrolysis of ATP (reaction II), yielding a 'net reaction' III that is favorable for synthesis of Glc-6-P:

$$\Delta G°'$$

I: $Glc + Pi \rightarrow Glc\text{-}6\text{-}P + H_2O$ $+3.3\,kcal/mol$

II: $ATP + H_2O \rightarrow ADP + Pi$ $-7.3\,kcal/mol$

Net: $Glc + ATP \rightarrow Glc\text{-}6\text{-}P + ADP$ $-4\,kcal/mol$

This is possible because of the high free energy or 'group transfer potential' of ATP. The physical transfer of the phosphate from ATP to glucose occurs in the active site of a kinase enzyme, such as glucokinase. This motif, in which ATP is used to drive biosynthetic reactions, transport processes or muscle activity, occurs commonly in metabolic pathways.

MITOCHONDRIAL SYNTHESIS OF ADENOSINE TRIPHOSPHATE FROM REDUCED COENZYMES

Metabolism of carbohydrates begins in the cytoplasm through the glycolytic pathway (see Chapter 12), whereas energy production from fatty acids occurs exclusively in the mitochondrion. Mitochondria are subcellular organelles, about the size of bacteria. They are essential for aerobic metabolism in eukaryotes. Their main function is to oxidize metabolic fuels and conserve free energy by synthesizing ATP.

Mitochondria are bounded by a dual membrane system (Fig. 9.3). The outer membrane (OMM) contains enzyme and transport proteins and via the pore-forming protein porin (P), it is permeable to virtually all ions, small molecules (S) and proteins less than 10 000 Da. Large proteins must be transported via the TOM (translocase in the outer mitochondrial membrane) and TIM (translocases in the inner mitochondrial membrane) complexes. This is especially vital to the cell, because almost all mitochondrial proteins are nuclear

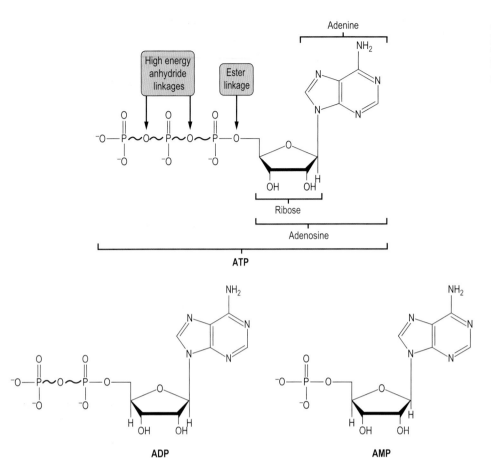

Fig. 9.2 **Structures of high-energy phosphates.** ATP is shown, together with its hydrolysis products, adenosine diphosphate (ADP) and adenosine monophosphate (AMP).

EXERCISE AND MITOCHONDRIAL BIOGENESIS

It has long been known that exercise increases the oxidative capacity of skeletal muscle by inducing mitochondrial biogenesis. Continued exercise results in energy consumption, and AMP accumulates. AMP-activated protein kinase (AMPK) is a fuel sensor, and it plays a critical role in initiating the production of new mitochondria and electron transport components such as heme. Such mechanisms are of importance not only in exercise training, but also in the regeneration of tissues after tissue injury, such as trauma, heart attacks and strokes.

encoded and must be transported into the mitochondrion. The mitochondrial genome, mtDNA, encodes 13 vital subunits of the proton pumps and ATP synthase. The inner membrane (IMM) is pleated with structures known as cristae, and is impermeable to most ions and small molecules, such as nucleotides (including ATP), coenzymes, phosphate, and protons. Transporter proteins are required to selectively facilitate translocation of specific molecules across the inner membrane. The inner membrane also contains components of oxidative phosphorylation – the process by which the oxidation of reduced nucleotide coenzymes is coupled to the synthesis of ATP.

Transduction of energy from reduced coenzymes to high-energy phosphate

NAD⁺, FAD, and FMN are the major redox coenzymes

The major redox coenzymes involved in transduction of energy from fuels to ATP are nicotinamide adenine dinucleotide (NAD⁺), flavin adenine dinucleotide (FAD) and flavin mononucleotide (FMN) (Fig. 9.4). During energy metabolism, electrons are transferred from carbohydrates and fats to these coenzymes, reducing them to NADH, FADH$_2$ and FMNH$_2$. In each case, two electrons are transferred, but the number of protons transferred differs. NAD⁺ accepts a hydride ion (H⁻) that consists of one proton and two electrons; the remaining proton is released into solution. FAD and FMN accept two electrons and two protons.

The oxidation of reduced nucleotides by the electron transport system produces a large amount of free energy. When the oxidation of 1 mole of NADH is coupled to the reduction of 0.5 mole of oxygen to form water, the energy produced is theoretically sufficient to synthesize seven moles of ATP:

$$NADH + H^+ + \tfrac{1}{2}O_2 \rightarrow NAD^+ + H_2O$$
$$\Delta G^{\circ\prime} = -220\,kJ/mol\ (-52.4\,kcal/mol)$$

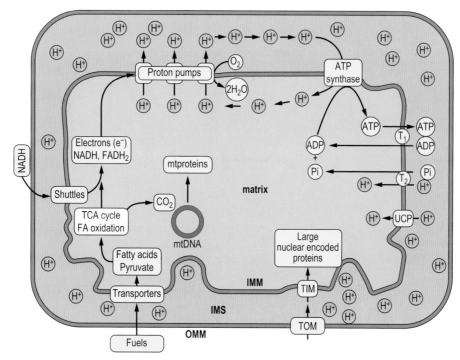

Fig. 9.3 **Mitochondrial structure and pathways of energy transduction: the mechanism of oxidative phosphorylation.** Major fuels, such as pyruvate and fatty acids (FA), are transported into the matrix where they are oxidized to generate CO_2 and the reduced nucleotide coenzymes NADH and $FADH_2$. Oxidation of these nucleotides via the electron transport system reduces oxygen to water and pumps protons by three proton pumps out of the matrix and into the intermembrane space (IMS), creating a pH gradient, which is the major contributor to the membrane potential. It should be noted that protons in the intermembrane space freely diffuse through the outer membrane via the protein porin, so the intermembrane space is roughly equivalent to the cytosol. Although the membrane potential is mostly composed of the proton gradient it actually consists of several electrochemical gradients and is expressed as a voltage. Controlled influx of protons through ATP synthase powers the synthesis of ATP by ATP synthase. Mitochondrial ATP is then exchanged for cytoplasmic ADP through the ADP-ATP translocase (T_1). Phosphate (Pi), which is also required for ATP synthesis, is transported by the phosphate translocase (T_2). The inner membrane also contains uncoupling proteins (UCP) that may be used to allow the controlled leakage of protons back into the matrix. OMM, outer mitochondrial membrane; IMM, inner mitochondrial membrane; mtproteins, mitochondrial proteins; mtDNA, mitochondrial DNA; TOM and TIM, protein translocase complexes in outer and inner mitochondrial membrane; TCA, tricarboxylic acid cycle.

METABOLIC FUNCTION OF ATP REQUIRES MAGNESIUM

ATP readily forms a complex with magnesium ion, and it is this complex that is required in all reactions in which ATP participates, including its synthesis. A magnesium deficiency impairs virtually all of metabolism, because ATP can neither be made nor utilized in adequate amounts.

$$ADP + Pi \rightarrow ATP + H_2O$$

$$\Delta G^{\circ\prime} = -30.5 \text{ kJ/mol } (-7.3 \text{ kcal/mol}) \text{ (see Table 9.2)}$$

Dividing 220 kJ/mol of $\Delta G^{\circ\prime}$ available from oxidation of NADH by $\Delta G^{\circ\prime}$ 30.5 required for synthesis of ATP yields theoretically ~ 7 mol ATP/mol NADH. As discussed below, the actual yield is closer to 2.5 mol ATP/mol NADH oxidized.

The free energy of oxidation of NADH is used via the electron transport system to pump protons into the intermembrane space. The energy produced when these protons reenter the mitochondrial matrix is used to synthesize ATP. This process is known as oxidative phosphorylation (see Fig. 9.3).

THE MITOCHONDRIAL ELECTRON TRANSPORT SYSTEM

The entire electron transport system, also known as the electron transport chain or respiratory chain, is located in the inner mitochondrial membrane (Fig. 9.5). It consists of several large protein complexes and two small, independent components – ubiquinone and cytochrome *c*. The protein components are each very complex; complex I, for example, contains at least 46 subunits. Each step in the electron transport chain involves a redox reaction where electrons

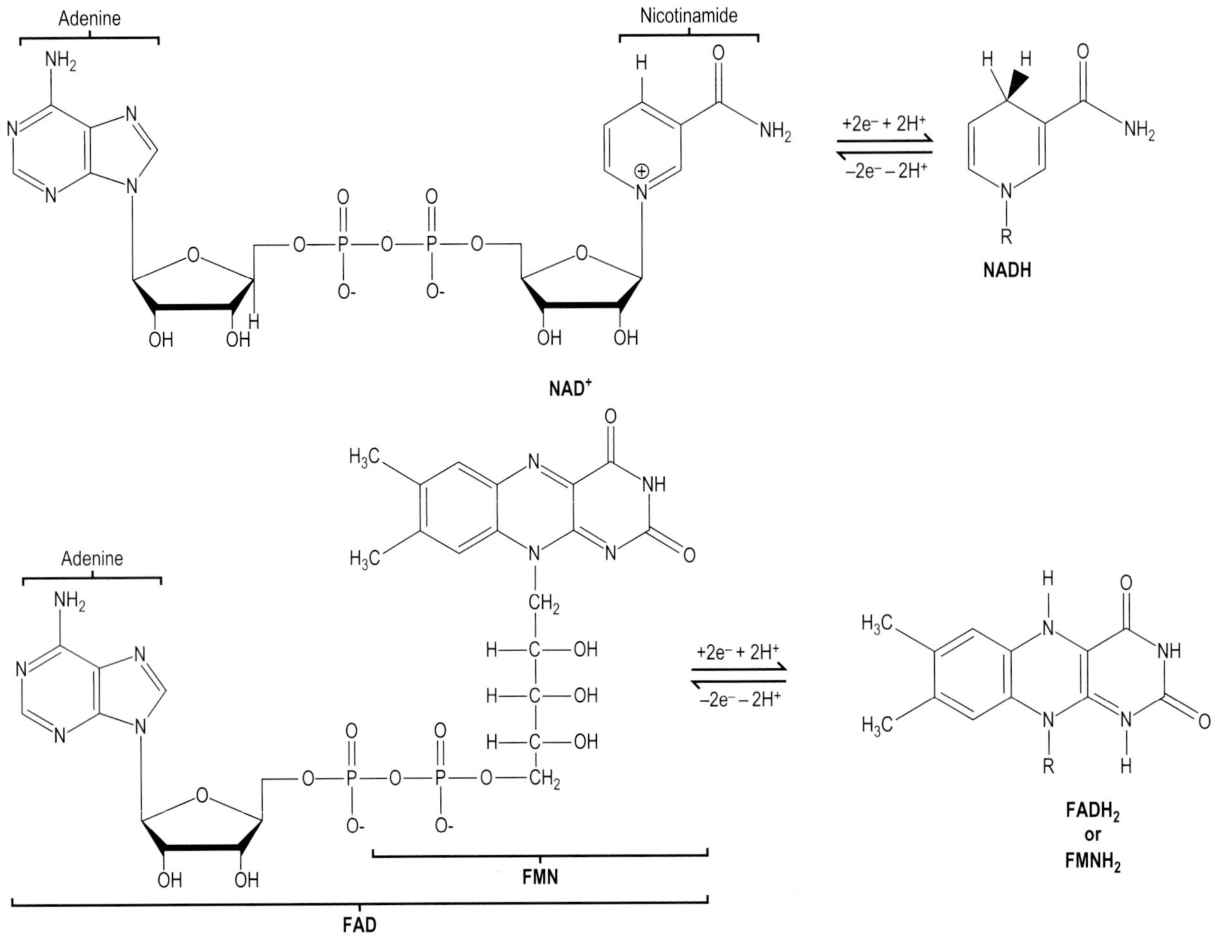

Fig. 9.4 **The structure of redox coenzymes.** NAD$^+$ and its reduced form, NADH (nicotinamide adenine dinucleotide), consists of adenine, two ribose units, two phosphates, and nicotinamide. FAD and its reduced form, FADH$_2$ (flavin adenine dinucleotide), consists of riboflavin, two phosphates, ribose and adenine. FMN and FMNH$_2$ consist of riboflavin phosphate. The nicotinamide and riboflavin components of these coenzymes are reversibly oxidized and reduced during electron transfer (redox) reactions. NADH and FADH$_2$ are often called reduced nucleotides or reduced coenzymes.

leave components with more negative reduction potentials and go to components with more positive reduction potentials. Electrons are conducted through this system in a defined sequence from reduced nucleotide coenzymes to oxygen, and the free energy changes drive the transport of protons from the matrix into the intermembrane space via the three proton pumps. After each step, the electrons are at a lower energy state.

Electrons are funneled into the electron transport chain by several flavoproteins. Of these, there are four major species, including complex I, which contains FMN, and three that contain FAD. These pathways all reduce the small, lipophilic molecule ubiquinone (Q or coenzyme Q_{10}), at the beginning of the common electron transport pathway, consisting of Q, complex III, cytochrome *c*, and complex IV.

$$\text{Flavoprotein}_{(reduced)} + Q \rightarrow \text{Flavoprotein}_{(oxidized)} + QH_2$$

Protons are pumped from the matrix into the intermembrane space by complexes I, III, and IV. Oxygen (O_2) is the final

electron acceptor at the end of the chain, and it is reduced to two water molecules by the transfer of four electrons from complex IV.

The efficiency of oxidative phosphorylation is measured by dividing the amount of phosphate incorporated into ADP by the amount of atomic oxygen reduced. One atom of oxygen is reduced by two electrons (one electron pair).

$$ADP + Pi + \tfrac{1}{2}O_2 + 2H^+ + 2e^- \rightarrow ATP + H_2O$$

For each pair of electrons transported through complexes I, III or IV, a sufficient number of protons is pumped by each complex for the synthesis of approximately one mole of ATP/complex. If electron transport begins with an electron pair from NADH, approximately 2.5 moles of ATP are synthesized, whereas an electron pair from any of the other three FADH$_2$-containing flavoproteins yields about 1.5 moles of ATP, because the proton-pumping capability of complex I is bypassed.

Flavoproteins contain FAD or FMN prosthetic groups

Complex I, also called NADH-Q reductase or NADH dehydrogenase, is a flavoprotein containing FMN. It oxidizes mitochondrial NADH, and transfers electrons through FMN and iron–sulfur (FeS) complexes to ubiquinone, providing enough energy to pump four protons from the matrix in the reaction:

$$NADH + Q + 5H^+_{matrix} \rightarrow NAD^+ + QH_2 + 4H^+_{intermembrane\ space}$$

Three other flavoproteins transfer electrons from oxidizable substrates via $FADH_2$ to ubiquinone (Q) (see Fig. 9.5):

- succinate – Q reductase (complex II or succinate dehydrogenase of the TCA cycle) (see Chapter 14) oxidizes succinate to fumarate and reduces FAD to $FADH_2$
- glycerol-3-phosphate – Q reductase, a part of the glycerol-3-P shuttle (see below), oxidizes cytoplasmic glycerol-3-P to dihydroxyacetone phosphate (DHAP) and reduces FAD to $FADH_2$
- fatty acyl CoA dehydrogenase catalyzes the first step in the mitochondrial oxidation of fatty acids and also produces $FADH_2$.

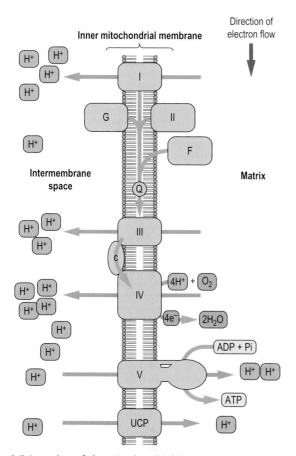

Fig. 9.5 **A section of the mitochondrial inner membrane with the electron transport system and ATP synthase.** I, complex I; II, complex II; III, complex III; IV, complex IV; V, complex V or ATP synthase; G, glycerol 3-phosphate dehydrogenase; F, fatty acyl CoA dehydrogenase; Q, ubiquinone; c, cytochrome c; UCP, uncoupling protein.

 IRON DEFICIENCY LEADS TO ANEMIA

A 45-year-old woman complains of tiredness and appears pale. She is a vegetarian and is experiencing a monthly menstrual flow that is heavy and prolonged. Her hematocrit is 0.32 (reference range 0.41–0.46) and her hemoglobin concentration 9 g/L (normal range 120–160 g/L; 12–16 g/dL).

Comment. Iron deficiency anemia is a common nutritional problem and is especially common in menstruating and pregnant women because of their increased dietary requirement for iron. Men require about 1 mg iron/day, menstruating women about 2 mg/day, and pregnant women about 3 mg/day. Iron is required to maintain normal amounts of hemoglobin, the cytochromes, and iron–sulfur complexes that are central to oxygen transport and energy metabolism. All these processes are impaired in iron deficiency. Heme iron, which is found in meats, is absorbed much more readily than inorganic iron such as that found in egg yolks, vegetables, and nuts.

 A RARE COENZYME Q$_{10}$ DEFICIENCY

A 4-year-old boy presented with seizures, progressive muscle weakness, and encephalopathy. Accumulation of lactate, a product of anaerobic metabolism of glucose, in the cerebrospinal fluid (CSF) suggested a defect in mitochondrial oxidative metabolism. Muscle mitochondria were isolated for study. The activities of the individual Complexes I, II, III, and IV were normal, but the combined activities of I + III and II + III were significantly decreased. Treatment with coenzyme Q$_{10}$ improved the muscle weakness, but not the encephalopathy.

Comment. Severe muscle weakness, encephalopathy, or both, may be caused in so-called mitochondrial myopathies by mitochondrial defects involving the electron transport system. The finding of increased lactate in the CSF suggests a defect in oxidative phosphorylation. The decreased activities of complexes I + III and II + III suggested a deficiency in coenzyme Q$_{10}$, which was confirmed by direct measurements.

✳ IRON–SULFUR COMPLEXES

Iron–sulfur complexes participate in redox reactions

Iron is an important constituent of heme proteins, such as hemoglobin, myoglobin, cytochromes, and catalase, but it is also associated with iron–sulfur (FeS) complexes or nonheme iron proteins that function as electron transporters in the mitochondrial electron transport system. The Fe_2S_2 and Fe_4S_4 types are shown in Figure 9.6. In each case, the iron–sulfur center is bound to a peptide through cysteine residues. The FeS complexes undergo one-electron redox reactions that induce reversible distortion and relaxation. The redox energy is said to be conserved in the 'conformational energy' of the protein (see Chapter 37).

Both FMN and FAD contain the water-soluble vitamin riboflavin. A dietary deficiency of riboflavin can severely impair the function of these and other flavoproteins.

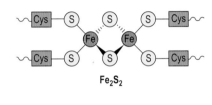

Fe_2S_2

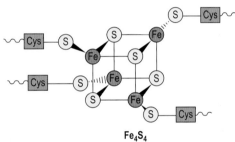

Fe_4S_4

Fig. 9.6 **Iron-sulfur complexes.** Cys, cysteine.

TRANSFER OF ELECTRONS FROM NADH INTO MITOCHONDRIA

Electron shuttles

NADH is produced in the cytosol during carbohydrate metabolism. NADH cannot cross the inner mitochondrial membrane, and therefore it cannot be oxidized by the electron transport system. Two redox shuttles permit the oxidation of cytosolic NADH without its physical transfer into the mitochondrion. A characteristic feature of these shuttles is that they are powered by cytoplasmic and mitochondrial isoforms of the same enzyme. The glycerol-3-P shuttle is the simpler of the two (Fig. 9.7A). It transfers the electrons of NADH from the cytoplasm to the mitochondrion by reducing FAD to $FADH_2$. Cytoplasmic glycerol-3-P dehydrogenase catalyzes reduction of DHAP with NADH to glycerol-3-P. The cytoplasmic glycerol-3-phosphate is oxidized back to DHAP by another glycerol-3-phosphate dehydrogenase isoform facing the outer surface of the inner mitochondrial membrane; this enzyme is a flavoprotein in which FAD is reduced to $FADH_2$. The electrons are then transferred to the common pathway via ubiquinone. The yield of ATP from cytoplasmic NADH by this pathway is approximately 1.5 moles, rather than the 2.5 moles available from mitochondrial NADH via the NADH-Q reductase complex (complex I).

Many cells, e.g. in skeletal muscle, use the glycerol 3-P shuttle, but heart and liver rely on the malate-aspartate shuttle (Fig. 9.7B), which yields 2.5 moles of ATP per mole of NADH. This shuttle is more complicated, because the substrate, malate, can cross the inner mitochondrial membrane, but the membrane is impermeable to the product, oxaloacetate – there is no oxaloacetate transporter. The exchange is therefore accomplished by interconversion between α-keto- and α-amino acids, involving cytoplasmic and mitochondrial glutamate and α-ketoglutarate, and isozymes of glutamate-oxaloacetate transaminase (aspartate aminotransferase).

Ubiquinone (coenzyme Q₁₀) transfers electrons to complex III

Ubiquinone is so named because it is ubiquitous in virtually all living systems. It is a small, lipid-soluble compound found in the inner membrane of animal and plant mitochondria and in the plasma membrane of bacteria. The primary form of mammalian ubiquinone contains a side chain of 10 isoprene units and is often called CoQ_{10}. It diffuses within the inner membrane, accepts electrons from the four major mitochondrial flavoproteins, and transfers them to complex III (QH₂-cytochrome *c* reductase). Ubiquinone

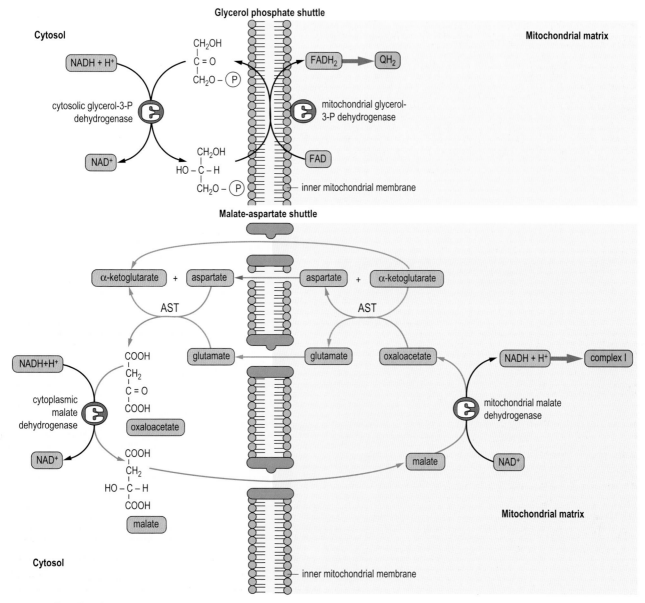

Fig. 9.7 **Redox shuttles in the inner mitochondrial membrane.** (Top) The glycerol phosphate shuttle. (Bottom) The malate-aspartate shuttles. AST, aspartate aminotransferase.

can carry either one or two electrons (Fig. 9.8) and is also thought to be a major source of superoxide radicals in the cell (see Chapter 37).

Complex III – cytochrome *c* reductase

This enzyme complex, also known as ubiquinone-cytochrome *c* reductase or QH$_2$-cytochrome *c* reductase, oxidizes ubiquinone and reduces cytochrome *c*. Reduced ubiquinone funnels electrons that it gathers from mitochondrial flavoproteins and transfers them to complex III. Electrons from ubiquinone are

transferred through two species of cytochrome *b*, to an FeS center, to cytochrome c_1, and finally to cytochrome *c*. Transport of two electrons to cytochrome *c* yields sufficient free energy change and protons pumped to synthesize about one mole of ATP. The overall reaction is:

$$QH_2 + 2cyt\ c_{oxidized} + 2H^+_{matrix} \rightarrow$$
$$2Q + 2cyt\ c_{reduced} + 4H^+_{intermembrane\ space}$$

Four protons are pumped during this reaction, two from fully reduced ubiquinone and two from the matrix.

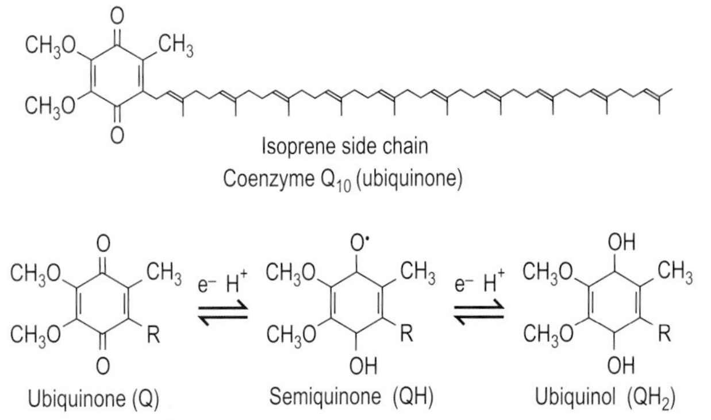

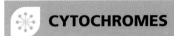

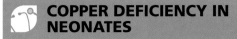

Fig. 9.8 **Coenzyme Q$_{10}$, or ubiquinone,** accepts one or two electrons, transferring them from flavoproteins to complex III. The semiquinone form is a free radical.

CYTOCHROMES

Cytochromes, found in the mitochondrion and endoplasmic reticulum, are proteins that contain heme groups, but which are not involved in oxygen transport (Fig. 9.9). The core structure of these heme groups is a tetrapyrrole ring similar to that of hemoglobin, sometimes differing only in the composition of the side chains. The heme group of cytochromes b and c$_1$ is known as iron protoporphyrin IX and is the same heme that is found in hemoglobin, myoglobin, and catalase. Cytochrome c contains heme C that is covalently bound to the protein through cysteine residues. Cytochromes a and a$_3$ contain heme A which, in common with ubiquinone, contains a hydrophobic isoprene side chain. In hemoglobin and myoglobin, heme must remain in the ferrous (Fe^{2+}) state; in cytochromes, the heme iron is reversibly reduced and oxidized between the Fe^{2+} and Fe^{3+} states as electrons are shuttled from one protein to another.

Cytochrome *c*

Cytochrome *c*, a small heme protein that is loosely bound to the outer surface of the inner membrane, shuttles electrons from complex III to complex IV. Each cytochrome *c* carries only one electron, so the reduction of O$_2$ to 2 H$_2$O by complex IV requires four reduced cytochrome *c* molecules. The binding of cytochrome *c* to complexes III and IV is largely electrostatic, involving a number of lysine residues on the protein surface. Reduction of ferricytochrome *c* (Fe^{3+}) to ferrocytochrome *c* (Fe^{2+}) by cytochrome *c*$_1$ leads to a change in the three-dimensional structure, charge distribution and dipole moment of the protein, promoting transfer of electrons to cytochrome *a* in complex IV (see Fig. 9.5). Under certain conditions (at low membrane potentials), cytochrome *c* may be released from the inner mitochondrial membrane and leak into the cytosol, inducing apoptosis (cell death).

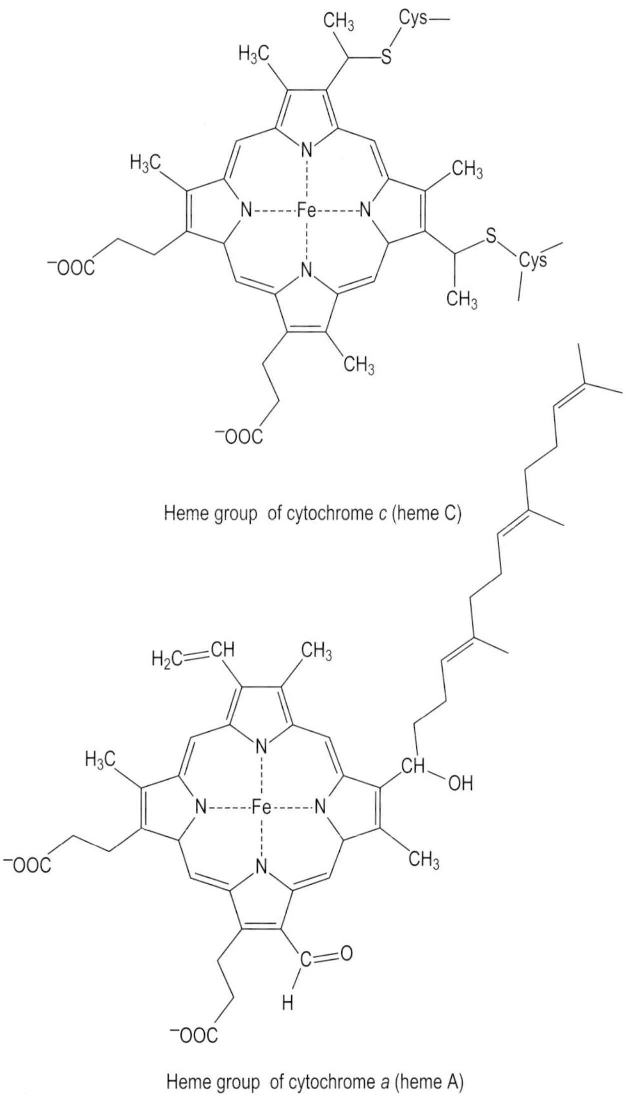

Heme group of cytochrome *c* (heme C)

Heme group of cytochrome *a* (heme A)

Fig. 9.9 **Variations in heme structures among cytochromes.** The cytochromes are proteins that contain heme groups.

COPPER DEFICIENCY IN NEONATES

Copper is required in trace amounts for optimal human nutrition. Although copper deficiency is rare in adults, premature infants have low stores of copper and may suffer from its deficiency. This may lead to anemia and cardiomyopathy, because of failure to synthesize adequate amounts of cytochrome c oxidase and other enzymes, including several cuproenzymes involved in the synthesis of heme.

Comment. Copper deficiency can impair ATP production by inhibiting the terminal reaction of the electron transport chain, leading to pathology in the heart, where energy demand is high. Dietary formulas for premature infants must contain adequate copper; cow's milk alone is unsuitable, because it is low in copper.

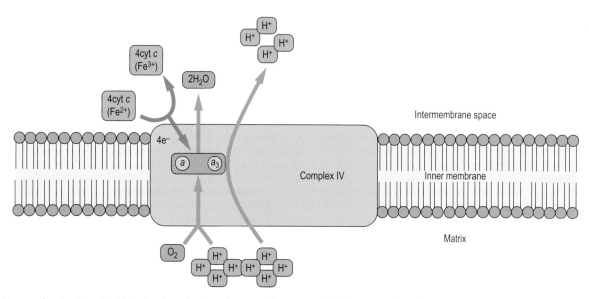

Fig. 9.10 **Complex IV.** Complex IV utilizes four electrons from cytochrome c and eight protons from the matrix. Four protons and electrons reduce oxygen to water. Four additional protons are pumped out of the matrix. Complex IV is regulated allosterically by ATP, by reversible phosphorylation/dephosphorylation, and by thyroid hormone (T_2 or diiodothyronine). *a*, cytochrome *a*; a_3, cytochrome a_3.

Complex IV

Complex IV, known as cytochrome *c* oxidase or cytochrome oxidase, exists as a dimer in the IMM. It oxidizes the mobile cytochrome *c*, and conducts electrons through cytochromes *a* and a_3, finally reducing oxygen to water in a four-electron transfer reaction (Fig. 9.10). Copper is a common component of this and other oxidase enzymes. Small molecule poisons, such as azide, cyanide, and carbon monoxide, bind to the heme group of cytochrome a_3 in cytochrome *c* oxidase and inhibit complex IV. In common with complexes I and III, the cytochrome oxidase complex pumps protons out of mitochondria, providing for the synthesis of about one mole of ATP per pair of electrons transferred to oxygen. The actual number of protons pumped is four. In addition, another four are required in the reduction of O_2 to water. The overall reaction catalyzed by complex IV is:

$$4\text{cyt c}_{\text{reduced}} + 4\text{H}^+_{(\text{matrix})} + O_2 \rightarrow 4\text{cyt c}_{\text{oxidized}} + 2\text{H}_2\text{O}$$

SYNTHESIS OF ADENOSINE TRIPHOSPHATE – THE CHEMIOSMOTIC HYPOTHESIS

According to the chemiosmotic hypothesis, mitochondria produce ATP using the free energy from the proton gradient generated during oxidation of NADH and $FADH_2$. This energy is described as a proton motive force, an electrochemical gradient created by the proton concentration gradient and a proton charge differential (outside positive) across

the inner mitochondrial membrane. To operate, it requires an inner membrane system that is impermeable to protons, except through ATP synthase or other complexes in a regulated fashion. When protons are pumped out of the matrix, the intermembrane space becomes more acidic and more positively charged than the matrix.

The ATP synthase complex (complex V) is an example of rotary catalysis

Lining the inner matrix face of the inner membrane of each mitochondrion are thousands of copies of the ATP synthase complex, also called complex V or F_0F_1-ATP synthase (F = coupling factor; see Inhibitors of ATP Synthase, below). ATP synthase is also called an ATPase, because it can hydrolyze ATP. ATP synthase consists of two major complexes (Fig. 9.11). The inner membrane component, termed F_0, is the proton-driven motor with the stoichiometry of *a*, b_2 and c_{10-14}. The *c*-subunits form the *c*-ring, which rotates in a clockwise direction in response to the flow of protons through the complex. Since the γ and ε-subunits are bound to the *c*-ring, they rotate with it, inducing large conformational changes in the three-αβ dimers. The two β proteins immobilize the second complex (F_1-ATP synthase).

F_1 has a stoichiometry of $α_3$, $β_3$, γ, δ, ε. The major part of F_1 consists of three αβ dimers arranged like slices of an orange, with the catalytic activity residing on the β-subunits. Each 120° rotation of the γ-subunit induces conformational changes in the αβ-dimeric subunits such that the nucleotide-binding sites alternate between three states: the first binds ADP and Pi, the second synthesizes ATP, and the third releases ATP, so each complete turn produces 3ATP. This is known as the binding-change mechanism (Fig. 9.12). Surprisingly, the proton-motive free energy

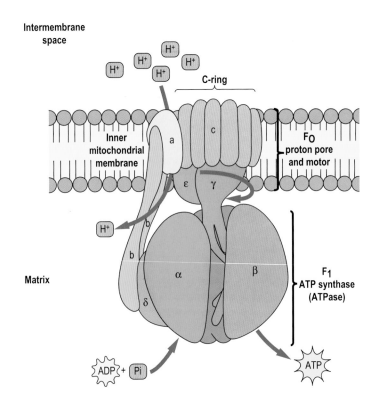

Fig. 9.11 **ATP synthase complex.** The ATP synthase complex consists of a motor (F_O) and generator (F_1). The proton pore involves the c-ring and the a-protein. The rotary component is the coiled-coil γ-subunit, which is bound to the ε-subunit and to the c-ring. The stationary component is the hexameric $\alpha_3\beta_3$ unit, which is held in place by the δ, b and a-proteins.

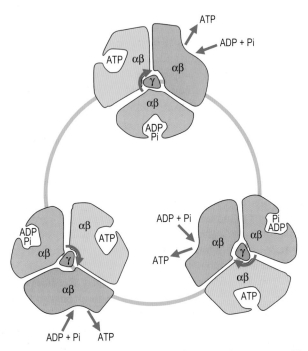

Fig. 9.12 **Binding-change mechanism of ATP synthase.** Powered by protons, the rotation of the γ-subunit of ATP synthase induces simultaneous conformational changes in all three αβ-dimers. Each 120° rotation results in ejection of an ATP, binding of ADP and Pi and ATP synthesis.

used by ATP synthase is not for ATP synthesis itself, but for its release; when the proton gradient is too low to support ATP release, ATP remains stuck to ATP synthase and further ATP production ceases. ADP and Pi are bound to the complex as soon as ATP leaves. The αβ-dimers are asymmetrical, because each is in a different conformation at any given moment. This complex is a proton-driven motor, and it is an example of rotary catalysis. About three protons are required for the synthesis of each ATP. This complex acts independently of the electron transport chain; addition of a weak acid, such as acetic acid, to a suspension of isolated mitochondria is sufficient to induce the biosynthesis of ATP in vitro.

P:O ratios

The P:O ratio is a measure of the number of high-energy phosphates (i.e. amount of ATP) synthesized per atom of oxygen ($\frac{1}{2}O_2$) consumed, or per mole of water produced. The P:O ratio can be calculated from the moles of ADP used to synthesize ATP and the atoms of oxygen taken up by mitochondria. For example, if 2 mmol of ADP is converted to ATP and 0.5 mmol of oxygen (1.0 milliatom of oxygen) is taken up, the P:O ratio is 2.0. As discussed earlier, the theoretical

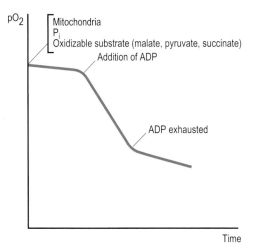

Fig. 9.13 **Effect of ADP on the uptake of oxygen by isolated mitochondria.** This may be studied in an isolated (sealed) system with an oxygen electrode and a recording device. The graph shows a typical recording of oxygen consumption (pO_2, partial pressure of oxygen) by normal mitochondria on introduction of ADP.

yield of ATP per mole of NADH is about seven moles; however, by actual measurement with isolated mitochondria, the P:O ratio for oxidation of metabolites that yield NADH is about 2.5 and the ratio for those that yield $FADH_2$ is about 1.5. The remainder of the energy available from the oxidation of NADH and $FADH_2$ is released in the form of heat.

'Respiratory control' is the dependence of oxygen uptake by mitochondria on the availability of ADP

Normally, oxidation and phosphorylation are tightly coupled: substrates are oxidized, electrons are transported, and oxygen is consumed only when synthesis of ATP is required (coupled respiration). Thus, resting mitochondria consume oxygen at a slow rate, which can be greatly stimulated by addition of ADP (Fig. 9.13). ADP is taken up by the mitochondria and stimulates ATP synthase, which lowers the proton gradient. Respiration increases, because the proton pumps are stimulated to reestablish the proton gradient. When the ADP is depleted, ATP synthesis terminates and respiration returns to the original rate. Oxygen uptake declines to the original rate when the concentration of ADP is depleted and ATP synthesis terminates.

Mitochondria can become partially uncoupled if the inner membrane loses its structural integrity. They are said to be 'leaky', because protons can diffuse through the inner membrane without involving ATP synthase. This occurs if isolated mitochondria are treated with mild detergents that disrupt the inner membrane, or if they have been stored for a period of time. Such mitochondria are said to be 'uncoupled'; oxidation proceeds without production of ATP and uncoupled mitochondria lose respiratory control because protons pumped by the electron chain bypass the ATPase and leak unproductively back into the matrix. The P:O ratio declines under these conditions.

The mechanism of respiratory control probably depends on the requirement for ADP and Pi binding to the ATP synthase complex: in the absence of ADP and Pi, protons cannot enter the mitochondrion through this complex and oxygen consumption markedly decreases, because the proton pumps cannot pump protons against a high proton back-pressure. This happens because the free energy of the electron transport reactions is sufficient to generate a pH gradient of only two units across the membrane. If the pH gradient cannot be discharged for production of ATP, the two pH unit gradient is established and the pumps grind to a halt and stall. The electron transport chain becomes reduced and substrate oxidation and oxygen consumption decrease. A little physical activity, with consumption of ATP and generation of ADP and Pi, opens up the ATPase channels, discharging the proton gradient and activating the electron transport chain, and fuel and oxygen consumption. At a whole-body level, we breathe faster during exercise to provide the additional oxygen needed for increased oxidative phosphorylation.

Uncouplers

Uncouplers of oxidative phosphorylation dissipate the proton gradient by transporting protons back into mitochondria, bypassing the ATP synthase. Uncouplers stimulate respiration, because the system makes a futile attempt to restore the proton gradient by oxidizing more fuel and pumping more protons out of mitochondria. Uncouplers are typically hydrophobic compounds and either weak acids or bases, with pK_a near pH 7. The classic uncoupler, 2,4-dinitrophenol (DNP) (Fig. 9.14), is protonated in solution on the outer, more acidic side of the inner mitochondrial membrane. Because of its hydrophobicity, it may then freely diffuse through the inner mitochondrial membrane. When it reaches the matrix side, it encounters a more basic pH and the proton is released, effectively discharging the pH gradient. Other uncouplers include preservatives and antimicrobial agents, such as pentachlorophenol and *p*-cresol.

Uncoupling proteins (UCP)

According to the chemiosmotic hypothesis, the inner mitochondrial membrane is topologically closed. However, it has long been known that protons are transported into the matrix from the intermembrane space by routes other than the ATP synthase complex and inner membrane transporters. Much of the BMR is now thought to be mainly due to inner membrane components called uncoupling proteins (UCP). The first discovered was uncoupling protein-1 (UCP1), formerly known as thermogenin, which is found exclusively in brown adipose tissue. Brown adipose tissue is abundant in the newborn and in some adult mammals, and it is brown because of its high content of mitochondria. In humans,

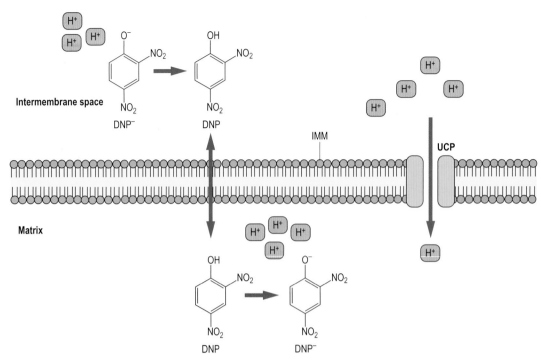

Fig. 9.14 **Proton transport by uncouplers.** Uncouplers transport protons into the mitochondrion, dissipating the proton gradient. DNP is an example of an exogenous uncoupler. The uncoupling proteins (UCP) are endogenous uncouplers in the IMM and are regulated by hormones. The gradient consisting of protons and other factors constitute the mitochondrial membrane potential (MMP), which is expressed in millivolts (mV). DNP, 2,4-dinitrophenol; IMM, inner mitochondrial membrane.

 ## 2,4-DINITROPHENOL POISONING

An unresponsive 25-year-old woman is carried into the emergency room by her boyfriend, because after taking two doses of 'weight loss' pills, she complained of headache, fever, chest pain, profuse sweating, and weakness. Initial findings were: rectal temperature, 40.8°C (105.5°F), pulse 151 beats per minute, respiratory rate 56 per minute, blood pressure 40/10. In 15 minutes she died and could not be resuscitated. After death, rigor mortis set in after 10 minutes and her temperature rose to 46°C (115°F) in 10 additional minutes. It was found that she was a body builder and that she took 'weight loss' capsules purchased from a friend, because she wanted to have a leaner body for a show. Among her personal effects was a plastic bottle containing capsules that proved to contain 2,4-dinitrophenol.

Comment. Dinitrophenol (DNP) is an uncoupler of oxidative phosphorylation (see Fig. 9.14). It was first discovered to induce weight loss during World War I when it was noticed that French munitions workers who were exposed to dinitrophenol during the synthesis of dynamite (trinitrotoluene, TNT) rapidly lost weight. In the 1930s it was prescribed by physicians for weight loss and was also available over the counter, but because people suffered significant side effects, such as cataracts, blindness, kidney and liver damage and death, it was banned for medical use in the United States after a congressional investigation. The case above was adapted from those hearings. Dinitrophenol is currently used industrially in the manufacture of dyes, explosives, herbicides, insecticides and lumber preservatives. DNP kills bacteria and fungi by uncoupling phosphorylation. Unfortunately, DNP has resurfaced as an illegal weight loss product. It radically increases consumption of oxygen and metabolic fuels, and nearly all metabolic energy is wasted as heat. Cells die because of both excess temperature and lack of ATP.

brown adipose tissue is abundant in infants, but it gradually diminishes and is barely detectable in adults. The sole function of UCP1 is to provide body heat during cold stress in the young and in some adult animals. It accomplishes this by uncoupling the proton gradient, thereby generating heat (thermogenesis) instead of ATP. Uncoupling proteins are expressed at high levels in hibernating animals, permitting them to maintain body temperature without movement or exercise.

Four additional uncoupling proteins are expressed by the human genome: UCP2, UCP3, UCP4 and UCP5. While UCP1 is exclusive to brown adipose tissue, UCP2 is expressed ubiquitously, UCP3 is mainly expressed in skeletal muscle, and UCP4 and UCP5 are expressed in the brain. Except for UCP1, the physiological functions of these proteins are not well understood, but could be of profound significance in our understanding of such health issues as diabetes, obesity, cancer, thyroid disease and aging. As uncouplers, they have been linked to a number of fundamental functions. For example, there is strong evidence that obesity induces the synthesis of UCP2 in β-cells of the pancreas. This may play a role in the β-cell dysfunction found in type 2 diabetes, because it lowers the intracellular concentration of ATP, which is required for secretion of insulin. The thyroid hormone (T_3) has been shown to stimulate thermogenesis in rats by promoting the synthesis of UCP3 in skeletal muscle. Of course, the common fever that is induced by infectious organisms is probably due to uncoupling by UCPs, but the mechanism is unknown. The UCP system is important in regulating the membrane potential. For example, UCP2 is upregulated by high membrane potentials to decrease production of reactive oxygen species (see Chapter 37).

INHIBITORS OF OXIDATIVE METABOLISM

Electron transport system inhibitors

Inhibitors of electron transport selectively inhibit complexes I, III or IV, interrupting the flow of electrons through the respiratory chain. This stops proton pumping, ATP synthesis, and oxygen uptake. Several inhibitors are readily available poisons that could be encountered in the practice of medicine. It is noteworthy that genetic defects in respiratory chain components often mimic the effects of these inhibitors.

Rotenone inhibits complex I (NADH-Q reductase)

Rotenone, a common insecticide, and some barbiturates (e.g. amytal) inhibit complex I. Because malate and lactate are oxidized by NAD^+, their oxidation will be decreased by rotenone. However, substrates yielding $FADH_2$ can still be oxidized, because complex I is bypassed and electrons are donated to ubiquinone. Addition of ADP to a suspension of mitochondria supplemented with malate and phosphate (Fig. 9.15) markedly stimulates oxygen uptake as ATP synthesis occurs. Oxygen uptake is markedly inhibited by rotenone, but when succinate is added, ATP synthesis and oxygen consumption resume until the supply of ADP is exhausted. Rotenone inhibition of complex I causes reduction of all components prior to the point of inhibition, because they cannot be oxidized, whereas those after the point of inhibition become fully oxidized. This is known as a crossover point, and it can be determined spectrophotometrically, because light absorption by respiratory chain components changes according to redox

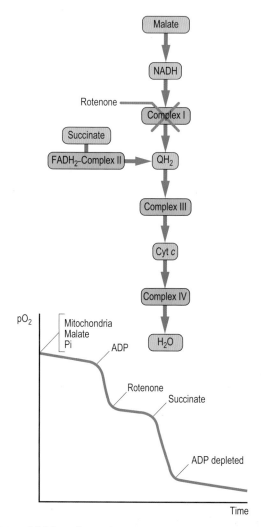

Fig. 9.15 **Inhibition of complex I**. Inhibitors such as rotenone, retard oxygen uptake by mitochondria when NADH-producing substrates are being oxidized.

state. Such analyses were used to define the sequence of components in the respiratory chain.

Antimycin A inhibits complex III (QH₂-cytochrome c reductase)

The inhibition of complex III by antimycin A prevents transfer of electrons from either complex I or $FADH_2$-containing flavoproteins to cytochrome c. In this case, components preceding complex III become fully reduced, and those after it become oxidized. The oxygen uptake curve (Fig. 9.16) shows that the stimulation of respiration by ADP is inhibited by antimycin A, but that the addition of succinate does not relieve the inhibition. Ascorbic acid can reduce cytochrome c, and addition of ascorbic acid restores respiration, illustrating that complex IV is unaffected by antimycin A.

Cyanide and carbon monoxide inhibit complex IV

Azide (N_3^-), cyanide (CN^-), and carbon monoxide (CO) inhibit complex IV (cytochrome c oxidase) (Fig. 9.17). Because

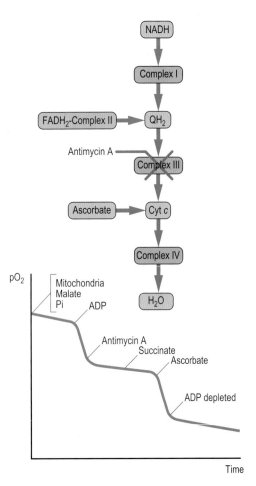

Fig. 9.16 **Inhibition of complex III by antimycin.** Antimycin A inhibits complex III, blocking transfer of electrons from both complex I and flavoproteins, such as complex II.

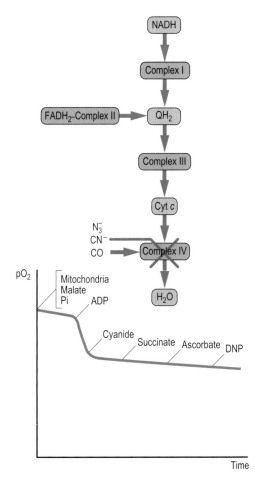

Fig. 9.17 **Inhibition of complex IV.** The inhibition of complex IV interrupts the transfer of electrons, in the final step of electron transport. Electrons cannot be transferred to oxygen, and the synthesis of ATP is halted.

complex IV is the terminal electron transfer complex, its inhibition cannot be bypassed. All components preceding complex IV become reduced, oxygen cannot be reduced, none of the complexes can pump protons, and ATP is not synthesized. Uncouplers such as DNP have no effect, because there is no proton gradient. Cyanide and carbon monoxide also bind to hemoglobin, and it cannot carry oxygen (see Chapter 5). In these poisonings, both the ability to transport oxygen and to synthesize ATP are impaired. The administration of oxygen is used for the treatment of such poisonings. It is of interest that sodium azide is the nitrogen source for the inflation of air bags; it may pose an environmental problem if it is accidentally released, i.e. nonexplosively.

Inhibitors of ATP synthase

Oligomycin inhibits respiration but, in contrast to electron transport inhibitors, it is not a direct inhibitor of the electron transport system. Instead, it inhibits the proton channel of ATP synthase. It causes an accumulation of protons outside the mitochondrion, because the proton pumping system is still intact but the proton channel is blocked. The addition of the uncoupler DNP after oxygen uptake has been inhibited by oligomycin illustrates this point: DNP dissipates the proton gradient and stimulates oxygen uptake as the electron transport system attempts to reestablish the proton gradient (Fig. 9.18).

Inhibitors of the ADP–ATP translocase

Most ATP is synthesized in the mitochondrion, but used in the cytosol for biosynthetic reactions. Newly synthesized mitochondrial ATP and spent cytosolic ADP are exchanged by a mitochondrial ADP–ATP translocase, representing about 10% of the protein in the inner mitochondrial membrane (see Fig. 9.3). This translocase can be inhibited by unusual plant and mold toxins, such as bongkrekic acid and atractyloside. Their effects are similar to those of oligomycin in vitro – a proton gradient builds up and electron transport stops, but, as with oligomycin, respiration can be reactivated by uncouplers.

CYANIDE AND CARBON MONOXIDE ARE MITOCHONDRIAL POISONS

Both cyanide and carbon monoxide bind to hemoglobin and inhibit oxygen transport. They also inhibit electron transport and production of ATP.

Comment. Cells respond to cyanide or carbon monoxide poisoning by switching to anaerobic metabolism, resulting in lactic acidosis and ultimate death, unless immediate measures are taken. Carbon monoxide poisoning is treated with oxygen. In both cyanide and carbon monoxide poisoning, methylene blue can be administered: it alleviates the inhibition of complex IV by accepting electrons from complex III (cytochrome c reductase), allowing both complex I and complex III to pump protons, so that ATP can continue to be synthesized. Cyanide can also be converted to the relatively harmless thiocyanate ion by the administration of thiosulfate.

 ## MITOCHONDRIAL ENCEPHALOMYOPATHY

A 16-year-old boy presented with headache, seizures and visual loss. There was a long history of inability to exercise due to muscle weakness. There have been episodes of hemianopia and mild hemiparesis lasting several days. His maternal aunt had a similar illness. Accumulation of lactate during and after exercise suggested a defect in mitochondrial oxidative metabolism. Muscle mitochondria were isolated for study. Respiratory Complex I activity was reduced. A point mutation in mitochondrial DNA was identified.

Comment. A diagnosis of mitochondrial myopathy, encephalopathy, lactic acidosis and stroke-like episodes (MELAS) was made. MELAS is one of a group of conditions caused by defects in oxidative phosphorylation and characterized by defects in the process whereby NADH drives electrons along the mitochondrial respiratory chain complex and generates ATP.

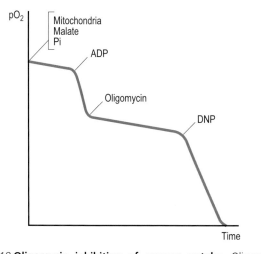

Fig. 9.18 **Oligomycin inhibition of oxygen uptake.** Oligomycin inhibits oxygen uptake in ATP-synthesizing mitochondria. Oligomycin inhibits ATP synthase and oxygen uptake in coupled mitochondria. However, DNP stimulates oxygen uptake after oligomycin inhibition, by dissipating the proton gradient.

REGULATION OF OXIDATIVE PHOSPHORYLATION

Respiratory control and feedback regulation

The oldest and simplest known mechanism of respiratory control is accomplished by the supply of ADP. This is based on the fact that when added to isolated mitochondria, ADP stimulates respiration and ATP synthesis. When ADP is completely converted to ATP, respiration returns to the initial rate. Oxidative phosphorylation is also tightly coupled to other fundamental pathways such as glycolysis, fatty acid oxidation and the tricarboxylic acid cycle (see Chapters 12, 14 and 15) through feedback regulatory mechanisms. The ratios of NADH/NAD and ATP/ADP feedback on key enzymes, such as PFK-1, pyruvate dehydrogenase and isocitrate dehydrogenase. If, for example, oxidative phosphorylation is switched off because of high ATP, both NADH and ATP will negatively feedback on other extramitochondrial pathways, limiting the flux of fuel to mitochondria. Since oxidative phosphorylation responds to the supply of $FADH_2$, NADH, ADP, and Pi as well as the ATP/ADP ratio, magnitude of the membrane potential, uncoupling and hormonal factors, its modes of regulation are clearly complex.

Regulation by covalent modification and allosteric effectors (ATP-ADP)

The main target for regulating oxidative phosphorylation appears to be complex IV. It is phosphorylated in response to hormone action (see Chapter 13) by cyclic-3′5′-adenosine monophosphate (*c*AMP)-dependent protein kinase (PKA) and dephosphorylated by a Ca^{2+}-stimulated protein phosphatase. Phosphorylation enables allosteric regulation by ATP (ATP/ADP ratio). A high ATP/ADP ratio inhibits and a low ratio stimulates oxidative phosphorylation. It is thought that the complex is normally phosphorylated and inhibited by ATP. With high Ca^{2+} levels, e.g. in muscle during exercise (see Chapter 20), the enzyme is dephosphorylated, the inhibition by ATP is abolished, and its activity greatly stimulated, increasing ATP production, as well as the membrane potential and production of reactive oxygen species (Chapter 37).

Based on the observation that in type 2 diabetes, ATP production is decreased when the β-subunit of ATP synthase is phosphorylated, it has been proposed that this complex is also regulated by phosphorylation/dephosphorylation. Note that the secretion of insulin in β-cells of the pancreas is ATP dependent, because ATP binds to the ATP-sensitive potassium channel (see Insulin Secretion, Chapter 21 and box on p. 95).

Regulation by thyroid hormones

Thyroid hormones act at two levels in mitochondria. In rats, T_3 stimulates the synthesis of UCP2 and UCP3, which can uncouple the proton gradient, but this has not been documented in humans. Additionally, T_2 binds to complex IV on the matrix side, inducing slip in cytochrome *c* oxidase. The term 'slip' means that complex IV pumps fewer protons per electron transported through the complex, resulting in thermogenesis. The action of T_3 could explain, in part, the long-term and T_2 the short-term thermogenic effects of thyroid hormones (see also Chapter 39).

Summary

The electron transport system consists of electron carriers that are located in the inner mitochondrial membrane, each of which is isolable as a complex or as a single molecule. Electrons from four major flavoproteins feed electrons to ubiquinone, the first member of the common pathway. Energy derived from the conductance of electrons through the electron transport system is used by three of the complexes to pump protons into the intermembrane space, creating an electrochemical gradient or proton motive force. The proton gradient is used to power ATP synthase for synthesis of ATP by rotary catalysis as well as transport of intermediates across the inner membrane. Numerous toxins can severely impair the electron transport system, the ATP synthase and the translocase that exchanges ATP and ADP across the inner mitochondrial membrane. The rate of ATP production by the electron transport system is regulated by modulation of the proton gradient, by allosteric modification and phosphorylation-dephosphorylation and by thyroid hormones. At least five UCP with specific tissue distributions occur in the inner mitochondrial membrane, and they all regulate the membrane potential and thermogenesis. Chronic diseases or conditions such as diabetes, cancer, obesity, and aging all have metabolic links to dysregulation of oxidative phosphorylation through effects on the electron transport system and ATP synthase.

ACTIVE LEARNING

Test your knowledge

1. The glycerol-3-phosphate and malate-aspartate shuttles both transport electrons into the mitochondria from cytoplasmic NADH. Explain how the glycerol-3-phosphate shuttle is more thermogenic than the malate-aspartate shuttle. Why are there two separate transport systems? How are they distributed among tissues?
2. Describe how increased synthesis of a UCP could decrease ATP synthesis.
3. How many 360° rotations of ATP synthase occur as a result of one turn of the TCA cycle if all components are fully coupled?
4. Which type of inhibitors would mimic a genetic defect in cytochrome oxidase?
5. Describe how a deficiency in riboflavin could severely impair ATP synthesis.

Further reading

Argyropoulos G, Harper ME. Uncoupling proteins and thermoregulation. *J Appl Physiol* 2002;**92**:2187–2198.

Crompton M. Mitochondria and aging: a role for the permeability transition? *Aging Cell* 2004;**3**:3–6.

Dimauro S, Schon EA. Mitochondrial respiratory chain diseases. *N Engl J Med* 2003;**348**:2656–2668.

Fearnley IM et al. Proteomic analysis of the subunit composition of complex I (NADH:ubiquinone oxidoreductase) from bovine heart mitochondria. *Methods Mol Biol* 2007;**357**:103–125.

Gambert S, Ricquier D. Mitochondrial thermogenesis and obesity. *Curr Opin Clin Nutr Metab Care* 2007;**10**:664–670.

Harper ME, Seifert EL. Thyroid hormone effects on mitochondrial energetics. *Thyroid* 2008;**18**:145–156.

Kadenbach B. Instrinsic and extrinsic uncoupling of phosphorylation. *Biochim Biophys Acta – Bioenergetics* 2003;**1604**:77–94.

Soane L et al. Mechanisms of impaired mitochondrial energy metabolism in acute and chronic neurodegenerative disorders. *J Neurosci Res* 2007;**85**:3407–3415.

Websites

ATP synthase movies: www.cnr.berkeley.edu/~hongwang/Project/ATP_synthase/
ATP synthase:
- http://vcell.ndsu.nodak.edu/animations/atpgradient/index.htm
GOOGLE: 'ATP synthase movies'
Oxidative phosphorylation: www.sp.uconn.edu/~terry/images/anim/ETS.html
  http://bcs.whfreeman.com/thelifewire/content/chp07/0702001.html
Bioenergetics: www.bmb.leeds.ac.uk/illingworth/oxphos/
Neuromuscular Disease Center: www.neuro.wustl.edu/neuromuscular/mitosyn.html
The Children's Mitochondrial Disease Network: www.emdn-mitonet.co.uk/
Mitochondrial diseases:
- www.umdf.org/mitodisease/
- www.neuro.wustl.edu/neuromuscular/mitosyn.html

10. Function of the Gastrointestinal Tract

U V Kulkarni and I Broom

LEARNING OBJECTIVES

After reading this chapter you should be able to:

- Describe the main stages of digestion.
- Discuss mechanisms involved in the absorption of nutrients from the digestive tract.
- Discuss the role of digestive enzymes.
- Discuss digestion of the main classes of nutrients: carbohydrates, proteins and fats.
- Identify compounds arising from the digestion of carbohydrates, proteins and fats that become substrates for further metabolism.

INTRODUCTION

Food provides an organism with sources of energy and with materials for building up or renewing body structures. The survival of the organism is dependent on its ability to extract these resources from the food taken in.

Food that is eaten enters the gastrointestinal (GI) tract. The GI tract and organs functionally associated with it, principally the liver and pancreas, are responsible for digestion and absorption. Digestion is the process by which nutrient molecules are transformed into components simple enough to be absorbed in the intestine. Absorption is the process of uptake of these products of digestion by intestinal cells (enterocytes) and thence into the body. Digestion and absorption of nutrients are closely linked. Digestion is regulated by the nervous system, several hormones and paracrine factors. The physical presence of food particles in the GI tract also stimulates these processes.

The main classes of macromolecules contained in food are carbohydrates, proteins and lipids

Carbohydrates and lipids serve primarily as sources of energy (metabolic fuels; see Table 9.1 for energy yields) but also have a nonfuel function in the body. Protein, on the other hand, is primarily used for nonfuel purposes but can, under certain circumstances, serve as an energy source. The composition of different foods varies in their proportions of carbohydrate, protein and fats. In addition, some ingested material, such as complex carbohydrates of plant origin, are indigestible and constitute what is termed 'fiber'.

THE GASTROINTESTINAL TRACT

The GI tract is effectively a long coiled tube with the liver and pancreas draining into it through secretory ducts. Its function is to transfer the components of food from the outside to the inside of the body (Fig. 10.1). To optimize this function, its different anatomical parts have specific functions relating to digestion and absorption:

- the stomach and duodenum deal with the initial process of mixing ingested food and initiating digestion
- the jejunum continues the digestive process and begins the absorptive process
- the ileum absorbs digested nutrients; and the large intestine is involved in the absorption of fluid and electrolytes.

Along the lengths of the GI tract various fluids, electrolytes and proteins are added to aid in the mixing, hydration and digestion of the food. The gut does more than simply pass all digested food to other organs, such as the liver. It will, for example, treat the simple monosaccharide glucose differently when this is received from the lumen or via the mesenteric blood supply. Glucose absorbed from the lumen is transferred directly to the liver unaltered, whereas glucose received via the blood supply is metabolized to lactate prior to passage to the liver. The amino acid glutamine, derived from dietary protein, is used by the enterocytes as a major energy source and does not enter the portal blood supply, which goes to the liver (see below).

Mechanical and anatomical basis of digestion

There is a purely mechanical component to digestion. Mastication (chewing) and preliminary digestion of food take place in the mouth. The food is then swallowed into the esophagus by a process driven by the esophageal reflex. Food is broken down into smaller particles as it travels along the upper GI tract, e.g. in the stomach, and its presence itself triggers peristalsis, which further helps mixing and stimulates

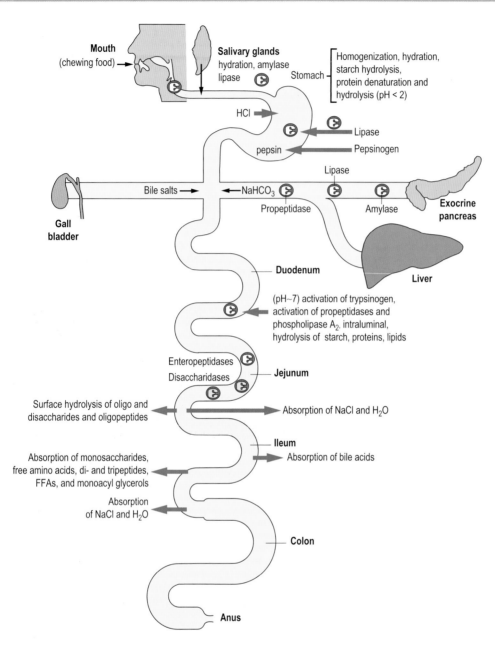

Fig. 10.1 **The gastrointestinal (GI) tract.** The digestion and absorption of nutrients requires integrated function of several organs. Mixing of food and initiation of digestion take place in the stomach. Digestion continues in the jejunum, where the absorptive processes start. The bulk of nutrients are absorbed in the ileum. The large intestine is involved in the absorption of water and electrolytes, and participates in the recirculation of the bile acids to the liver (see Chapter 29). Taking into account all intake and secretions, a large amount of fluid (approximately 7 liters) passes through the GI tract every day. FFA, free fatty acids.

digestive secretions. Major stimuli to peristalsis are mediated through the parasympathetic nervous system. The stomach and intestines are lined by epithelium which has an invaginated surface, which greatly increases its surface area. The small intestine, which contains the main absorptive surfaces, is lined by mucosal folds, enterocytes arranged in intestinal villi and microvilli on the cells.

Volume and pH of intestinal secretions

The maintenance of an appropriate hydrogen ion concentration in different parts of the GI tract is crucial for the digestive process and for preservation of the underlying tissues of the stomach and intestines. Saliva secreted into the mouth is alkaline due to its bicarbonate content. The contents of the lumen of the stomach are strongly acidic, but the mucus protecting its walls is alkaline. The acidic contents of the stomach are neutralized by strongly alkaline pancreatic secretions when they enter the duodenum.

Intestinal secretions total about 7.5 liters every day, over and above an average water intake of about 1.5 liters. Most of this fluid is absorbed back by the lower GI tract, and normally only about 150–250 mL of water is contained in the stool.

Excessive loss of fluid from the gastrointestinal tract may lead to disturbances of fluid, electrolyte and acid–base balance

Prolonged vomiting, i.e. the loss of primarily stomach contents, causes the direct loss of water, hydrogen and chloride ions, and a further loss of potassium due to the body's compensatory mechanisms. Diarrhea may be caused by increased intestinal secretion due to, for instance, inflammation or may be caused by malabsorption of nutrients. Severe diarrhea, leading to the loss of alkaline intestinal contents in large amounts, may lead to dehydration and metabolic acidosis. It also results in the loss of sodium, potassium and other minerals (see Chapters 11, 23 and 24).

DIGESTION

Digestion is a sequential, ordered series of processes

The process of digestion is characterized by a number of specific stages which occur in a sequence, allowing the interaction of fluid, pH, emulsifying agents and enzymes. This, in turn, requires concerted secretory action from the salivary glands, liver and gall bladder, the pancreas, and the intestinal mucosa. The processes involved are outlined in Figure 10.1 and can be summarized as follows:

- Lubrication and homogenization of food with fluids secreted by glands of the intestinal tract, starting in the mouth.
- Secretion of enzymes whose prime function is to breakdown macromolecules to a mixture of oligomers, dimers and monomers.
- Secretion of electrolytes, hydrogen ions and bicarbonate within different parts of the GI tract to optimize the environmental conditions for enzymic hydrolysis specific to that region.
- Secretion of bile acids to emulsify dietary lipid, thus allowing appropriate enzymic hydrolysis and absorption.
- Further hydrolysis of oligomers and dimers within the jejunum by membrane-bound surface enzymes.
- Specific transport of digested material into enterocytes and thence to blood or lymph.

Numerous secretions from the GI tract and its associated organs are involved in these processes and each area contains specialized glands and unique surface epithelial properties (Table 10.1).

In general, there is considerable functional reserve in all aspects of digestion and absorption. Minor functional loss may go unnoticed by the individual, allowing pathology to progress for some time before being diagnosed. Signs and symptoms of GI maldigestion or malabsorption therefore require considerable impairment of structure/function relationships to be manifest. Each of the organs involved in digestion and absorption has the capacity to increase its activity severalfold in response to specific stimulation; this adds greatly to the gut's reserve capacity. For example, pancreatic disease manifests itself only after 90% of the pancreatic function is destroyed. In addition, the GI tract can accommodate loss of function of one particular constituent organ. For example, if the stomach

Organization of the gastrointestinal tract by functional requirements	
Gastrointestinal organ	**Primary function in absorption of foodstuffs**
Salivary glands	Production of fluid and digestive enzymes for homogenization, lubrication and digestion of carbohydrate (amylase) lipid (lingual lipases)
Stomach	Secretion of HCl and proteases to initiate hydrolysis of proteins
Pancreas	Secretion of bicarbonate, proteases and lipases to continue digestion of protein and lipids; and amylase to continue digestion of starch
Liver and gall bladder	Secretion and storage of bile acids for release into the small intestine
Small bowel	Final intraluminal digestion of foodstuffs, digestion of carbohydrate dimers and specific absorptive pathways for digested material
Large bowel	Absorption of fluid and electrolytes and products of bacterial action in the colon

Table 10.1 **Organization of the gastrointestinal tract by functional requirements.**

is surgically removed, because of cancer, both the pancreas and small intestine can compensate for the total loss of gastric digestion. In pancreatic disease, lingual lipases can accommodate, in part, some loss of pancreatic lipase production.

Digestive enzymes and zymogens

Most digestive enzymes in the GI tract are secreted as inactive precursors

With the exception of salivary amylase and lingual (associated with the tongue; hence oral) lipases, digestive enzymes are secreted into the gut lumen as inactive precursors termed zymogens (see also Chapter 6). The secretion of gut enzymes is similar in the salivary glands, gastric mucosa and pancreas. These organs contain specialized cells for the synthesis, packaging and transport of enzymes to the cell surface and thence to the intestinal lumen. These secretions are termed exocrine, i.e. 'secreting to the outside', as opposed to the endocrine secretion of hormones.

Enzymes involved in protein digestion (proteases) and the lipase phospholipase A_2 are synthesized as inactive zymogens and are only activated on their release to the gut lumen. In general, these enzymes, once in their active form, can activate their own precursors. Activation of their precursors can occur by change in pH (e.g. pepsinogen in the stomach is converted at pH below 4.0 into pepsin, the active enzyme) or by the action of specific enteropeptidases bound to the mucosal membrane of the duodenum (see Fig. 10.1).

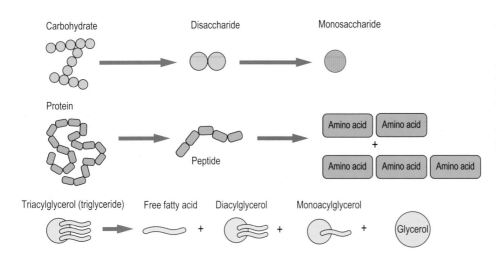

Fig. 10.2 **Digestion of dietary polymers.** Polysaccharides are digested to yield di- and monosaccharides and proteins to yield the component amino acids. Fat is ingested mostly as triacylglycerols (triglycerides), the esters of glycerol and fatty acids. During digestion a stepwise removal of fatty acid molecules takes place yielding di- and monoacylglycerols.

All digestive enzymes are hydrolases

All digestive enzymes hydrolyze their substrates. The products of such hydrolytic procedures are oligomers, dimers and monomers of the parent macromolecule. Thus, carbohydrates are hydrolyzed into a mixture of dissacharides and monosaccharides. Proteins are broken down to a mixture of di- and tripeptides and amino acids. Lipids, however, are treated differently – they are broken down to a mixture of fatty acids (FA), glycerol and mono- and diacyl glycerols (Fig. 10.2).

DIGESTION AND ABSORPTION OF CARBOHYDRATES

Dietary carbohydrates enter the GI tract as mono-, di- and polysaccharides

Dietary carbohydrates consist of mainly plant and animal starches (polysaccharides), the disaccharides sucrose and lactose, and monosaccharides (Fig. 10.3). Monosaccharides include glucose, fructose and galactose, which are either present as such in the diet or are generated by digestion of di- and polysaccharides, e.g. galactose is derived mainly from dairy products. These sugar monomers require no further digestion to be absorbed from the GI tract.

Monosaccharides exist in several isomeric forms. Their classification into D- and L-forms is based on the orientation of the hydrogen and hydroxyl groups at the asymmetric carbon atom adjacent to the terminal alcohol group. These isomers rotate the polarized light to the right (D) or left (L). The reference molecule for this system of classification is the simplest monosaccharide (triose), glyceraldehyde. In the ring forms of pentoses and higher sugars the carbon atom at position 1 also becomes asymmetric (anomeric). Different steric arrangements in this position result in either α- or β-anomers. α-Anomers have a hydroxyl group pointing below the plane of the ring structure, and β-anomers have a hydroxyl group pointing above the plane (see Chapter 3).

Disaccharides, and polysaccharides such as starch and glycogen, require hydrolytic cleavage into monosaccharides before absorption

Disaccharides are broken down by membrane-bound disaccharidases present on the intestinal mucosal surface. Starch and glycogen require the additional hydrolytic capacity of the enzyme amylase found in the secretions of the salivary glands and pancreas (Fig. 10.4).

Starch is a plant polysaccharide and glycogen is its animal equivalent. Both contain a mixture of linear chains of glucose molecules linked by α-1,4 glycosidic bonds (amylose) and by branched glucose chains with α-1,6 linkages (amylopectin). Glycogen has a far more branched structure than starch. The digestion of these polysaccharides is promoted by the endosaccharidases and amylase produced by the salivary glands and pancreas. Amylase in the gut lumen is not bound to enterocytes forming the mucosal membrane lining.

The products of hydrolysis of starch are the disaccharide maltose, the trisaccharide maltotriose and a branched unit, termed the α-limit dextrin. These products are further hydrolyzed by enzymes bound to the enterocytes of the mucosal membrane for the final formation of the monosaccharide glucose (Fig. 10.5A).

Dietary disaccharides such as lactose, sucrose and trehalose (a disaccharide made up of two glucose molecules in a 1,1 linkage) are hydrolyzed to their constituent monomeric sugars by specific disaccharidases attached to the small intestinal brush border membrane. The catalytic domains of these enzymes project into the gut lumen to react with their specific substrates, whilst their noncatalytic, structural domain(s) are attached to the enterocyte cell membrane.

With the exception of lactase, all disaccharidases are inducible

The greater the amount of a disaccharide (e.g. sucrose) present in the diet or produced by digestion, the greater is the amount of the relevant specific disaccharidase (e.g. sucrase)

Carbohydrate	Food source	Structure
Starch (amylose) [plant]	Potatoes, rice, bread, onions	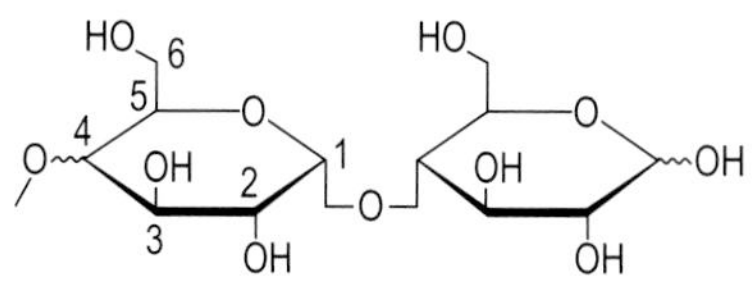
Amylopectin (glycogen) [plant, animal]	Potatoes, rice, bread, muscle, liver	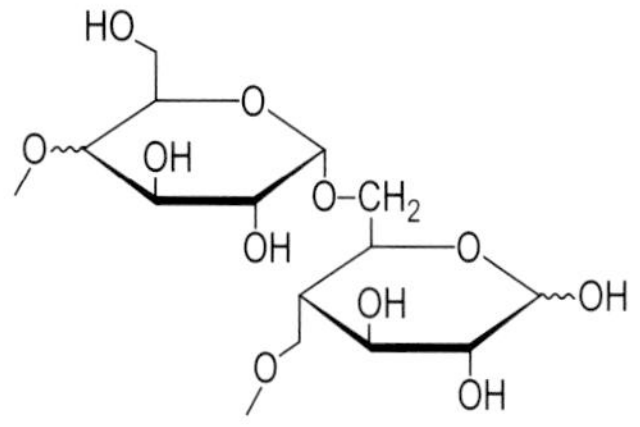
Sucrose	Desserts, sweets, 'sugar'	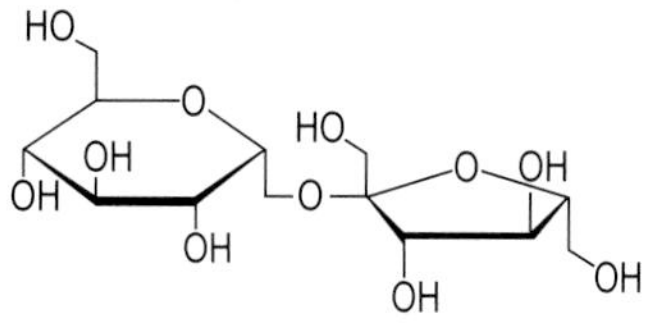
Lactose	Milk	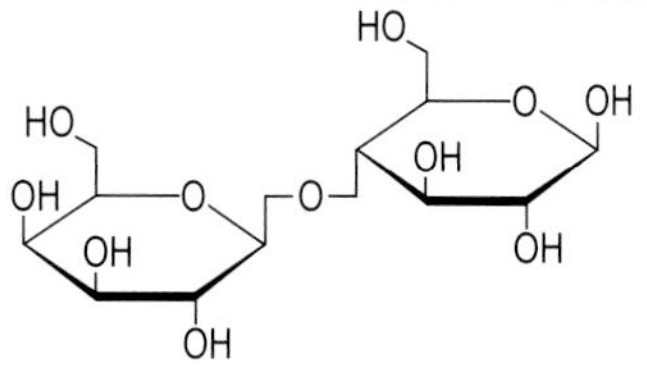
Fructose	Fruits, honey	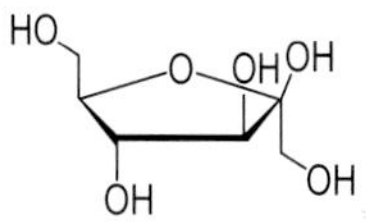
Glucose	Fruits, honey	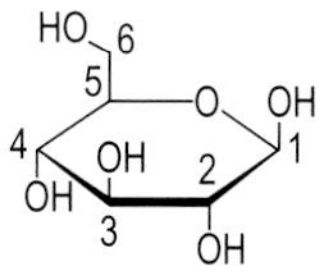

Fig. 10.3 **Structure of main dietary carbohydrates.** Starch and amylopectin are polysaccharides and only two component sugar molecules are shown for each to illustrate the intermolecular linkages. Sucrose and lactose are the most common disaccharides, and fructose and glucose the most common monosaccharides. Monosaccharides require no further digestion. Refer to the glucose molecule for the standard numbering of carbon atoms (see also Chapter 3).

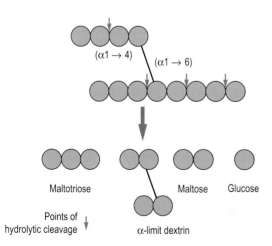

Fig. 10.4 **Hydrolytic cleavage of polysaccharides.** Enzymatic hydrolysis is the mechanism of digestion of polysaccharides and disaccharides. The arrows illustrate points of cleavage and the type of hydrolyzed bond. Note that α-limit dextrin still contains both α1–4 and α1–6 bonds.

produced by the enterocyte. The rate-limiting step in the absorption of dietary disaccharides is thus the transport of the resultant monomeric sugars. Lactose is a noninducible brush border disaccharidase and therefore the rate-limiting factor in lactose absorption is its hydrolysis and not the transport of glucose and galactose.

There are passive and active transport systems that move carbohydrate monomers across the brush border membrane

The process of digestion results in a great increase in the number of osmotically active monosaccharide particles within the gut lumen. Water will therefore be drawn from the GI tract mucosa and vascular compartment into the lumen. Increased brush border hydrolysis will thus increase the osmotic load, while increased monosaccharide transport across the enterocyte brush border will decrease it. As discussed above, for most oligo- and disaccharidases, the transport

A Luminal digestion

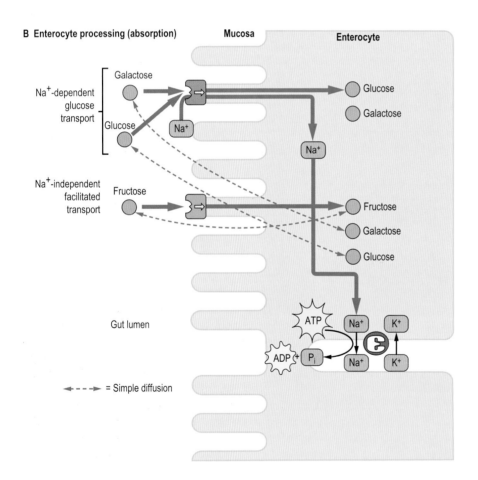

Fig. 10.5 **Digestion and absorption of dietary carbohydrates.** (A) Monosaccharides are generated as a result of hydrolysis of different polysaccharides. Note that preliminary digestion occurs in the gut lumen, and the final stage takes place on the mucosal surface. (B) Links between absorption of monosaccharides and sodium, and their relationship to the activity of Na-K-ATPase (see also Chapter 8). ADP, adenosine diphosphate; ATP, adenosine triphosphate; Pi, inorganic phosphate. Compare Fig. 8.5.

B Enterocyte processing (absorption)

of the resulting monomers is rate limiting. Therefore compensatory mechanisms exist to avoid accumulation of fluid in the gut. As monomeric sugar concentrations increase in the gut lumen, the osmolality increases and there is a compensatory decrease in the activity of brush border disaccharidases. This controls the osmotic load and prevents fluid shifts.

Glucose, fructose and galactose are the primary monosaccharides resulting from the digestion of dietary carbohydrates. Absorption of these sugars and other minor monosaccharides occurs by means of specific carrier-mediated mechanisms (Fig. 10.5B), all of which demonstrate substrate specificity and stereospecificity, show saturation kinetics and can be specifically inhibited. In addition, all monosaccharides can cross

POLYSACCHARIDE DIGESTION

During eating, homogenization occurs with mastication in the mouth and the action of stomach wall muscles and gastric folds. One consequence of this is that dietary polysaccharides become hydrated. Hydration of polysaccharides is essential for the action of amylase. This enzyme is specific for internal α1,4-glycosidic linkages and is totally inert towards α1,6-linkages. In addition, amylase does not act on α1,4-linkages of glycosyl residues serving as branching units. The cleaved units thus formed by its action are the disaccharide maltose, the trisaccharide maltotriose, and an oligosacchide with one or more α1,6-branches and containing on average eight glycosyl units termed the 'α-limit dextrin'. These compounds are then further cleaved to glucose units by oligosaccharidase and α-glucosidase, the latter removing single glucose residues from α1,4-linked oligosaccharides (including maltose) from the non-reducing end of the oligomer. A sucrase–isomaltase complex is secreted as a single polypeptide precursor molecule and then activated into two separate active polypeptide enzymes, one of which (isomaltase) is responsible for the hydrolytic cleavage of α1,6 glycosidic linkages. The final product of digestion of starches is thus glucose, but it only emerges from a complex series of linked enzyme reactions. The initial digestion involves amylase, which occurs free in the lumen, whereas the final processes involve α-glucosidases and isomaltase, which are attached to the mucosal membrane of the enterocyte.

THE STOMACH

There are different cell types in the mucosal wall of the stomach, which perform different digestive functions. Cells called 'chief cells' secrete pepsinogen, which is a precursor to pepsin, a peptidase. Pepsinogen is activated to pepsin in the acidic environment of the stomach lumen. The acidity is maintained by hydrogen ion secretion. This is done by the parietal cells, which generate the hydrogen ions using carbonic anhydrase and then pump it into the lumen by an ATP-dependent proton pump on the luminal cell membrane. Parietal cell activity is stimulated by the action of histamine, produced by histamine-secreting cells, acting on H_2 receptors. The hormone gastrin is secreted by G-cells in the stomach, triggered by food entering the stomach. Stomach cells also secrete the intrinsic factor (IF), which facilitates absorption of vitamin B_{12} in the intestine (Chapter 11). Last but not least, stomach cells secrete alkaline mucus, which protects the stomach lining from the effects of the strong acid. Ulcers can result from damage to the lining of the stomach or duodenum. Treatment of such ulcers focuses on neutralizing the acid by drinking alkaline suspensions; by blocking the H_2 receptors (see Fig. 8.6) and thus the main stimulus to acid secretion; or by inhibiting the proton pump.

GLUT-2, a protein which transports monosaccharides out of the enterocyte into the circulation (see also Table 8.2).

DIGESTION AND ABSORPTION OF LIPIDS

Globules of dietary fat need to be emulsified before enzymatic digestion can take place

Approximately 90% of fat in the diet is triacylglycerol (TAG), also termed triglyceride. The remainder consists of cholesterol, cholesteryl ester, phospholipids and nonesterified fatty acids (NEFA). The hydrophobic nature of fats excludes water-soluble digestive enzymes. Furthermore, fat globules present only a limited surface area for enzyme action. These issues are overcome by the emulsification process.

The change in the physical nature of lipids begins in the stomach: the core body temperature within the stomach helps to liquefy dietary lipids, and peristaltic movements aid in the formation of a lipid emulsion. The emulsification pro-cess is also aided by acid-stable salivary and gastric lipases. The initial rate of hydrolysis is slow, due to the separate aqueous and lipid phases and relatively small lipid–water interface. Once hydrolysis begins, however, the water-immiscible TAGs are degraded to fatty acids, which act as surfactants. They confer a hydrophilic surface to lipid droplets and break them down into smaller particles, thus increasing the lipid–water interface and facilitating rapid hydrolysis. The lipid phase therefore becomes dispersed throughout the aqueous phase as an emulsion.

the brush border membrane by a simple diffusion process although this is extremely slow.

At least two carrier-mediated transport mechanisms for monosaccharides exist: a sodium-dependent co-transporter and a sodium-independent transporter

At the brush border membrane both glucose and galactose are transported by the sodium-dependent glucose transporter. This membrane-linked protein binds with glucose or galactose and Na^+ at separate sites and transports both into the enterocyte cytosol. Na^+ is thus transported down its concentration gradient (the concentration within the gut lumen being higher than that inside cells), carrying glucose along against its concentration gradient. This transport mechanism is linked to Na/K-ATPase which then removes Na^+ from the cell in exchange for K^+ with the concomitant hydrolysis of ATP (see Chapter 8). The transport of glucose or galactose is thus an indirect active process. The interesting consequence of this mechanism is that sodium absorption from the gut is facilitated when some carbohydrates are present in the lumen.

Fructose is transported across the brush border membrane by a sodium-independent facilitated diffusion involving the membrane-associated glucose transporter GLUT-5, which is present on the brush border side of the enterocyte, and

Other dietary factors also act as surfactants. These include phospholipids, fatty acids and monoacyl glycerols. They aid the emulsification process and promote the binding of acid-stable lipases to the lipid–water interface. This in turn facilitates hydrolysis of TAGs and emulsification of lipid droplets.

 ## THE PANCREAS

The pancreas lies retroperitoneally, posterior to the stomach and contains two functionally distinct parts: an exocrine part which secretes digestive enzymes, and an endocrine part, the islets of Langerhans, which secrete insulin, glucagon and other hormones such as somatostatin (see Chapter 21).

The exocrine part is made up of groups of cells called acini. Exocrine secretions flow into the pancreatic duct, which empties into the duodenum along with the common bile duct from the liver and gall bladder. Food entering the duodenum stimulates the secretion of cholecystokinin and this in turn stimulates pancreatic enzyme production and secretion. The acidity of stomach contents entering the duodenum stimulates the release of another hormone, secretin, which triggers the secretion of bicarbonate-rich pancreatic fluid, which neutralizes the acidity in the duodenum.

The pancreas secretes enzymes, which digest carbohydrates, lipids and proteins. Pancreatic amylase digests carbohydrates to oligo- and monosaccharides; lipase digests triacylglycerols while cholesteryl esterase yields free cholesterol and fatty acids; finally, proteases and peptidases break down proteins and peptides. To prevent the powerful proteases breaking down the pancreas itself (autodigestion), they are secreted as proenzymes (see Chapter 6) and activated in the intestinal lumen.

 ## PANCREATITIS

Inflammation of the pancreas is a potentially life-threatening disease. Acute pancreatitis may be caused by gall stones blocking the duct outlet into the duodenum, by excessive alcohol intake, by some drugs or viruses, or it may be seen in association with high concentrations of plasma triacylglycerols. Patients present with severe abdominal pain, nausea and vomiting. The most important biochemical marker of pancreatitis is increased activity of the enzyme amylase in serum, but increased activity of lipase and a decrease in serum calcium can also occur. In a proportion of patients, the amylase remains normal, and therefore other tests such as ultrasound or computed tomography imaging (CT) may be essential for diagnosis alongside biochemical tests. Long-term inflammation, lasting months to years, is called chronic pancreatitis and leads to metabolic complications such as hyperglycemia, malnutrition and, characteristically, an increase in fat excretion in the stool (steatorrhea).

In the duodenum, bile salts and pancreatic enzymes act on the lipid emulsion

The lipid emulsion is ejected from the stomach into the duodenum where dietary lipid undergoes its major digestive process using enzymes secreted by the pancreas. Solubilization is aided by the release of bile salts from the gall bladder. The secretion of bile from the gall bladder is stimulated by the hormone cholecystokinin.

The major enzyme secreted by the pancreas is pancreatic lipase. This enzyme is, however, inactivated in the presence of bile salts normally secreted during lipid digestion into the small intestine. This inhibition is overcome by the concomitant secretion of co-lipase by the pancreas. Co-lipase binds to both the water–lipid interface and to pancreatic lipase, simultaneously anchoring and activating the enzyme. As indicated in Figure 10.6, only a small proportion of dietary TAGs is completely hydrolyzed to glycerol and fatty acids. The second and third fatty acids in TAGs are hydrolyzed with increasing difficulty; therefore the action of pancreatic lipase produces mainly 2-monoacyl glycerols (2-MAGs) for absorption into enterocytes.

Bile salts are essential for solubilizing lipids during the digestive process

Without bile salts acting as detergents, digested lipids would not be in a form suitable for absorption from the gut. The structure of bile acids is demonstrated by cholic acid (Fig. 10.7; see also Chapter 29). Its structure is planar, with hydrophobic and hydrophilic surfaces. The hydrophobic region is formed by the upper surface of the fused ring system, whilst the carboxyl group and all hydroxyl groups are on the opposite surface, giving it hydrophilic properties. Bile acids, which are bile salts at the alkaline pH of the intestine, reversibly form aggregates at concentrations above a critical level, termed the critical micellar concentration. Such aggregates are termed 'micelles' and their constituent bile acids are in equilibrium with free bile acids (salts). Micelles are thus equilibrium structures of well-defined size, considerably smaller than lipid emulsion droplets. The size of these micelles is dependent on bile acid concentration and the ratio of bile acid to lipid.

The conversion of fat emulsion into micellar structures facilitates transport of lipid through the aqueous environment of the lumen of the GI tract. Bile salt micelles can solubilize other lipids too, and these mixed micelles have disk-like shapes. During digestion of TAGs, the lipid digest changes from fat emulsion droplets into micellar structures. These micelles allow the transport of lipids to the brush border of the enterocyte where the lipids are absorbed.

The absorption of lipids into the epithelial cells lining the small intestine occurs by diffusion through the plasma membrane. Almost all the fatty acids and 2-MAGs are absorbed, as both are slightly water soluble. Water-insoluble lipids are poorly absorbed, e.g. only 30–40% of dietary cholesterol is

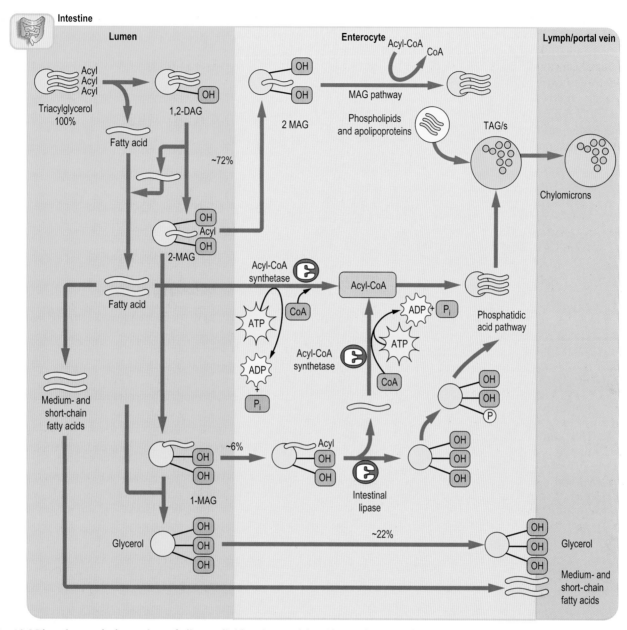

Fig. 10.6 **Digestion and absorption of dietary lipids.** Dietary triglycerides undergo variable degrees of hydrolysis in the intestinal lumen. Subsequently, medium and short fatty acids are absorbed as such into the portal blood. However, long-chain fatty acids (C > 12) are resynthesized into triacylglycerols before being incorporated into chylomicrons for transport from the gut. The fatty acids need to be activated by acetyl-CoA before the synthesis of acylglycerols can take place. This diagram does not take into account the solubilization factors involved or micelle formation. Note that enterocytes do not possess glycerol kinase: the formation of glycerol phosphate requires the presence of glucose. TAG, triacylglycerol; DAG, diacylglycerol; MAG, monoacylglycerol; CoA, coenzyme A.

absorbed. The bile salts pass into the ileum where themselves are absorbed and passed back to the liver; this circuit is called the enterohepatic circulation (see also Chapter 29).

The fate of fatty acids entering enterocytes is dependent on their chain length

Medium and short-chain fatty acids (less than 10 carbon atoms) pass directly through the epithelial cells into the hepatic portal blood supply. In contrast, fatty acids of more than 12 carbon atoms are bound to a fatty acid binding protein and transferred to the rough endoplasmic reticulum of the enterocyte for resynthesis into TAGs. The glycerol for this process is obtained either from absorbed 2-MAGs (the MAG pathway; see Fig. 10.6), from hydrolysis of 1-MAG producing free glycerol or via glycerol-3-phosphate produced during glycolysis (the phosphatidic acid pathway; see Fig. 10.6). Glycerol produced in the intestinal lumen is not reutilized in the enterocyte for TAG synthesis but passes directly to the portal system.

Triacylglycerol synthesis requires activation of fatty acids

Fatty acid activation is accomplished by the production of acyl-CoA derivatives by acyl-CoA synthase. All long-chain fatty acids absorbed by the intestinal epthelial cell are thus reutilized to form TAG before being transferred to the lymphatic system as chylomicrons. Chylomicrons are large particles containing 99% lipid and 1% protein. They are assembled within enterocytes on the rough endoplasmic reticulum before being released into the intercellular space by exocytosis, and finally leave the intestine via the lymphatic system (see Chapter 18).

DIGESTION AND ABSORPTION OF PROTEINS

The total protein load received by the gut is derived from two sources: 70–100 g dietary protein per day and 35–200 g of endogenous protein. The latter is either secreted into the gut (mostly enzymes) or shed from the epithelium as a result of cell turnover. The digestion and absorption of protein is extremely efficient: of this large load, only 1–2 g of nitrogen, equivalent to 6–12 g of protein, are lost in the feces daily.

Proteins are hydrolyzed by peptidases

Proteins are broken down by hydrolysis of peptide bonds and hence the enzymes involved are termed peptidases. These enzymes can either cleave internal peptide bonds (endopeptidases) or cleave off one amino acid at a time from either the —COOH or —NH$_2$ terminal of the polypeptide (exopeptidases, subclassified into carboxypeptidases and aminopeptidases respectively). Endopeptidases break down large polypeptides to smaller oligopeptides which can be acted upon by the exopeptidases to produce the final products of protein digestion, amino acids and di- and tripeptides which are then absorbed by the enterocytes. Depending on the source of the peptidases, the protein digestive process can be divided into gastric, pancreatic and intestinal phases (Fig. 10.8, Table 10.2).

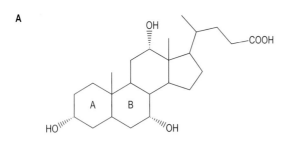

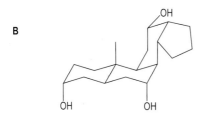

Fig. 10.7 **Bile acid.** Cholic acid is formed in the liver. It is subsequently conjugated with the amino acids glycine or taurine, forming glycocholic or taurocholic acid which is excreted into the bile (see Chapter 17).

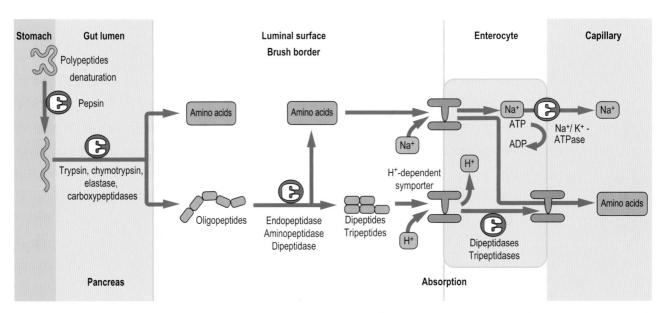

Fig. 10.8 **Digestion and absorption of dietary proteins.** The preliminary stage for digestion is protein denaturation which takes place in the stomach. The peptide bonds between amino acids are hydrolyzed by endo- and exopeptidases. Single amino acids and di- and tripeptides are absorbed by several specific transport systems located in the enterocyte membrane.

Protein digestion begins in the stomach

In the stomach, secreted HCl reduces the pH to 1–2 with consequent denaturation of dietary proteins. Denaturation unfolds polypeptide chains, making proteins more accessible to protease activity. In addition, pepsins are secreted by the chief cells of the gastric mucosa. These are unique proteins relative to their acid stability. They are released as inactive precursors, pepsinogens I and II, and are activated by either an intramolecular reaction (autoactivation) at pH below 5.0 or by active pepsin (autocatalysis). At pH above 2.0 the liberated peptide remains bound to pepsin and acts as an inhibitor of pepsin activity. This inhibition is removed by either a drop in pH below 2.0 or by further pepsin action. The major products of digestion of proteins by pepsin are large peptide fragments and some free amino acids. Gastric protein digests stimulate cholecystokinin release in the duodenum, triggering the release of the main digestive enzymes by the pancreas.

Proteolytic enzymes released from the pancreas are all released as inactive zymogens, in a manner similar to pepsinogen. Duodenal enteropeptidase converts trypsinogen to the active form trypsin. This enzyme is then capable of autoactivation and the activation of all other pancreatic zymogens, thus activating chymotrypsin, elastase and carboxypeptides A and B. Because of this prime role of trypsin in activating other pancreatic enzymes, its activity is controlled within the pancreas and pancreatic ducts by a small molecular weight inhibitory peptide.

Enzymes that digest proteins				
Source	**Zymogen/enzyme**	**Activation**	**Substrate**	**Endproduct**
stomach (fundus)	pepsinogen A	HCl	protein	peptides
stomach (pylorus)	pepsinogen B	pH 1–2 autoactivation	protein	peptides
pancreas	trypsinogen	enteropeptidase, trypsin	protein, peptides	dipeptides, polypeptides
	chymo-trypsinogen	trypsin	protein, peptides	dipeptides, polypeptides
	proelastase	trypsin	protein, peptides	dipeptides, polypeptides
	procarboxy-peptidases	trypsin	polypeptides at COOH end	small peptides, amino acids
small intestine	aminopeptidase	no inactive precursor	polypeptide at NH_2 end, dipeptides	small peptides, amino acids
	dipeptidases, endopeptidases	no inactive precursor	polypeptides	small peptides, dipeptides

Table 10.2 **Enzymes that digest proteins.**

 ## ACTIVE TRANSPORT OF AMINO ACIDS INTO INTESTINAL EPITHELIAL CELLS

Mechanisms of active transport of amino acids and di- or tripeptides into intestinal epithelial cells are similar to those described for glucose uptake. At the brush border membrane Na^+-dependent symporters mediating amino acid uptake are linked to ATP-dependent pumping out of Na^+ at the contraluminal membrane. A similar H^+-dependent symporter is present on the brush border surface for di- and tripeptide active transport into the cell. Na^+-independent transporters are present on the contraluminal surface, allowing facilitated transport of amino acids to the hepatic portal system (see Chapter 8).

From both genetic and transporter studies at least six specific symporter systems have been identified for the uptake of L-amino acids from the intestinal lumen.

- Neutral amino acid symporter for amino acids with short or polar side chains (Ser, Thr, Ala)

- Neutral amino acid symporter for aromatic or hydrophobic side chains (Phe, Tyr, Met, Val, Leu, Ileu)
- Imino acid symporter (Pro, OH-Pro)
- Basic amino acid symporter (Lys, Arg, Cys)
- Acidic amino acid symporter (Asp, Glu)
- β-amino acid symporter (β-Ala, Tau)

These transport systems are also present in the renal tubules and defects in their molecular structure can lead to disease (e.g. Hartnup disease, an inherited disorder with intestinal defects of amino acid absorption and urinary wastage of neutral amino acids described in box on p. 90).

CELIAC DISEASE

A 22-year-old man presented with a history of weight loss, diarrhea, abdominal bloating and anemia. He described his stools as pale and bulky. Laboratory features included hemoglobin of 90 g/L (9 g/dL) (reference range 130–180 g/L; 13–18 g/dL). Biopsy of his small bowel demonstrated flattening of the mucosal surface, villous atrophy and disappearance of microvilli. A diagnosis of gluten-induced enteropathy or celiac disease was made. All wheat products were removed from the patient's diet and the symptoms resolved.

Comment. Celiac disease is an autoimmune condition characterized by malabsorption and specific diagnostic features exhibited by the intestinal mucosa. Since the absorptive surface is markedly reduced, the resulting indigestion/malabsorption is severe. The histologic changes are due to the interaction of gluten, the principal protein of wheat, with the epithelium. There is evidence to suggest that the deficit is located within the mucosal cells of the intestine and permits polypeptides, resulting from peptic and tryptic digestion of gluten, not only to exert local harmful effects within the intestine but also to be absorbed and to induce an antibody response. Circulating antibodies to wheat gluten and its fractions are frequently present in cases of celiac disease. The use of sensitive and specific serologic screening tests, such as endomysial antibodies of IgA subclass, has shown that celiac disease is underdiagnosed, especially in patients with unexplained anemia.

For hematology reference values, refer to Table 5.2 on p. 56.

LACTOSE INTOLERANCE

A 15-year-old African-American boy came across to the UK on an exchange visit for 2 months. After 2 weeks in the UK, he complained of abdominal discomfort, a feeling of being bloated, increased passage of urine and, more recently, the development of diarrhea. His only change in diet noted at the time was the introduction of milk. He had developed a considerable liking for milk and was consuming 1–2 large cartons per day. A lactose tolerance test was performed, whereby the young man was given 50 g lactose in an aqueous vehicle to drink. Plasma glucose levels did not rise by more than 1 mmol/L (18 mg/dL) over the next 2 hours, with sampling at 30-minute intervals. A diagnosis of lactose intolerance was made.

Comment. Lactose intolerance is a physiologic change resulting from acquired lactase deficiency. Lactase activity decreases with increasing age in children but the extent of the decline in activity is genetically determined and demonstrates ethnic variation. Lactase deficiency in the adult black population varies from 45% to 95%. If symptoms of malabsorption occur after the introduction of milk to adult diets, the diagnosis of acquired lactase deficiency should be considered. A diagnosis is made by challenging the small bowel with lactose and monitoring the rise in plasma glucose. An increase of more than 1.7 mmol/L (30 mg/dL) is considered normal. A rise of less than 1.1 mmol/L (20 mg/dL) is diagnostic of lactase deficiency. A rise of 1.1–1.7 mmol/L (20–30 mg/dL) is inconclusive.

Pancreatic proteases have different substrate specificity with respect to peptide bond cleavage

Trypsin cleaves proteins at arginine and lysine residues, chymotrypsin at aromatic amino acids and elastase at hydrophobic amino acids. The combined effect of these pancreatic enzymes is to produce an abundance of free amino acids and small molecular weight peptides of 2–8 residues in length.

Alongside protease secretion, the pancreas also produces copious amounts of sodium bicarbonate. This results in the neutralization of the acid contents of the stomach as they pass into the duodenum, thus promoting pancreatic protease activity.

Final digestion of peptides is dependent on small intestinal peptidases

The final digestion of di- and oligopeptides is carried out by small intestinal membrane-bound endopeptidases, dipeptidases and aminopeptidases. The endproducts of this surface enzyme activity are free amino acids, and di- and tripeptides which can then be absorbed across the enterocyte membrane by specific carrier-mediated transport. Di- and tripeptides are further hydrolyzed to their constituent amino acids within the enterocyte. The final step is therefore the transfer of free amino acids out of the enterocyte into the portal blood.

Summary

- Digestion and absorption of foods make the metabolic fuels available to the organism.
- Carbohydrates are digested to simple sugars.
- Fats are hydrolyzed to di- and monoglycerides.
- Proteins are hydrolyzed to di- and tripeptides and free amino acids.
- Digestion is a series of processes which prepare food for absorption.
- Defects in these mechanisms result in a variety of malabsorption and food intolerance syndromes.

ACTIVE LEARNING

1. Describe the process of digestion of starch.
2. Discuss the possible complications of persistent vomiting.
3. Which hormones aid digestion?
4. List the secretory products of the stomach.
5. Outline the mechanisms of sugar transport in the small intestine.
6. What is the role of micelles in the digestion of fat?

Further reading

Baumgart D, Carding SR. Inflammatory bowel disease: cause and immunobiology. *Lancet* 2007;**369**:1627–1640.

Broer A, Cavanaugh JA, Rasko JEJ, Broer S. The molecular basis of neutral aminoacidurias. *Pflugers Arch Eur J Physiol* 2006;**451**:511–517.

Drozdowski LA, Thomson ABR. Intestinal sugar transport. *World J Gastroenterol* 2006;**12**:1657–1670.

Hou W, Schubert ML. Gastric secretion. *Curr Opin Gastroenterol* 2006;**22**:593–598.

11. Micronutrients: Vitamins and Minerals

M H Dominiczak and I Broom

LEARNING OBJECTIVES

After reading this chapter you should be able to:

- Describe fat-soluble and water-soluble vitamins.
- Discuss the actions and sources of vitamins.
- Discuss signs and symptoms of vitamin deficiencies.
- Describe the role of trace metals in metabolism.

INTRODUCTION

Many vitamins and trace metals are essential nutrients. Deficiencies of micronutrients lead to specific clinical syndromes. They may be part of general malnutrition or may become manifested during illness. They are closely linked to malabsorption syndromes and also occur as a complication of gastrointestinal tract surgery. Multiple micronutrient deficiencies are much more common than single deficiencies. This chapter should be read in conjunction with Chapter 22.

Vitamins act as coenzymes, e.g. riboflavin in oxidoreductase reactions and biotin in carboxylation reactions. We classify the vitamins into fat-soluble and water-soluble. Fat-soluble vitamins are A, D, E, and K, and water-soluble vitamins are B_1, B_2, B_3, B_5, B_6, B_{12}, folate, biotin and vitamin C.

Several trace metals are also essential nutrients

Many of the trace metals, e.g. zinc, manganese or magnesium, are components of metalloenzymes. These enzymes lose their biological function without their trace metal prosthetic groups. Some trace elements such as cadmium, mercury, and aluminum find their way into the food chain and are cytotoxic. Essential trace elements, e.g. copper and manganese, may be toxic in excess.

To prevent the development of pathologies caused by vitamin or trace metal deficiencies, certain levels of intake have been recommended for healthy people. The requirement for vitamins depends, to some extent, on the macronutrient intake (Chapter 22).

Malnutrition is usually associated with multiple nutrient deficiencies

The assessment of micronutrient status is difficult for several reasons. Measurements of concentrations of circulating vitamins are inappropriate in the case of water-soluble vitamins, because these levels relate to the recent intake and do not reflect overall body status. Measurement of activities of enzymes associated with particular vitamins has been suggested as the most appropriate assessment. This is usually carried out as stimulation tests, i.e. enzyme activity is measured in the absence and in the presence of the vitamin. A deficit is recognized if the enzyme activity is stimulated in the presence of added vitamin.

There are also problems with interpretation of circulating concentrations of fat-soluble vitamins. They are associated with body fat and are often stored in tissues with circulating concentrations being kept relatively constant; for example, vitamin A is stored in the liver and is transported in plasma by specific binding proteins. A decrease in level of a nutrient within blood or plasma does not necessarily indicate a deficiency; it could be simply reflecting a metabolic response to stress or a change in physiologic status, such as pregnancy. Similarly, the circulating concentrations of trace metals bear little relation to nutrient status. For evaluation of trace element toxicity, tissues other than blood may need to be analyzed before a diagnosis of metal poisoning can be made.

FAT-SOLUBLE VITAMINS

Fat-soluble vitamins are stored in tissues

Fat-soluble vitamins are not as readily absorbed or extracted from the diet as water-soluble vitamins but ample amounts are stored in tissues. With the exception of vitamin K they do not act as coenzymes. Vitamins A and D behave more like hormones. Note that vitamin A and vitamin D but not vitamin E or K can be toxic in excess.

Vitamin A

'Vitamin A' is a generic term for three compounds, retinol, retinal and retinoic acid, all of which are found in animals. The most active of these derivatives is the retinoic acid.

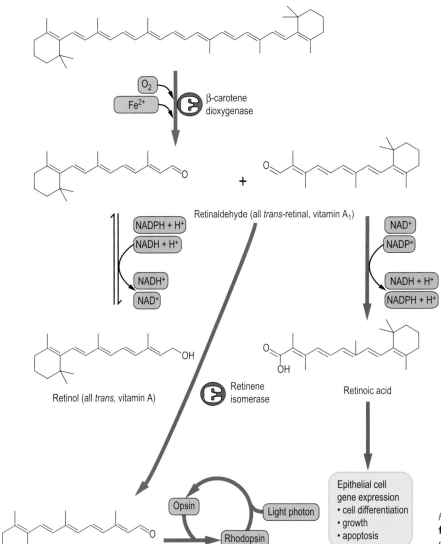

Fig. 11.1 **Structure, metabolism and function of vitamin A.** Conversion of retinaldehyde to retinoic acid is irreversible. (See also Chapter 40.)

The term 'retinoids' has been used to define these three substances as well as other synthetic compounds associated with vitamin A-like activity. The provitamin of vitamin A is β-carotene, which is water soluble and is found in plant food. β-Carotene is converted to all-*trans* retinal by the action of β-carotene dioxygenase in the small bowel. Further metabolism in the enterocytes produces retinol and retinoic acid (Fig. 11.1), which are transported to the liver for storage.

Vitamin A is stored in the liver and needs to be transported to its sites of action

Vitamin A is stored in the liver in the form of retinol and retinyl esters (retinol palmitate), bound to the cytosolic retinol-binding proteins (CRBP). Retinol is excreted from the liver bound to serum retinol-binding protein (RBP). Retinoic acid is thought to be transported to cells bound to either albumin or to a specific retinoic acid-binding protein (RABP). Retinol is taken up by cells via a membrane receptor.

Retinoic acid is a signaling molecule which interacts with ligand-activated transcription factors, the nuclear retinoid receptors. The retinoid acid receptors (RAR) bind all-*trans* and 9-*cis* retinoic acid, while the so-called rexinoid receptors (RXR) bind the 9-*cis* isomer only. These receptors can form heterodimers. RXR-type receptors can also interact with other nuclear receptors such as those for vitamin D_3, thyroid hormones or peroxisome proliferator-activated receptors (PPARs). Retinoic acid also has a role in the growth and development of the central nervous system.

Dark-green and yellow vegetables are good sources of β-carotene. Conversion of carotenoids to vitamin A is rarely 100% efficient and the potency of foods is described in retinol equivalents (RE; 1 RE equals 1 mg of retinol or 6 mg β-carotene, or 12 mg of other carotenes). The stores in the liver comprise approximately 1 year's supply. Liver, egg yolk, butter, and milk are good sources of preformed vitamin A.

Vitamin A deficiency presents as night blindness

The visual pigment rhodopsin is found in the rod cells of the retina and is formed by the binding of 11-*cis*-retinal to the apoprotein opsin. When rhodopsin is exposed to light, it is bleached, and retinal dissociates and is isomerized and reduced to all-*trans*-retinol (see Fig. 11.1). This reaction is accompanied by a conformational change and elicits a nerve impulse perceived by the brain as light (see also Chapter 41). Rod cells are responsible for vision in poor light.

Vitamin A deficiency presents as defective night vision or night blindness. Vitamin A also affects growth and differentiation of epithelial cells; thus its deficiency produces defective epithelialization and keratomalacia – corneal softening and opacity. Severe vitamin A deficiency leads to progressive keratinization of the cornea and to permanent blindness. In fact, vitamin A deficiency is the commonest cause of blindness in the world. Subclinical vitamin A deficiency may lead to increased susceptibility to infection. Severe vitamin A deficiency occurs mostly in the developing world but it is also fairly common in patients with severe liver disease or fat malabsorption.

Vitamin A is toxic in excess

Vitamin A is toxic in excess, with symptoms including bone pain, hair loss, dermatitis, hepatosplenomegaly, nausea, vomiting, double vision, headaches and diarrhea. It is virtually impossible to develop vitamin A toxicity by ingesting normal foods; however, toxicity may result from the use of vitamin A supplements. Increased intake of vitamin A is also associated with teratogenicity and should be avoided during pregnancy.

Vitamin D

Vitamin D (calciol) is really a hormone; it is only under conditions of inadequate exposure to sunlight that dietary intake is required. Vitamin D is the only vitamin that is not usually required in the diet. It is, in fact, a group of closely related sterols produced by the action of ultraviolet light (wavelength 290–310nm) on provitamins (ergosterol in plants and 7-dehydrocholesterol in animals; Fig. 11.2). 7-Dehydrocholesterol is synthesized in the liver and is found in the skin. The products of the photolytic reaction are ergocalciferol (vitamin D_2) and cholecalciferol (vitamin D_3), respectively. They are equipotent. Both are converted to a series of hydroxylated derivatives, firstly at the 25-position in the liver producing 25-hydroxycholecalciferol (25(OH)D_3; calcidiol) and at the 1-position in the kidney, producing the active compound 1α-,25-dihydroxycholecalciferol (1,25(OH)$_2D_3$; calcitriol). Details of of vitamin D metabolism and action are described in Chapter 25.

Most of the vitamin intake is via milk and other fortified foodstuffs. Fish oils, egg yolks and liver are also rich in vitamin D. Insufficient sunlight and increased metabolism of vitamin D due to low calcium intake or absorption may lead to deficiency. Vitamin D requirements are greater in winter due to lower exposure to sunlight.

Deficiency of vitamin D produces rickets in children and osteomalacia in adults

Rickets is characterized by soft pliable bones due to defective mineralization secondary to calcium deficiency. The characteristic bowing of the leg bones and the formation of the 'rickety rosary' around costochondral junctions result. In the adult, demineralization of preexisting bones takes place, increasing susceptibility to fractures. Vitamin D deficiency is also characterized by low circulating concentrations of calcium and an increased serum alkaline phosphatase activity (see Chapter 25).

Vitamin D is toxic in excess

Vitamin D excess causes enhanced calcium absorption and bone reabsorption, leading to hypercalcemia and metastatic calcium deposition. There is also a tendency to develop kidney stones because of the hypercalciuria secondary to hypercalcemia.

Vitamin E

Dietary vitamin E is a mixture of several compounds, called tocopherols. Ninety percent of vitamin E present in human tissues is in the form of the natural isomer, α-tocopherol (Fig. 11.3). The richest sources of naturally occurring vitamin E are vegetable oils and nuts. In European folklore, vitamin E has been associated with fertility and sexual activity. This is certainly true in other animal species where vitamin E plays a role in sperm production and egg implantation, but it is not the case in man.

Vitamin E is a membrane antioxidant

Vitamin E is the most abundant natural antioxidant and, owing to its lipid solubility, it is associated with all lipid-containing structures: membranes, lipoproteins and fat deposits (see Fig. 37.9). It is absorbed from the diet with other lipid components and there is no specific transport protein. In the circulation it is associated with lipoproteins. Fat malabsorption reduces the body fat content of vitamin E and, after a prolonged period, neurologic symptoms related to vitamin E deprivation have been reported. Low vitamin E intake in pregnancy and newborn infants may be associated with deficiency. This is usually found only in preterm infants fed on formula milk with low vitamin E content. Deficiency of vitamin E in premature infants causes hemolytic anemia, thrombocytosis and edema. There is little evidence in support of vitamin E toxicity.

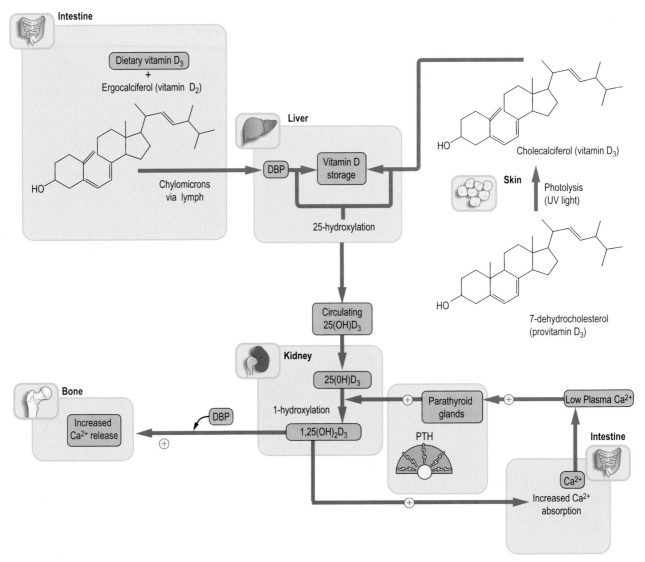

Fig. 11.2 **Structure, function and metabolism of vitamin D.** PTH, parathyroid hormone. DBP, vitamin D-binding protein.

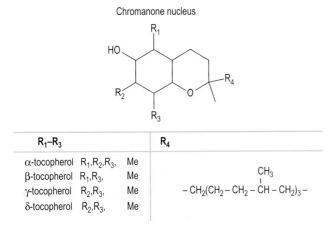

Chromanone nucleus

R$_1$–R$_3$		R$_4$
α-tocopherol	R$_1$,R$_2$,R$_3$, Me	
β-tocopherol	R$_1$,R$_3$, Me	
γ-tocopherol	R$_2$,R$_3$, Me	$-CH_2(CH_2-CH_2-\overset{CH_3}{\underset{|}{CH}}-CH_2)_3-$
δ-tocopherol	R$_2$,R$_3$, Me	

Fig. 11.3 **Structure of vitamin E family (tocopherols).** R$_1$-R$_3$ can be methylated in a variety of combinations. The polyisoprenoid side chain occurs at R$_4$. Me, methyl.

Vitamin K

Vitamin K is necessary for blood coagulation

Vitamin K is a group of related compounds, varying in the number of isoprenoid units in their side chain. Like vitamin E, the absorption of vitamin K depends on appropriate fat absorption. The structure, nomenclature and sources of the vitamin Ks are outlined in Figure 11.4. Vitamin K circulates as phylloquinone and its hepatic stores are in the form of manaquinones. It is required for the posttranslational modification of several proteins (factors II, VII, IX, and X) in the coagulation cascade (see Fig. 7.3). All these proteins are synthesized by the liver as inactive precursors and are activated by the carboxylation of specific glutamic acid (Gla) residues by a vitamin K-dependent enzyme (Fig. 11.5). Prothrombin

Source	Structure	Group
Plants	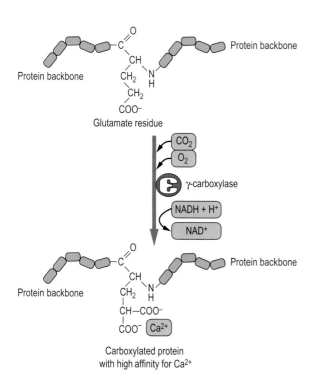	Phylloquinone (vitamin K_1)
Animal tissue Bacteria		Menaquinones (vitamin K_2)

Fig. 11.4 **Structure of the different forms of vitamin K.**

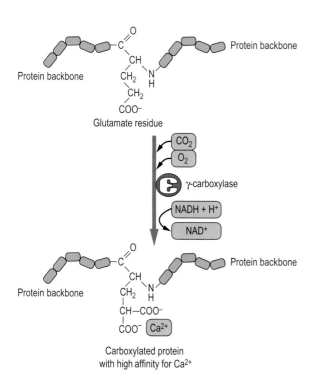

Fig. 11.5 **Vitamin K-mediated carboxylation of glutamate residues.** This reaction produces carboxylated residues, which are required for Ca^{2+} chelation.

(factor II) contains 10 of these carboxylated residues and all are required for this protein's specific chelation of Ca^{2+} ions during its function in coagulation. Recently, other proteins containing vitamin K-dependent Gla residues, such as osteocalcin, have been identified in tissues. Vitamin K is widely distributed in nature: its dietary sources are green leafy vegetables, fruits, dairy products, vegetable oils, cereals, and meats.

Vitamin K deficiency causes bleeding disorders

Vitamin K production by the intestinal microflora virtually ensures that dietary deficiency does not occur in man. However, rare deficiency may develop in those with liver disease or fat malabsorption, or in the newborn, and it is associated with bleeding disorders. Premature infants are especially at risk and may suffer from hemorrhagic disease of the newborn. The placental transfer of maternal vitamin K to the fetus is inefficient. Immediately after birth the circulating concentration decreases. Normally, it recovers on absorption of food but this might be delayed in preterm infants. In addition, the gut of the newborn is sterile, and therefore for several days after birth there is no source of vitamin K later provided by the intestinal microflora.

Inhibitors of vitamin K action are valuable antithrombotic drugs

Specific inhibitors of vitamin K-dependent carboxylation are used in the treatment of thrombosis-related diseases, e.g. in patients with deep vein thrombosis and pulmonary thromboembolism, or those with atrial fibrillation who are at risk of thrombosis. These are drugs of the dicoumarin group, e.g. warfarin, which inhibit the action of vitamin K. This drug is also used as rat poison and vitamin K is thus the antidote for human poisoning by this agent.

WATER-SOLUBLE VITAMINS

B-complex vitamins

B-complex vitamins act as coenzymes in many metabolic pathways

With the exception of vitamin B_{12} the body has no storage capacity for water-soluble vitamins. As a consequence, all water-soluble vitamins must be regularly supplied in the diet.

Vitamin	Structure	Deficiency disease	Food source
Thiamin (vit B₁)	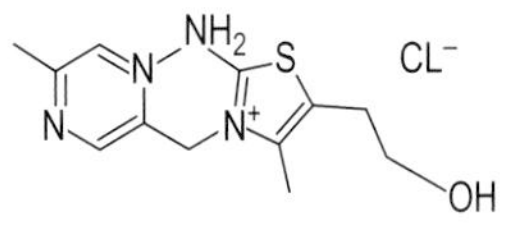	Beri-beri	Seeds, nuts, wheatgerms, legumes, lean meat
Riboflavin (vit B₂)	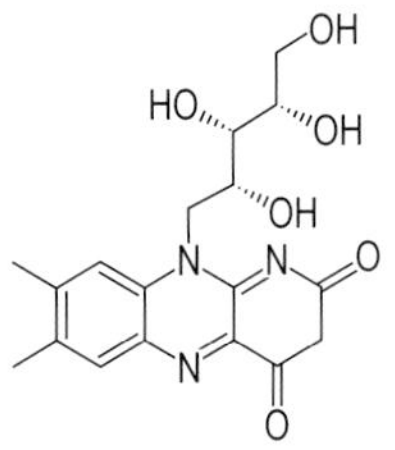	Pellagra	Meats, nuts, legumes
Niacin (vit B₃)	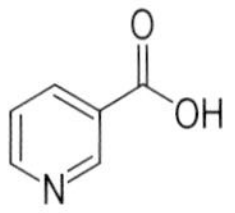	Pellagra	Meats, nuts, legumes
Panthothenic acid (vit B₅)	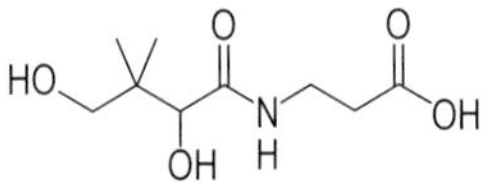		Yeast, grains, egg yolk, liver
Pyridoxine (vit B₆)	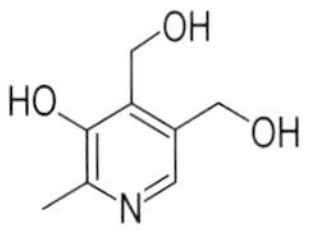	Neurologic disease	Yeast, liver, wheatgerm, nuts beans, bananas
Biotin	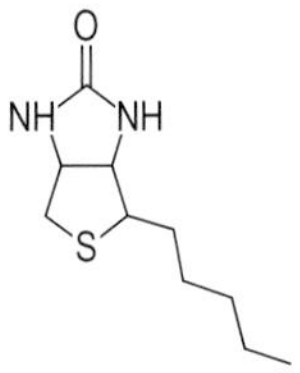	Widespread injury	Corn, soy, egg yolk, liver, kidney, tomatoes
Folate	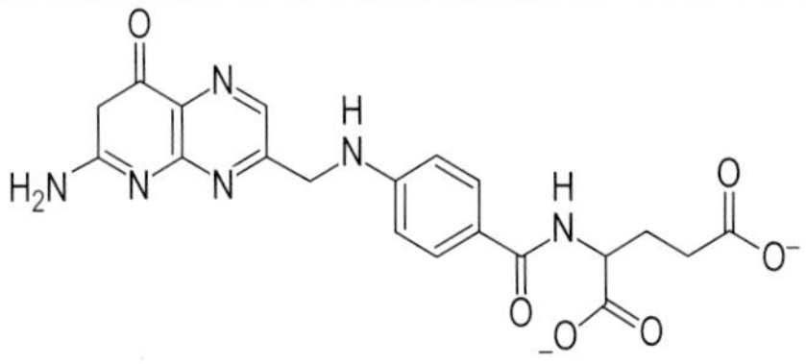	Anemia	Yeast, liver, leafy vegetables
Cobalamin (vit B₁₂)	Complex	Pernicious anemia	Liver, kidney, egg, cheese

Fig. 11.6 **Structure, sources and deficiency diseases of B vitamins.**

Any excess of these vitamins is excreted in the urine. In contrast to the fat-soluble vitamins there is no toxicity associated with excess of these vitamins.

B-complex vitamins are essential to the normal metabolism and are involved as coenzymes in many reactions. The B vitamins and their deficiency states are listed in Figure 11.6. Patients often present with multiple deficiencies; a deficiency of a single B vitamin is rare.

Thiamin (vitamin B₁)

Thiamin is essential for carboxylation reactions

Thiamin, in its active form as thiamin pyrophosphate, is essential for carboxylation reactions and some reactions catalyzed by transferases, and for normal carbohydrate energy metabolism. Thiamin is required for the transketolase reaction in the hexose monophosphate pathway (see Chapter 12). Although the pathways which require thiamin are well characterized, their failure in deficiency states and the signs and symptoms of deficiency are not clearly related.

Thiamin deficiency is associated with alcoholism

The early symptoms of thiamin deficiency are loss of appetite, constipation and nausea. They may progress to depression, peripheral neuropathy and unsteadiness, the latter related to impaired nerve cell function. Further deterioration in thiamin status results in mental confusion (loss of short-term memory), ataxia and loss of eye coordination. This combination, often seen in alcoholic patients, is the Wernicke–Korsakoff psychosis. Severe thiamin deficiency results in beri-beri, either 'dry' (without fluid retention) or 'wet' (associated with cardiac failure with edema). Beri-beri is characterized primarily by neuromuscular symptoms, and occurs in populations relying exclusively on polished rice for food. Wet beri-beri is particularly associated with alcoholism. The signs and symptoms of deficiency may also be seen in the elderly or in low-income groups with poor diet. The tests used to assess the thiamin status include measurement of erythrocyte transketolase activity and direct measurement by high-pressure liquid chromatography.

The greater the caloric intake, the larger the requirement for B vitamins

Diseases associated with high caloric requirement require greater intake of thiamin and other B vitamins. Increased energy supply, in particular from carbohydrates, requires increased amounts of B vitamins. Therefore, beri-beri might develop on a high-carbohydrate diet.

Riboflavin (vitamin B$_2$)

Riboflavin is associated with oxidoreductases

Riboflavin is attached to the sugar alcohol ribitol. The molecule is colored, fluorescent and decomposes in visible light but is heat stable. It is found in the oxidoreductases as flavin mononucleotide (FMN) and flavin adenine dinucleotide (FAD), and is required for the energy metabolism of both sugars and lipids (see Chapter 9). The activation of riboflavin is via an ATP-dependent enzyme system resulting in the production of FMN and FAD.

Lack of riboflavin in the diet causes a deficiency syndrome of inflammation of the corners of the mouth (angular stomatitis), the tongue (glossitis) and scaly dermatitis. A degree of photophobia may also exist. Owing to its light sensitivity, riboflavin deficiency may occur in newborn infants with jaundice, who are treated by phototherapy. Hypothyroidism is also known to affect the conversion of riboflavin to FMN and flavin adenine FAD. The measurements of erythrocyte glutathione reductase activity are used to determine the riboflavin status.

Niacin (vitamin B$_3$)

Niacin is required for NAD$^+$ and NADP$^+$ synthesis

Niacin is a generic name for nicotinic acid or nicotinamide, both of which are essential nutrients.

Niacin is active as part of the coenzyme nicotinamide adenine dinucleotide (NAD$^+$) and nicotinamide adenine dinucleotide phosphate (NADP$^+$), which participate in oxidoreductase reactions. The active form of the vitamin required for synthesis of NAD$^+$ and NADP$^+$ is nicotinate, and therefore nicotinamide must be deamidated before becoming available for synthesis of these coenzymes. Niacin can be synthesized from tryptophan and hence, in the truest sense, is not a vitamin. The conversion is, however, very inefficient and cannot supply sufficient amounts of niacin. In addition, the conversion requires thiamin, pyridoxine, and riboflavin, and on marginal diets such a synthesis would be problematic. The requirement for niacin is also related to energy expenditure.

Severe niacin deficiency produces dermatitis, diarrhea and dementia

Niacin deficiency initially produces a superficial glossitis but may progress to pellagra, which is characterized by dermatitis, sunburn-like skin lesions in areas of body exposed to sunlight and to pressure, and also by diarrhea, and dementia. Untreated pellagra is fatal. Certain drugs, e.g. the antituberculosis drug isoniazid, predispose to niacin deficiency. Very high doses of niacin can cause hepatotoxicity which is reversible on withdrawal. In the modern world pellagra is a medical curiosity.

Pyridoxine (vitamin B$_6$)

Pyridoxine is important in amino acid metabolism

Vitamin B$_6$ is a mixture of pyridoxine, pyridoxal, pyridoxamine, and their 5′-phosphates. Pyridoxine is the major form of vitamin B$_6$ in the diet, and pyridoxal phosphate is the active form of the vitamin. Pyridoxal phosphate participates as a cofactor in amino acid metabolism, and also in the glycogen phosphorylase reaction (see Fig. 19.2).

All forms of the vitamin are absorbed from the gut and during that time some hydrolysis of the phosphates occurs. Most tissues, however, contain pyridoxal kinase, which resynthesizes the phosphorylated forms required for the synthesis, catabolism and interconversion of amino acids (see Chapter 19). Pyridoxine is also required for synthesis of the neurotransmitters, serotonin and noradrenaline (see Chapter 42 and boxes on p. 590), the synthesis of sphingosine, and a component of sphingomyelin and sphingolipids (see Chapter 27). It is also required for the synthesis of heme (see Chapter 29).

Vitamin B₆ requirements increase with high protein intake

Because of its role in amino acid metabolism, vitamin B_6 requirements increase with protein intake. Vitamin B_6 deficiency in its mild form causes irritability, nervousness and depression, progressing in severe deficiency to peripheral neuropathy, convulsions and coma. Severe deficiency is also associated with a sideroblastic anemia. The drug isoniazid, by binding to pyridoxine, and the oral contraceptive pill, by increasing the synthesis of enzymes requiring the vitamin, may precipitate deficiency. Peripheral neuropathy is also associated with isoniazid treatment. The debate concerning the contraceptive pill continues but it is generally accepted that there is an increased requirement for pyridoxine. Assessment of pyridoxine status is based on the measurement of erythrocyte aspartate aminotransferase.

Biotin

Biotin is important for carboxylation reactions

Biotin is normally synthesized by the intestinal flora. It serves as a coenzyme in multienzyme complexes involved in carboxylation reactions (see Fig. 14.4). It is important in lipogenesis, gluconeogenesis, and the catabolism of the branched-chain amino acids. Most of the requirement for biotin is met from the synthesis by intestinal bacteria. Consumption of raw eggs can cause biotin deficiency because the egg-white protein, avidin, combines with biotin, preventing its absorption. Interestingly, certain inherited single or multiple carboxylase deficiencies can also lead to apparent biotin deficiency syndrome. Symptoms of biotin deficiency include depression, hallucinations, muscle pain and dermatitis. Children with multiple decarboxylase deficiency also demonstrate immunodeficiency disease.

Panthotenic acid

Panthotenic acid is a part of the coenzyme A (CoA) molecule

It is widely distributed in animals and plants. There is no evidence of deficiency in man, except on experimental diets.

Folic acid

Folic acid derivatives are important in single carbon transfer reactions

Folic acid (pteroyl glutamic acid) has a number of derivatives known collectively as folates. It participates in single carbon transfer reactions (e.g. methylation reactions important in both metabolism and regulation of gene expression) in numerous pathways including the synthesis of choline, serine, glycine, methionine and nucleic acids. Deficiency of folate contributes to hyperhomocysteinemia, which has been associated with the increased risk of cardiovascular disease. Folic acid is physiologically inactive until reduced to dihydrofolic acid. Its main forms are tetrahydrofolate, 5-methyl tetrahydrofolate (N^5MeTHF) and N^{10}-formyltetrahydrofolate-polyglutamate derived from 5MeTHF predominant in fresh food. Before polyglutamates can be absorbed, they must be hydrolyzed by glutamyl hydrolase (conjugase) in the small intestine. The main circulating form of folate is the monoglutamate N^5-THF. Polymorphisms associated with variants of 5,10-methylenetetrahydrofolate reductase gene, a key enzyme in folate metabolism, are associated with conditions such as colon cancer, spina bifida and adult acute lymphocytic leukemia.

Folic acid is necessary for the synthesis of DNA

Rapidly dividing cells have high requirements for this vitamin since its role is in the synthesis of purines and pyrimidine thymine required for DNA synthesis (see Chapter 31 and box on p. 413). On the basis of selective toxicity in rapidly growing cells, e.g. bacteria and cancer cells, this function of folate was the principle behind the development of structural analogs of folate (folic acid antagonists), which are used as antibiotics (e.g. trimethoprim) and anticancer agents (methotrexate). Folic acid is present in liver, yeast, and green leafy vegetables. It is measured by high pressure liquid chromato-graphy (HPLC).

Folate deficiency causes megaloblastic anemia

Failure to synthesize methionine and nucleic acids in folate deficiency states accounts for the signs and symptoms of megaloblastic anemia, i.e. the presence of enlarged blast cells in the bone marrow. Deficiency of folate is one of the commonest vitamin deficiencies and the hematologic abnormalities associated with this cannot be distinguished from those of vitamin B_{12} deficiency (see below). The neurologic changes are also similar. The block in synthesis slows down the production of erythrocytes, causing the appearance of macrocytic erythrocytes with fragile membranes and a tendency to hemolyze. A macrocytic anemia thus ensues in association with a megaloblastic bone marrow.

There are many causes of folate deficiency, including inadequate intake, impaired absorption, impaired metabolism, and increased demand. The most common examples of increased demand are pregnancy and lactation. Folic acid requirements increase dramatically as the blood volume and number of erythrocytes increase in pregnancy. By the third trimester of pregnancy folic acid requirements double. However, megaloblastic anemias in pregnancy, other than multiple pregnancy, are rare. The common practice is to provide folate supplements during pregnancy. Folate supplementation during the periconception period (definitions of that period are variable: the one used in clinical studies is 4 weeks before and 8 weeks after conception) prevents spina bifida; the closure of the neural tube occurs between 22–28 days

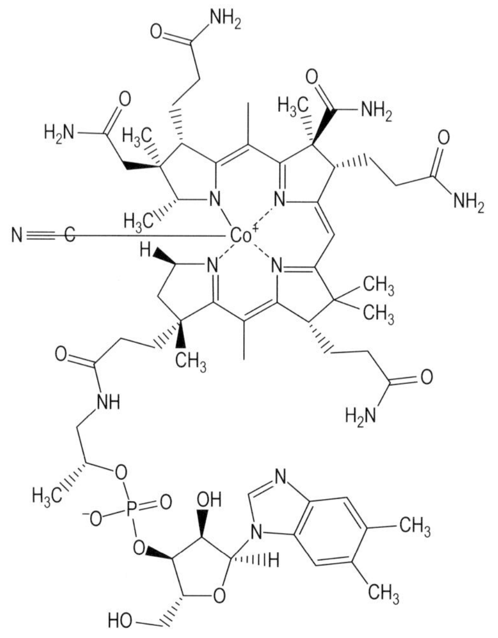

Fig. 11.7 **Vitamin B$_{12}$.** There is a cyano-group (CN) attached to the cobalt: this is an artifact of extraction but it is also the most stable form of the vitamin and indeed is the commercially available product for treatment. The cyano group does require removal for conversion to the active form of the vitamin.

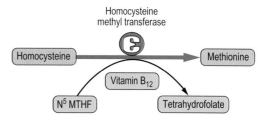

Fig. 11.8 **The 'tetrahydrolate trap'.** Vitamin B$_{12}$ and folate are involved in the conversion of homocysteine to methionine. An absence of vitamin B$_{12}$ inhibits the reaction and leads to the build-up of N^5-methyltetrahydrofolate (N^{5}MeTHF). This is known as the 'tetrahydrofolate trap'.

after conception. Folate deficiencies are seen in the elderly as a result of poor diet and poor absorption.

Vitamin B$_{12}$

Vitamin B$_{12}$ is part of the structure of heme

Vitamin B$_{12}$ (cobalamin) has a complex ring structure similar to the porphyrin system of heme (see Chapter 29) but is more hydrogenated. The iron at the center of the heme ring is replaced by a cobalt ion (Co^{3+}). This is the only known function of cobalt in the body. In addition, and essential for the chelation of the cobalt ion, a dimethylbenzimidazole ring is also part of the active molecule (Fig. 11.7). Vitamin B$_{12}$ participates in the recycling of folates, and in methionine synthesis.

Vitamin B$_{12}$ is synthesized solely by bacteria. It is absent from all plants but is concentrated in the livers of animals in three forms: methylcobalamin, adenosylcobalamin, and hydroxycobalamin. Liver is a useful source of this vitamin and in the past was used in the treatment of deficiency states.

It is impossible to consider the function of vitamin B$_{12}$ in isolation from folate

The functions of vitamin B$_{12}$ and folate are interrelated and deficiency of either produces the same signs and symptoms. The reaction involving both these vitamins is a methylation

reaction, the conversion of homocysteine to methionine (Fig. 11.8).

Vitamin B$_{12}$ is required in only one further reaction, that is the conversion of methylmalonyl-CoA to succinyl-CoA. The coenzyme form of the vitamin in this case is 5′-deoxyadenosyl cobalamin. Specific mechanisms exist for the absorption and transport of cobalamin (Fig. 11.9).

Megaloblastic anemia characteristic of vitamin B$_{12}$ deficiency is probably due to a secondary deficiency of reduced folate and a consequence of the accumulation of N^5-methyltetrahydrofolate; therefore, the folate/B$_{12}$-associated syndrome. A neurologic presentation can also develop in the absence of anemia. This is known as subacute combined degeneration of the cord and is probably secondary to a relative deficiency of methionine in the cord. Since vitamin B$_{12}$ is required in only two reactions, deficiency of this vitamin results in an accumulation of methylmalonic acid and homocysteine and consequent methylmalonic aciduria and homocystinuria.

Vitamin B$_{12}$ deficiency causes pernicious anemia

Vitamin B$_{12}$ deficiency can occur through several mechanisms. The most common one is pernicious anemia, and it is due to lack of intrinsic factor (IF) in the stomach; this prevents the vitamin absorption in the terminal ileum. IF lack can also be caused by gastric surgery. A similar situation, albeit caused through a different mechanism, arises upon surgical removal of the ileum, for instance in Crohn's disease (see Chapter 10). Vegans are at risk of developing a dietary deficiency of vitamin B$_{12}$ since it is found only in foods of animal origin (the vegetable diet may contain some vitamin only if it is contaminated with microorganisms, such as yeasts). Vitamin B$_{12}$ is secreted in the bile and there is a marked enterohepatic circulation. Disturbances of this circulation can have major effects on vitamin B$_{12}$ status (Table 11.1).

Vitamin B$_{12}$ must be supplemented when folate treatment is given

Importantly, giving folate alone in a case of vitamin B$_{12}$ deficiency aggravates the neuropathy. Therefore, if supplementation is required during investigation of the cause of

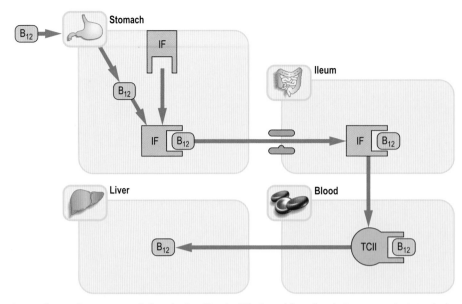

Fig. 11.9 **Digestion, absorption and transport of vitamin B$_{12}$.** Simple diffusion of free vitamin B$_{12}$ across the intestinal membrane accounts for 3% of transported vitamin, and complexing with intrinsic factor (IF) accounts for 97%. Vitamin B$_{12}$ derivatives are released from food by peptic digestion in the stomach and become attached to specific binding on IF, secreted by the parietal cells of the gastric mucosa. IF–B$_{12}$ complex is required for absorption by specific receptor sites on the ileal mucosa. The rate-limiting factor in this process is the number of ileal receptor sites. Other transport proteins (transcobalamin I, II and III (TC I, II and III) and R-proteins) are involved in the delivery or storage of the cobalamins. The latter are secreted by the salivary glands and gastric mucosa.

Causes of vitamin B$_{12}$ deficiency	
Mechanism	**Time to develop clinical deficiency (years)**
vegan diet	10–12
intrinsic factor failure	1–4
ileal dysfunction	rapid

Table 11.1 **Causes of vitamin B$_{12}$ deficiency.**

megaloblastic anemia, folate needs to be given together with vitamin B$_{12}$ (after blood and bone marrow specimens have been taken to confirm the diagnosis).

Vitamin C

Vitamin C is a reducing agent

Vitamin C, ascorbic acid, is an essential nutrient in humans, higher primates, guinea pigs and fruit-eating bats. In all other animals, a specific pathway exists for its synthesis. The synthetic pathway and structure of vitamin C are shown in Figure 11.10. Vitamin C is labile: it is easily destroyed by oxygen, metal ions, increased pH, heat and light. Vitamin C serves as a reducing agent and its active form is ascorbic acid, which is oxidized during the transfer of reducing equivalents

to dehydroascorbic acid (which also can act as a source of the vitamin). Antioxidant activity of vitamin C is illustrated in Figure 37.8. Vitamin C participates in the synthesis of collagen and adrenaline, in steroidogenesis, degradation of tyrosine, bile acid formation, in the absorption of iron and in bone mineral metabolism. The prime function of this compound is to maintain metal cofactors in their lower valence state, e.g. Fe^{2+} and Cu^{2+}. This is the case in the synthesis of collagen where it is required specifically for the hydroxylation of proline (see Chapter 28).

Vitamin C deficiency causes scurvy and compromises immune function

Vitamin C deficiency causes scurvy characterized by a defective collagen synthesis. It is characterized by subcutaneous and other hemorrhages, muscle weakness, soft, swollen, bleeding gums, osteoporosis, poor wound healing and anemia. The osteoporosis results from the inability to maintain bone matrix in association with demineralization. This latter aspect results in the appearance of Looser's zones on radiography, especially in the hands.

Except in older individuals, vitamin C deficiency resulting in the full clinical picture of scurvy is rare.

Milder forms of vitamin C deficiency are more common and the manifestation of such includes easy bruising and the formation of petechiae (small, pinpoint hemorrhages under the skin) both due to increased capillary fragility. Immune function is also compromised. This reduction in immuno-competence has been the basis for providing megadoses of

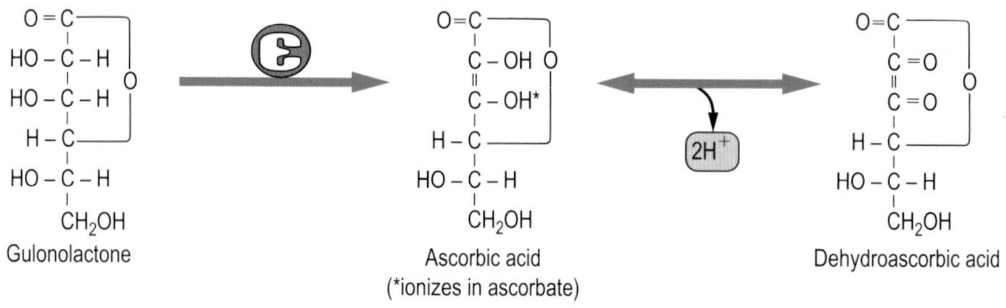

Fig. 11.10 **Structure and synthesis of vitamin C (ascorbic acid).** Note that the enzyme that converts gulonolactone to ascorbic acid is absent in man, higher primates, guinea pigs and fruit-eating bats.

the vitamin to prevent the common cold and also for its role in cancer prevention. No clear evidence exists, however, to substantiate these claims first made by Linus Pauling in the 1970s. Vitamin C is certainly required for normal leukocyte function, and leukocyte vitamin C levels drop precipitously after stress caused by either trauma or infection.

VITAMIN B$_{12}$ TRANSPORT PROTEINS

The intrinsic factor (IF) is a highly specific glycoprotein. Other cobalamin-binding proteins, R-proteins, secreted by the salivary glands and stomach, are also glycoproteins and along with trans-cobalamin (TC)I and III are now termed cobalaphilins. The third type of cobalamic protein, also a glycoprotein, is TCII. All three classes of B$_{12}$-transport proteins are glycoproteins, are single polypeptide chains (340–375 amino acid residues), and have a single binding site for cobalamin. They do not, however, cross-react with each other immunologically, and are coded for by different genes.

At acid pH, R-proteins bind cobalamin more strongly than IF. In contrast to IF, they are normally degraded by pancreatic proteinases. Thus, in pancreatic disease where R-proteins are not degraded, there is less cobalamin available to bind to IF, with loss of absorptive capacity for this vitamin.

In the final stages of the absorption process, a specific site on the IF molecule binds to the ileal receptor in the presence of Ca^{2+} and at neutral pH. As the IF–B$_{12}$ complex crosses the ileal mucosa, IF is released and the B$_{12}$ is transferred to a plasma transport protein TCII. Other cobalamin-binding proteins, TCI and possibly TCIII, exist in the plasma and liver. In the liver, these provide excellent storage forms of the vitamin, a situation that is unique for water-soluble vitamins.

Once cobalamin is bound to TCII in portal blood, it disappears from plasma in a few hours. The major circulating form is methylcobalamin. In the liver, 5'-deoxyadenosyl cobalamin accounts for 70% and methylcobalamin for only 3% of the total amount.

The TCII–cobalamin complex delivers exogenous cobalamin to the tissues, where it binds to specific cell surface receptors. It enters the cell by endocytosis, ultimately releasing the cobalamin as hydroxycobalamin. Conversion of hydroxycobalamin to methylcobalamin occurs in the cytosol. TCII is also thought to be necessary for the delivery of vitamin B$_{12}$ to the central nervous system.

Citrus and soft fruits and growing points of vegetables are rich sources of vitamin C. There is no evidence that vitamin C taken in excess is toxic. Theoretically, since it is metabolized to oxalate, there is a risk of the development of renal oxalate stones in susceptible individuals. However, this has not been substantiated in practice.

Dietary supplementation of vitamins

Supplementation of some vitamins provides clear health benefit.

Areas where the benefits of vitamin supplementation are clear include supplementation of folic acid to women who are pregnant or are planning pregnancy, to prevent neural tube defects. Vitamin D provision to people living in areas of low sunlight has also been beneficial.

Benefits of vitamin supplementation in cancer and cardiovascular disease are uncertain

Because the supplementation of folic acid and vitamin B$_6$ and B$_{12}$ lowers plasma homocysteine concentration, it has been suggested that it could be beneficial for the prevention of cardiovascular disease. There also were suggestions that supplementation of vitamins A, C and E is protective against cancer. Some observational studies suggested that the supplementation of vitamins C and E could also be useful in the prevention of cardiovascular disease. However, prospective studies of this yielded controversial results. The recommendations of the US Preventive Services Task Force published in 2003 (www.preventiveservices.ahrq.gov) say that 'current evidence is insufficient to recommend for or against the use of supplements of vitamins A, C, or E , multivitamins with folic acid, or antioxidant combinations for the prevention of cancer or cardiovascular disease'. Note that these recommendations do not apply to people with nutritional deficiencies, pregnant and lactating women, children, elderly persons and people with chronic illnesses.

As mentioned above, high-dose vitamin supplementation may be harmful: the example is the reduction of bone mineral density, hepatotoxicity, and teratogenicity associated with high doses of vitamin A. β-Carotene supplementation to smokers was also harmful, resulting in an increase in lung cancer mortality.

Fruit and vegetables are the best sources of vitamins

In the clinical studies mentioned above, the vitamins were supplemented in a pure form, rather than as complete food-stuffs, and it might be that this is why the benefit of supplementation was not evident. Clearly, there are benefits of eating diets rich in vegetables and fruit, which are the most important sources of vitamins. There is no reason to discourage people from taking vitamin supplements apart from proven instances of toxicity associated with excessive supplementation.

TRACE ELEMENTS

Metal ions are required as active components of proteins

The most obvious of these is iron. It forms part of the proteins involved in the transfer of molecular oxygen (see Chapter 5). Other metals have been found to be essential for normal biological function. These include metals previously thought to be toxic; indeed, environmental excesses of these do result in toxicity. Such elements include chromium, selenium, manganese, copper and zinc, and are called essential trace elements.

Zinc

Zinc is a component of numerous enzymes associated with carbohydrate and energy metabolism, protein synthesis and degradation, nucleic acid synthesis, cellular transport functions and protection from oxidative damage. Spermatogenesis is also a zinc-dependent process based on the metal's role in testosterone metabolism. It plays a role in maintaining exocrine and endocrine pancreatic function. Its effects, however, are most obviously seen in the maintenance of skin integrity and in wound healing.

Absorption of zinc from the diet is an active process and shares gut transport mechanisms with copper and iron

On absorption, zinc is found bound to the protein metallothioneine, a cysteine-rich protein, which is also associated with the binding of other divalent metal ions such as copper. Its synthesis is dependent on the amount of trace metals present in the diet. Its excess may interfere with copper absorption. Zinc is probably the least toxic of the trace metals but increased oral intake interferes with copper absorption, leading to deficiency of the latter.

Zinc deficiency affects growth, skin integrity and wound healing

ZINC DEFICIENCY

A 34-year-old man who required total intravenous feeding had been receiving the same prescription for some 4 months, with no assessment of his trace metal status. During this time, he continued to have major gastrointestinal losses and intermittent pyrexia. Initially, he developed a rash across his face, head, and neck, with accompanying hair loss and, by the end of the 4-month period, was clearly zinc deficient. He had a widespread acne-type rash and was virtually devoid of hair. His serum zinc concentration at that time was less than 1 μmol/L (range: 9–20 μmol/L; 60–130 μg/dL).

Comment. Patients with major catabolic illness and increased gastrointestinal losses have markedly increased zinc requirements. The zinc-depleted state this patient developed would aggravate his illness by preventing healing of his gastrointestinal lesions and by making him more susceptible to infection due to defects in his immune competence. Patients receiving intravenous feeding need to have their micronutrient status checked regularly.

Zinc deficiency is not uncommon: in children it is characterized by growth retardation, skin lesions, and impairment of sexual development. A specific inherited defect in the absorption of zinc from the gut was identified in the 1970s; it was termed acrodermatitis enteropathica with the clinical appearance of severe skin lesions, diarrhea and loss of hair (alopecia). Its deficiency also leads to impairment in taste and smell and to delayed wound healing.

Increased losses of zinc occur in patients with major burns and in those with renal damage. Zinc loss in renal disease is due to its association with plasma albumin, and it accompanies urinary protein loss. Substantial amounts of zinc may also be lost during dialysis. Increased metallothioneine synthesis is part of the metabolic response to trauma and results in a reduction of serum zinc concentration. During intravenous feeding, in situations where there is frequently an increased demand, failure to replace it may produce a symptomatic deficiency.

Measurement of serum zinc concentration is the usual method of assessing zinc status. However, many conditions and environmental factors affect its concentration in plasma, including inflammation, stress, cancer, smoking, steroid administration and hemolysis.

Copper

Copper scavenges superoxide and other reactive oxygen species

Copper is associated with several oxygenase enzymes including cytochrome oxidase and superoxide dismutase (the latter also requires zinc for activity). One of the main roles of copper, especially in superoxide dismutase but also in association with the plasma copper-carrying protein ceruloplasmin, is the scavenging of superoxide and other reactive oxygen species. Copper is also required for the crosslinking of collagen, being an essential component of lysyl oxidase. The only mechanism of copper excretion is elimination through bile.

Absorption of copper from the gut is, similarly to zinc, associated with metallothioneine. Copper availability in the diet is less affected by dietary constituents than zinc, although high fiber intake reduces availability by complexing with copper.

In plasma, the absorbed copper is bound to albumin. Copper–albumin complex is quickly taken up by the liver. Within the hepatocyte copper is associated with intracellular metallothioneines which are also capable of binding zinc and cadmium. Copper is transported within the hepatocyte to sites of protein synthesis by a chaperone protein and it is incorporated into apoceruloplasmin. This incorporation is catalyzed by an ATPase called ATP7B. Ceruloplasmin is released into circulation.

Copper excess causes liver cirrhosis

When taken orally, copper is generally nontoxic but in large doses it accumulates in tissues. Chronic excessive intake, however, results in liver cirrhosis. Acute toxicity is manifested by marked hemolysis and damage to both liver and brain cells. The latter is seen in the autosomal dominant inherited metabolic defect of Wilson's disease, where the liver's capacity to synthesize ceruloplasmin is compromised. The cause are mutations in the gene coding for the ATP7B ATPase. This results in a reduced incorporation of copper into ceruloplasmin, and in cellular accumulation. Excess of apoceruloplasmin is degraded. Copper accumulates in tissues such as the brain and cornea. Patients present with neurological symptoms or liver cirrhosis and have typical Kaiser–Fleischer rings in the cornea. Typically, there is also a low concentration of ceruloplasmin and high urinary copper excretion (see box on p. 92).

Copper deficiency is rare

Rare copper deficiency leads to an anemia; skin and hair may also be affected. Copper deficiency is most likely to occur from reduced intake or excess loss, e.g. during renal dialysis. Deficiency manifests itself as a microcytic hypochromic anemia (characterized by pale erythrocytes) that is resistant to iron therapy. There is also a reduction in the number of leukocytes in the blood (neutropenia) and degeneration of vascular tissue with bleeding, due to defects in the synthesis of elastin and collagen. In severe deficiency, skin depigmentation and alteration in hair structure also occur.

Selenium

Selenium occurs in all cells as amino acids selenomethionine and selenocysteine

Selenium forms a part of an antioxidant enzyme glutathione peroxidase. It is also a part of type I iodothyronine 5-deiodinase which participates in the hepatic deiodination of thyroxine; in animals it is a component of muscle proteins selenoprotein P and selenoprotein W. Selenium is absorbed from the small intestine. It is protein bound in circulation, and is excreted in urine.

Selenium is present in diet as selenomethionine and selenocysteine. Its content in plant food depends on the content in the the soil. Its dietary sources include organ meats, fish (tuna) and shellfish, and cereals.

Increased intake of selenium might be required during lactation. There is a rare selenium-responsive cardiomyopathy (Keshan disease), which is endemic in China in areas of very low selenium intake. Deficiency of selenium can also develop during total parenteral nutrition and may result in chronic muscle pain, abnormal nail beds, and cardiomyopathy. Excess of selenium leads to liver cirrhosis, splenomegaly, gastrointestinal bleeding and depression.

Other metals

Numerous other trace metals are required for normal biologic function, for example manganese, molybdenum, vanadium, nickel, and even cadmium. The latter is probably better known for its renal toxic effects and has been seen especially in shipyard workers exposed to this metal over long periods of time. No doubt, as techniques for separation and analysis develop, other metals and other functions of known essential minerals will become known. This will lead to a better understanding of the epidemiology of certain diseases which may have, at least in part, an environmental etiology.

Summary

- Vitamins function mostly as cofactors to enzymes.
- Fat-soluble vitamins can be stored in the adipose tissue but there usually is only a short-term supply of the water-soluble ones.
- Dietary micronutrient deficiencies are most likely to occur in susceptible groups with increased demand, or in people unable to maintain sufficient intake. Children, pregnant women, the elderly and low-income groups are particularly vulnerable.
- Gastrointestinal disease and gastrointestinal surgery are potential causes of micronutrient deficiencies.

■ Vitamin and trace metal supplements are particularly important in patients who remain on artificial diets and on parenteral nutrition.

■ While there are controversies regarding some vitamin supplementation, the intake of fruit and vegetables as sources of micronutrients is unequivocally recommended.

ACTIVE LEARNING

1. Compare and contrast the deficiencies of vitamin B_{12} and folic acid.
2. When may an increased intake of a nutrient or energy precipitate vitamin deficiencies?
3. Is vitamin A supplementation safe?
4. Describe the clinical importance of copper.
5. Which vitamins play a role in the development of hyperhomocysteinemia?

Further reading

Asplund K. Antioxidant vitamins in the prevention of cardiovascular disease: a systematic review. *J Int Med* 2002;**251**:372–392.

El-Youssef M. Wilson disease. *Mayo Clin Proc* 2003;**78**:1126–1136.

Fairfield KM, Fletcher RH. Vitamins for chronic disease prevention in adults: scientific review. *JAMA* 2002;**287**:3116–3126.

Ferenci P. Diagnosis and current therapy of Wilson's disease. *Aliment Pharmacol Therapeut* 2004;**19**:157–165.

Fletcher RH, Fairfield KM. Vitamins for chronic disease prevention in adults: clinical applications. *JAMA* 2002;**287**:3127–3129.

Jones G. Eating fruit and vegetables. *BMJ* 2003;**326**:888.

Lucock M. Is folic acid the ultimate functional food component for disease prevention?. *BMJ* 2004;**328**:211–214.

Panel on Dietary Reference Values of the Committee on Medical Aspects of Food Policy. *Dietary reference values for food energy and nutrients for the United Kingdom* London: TSO, 2003.

Websites

National Guideline Clearinghouse: www.guideline.gov
US Preventive Services Task Force: www.preventiveservices.ahrq.gov

12. Anaerobic Metabolism of Glucose in the Red Blood Cell

J W Baynes

LEARNING OBJECTIVES

After reading this chapter you should be able to:

- Outline the sequence of reactions in anaerobic glycolysis, the central pathway of carbohydrate metabolism in all cells.
- Summarize the energetics of anaerobic glycolysis, including the reactions involved in the utilization and formation of ATP, and the net yield of ATP during glycolysis.
- Identify the primary site of allosteric regulation of glycolysis and the mechanism of regulation of this enzyme.
- Identify steps in glycolysis that illustrate the use of coupled reactions to drive thermodynamically unfavored processes, including substrate-level phosphorylation.
- Describe the major roles of the pentose phosphate pathway in erythrocytes and nucleated cells.
- Describe the role of anaerobic glycolysis in development of dental caries.
- Explain why glycolysis is essential for normal red cell functions, including consequences of deficiencies in glycolytic enzymes and the role of glycolysis in adaptation to high altitude.
- Explain the origin of drug-induced hemolytic anemia in persons with G6PD deficiency.

INTRODUCTION

Glucose is the major carbohydrate on Earth, the backbone and monomer unit of cellulose and starch. It is also the only fuel that is used by all cells in our body. All of these cells, even the microbes in our intestines, begin the metabolism of glucose by a pathway termed glycolysis, i.e. carbohydrate (glyco) splitting (lysis). Glycolysis is catalyzed by soluble cytosolic enzymes and is the ubiquitous, central metabolic pathway for glucose metabolism. The erythrocyte, commonly known as the red blood cell (RBC), is unique among all cells in the body – it uses glucose and glycolysis as its sole source of energy. Thus, the RBC is a useful model for an introduction to glycolysis.

Pyruvate, a three-carbon carboxylic acid, is the endproduct of glycolysis; 2 moles of pyruvate are formed per mole of glucose. In cells with mitochondria and oxidative metabolism, pyruvate is converted completely into CO_2 and

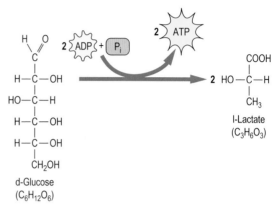

Fig. 12.1 **Conversion of glucose to lactate during anaerobic glycolysis.** One mole of glucose is converted to 2 moles of lactate during anaerobic glycolysis. No oxygen is consumed, nor is CO_2 produced in this pathway. There is a net yield of 2 mol ATP per mol glucose converted to lactate.

H_2O – glycolysis in this setting is termed aerobic glycolysis. In RBCs, which lack mitochondria and oxidative metabolism, pyruvate is reduced to lactic acid, a three-carbon hydroxy-acid, the product of anaerobic glycolysis. Each mole of glucose yields 2 moles of lactate, which are then excreted into blood. Two molecules of lactic acid contain exactly the same number of carbons, hydrogens, and oxygens as one molecule of glucose (Fig. 12.1); however, there is sufficient free energy available from the cleavage and rearrangement of the glucose molecule to produce 2 moles of ATP per mole of glucose converted into lactate. The RBC uses most of this ATP to maintain electrochemical and ion gradients across its plasma membrane.

In the red cell, 10–20% of the glycolytic intermediate, 1,3-bisphosphoglycerate, is diverted to the synthesis of 2,3-bisphosphoglycerate (2,3-BPG), an allosteric regulator of the O_2 affinity of Hb. The pentose phosphate pathway, a shunt from glycolysis, accounts for about 10% of glucose metabolism in the red cell. In the red cell, this pathway has a special role in protection against oxidative stress, while in nucleated cells it also serves as a source of NADPH for biosynthetic reactions and pentoses for nucleic acid synthesis.

THE ERYTHROCYTE

The erythrocyte, or red blood cell (RBC), represents 40–45% of blood volume and over 90% of the formed elements (erythrocytes, leukocytes, and platelets) in blood. The RBC is, both structurally and metabolically, the simplest cell in the body – the endproduct of the maturation of bone marrow reticulocytes. During its maturation, the RBC loses all its subcellular organelles. Without nuclei, it lacks the ability to synthesize DNA or RNA. Without ribosomes or an endoplasmic reticulum, it cannot synthesize or secrete protein. Because it cannot oxidize fats, a process requiring mitochondrial activity, the RBC relies exclusively on blood glucose as a fuel. Metabolism of glucose in the RBC is entirely anaerobic, consistent with the primary role of the RBC in oxygen transport and delivery, rather than its utilization.

GLYCOLYSIS

Overview

Glucose enters the RBC by facilitated diffusion, via the insulin-independent glucose transporter, GLUT-1. The glucose concentration in the RBC is not significantly different from that in plasma. Thus, clinical laboratory measurements of glucose concentration in plasma, serum and whole blood are essentially identical.

Glycolysis proceeds through a series of phosphorylated intermediates, starting with the synthesis of glucose-6-phosphate (Glc-6-P). During this process, which involves 10 enzymatically catalyzed steps, two molecules of ATP are expended (*investment* stage) to build up a nearly symmetric intermediate, fructose-1,6-bisphosphate (Fru-1,6-BP), which is then cleaved (*splitting* stage) to two three-carbon triose phosphates. These are eventually converted into lactate, with production of ATP, during the *yield* stage of glycolysis. The yield stage includes both redox and phosphorylation reactions, leading to formation of four molecules of ATP during the conversion of the two triose phosphates into lactate. The outcome is a net 2 moles of ATP per mole of glucose converted into lactate.

Glycolysis is a relatively inefficient pathway for extracting energy from glucose: the yield of 2 moles of ATP per mole of glucose is only about 5% of the 36–37 ATP that are available by complete oxidation of glucose to CO_2 and H_2O by mitochondria in other tissues.

One might ask why a 10-step pathway is required to convert glucose to lactate; couldn't it have been done in fewer steps or by cleavage of one carbon at a time? The answer, from a metabolic point of view, is that glycolysis is not an isolated pathway; most glycolytic intermediates serve as branch points to other metabolic pathways. In this way, the metabolism of glucose intersects with the metabolism of fats, proteins and nucleic acids, as well as other pathways of carbohydrate metabolism. Some of these metabolic interactions are shown in Figure 12.2.

The investment stage of glycolysis

Glucose-6-phosphate

Glucose is taken up into the red cell via the facilitated transporter, GLUT-1 (Chapter 8); this protein accounts for about 5% of total red cell membrane protein, so that glucose transport is not rate limiting for glycolysis. The first step in the commitment of glucose to glycolysis is the phosphorylation of glucose to Glc-6-P, catalyzed by the enzyme hexokinase (Fig. 12.3, top). The formation of Glc-6-P from free glucose and inorganic phosphate is energetically unfavorable, so that a molecule of ATP must be expended or *invested* in the phosphorylation reaction; the hydrolysis of ATP is coupled to the synthesis of Glc-6-P. Glc-6-P is trapped in the RBC, along with other phosphorylated intermediates in glycolysis, because there are no transport systems for sugar phosphates in the plasma membranes of mammalian cells.

Fructose-6-phosphate

The second step in glycolysis is the conversion of Glc-6-P into Fru-6-P by phosphoglucose isomerase (Fig. 12.3, middle). Isomerases catalyze freely reversible equilibrium reactions, in this case an aldose–ketose interconversion. The Fru-6-P is now phosphorylated at C-1 by phosphofructokinase-1 (PFK-1) to yield the pseudosymmetric intermediate, fructose 1,6-bisphosphate (Fru-1,6-BP), which has a phosphate ester on each end of the molecule. Like hexokinase, PFK-1 requires ATP as a substrate and catalyzes an essentially irreversible reaction (K_{eq} ~500). Both hexokinase and PFK-1 are important regulatory enzymes in glycolysis, but PFK-1 is the critical, commitment step. This reaction directs glucose to glycolysis, the only pathway for metabolism of Fru-1,6-BP.

 GLUCOSE UTILIZATION IN THE RED CELL

In a 70 kg person, there are about 5 L of blood and a little over 2 kg (2 L) of RBCs. These cells constitute about 3% of total body mass and consume about 20 g (0.1 mole) of glucose per day, representing about 10% of total body glucose metabolism. The RBC has the highest specific rate of glucose utilization of any cell in the body, approximately 10 g of glucose/kg of tissue/day, compared with ~2.5 g of glucose/kg of tissue/day for the whole body.

In the RBC, about 90% of glucose is metabolized via glycolysis, yielding lactate, which is excreted into blood. Despite its high rate of glucose consumption, the RBC has one of the lowest rates of ATP synthesis of any cell in the body, ~0.1 mole of ATP/kg tissue/day, reflecting the fact that anaerobic glycolysis recovers only a fraction of the energy available from complete combustion of glucose to CO_2 and H_2O.

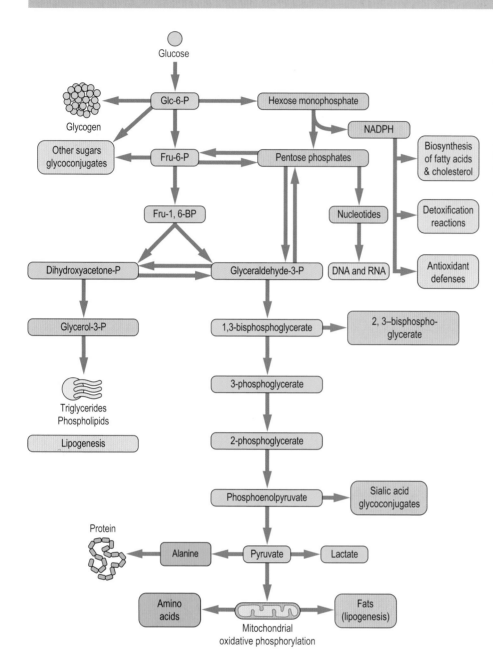

Fig. 12.2 **Interactions between glycolysis and other metabolic pathways.** The green colored boxes indicate intermediates involved in the pathway of glycolysis. Other boxes illustrate some of the metabolic interactions between glycolysis and other metabolic pathways in the cell. Not all of these pathways are active in the red cell which has limited biosynthetic capacity and lacks mitochondria. Glc-6-P, glucose-6-phosphate; Fru-6-P, fructose-6-phosphate; Fru-1,6-BP, fructose-1,6-bisphosphate.

The splitting stage of glycolysis

In the splitting stage of glycolysis, Fru-1,6-BP is cleaved in the middle by a reverse-aldol reaction (Fig. 12.3, bottom), thus the name aldolase. The aldolase reaction is a freely reversible equilibrium reaction, yielding two triose phosphates, dihydroxyacetone phosphate and glyceraldehyde-3-phosphate, from the top and bottom halves of the Fru-1,6-BP molecule, respectively. Only the glyceraldehyde-3-phosphate continues through the yield stage of glycolysis, but triose phosphate isomerase catalyzes the interconversion of dihydroxyacetone phosphate into glyceraldehyde-3-phosphate, so that both halves of the glucose molecule are eventually metabolized to lactate.

The yield stage of glycolysis – synthesis of ATP by substrate-level phosphorylation

The yield stage of glycolysis produces 4 moles of ATP, yielding a net of 2 moles of ATP per mole of glucose converted into lactate (Fig. 12.4). The synthesis of ATP is accomplished by kinases that catalyze *substrate-level phosphorylation*, a process in which a high-energy phosphate compound transfers its phosphate to ADP, yielding ATP.

Substrate-level phosphorylation: $X{\sim}P + ADP \rightarrow X + ATP$

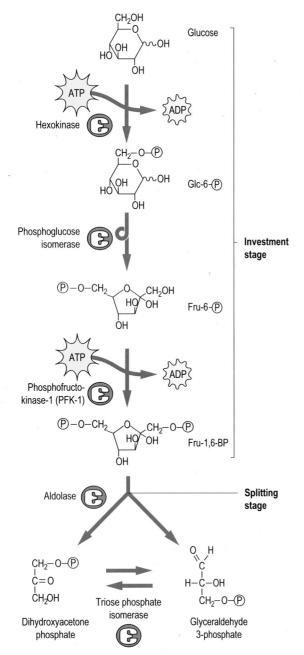

Fig. 12.3 **The investment and splitting stages of glycolysis.** Note the consumption of ATP at the hexokinase and phosphofructokinase-1 reactions.

Glyceraldehyde-3-phosphate dehydrogenase

To set the stage for substrate-level phosphorylation, the aldehyde group of glyceraldehyde-3-phosphate is oxidized to a carboxylic acid and the energy available from the oxidation reaction is used, in part, to trap a phosphate from the cytoplasmic pool as an acyl phosphate. This reaction is catalyzed by glyceraldehyde-3-phosphate dehydrogenase (GAPDH),

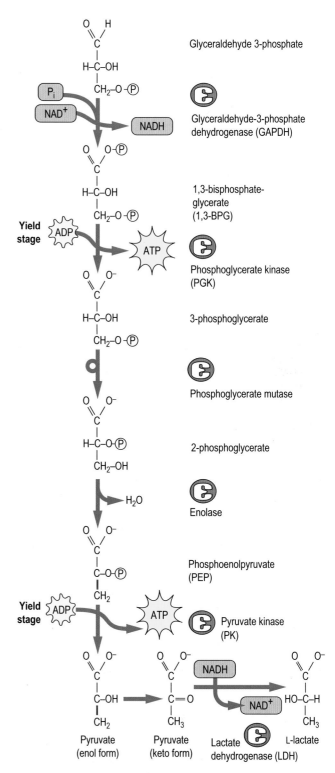

Fig. 12.4 **The yield stage of glycolysis.** Substrate-level phosphorylation reactions catalyzed by phosphoglycerate kinase and pyruvate kinase produce ATP, using the high-energy compounds, 1,3-bisphosphoglycerate and phosphoenolpyruvate, respectively. Note that NADH produced during the glyceraldehyde-3-phosphate dehydrogenase reaction is recycled back to NAD^+ during the lactate dehydrogenase reaction, permitting continued glycolysis in the presence of only catalytic amounts of NAD^+.

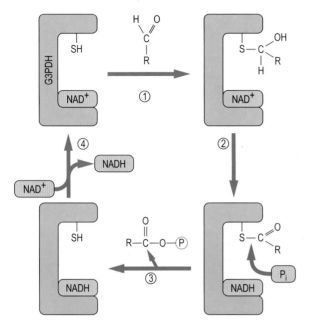

Fig. 12.5 **Mechanism of the glyceraldehyde-3-phosphate dehydrogenase (GAPDH) reaction.** In Step 1, the active-site sulfhydryl group of G3PDH forms a thiohemiacetal adduct with an active-site cysteine residue in GAPDH. In Step 2, the thiohemiacetal is oxidized to a thioester by NAD$^+$, also bound in the active site of the enzyme. In Step 3, phosphate enters the active site and, in a phosphorylase reaction, cleaves the carbon–sulfur bond, displacing the 3-phosphoglycerate group, producing 1,3-bisphosphoglycerate and regenerating the sulfhydryl group. In Step 4, the enzyme exchanges NADH for NAD$^+$, completing the catalytic cycle.

yielding the high-energy compound (X~P), 1,3-bisphosphoglycerate (1,3-BPG). The coenzyme NAD$^+$ is simultaneously reduced to NADH (Figs 12.4, 12.5).

The GAPDH reaction provides an interesting illustration of the role of enzyme-bound intermediates in the formation of high-energy phosphates. How does the oxidation of an aldehyde and the reduction of NAD$^+$ lead to the formation of an acyl phosphate bond in 1,3-BPG? How does the phosphate enter the picture, and become activated to a high-energy state? The inhibition of GAPDH by thiol reagents such as iodoacetamide, *p*-chloromecuribenzoate and *N*-ethylmaleimide pointed to involvement of an active-site sulfhydryl residue. The mechanism of action of this enzyme is described in Figure 12.5.

Substrate-level phosphorylation

Phosphoglycerate kinase (PGK) catalyzes transfer of the phosphate group from the high-energy acyl phosphate of 1,3-BPG to ADP, forming ATP. This substrate-level phosphorylation reaction yields the first ATP produced in glycolysis. The remaining phosphate group in 3-phosphoglycerate is an ester phosphate and does not have enough energy to phosphorylate ADP, so a series of isomerization and dehydration reactions is enlisted to convert the ester phosphate into a high-energy enol phosphate. The first step is to shift the

phosphate to C-2 of glycerate, converting 3-phosphoglycerate into 2-phosphoglycerate, catalyzed by the enzyme phosphoglycerate mutase (see Fig. 12.4). Mutases catalyze the transfer of functional groups within a molecule. Phosphoglycerate mutase has an active-site histidine residue, and a phosphohistidine adduct is formed as an enzyme-bound intermediate during the phosphate transfer reaction.

2-Phosphoglycerate then undergoes a dehydration reaction, catalyzed by enolase, a hydratase, to yield the high-energy phosphate compound, phosphoenolpyruvate (PEP). PEP is used by pyruvate kinase to phosphorylate ADP, yielding pyruvate and the second ATP, again by substrate-level phosphorylation. It seems strange that the high-energy phosphate bond in PEP can be formed from the low-energy phosphate compound 2-phosphoglycerate by a simple sequence of isomerization and dehydration reactions. However, the thermodynamic driving force for these reactions is probably derived from charge–charge repulsion between the phosphate and carboxylate groups of 2-phosphoglycerate and the isomerization of enolpyruvate to pyruvate following the phosphorylation reaction.

Phosphoglycerate kinase and pyruvate kinase catalyze the substrate-level phosphorylation, ATP-generating reactions of glycolysis, yielding 2 moles of ATP per mole of triose phosphate, or a total of 4 moles of ATP per mole of Fru-1,6-BP. After adjustment for the ATP invested in the hexokinase and PFK-1 reactions, the net energy yield is 2 moles of ATP per mole of glucose converted into pyruvate.

Lactate dehydrogenase (LDH)

Two molecules of pyruvate have exactly the same number of carbons and oxygens as one molecule of glucose; however, there is a deficit of four hydrogens – each pyruvate has four hydrogens, a total of eight hydrogens for two pyruvates, compared with 12 in a molecule of glucose. The 'missing' four hydrogens remain in the form of the 2NADH and 2H$^+$ formed in the G3PDH reaction. Since NAD$^+$ is present in only catalytic amounts in the cell and is an essential cofactor for glycolysis (and other reactions), there must be a mechanism for regeneration of NAD$^+$ if glycolysis is to continue.

The oxidation of NADH is accomplished under anaerobic conditions by lactate dehydrogenase (LDH) which catalyzes reduction of pyruvate to lactate by NADH + H$^+$ and regenerates NAD$^+$. In mammals, all cells have LDH, and lactate is the endproduct of glycolysis under anaerobic conditions. Under aerobic conditions, mitochondria oxidize NADH to NAD$^+$ and convert pyruvate to CO$_2$ and H$_2$O, so that lactate is not formed. Despite their capacity for oxidative metabolism, however, some cells may at times 'go glycolytic', forming lactate, e.g. in muscle during oxygen debt and in phagocytes in pus or in poorly perfused tissues. Most of the lactate excreted into blood is retrieved by the liver for use as a substrate for gluconeogenesis (Chapter 13).

INHIBITION OF SUBSTRATE-LEVEL PHOSPHORYLATION BY ARSENATE

Arsenic is just below phosphorus in the Periodic Chart of the Elements, and it might be expected to share some of the properties and reactivity of phosphate. In fact, arsenate has pK_a values similar to those of phosphate and can actually be used by GAPDH, producing 1-arsenato-3-phosphoglycerate. However, the acyl–arsenate bond is unstable and hydrolyzes rapidly, and ATP is not generated by substrate-level phosphorylation. While arsenate does not inhibit any of the enzymes of glycolysis, it dissipates the redox energy available from the GAPDH reaction and prevents the formation of ATP by substrate-level phosphorylation at the PGK reaction. In effect, arsenate *uncouples* the GAPDH and PGK reactions. Note that arsenic and arsenite are also toxic, but have a different mechanism of action: they react with thiol groups in sulfhydryl enzymes, such as GAPDH (See Fig. 12.5), irreversibly inhibiting their activity.

INHIBITION OF ENOLASE BY FLUORIDE

Measurements of blood glucose concentration are used for the diagnosis and management of diabetes. Frequently, these measurements are made in the clinical laboratory more than 1 h after the collection of the blood sample. Because RBCs can metabolize glucose to lactate, even in a sealed, anoxic container, glucose in blood will be consumed and lactate will be produced, which will lead to acidification of the blood sample. These reactions proceed in RBCs, even at room temperature, so that both blood glucose concentration and pH will decrease during standing, possibly leading to false diagnosis of hypoglycemia and acidemia. Anaerobic metabolism of glucose can be prevented by adding an inhibitor of glycolysis to the blood collection tube. Sulfhydryl reagents would work as they are inhibitors of GAPDH; however, most blood samples are collected with a small amount of a much cheaper reagent, sodium fluoride, in the sample-collection vial. Fluoride is a strong competitive inhibitor of enolase, blocking glycolysis and lactate production in the RBC. It is an unusual competitive inhibitor, since fluoride bears little resemblance to 2-phosphoglycerate. In this case, fluoride forms a complex with phosphate and Mg^{2+} in the active site of the enzyme, blocking access of substrate.

Fermentation

Fermentation is a general term for anaerobic metabolism of glucose, usually applied to monocellular organisms. Some anaerobic bacteria, such as lactobacilli, produce lactate, while others have alternative pathways for anaerobic oxidation of NADH formed during glycolysis. During fermentation in yeast, the pathway of glycolysis is identical with that

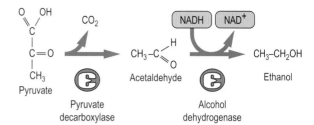

Fig. 12.6 **Anaerobic glycolysis in yeast.** Formation of ethanol by anaerobic glycolysis during fermentation. Pyruvate is decarboxylated by pyruvate decarboxylase, yielding acetaldehyde and CO_2. Alcohol dehydrogenase uses NADH to reduce acetaldehyde to ethanol, regenerating NAD^+ for glycolysis.

GLYCOLYSIS AND DENTAL CARIES

Streptococcus mutans and *lactobacillus* are anaerobic bacteria that colonize the oral cavity and contribute to the development of dental caries. These bacteria grow optimally on refined, fermentable carbohydrates in the diet and excrete organic acids, such as lactate. They thrive in acidic, anaerobic microenvironments in fissures in the teeth and in gingival pockets. The organic acids gradually erode tooth enamel and dentin, and the chronic dissolution of the calcium phosphate (hydroxyapatite) matrix of the teeth sets the stage for cavity formation. Fluoride, provided either topically or in toothpaste, at levels too low to inhibit enolase, integrates into the tooth surface, forming fluoroapatite, which is more resistant to demineralization.

in the RBC, except that pyruvate is converted into ethanol (Fig. 12.6). The pyruvate is first decarboxylated by pyruvate decarboxylase to acetaldehyde, releasing CO_2. The NADH produced in the GAPDH reaction is then reoxidized by alcohol dehydrogenase, regenerating NAD^+ and producing ethanol. Ethanol is a toxic compound and yeasts die when the ethanol concentration in their medium reaches about 12%, which is the approximate concentration of alcohol in natural wines.

Regulation of glycolysis in erythrocytes

Hexokinase

RBCs consume glucose at a fairly steady rate. They are not physically active like muscle, and do not require energy for transport of O_2 or CO_2. Glycolysis in red cells appears to be regulated simply by the energy needs of the cell, primarily for maintenance of ion gradients. The balance between ATP consumption and production is controlled allosterically at three sites: the hexokinase, phosphofructokinase-1, and pyruvate kinase reactions (see Fig. 12.2). Based on measurements

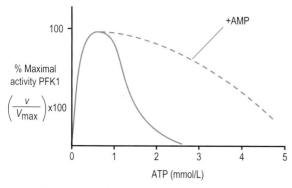

Fig. 12.7 **Allosteric regulation of phosphofructokinase-1 (PFK-1) by ATP.** AMP is a potent activator of PFK-1 in the presence of ATP.

Regulation of glycolysis in the red cell	
Enzyme	**Regulator**
Hexokinase	inhibited by glucose-6-P
Phosphofructokinase-1	inhibited by ATP; activated by AMP
Pyruvate kinase	activated by fructose-1,6-BP

Table 12.1 **Regulation of glycolysis in the red cell.**

of the V_{max} of the various enzymes in RBC lysates in vitro, hexokinase is present at the lowest activity of all glycolytic enzymes. Its maximal activity is about five times the rate of glucose consumption by the RBC, but it is subject to feedback (allosteric) inhibition by its product Glc-6-P. Hexokinase has 30% homology between its *N*- and *C*-terminal domains, the result of duplication and fusion of a primordial gene; binding of Glc-6-P to the *N*-terminal domain inhibits the activity of the enzyme and production of Glc-6-P at the active site in the *C*-terminal domain.

Phosphofructokinase-1 (PFK-1)

PFK-1 is the primary site of regulation of glycolysis, controlling the flux of Fru-6-P to Fru-1,6-BP and, indirectly through the phosphoglucose isomerase reaction, the level of Glc-6-P and inhibition of hexokinase. Although present at 20 times higher activity than hexokinase, PFK-1 is strongly inhibited by ambient ATP, so that its activity varies with the energy status of the cell. Amazingly, ATP is both a substrate (see Fig. 12.3) and an allosteric inhibitor (Fig. 12.7) of PFK-1, a dual function that permits fine control over the activity of the enzyme.

As shown in Figure 12.7, the concentration of ATP in the RBC (~2 mmol/L) normally suppresses the activity of PFK-1. AMP, which is present at much lower concentration (~0.05 mmol/L), relieves this inhibition. Because of their relative concentrations, a small fractional conversion of ATP to AMP in the RBC yields a large relative increase in AMP concentration, which activates PFK-1. ADP also relieves the inhibition of PFK-1 by ATP, but its concentration does not change as much with energy utilization. AMP (and ADP) not only relieves the inhibition of PFK-1 by ATP, but also decreases the K_m for the substrate Fru-6-P, further increasing the catalytic efficiency of the enzyme.

Through allosteric mechanisms, the activity of PFK-1 in the red cell is exquisitely sensitive to changes in the energy status of the cell, as measured by the relative concentrations of ATP, ADP and AMP. In effect, the overall activity of PFK-1, and thus the rate of glycolysis, depends on the cell's (AMP +

ADP)/ATP concentration ratio. These products are interconvertible by the adenylate kinase reaction:

$$2\,ADP \rightleftharpoons ATP + AMP$$

When ATP is consumed and ADP increases, AMP is formed by the adenylate kinase reaction. The increase in AMP concentrations relieves the inhibition of PFK-1 by ATP, activating glycolysis. The phosphorylation of ADP during glycolysis and then of AMP by the adenylate kinase reaction gradually restores the ATP concentration or *energy charge* of the cell and, as the AMP concentration declines, the rate of glycolysis decreases to a steady-state level. Glycolysis operates at a fairly constant rate in the red cell, where ATP consumption is steady, but the activity of this pathway changes rapidly in response to ATP utilization in muscle during exercise.

Pyruvate kinase (PK)

In addition to regulation by hexokinase and PFK-1, pyruvate kinase in liver is allosterically activated by Fru-1,6-BP, the product of the PFK-1 reaction. This process, known as feedforward regulation, may be important in the RBC to limit the accumulation of reactive triose phosphate intermediates in the cytosol.

Characteristics of regulatory enzymes

Each of the three enzymes involved in regulation of glycolysis – hexokinase, PFK-1, and pyruvate kinase – has the characteristic features of a regulatory enzyme: they are dimeric or tetrameric enzymes whose structure and activity are responsive to allosteric modulators; they are present at low V_{max} in comparison with other enzymes in the pathway; and they catalyze irreversible reactions. The regulation of glycolysis in liver, muscle, and other tissues is more complicated than in the RBC (Table 12.1) because of greater variability in the rate of fuel consumption and the interplay between carbohydrate and lipid metabolism during aerobic metabolism. In these tissues, the amount and activity of the regulatory enzymes are regulated by other allosteric effectors, by covalent modification, and by induction or repression of enzyme activity.

SYNTHESIS OF 2,3-BISPHOSPHOGLYCERATE

2,3-Bisphosphoglycerate (2,3-BPG) (Fig. 12.8) is an important by-product of glycolysis in the RBC, sometimes reaching 5 mmol/L concentration, which is comparable to the molar concentration of hemoglobin (Hb) in the RBC. 2,3-BPG is in fact the major phosphorylated intermediate in the erythrocyte, present at even higher concentrations than ATP (1–2 mmol/L) or inorganic phosphate (1 mmol/L). 2,3-BPG is a negative allosteric effector of the O_2 affinity of Hb. It decreases the O_2 affinity of hemoglobin, promoting the release of O_2 in peripheral tissue. The presence of 2,3-BPG in the RBC explains the observation that the O_2 affinity of purified HbA is greater than that of whole RBCs. 2,3-BPG concentration increases in the RBC during adaptation to high altitude, in chronic obstructive pulmonary disease and in anemia, promoting the release of O_2 to tissues when the O_2 tension and saturation of hemoglobin is decreased in the lung. Fetal Hb (HbF) is less sensitive than adult Hb (HbA) to the effects of 2,3-BPG; the higher oxygen affinity of HbF, even in the presence of 2,3-BPG, promotes efficient transfer of O_2 across the placenta from HbA to HbF (see Chapter 5).

 PYRUVATE KINASE DEFICIENCY

A child presented with jaundice and abdominal (splenic) tenderness. Laboratory tests revealed a low hematocrit and hemoglobin concentration, normochromatic erythrocytes with normal morphology, and mild reticulocytosis. Serum bilirubin was increased.

Comment. Pyruvate kinase deficiency is the most common of the hemolytic anemias that result from a deficiency in a glycolytic enzyme. It is an autosomal recessive disorder that occurs with a frequency of 1/10 000 (~1% gene frequency) in the world population. It is second only to G6PDH deficiency as an enzymatic cause of hemolytic anemia. These diseases are diagnosed by measurement of erythrocyte levels of enzymes or metabolites, by demonstrating abnormalities in enzymatic activities or by genetic analysis. Enzymatic defects in pyruvate kinase that have been characterized include thermal lability, increased K_m for PEP, and decreased activation by Fru-1,6-BP.

Pyruvate kinase deficiency varies significantly in severity, from a mild, compensated condition requiring little intervention to a severe disease requiring transfusions. The anemia results from inability to synthesize ATP, required for maintenance of RBC metabolism, ion gradients and cell shape. Interestingly, patients may tolerate the anemia quite well. Even with mild anemia, the accumulation of 2,3-bisphosphoglycerate in their RBCs decreases the oxygen affinity of hemoglobin, promoting oxygen delivery to muscle during exercise and even to the fetus during pregnancy.

THE PENTOSE PHOSPHATE PATHWAY

Overview

The pentose phosphate pathway is a cytosolic pathway present in all cells, so named because it is the primary pathway for formation of pentose phosphates for synthesis of nucleotides for incorporation into DNA and RNA. This pathway branches from glycolysis at the level of Glc-6-P, thus its alternative designation, the hexose monophosphate shunt. The pentose phosphate pathway is sometimes described as a shunt, rather than a pathway, because when pentoses are not needed for biosynthetic reactions, the pentose phosphate intermediates are recycled to the mainstream of glycolysis by

 GLYCOLYSIS IN TUMOR CELLS

Tumors are often said to 'go glycolytic', i.e. to increase their reliance on glycolysis as a source of energy. The increase in glycolysis might result from mitochondrial dysfunction as a result of hypoxia, possibly because the metabolic requirements of rapidly dividing tumor cells exceed the supply of oxygen and nutrients from blood. In these cases, the production and accumulation of lactate may become toxic to the tumor cell, contributing to necrosis and formation of a necrotic core in the tumor. Some tumors secrete cytokines that promote angiogenesis (neovascularization), thereby increasing their fuel and oxygen supply and enhancing tumor growth. Angiogenesis inhibitors, designed to inhibit the vascularization of the tumor, are being evaluated as a nonsurgical approach to tumor therapy. The ability to survive by relying on glycolysis in hypoxic environments may be an important factor in tumor survival and growth.

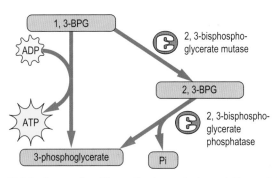

Fig. 12.8 **Pathway for biosynthesis and degradation of 2,3-bisphosphoglycerate (2,3-BPG).** BPG mutase catalyzes the conversion of 1,3-BPG into 2,3-BPG. This same enzyme has bisphosphoglycerate phosphatase activity, so that it controls both the synthesis and hydrolysis of 2,3-BPG. Note that this pathway bypasses the phosphoglycerate kinase reaction, so that the overall yield of ATP per mol of glucose is decreased to zero.

conversion into Fru-6-P and glyceraldehyde-3-phosphate. This rerouting is especially important in the RBC and in non-dividing or quiescent cells, where there is limited need for synthesis of DNA and RNA.

NADPH is a major product of the pentose phosphate pathway in all cells. In tissues with active lipid biosynthesis, e.g. liver, adrenal cortex or lactating mammary glands, the NADPH is used in redox reactions required for biosynthesis of cholesterol, bile salts, steroid hormones and triglycerides. The liver also uses NADPH for hydroxylation reactions involved in the detoxification and excretion of drugs. The RBC has little biosynthetic activity, but still shunts about 10% of glucose through the pentose phosphate pathway, in this case almost exclusively for the production of NADPH. The NADPH is used primarily for the reduction of a cysteine-containing tripeptide glutathione (GSH), an essential cofactor for antioxidant protection (Chapter 37).

The pentose phosphate pathway is divided into an irreversible redox stage, which yields both NADPH and pentose phosphates, and a reversible interconversion stage, in which excess pentose phosphates are converted into glycolytic intermediates. Both stages are important in the RBC, since it needs NADPH for reduction of glutathione, but has limited need for de novo synthesis of pentoses.

The redox stage of the pentose phosphate pathway – synthesis of NADPH

NADPH is synthesized by two dehydrogenases, in the first and third reactions of the pentose phosphate pathway (Fig. 12.9). In the first step of the pathway, the Glc-6-P dehydrogenase (G6PDH) reaction produces NADPH by oxidation of Glc-6-P to 6-phosphogluconic acid lactone, a cyclic sugar ester. The lactone is hydrolyzed to 6-phosphogluconic acid by lactonase. Oxidative decarboxylation of 6-phosphogluconate, catalyzed by 6-phosphogluconate dehydrogenase, then yields the ketose sugar, ribulose 5-phosphate, plus 1 mole of CO_2, and the second mole of NADPH.

G6PDH and 6-phosphogluconate dehydrogenase maintain a cytoplasmic ratio of $NADPH/NADP^+ \sim 100$. Interestingly, because NAD^+ is required for glycolysis, the ratio of $NADH/NAD^+$ in the cytoplasm is nearly the inverse, less than 0.01. Although the total concentrations (oxidized plus reduced forms) of NAD(H) and NADP(H) in the RBC are similar ($\sim 25 \mu mol/L$), the cell maintains these two redox systems with similar redox potentials at such different set-points in the same cell by isolating their metabolism through the specificity of cytoplasmic dehydrogenases. The glycolytic enzymes (GAPDH and LDH) use only NAD(H), while pentose phosphate pathway enzymes use only NADP(H). There are no enzymes in the RBC that catalyze the reduction of NAD^+ by NADPH, so that high levels of both NAD^+ and NADPH can exist simultaneously in the same compartment.

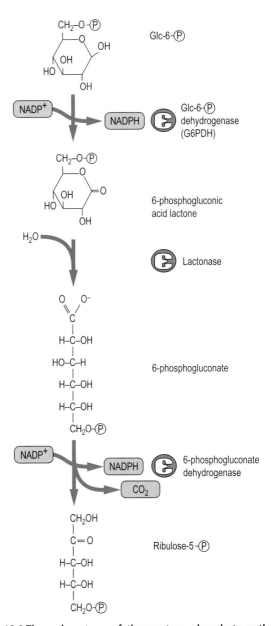

Fig. 12.9 **The redox stage of the pentose phosphate pathway.** A sequence of three enzymes forms 2 moles of NADPH per mole of Glc-6-P, which is converted into ribulose-5-phosphate, with evolution of CO_2.

The interconversion stage of the pentose phosphate pathway

In cells with active nucleic acid synthesis, ribulose-5-phosphate from the 6-phosphoglucose dehydrogenase reaction is isomerized to ribose-5-phosphate for synthesis of ribo- and deoxyribonucleotides for RNA and DNA (Fig. 12.10). In non-dividing cells, the pentose phosphates are routed back to glycolysis. This is accomplished by a series of equilibrium reactions in which 3 moles of ribulose-5-phosphate are converted into 2 moles of Fru-6-P and 1 mole of glyceraldehyde-3-phosphate.

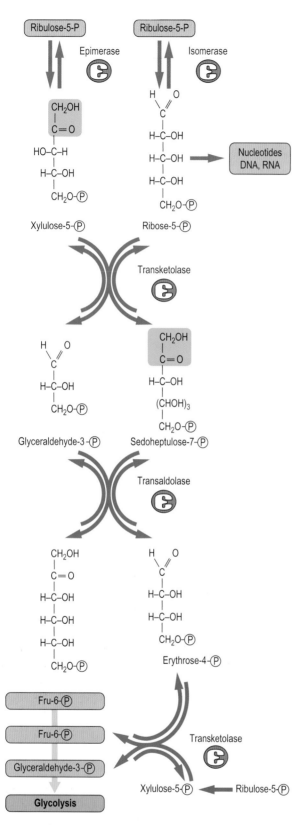

Fig. 12.10 **The interconversion stage of the pentose phosphate pathway.** The carbon skeletons of three molecules of ribulose-5-phosphate are shuffled to form two molecules of Fru-6-P and one molecule of glyceraldehyde 3-phosphate, which enter into glycolysis.

Certain restrictions are imposed on the interconversion reactions – they may be carried out only by transfer of two or three carbon units between sugar phosphates. Each reaction must also involve a ketose donor and an aldose receptor. Isomerases and epimerases convert ribulose-5-phosphate to the aldose- and ketose-phosphate substrates for the interconversion stage. Transketolase, a thiamine-dependent enzyme, catalyzes the two-carbon transfer reactions. Transaldolase acts similarly to the aldolase in glycolysis, except that the three-carbon unit is transferred to another sugar, rather than released as a free triose phosphate for glycolysis.

As shown in Figure 12.10 and Table 12.2, two molecules of ribulose 5-phosphate, the first pentose product of the redox stage, are converted into separate products: one molecule is isomerized to the aldose sugar ribose-5-phosphate, and the other is epimerized to xylulose-5-phosphate. Transketolase then catalyzes transfer of two carbons from xylulose-5-phosphate to ribose-5-phosphate, yielding a seven-carbon ketose sugar, sedoheptulose-7-phosphate, and the three-carbon glyceraldehyde-3-phosphate. Transaldolase then catalyzes a three-carbon transfer between the two transketolase products, from sedoheptulose-7-phosphate to glyceraldehyde-3-phosphate, yielding the first glycolytic intermediate, Fru-6-P, and a residual erythrose-4-phosphate. A third molecule of xylulose-5-phosphate donates two carbons to erythrose-4-phosphate in a second transketolase reaction, yielding a second molecule of Fru-6-P and a molecule of glyceraldehyde-3-phosphate, both of which enter glycolysis.

Thus, three five-carbon sugar phosphates (ribulose-5-phosphate) formed in the redox stage of the pentose phosphate pathway are converted into one three-carbon (glyceraldehyde-3-phosphate) and two six-carbon (fructose-6-phosphate) intermediates for glycolysis. In the RBC, these glycolytic intermediates normally continue through glycolysis to lactate, illustrating that glucose is only temporarily shunted away from the mainstream of glycolysis.

Function of the pentose phosphate pathway in the red cell

Glutathione (GSH) is a tripeptide γ-glutamyl-cysteinyl-glycine (Fig. 12.11). It is present in cells at 2–5 mmol/L, 99% in the reduced (thiol) form, and is an essential coenzyme for protection of the cell against a range of oxidative and chemical insults (Chapter 37). Most of the NADPH formed in the red cell is used by glutathione reductase to maintain GSH in the reduced state. During its function as a coenzyme for antioxidant activities, GSH is oxidized to the disulfide form, GSSG, which is then regenerated by the action of glutathione reductase (Fig. 12.12).

GSH has a range of protective functions in the cell. Glutathione peroxidase (GPx) is found in all cells and uses GSH for detoxification of hydrogen peroxide and organic (lipid)

The pentose phosphate pathway

Substrate(s)		Product(s)	Enzyme
Ribulose-5-P	⇌	Ribose-5-P	isomerase
2 Ribulose-5-P	⇌	2 Xylulose-5-P	epimerase
Xylulose-5-P + Ribose-5-P	⇌	Glyceraldehyde-3-P + Sedoheptulose-7-P	transketolase
Sedoheptulose-7-P + Glyceraldehyde-3-P	⇌	Erythrose-4-P + Fructose-6-P	transaldolase
Xylulose-5-P + Erythrose-4-P	⇌	Glyceraldehyde-3-P + Fructose-6-P	transketolase
3 Ribulose-5-P	⇌	Glyceraldehyde-3-P + 2 Fructose-6-P	

Table 12.2 **Summary of equilibrium reactions in the pentose phosphate pathway.**

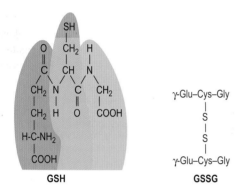

GSH   **GSSG**

Fig. 12.11 **Glutathione.** Structure of reduced glutathione (GSH) and oxidized glutathione (GSSG).

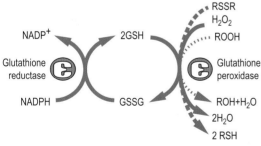

Fig. 12.12 **Antioxidant activities of glutathione.** GSH is the coenzyme for glutathione peroxidase which detoxifies hydrogen peroxide and organic (lipid) hydroperoxides. Hydrogen peroxide and lipid peroxides are formed spontaneously in the red cell, catalyzed by side reactions of heme iron during oxygen transport on hemoglobin (Chapter 37). GSH also reduces disulfide bonds in proteins, formed during oxidative stress.

peroxides in the cytosol and cell membranes (see Fig. 12.12). Because GPx contains a selenocysteine residue in its active site, selenium, which is required in trace amounts in the diet, is often described as an antioxidant nutrient (see Chapter 11).

GLUCOSE-6-PHOSPHATE DEHYDROGENASE DEFICIENCY CAUSES HEMOLYTIC ANEMIA

Just prior to a planned departure to the tropics, a patient visited his physician, complaining of weakness and noting that his urine had recently become unexplainably dark. Physical examination revealed slightly jaundiced (yellow, icteric) sclera. Laboratory tests indicated a low hematocrit, a high reticulocyte count, and a significantly increased blood level of bilirubin. The patient had been quite healthy during a previous visit a month ago when he received immunizations and prescriptions for antimalarial drugs.

Comment. A number of drugs, particularly primaquine and related antimalarials, undergo redox reactions in the cell, producing large quantities of reactive oxygen species (ROS) (Chapter 37). The ROS cause oxidation of −SH groups in hemoglobin and peroxidation of membrane lipids. Some persons have a genetic defect in G6PDH, typically yielding an unstable enzyme that has a shorter half-life in the RBC or is unusually sensitive to inhibition by NADPH. In either case, because of the decreased activity of this enzyme and insufficient production of NADPH under stress, the cell's ability to recycle GSSG to GSH is impaired, and drug-induced oxidative stress leads to excessive damage and lysis of RBCs (hemolysis) and hemolytic anemia. Bilirubin, a product of heme metabolism, overloads hepatic detoxification pathways, and also accumulates in plasma and tissues, causing jaundice. If the hemolysis is severe enough, Hb spills over into the urine, resulting in hematuria and dark-colored urine. Heinz bodies, disulfide crosslinked aggregates of hemoglobin, are also apparent in blood smears. G6PDH deficiency is asymptomatic, except in response to an oxidative challenge, which may be induced by drugs (antimalarials, sulfa drugs), diet (fava beans) or severe infection.

There are over 200 known mutations of the G6PDH gene, yielding a wide variation in severity of disease. The RBC appears to be especially sensitive to oxidative stress because, unlike other cells, it cannot synthesize and replace enzymes. Older cells, which have lower G6PDH activity, are therefore particularly affected. The activity of all enzymes in the RBC declines with the age of the cell, and cell death eventually results from inability of the cells to produce sufficient ATP for maintenance of cellular ion gradients. The gradual decline in activity of the pentose phosphate pathway in older cells is one mechanism leading to oxidative crosslinking of membrane proteins and turnover of the RBC in the spleen.

GSH also acts as an intracellular sulfhydryl buffer, maintaining exposed -SH groups on proteins and enzymes in the reduced state. Under normal circumstances, when proteins are exposed to O_2, their free sulfhydryl groups gradually oxidize to form disulfides, either intramolecularly or by intermolecular crosslinking with other protein molecules. In the red cell, GSH maintains the -SH groups of hemoglobin in the reduced state, inhibiting oxidative crosslinking of the protein.

Summary

This chapter describes two ancient metabolic pathways common to all cells in the body: glycolysis and the pentose phosphate pathway. The RBC, which lacks mitochondria and the capability for oxidative metabolism and obtains all of its ATP energy by glycolysis, is used as a model for introducing these pathways. Anaerobic glycolysis in the RBC provides a limited amount of ATP by conversion of the six-carbon sugar glucose to two molecules of the three-carbon hydroxyacid lactate. Through a series of sugar phosphate intermediates, glycolysis provides metabolites for branch points to numerous other metabolic pathways, including the pentose phosphate pathway. This pathway provides pentoses for synthesis of DNA and RNA in nucleated cells, and NADPH for biosynthetic reactions. NADPH is also required for maintenance of reduced glutathione, which is an essential cofactor for antioxidant defense systems that protect the cell against oxidative stress.

ACTIVE LEARNING

1. Why was glucose selected as blood sugar during evolution, rather than other sugars, e.g. galactose, fructose or sucrose?
2. Describe coupled enzymatic reactions, using only red cell enzymes and a spectrometer for measuring NAD(P)(H) production or consumption, that could be used to measure blood glucose and lactate concentrations.
3. Explain the metabolic origin of acidosis in chronic obstructive pulmonary disease.

Further reading

Gatenby RA, Gillies RJ. Glycolysis in cancer: a potential target for therapy. *Int J Biochem Cell Biol* 2007;**39**:1358–1366.

Krol DM, Nedley MP. Dental caries: state of the science for the most common chronic disease of childhood. *Adv Pediatr* 2007;**54**:215–239.

Mason PJ, Bautista JM, Gilsanz F. G6PD deficiency: the genotype-phenotype association. *Blood Rev* 2007;**21**:267–283.

Tozzi MG, Camici M, Mascia L, Sgarrella F, Ipata PL. Pentose phosphates in nucleoside interconversion and catabolism. *FEBS J* 2006;**273**:1089–1101.

van Wijk R, van Solinge WW. The energy-less red blood cell is lost: erythrocyte enzyme abnormalities of glycolysis. *Blood* 2005;**106**:4034–4042.

Zanella A, Fermo E, Bianchi P, Chiarelli LR, Valentini G. Pyruvate kinase deficiency: the genotype-phenotype association. *Blood Rev* 2007;**21**:217–231.

Websites

American Society of Hematology, case studies on anemia: www.ashteachingcases.org

National Institutes of Health: www.nlm.nih.gov/medlineplus/ency/article/000528.htm

E-Medicine: www.emedicine.com/med/topic1980.htm and topic900.htm

Glucose-6-P dehydrogenase deficiency: www.rialto.com/g6pd/

Animations – glycolysis:
- www.tcd.ie/Biochemistry/IUBMB-Nicholson/swf/glycolysis.swf
- http://trc.ucdavis.edu/biosci10v/bis10v/media/ch06/glycolysis.swf
- www.northland.cc.mn.us/biology/Biology1111/animations/glycolysis.html

Animation – pentose phosphate pathway:
- www.uwsp.edu/chemistry/tzamis/p3animrunP.gif

13. Carbohydrate Storage and Synthesis in Liver and Muscle

J W Baynes

LEARNING OBJECTIVES

After reading this chapter you should be able to:

- Describe the structure of glycogen.
- Identify the primary sites of glycogen storage in the body and the function of glycogen in these tissues.
- Outline the metabolic pathways for synthesis and degradation of glycogen.
- Describe the mechanism by which glycogen is mobilized in liver in response to glucagon, in muscle during exercise, and in both tissues in response to epinephrine.
- Explain the origin and consequences of glycogen storage diseases in liver and muscle.
- Describe the mechanism for counterregulation of glycogenolysis and glycogenesis in liver.
- Outline the pathway of gluconeogenesis, including substrates, unique enzymes and regulatory mechanisms.
- Describe the complementary roles of glycogenolysis and gluconeogenesis in maintenance of blood glucose concentration.

INTRODUCTION

The red cell and the brain have an absolute requirement for blood glucose for energy metabolism. These cells consume about 80% of the 200 g of glucose consumed in the body per day. There is only about 10 g of glucose in the plasma and extracellular fluid volume, so that blood glucose must be replenished constantly. Otherwise, hypoglycemia develops and compromises brain function, leading to confusion and disorientation, and possibly life-threatening coma at blood glucose concentrations below 2.5 mmol/L (45 mg/dL). We absorb glucose from our intestines for only 2–3 h following a carbohydrate-containing meal, so there must be a mechanism for maintenance of blood glucose between meals.

Glycogen, a polysaccharide storage form of glucose, is our first line of defense against declining blood glucose concentration. During and immediately following a meal, glucose is converted into glycogen, a process known as glycogenesis, in both liver and muscle. The tissue concentration of glycogen is higher in liver than in muscle but because of the relative masses of muscle and liver, the majority of glycogen in the body is stored in muscle (Table 13.1).

Hepatic glycogen is gradually degraded between meals, by the pathway of glycogenolysis, releasing glucose to maintain blood glucose concentration. However, total hepatic glycogen stores are barely sufficient for maintenance of blood glucose concentration during a 12-h fast.

During sleep, when we are not eating, there is a gradual shift from glycogenolysis to de novo synthesis of glucose, also an hepatic pathway, known as gluconeogenesis (Fig. 13.1).

Glucose and glycogen stores in the body (70 kg adult)

Tissue	Type	Amount	% of tissue mass	Calories
liver	glycogen	75 g	3–5%	300
muscle	glycogen	250 g	0.5–1.0%	1000
blood and extracellular fluid	glucose	10 g	–	40

Table 13.1 **Tissue distribution of carbohydrate energy reserves (70 kg adult).**

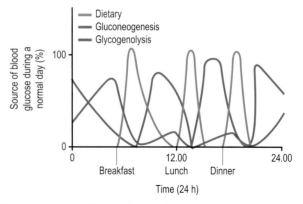

Fig. 13.1 **Sources of blood glucose during a normal day.** Between meals, blood glucose is derived primarily from hepatic glycogen. Depending on the frequency of snacking, glycogenolysis and gluconeogenesis may be more or less active during the day. Late in the night or in early morning, following depletion of a major fraction of hepatic glycogen, gluconeogenesis becomes the primary source of blood glucose.

Gluconeogenesis is essential for survival during fasting or starvation, when glycogen stores are negligible. The liver uses amino acids from muscle protein as the primary precursor of glucose, but also makes use of lactate from glycolysis and glycerol from fat catabolism. Fatty acids, mobilized from adipose tissue triglyceride stores, provide the energy for gluconeogenesis.

Muscle glycogen is not available for maintenance of blood glucose. Glucose obtained from blood and glycogen is used exclusively for energy metabolism in muscle, especially during bursts of physical activity. Although cardiac and skeletal muscles rely on fats as their primary source of energy, some glucose metabolism is essential for efficient fat metabolism in these tissues.

This chapter describes the pathways of glycogenesis and glycogenolysis in liver and muscle, and the pathway of gluconeogenesis in liver.

STRUCTURE OF GLYCOGEN

Glycogen is a branched polysaccharide of glucose, a homoglucan. It contains only two types of glycosidic linkages, chains of $\alpha1{\rightarrow}4$-linked glucose residues with $\alpha1{\rightarrow}6$ branches spaced about every 4–6 residues along the $\alpha1{\rightarrow}4$ chain (Fig. 13.2). Glycogen is closely related to starch, the storage polysaccharide of plants, but starch consists of a mixture of amylose and amylopectin. The amylose component contains only linear $\alpha1{\rightarrow}4$ chains; the amylopectin component is more glycogen-like in structure but with fewer $\alpha1{\rightarrow}6$ branches, about one per 12 $\alpha1{\rightarrow}4$-linked glucose residues. The gross structure of glycogen is dendritic in nature, expanding from a core sequence bound to a tyrosine residue in the protein glycogenin and developing into a final structure

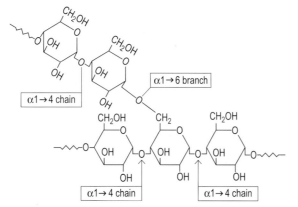

Fig. 13.2 **Close-up of the structure of glycogen.** The figure shows $\alpha1{\rightarrow}4$ chains and an $\alpha1{\rightarrow}6$ branch point. Glycogen is stored as granules in liver and muscle cytoplasm.

resembling a head of cauliflower. The enzymes of glycogen metabolism are bound to the surface of the glycogen particle; many terminal glucose molecules on the surface of the molecule provide ready access for rapid release of glucose from the glycogen polymer.

PATHWAY OF GLYCOGENESIS FROM BLOOD GLUCOSE IN LIVER

The liver is rich in the high-capacity, low-affinity ($K_m > 10$ mmol/L) glucose transporter GLUT-2, making it freely permeable to glucose delivered at high concentration in portal blood during and following a meal (see Table 8.2). The liver is also rich in glucokinase, an enzyme that is specific for glucose and converts it into glucose 6-phosphate (Glc-6-P). Glucokinase (GK) is inducible by continued consumption of a high-carbohydrate diet. It has a high K_m, about 5–7 mmol/L, so that it is poised to increase in activity as portal glucose increases above the normal 5 mmol/L (100 mg/dL) blood glucose concentration. Unlike hexokinase, GK is not inhibited by Glc-6-P, so that the concentration of Glc-6-P increases rapidly in liver following a carbohydrate-rich meal, forcing glucose into all the major pathways of glucose metabolism: glycolysis, the pentose phosphate pathway, and glycogenesis (see Fig. 12.2). Glucose is channeled into glycogen, providing a carbohydrate reserve for maintenance of blood glucose during the postabsorptive state. Excess Glc-6-P in liver, beyond that needed to replenish glycogen reserves, is then funneled into glycolysis, in part for energy production but primarily for conversion into fatty acids and triglycerides, which are exported for storage in adipose tissue. Glucose that passes through the liver causes an increase in peripheral blood glucose concentration following carbohydrate-rich meals. This glucose is used in muscle for synthesis and storage of glycogen and in adipose tissue as a source of glycerol for triglyceride biosynthesis.

The pathway of glycogenesis from glucose (Fig. 13.3A) involves four steps:

- conversion of Glc-6-P into glucose-1-phosphate (Glc-1-P) by phosphoglucomutase
- activation of Glc-1-P to the sugar nucleotide uridine diphosphate (UDP)-glucose by the enzyme UDP-glucose pyrophosphorylase
- transfer of glucose from UDP-Glc to glycogen in $\alpha1{\rightarrow}4$ linkage by glycogen synthase, a member of the class of enzymes known as glycosyl transferases
- when the $\alpha1{\rightarrow}4$ chain exceeds eight residues in length, glycogen branching enzyme, a transglycosylase, transfers some of the $\alpha1{\rightarrow}4$-linked sugars to an $\alpha1{\rightarrow}6$ branch, setting the stage for continued elongation of both $\alpha1{\rightarrow}4$ chains until they, in turn, become long enough for transfer by branching enzyme.

Glycogen synthase is the regulatory enzyme for glycogenesis, rather than UDP-glucose pyrophosphorylase, because UDP-glucose is also used for synthesis of other sugars, and as a glycosyl donor for synthesis of glycoproteins, glycolipids and proteoglycans (Chapters 26–28). Pyrophosphate (PPi), the other product of the pyrophosphorylase reaction, is rapidly hydrolyzed to inorganic phosphate by pyrophosphatase; this reaction provides the thermodynamic driving force for biosynthesis of glycogen.

PATHWAY OF GLYCOGENOLYSIS IN LIVER

As with most metabolic pathways, separate enzymes, sometimes in separate subcellular compartments, are required for the forward and reverse pathways. The pathway of glycogenolysis (Fig. 13.3B) begins with removal of the abundant, external $\alpha 1{\rightarrow}4$-linked glucose residues in glycogen. This is accomplished not by a hydrolase but by glycogen phosphorylase, an enzyme that uses cytosolic phosphate and releases glucose from glycogen in the form of Glc-1-P. The Glc-1-P is isomerized by phosphoglucomutase to Glc-6-P, placing it at the top of the glycolytic pathway; the phosphorylase

reaction, in effect, bypasses the requirement for ATP in the hexokinase or glucokinase reactions. In liver, the glucose is released from Glc-6-P by glucose-6-phosphatase (Glc-6-Pase), and the glucose exits via the GLUT-2 transporter into blood. The rate-limiting, regulatory step in glycogenolysis is catalyzed by phosphorylase, the first enzyme in the pathway.

Phosphorylase is specific for $\alpha 1{\rightarrow}4$ glycosidic linkages; it cannot cleave $\alpha 1{\rightarrow}6$ linkages. Further, this large enzyme cannot approach the branching glucose residues efficiently. Thus, as shown in Figure 13.3B, phosphorylase cleaves the external glucose residues until the branches are three or four residues long, then debranching enzyme, which has both transglycosylase and glucosidase activity, moves a short segment of glucose residues bound to the $\alpha 1{\rightarrow}6$ branch to the end of an adjacent $\alpha 1{\rightarrow}4$ chain, leaving a single glucose residue at the branch point. This glucose is then removed by the exo-1,6-glucosidase activity of branching enzyme, allowing glycogen phosphorylase to proceed with degradation of the extended $\alpha 1{\rightarrow}4$ chain until another branch point is approached, setting the stage for a repeat of the transglycosylase and glucosidase reactions. About 90% of the glucose is released from glycogen as Glc-1-P, and the remainder, derived from the $\alpha 1{\rightarrow}6$ branching residues, as free glucose.

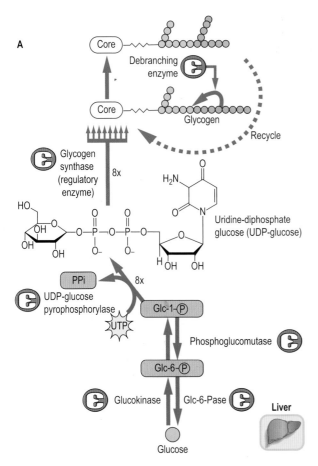

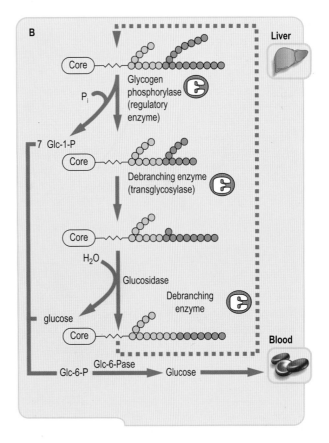

Fig. 13.3 **Pathways of glycogenesis (A) and glycogenolysis (B).**

VON GIERKE'S DISEASE: GLYCOGEN STORAGE DISEASE CAUSED BY GLC-6-PASE DEFICIENCY

A baby girl was chronically cranky, irritable, sweaty, and lethargic, and demanded food frequently. Physical evaluation indicated an extended abdomen, resulting from an enlarged liver. Blood glucose, measured 1 h after feeding, was 3.5 mmol/L (70 mg/dL); normal value ≈5 mmol/L (100 mg/dL). After 4 h, when the child was exhibiting irritability and sweating, her heart rate was increased (pulse = 110), and blood glucose had declined to 2 mmol/L (40 mg/dL). These symptoms were corrected by feeding. A liver biopsy showed massive deposition of glycogen particles in the liver cytosol.

Comment. This child cannot mobilize glycogen. Because of the severity of hypoglycemia, the most likely mutation is in hepatic Glc-6-Pase, which is required for glucose production by both glycogenolysis and gluconeogenesis. Treatment involves frequent feeding with slowly digested carbohydrate, e.g. uncooked starch, and nasogastric drip-feeding during the night.

HORMONAL REGULATION OF HEPATIC GLYCOGENOLYSIS

Glycogenolysis is activated in liver in response to a demand for blood glucose, either because of its utilization during the postabsorptive state or in preparation for increased glucose utilization in response to stress. There are three major hormonal activators of glycogenolysis: glucagon, epinephrine (adrenaline), and cortisol (Table 13.2).

Glucagon is a peptide hormone (3500 Da), secreted from the α-cells of the endocrine pancreas. Its primary function is to activate hepatic glycogenolysis for maintenance of normal blood glucose concentration (normoglycemia). Glucagon has a short half-life in plasma, about 5 min, as a result of receptor binding, renal filtration, and proteolytic inactivation in liver. Glucagon concentration in plasma therefore changes rapidly in response to the need for blood glucose. Blood glucagon increases between meals, decreases during a meal, and is chronically increased during fasting or on a low-carbohydrate diet (Chapter 21).

Glycogenolysis is also activated in response to both acute and chronic stress. The stress may be:

■ physiologic, e.g. in response to increased blood glucose utilization during exercise
■ pathologic, e.g. as a result of blood loss (shock)
■ psychological, e.g. in response to acute or chronic threats.

Acute stress, regardless of its source, causes an activation of glycogenolysis through the action of the catecholamine hormone epinephrine, released from the adrenal medulla.

Hormonal control of glycogenolysis			
Hormone	**Source**	**Initiator**	**Effect on glycogenolysis**
glucagon	pancreatic α-cells	hypoglycemia	rapid activation
epinephrine	adrenal medulla	acute stress, hypoglycemia	rapid activation
cortisol	adrenal cortex	chronic stress	chronic activation
insulin	pancreatic β-cells	hyperglycemia	inhibition

Table 13.2 **Hormones involved in control of glycogenolysis.**

During prolonged exercise, both glucagon and epinephrine contribute to the stimulation of glycogenolysis and maintenance of blood glucose concentration.

Increased blood concentrations of the adrenocortical steroid hormone cortisol also induce glycogenolysis. Levels of the glucocorticoid cortisol vary diurnally in plasma, but may be chronically elevated under continuously stressful conditions, including psychological and environmental (e.g. cold) stress.

Glucagon serves as a general model for the mechanism of action of hormones that act by way of cell surface receptors. Cortisol, which acts at the level of gene expression, will be discussed later in Chapters 34 and 39.

MECHANISM OF ACTION OF GLUCAGON

Glucagon binds to an hepatic plasma membrane receptor and initiates a cascade of reactions that lead to mobilization of hepatic glycogen (Fig. 13.4) during the postabsorptive state. On the inside of the plasma membrane there is a class of signal transduction proteins, known as G-proteins, that bind guanosine triphosphate (GTP) and guanosine diphosphate (GDP), nucleotide analogs of ATP and ADP. GDP is bound in the resting state. Binding of glucagon to the plasma membrane receptor stimulates exchange of GDP for GTP on the G-protein, and the G-protein then undergoes a conformational change that leads to dissociation of one of its subunits, which then binds to and activates the plasma membrane enzyme adenylate cyclase. This enzyme converts cytoplasmic ATP into cyclic-3′,5′-AMP (cAMP), a soluble mediator that is described as the 'second messenger' for action of glucagon (and other hormones). Cyclic AMP binds to the cytoplasmic enzyme protein kinase A (PKA), causing dissociation of inhibitory (regulatory) subunits from the catalytic subunits of the heterodimeric enzyme, relieving inhibition of PKA (see Chapters 21 and 40), which then phosphorylates serine and threonine residues on target proteins and enzymes.

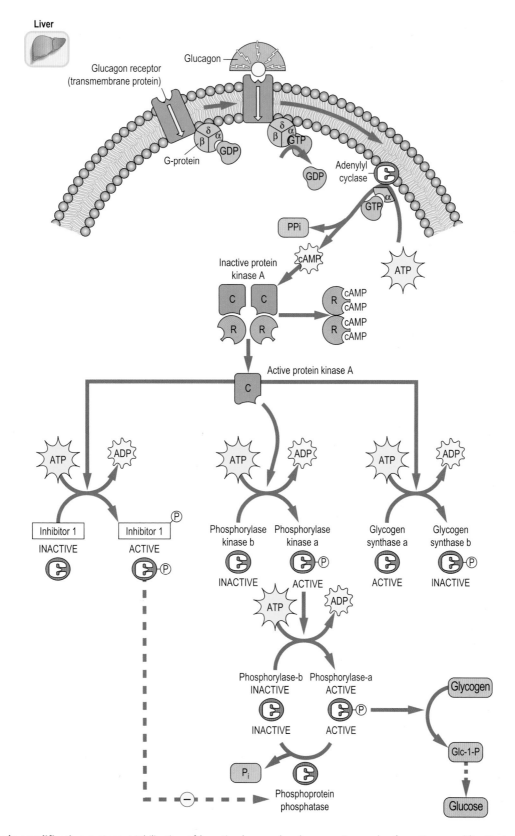

Fig. 13.4 **Cascade amplification system.** Mobilization of hepatic glycogen by glucagon. A cascade of reactions amplifies the hepatic response to glucagon binding to its plasma membrane receptor. cAMP is known as the second messenger of glucagon action. PKA indirectly activates phosphorylase via phosphorylase kinase and directly inactivates glycogen synthase. C, catalytic subunits; R, regulatory (inhibitory) subunits; PKA, protein kinase A. (Compare Fig. 21.6.)

G-PROTEINS

G-proteins are plasma membrane, guanosine nucleotide-binding proteins that are involved in signal transduction for a wide variety of hormones (Fig. 13.4; see also Chapter 40). In some cases they stimulate (Gs) and in other cases they inhibit (Gi) protein kinases and protein phosphorylation. G-proteins are closely associated with hormone receptors in plasma membranes and consist of α, β, and γ subunits. The G_α-subunit binds GDP in the resting state. Following hormone binding (ligation), the receptor recruits G-proteins, stimulating exchange of GDP for GTP on the G_α-subunit. GTP binding leads to release of the β- and γ-subunits, and the α-subunit is then free to bind to and activate adenylate cyclase. The hormonal response is amplified following receptor binding, because a single receptor can activate many α-subunits. Hormonal responses are also turned off at the level of receptors and G-proteins by two mechanisms:

- the G_α-subunit has a sluggish guanosine triphosphate phosphatase (GTPase) activity that hydrolyzes GTP, with a half-time measured in minutes, so that it gradually dissociates from, and thereby ceases to activate, adenylate cyclase
- phosphorylation of the hormone receptor by protein kinase A decreases its affinity for the hormone, a process described as desensitization or hormone resistance.

PROTEIN KINASE A IS VERY SENSITIVE TO SMALL CHANGES IN cAMP CONCENTRATION

As illustrated in Figure 13.4, cAMP-dependent PKA is a tetrameric enzyme with two different types of subunits (R_2C_2); the catalytic C-subunit has protein kinase activity, and the regulatory R-subunit inhibits the protein kinase activity. The R-subunit has a sequence of amino acids that would normally be recognized and phosphorylated by the C-subunit, except that this sequence in R contains an alanine, rather than a serine or threonine, residue. Binding of two molecules of cAMP to each R-subunit results in conformational changes that lead to dissociation of a ($cAMP_2$-R)$_2$ dimer from the C-subunits. The monomeric, active C-subunits then proceed to phosphorylate serine and threonine residues in target enzymes. PKA is not a typical allosteric enzyme, in that the binding of the allosteric effector (cAMP) causes subunit dissociation; however, the complete activation of PKA involves cooperative binding of four molecules of cAMP to two R-subunits. PKA is fully activated at submicromolar concentrations of cAMP, so that it is exquisitely sensitive to small changes in adenylate cyclase activity in response to glucagon.

The pathway for activation of glycogen phosphorylase (see Fig. 13.4) involves phosphorylation of many molecules of phosphorylase kinase by PKA, which then phosphorylates and activates many molecules of glycogen phosphorylase. The net effect of these sequential steps, beginning with activation of many molecules of adenylate cyclase by G-proteins, is a 'cascade amplification' system, not unlike that of a series of amplifiers in a radio or stereo set, resulting in a massive increase in signal strength within seconds after glucagon binding to the hepatocyte plasma membrane. Phosphorylation of phosphorylase activates glycogenolysis, leading to production of Glc-6-P in liver, which is then hydrolyzed to glucose and exported into blood. Another target of PKA is inhibitor-1, a protein phosphatase inhibitor protein, which is activated by phosphorylation. Phosphorylated inhibitor-1 inhibits cytoplasmic phosphoprotein phosphatases, which would otherwise reverse the phosphorylation of enzymes and quench the response to glucagon (see Fig. 13.4).

Glycogenolysis and glycogenesis are opposing pathways. Theoretically, Glc-1-P produced by phosphorylase could be rapidly activated to UDP-glucose and reincorporated into glycogen. To prevent this wasteful or *futile cycle*, PKA also acts directly on glycogen synthase, in this case inactivating the enzyme. Thus, the activation of phosphorylase (glycogenolysis) is coordinated with inactivation of glycogen synthase (glycogenesis). Other hepatic biosynthetic pathways, including protein, cholesterol, fatty acid, and triglyceride synthesis, as well as glycolysis, are also regulated by phosphorylation of key regulatory enzymes, focusing liver metabolism in response to glucagon on the provision of glucose to blood for maintenance of vital body functions (see Chapter 21).

Perhaps in order to balance the cascade of events amplifying the response to glucagon, there are multiple, redundant mechanisms to insure rapid termination of the hormonal response (Table 13.3). In addition to the slow GTPase activity of the G_α-subunit, there is also a phosphodiesterase activity in the cell that hydrolyzes cAMP to AMP, permitting reassociation of the inhibitory and catalytic subunits of PKA, decreasing its protein kinase activity. There are also phosphoprotein phosphatases that remove the phosphate groups from the active, phosphorylated forms of phosphorylase kinase and phosphorylase. The decrease in cAMP concentration

Mechanisms of termination of hormonal response to glucagon
Hydrolysis of GTP on G_α-subunit
Hydrolysis of cAMP by phosphodiesterase
Protein phosphatase activity

Table 13.3 **Several mechanisms are involved in terminating the hormonal response to glucagon**.

and PKA activity also leads to decreased phosphorylation of inhibitor-1, permitting increased activity of phosphoprotein phosphatases. Thus, an array of mechanisms acts in concert to insure that hepatic glycogenolysis declines rapidly in response to increasing blood glucose and decreasing blood glucagon concentrations following a meal.

There are a number of autosomal recessive genetic diseases affecting glycogen metabolism (Table 13.4). These

Glycogen storage diseases			
Type	Name	Enzyme deficiency	Structural or clinical consequences
I	von Gierke's	Glc-6-Pase	severe postabsorptive hypoglycemia, lactic acidemia, hyperlipidemia
II	Pompe's	lysosomal α-glucosidase	glycogen granules in lysosomes
III	Cori's	debranching enzyme	altered glycogen structure, hypoglycemia
IV	Andersen's	branching enzyme	altered glycogen structure
V	McArdle's	muscle phosphorylase	excess muscle glycogen deposition, exercise-induced cramps and fatigue
VI	Hers'	liver phosphorylase	hypoglycemia, not as severe as Type I

Table 13.4 **Major classes of glycogen storage diseases**.

diseases, known as glycogen storage diseases, are characterized by accumulation of glycogen granules in tissues, which eventually compromises tissue function. Predictably, glycogen storage diseases affecting hepatic glycogen metabolism are characterized by fasting hypoglycemia and may be life-threatening, while defects in muscle glycogen metabolism are characterized by rapid muscle fatigue during exercise.

MOBILIZATION OF HEPATIC GLYCOGEN BY EPINEPHRINE

Epinephrine works through several distinct receptors on different cells. The best studied of these receptors are the α- and β-adrenergic receptors; they recognize different features of the epinephrine molecule, bind epinephrine with different affinities, work by different mechanisms, and are inhibited by different classes of drugs. During severe hypoglycemia, glucagon and epinephrine work together to magnify the glycogenolytic response in liver. However, even when blood glucose is normal, epinephrine is released in response to real or perceived threats, causing an increase in blood glucose to support a 'fight or flight' response. Caffeine in coffee and theophylline in tea are inhibitors of phosphodiesterase and also cause an increase in hepatic cAMP and blood glucose. Like epinephrine, caffeine, administered in the form of a few strong cups of coffee, can also make us alert, responsive, and aggressive.

Epinephrine action on hepatic glycogenolysis proceeds by two pathways. One of these, through the epinephrine β-adrenergic receptor, is similar to that for glucagon, involving a plasma membrane epinephrine-specific receptor, G-proteins, and cAMP. The epinephrine response augments the effects of

 McARDLE'S DISEASE: A GLYCOGEN STORAGE DISEASE THAT REDUCES CAPACITY FOR EXERCISE

A 30-year-old man consulted his physician because of chronic arm and leg muscle pains and cramps during exercise. He indicated that he had always had some muscle weakness and, for this reason, was never active in scholastic sports, but the problem did not become severe until he recently enrolled in an exercise program to improve his health. He also noted that the pain generally disappeared after about 15–30 min, and then he could continue his exercise without discomfort. His blood glucose concentration was normal during exercise, but serum creatine kinase (MM isoform from skeletal muscle) was elevated, suggesting muscle damage. Blood glucose declined slightly during 15 min of exercise, but unexpectedly blood lactate also declined, rather than increased, even when he was experiencing muscle cramps. A biopsy indicated an unusually high level of glycogen in muscle, suggesting a glycogen storage disease.

Comment. This patient suffers from McArdle's disease, a rare deficiency of muscle phosphorylase activity. The actual enzyme

deficiency must be confirmed by enzyme assay, since a number of other mutations could also affect muscle glycogen metabolism. During the early periods of intense exercise, the muscle obtains most of its energy by metabolism of glucose, derived from glycogen. During cramps, which normally occur during oxygen debt, most of the pyruvate produced by glycolysis is excreted into blood as lactate, leading to an increase in blood lactate concentration. In this case, however, the patient had cramps but did not excrete lactate, suggesting a failure to mobilize muscle glycogen to produce glucose. His recovery after 15–30 min results from epinephrine-mediated activation of hepatic glycogenolysis, which provides glucose to blood and relieves the deficit in muscle glycogenolysis. Treatment of McArdle's disease usually involves exercise avoidance or carbohydrate consumption prior to exercise. Otherwise, the course of the disease is uneventful.

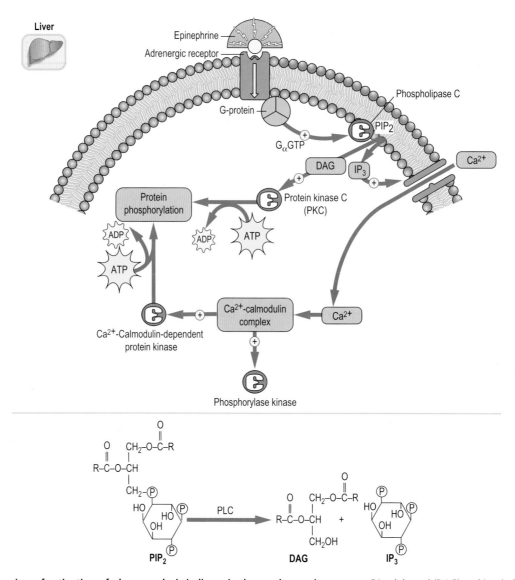

Fig. 13.5 **Mechanism of activation of glycogenolysis in liver via the α-adrenergic receptor.** Diacylglycerol (DAG) and inositol trisphosphate (IP$_3$) are second messengers mediating the adrenergic response. Both DAG and PKC remain associated with the plasma membrane. PIP$_2$, phosphatidylinositol bisphosphate; PKC, protein kinase C. See also Figures 13.8 and 13.9 and Chapter 40.

glucagon during severe hypoglycemia (metabolic stress) and also explains, in part, the rapid heartbeat, sweating, tremors, and anxiety associated with hypoglycemia. Epinephrine also works simultaneously through an α-receptor, but by a different mechanism. Binding to α-receptors also involves G-proteins, common elements in hormone signal transduction, but in this case, the G-protein is specific for activation of a membrane isozyme of phospholipase C (PLC), which is specific for cleavage of a membrane phospholipid, phosphatidylinositol bisphosphate (PIP$_2$) (Fig. 13.5). Both products of PLC action, diacylglycerol (DAG) and inositol trisphosphate (IP$_3$), act as second messengers of epinephrine action. DAG activates

protein kinase C (PKC) which, like PKA, initiates phosphorylation of serine and threonine residues on target proteins. IP$_3$ promotes the transport of Ca^{2+} into the cytosol. Ca^{2+} then binds to the cytoplasmic protein calmodulin, which binds to and activates phosphorylase kinase, leading to cAMP-independent phosphorylation and activation of phosphorylase. A Ca^{2+}–calmodulin-dependent protein kinase and other enzymes are also activated, either by phosphorylation or by association with the Ca^{2+}–calmodulin complex. Thus, a range of metabolic pathways is activated in response to stress, especially those involved in the mobilization of energy reserves.

CHILD BORN OF MALNOURISHED MOTHER MAY HAVE HYPOGLYCEMIA

A baby girl was born at 39 weeks of gestation to a young, malnourished mother. The child was also thin and weak at birth and within 1 h after birth was showing signs of distress, including rapid heartbeat and respiration. Her blood glucose was 3.5 mmol/L (63 mg/dL) at birth, and declined rapidly to 1.5 mmol/L (27 mg/dL) by 1 h, when she was becoming unresponsive and comatose. Her condition was markedly improved by infusion of a glucose solution, followed by a carbohydrate-rich diet. She improved gradually over the next 2 weeks before discharge from the hospital.

Comment. During development in utero, the fetus obtains glucose exogenously, from the placental circulation. However, following birth, the child relies at first on mobilization of hepatic glycogen and then on gluconeogenesis for maintenance of blood glucose. Because of the malnourished state of the mother, this child was born with negligible hepatic glycogen reserves. Thus, she was unable to maintain blood glucose homeostasis postpartum and rapidly declined into hypoglycemia, initiating a stress response. After surviving the transient hypoglycemia, she probably still lacked adequate muscle mass to provide a sufficient supply of amino acids for gluconeogenesis. Infusion of glucose, followed by a carbohydrate-rich diet, would address these deficits, but may not correct more serious damage from prolonged malnutrition during fetal development.

LARGE CHILD BORN OF A DIABETIC MOTHER

A baby boy, born of a poorly controlled, chronically hyperglycemic, diabetic mother, was large and chubby (macrosomic) at birth (5 kg) but appeared otherwise normal. He declined rapidly, however, and within 1 h showed all the symptoms of hypoglycemia, similar to the case of the baby girl born of a malnourished mother. The difference, in this case, was that the boy was obviously on the heavy side, rather than thin and malnourished.

Comment. This child has experienced a chronically hyperglycemic environment during uterine development. He adapted by increasing endogenous insulin production, which has a growth hormone-like activity, resulting in macrosomia. At birth, when placental delivery of glucose ceases, he has a normal blood glucose concentration and a substantial supply of hepatic glycogen. However, chronic hyperinsulinemia prior to birth probably represses gluconeogenic enzymes, and his high blood insulin concentration at birth promotes glucose uptake into muscle and adipose tissue. In the absence of a maternal source of glucose, insulin-induced hypoglycemia leads to a stress response, which was corrected by glucose infusion. After 1–2 days, his ample body mass will provide a good reservoir for synthesis of blood glucose from muscle protein.

GLYCOGENOLYSIS IN MUSCLE

The tissue localization of hormone receptors provides tissue specificity to hormone action. Thus, only those tissues with glucagon receptors respond to glucagon. Muscle may be rich in glycogen, even during hypoglycemia, but it lacks both the glucagon receptor and Glc-6-Pase. Therefore muscle glycogen cannot be mobilized to replenish blood glucose. Muscle glycogenolysis is activated in response to epinephrine through the cAMP-dependent β-adrenergic receptor, but the glucose is metabolized through glycolysis for energy production. This occurs not only during 'fight or flight' situations, but also in response to metabolic demands during prolonged exercise. There are also two important hormone-independent mechanisms for activation of glycogenolysis in muscle (Fig. 13.6). First, the influx of Ca^{2+} into the muscle cytoplasm in response to nerve stimulation activates the basal, unphosphorylated form of phosphorylase kinase by action of the Ca^{2+}–calmodulin complex. This hormone-independent activation of phosphorylase provides for rapid activation of glycogenolysis during short bursts of exercise, even in the absence of epinephrine action. A second mechanism for activation of muscle glycogenolysis involves direct allosteric activation of phosphorylase by AMP. Increased usage of ATP during a rapid burst of muscle activity leads to rapid accumulation of ADP, which is converted in part into AMP by action of the enzyme myokinase (adenylate kinase), which catalyzes the reaction:

$$2\,ADP \rightleftarrows ATP + AMP$$

MAXIMAL INHIBITION OF GLYCOGEN SYNTHASE IS ACHIEVED ONLY THROUGH SEQUENTIAL ACTION OF SEVERAL KINASES

When both glucagon and epinephrine are acting on liver, the activation of glycogenolysis and inhibition of glycogenesis is mediated by at least three kinases: protein kinase A (PKA), protein kinase C (PKC), and Ca^{2+}-calmodulin activated protein kinase. All three of these protein kinases phosphorylate key serine and threonine residues in regulatory enzymes. These and other protein kinases work in concert with one another in a process known as sequential or hierarchical phosphorylation, leading to phosphorylation of up to nine amino acid residues on glycogen synthase. Maximal inhibition of glycogen synthase is achieved only through the sequential activity of several kinases. In some cases, certain serine or threonine residues must be phosphorylated in a specific sequence by cooperative action of different kinases, i.e. phosphorylation of one site by one enzyme requires prior phosphorylation of another site by a separate enzyme.

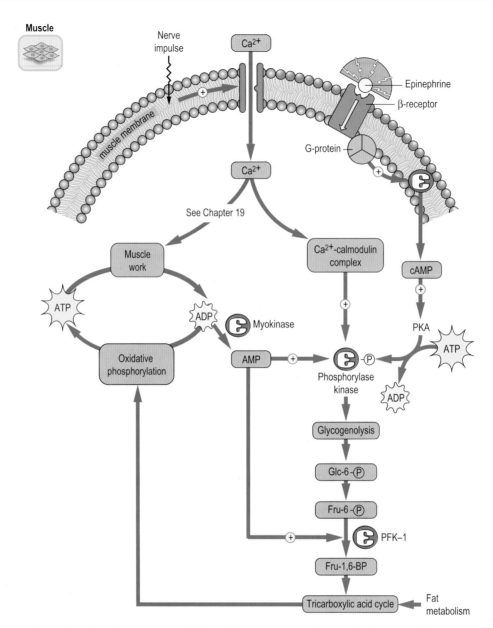

Fig. 13.6 **Regulation of protein kinase A in muscle.** Activation of glycogenolysis and glycolysis in muscle during exercise. PFK-1, phosphofruc-tokinase-1. Compare Figure 8.4.

AMP activates both the basal and phosphorylated forms of phosphorylase, enhancing glycogenolysis in either the absence or presence of hormonal stimulation. AMP also relieves inhibition of phosphofructokinase-1 (PFK-1) by ATP (see Chapter 12), stimulating the utilization of glucose through glycolysis for energy production. The stimulatory effects of Ca^{2+} and AMP insure that the muscle can respond to its energy needs, even in the absence of hormonal input.

REGULATION OF GLYCOGENESIS

Glycogenesis, and energy storage in general, occurs during and immediately following meals. Glucose and other carbohydrates, rushing into the liver from the intestines via the portal circulation, are efficiently trapped to make glycogen. Excess glucose proceeds to the peripheral circulation, where it is taken up into muscle and adipose tissue for energy reserves or storage. We normally eat sitting down, rather than during exercise, so that the opposing pathways of uptake and storage versus mobilization and utilization of energy supplies are temporally compartmentalized functions in our lives.

Energy storage is under the control of the polypeptide hormone insulin, which is stored in β-cells in the pancreatic islets of Langerhans (Chapter 21). Insulin is secreted into blood following a meal, tracking blood glucose concentration. It has two primary functions in carbohydrate metabolism: first, insulin reverses the actions of glucagon in

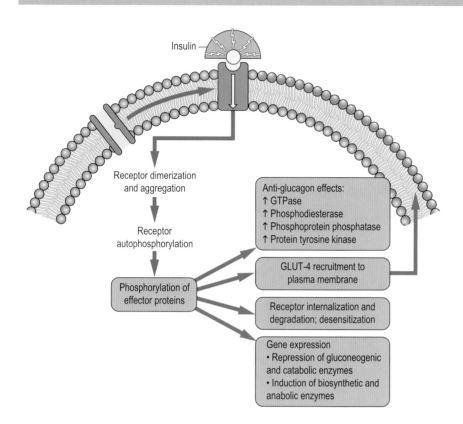

Fig. 13.7 **Mechanisms of insulin action.** Regulatory effects of insulin on hepatic and muscle carbohydrate metabolism. (See also Chapter 21.)

phosphorylation of proteins, turning off glycogen phosphorylase and activating glycogen synthase, promoting glucose storage; second, it stimulates the uptake of glucose into peripheral tissues (muscle and adipose tissue), facilitating synthesis and storage of glycogen and triglycerides. Insulin also acts at the level of gene expression, stimulating the synthesis of enzymes involved in carbohydrate metabolism and storage and conversion of glucose into triglycerides.

Protein tyrosine phosphorylation, rather than serine and threonine phosphorylation, is a characteristic feature of insulin and growth factor activity. Insulin binding to its transmembrane receptor (Fig. 13.7) stimulates aggregation of receptors and promotes tyrosine kinase activity in the intracellular domain of the receptor. The insulin receptor autophosphorylates its tyrosine residues, enhancing its protein tyrosine kinase activity, and phosphorylates tyrosine residues in other intracellular effector proteins, which then activate secondary pathways. Among these are kinases that phosphorylate serine and threonine residues on proteins, but at sites and on proteins distinct from those phosphorylated by PKA and PKC. Insulin-dependent activation of GTPase, phosphodiesterase and phosphoprotein phosphatases also checks the action of glucagon, which is typically present at high concentration in the blood at mealtimes, i.e. several hours since the last meal.

The liver also appears to be directly responsive to ambient blood glucose concentration, since hepatic glycogen synthesis increases following a meal, even in the absence of hormonal input. Thus, the increase in hepatic glycogenesis begins more rapidly than the increase in insulin concentration in blood. Perfusion of liver with glucose solutions in vitro, in the absence of insulin, also leads to inhibition of glycogenolysis and activation of glycogenesis. This appears to occur by direct allosteric inhibition of phosphorylase by glucose and secondary stimulation of protein phosphatase activity.

Most, if not all, cells in the body are responsive to insulin in some way, but the major sites of insulin action, on a mass basis, are muscle and adipose tissue. These tissues normally have low levels of cell surface glucose transporters, restricting the entry of glucose – they rely mostly on lipids for energy metabolism. In muscle and adipose tissue, insulin receptor tyrosine kinase activity induces movement of glucose transporter-4 (GLUT-4; see Table 8.2) from intracellular vacuoles to the cell surface, increasing glucose transport into the cell. The glucose is then used in muscle for synthesis of glycogen, and in adipose tissue to produce glyceraldehyde-3-phosphate which is converted to glycerol-3-phosphate for synthesis of triglycerides (Chapter 16). The insulin-stimulated, GLUT-4 mediated uptake of glucose into muscle and adipose tissue is the primary mechanism limiting the increase in blood glucose following a meal.

GLUCONEOGENESIS

During fasting and starvation, when hepatic glycogen is depleted, gluconeogenesis is essential for maintenance of blood glucose homeostasis. Unlike glycogenolysis, which can be turned on rapidly in response to hormonal stimulation, gluconeogenesis increases more slowly, depending on changes in gene expression, and reaches maximal activity over a period of hours (see Fig. 13.1); it becomes the primary source of our blood glucose concentration about 8 hours into the postabsorptive state (Chapter 21). Gluconeogenesis requires both a source of energy for biosynthesis and a source of carbons for formation of the backbone of the glucose molecule. The energy is provided by metabolism of fatty acids released from adipose tissue. The carbon skeletons are provided from three primary sources:

■ lactate produced in tissues such as the red cell and muscle
■ amino acids derived from muscle protein
■ glycerol released from triglycerides during lipolysis in adipose tissue.

Among these, muscle protein is the major precursor of blood glucose – the rate of gluconeogenesis is often limited by the availability of substrate, including the rate of proteolysis in muscle or, in some cases, muscle mass. During prolonged fasting, malnutrition or starvation, we lose both adipose and muscle mass. The fat is used both for the general energy needs of the body and to support gluconeogenesis, while most of the amino acids in protein are converted into glucose.

Gluconeogenesis from lactate

Gluconeogenesis is conceptually the opposite of anaerobic glycolysis but proceeds by a slightly different pathway, involving both mitochondrial and cytosolic enzymes (Fig. 13.8). During hepatic gluconeogenesis lactate is converted back into glucose, using, in part, the same glycolytic enzymes involved in conversion of glucose into lactate. The lactate cycle involving the liver, red cells, and muscle, known as the Cori cycle, is discussed in detail in Chapter 21. At this point, we focus on the metabolic pathway for conversion of lactate to glucose.

A critical problem in the reversal of glycolysis is overcoming the irreversibility of three kinase reactions: glucokinase (GK), phosphofructokinase-1 (PFK-1), and pyruvate kinase (PK). The fourth kinase in glycolysis, phosphoglycerate kinase (PGK), catalyzes a freely reversible, equilibrium reaction; a substrate-level phosphorylation reaction, transferring a high-energy acyl phosphate in 1,3-bisphosphoglycerate to an energetically similar pyrophosphate bond in ATP. To circumvent the three irreversible reactions, the liver uses four unique enzymes: pyruvate carboxylase (PC) in the mitochondrion and phosphoenolpyruvate carboxykinase (PEPCK) in the cytoplasm to bypass PK, fructose-1,6-bisphosphatase (Fru-1,6-BPase) to bypass PFK-1, and Glc-6-Pase to bypass GK (see Fig. 13.8). Gluconeogenesis from lactate involves,

first, its conversion into phosphoenolpyruvate (PEP), a process requiring investment of two ATP equivalents because of the high energy of the enol–phosphate bond in PEP. Lactate is first converted into pyruvate by lactate dehydrogenase (LDH), and then enters the mitochondrion, where it is converted to oxaloacetate by PC, using biotin and ATP. Oxaloacetate is reduced to malate by the TCA cycle enzyme, malate dehydrogenase, exits the mitochondrion, and is then reoxidized to oxaloacetate by cytosolic malate dehydrogenase. The cytosolic oxaloacetate is then decarboxylated by PEPCK, using GTP as a co-substrate, yielding PEP. The energy for synthesis of PEP from oxaloacetate is derived from both the GTP and the decarboxylation of oxaloacetate.

Glycolysis may now proceed backwards from PEP until it reaches the next irreversible reaction, PFK-1. This enzyme is bypassed by a simple hydrolysis reaction, catalyzed by Fru-1, 6-BPase without production of ATP, reversing the PFK-1 reaction and producing Fru-6-P. Similarly, the bypass of GK is accomplished by hydrolysis of Glc-6-P by Glc-6-Pase, without production of ATP. The free glucose is then released into blood.

Gluconeogenesis is fairly efficient – the liver can make a kilogram of glucose per day by gluconeogenesis, and actually does so in poorly controlled, hyperglycemic diabetic patients. Normal glucose production, in the absence of dietary carbohydrate, is ~200 g/day, almost a half-pound of glucose. Gluconeogenesis from pyruvate is moderately expensive, requiring a net expenditure of the equivalent of 4 moles of ATP per mole of pyruvate converted into glucose, i.e. 2 mol ATP at the PC reaction and 2 mol of GTP at the PEPCK reaction. This ATP is provided by oxidation of fatty acids (Chapter 15).

Gluconeogenesis from amino acids and glycerol

Most amino acids are glucogenic, i.e. following deamination, their carbon skeletons can be converted into glucose. Alanine and glutamine are the major amino acids exported from muscle for gluconeogenesis. Their relative concentrations in venous blood from muscle exceed their relative concentration in muscle protein, indicating considerable reshuffling of muscle amino acids to provide gluconeogenic substrates. As discussed in more detail in Chapter 19, alanine is converted directly into pyruvate by the enzyme alanine aminotransferase (alanine transaminase, ALT), and then gluconeogenesis proceeds as described for lactate. Other amino acids are converted into tricarboxylic acid cycle (TCA cycle) intermediates, then to malate for gluconeogenesis. Aspartate, for example, is converted into oxaloacetate by aspartate aminotransferase (aspartate transaminase, AST), and glutamate into α-ketoglutarate by glutamate dehydrogenase. Some glucogenic amino acids are converted by less direct routes into alanine or intermediates in the tricarboxylic acid cycle for gluconeogenesis. The amino groups of these amino

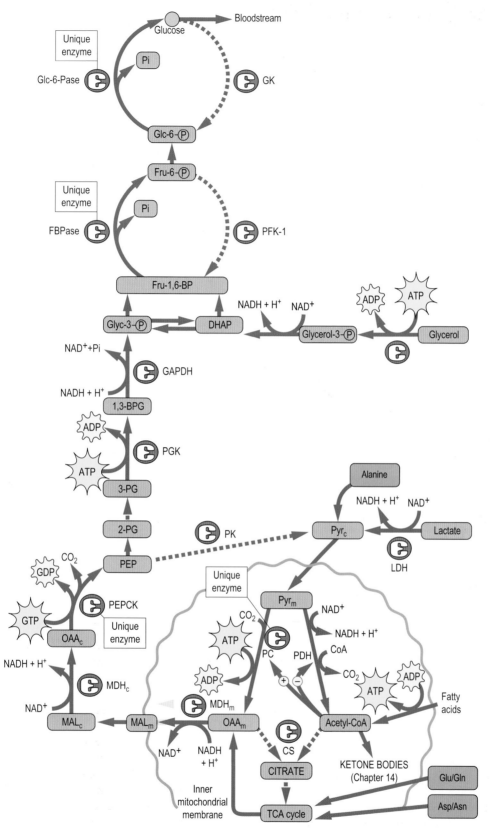

Fig. 13.8 **Pathway of gluconeogenesis.** Gluconeogenesis is the reverse of glycolysis. Unique enzymes overcome the irreversible kinase reactions of glycolysis. **Compartments:** c, cytoplasmic; imm, inner mitochondrial membrane; m, mitochondrial. **Enzymes:** CS, citrate synthase; Fru-1,6-BPase, fructose-1,6-bisphosphatase; GAPDH, glyceraldehyde-3-P dehydrogenase; Glc-6-Pase, glucose-6-phosphatase; GK, glucokinase; MDH, malate dehydrogenase; PC, pyruvate carboxylase; PDH, pyruvate dehydrogenase; PEP, phosphoenolpyruvate; PEPCK, PEP carboxykinase; PGK, phosphoglycerate kinase. **Substrates:** 2,3-BPG, bisphosphoglycerate; DHAP, dihydroxyacetone phosphate; Fru-1,6-BP, fructose-1,6-bisphosphate; Glyc-3-P, glyceraldehyde 3-phosphate; MAL, malate; OAA, oxaloacetate; Pyr, pyruvate; 3-PG, 3-phosphoglycerate. *Solid lines*: active during gluconeogenesis. *Dotted lines*: inactive during gluconeogenesis.

acids are converted into urea, via the urea cycle in hepatocytes, and the urea is excreted in urine (Chapter 19).

Glycerol enters gluconeogenesis at the level of triose phosphates (see Fig. 13.8). Following release of glycerol and fatty acids from adipose tissue into plasma, the glycerol is taken up into liver and phosphorylated by glycerol kinase, and then enters the gluconeogenic pathway as dihydroxyacetone phosphate. Only the glycerol component of fats can be converted into glucose. The incorporation of glycerol into glucose requires only 2 mol ATP per mol glucose produced.

Glucose cannot be synthesized from fatty acids

As discussed in Chapter 15, metabolism of fatty acids involves their conversion in two carbon oxidation steps to form acetyl-coA, which is then metabolized in the tricarboxylic acid cycle following condensation with oxaloacetate to form citrate. While the carbons of acetate are theoretically available for gluconeogenesis by conversion to malate, during the pathway from citrate to malate, two molecules of CO_2 are eliminated, at the isocitrate and α-ketoglutarate dehydrogenase reactions. Thus, although energy is produced in the tricarboxylic acid cycle, the two carbons invested for gluconeogenesis from acetyl-coA are lost as CO_2.

For this reason, acetyl-coA, and therefore even-chain fatty acids, cannot serve as substrates for *net* gluconeogenesis. However, odd-chain and branched-chain fatty acids, which form propionyl-coA, can serve as minor precursors for gluconeogenesis. Propionyl-coA is first carboxylated to methylmalonyl-coA, which undergoes racemase and mutase reactions to form succinyl-coA, a tricarboxylic acid cycle intermediate (see Chapter 15). Succinyl-coA is converted into malate, exits the mitochondrion and is oxidized to oxaloacetate. Following decarboxylation by PEPCK, the three carbons of propionate are conserved in PEP and glucose.

Regulation of gluconeogenesis

Like glycogen metabolism in liver, gluconeogenesis is regulated primarily by hormonal mechanisms. In this case, the regulatory process involves counterregulation of glycolysis and gluconeogenesis, largely by phosphorylation/dephosphorylation of enzymes, under control of glucagon and insulin. The primary control point is at the regulatory enzymes PFK-1 and Fru-1,6-BPase which, in liver, are exquisitely sensitive to the allosteric effector fructose 2,6-bisphosphate (Fru-2, 6-BP). Fru-2,6-BP is an activator of PFK-1 and an inhibitor

 EXCESS ALCOHOL CONSUMPTION CAN LEAD TO HYPOGLYCEMIA

A middle-aged, emaciated, chronic alcoholic man collapsed in a bar at about 11 a.m. and was transported to the emergency room by ambulance. Another patron noted that the man had had only a few shots of vodka and did not appear to be unusually drunk, although he was a little confused, at the time that he fainted. The bartender suggested that the man might have had a heart attack. Physical examination revealed a somewhat clammy skin, unusual for a winter morning, rapid breathing, and a rapid heartbeat. Laboratory tests indicated a blood glucose of 2.5 mmol/L (50 mg/dL), in the hypoglycemic range, and a blood alcohol level of 0.2%, suggesting intoxication. Other tests indicated a normal level of troponin T, a protein measured for early diagnosis of myocardial infarction, high serum aspartate aminotransferase activity, indicative of liver damage (hepatitis or cirrhosis), a slightly acidic blood pH (7.29 versus normal 7.35), low pCO_2, and high blood lactate. The man responded to an infusion of a glucose solution, regained consciousness, had brunch and a few hours later, after a miraculous recovery, was referred to a counselor for treatment. What happened?

Comment. This patient probably had not eaten breakfast before starting his morning binge. His glycogen stores were negligible, so he was dependent on gluconeogenesis for maintenance of blood glucose concentration, but gluconeogenesis may be compromised both by liver disease and by the limited muscle mass available to mobilize amino acids for gluconeogenesis. The

consumption of alcohol places additional stress on gluconeogenesis, since alcohol is metabolized primarily in the liver. The two-step metabolism of alcohol is relatively unregulated, leading to a rapid increase in hepatic NADH

Alcohol dehydrogenase:

$$CH_3CH_2OH + NAD^+ + H^+ \rightarrow CH_3CHO + NADH$$

Aldehyde dehydrogenase:

$$CH_3CHO + NAD^+ + H^+ \rightarrow CH_3COOH + NADH$$

The increase in hepatic NADH shifts the equilibrium of the LDH reaction toward lactate, limiting gluconeogenesis from pyruvate derived from lactate (or alanine), leading to accumulation of lactic acid in blood (lacticacidemia). It also shifts cytosolic oxaloacetate toward malate, reducing gluconeogenesis from citric acid cycle intermediates, and shifts dihydroxyacetone phosphate toward glycerol-3-phosphate, reducing gluconeogenesis from glycerol. Thus, the redox imbalance induced by alcohol consumption leads to a large increase in NADH in the cytoplasm, inhibiting the flux of all major substrates (lactate, amino acids and glycerol) into gluconeogenesis. The low blood glucose leads to a stress response (rapid heart beat, clammy skin), an effort to enhance stimulation of gluconeogenesis by combined action of glucagon and epinephrine. The rapid breathing is a physiologic response to metabolic acidosis, resulting from the excess of lactic acid in blood.

of Fru-1,6-BPase, counterregulating the two opposing pathways. As shown in Figure. 13.9, Fru-2,6-BP is synthesized by an unusual, bifunctional enzyme, phosphofructokinase-2/fructose-2,6-bisphosphatase (PFK-2/Fru-2,6-BPase) which has both kinase and phosphatase activities. In the phosphorylated state, effected by glucagon through protein kinase A, this enzyme displays Fru-2,6-BPase activity, which reduces the level of Fru-2,6-BP. The decrease in Fru-2, 6-BP simultaneously decreases the stimulation of glycolysis at PFK-1 and relieves inhibition of gluconeogenesis at Fru-1,6-BPase. In this way, glucagon-mediated phosphorylation of PFK-2/Fru-2,6-BP places the liver cell in a gluconeogenic mode. The coordinate, allosterically mediated increase in Fru-1,6-BPase and decrease in PFK-1 activities ensure that glucose made by gluconeogenesis is not consumed by glycolysis in a futile cycle, but released into blood by Glc-6-Pase. Similarly, any flux of glucose from glycogen through glycogenolysis, also induced by glucagon, is diverted to blood, rather than to glycolysis, by inhibition of PFK-1. PK is also inhibited by phosphorylation by protein kinase A (PKA), providing an additional site for inhibition of glycolysis.

When glucose enters the liver following a meal, insulin mediates the dephosphorylation of PFK-2/Fru-2,6-BPase, turning on its PFK-2 activity. The resultant increase in

Fru-2,6-BP activates PFK-1 and inhibits Fru-1,6-BPase activity. Gluconeogenesis is inhibited and glucose entering the liver is then incorporated into glycogen or routed into glycolysis for lipogenesis. Thus, liver metabolism following a meal is focused on synthesis and storage of both carbohydrate and lipid energy reserves, which are used later, in the postabsorptive state, for maintenance of blood glucose and fatty acid homeostasis.

Gluconeogenesis is also regulated in the mitochondrion by acetyl-coA. The influx of fatty acids from adipose tissue, stimulated by glucagon to support gluconeogenesis, leads to an increase in hepatic acetyl-coA, which is both an inhibitor of pyruvate dehydrogenase (PDH) and an essential allosteric activator of pyruvate carboxylase (PC) (see Fig. 13.8). In this way, fat metabolism inhibits the oxidation of pyruvate and favors its use for gluconeogenesis in liver. In muscle during the fasting state, glucose utilization for energy metabolism is limited both by the low level of GLUT-4 in the plasma membranes (because of the low plasma insulin concentration) and by inhibition of PDH by acetyl-coA. Active fat metabolism and high levels of acetyl-coA in muscle promote the excretion of a significant fraction of pyruvate as lactate, even in the resting state. The carbon skeleton of glucose is returned to the liver via the Cori Cycle (Chapter 21), and recycling of pyruvate into glucose, in effect, conserves muscle protein.

Conversion of fructose and galactose to glucose

As discussed in detail in Chapter 26, fructose is metabolized almost exclusively in the liver. It enters glycolysis at the level of triose phosphates, bypassing the regulatory enzyme,

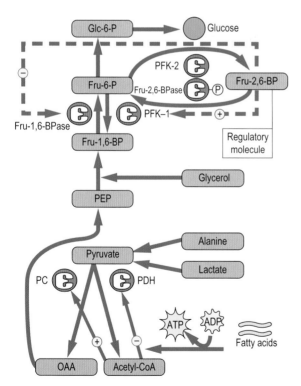

Fig. 13.9 **Regulation of gluconeogenesis.** Gluconeogenesis is regulated by hepatic levels of Fru-2,6-BP and acetyl-coA. The upper part of the diagram focuses on the reciprocal regulation of Fru-1,6-BPase and PFK-1 by Fru-2,6-BP and the lower part on the reciprocal regulation of pyruvate dehydrogenase (PDH) and pyruvate carboxylase (PC) by acetyl-coA.

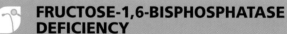

🏊 FRUCTOSE-1,6-BISPHOSPHATASE DEFICIENCY

A 3-day-old child was screened for sepsis because of apparent hyperventilation and recurrent spells of apnea. Blood glucose was low (2 mmol/L; hypoglycemia), and lactate was grossly elevated at 15 mmol/L. Feeding every 2 h stopped further attacks, but the liver was noted to be slightly enlarged.

Comment. About half the cases of fructose-1,6-bisphosphatase deficiency present with hypoglycemia and severe lactic acidosis in the first few days of life. Frequent feeding with carbohydrate prevents further problems. FBPase deficiency impairs the formation of glucose from all gluconeogenic precursors, and normoglycemia is dependent on glucose intake, and on degradation of hepatic glycogen. The frequency of attacks decreases with age and the majority of affected children have normal psychomotor development.

PFK-1, so that large amounts of pyruvate may be forced on the mitochondrion for use in energy metabolism or fat biosynthesis. During a gluconeogenic state, this fructose may also proceed toward Glc-6-P, providing a convenient source of blood glucose. Gluconeogenesis from galactose is equally efficient, since Glc-1-P, derived from galactose 1-phosphate (Chapter 26), is readily isomerized to Glc-6-P by phosphoglucomutase. Fructose and galactose are good sources of glucose, independent of glycogenolysis and gluconeogenesis.

Summary

Glycogen is stored in two tissues in the body for different reasons: in liver for short-term maintenance of blood glucose homeostasis, and in muscle as a source of energy. Glycogen metabolism in these tissues responds rapidly to both allosteric and hormonal control. In liver, the balance between glycogenolysis and glycogenesis is regulated by the balance between concentrations of glucagon and insulin in the circulation, which controls the state of phosphorylation of enzymes. Phosphorylation of enzymes under the influence of glucagon directs glycogen mobilization and is the most common condition in the liver, e.g. during sleep. Increases in blood insulin during and after meals promote dephosphorylation of the same enzymes, leading to glycogenesis. Insulin also promotes glucose uptake into muscle and adipose tissue for glycogen and triglyceride synthesis following a meal. Epinephrine increases phosphorylation of liver enzymes, enabling a burst in hepatic glycogenolysis and an increase in blood glucose for stress responses. Muscle is also responsive to epinephrine, but not to glucagon; in this case the glucose produced by glycogenolysis is used for muscle energy metabolism – fight or flight. In addition, muscle glycogenolysis is responsive to intracellular Ca^{2+} and AMP concentrations, providing a mechanism for coupling glycogenolysis to normal energy consumption during exercise. The actions of insulin, glucagon, and epinephrine illustrate many of the fundamental principles of hormone action (Table 13.5).

Gluconeogenesis takes place primarily in liver, and is designed for maintenance of blood glucose during the fasting state. It is essential after 12 h of fasting, when the majority of hepatic glycogen has been consumed. The major substrates for gluconeogenesis are lactate, amino acids, and glycerol; fatty acid metabolism provides the energy. The major control point is at the level of phosphofructokinase-1 (PFK-1), which is activated by the allosteric effector Fru-2,6-BP. The synthesis of Fru-2,6-BP is under control of the bifunctional enzyme, PFK-2/Fru-2,6-BPase, whose kinase and phosphatase activities are regulated by phosphorylation/dephosphorylation, under hormonal control by insulin and glucagon. During fasting and active gluconeogenesis, glucagon mediates phosphorylation and activation of the phosphatase activity of this enzyme, leading to a decrease in the level of Fru-2,6-BP and a corresponding decrease in glycolysis; carbohydrate degradation

General features of hormone action
Tissue specificity, determined by receptor distribution
Multistep, cascade amplification
Intracellular second messengers
Coordinate counterregulation of opposing pathways
Augmentation and/or opposition by other hormones
Multiple mechanisms of termination of response

Table 13.5 **General features of hormone action.** Hormonal regulation of glucose metabolism illustrates fundamental principles of hormone action (see Chapter 39).

ACTIVE LEARNING

1. The inactivation of glycogenesis in response to epinephrine occurs in a single-step by action of PKA on glycogen synthase, while the activation of glycogenolysis involves an intermediate enzyme, phosphorylate kinase, which phosphorylates phosphorylase. Discuss the metabolic advantages of the two-step activation of glycogenolysis.
2. Investigate the use of inhibitors of gluconeogenesis for treatment of type 2 diabetes.
3. Glucose-6-phosphatase is essential for production of glucose in liver, but is not a cytosolic enzyme. Describe the activity and subcellular localization of this enzyme and the final stages of the pathway for production of glucose in liver.

is inhibited and fats become the primary energy source during fasting and starvation. Oxidation of pyruvate is also inhibited in the mitochondrion by inhibition of PDH by acetyl-coA, derived from fat metabolism. Following a meal, the decrease in phosphorylation of enzymes enhances PFK-2 activity; the increase in Fru-2,6-BP concentration activates PFK-1 and promotes glycolysis, providing pyruvate, which is converted to acetyl-coA for lipogenesis.

Further reading

Beale EG, Harvey BJ, Forest C. PCK1 and PCK2 as candidate diabetes and obesity genes. *Cell Biochem Biophys* 2007; **48**:89–95.

Boden G. Gluconeogenesis and glycogenolysis in health and diabetes. *J Invest Med* 2004;**52**:375–378.

Bongaerts GP, van Halteren HK, Verhagen CA, Wagener DJ. Cancer cachexia demonstrates the energetic impact of gluconeogenesis in human metabolism. *Med Hypotheses* 2006;**67**:213–1222.

de Lonlay P, Giurgea I, Touati G, Saudubray JM. Neonatal hypoglycaemia: aetiologies. *Semin Neonatol* 2004;**9**:49–58.

Geel TM, McLaughlin PM, de Leij LF, Ruiters MH, Niezen-Koning KE. Pompe disease: current state of treatment modalities and animal models. *Mol Genet Metab* 2007;**92**:299–307.

Hume R, Burchell A, Williams FL, Koh DK. Glucose homeostasis in the newborn. *Early Hum Dev* 2005;**81**:95–101.

Lomako J, Lomako WM, Whelan WJ. Glycogenin: the primer for mammalian and yeast glycogen synthesis. *Biochim Biophys Acta* 2004;**1673**:45–55.

Ozen H. Glycogen storage diseases: new perspectives. *World J Gastroenterol* 2007; **13**(18):2541–2553.

Wu C, Okar DA, Kang J, Lange AJ. Reduction of hepatic glucose production as a therapeutic target in the treatment of diabetes. *Curr Drug Targets Immune Endocr Metabol Disord* 2005; **5**:51–59.

Websites

Gluconeogenesis: www.wiley.com/legacy/college/boyer/0470003790/animations/gluconeogenesis/gluconeogenesis.htm

Glycogen:
- http://bip.cnrs-mrs.fr/bip10/glycogen.htm
- www.rpi.edu/dept/bcbp/molbiochem/MBWeb/mb1/part2/9-glycogen.ppt

Hypoglycemia: http://diabetes.niddk.nih.gov/dm/pubs/hypoglycemia/index.htm

14. The Tricarboxylic Acid Cycle

L W Stillway

LEARNING OBJECTIVES

After reading this chapter you should be able to:

- Outline the sequence of reactions in the tricarboxylic acid (TCA) cycle and explain the purpose of the cycle.
- Identify the four oxidative enzymes in the TCA cycle and their products.
- Identify the two intermediates required in the first step of the TCA cycle and their metabolic sources.
- Identify four major metabolic intermediates synthesized from TCA cycle intermediates.
- Describe how the TCA cycle is regulated by substrate supply, allosteric effectors, covalent modification, and protein synthesis.
- Explain why there is no net synthesis of glucose from acetyl-CoA.
- Explain the concept of 'suicide substrate' as applied to the TCA cycle.

INTRODUCTION

Located in the mitochondrion, the tricarboxylic acid (TCA) cycle, also known as the Krebs or citric acid cycle, is a common pathway for metabolism of all fuels. It oxidatively strips electrons from fat, carbohydrate and protein fuels, producing the majority of the reduced coenzymes that are used for the generation of adenosine triphosphate (ATP) in the electron transport chain. Although the TCA cycle does not use oxygen in any of its reactions, it requires oxidative metabolism in the mitochondrion for reoxidation of reduced coenzymes. The TCA cycle has two major functions: energy production and biosynthesis (Figure 14.1).

FUNCTIONS OF THE TRICARBOXYLIC ACID CYCLE

Four oxidative steps provide free energy for ATP synthesis

A common endproduct of carbohydrate, fatty acid and amino acid metabolism, acetyl-CoA is oxidized in the TCA cycle to produce reduced coenzymes by four redox reactions per turn of the cycle. Three produce reduced nicotinamide adenine dinucleotide (NADH) and another produces reduced flavin adenine dinucleotide ($FADH_2$). These reduced nucleotides provide energy for ATP synthesis by the electron transport system (see Chapter 9). One high-energy phosphate, guanosine triphosphate (GTP), is also produced in the cycle by substrate-level phosphorylation. Nearly all metabolic carbon dioxide is produced by decarboxylation reactions catalyzed by pyruvate dehydrogenase and TCA cycle enzymes in the mitochondrion.

The TCA cycle provides a common ground for interconversion of fuels and metabolites

The TCA cycle (see Figure 14.1) participates in the synthesis of glucose from amino acids and lactate during starvation and fasting (gluconeogenesis; Chapter 13). It is also involved in the conversion of carbohydrates to fat following a carbohydrate-rich meal (Chapter 16). It is a source of nonessential amino acids, such as aspartate and glutamate, which are synthesized directly from TCA cycle intermediates. One TCA cycle intermediate, succinyl-coenzyme A (succinyl-CoA), serves as a precursor to porphyrins (heme) in all cells, but especially in bone marrow and liver (Chapter 29). Biosynthetic reactions proceeding from the TCA cycle require the input of carbons from intermediates other than acetyl-CoA. Such reactions are known as anaplerotic (building up) reactions.

Acetyl-CoA is a common product of many catabolic pathways

The TCA cycle begins with acetyl-CoA, which has three major metabolic precursors (Figure 14.2). Carbohydrates undergo glycolysis to yield pyruvate (Chapter 12), which can be taken up by mitochondria and oxidatively decarboxylated to acetyl-CoA by the pyruvate dehydrogenase complex. During lipolysis, triacylglycerols are converted to glycerol and free fatty acids, which are taken up by cells and transported into mitochondria where they undergo oxidation to acetyl-CoA (Chapter 15). Lastly, proteolysis of tissue proteins releases constituent amino acids, many of which are metabolized to acetyl-CoA and TCA cycle intermediates (Chapter 19).

The first version of the TCA cycle, proposed by Krebs in 1937, began with pyruvic acid, not acetyl-CoA. Pyruvic acid was decarboxylated and condensed with oxaloacetic acid through an unknown mechanism to form citric acid. The key intermediate, acetyl-CoA, was not identified until years

Energy production

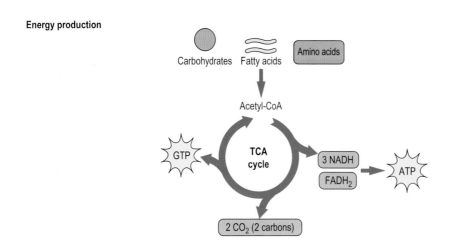

Fig. 14.1 **Amphibolic nature of the TCA cycle.** The TCA cycle provides energy and metabolites for cellular metabolism. Because of the catabolic and anabolic nature of the TCA cycle, it is described as amphibolic. FAD, flavin adenine dinucleotide; GDP, guanosine diphosphate; NADH, nicotinamide adenine dinucleotide; Pi, inorganic phosphate.

Biosynthesis

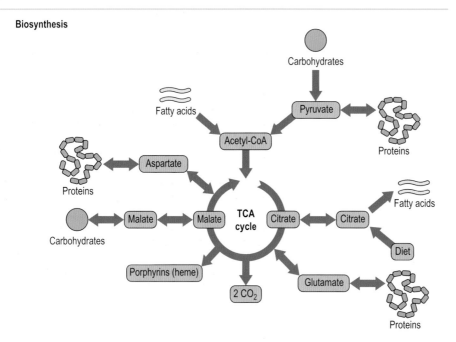

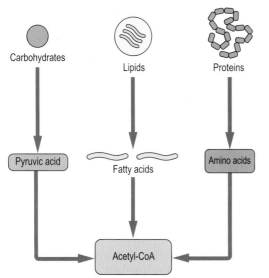

Fig. 14.2 **Metabolic sources of acetyl-CoA.** Carbohydrates, lipids and amino acids are precursors of mitochondrial acetyl-CoA necessary for operation of the TCA cycle.

later. It is tempting to begin the TCA cycle with pyruvic acid, unless it is recognized that fatty acids and many amino acids form acetyl-CoA by pathways that bypass pyruvate. It is for this reason that the TCA cycle is said to begin with acetyl-CoA, not pyruvic acid.

The TCA cycle is located in mitochondria

Localization of the TCA cycle in the mitochondrial matrix is important metabolically; this allows identical intermediates to be used for different purposes inside and outside mitochondria. Acetyl-CoA, for example, cannot cross the inner mitochondrial membrane. The main fate of mitochondrial acetyl-CoA is oxidation in the TCA cycle but, in the cytoplasm, it is used for biosynthesis of fatty acids and cholesterol.

Metabolic defects in the TCA cycle are rare

Metabolic defects involving enzymes of the TCA cycle are rare, because normal functioning of the cycle is absolutely essential to sustain life. Products of energy-producing pathways must be metabolized in the TCA cycle for efficient production of ATP. Any defect in the TCA cycle will limit ATP production, and cells deprived of ATP either die rapidly or are severely impaired functionally. Tissues that use oxygen at rapid rates, such as the central nervous system and muscle, are most susceptible to such defects.

PYRUVATE CARBOXYLASE

Pyruvate may be directly converted to four different metabolites

Pyruvate is at a crossroads in metabolism. It may be converted in one step to lactate (lactate dehydrogenase), to alanine (alanine aminotransferase, ALT), to oxaloacetate (pyruvate carboxylase), and to acetyl-CoA (pyruvate dehydrogenase complex) (Figure 14.3). Depending on metabolic circumstances, pyruvate may be routed toward gluconeogenesis (Chapter 13), fatty acid biosynthesis (Chapter 16) or the TCA cycle itself. Pyruvate carboxylase, like most other carboxylases, uses CO_2 and the coenzyme biotin (Figure 14.4), a water-soluble vitamin, and ATP to drive the carboxylation reaction. The enzyme is a tetramer of identical

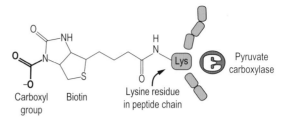

Fig. 14.4 **The carboxy-biotin intermediate.** Pyruvate carboxylase catalyzes carboxylation of pyruvate to oxaloacetate. The coenzyme, biotin, is covalently bound to pyruvate carboxylase, and transfers the carbon originating from CO_2 to pyruvate (see Chapter 11).

MEASURING LACTATE

Lactic acid is measured in a clinical setting, because its accumulation can result in rapid death. Lactic acid is produced metabolically by the reversible reduction of pyruvate with NADH by the enzyme lactate dehydrogenase (LDH). Both lactate and pyruvate coexist in metabolic systems, and the ratio of pyruvate:lactate is roughly proportional to the cytosolic ratio of $NAD^+/NADH$. Both lactate and pyruvate contribute to the acidity of biologic fluid; however, lactate is usually present at higher concentrations and is more easily measured. Blood lactate may increase in chronic obstructive lung disease and during intense exercise. Its measurement is usually indicated when there is metabolic acidosis, characterized by an elevated anion gap, $[Na^+] - ([Cl^-] + [HCO_3^-])$, indicating the presence of an unknown anion(s) in plasma. Although rare, lactic acidosis can be caused by metabolic defects in energy-producing pathways, such as some of the glycogen storage diseases or in any enzyme in the pathways from pyruvate to the generation of ATP, including the pyruvate dehydrogenase complex, TCA cycle, electron transport system or ATP synthase.

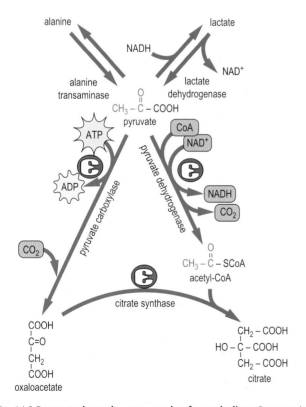

Fig. 14.3 **Pyruvate is at the crossroads of metabolism.** Pyruvate is readily formed from lactate or alanine. Acetyl-CoA and oxaloacetate are derived from pyruvate through the catalytic action of pyruvate dehydrogenase and pyruvate carboxylase, respectively. ADP, adenosine diphosphate.

subunits, each of which contains an allosteric site that binds acetyl-CoA, a positive heterotropic modifier. In fact, pyruvate carboxylase has an absolute requirement for acetyl-CoA; the enzyme does not work in its absence. An abundance of mitochondrial acetyl-CoA acts as a signal for the generation of additional oxaloacetate. For example, when lipolysis is stimulated, intramitochondrial acetyl-CoA levels rise, allosterically activating pyruvate carboxylase to produce additional oxaloacetate for gluconeogenesis (Chapter 13).

THE PYRUVATE DEHYDROGENASE COMPLEX

The pyruvate dehydrogenase complex (PDC) serves as a bridge between carbohydrates and the TCA cycle (Figure 14.5). PDC is one of several α-ketoacid dehydrogenases having analogous reaction mechanisms, including α-ketoglutarate

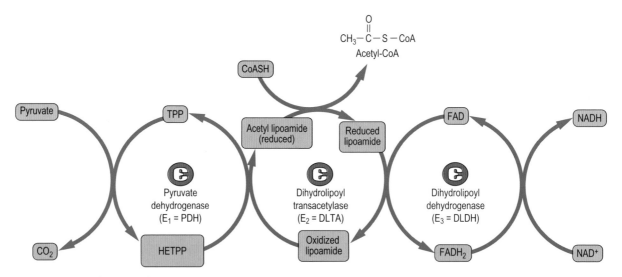

Fig. 14.5 **Mechanism of action of the pyruvate dehydrogenase complex.** The three enzyme components of the pyruvate dehydrogenase complex are pyruvate dehydrogenase (E_1 = PDH), dihydrolipoyl transacetylase (E_2 = DLTA) and dihydrolipoyl dehydrogenase (E_3 = DLDH). Pyruvate is first decarboxylated by the thiamine pyrophosphate-containing enzyme (E_1), forming CO_2 and hydroxyethyl-thiamine pyrophosphate (HETPP). Lipoamide, the prosthetic group on E_2, serves as a carrier in the transfer of the 2-carbon unit from HETPP to coenzyme A (CoA). The oxidized, cyclic disulfide form of lipoamide accepts the hydroxyethyl group from HETPP. The lipoamide is reduced and the hydroxyethyl group converted to an acetyl group during this transfer reaction, forming acetyldihydrolipoamide. Following transfer of the acetyl group to CoA, E_3 reoxidizes the lipoamide, using FAD, and the $FADH_2$ is in turn oxidized by NAD^+, yielding NADH.

dehydrogenase in the TCA cycle and α-ketoacid dehydrogenases associated with the catabolism of leucine, isoleucine and valine. Its irreversibility explains in part why acetyl-CoA cannot yield a net synthesis of glucose. The complex functions as a unit consisting of three principal enzymes:

- pyruvate dehydrogenase
- dihydrolipoyl transacetylase
- dihydrolipoyl dehydrogenase.

Intermediates are tethered to the transacetylase component of the complex during the reaction sequence (Figures 14.5 and 14.6). This optimizes the catalytic efficiency of the enzyme since substrate does not equilibrate into solution.

Two additional enzymes of the complex, pyruvate dehydrogenase kinase and pyruvate dehydrogenase phosphatase, regulate its activity by covalent modification via reversible phosphorylation/dephosphorylation. There are four known isoforms of the kinase, and two of the phosphatase; the relative amounts of each are cell specific.

Five coenzymes are required for PDC activity: thiamine pyrophosphate, lipoamide (lipoic acid bound in amide linkage to protein), CoA, FAD, and NAD^+. Four vitamins are required for their synthesis: thiamin, pantothenic acid, riboflavin and nicotinamide. Deficiencies in any of these vitamins have obvious effects on energy metabolism. For example, increases in cellular concentrations of pyruvate and α-ketoglutarate are found in beri-beri because of thiamin deficiency (Chapter 11). In this case, all the proteins are available but the relevant coenzyme is not, and the conversions of pyruvate to acetyl-CoA and α-ketoglutarate to succinyl-CoA are significantly decreased. Symptoms include cardiac and skeletal muscle weakness and neurologic disease. Thiamin deficiency is common in alcoholism, because distilled spirits are devoid of vitamins, and symptoms of beri-beri are often observed.

PYRUVATE DEHYDROGENASE COMPLEX DEFICIENCY

Most children with this enzyme deficiency present in infancy with delayed development and reduced muscle tone often associated with ataxia and seizures. Some infants have congenital malformations of the brain.

Comment. Without mitochondrial oxidation, pyruvate is reduced to lactate. The ATP yield from anaerobic glycolysis is less than a tenth of that produced from complete oxidation of glucose via the tricarboxylic acid cycle. The diagnosis is suggested by elevated lactate, but with a normal lactate/pyruvate ratio, i.e. no evidence of hypoxia. A ketogenic diet and severe restriction of protein (<15%) and carbohydrate (<5%) improve mental development. Such treatment ensures that the cells use acetyl-CoA from fat metabolism. A few children show a reduction in plasma lactate on treatment with large doses of thiamine, but the outlook is generally poor.

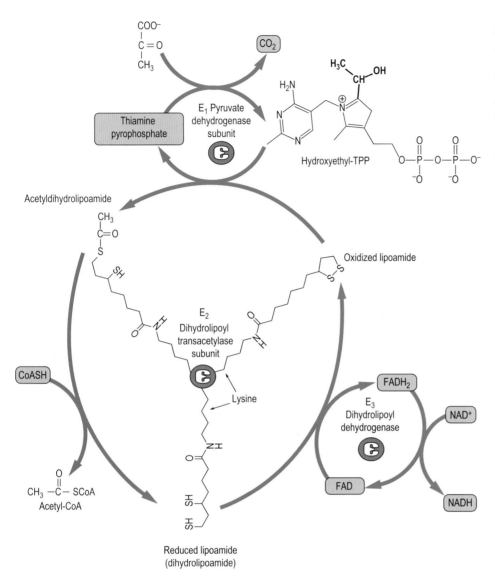

Fig. 14.6 **Lipoic acid in the pyruvate dehydrogenase complex.** The coenzyme lipoamide is attached to a lysine residue in the transacetylase subunit of pyruvate dehydrogenase. Lipoamide moves from one active site to another on the transacetylase subunit in a 'swinging arm' mechanism. The structures of thiamine pyrophosphate (TPP) and lipoamide are shown.

ENZYMES AND REACTIONS OF THE TRICARBOXYLIC ACID CYCLE

The TCA cycle is a sequence of eight enzymatic reactions (Figure 14.7), beginning with condensation of acetyl-CoA with oxaloacetate (OAA) to form citrate. The oxaloacetate is regenerated on completion of the cycle. Of the four oxidations in the cycle, two involve decarboxylations. Three produce NADH and one produces $FADH_2$. GTP, a high-energy phosphate, is produced at one step by substrate-level phosphorylation.

Citrate synthase

Citrate synthase begins the TCA cycle by catalyzing the condensation of acetyl-CoA and oxaloacetate to form citric acid. The reaction is driven by cleavage of the high-energy

 TOXICITY OF FLUOROACETATE – A SUICIDE SUBSTRATE

Fluoroacetate, originally isolated from plants, is a potent toxin. It is activated as fluoroacetyl-CoA and then condenses with oxaloacetate to form fluorocitrate (Figure 14.8). Death results from inhibition of the TCA cycle by 2-fluorocitrate, a strong inhibitor of aconitase. Fluoroacetate is an example of a 'suicide substrate', a compound that is not toxic per se but is metabolically activated to a toxic product. Thus, the cell is said to commit suicide by converting an apparently harmless substrate to a lethal toxin. Similar processes are involved in the activation of many environmental procarcinogens to carcinogens that induce mutations in DNA.

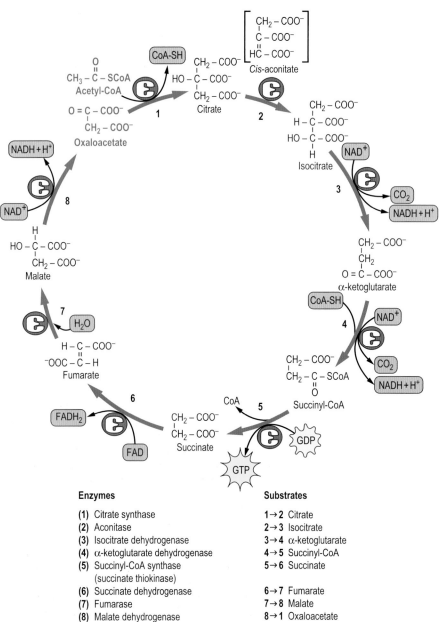

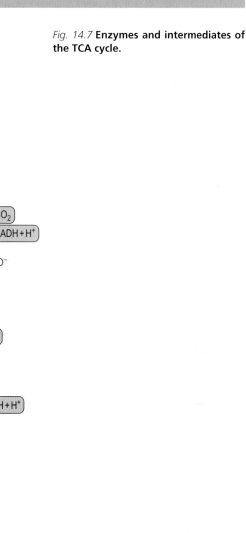

Fig. 14.7 **Enzymes and intermediates of the TCA cycle.**

Enzymes

(1) Citrate synthase
(2) Aconitase
(3) Isocitrate dehydrogenase
(4) α-ketoglutarate dehydrogenase
(5) Succinyl-CoA synthase
    (succinate thiokinase)
(6) Succinate dehydrogenase
(7) Fumarase
(8) Malate dehydrogenase

Substrates

1→2 Citrate
2→3 Isocitrate
3→4 α-ketoglutarate
4→5 Succinyl-CoA
5→6 Succinate

6→7 Fumarate
7→8 Malate
8→1 Oxaloacetate

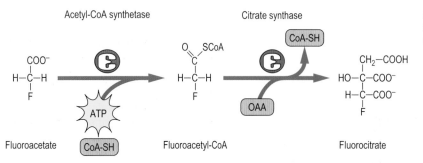

Fig. 14.8 **Toxicity of fluoroacetate – a suicide substrate.** Fluoroacetate is a competitive inhibitor of aconitase. OAA, oxaloacetate.

thioester bond of citroyl-CoA, an intermediate in the reaction. A later TCA cycle enzyme, succinyl-CoA synthetase, utilizes the high-energy thioester bond in succinyl-CoA to produce GTP, a high-energy phosphate.

Aconitase

Aconitase is an iron-sulfur protein (Chapter 9) that isomerizes citrate to isocitrate through the enzyme-bound intermediate

cis-aconitate. The two-step reaction is reversible and involves dehydration followed by hydration. Although citrate is a symmetric molecule, aconitase works specifically on the oxaloacetate end of citrate, not the end derived from acetyl-CoA (Figure 14.9). Such stereochemical specificity occurs because of the geometry of the active site of aconitase (Figure 14.10). A cytosolic protein with aconitase activity, known as IRE-BP (iron-response element binding protein), functions in the regulation of iron storage.

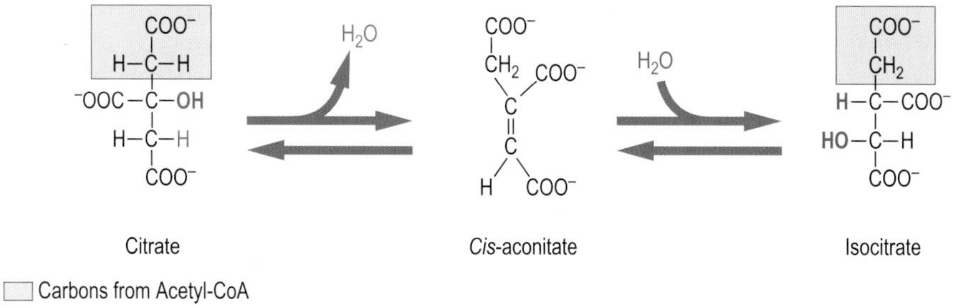

Fig. 14.9 **Specificity of isomerization during the aconitase reaction.**

Citrate   Cis-aconitate   Isocitrate

☐ Carbons from Acetyl-CoA

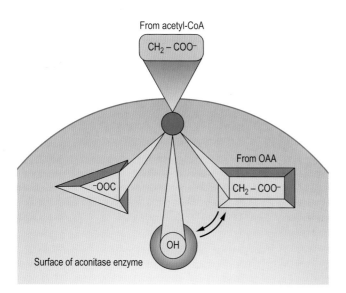

Fig. 14.10 **Stereochemistry of the aconitase reaction.** Aconitase converts achiral citrate to a specific chiral form of isocitrate. Binding of the C-3 hydroxyl (OH) and carboxylate (COO⁻) groups of citrate on the enzyme surface places the carboxymethyl (—CH₂—COO⁻) group, derived from the oxaloacetate end of the molecule, in touch with the third binding locus in the active site of aconitase. This assures the transfer of the OH group to the CH₂ group derived from oxaloacetate, indicated by arrows, rather than that derived from the acetyl group. OAA, oxaloacetate.

STEREOSPECIFICITY OF ENZYMES

Aconitase catalyzes isomerization at the oxaloacetate end of the citrate molecule. However, citrate has no asymmetric centers; it is achiral. How does aconitase know 'which end is up'? The answer lies in the nature of citrate binding to the active site of aconitase, a process known as three-point attachment. As shown in Figure 14.10, because of the geometry of the active site of aconitase, there is only one way for citrate to bind. This 'three-point binding' places the oxaloacetate carbons in the proper orientation for the isomerization reaction, while the carbons derived from acetyl-CoA are excluded from the active site. Although citrate is a symmetric or achiral molecule, it is termed 'prochiral' because it is converted to a chiral molecule, isocitrate. Similar types of three-point binding processes are involved in transaminase reactions that produce exclusively L-amino acids from ketoacids. The reduction of the nicotinamide ring by NAD(H)-dependent dehydrogenases is also stereospecific. Some dehydrogenases place the added hydrogen exclusively on the front face of the nicotinamide ring (viewed with the amide group to the right), while others add hydrogen only to the back face (see Figure 14.11 and Chapter 6).

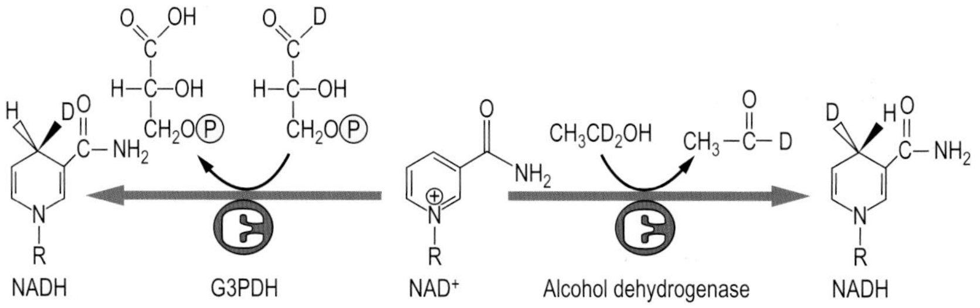

Fig. 14.11 **Stereochemistry of the reduction of NAD⁺ by dehydrogenases.** Alcohol dehydrogenase places the hydrogen ion on the front face of the nicotinamide ring, while glyceraldehyde-3-phosphate dehydrogenase (G3PDH) places the hydrogen on the back face of the ring. The two positions can be discriminated using deuterated (D) substrates.

NADH   G3PDH   NAD⁺   Alcohol dehydrogenase   NADH

Isocitrate dehydrogenase and α-ketoglutarate dehydrogenase

Isocitrate dehydrogenase and the α-ketoglutarate dehydrogenase complex catalyze two sequential oxidative decarboxylation reactions in which NAD^+ is reduced to NADH, and CO_2 is released. The first of these enzymes, isocitrate dehydrogenase, catalyzes the conversion of isocitrate to α-ketoglutarate.

It is an important regulatory enzyme that is inhibited under energy-rich conditions by high levels of NADH and ATP, and is activated when NAD^+ and ADP are produced by metabolism. Inhibition of this enzyme following a carbohydrate meal causes intramitochondrial accumulation of citrate, which is then exported to the cytosol for lipogenesis (Chapter 16). Citrate is also an important allosteric effector, inhibiting phosphofructokinase-1 (Chapter 12) and activating acetyl-CoA carboxylase.

 DEFICIENCIES IN PYRUVATE METABOLISM IN THE TCA CYCLE

A 7-month-old-child showed progressive neurologic deterioration characterized by loss of coordination and muscle tone. He was unable to keep his head upright and had great difficulty moving his limbs, which were limp. He also suffered from unrelenting acidosis. Administration of thiamine had no effect. Measurements showed that he had elevated blood levels of lactate, α-ketoglutarate and branched-chain amino acids. The child died a week later. Liver, brain, kidney, skeletal muscle, and heart were examined postmortem, and all gluconeogenic enzymes were shown to have normal activities, but both pyruvate dehydrogenase and α-ketoglutarate dehydrogenase were deficient. The defective component was shown to be dihydrolipoyl dehydrogenase (E_3), which is a single gene component required by all of the α-ketoacid dehydrogenases.

Comment. This is an example of one of the many variants of Leigh's disease, which is a group of disorders that are all characterized

by lactic acidosis. Lactic acid accumulates under anaerobic conditions or because of any enzyme defect in the pathway from pyruvate to the synthesis of ATP. In this case, there are defects in both the pyruvate dehydrogenase and α-ketoglutarate complexes, as well as other α-keto acid dehydrogenase complexes required for the catabolism of branched-chain amino acids. The failure of aerobic metabolism leads to increases in blood levels of lactate, α-ketoglutarate and branched-chain amino acids. Tissues dependent on aerobic metabolism, such as brain and muscle, are most severely affected, so that the clinical picture includes impaired motor function, neurologic disorders and mental retardation. These diseases are rare, but deficiencies in pyruvate carboxylase and all the components of the pyruvate dehydrogenase complex (PDH) have been described, including the associated kinase and phosphatase enzymes (Figure 14.12).

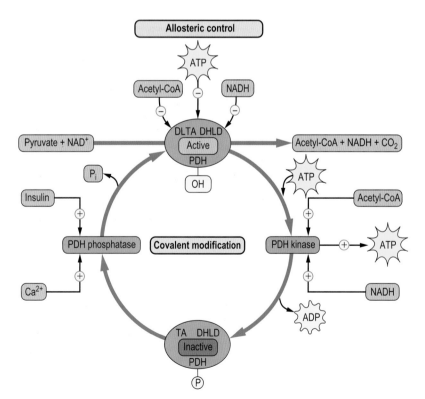

Fig. 14.12 **Regulation of the pyruvate dehydrogenase complex.** The pyruvate dehydrogenase complex regulates the flux of pyruvate into the TCA cycle. NAD(H), ATP and acetyl-CoA exert both allosteric and covalent control of enzyme activity. PDH, pyruvate dehydrogenase; TA, dihydrolipoyl transacetylase; DHLD, dihydrolipoamide dehydrogenase subunit.

The second dehydrogenase, the α-ketoglutarate dehydrogenase complex, catalyzes the oxidative decarboxylation of α-ketoglutarate to NADH, CO_2 and succinyl-CoA, a high-energy thioester compound. Like the pyruvate dehydrogenase complex, this enzyme complex contains three subunits having the same designations as pyruvate dehydrogenase (E_1, E_2 and E_3). E_3 is identical in the two complexes and is encoded by the same gene. The reaction mechanisms and the cofactors thiamine pyrophosphate, lipoate, CoA, FAD and NAD^+ are the same. Both enzymes begin with an α-keto acid, pyruvate or α-ketoglutarate, and both form the CoA esters, acetyl-CoA or succinyl-CoA, respectively.

At this point, the net carbon yield of the TCA cycle is zero, i.e. two carbons were introduced as acetyl-CoA and two carbons were liberated as CO_2. Note, however, that because of the asymmetry of the aconitase reaction, neither of the CO_2 molecules produced in this first round trip through the TCA cycle originates from the carbons of the acetyl-CoA, because they are derived from the oxaloacetate end of the citrate molecule. Both of the carbons that originated from acetyl-CoA remain in the TCA cycle intermediates, and may appear in compounds produced in biosynthetic reactions branching from the TCA cycle, including glucose, aspartic acid and heme. However, because of the loss of two CO_2 molecules at this point, there is no net synthesis of these metabolites from acetyl-CoA.

Animals cannot perform net synthesis of glucose from acetyl-CoA. This is an especially important concept in the understanding of starvation, diabetes and ketogenesis, because large amounts of acetyl-CoA are generated from fatty acids, but it does not yield a net synthesis of glucose. 'Net' synthesis is invoked, because labeled carbons from acetyl-CoA eventually appear in glucose, making it appear that glucose is synthesized from acetyl-CoA. However, the investment of the two carbons of acetyl-CoA is dissipated by the two decarboxylation reactions in the TCA cycle. Net synthesis also means that in order for continued operation of the TCA cycle, as well as glucose production, anaplerotic reactions must supply carbons to the cycle in forms other than acetyl-CoA. In this case, the most immediate anaplerotic reaction involves production of oxaloacetate from pyruvate (pyruvate carboxylase) or from aspartate (aspartate aminotransferase, AST; Chapter 19).

Succinyl-CoA synthetase

Succinyl-CoA synthetase (succinate thiokinase) catalyzes the conversion of energy-rich succinyl-CoA to succinate and free CoA. The free energy of the thioester bond in succinyl-CoA is conserved by formation of GTP from GDP and inorganic phosphate (Pi). Because a high-energy compound serves as the driving force for the synthesis of GTP, this is a substrate-level phosphorylation reaction, like the reactions catalyzed by phosphoglycerate kinase and pyruvate kinase in glycolysis

(Chapter 12). GTP is used by enzymes such as phosphoenolpyruvate carboxykinase (PEPCK) in gluconeogenesis (Chapter 13), but is also readily equilibrated with ATP by the enzyme nucleoside diphosphate kinase:

$$GTP + ADP \rightleftharpoons GDP + ATP$$

The next three reactions in the TCA cycle illustrate a common theme in metabolism for introducing a carbonyl group into a molecule:

- introduction of a double bond
- addition of water across the double bond to form an alcohol
- oxidation of the alcohol to a ketone.

This same sequence occurs in the form of enzyme-bound intermediates during conversion of citrate to α-ketoglutarate and in the oxidation of fatty acids.

Succinate dehydrogenase

Succinate dehydrogenase is a flavoprotein containing the prosthetic group FAD. As described in Chapter 9, this enzyme

 THE MALONATE BLOCK

The malate dehydrogenase reaction played an important role in the elucidation of the cyclic nature of the TCA cycle. Addition of tricarboxylic acids (citrate, aconitate) and α-ketoglutarate was known to catalyze pyruvate metabolism – we now know that this is the result of formation of catalytic amounts of oxaloacetate from these intermediates. In 1937, Krebs found that malonate, the 3-carbon dicarboxylic acid homolog of succinate and competitive inhibitor of succinate dehydrogenase, blocked metabolism of pyruvate by minced muscle preparations. He also showed that malonate inhibition of pyruvate metabolism led to accumulation not only of succinate but also of citrate and α-ketoglutarate, suggesting that succinate was a product of pyruvate metabolism and that the tricarboxylic acids might be intermediates in this process. Interestingly, fumarate and oxaloacetate also stimulated pyruvate oxidation and led to accumulation of citrate and succinate during malonate block, suggesting that the 3- and 4-carbon acids might combine to form the tricarboxylic acids. The experiments with fumarate indicated that there were two paths between fumarate and succinate, one involving reversal of the succinate dehydrogenase reaction, which was inhibited during malonate block, and the other involving conversion of fumarate to succinate through a series of organic acids. These observations, combined with Krebs' experience a few years earlier in characterization of the urea cycle (Chapter 19), led to his description of the TCA cycle.

is embedded in the inner mitochondrial membrane where it is a part of Complex II (succinate-Q reductase). The reaction involves oxidation of succinate to the *trans*-dicarboxylic acid, fumarate, with reduction of FAD to $FADH_2$.

Fumarase

Fumarase stereospecifically adds water across the trans double bond of fumarate to form the α-hydroxy acid, L-malate.

Malate dehydrogenase

Malate dehydrogenase catalyzes the oxidation of L-malate to oxaloacetate, producing NADH, completing one round trip through the TCA cycle. The oxaloacetate may then react with acetyl-CoA, continuing the cycle of reactions.

ENERGY YIELD FROM THE TRICARBOXYLIC ACID CYCLE

During the course of the TCA cycle, each mole of acetyl-CoA generates sufficient reduced nucleotide coenzymes for synthesis of $\sim$9 moles ATP by oxidative phosphorylation.

$$3 \text{ NADH} \rightarrow 7.5 \text{ ATP}$$

$$1 \text{ FADH}_2 \rightarrow 1.5 \text{ ATP}$$

Together with the GTP synthesized by substrate-level phosphorylation in the succinyl-CoA synthetase (succinate thiokinase) reaction, a total of $\sim$10 ATP equivalents is available per mole of acetyl-CoA. Thus, complete metabolism of a mole of glucose through glycolysis, the pyruvate dehydrogenase complex and the TCA cycle yields $\sim$30–32 moles ATP (Table 14.1). (The actual ATP yield depends on the route

Energetics of glucose oxidation		
Reaction	Mechanism	Moles ATP/mol Glc
hexokinase	phosphorylation	−1
phosphofructokinase	phosphorylation	−1
G3PDH	NADH, oxidative phosphorylation	+5(+3)*
phosphoglycerate kinase	substrate-level phosphorylation	+2
pyruvate kinase	substrate-level phosphorylation	+2
pyruvate dehydrogenase	NADH, oxidative phosphorylation	+5
isocitrate dehydrogenase	NADH, oxidative phosphorylation	+5
α-ketoglutarate dehydrogenase	NADH, oxidative phosphorylation	+5
succinyl-CoA synthetase	substrate-level phosphorylation (GTP)	+2
succinate dehydrogenase	$FADH_2$, oxidative phosphorylation	+3
malate dehydrogenase	NADH, oxidative phosphorylation	+5
TOTAL		**32 (30)***

Electrons from cytosolic NADH can result in the synthesis of about 5 moles of ATP per mole of glucose via the malate–aspartate shuttle, but only about 3 via the glycerol 3-phosphate shuttle per mole of glucose (Chapter 9).

Table 14.1 **ATP yield from glucose during oxidative metabolism.** The yields of ATP shown are approximate, because they are measured experimentally with live, isolated mitochondria and there is some variability. Recent work suggests that the actual yields of ATP from NADH and $FADH_2$ are about 2.5 and 1.5 respectively, yielding approximately 30–32 moles of ATP per mole of glucose. The oxidation of glucose in a bomb calorimeter yields 2870 kJ/mol (686 cal/mol), while the synthesis of ATP requires 31 kJ/mol (7.3 kcal/mol). Aerobic metabolism of glucose is therefore about 40% efficient (2870 kJ/mol glucose / 31 kJ/mole ATP = 93 theoretical moles of ATP/mol glucose; 36/93 = 39%).

of transport of redox equivalents to the mitochondrion, i.e. about 5 moles of ATP by the malate aspartate shuttle and about 3 moles of ATP by the glycerol phosphate shuttle (Chapter 9).) In contrast, only 2 moles of ATP (net) are recovered by anaerobic glycolysis in which glucose is converted to lactate.

REGULATION OF THE TRICARBOXYLIC ACID CYCLE

There are several levels of control of the TCA cycle. In general, the overall activity of the cycle depends on the availability of NAD^+ for the dehydrogenase reactions. This, in turn, is linked to the rate of NADH consumption by the electron transport system, which ultimately depends on the rate of ATP utilization and production of ADP by metabolism (see Table 14.1). Thus, as ATP is used for metabolic work, ADP is produced, then NADH is consumed by the electron transport system for ATP production, and NAD^+ is produced. The TCA cycle is activated, fuels are consumed, and more NADH is produced so that more ATP may be made. The mitochondrial level of NAD^+ provides a link between work (ATP utilization) and fuel consumption (Chapter 9).

There are several regulatory enzymes that affect the activity of the TCA cycle. The activity of the pyruvate dehydrogenase complex, and therefore the supply of acetyl-CoA from glucose, lactate and alanine, is regulated by allosteric and covalent modifications (see Fig. 14.12). The products of the pyruvate dehydrogenase reaction, NADH and acetyl-CoA, as well as ATP, act as negative allosteric effectors of the enzyme complex. In addition, the pyruvate dehydrogenase complex has associated kinase and phosphatase enzymes that modulate the degree of phosphorylation of regulatory serine residues in the complex. NADH, acetyl-CoA and ATP activate the kinase, which phosphorylates and inactivates the enzyme complex. In contrast, when these three compounds are low in concentration, the enzyme complex is activated allosterically and by dephosphorylation by the phosphatase. This is an important regulatory process during fasting and starvation, when gluconeogenesis is essential to maintain blood glucose concentration. Active fat metabolism during fasting leads to increased NADH and acetyl-CoA in the mitochondrion, which leads to inhibition of pyruvate dehydrogenase and blocks the utilization of carbohydrate for energy metabolism in the liver. Under this condition, pyruvate, from such intermediates as lactate and alanine, is directed toward gluconeogenesis. Conversely, insulin stimulates pyruvate dehydrogenase by activating the phosphatase in response to dietary carbohydrates. This directs carbohydrate-derived carbons into fatty acids via citrate synthase. Ca^{2+} also affects PDC phosphatase activity, in response to the increase in intracellular Ca^{2+} during muscle contraction (see Chapter 20).

Oxaloacetate is required for entry of acetyl-CoA into the TCA cycle but, at times, the availability of oxaloacetate appears to regulate the activity of the cycle. This occurs especially during fasting when levels of ATP and NADH, derived from fat metabolism, are increased in the mitochondrion. The increase in NADH shifts the malate:oxaloacetate equilibrium toward malate, directing TCA cycle intermediates toward malate, which is exported to the cytosol for gluconeogenesis (Chapter 13). Meanwhile, acetyl-CoA derived from fat metabolism is directed toward synthesis of ketone bodies because of the lack of oxaloacetate, regenerating CoASH and leading to the increase in ketone bodies in plasma during fasting (Chapter 15).

Isocitrate dehydrogenase is a major regulatory enzyme within the TCA cycle. It is subject to allosteric inhibition by ATP and NADH and stimulation by ADP and NAD^+. During consumption of a high carbohydrate diet under resting conditions, the demand for ATP is diminished and the level of carbohydrate-derived intermediates increases. Under these circumstances, increased insulin levels stimulate the pyruvate dehydrogenase complex, and the accumulation of ATP and NADH inhibits isocitrate dehydrogenase, causing a mitochondrial accumulation of citrate. The citrate is then exported to the cytosol for synthesis of fatty acids, which are exported from the liver for storage in adipose tissue as triglycerides. With an increase in energy demand, e.g. during muscle contraction, NAD^+ and ADP accumulate, and they stimulate isocitrate dehydrogenase.

Induction and repression, as well as proteolysis of enzyme proteins, such as pyruvate carboxylase and those in the pyruvate dehydrogenase complex and the TCA cycle, also play an important regulatory role. In fact, all of the TCA cycle and associated enzymes are synthesized in the cytoplasm and transported through a complex series of steps into the mitochondrion. Regulation can occur at the level of translation, transcription and intracellular transport. Diet, for example, is known to control expression of four pyruvate dehydrogenase kinases; one of them is induced in response to a high-fat diet and is repressed in response to a high-carbohydrate diet. Unfortunately, the regulation of the TCA cycle at genetic and transport levels is not as well understood, although it is clearly important for understanding the pathogenesis of a wide range of contemporary health problems, such as diabetes and obesity.

ANAPLEROTIC ('BUILDING UP') REACTIONS

As shown in Figure 14.1, many TCA cycle intermediates participate in biosynthetic processes, which deplete TCA cycle intermediates. For example, the synthesis of 1 mole of heme requires 8 moles of succinyl-CoA. The TCA cycle would cease to function if the intermediates were not replenished, because acetyl-CoA cannot yield a net synthesis of oxalo-acetate. Anaplerotic (building up) reactions provide the TCA cycle with intermediates other than acetyl-CoA to maintain activity of the cycle. Pyruvate carboxylase is a prime example of an enzyme that catalyzes an anaplerotic reaction. It converts pyruvate to malate, a precursor of oxaloacetate, which is required for initiation of the cycle. Malic enzyme in the cytoplasm also converts pyruvate to malate, which can enter the mitochondrion as a substrate for the TCA cycle. α-Ketoglutarate can be produced through an aminotransferase reaction from glutamate, as well as by the glutamate dehydrogenase reaction. Several other 'glucogenic' amino acids (Chapter 19) may also serve as sources of pyruvate or TCA cycle intermediates, guaranteeing that the cycle never stalls because of a lack of intermediates.

Summary

Located in the mitochondrion, the TCA cycle is closely associated with the pyruvate dehydrogenase complex, the electron transport system and other pathways, all of which function as a highly coordinated unit. The TCA cycle is the central, common pathway by which fuels are oxidized, and it also participates in major biosynthetic pathways. In its oxidative role, its major products are GTP and the reduced coenzymes NADH and $FADH_2$, which furnish large amounts of free energy for the synthesis of ATP by oxidative phosphorylation. In its biosynthetic role, it provides essential intermediates for the synthesis of glucose, fatty acids, amino acids and heme, as well as the ATP required for their biosynthesis. The activity of the TCA cycle is tightly regulated by substrate supply, by allosteric effectors and control of gene expression so that fuel consumption is coordinated with energy production.

ACTIVE LEARNING

1. In beri-beri, the vitamin thiamine is deficient. Which intermediates would accumulate, and why?
2. Based on rates of oxygen consumption, which tissues would be the most critically impaired because of genetically defective enzymes of the TCA cycle?
3. Compare the regulation of the pyruvate dehydrogenase complex to the regulation of cytosolic enzymes by phosphorylation/dephosphorylation reactions.
4. Predict the consequences of deficiencies in TCA cycle enzymes such as succinate dehydrogenase, fumarase or malate dehydrogenase.

Further reading

De Meirleir L. Defects of pyruvate metabolism and the Krebs cycle. *J Child Neurol* 2002; **17**(suppl 3): 3S26–S33; discussion 3S33–34.

Haggie PM, Verkman AS. Diffusion of tricarboxylic acid cycle enzymes in the mitochondrial matrix *in vivo*. Evidence for restricted mobility of a multienzyme complex. *J Biol Chem* 2002;**277**:40782–40788.

Kohanski MA, Dwyer DJ, Hayete B et al. A common mechanism of cellular death induced by bactericidal antibiotics. *Cell* 2007;**130**:797–810.

McCammon MT, Epstein CB, Przybyla-Zawislak B, McAlister-Henn L, Butow RA. Global transcription analysis of Krebs tricarboxylic acid cycle mutants reveals an alternating pattern of gene expression and effects on hypoxic and oxidative genes. *Mol Biol Cell* 2003;**14**:958–972.

Owen OE, Kalhan SC, Hanson RW. The key role of anaplerosis and cataplerosis for citric acid cycle function. *J Biol Chem* 2002;**277**:30409–30412.

Sharma N, Okere IC, Brunengraber DZ et al. Regulation of pyruvate dehydrogenase activity and citric acid cycle intermediates during high cardiac power generation. *J Physiol* 2005;**562**:593–603.

Sugden MC, Holness MJ. Recent advances in mechanisms regulating glucose oxidation at the level of the pyruvate dehydrogenase complex by PDKs. *Am J Physiol* 2003;**284**:E855–E862.

Walton ME, Ebert D, Haller RG. Relative rates of anaplerotic flux in rested and contracted rat skeletal muscle measured by 13C NMR spectroscopy. *J Physiol* 2003;**548**:541–548.

Websites

TCA cycle:
- www.johnkyrk.com/krebs.html
- www.wiley.com/legacy/college/boyer/0470003790/animations/tca/tca.htm

Causes of Leigh's disease: www.ninds.nih.gov/health_and_medical/disorders/leighsdisease_doc.htm

Listing of genetic disorders: www.ncbi.nlm.nih.gov/sites/entrez?db=omim-SEARCH:KREBS CYCLE

15. Oxidative Metabolism of Lipids in Liver and Muscle

J W Baynes

LEARNING OBJECTIVES

After reading this chapter you should be able to:

- Describe the pathway for activation and transport of fatty acids to the mitochondrion for catabolism.
- Outline the sequence of reactions involved in oxidation of fatty acids in the mitochondrion.
- Describe the general features of pathways for oxidation of unsaturated, odd-chain and branched-chain fatty acids.
- Explain the rationale for the pathway of ketogenesis and identify the major intermediates and products of this pathway.
- Describe the mechanism by which hormonal activation of lipolysis in adipose tissue is coordinated with activation of gluconeogenesis in liver during fasting.

INTRODUCTION

Fats are normally the major source of energy in liver and in muscle, and in human tissues in general, except for red cells and brain. Triglycerides are the storage and transport form of fats; fatty acids are the immediate source of energy. They are released from adipose tissue, transported in association with plasma albumin, and delivered to cells for metabolism. The catabolism of fatty acids is entirely oxidative; after they have been transported through the cytoplasm, their oxidation proceeds in both the peroxisome and the mitochondrion, primarily by a cycle of reactions known as β-oxidation. Carbons are released, two at a time, from the carboxyl end of the fatty acid; the major endproducts are acetyl-coenzyme A (acetyl-CoA) and the reduced forms of the nucleotides, $FADH_2$ and NADH. In muscle, the acetyl-CoA is metabolized via the tricarboxylic acid cycle and oxidative phosphorylation to produce ATP. In liver, acetyl-CoA is converted largely to ketone bodies (ketogenesis), which are water-soluble lipid derivatives that, like glucose, are exported for use in other tissues. Fat metabolism is controlled primarily by the rate of triglyceride hydrolysis (lipolysis) in adipose tissue, which is regulated by hormonal mechanisms involving insulin and glucagon, epinephrine, and cortisol.

These hormones coordinate the metabolism of carbohydrate, lipid and protein throughout the body (see Chapter 21).

ACTIVATION OF FATTY ACIDS FOR TRANSPORT INTO THE MITOCHONDRION

Fatty acids do not exist to a significant extent in free form in the body – salts of fatty acids are soaps; they would dissolve cell membranes. In blood, fatty acids are bound to albumin, which is present at ~0.5 mmol/L concentration (35 mg/mL) in plasma. Each molecule of albumin can bind 6–8 fatty acid molecules. In the cytosol, fatty acids are bound to a series of fatty acid-binding proteins and enzymes. As the priming step for their catabolism, the fatty acids are activated to their CoA derivative, using ATP as the energy source (Fig. 15.1). The carboxyl group is first activated to an enzyme-bound, high-energy acyl-adenylate intermediate, formed by reaction

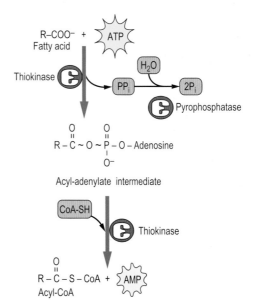

Fig. 15.1 **Activation of fatty acids by fatty acyl-CoA synthetase (thiokinase).** ATP forms an enzyme-bound acyl-adenylate intermediate, which is discharged by CoASH to form acyl-CoA. AMP, adenosine monophosphate; CoASH, coenzyme A; PPi, inorganic pyrophosphate.

Metabolism of fatty acids			
Size class	Number of carbons	Site of catabolism	Membrane transport
Short-chain	2–4	mitochondrion	diffusion
Medium-chain	4–12	mitochondrion	diffusion
Long-chain	12–20	mitochondrion	carnitine cycle
Very long-chain	>20	peroxisome	unknown

Table 15.1 **Metabolism of the four classes of fatty acids**. Compare Table 3.20.

of the carboxyl group of the fatty acid with ATP. The acyl group is then transferred to CoA by the same enzyme, fatty acyl-CoA synthetase. This enzyme is commonly known as fatty acid thiokinase, because ATP is consumed in the formation of the thioester bond in acyl-CoA.

The length of the fatty acid dictates where it is activated to CoA

Short- and medium-chain fatty acids (Table 15.1) can cross the mitochondrial membrane by passive diffusion, and are activated to their CoA derivative within the mitochondrion. Very long-chain fatty acids from the diet are shortened to long-chain fatty acids in peroxisomes. Long-chain fatty acids are the major components of storage triglycerides and dietary fats. They are activated to their CoA derivatives in the cytoplasm and are transported into the mitochondrion via the carnitine shuttle.

The carnitine shuttle

CoA is a large, polar, nucleotide derivative, and cannot penetrate the mitochondrial inner membrane. Thus, for the transport of long-chain fatty acids, the fatty acid is first transferred to the small molecule, carnitine, by carnitine palmitoyl transferase-I (CPT-I), located in the outer mitochondrial membrane. An acyl-carnitine transporter or translocase in the inner mitochondrial membrane mediates transfer of the acyl-carnitine into the mitochondrion, where CPT-II regenerates the acyl-CoA, releasing free carnitine. The carnitine shuttle (Fig. 15.2) operates by an antiport mechanism in which free carnitine and the acyl-carnitine derivative move in opposite directions across the inner mitochondrial membrane. The shuttle is an important site in the regulation of fatty acid oxidation. As discussed in the next chapter, the carnitine shuttle is inhibited by malonyl-CoA after the ingestion of carbohydrate-rich meals. Malonyl-CoA prevents the futile cycle in which newly synthesized fatty acids would be oxidized in the mitochondrion.

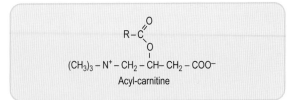

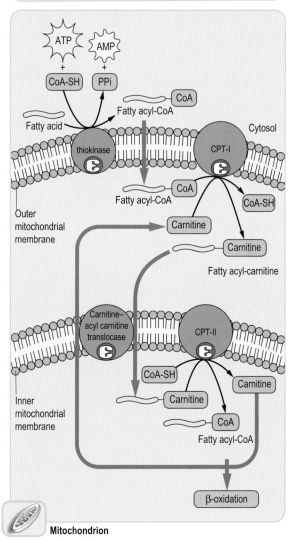

Fig. 15.2 **Transport of long-chain fatty acids into the mitochondrion.** The three components of the carnitine pathway include carnitine palmitoyl transferases (CPTs) in the outer and inner mitochondrial membranes and the carnitine-acyl carnitine translocase.

OXIDATION OF FATTY ACIDS

Mitochondrial β-oxidation

Fatty acyl-CoAs are oxidized in a cycle of reactions involving oxidation of the β-carbon to a ketone; hence the term β-oxidation (Figs 15.3 and 15.4). The oxidation is followed by cleavage between the α- and β-carbons by a thiolase

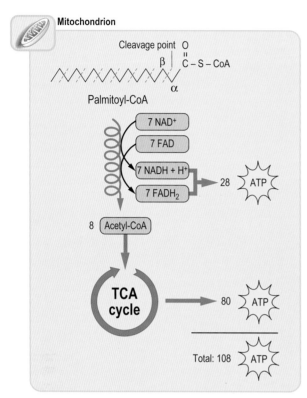

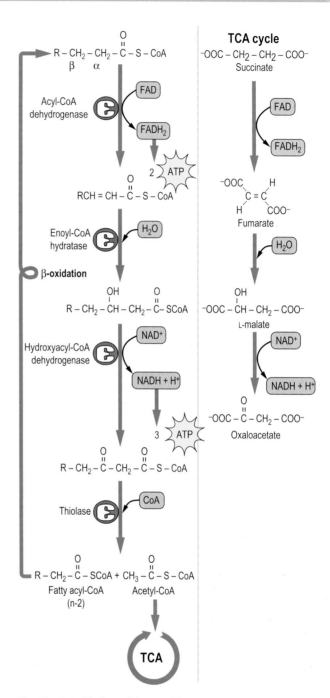

Fig. 15.3 **Overview of β-oxidation of palmitate.** In a cycle of reactions, the carbons of the fatty acyl-CoA are released in two-carbon acetyl-CoA units; the yield of 28 ATP from this β-oxidation is nearly equivalent to that from complete oxidation of glucose. In liver, the acetyl-CoA units are then used for synthesis of ketone bodies, and in other tissues they are metabolized in the TCA cycle to form ATP. The complete oxidation of palmitate yields a net 106 moles of ATP, after correction for the 2-mole equivalents of ATP invested at the thiokinase reaction. The overall production of ATP per gram of palmitate is about twice that per gram of glucose, because glucose is already partially oxidized in comparison with palmitate. For this reason, the caloric value of fats is about twice that of sugars (Table 15.2).

reaction. One mole each of acetyl-CoA, FADH$_2$ and NADH is formed during each cycle, along with a fatty acyl-CoA with two fewer carbon atoms. For a 16-carbon fatty acid, such as palmitate, the cycle is repeated seven times, yielding 8 moles of acetyl-CoA (see Fig. 15.3 and Table 15.1), plus 7 moles of FADH$_2$ and 7 moles of NADH + H$^+$. This process occurs in the mitochondrion, and the reduced nucleotides are used directly for synthesis of ATP by oxidative phosphorylation (Table 15.2).

The four steps in the cycle of β-oxidation are shown in detail in Figure 15.3. Note the similarity between the sequence of these reactions and those from succinate to oxaloacetate in the TCA cycle. In common with succinate dehydrogenase, acyl-CoA dehydrogenase uses FAD as a coenzyme, and is an integral protein in the inner mitochondrial membrane. Even the *trans* geometry of fumarate and the stereochemical configuration of L-malate in the TCA cycle are mirrored by the *trans* geometry of the trans-enoyl-CoA and L-hydroxy-acyl-CoA intermediates in β-oxidation. The last step of the

Fig. 15.4 **β-Oxidation of fatty acids**. Oxidation occurs in a series of steps at the carbon that is β to the keto group. Thiolase cleaves the resultant β-ketoacyl-CoA derivative to give acetyl-CoA and a fatty acid with two fewer carbon atoms, which then re-enters the β-oxidation cascade. Note the similarity between these reactions and those of the TCA cycle, shown on the right.

β-oxidation cycle is catalyzed by thiolase, which traps the energy obtained from the carbon–carbon bond cleavage as acyl-CoA, allowing the cycle to continue without the necessity of reactivating the fatty acid. The cycle continues until all the fatty acid has been converted to acetyl-CoA, the common intermediate in the oxidation of carbohydrates and lipids.

Caric value of glucose and palmitate				
Substrate	Molecular weight	Net ATP yield (mol/mol)	ATP (mol/g)	Caloric value Cal/g (kJ)
glucose	180	36–38	0.2	4 (17)
palmitate	256	129	0.5	9 (37)

Table 15.2 **Comparative energy yield from glucose and palmitate.** Compare Table 9.1.

CONSEQUENCES OF IMPAIRED OXIDATION OF MEDIUM-CHAIN FATTY ACIDS

Fatty acyl-CoA dehydrogenase deficiency

Fatty acyl-CoA dehydrogenase is not a single enzyme, but a family of enzymes with chain-length specificity for oxidation of short-, medium- and long-chain fatty acids; fatty acids are transferred from one enzyme to the other during chain-shortening β-oxidation reactions. Medium-chain fatty acyl-CoA dehydrogenase (MCAD) deficiency is an autosomal recessive disease characterized by hypoketotic hypoglycemia. It presents in infancy and is characterized by high concentrations of medium-chain carboxylic acids, acyl carnitines, and acyl glycines in plasma and urine. Hyperammonemia may also be present, as a result of liver damage. Concentrations of hepatic mitochondrial medium-chain acyl-CoA derivatives are also increased, limiting β-oxidation and recycling of CoA during ketogenesis. The inability to metabolize fats during fasting is life threatening because it limits gluconeogenesis and causes hypoglycemia. MCAD deficiency is treated by frequent feeding, avoidance of fasting, and carnitine supplementation. Deficiencies in short- and long-chain fatty acid dehydrogenases have similar clinical features.

Peroxisomal catabolism of fatty acids

Peroxisomes are subcellular organelles found in all nucleated cells. They are involved in the oxidation of a number of substrates, including urate, and long-, very long- and branched-chain fatty acids. They are also the principal sites of production of hydrogen peroxide (H_2O_2) in the cell, and account for nearly 20% of oxygen consumption in hepatocytes. Peroxisomes have a carnitine shuttle and conduct β-oxidation by a pathway similar to the mitochondrial pathway, except that their acyl-CoA dehydrogenase is an oxidase, rather than a dehydrogenase. $FADH_2$ produced in this and other oxidation reactions, including α- and ω-oxidation, is oxidized by molecular oxygen to produce H_2O_2. This pathway is energetically less efficient than β-oxidation in the mitochondrion because no ATP is produced by oxidative phosphorylation. Peroxisomal enzymes cannot oxidize short-chain fatty acids, so products such as butanoyl-, hexanoyl- and octanoyl-carnitine are exported for further catabolism in the mitochondrion.

The fibrates are a class of hypolipidemic drugs that act by inducing peroxisomal proliferation in liver. Zellweger syndrome, resulting from defects in import of enzymes into peroxisomes, is a severe multiorgan disorder, leading to death usually at about 6 months of age; it is characterized by accumulation of long-chain fatty acids in neuronal tissue, most likely because of the inability to turn over neuronal fatty acids. Peroxisomes also have anabolic functions. They are thought to have a role in production of acetyl-CoA for biosynthesis of cholesterol and polyisoprenoids (Chapter 17), and they contain the dihydroxyacetone-phosphate acyltransferase required for synthesis of plasmalogens (Chapter 27).

Alternative pathways of oxidation of fatty acids

Unsaturated fatty acids yield less $FADH_2$ when they are oxidized

Unsaturated fatty acids are already partially oxidized, so less $FADH_2$, and correspondingly less ATP, is produced by their oxidation. The double bonds in polyunsaturated fatty acids have *cis* geometry and occur at three-carbon intervals, whereas the intermediates in β-oxidation have *trans* geometry and the reactions proceed in two-carbon steps. The metabolism of unsaturated fatty acids therefore requires several additional enzymes, both to shift the position and to change the geometry of the double bonds.

Odd-chain fatty acids produce succinyl-CoA from propionyl-CoA

The oxidation of fatty acids with an odd number of carbons proceeds from the carboxyl end, like that of normal fatty acids, except that propionyl-CoA is formed by the last thiolase cleavage reaction. The propionyl-CoA is converted to succinyl-CoA by a multistep process involving three enzymes and the vitamins biotin and cobalamin (Fig. 15.5). The succinyl-CoA enters directly into the TCA cycle.

α-Oxidation initiates oxidation of branched-chain fatty acids to acetyl-CoA and propionyl-CoA

Phytanic acids are branched-chain polyisoprenoid lipids found in plant chlorophylls. Because the β-carbon of phytanic acids is at a branch point, it is not possible to oxidize this carbon to a ketone. The first and essential step in catabolism of phytanic acids is α-oxidation to a pristanic acid, releasing the α-carbon as carbon dioxide. Thereafter, as shown in Figure 15.6, acetyl-CoA and propionyl-CoA are released alternately and in equal amounts. Refsum's disease is a rare neurologic disorder, characterized by accumulation of phytanic acid deposits in nerve tissues as a result of a genetic defect in α-oxidation.

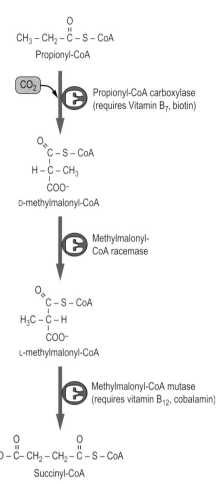

Fig. 15.5 **Metabolism of propionyl-CoA to succinyl-CoA.** Propionyl-CoA from odd-chain fatty acids is a minor source of carbons for gluconeogenesis. The intermediate, methylmalonyl-CoA, is also produced during catabolism of branched-chain amino acids. Defects in methylmalonyl-CoA mutase or deficiencies in vitamin B_{12} lead to methylmalonic aciduria.

Fig. 15.6 **α-Oxidation of branched-chain phytanic acids.** The first carbon of phytanic acids is removed as carbon dioxide. In subsequent cycles of β-oxidation, acetyl-CoA and propionyl-CoA are released alternately.

KETOGENESIS – A METABOLIC PATHWAY UNIQUE TO LIVER

Gluconeogenesis in fasting and starvation

The liver uses fatty acids as its source of energy for gluconeogenesis during fasting and starvation. Fats are a rich source of energy and, under conditions of fasting or starvation, liver mitochondrial concentrations of fat-derived ATP and NADH are high, inhibiting isocitrate dehydrogenase and shifting the oxaloacetate–malate equilibrium toward malate. TCA cycle intermediates that are formed from amino acids released from muscle as part of the response to fasting and starvation (see Chapter 21) are converted to malate in the TCA cycle. The malate exits the mitochondrion to take part in gluconeogenesis (Chapter 13). The resulting low level of oxaloacetate in hepatic mitochondria limits the activity of the TCA cycle,

DEFECTS IN β-OXIDATION

Dicarboxylic aciduria and β-oxidation of fatty acids

Several disorders of lipid catabolism, including alterations in the carnitine shuttle, acyl-CoA dehydrogenase deficiencies, and Zellweger syndrome (a defect in peroxisome biogenesis), are associated with the appearance of medium-chain dicarboxylic acids in urine. When β-oxidation of fatty acids is impaired, fatty acids are oxidized, one carbon at a time, by α-oxidation or from the ω-carbon by microsomal cytochrome P-450 dependent hydroxylases and dehydrogenases. These dicarboxylic acids are substrates for peroxisomal β-oxidation, which continues to the level of short-chain dicarboxylic acids, which are then excreted from the peroxisome and eventually appear in urine.

resulting in an inability to metabolize acetyl-CoA efficiently in the TCA cycle. Although the liver could obtain sufficient energy to support gluconeogenesis simply by the enzymes of β-oxidation, which generate both $FADH_2$ and NADH, the accumulation of acetyl-CoA, with concomitant depletion of CoA, limits β-oxidation.

What does the liver do with the excess acetyl-CoA that accumulates in fasting or starvation?

The problem of dealing with excess acetyl-CoA is a critical one because CoA is present in only catalytic amounts in tissues, and free CoA is required to initiate and continue the cycle of β-oxidation which is the primary source of ATP in liver. To recycle the acetyl-CoA, the liver uses a pathway known as ketogenesis, in which free CoA is regenerated and the acetate group appears in blood in the form of three water-soluble lipid-derived products: acetoacetate, β-hydroxybutyrate, and acetone. The pathway of formation of these 'ketone bodies' (Fig. 15.7) involves the synthesis and decomposition of hydroxymethylglutaryl (HMG)-CoA in the mitochondrion. The liver is unique in its content of HMG-CoA synthase and lyase, but is deficient in enzymes required for metabolism of ketone bodies, which explains their export into blood.

Ketone bodies are taken up in extrahepatic tissues, including skeletal and cardiac muscle, where they are converted to CoA derivatives for metabolism (Fig. 15.8). Ketone bodies increase in plasma during fasting and starvation (Table 15.3) and are a rich source of energy. They are used in cardiac and

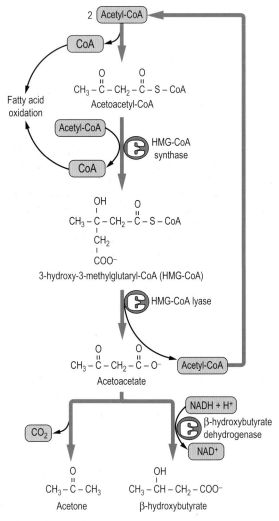

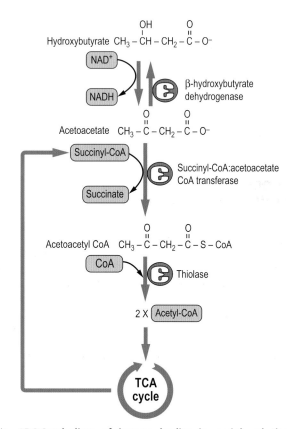

Fig. 15.8 **Catabolism of ketone bodies in peripheral tissues.** Succinyl-CoA:acetoacetate CoA transferase catalyzes the conversion of acetoacetate to acetoacetyl-CoA. A thiokinase-type enzyme may also directly activate acetoacetate in some tissues.

Fig. 15.7 **Pathway of ketogenesis from acetyl-CoA.** Ketogenesis generates ketone bodies from acetyl-CoA, releasing the CoA to participate in β-oxidation. The enzymes involved, HMG-CoA synthase and lyase, are unique to hepatocytes; mitochondrial HMG-CoA is an essential intermediate. The initial product is acetoacetic acid, which may be enzymatically reduced to β-hydroxybutyrate by β-hydroxybutyrate dehydrogenase, or may spontaneously (nonenzymatically) decompose to acetone, which is excreted in urine or expired by the lungs.

Plasma concentrations of fatty acids and ketone bodies			
Substrate	**Plasma concentration (mmol/L)**		
	Normal	**Fasting**	**Starvation**
Fatty acids	0.6	1.0	1.5
Acetoacetate	<0.1	0.2	1–2
β-Hydroxybutyrate	<0.1	1	5–10

Table 15.3 **Plasma concentrations of fatty acids and ketone bodies in different nutritional states.**

KETONE BODIES IN URINE (KETONURIA) AND WEIGHT LOSS PROGRAMS

The appearance of ketone bodies in the urine is an indication of active fat metabolism and gluconeogenesis. Ketonuria may also occur normally in association with a high-fat, low-carbohydrate diet. Some weight loss programs encourage gradual reduction in carbohydrate and total caloric intake until ketone bodies appear in urine (measured with Keto-Stix). Dieters are urged to maintain this level of caloric intake, checking urinary ketones regularly to confirm the consumption of body fat.

Comment. Keto-Stix and similar 'dry chemistry' tests are convenient test strips for urinary ketone bodies. They contain a chemical reagent, such as nitroprusside, which reacts with acetoacetate in urine to form a lavender color, graded on a scale with a maximum of '4+'. A reaction of '1+' (representing 5–10 mg ketone bodies/100 mL) or '2+' (10–20 mg/100 mL) on the test strip was established as a goal to assure continued fat metabolism, and therefore weight loss. This type of diet is discouraged today, because the appearance of ketone bodies in the urine indicates greater concentrations in the plasma, and may cause metabolic acidosis.

DEFECTIVE KETOGENESIS

Ketogenesis as a result of a deficiency in carnitine metabolism

The clinical presentation of deficiencies in carnitine metabolism occurs in infancy and is often life threatening. Characteristic features include hypoketotic hypoglycemia, hyperammonemia, and altered plasma free carnitine concentration. Hepatic damage, cardiomyopathy, and muscle weakness are common.

Comment. Carnitine is synthesized from lysine and α-ketoglutarate, primarily in liver and kidney, and is normally present in plasma in a concentration of about 50 μmol/L (1 mg/dL). There are high-affinity uptake systems for carnitine in most tissues, including the kidney, which resorbs carnitine from the glomerular filtrate, limiting its excretion in urine. Homozygous deficiencies in carnitine transporters, CPT-I and -II, and the translocase result in defects in long-chain fatty acid oxidation. Plasma and tissue carnitine concentrations decrease to <1 μmol/L in carnitine transport deficiency, because of both defective uptake into tissues and excessive loss in urine. On the other hand, plasma free carnitine may exceed 100 μmol/L (2 mg/dL) in CPT-I deficiency. In both translocase and CPT-II deficiency, total plasma carnitine may be normal, but is mostly in the form of acyl carnitine esters of long-chain fatty acids – in the former case because they cannot be transported into the mitochondrion, and in the latter because of backflow out from mitochondria. These diseases are treated by carnitine supplementation, by frequent high-carbohydrate feeding, and by avoidance of fasting.

skeletal muscle in proportion to their plasma concentration. During starvation, the brain also converts to the use of ketone bodies for more than 50% of its energy metabolism, sparing glucose and reducing the demand on degradation of muscle protein for gluconeogenesis (see Chapter 21).

Mobilization of lipids during gluconeogenesis and work

Insulin, glucagon, epinephrine, and cortisol control the direction and rate of glycogen and glucose metabolism in liver. During fasting and starvation, hepatic gluconeogenesis is activated by glucagon and requires the coordinated degradation of proteins and release of amino acids from muscle, and the degradation of triglycerides and release of fatty acids from adipose tissue. The latter process, known as lipolysis, is controlled by the adipocyte enzyme hormone-sensitive lipase, which is activated by phosphorylation by cAMP-dependent protein kinase A in response to increasing plasma concentrations of glucagon (Chapter 21). Like gluconeogenesis, lipolysis is inhibited by insulin.

The activation of hormone-sensitive lipase has predictable effects – increasing the concentration of free fatty acids and glycerol in plasma during fasting and starvation (Fig. 15.9); similar effects are observed in response to epinephrine during the stress response. Epinephrine activates both glycogenolysis in the liver and lipolysis in adipose tissue so that both fuels, glucose and fatty acids, increase in blood during stress. Cortisol exerts a more chronic effect on lipolysis and also causes insulin resistance. Cushing's syndrome (Chapter 39), in which there are high blood concentrations of cortisol, is characterized by hyperglycemia, muscle wastage, and redistribution of fat from glucagon-sensitive adipose

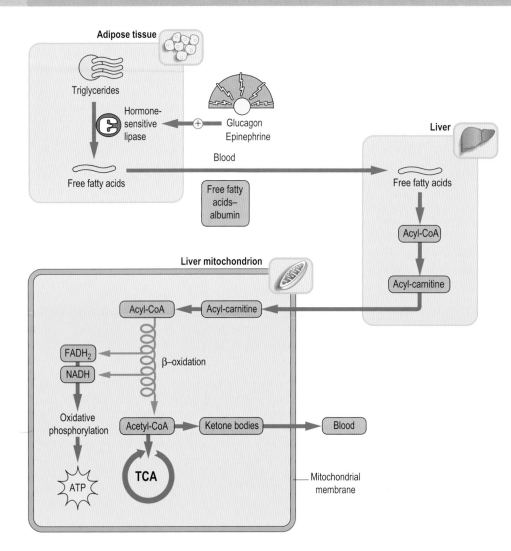

Fig. 15.9 **Regulation of lipid metabolism by glucagon and epinephrine.** Glucagon and epinephrine activate hormone-sensitive lipase in adipose tissue, in coordination with activation of proteolysis in muscle and gluconeogenesis in liver. Metabolism of fatty acids through β-oxidation in liver yields ATP for gluconeogenesis. The acetyl-CoA is converted to and released to blood as ketone bodies. These effects are reversed by insulin following a meal.

 HELLP AND AFLP SYNDROMES IN MOTHERS OF CHILDREN BORN WITH LCHAD (INCIDENCE 1 IN 200 000)

Long-chain L-3-hydroxy-acyl-CoA dehydrogenase deficiency (LCHAD) can present in a wide variety of ways. Those affected are prone to episodes of nonketotic hypoglycemia, but may develop fulminant hepatic failure, cardiomyopathy, rhabdomyolysis, and occasionally neuropathy and retinopathy. As with deficiencies in medium chain-(MCAD) or long-chain fatty acyl-CoA dehydrogenase (LCAD), treatment involves avoidance of fasting and diets enriched in medium chain fatty acids.

Perhaps the most striking feature of this rare defect in fatty acid metabolism is the association with maternal HELLP (**h**emolysis, **e**levated **l**iver enzymes and **l**ow **p**latelets) and AFLP (**a**cute **f**atty **l**iver of **p**regnancy). These potentially fatal obstetric emergencies may occur in mothers who are heterozygotes for LCHAD, especially if the child has LCHAD. These syndromes are also associated with another recessive fatty acid defect, carnitine palmitoyl-transferase-I deficiency.

depots to atypical sites, such as the cheeks, upper back, and trunk.

Summary

Unlike carbohydrate fuels, which enter the body primarily as glucose or sugars that are converted to glucose, lipid fuels are heterogeneous with respect to chain length, branching, and unsaturation. The catabolism of fats is primarily a mitochondrial process, but also occurs in peroxisomes. Using a variety of chain length-specific transport processes and catabolic enzymes, the primary pathways of catabolism of fatty acids involve their oxidative degradation in two-carbon units, a process known as β-oxidation, which produces acetyl-CoA. In most tissues, the acetyl-CoA units are used for ATP production in the mitochondrion. In the liver, the acetyl-CoA is catabolized to ketone bodies, primarily acetoacetate and β-hydroxybutyrate, by a mitochondrial pathway termed ketogenesis. The ketone bodies are exported from liver for energy metabolism in peripheral tissue.

ACTIVE LEARNING

1. Compare the metabolism of acetyl-CoA in liver and muscle. Explain why the liver produces ketone bodies during gluconeogenesis. What prevents hepatic oxidation of acetyl-CoA?
2. Review the merits of carnitine usage as a performance enhancer during exercise and as a supplement for geriatric patients.
3. Review the current use and mechanism of action of peroxisome proliferator drugs for treatment of dyslipidemia and diabetes.

Further reading

Cahill GF Jr. Fuel metabolism in starvation. *Annu Rev Nutr* 2006;**26**:1–22.
Charfen MA. Fernández-Frackelton M. Diabetic ketoacidosis. *Emerg Med Clin North Am* 2005;**23**:609–628.
Freeland BS. Diabetic ketoacidosis. *Diabetes Educator* 2003;**29**:384–395.

Klepper J, Leiendecker B. GLUT1 deficiency syndrome – 2007 update. *Dev Med Child Neurol* 2007;**49**:707–716.
Longo N, Amat di San Filippo C, Pasquali M. Disorders of carnitine transport and the carnitine cycle. *Am J Med Genet C Semin Med Genet* 2006;**142**:77–85.
Solis JO, Singh RH. Management of fatty acid oxidation disorders: a survey of current treatment strategies. *J Am Diet Assoc* 2002;**102**:1800–1803.
Wanders RJ, Waterham HR. Peroxisomal disorders: the single peroxisomal enzyme deficiencies. *Biochim Biophys Acta* 2006;**1763**:1707–1720.
Wanders RJ, Jansen GA, Lloyd MD. Phytanic acid alpha-oxidation, new insights into an old problem: a review. *Biochim Biophys Acta* 2003;**1631**:119–135.
Wierzbicki AS, Lloyd MD, Schofield CJ, Feher MD, Gibberd FB. Refsum's disease: a peroxisomal disorder affecting phytanic acid alpha-oxidation. *J Neurochem* 2002;**80**:727–735.
Wood PA. Defects in mitochondrial beta-oxidation of fatty acids. *Curr Opin Lipidol* 1999;**10**:107–112.

Websites

Acyl-CoA dehydrogenase deficiency: www.cdc.gov/genomics/hugenet/reviews/MCAD.htm
Carnitine: http://lpi.oregonstate.edu/infocenter/othernuts/carnitine/
Lipids OnLine – slide library: www.lipidsonline.org/slides/
Peroxisomes: www.kcl.ac.uk/kis/schools/life_sciences/biomed/bscb/softcell/peroxi.html
Peroxisomal disorders: www.emedicine.com/neuro/topic309.htm
α-Oxidation: www.uwsp.edu/chemistry/tzamis/boxanim.gif

16. Biosynthesis and Storage of Fatty Acids

U V Kulkarni and I Broom

LEARNING OBJECTIVES

After reading this chapter you should be able to:

- Describe the pathway of fatty acid synthesis, and in particular the roles of malonyl-CoA carboxylase and the multifunctional enzyme fatty acid synthase.
- Outline short-term and long-term regulation of fatty acid synthesis.
- Explain the concepts of elongation and desaturation of the fatty acid chain.
- Describe the synthesis of triglycerides.
- Discuss endocrine function of adipose tissue.

INTRODUCTION

The majority of fatty acids required by humans are supplied in the diet; however, the pathway for their de novo synthesis (lipogenesis) from two-carbon compounds is present in many tissues such as liver, brain, kidney, mammary gland and adipose tissue. In general, the pathway of de novo synthesis is primarily active in situations of excess energy intake, specifically in the form of excess carbohydrate. In this situation, carbohydrate is converted to fatty acids in the liver and stored as triacylglycerol (TAG, also known as triglycerides) in adipose tissue. In humans, adipose tissue is not an important site of fatty acid synthesis: the main lipogenic organ is the liver. Lipogenesis does not appear to be a critical requirement in humans, and no life-threatening illnesses associated with its malfunction have been identified. It does, however, have an important bearing on the development of obesity.

The pathway for lipogenesis is not simply the reverse of oxidation of fatty acids seen in oxidative pathways (Chapter 15). Lipogenesis requires a completely different set of enzymes and is located in a different cellular compartment, the cytosol. Furthermore, it uses nicotinamide dinucleotide phosphate ($NADP^+$) as a source of reductive power, as opposed to nicotinamide dinucleotide (NAD^+) required for β-oxidation.

FATTY ACID SYNTHESIS

Fatty acids are synthesized from acetyl-CoA

The synthesis of fatty acids in mammalian systems can be considered as a two-stage process, both stages requiring acetyl-CoA units and both employing multifunctional proteins in multienzyme complexes.

- Stage 1: formation of the key precursor malonyl-CoA from acetyl-CoA by acetyl-CoA carboxylase
- Stage 2: elongation of the fatty acid chain in two-carbon increments by fatty acid synthase.

The preparatory stage: acetyl-CoA carboxylase

Carboxylation of acetyl-CoA to malonyl-CoA is the committed step of fatty acid synthesis

In the first stage of fatty acid biosynthesis, acetyl-CoA, mostly derived from carbohydrate metabolism, is converted to malonyl-CoA by the action of the enzyme acetyl-CoA carboxylase (Fig. 16.1). This is a biotin-dependent enzyme with distinct enzymatic functions and a carrier protein function: its subunits serve as a biotin carboxylase, a transcarboxylase and biotin carboxyl carrier protein. The enzyme is synthesized in an inactive protomer form, each protomer containing all the above subunits, a molecule of biotin, and a regulatory allosteric site for the binding of citrate (a Krebs cycle metabolite) or palmitoyl-CoA (the endproduct of the fatty acid biosynthetic pathway). The reaction itself takes place in stages: first, there is the carboxylation of biotin, involving adenosine triphosphate (ATP), followed by the transfer of this carboxyl group to acetyl-CoA to produce the endproduct of the reaction: malonyl-CoA. At this stage, the free enzyme–biotin complex is released.

This process allows the building up of fatty acids with even numbers of carbon atoms in the next stage. Propionyl-CoA is a substrate for the synthesis of fatty acids with an odd number of carbon atoms.

Acetyl-CoA carboxylase is subject to strict regulation

The protomers of acetyl-CoA carboxylase polymerize in the presence of citrate or isocitrate, producing the active form of the enzyme. The polymerization process is also inhibited by

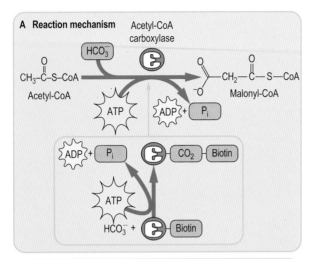

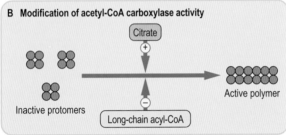

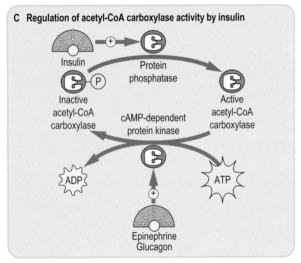

Fig. 16.1 **Conversion of acetyl-CoA to malonyl-CoA.** (A) The reaction catalyzed by the acetyl-CoA carboxylase. The enzyme has covalently attached biotin, which is carboxylated using a molecule of ATP. (B) Acetyl-CoA carboxylase requires presence of citrate for polymerization to its active form. (C) The activity of acetyl-CoA carboxylase is regulated by phosphorylation–dephosphorylation mechanism. This in turn is controlled by hormones that regulate fuel metabolism: insulin, glucagon and epinephrine. cAMP, cyclic adenosine monophosphate.

palmitoyl-CoA at the same allosteric site. The respective stimulatory and inhibitory effects of citrate and palmitoyl-CoA are entirely logical: under conditions of high citrate concentration, energy storage is desirable but when palmitoyl-CoA, the product of the pathway, accumulates, a decrease in the

synthesis of fatty acids is appropriate. There is an additional control mechanism, independent of the citrate or palmitoyl-CoA, involving phosphorylation and dephosphorylation of the enzyme molecule. This involves hormone-dependent protein phosphatase/kinase (see Fig. 16.1). Phosphorylation inhibits the enzyme and dephosphorylation activates it. Phosphorylation of the enzyme is promoted by glucagon or epinephrine and the active dephosphorylated form is promoted by the insulin, which is a lipogenic hormone.

The carboxylation of acetyl-CoA to malonyl-CoA commits the pathway to fatty acid synthesis. This is why this enzyme is under such strict short-term control. Longer term control also exists and is exerted by the induction or repression of enzyme synthesis effected by diet: synthesis of acetyl-CoA carboxylase is upregulated under conditions of high-carbohydrate/low-fat intake, whilst starvation or high-fat/low-carbohydrate intake leads to downregulation of synthesis of the enzyme.

Synthesizing a fatty acid chain: fatty acid synthase

The second major step in fatty acid synthesis also involves a multienzyme complex, the fatty acid synthase. This enzyme system is much more complex than acetyl-CoA carboxylase. The protein contains seven distinct enzyme activities and an acyl carrier protein (ACP). ACP, a highly conserved protein, replaces CoA as the entity that binds to the elongating fatty acid chain. The structure of this molecule is shown in Figure 16.2 and consists of a dimer of large identical polypeptides arranged head to tail. Each monomer contains all seven enzyme activities and the ACP. It also contains a long pantetheine group which acts as a flexible 'arm', making the molecule being synthesized available to different enzymes in the fatty acid synthesis complex. The function in fatty acid synthesis is shared between the two polypeptide chains.

Fatty acid synthase builds the fatty acid molecule up to 16-carbon length

The reaction proceeds after an initial priming of the cysteine (Cys-SH) group with acetyl-CoA, a reaction catalyzed by acetyl transacylase (Fig. 16.3). Then malonyl-CoA is transferred by malonyl transacylase to the -SH residue of the pantetheine group attached to the ACP in the other subunit. Next, 3-ketoacyl synthase (the condensing enzyme) catalyzes the reaction between the previously attached acetyl group and the malonyl residue, liberating CO_2 and forming the 3-ketoacyl enzyme complex. This frees the cysteine residue on chain 1 that had been occupied by the acetyl-CoA. The 3-ketoacyl group subsequently undergoes sequential reduction, dehydration and again reduction to form a saturated acyl–enzyme complex. The next molecule of malonyl-CoA displaces the acyl group from the pantetheine-SH group to the now free cysteine group, and the reaction sequence is

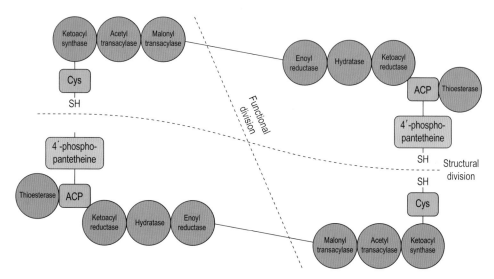

Fig. 16.2 **Structure of fatty acyl synthase.** Fatty acid synthase is a dimer consisting of two large subunits arranged head to tail. It contains seven distinct enzyme activities and an acyl-carrier protein (ACP). Cys, cysteine.

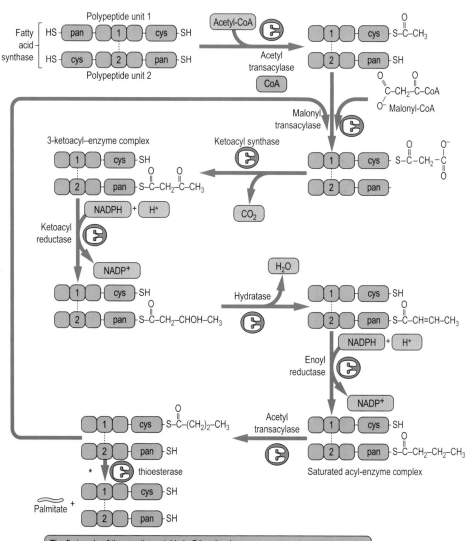

Fig. 16.3 **Reactions catalyzed by fatty acid synthase.** The synthesis of fatty acid chain is initiated by a molecule of malonyl-CoA (C3) which reacts with first molecule of acetyl-CoA (C2); this produces a C4 molecule (1 carbon is lost as CO_2 during condensation of malonyl-CoA and acetyl-CoA). There are six more cycles, each adding 2C to the fatty acid chain (seven cycles altogether), and the result is a 16-carbon molecule of palmitate. NADPH, reduced nicotinamide dinucleotide phosphate; pan, pantetheine.

*This reaction occurs once 16-carbon fatty acyl chain has been formed.

repeated through six more cycles (seven cycles altogether). Once the 16-carbon chain (palmitate) is formed, the saturated acyl–enzyme complex activates the thioesterase, releasing the molecule of palmitate from the enzyme complex. The two -SH sites are now free, allowing another cycle of palmitate synthesis to be initiated.

The synthesis of one palmitate molecule requires 8 molecules of acetyl-CoA, 7 ATP and 14 NADH:

$$8\,AcCoA + 7\,ATP + 14\,NADPH + 6\,H^+ = CH_3(CH_2)_{14}COO^-$$
$$\text{(palmitate)} + 14\,NADP^+ + 8\,CoA + 6\,H_2O + 7\,ADP + 7\,Pi$$

In common with the acetyl-CoA carboxylase system, fatty acid synthase is also regulated by substrate flux (the presence of phosphorylated sugars) via an allosteric effect, and also by induction and repression of the enzyme.

Alteration in the amount of enzyme protein is effected by the nutritional state of the individual; consequently, this is the main factor controlling the rate of lipogenesis. Rates of fatty acid synthesis are greatest when an individual follows a high-carbohydrate/low-fat diet and are low during fasting/starvation or when eating a high-fat diet. Situations where there are high circulating concentrations of fatty acids lead to marked inhibition of lipogenesis.

The malate shuttle

The malate shuttle allows recruitment of two-carbon units from the mitochondrion to the cytoplasm

The primary molecule required for the synthesis of fatty acids is acetyl-CoA. However, acetyl-CoA is generated in the mitochondria and cannot freely cross the inner mitochondrial membrane. As said above, fatty acid biosynthesis occurs in the cytosol. The malate shuttle is a mechanism allowing the transfer of two-carbon units from the mitochondria to the cytosol: it involves the malate-citrate antiporter (Fig. 16.4). Pyruvate derived from glycolysis is decarboxylated to acetyl-CoA in the mitochondria; it subsequently reacts with oxaloacetate in the tricarboxylic acid (TCA) cycle (see Chapter 14) to form citrate. Translocation of a molecule of citrate to the cytosol via the antiporter is accompanied by transfer of a molecule

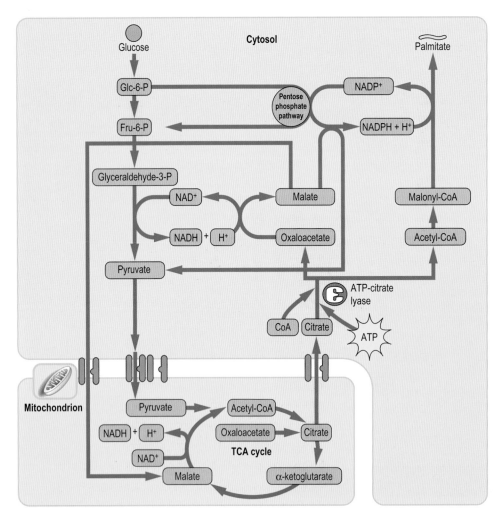

Fig. 16.4 **The malate shuttle.** Acetyl-CoA is generated in the mitochondria and cannot cross the mitochondrial membrane. The malate shuttle facilitates the transport of two-carbon units from the mitochondria to cytoplasm. Acetyl-CoA is resynthesized in the cytoplasm and enters lipogenesis. Fru-6-P, fructose-6-phosphate; Glc-6-P, glucose-6-phosphate; NADH, reduced nicotinamide dinucleotide. (See also Fig. 9.7.)

of malate to the mitochondrion. In the cytosol, citrate, in the presence of ATP and CoA, undergoes cleavage to acetyl-CoA and oxaloacetate by citrate lyase. This makes acetyl-CoA available for carboxylation to malonyl-CoA and for the synthesis of fatty acids. The synthesis of fatty acids is also linked to glucose metabolism through the pentose phosphate pathway which is the main provider of NADPH required for lipogenesis. Some NADPH is also generated by the $NADP^+$-linked decarboxylation of malate to pyruvate by malic enzyme:

$$Malate + NADP^+ + pyruvate + CO_2 + NADPH + H^+$$

FATTY ACID ELONGATION

The elongation of a fatty acid chain beyond 16-carbon length requires another set of enzymes.

Palmitate released from fatty acid synthase becomes a substrate for the synthesis of longer chain fatty acids, with the exception of certain essential fatty acids (see below). Chain elongation occurs by the addition of further two-carbon fragments derived from malonyl-CoA (Fig. 16.5). This process occurs on the endoplasmic reticulum by the action of yet

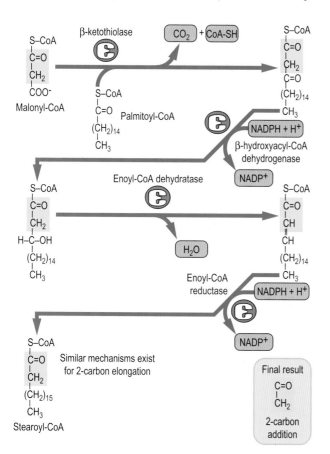

Fig. 16.5 Elongation of fatty acids. Fatty acid elongation occurs on the endoplasmic reticulum and is carried out by a multienzyme complex, fatty acid elongase.

another multienzyme complex – fatty acid elongase. The reactions occurring during chain elongation are similar to those involved in fatty acid synthesis, except that the fatty acid is attached to CoA, rather than to the ACP.

The substrates for the cytosolic fatty acid elongase include saturated fatty acids with a chain length from 10-carbon upwards, and also unsaturated fatty acids. Very long-chain (22–24-carbon) fatty acids are produced in the brain, and elongation of stearoyl-CoA (C_{18}) in the brain increases rapidly during myelination, producing fatty acids required for the synthesis of sphingolipids.

Fatty acids can also be elongated in the mitochondria, where yet another system is used: it is NADH-dependent and uses acetyl-CoA as a source of two-carbon fragments. It is simply the reverse of β-oxidation (see Chapter 15) and the substrates for chain elongation are short- and medium-chain fatty acids containing fewer than 16 carbon atoms. During fasting and starvation, elongation of fatty acids is greatly reduced.

DESATURATION OF FATTY ACIDS

Desaturation reactions require molecular oxygen

The body has a requirement for mono- and polyunsaturated fatty acids, in addition to saturated fatty acids. Some of these

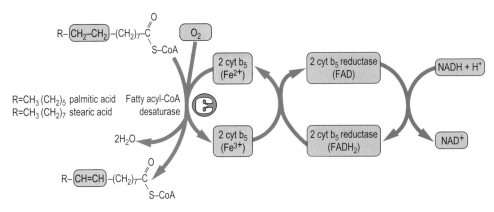

Overall reaction: $(-CH_2-CH_2-) + O_2 + NADH + H^+ \rightarrow (-CH_2=CH-) + 2H_2O + NAD^+$

Fig. 16.6 **Desaturation of fatty acids.** Desaturation of the fatty acids takes place in the endoplasmic reticulum. The reaction requires molecular oxygen, NADH$_2$, FADH$_2$ and cytochrome b$_5$. cyt b$_5$, cytochrome b$_5$; FAD, flavin adenine dinucleotide; FADH$_2$, reduced flavin adenine dinucleotide; Fe^{3+}, ferric ion.

CHANGES IN ENZYME EXPRESSION IN RESPONSE TO FOOD INTAKE REGULATE STORAGE OF ENERGY SUBSTRATES

The fed state is associated with the induction of enzymes that increase fatty acid synthesis in the liver. A wide range of enzymes are induced, including those involved in glycolysis, e.g. glucokinase (the hepatic form of hexokinase) and pyruvate kinase, as well as enzymes linked to increased production of NADPH (Glc-6-P dehydrogenase, 6-phosphogluconate dehydrogenase, and malic enzyme). Further, there is an increased expression of citrate lyase, acetyl-CoA carboxylase, fatty acid synthase, and Δ^9 desaturase.

Further, in the fed state, there is a concomitant repression of the key enzymes involved in gluconeogenesis. Phosphoenolpyruvate carboxykinase, glucose-6-phosphatase (Glc-6-P-ase), and some aminotransferases are reduced in amount, either by reduction in synthesis or by increased degradation (see Chapter 21).

need to be supplied in the diet; these two unsaturated fatty acids, linoleic and linolenic, are known as the essential fatty acids (EFA; see below). The desaturation system requires molecular oxygen, NADH, and cytochrome b$_5$. The process of desaturation, like that of chain elongation, occurs on the endoplasmic reticulum and results in the oxidation of both the fatty acid and NADH (Fig. 16.6).

In man, the desaturase system is unable to introduce double bonds between carbon atoms beyond carbon-9 and the ω (terminal methyl) carbon atom. Most desaturations occur between carbon atoms 9 and 10 (annotated as Δ^9 desaturations), e.g. those with palmitic acid producing palmitoleic acid (C-16:1, Δ^9), and those with stearic acid producing oleic acid (C-18:1, Δ^9).

ESSENTIAL FATTY ACIDS

The ω-3 and ω-6 fatty acids (or their precursors) must be supplied with diet

As discussed above, the human desaturase is unable to introduce double bonds beyond C-9. On the other hand, two types of fatty acids – those having double bonds 3 carbons from the methyl end (ω-3 fatty acids) and 6 carbons from the methyl end (ω-6 fatty acids) – are required for the synthesis of eicosanoids (C-20 fatty acids), precursors of important molecules such as prostaglandins, thromboxanes and leukotrienes. Therefore, the ω-3 and ω-6 fatty acids (or their precursors) must be supplied in the diet. As it happens, they are obtained from dietary vegetable oils which contain the ω-6 fatty acid, linoleic acid (C-18:2, $\Delta^{9,12}$) and the ω-3 fatty acid, linolenic acid (C-18:3, $\Delta^{9,12,15}$). Linoleic acid is converted in a series of elongation and desaturation reactions to arachidonic acid (C-20:4, $\Delta^{5,8,11,14}$), the precursor for the synthesis of other eicosanoids in man. Elongation and desaturation of linolenic acid produce eicosapentaenoic acid (EPA; C-20:5, $\Delta^{5,8,11,14,17}$), which is a precursor of yet another series of eicosanoids (see Table 3.2).

STORAGE AND TRANSPORT OF FATTY ACIDS: THE SYNTHESIS OF TRIACYLGLYCEROLS

Fatty acids, derived from endogenous synthesis or from diet, are stored and transported as triacylglycerols

In both liver and fat triacylglycerols are produced by a pathway involving phosphatidic acid as an intermediate (Fig. 16.7). The source of glycerol phosphate is, however, different in the two tissues. Glycerol itself is the source of phosphatidic

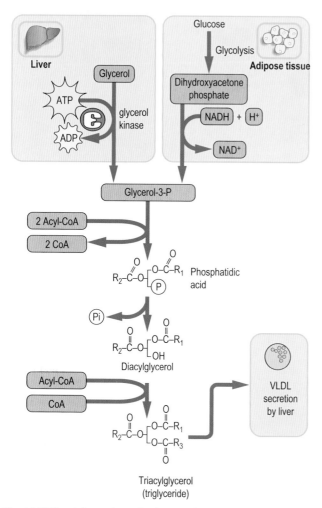

Fig. 16.7 **Triacylglycerol synthesis.** Triacylglycerols (triglycerides) are synthesized in the liver and in adipose tissue. The source of glycerol-3-P is different in the two tissues. In the liver it is glycerol but adipose tissue has no glycerol kinase activity. There, glycerol-3-P is generated from the glycolytic intermediate, dihydroxyacetone phosphate.

acid in the liver. However, in the adipose tissue, due to the lack of expressed glycerol kinase, glucose is the indirect source of glycerol, with the glycolytic metabolite dihydroxy acetone phosphate being its immediate precursor (see Fig. 16.7). The storage of fatty acids in adipose tissue can therefore only occur when glycolysis is activated, i.e. in the fed state.

Triacylglycerols produced in the liver on the smooth endoplasmic reticulum are not stored there but are complexed with cholesterol, phospholipids and apolipoproteins (also synthesized on the endoplasmic reticulum) for export to form very low-density lipoprotein (VLDL). The VLDL is then processed in the Golgi apparatus and released into the bloodstream for uptake by other tissues.

VLDL, once released into the bloodstream is acted upon by lipoprotein lipase (LPL). This enzyme is found attached to the basement membrane glycoproteins of capillary endothelial cells and is active against both VLDL and chylomicrons, the latter arising from the intestine after food intake (see Chapter 18). The nature of this enzyme differs from tissue to tissue: the muscle isoenzyme has a very low K_m for substrate and thus allows the usage of fatty acids for energy transduction from VLDL even at very low concentrations. In the adipocyte, however, the isoenzyme has a high K_m value for substrate and is thus only active, in terms of adipose tissue uptake of fatty acids, when VLDL or chylomicrons concentrations are elevated.

In the fed state, when adipose tissue is actively taking up fatty acids from the lipoproteins and storing this as triacylglycerols, the adipocytes synthesize LPL and secrete it into the capillaries of the adipose tissue. This increased synthesis and secretion of LPL is stimulated by the high insulin: glucagon ratio seen on feeding. Increased insulin levels also stimulate the uptake of glucose by adipose tissue and promote glycolysis. This has the net effect of producing increasing amounts of glycerol, and it facilitates the synthesis of triacylglycerols within the adipocyte.

Insulin is an important hormone in relation to fatty acid synthesis and storage (Fig. 16.8). It promotes glucose uptake in both the liver and adipose tissue. In the liver, by increasing fructose-2,6-bisphosphate levels, it stimulates glycolysis, thus increasing pyruvate production. By stimulating dephosphorylation of pyruvate dehydrogenase complex and activating this enzyme, insulin promotes production of acetyl-CoA, thus stimulating the TCA cycle and increasing citrate levels which in turn, through stimulation of the acetyl-CoA carboxylase, increase the rate of fatty acid synthesis (see also Chapter 21).

REGULATION OF TOTAL BODY FAT STORES

Adipose tissue is an active endocrine organ

It has long been understood that increased energy intake without appropriate increase in energy expenditure is associated with obesity, which is characterized by increased adiposity, in terms of both the numbers of adipocytes and their fat content. It is clear that adipose tissue, far from being an inert storage reservoir, is hormonally active. Hormones such as leptin, adiponectin and resistin (collectively known as adipokines), growth factors such as vascular endothelial growth factor, and proinflammatory cytokines such as tumor necrosis factor α (TNF-α) and interleukin 6 (IL-6) are all produced by adipocytes (see Chapter 22).

The amount of leptin present in blood is proportional to the body fat content

The main molecule shown so far to carry information about the fat stores in an individual is leptin. Leptin levels signal the amount of adipose tissue that is present. It crosses the blood–brain barrier, reduces appetite and causes an increase in

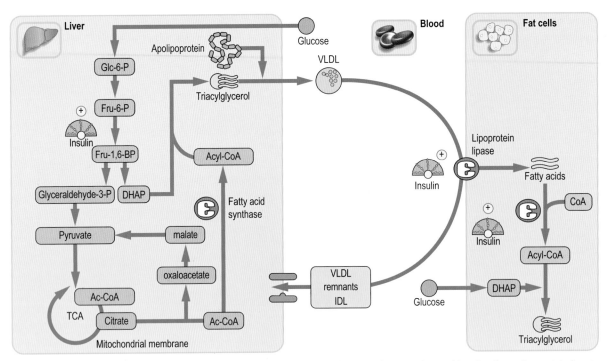

Fig. 16.8 **Transport and storage of fat in response to feeding.** A meal stimulates insulin secretion and insulin directs fat metabolism towards synthesis and storage. Insulin stimulates glycolysis in the liver, thereby increasing pyruvate production. Further, it activates the pyruvate dehydrogenase complex (by dephosphorylation of the enzyme), and thus promotes the synthesis of acetyl-CoA from pyruvate. This stimulates the TCA cycle and generates citrate. Citrate in turn stimulates acetyl-CoA carboxylase, increasing the rate of fatty acid biosynthesis. DHAP, dihydroacetone phosphate; Fru-1,6-BP, fructose-1,6 biphosphate; Glc-6-P, glucose-6-phosphate; IDL, intermediate-density lipoprotein; TCA, tricarboxylic acid cycle; VLDL, very low-density lipoprotein. (See also Chapter 18 for details of lipoprotein metabolism; compare also Fig. 21.11.)

LIFESTYLE AND OBESITY

A 48-year-old ex-Army infantryman (height 1.91 m) presented with the problem of increasing weight over the previous 8 years since leaving the Army. At the time of his retirement from active service, he had weighed 95 kg (209 lb) but at presentation weighed 193 kg (424.6 lb). His current occupation was that of truck driver. He denied any change in food intake since leaving the Army, but admitted to taking little or no exercise. Detailed enquiry indicated that his daily dietary intake provided between 12 600 and 16 800 kJ (3000 and 4000 kcal), with a fat intake approaching 40%. The patient was initially placed on a healthy eating plan, with fat intake reduced to 35% of total calories. He was advised to exercise and proceeded to swim three or four times per week. His weight immediately began to decrease, rapidly at first and then at 3–4 kg (6.6–8.8 lb) each month until it stabilized at 145–150 kg (319–330 lb). He was then placed on a high-protein/low-carbohydrate/low-fat diet, which induced a return of weight loss that continued for a further year, resulting in a final weight of 93 kg (204.6 lb).

Comment. Obesity is increasingly prevalent in many parts of the world. Clinical obesity is now clearly defined in terms of height and weight through the body mass index (BMI), which is calculated as the weight in kilograms divided by the height in meters[2] (see Chapter 13 for details):

$$\text{BMI (kg/m}^2) = \rightarrow \frac{\text{weight (kg)}}{(\text{height [m]})^2}$$

BMI 25–30 kg/m^2 is classified as overweight or grade I obesity, BMI >30 kg/m^2 is clinical or grade II obesity, and BMI >40 kg/m^2 is classified as morbid or grade III obesity. Our patient had a BMI of 53 at presentation falling to 26 after prolonged diet. If energy input exceeds output over time then weight will increase. Obesity predisposes to several diseases. The most important is type 2 diabetes mellitus: 80% of this type of diabetes is associated with the obese state. Other associated illnesses include coronary heart disease, hypertension, stroke, arthritis, and gall bladder disease. (See also Chapter 22.)

energy expenditure. Leptin-deficient animals are obese and lethargic; replacing leptin in these animal models reverses these features. However, the majority of obese individuals have high levels of leptin without this limiting their weight. They seem to be resistant to the central nervous system effect of leptin, and administering additional leptin does not result in resolution of the clinical and metabolic features of obesity.

A number of hormone-like agents are involved in total body fat stores

Insulin levels are also affected by the amount of body fat, with the endocrine pancreas secreting higher levels to compensate for the phenomenon of insulin resistance (see Chapter 21), which is particularly seen in abdominal obesity. There is a complex relationship between insulin, weight and fat stores; insulin has been shown to exert an appetite-suppressant effect on the central nervous system, but often causes weight gain in people with diabetes who begin treatment with insulin injections. Physiologically, insulin inhibits lipolysis, and its actions are influenced by other hormones released from adipose tissue, such as adiponectin.

The number of hormones and cellular markers involved in the interplay of energy balance and adipose tissue stores is increasing, and the interrelationships are complex (see Chapters 21 and 22). This is compounded by the fact that these physiologic mechanisms integrate with, and may be overridden by, environmental, societal and behavioral factors.

Summary

- Fatty acid synthesis and storage are essential components of body energy homeostasis.
- Lipogenesis takes place in the cytosol. Its committed step is the reaction catalyzed by acetyl-CoA carboxylase.
- Elongation of the fatty acid chain (up to the length of 16 carbon atoms) is carried out by the dimeric fatty acid synthase, which possesses several enzyme activities. Both are subject to a complex regulation.

ACTIVE LEARNING

1. Describe how a growing fatty acid chain is transferred between the subunits of fatty acid synthase.
2. How are eicosanoids synthesized?
3. Explain why the rate of lipolysis in the fed state is low.
4. What is the role of adipokines?
5. Describe the committed step of lipogenesis and its regulation.
6. What are the sources of acetyl-CoA for fatty acid synthesis?
7. Compare and contrast lipogenesis and lipolysis.

- The malate shuttle facilitates the transfer of two-carbon units from the mitochondria to cytoplasm for use in lipogenesis.
- The reducing power in the form of NADPH is supplied by the pentose phosphate pathway and also by the malate shuttle.
- The essential unsaturated fatty acids are linoleic and linolenic acid. Linoleic acid is converted to arachidonic acid, which in turn serves as the precursor of prostaglandins.
- Adiposity signals are provided by adipokines, particularly leptin. Insulin is also important in the regulation of food intake.

Further reading

Angulo P. Nonalcoholic fatty liver disease. *N Engl J Med* 2002;**346**: 1221–1231.

Lenz A, Diamond FB. Obesity: the hormonal milieu. *Curr Opin Endocrinol Diabetes Obesity* 2008;**15**:9–20.

Wynne K, Stanley S, McGowan B, Bloom S. Apetite control. *J Endocrinol* 2005; **184**:291–318.

17. Biosynthesis of Cholesterol and Steroids

M H Dominiczak and A M Wallace

LEARNING OBJECTIVES

After reading this chapter you should be able to:

- List the main steps involved in the synthesis of the cholesterol molecule.
- Discuss the regulation of intracellular cholesterol concentration.
- Explain mechanisms governing cholesterol metabolism and excretion.
- Describe bile acids and their enterohepatic circulation.
- Outline the main pathways of synthesis of steroid hormones.

INTRODUCTION

Cholesterol is an essential component of mammalian cell membranes. It is also a precursor of important biologically active compounds such as the bile acids, the steroid hormones, and vitamin D. Cholesterol homeostasis is important in the etiology of atherosclerosis (Chapter 18), and it is a major component of gall stones.

Humans synthesize 1 g cholesterol each day, mainly in the liver. The rate of endogenous cholesterol synthesis and the dietary intake determine its concentration in plasma. The typical daily Western diet contains approximately 500 mg (1.2 mmol) of cholesterol daily, mainly in meat, eggs, and dairy products (see Chapter 22). Under normal circumstances, 30–60% of this is absorbed during passage through the gut. Following intestinal absorption, cholesterol is transported to the liver and to peripheral tissues as a component of lipoprotein particles, chylomicrons. They are taken up by the liver. The liver repackages cholesterol and triglycerides into another, smaller lipoprotein – VLDL (Chapter 18). Triacylglycerols contained in the VLDL undergo sequential hydrolysis in the peripheral tissues, transforming the particles into VLDL remnants and then, after more extensive hydrolysis, into LDL. VLDL remnants and LDL deliver cholesterol back to the liver by binding to the apoB/E membrane receptor (LDL receptor). However, they may also enter the vascular wall.

Humans cannot metabolize the sterol ring of cholesterol – it is excreted in bile either as free cholesterol or in the form of bile acids. Most bile acids are reabsorbed in the terminal ileum and cycle back to the liver. This cycle is known as the enterohepatic circulation.

In its early steps, the pathway of cholesterol synthesis provides substrates for the synthesis of compounds important in cell proliferation and tumor growth, in electron transport and in ameliorating oxidative stress. Oxysterols generated at later stages of the pathway are signaling molecules that take part in the regulation of cholesterol homeostasis (Fig. 17.1).

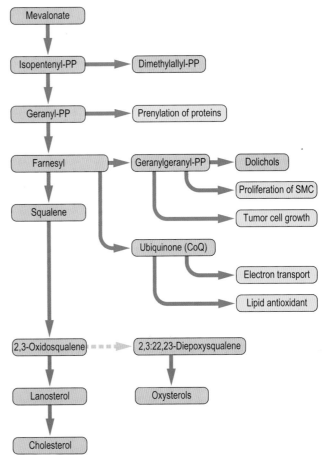

Fig. 17.1 **Cholesterol synthesis and related pathways** (modified from Charlton-Menys V, Durrington PN. *Exp Physiol* 2007; **93**: 27–42, with permission). SMC, smooth muscle cells; CoQ, coenzyme Q.

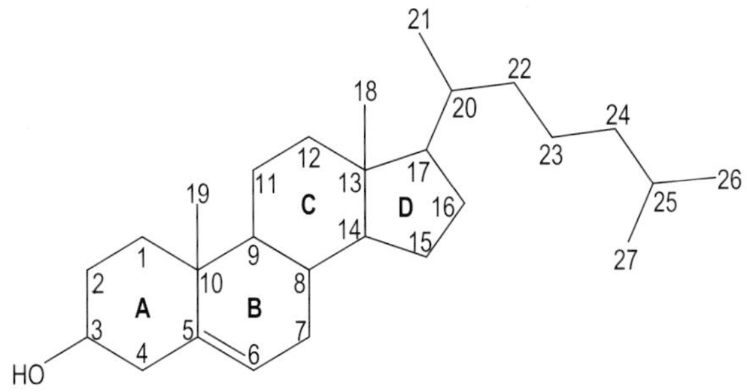

Fig. 17.2 **Structure of cholesterol.** A–D is the conventional notation used to describe the four rings. Numbers 1–27 describe the carbon atoms.

STRUCTURE OF CHOLESTEROL

The structure of cholesterol is shown in Figure 17.2. It has a molecular weight of 386 Da and contains 27 carbon atoms, of which 17 are incorporated into four fused rings (the cyclopentanoperhydrophenanthrene nucleus), two are in angular methyl groups attached at the junctions of rings AB and CD, and eight are in the peripheral side chain. Cholesterol is almost entirely composed of carbon and hydrogen atoms; there is a solitary hydroxyl group attached to carbon 3. Cholesterol is also almost completely saturated, having just one double bond between carbon atoms 5 and 6.

Cholesterol decreases membrane fluidity

Cholesterol (mostly free cholesterol) is an essential component of cell membranes. It is found in the highest concentrations in plasma membranes (up to 25% of the lipid content), while it is virtually absent from inner mitochondrial membranes. It is held in the lipid bilayer by physical interactions between the planar steroid ring and the fatty acid chains. The absence of covalent bonding means that it may transfer in and out of the membrane. Membranes are fluid structures in which both the lipid and protein molecules move and undergo conformational change (see Chapter 8). The more fluid the phospholipid bilayer becomes, the more permeable is the membrane. At body temperature, the long hydrocarbon chains of the lipid bilayer are capable of considerable motion. Cholesterol is located between these hydrocarbon chains, forming a loose crosslink and so reducing fluidity. This relative rigidity is increased still further if cholesterol is adjacent to saturated fatty acids. Cholesterol forms clustered regions within the lipid bilayer. In areas of a cholesterol cluster, there may be 1 mole of cholesterol per mole of phospholipid, while in adjacent areas there may be no cholesterol. Thus, the membrane contains cholesterol-rich impermeable patches and more permeable cholesterol-free areas.

FREE AND ESTERIFIED CHOLESTEROL

Cholesterol is poorly soluble in water. Only about 30% of circulating cholesterol occurs in the free form, the majority being esterified through the hydroxyl group to long-chain fatty acids including oleic and linoleic acids. Cholesterol esters are even less soluble in water than free cholesterol.

Dietary cholesterol brought to the liver is mostly in the free form. In the plasma, cholesterol is incorporated into the range of lipoproteins (see Chapter 18) and is present there mostly in the form of cholesteryl esters. Esters are also the tissue storage form of cholesterol. Cholesterol is esterified in the plasma by the enzyme cholesterol-lecithin acyltransferase and in the cells by the acyl-CoA:cholesterol acyltransferase (ACAT). Sixty to eighty percent of cholesteryl esters present in plasma is taken up by the liver.

INTESTINAL ABSORPTION OF CHOLESTEROL

Dietary cholesterol is absorbed from the intestine via a membrane transporter known as the Nieman-Pick C1-like (NPC1L1) protein. Another transporter present in the apical side of enterocytes is the ATP binding cassette G5/G8, comprising two half-transporters – ABCG5 and ABCG8. These transport cholesterol back to the intestine and are also involved in secretion of noncholesterol sterols into the bile. These transporters are upregulated by the nuclear receptor, liver X receptor (see below). Mutations of gene coding for these transporters result in tissue accumulation of plant sterols (sitosterolemia). The drug ezetimibe suppresses the NPC1L1-mediated cholesterol transport and has been used in the treatment of hypercholesterolemia.

BIOSYNTHESIS OF CHOLESTEROL

Cholesterol is synthesized from acetyl-coenzyme A. HMG-CoA reductase is the rate-limiting enzyme in the pathway

Virtually all human cells have the capacity to make cholesterol. Liver is the major site of cholesterol biosynthesis and smaller amounts are synthesized in the intestine, adrenal cortex and gonads. Generation of the many carbon–carbon and carbon–hydrogen bonds contained in cholesterol structure requires a source of carbon atoms, a source of reducing power and significant amounts of energy. Acetyl-coenzyme A (acetyl-CoA) provides a high-energy starting point. It may be derived from several sources, including the β-oxidation of long-chain fatty acids, dehydrogenation of pyruvate

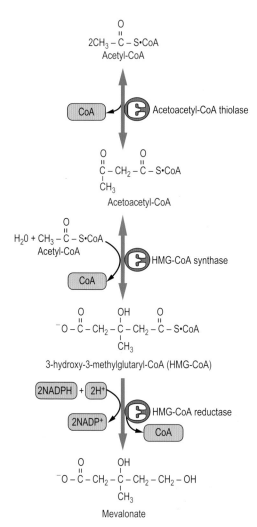

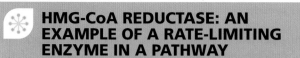

Fig. 17.3 **Biosynthesis of mevalonic acid.** Mevalonic acid contains six carbon atoms, which are derived from three molecules of acetyl-CoA.

✴ HMG-CoA REDUCTASE: AN EXAMPLE OF A RATE-LIMITING ENZYME IN A PATHWAY

HMG-CoA reductase is the rate-limiting enzyme in the pathway of cholesterol synthesis. It is a microsomal enzyme active in a nonphosphorylated state. Phosphorylation by a kinase inhibits its activity. Its synthesis is stimulated by fasting and inhibited by dietary cholesterol. Importantly, HMG-CoA reductase activity is controlled by the intracellular cholesterol concentration. It is also affected by several hormones: insulin and tri-iodothyronine increase its activity, while glucagon and cortisol inhibit it.

---

and oxidation of ketogenic amino acids such as leucine and isoleucine. The reducing power is provided by reduced nicotinamide dinucleotide phosphate (NADPH), which is generated in the pentose phosphate pathway (see Chapter 12).

Additional energy is provided by the breakdown of adenosine triphosphate (ATP). Overall, the production of 1 mole of cholesterol requires 18 moles of acetyl-CoA, 36 moles of ATP and 16 moles of NADPH. All the biosynthetic reactions occur within the cytoplasm, although some of the required enzymes are bound to membranes of the endoplasmic reticulum.

Mevalonic acid is the first unique compound in the pathway of cholesterol synthesis

Three molecules of acetyl-CoA are converted into the 6-carbon mevalonic acid (Fig. 17.3). The first two steps are condensation reactions leading to the formation of the 3-hydroxy-3-methylglutaryl-CoA (HMG-CoA). These reactions, catalyzed by acetoacetyl-CoA thiolase and HMG-CoA synthase, are common to the formation of ketone bodies, although the latter process occurs within mitochondria rather than the cytosol. These reactions are also favored energetically since they involve cleavage of a thioester bond and liberation of the free coenzyme-A. The rate-limiting reaction in cholesterol biosynthesis is that catalyzed by the microsomal enzyme HMG-CoA reductase which leads to the irreversible formation of mevalonic acid.

Drugs that inhibit hmg-coa reductase (statins)

HMG-CoA reductase inhibitors, known as statins, are lipid-lowering drugs that are used to lower circulating LDL-cholesterol concentrations in patients with, or at the risk of, atherosclerotic cardiovascular disease. They lower cholesterol by competitively inhibiting the liver enzyme. This causes a decrease in the intracellular cholesterol concentration and as a result, increase in the expression of LDL receptors. LDL clearance increases and the circulating LDL-cholesterol (and total plasma cholesterol) decreases. Hepatic HMG-CoA reductase activity is at a peak about 6 hours after dark and at a minimum some 6 hours after exposure to light. Therefore, statins are usually taken at night to ensure maximal effect.

Farnesyl pyrophosphate is made up of three isoprene units

Three molecules of mevalonic acid are each decarboxylated into 5-carbon atom isoprene units, which are sequentially condensed to produce the 15-carbon atom molecule farnesyl pyrophosphate (Fig. 17.4). The first two reactions require kinases and ATP to generate pyrophosphate. Further, decarboxylation results in the isomeric isoprene units isopentenyl pyrophosphate and dimethylallyl pyrophosphate, which condense together to form ger anyl pyrophosphate. Still further condensation with isopentenyl pyrophosphate produces farnesyl pyrophosphate. As well as being an intermediate in cholesterol biosynthesis, farnesyl pyrophosphate is the branching point for the synthesis of dolichol and ubiquinone (see Fig. 17.1).

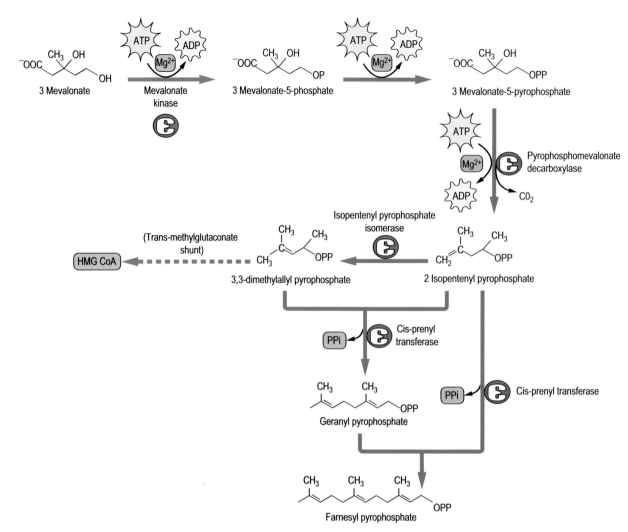

Fig. 17.4 **Biosynthesis of farnesyl pyrophosphate.** Farnesyl pyrophosphate is made up of three isoprene units. ADP, adenosine diphosphate; Mg^{2+}, magnesium; PPi, pyrophosphate. For trans-methylglutaconate shunt, see box on p. 209.

Squalene is a linear molecule capable of a ring formation

Squalene synthase is an enzyme present in the endoplasmic reticulum that facilitates condensation of two molecules of farnesyl pyrophosphate (Fig. 17.5). Several intermediates are involved and the resulting product is squalene, a 30-carbon hydrocarbon containing six double bonds, which enable it to fold into a ring similar to the steroid nucleus.

Squalene cyclizes to lanosterol

Before ring closure, squalene is converted to squalene 2,3-oxide by squalene monooxygenase in the endoplasmic reticulum. Thereafter, cyclization occurs under the action of the enzyme oxidosqualene cyclase (Fig. 17.6). It is interesting that, in plants, there is a different product of squalene cyclization, known as cycloartenol, which is further metabolized to a range of phytosterols, including β-sitosterol, rather than to cholesterol.

Final stages of cholesterol biosynthesis occur on a carrier protein

Squalene, lanosterol and all the further intermediates are hydrophobic molecules. In order for the final steps of the pathway to occur in an aqueous-medium, the intermediates react while bound to a squalene- and sterol-binding protein. The conversion from the 30-carbon lanosterol into the 27-carbon cholesterol involves three decarboxylation reactions, an isomerization and a reduction (see Fig. 17.6). NADPH is consumed in four of these reactions.

Regulation of cholesterol biosynthesis

Many factors are involved in the regulation of the intracellular concentration of cholesterol (Table 17.1). Under normal circumstances, there is an inverse relationship between dietary cholesterol intake and cholesterol biosynthesis. This ensures a relatively constant daily supply of cholesterol. It

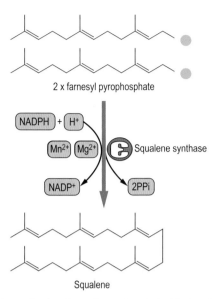

Fig. 17.5 **Biosynthesis of squalene.** The six double bonds enable the structure to fold into a ring similar to the steroid nucleus.

THE TRANS-METHYLGLUTACONATE SHUNT

The dimethylallyl pyrophosphate, one of the isoprene units formed from mevalonate (Fig. 17.4), can be dephosphorylated and broken down into acetoacetate and acetyl-CoA, which may then be diverted into other pathways, such as fatty acid biosynthesis. This mechanism is known as the trans-methylglutaconate shunt. Thus, high-energy compounds once destined to be converted into cholesterol may be redeployed to meet a higher priority need. Incidentally, an increase in fatty acid synthesis will increase the amount of substrate for cholesterol esterification.

DEFECT IN CHOLESTEROL BIOSYNTHESIS (INCIDENCE 1 IN 20 000–40 000)

Smith–Lemli-Opitz syndrome presents at birth with microencephaly, short nasal root, small chin, high arched palate, and often with midline cleft. There are often accompanying central nervous system (CNS) defects, polydactyly, and in males, ambiguous genitalia. Despite the pathway of cholesterol synthesis and metabolism being well understood, a defect in 7-dehydrocholesterol reductase was only identified in 1993. While some of these children die in infancy, the rest, if assisted in feeding, survive with severe mental retardation (IQ 20–40). Most develop growth retardation. The pathophysiology involves incomplete processing of embryonic signaling proteins (HH proteins) resulting in variable defects in different tissues. Treatment involves giving additional cholesterol to the child. This improves growth but it appears to have no CNS benefits, due to the embryonic microencephaly and other CNS defects.

TREATMENT OF HYPERCHOLESTEROLEMIA

Despite strict dietary control, a 50-year-old man, who had a family history of early cardiovascular disease, had a serum cholesterol result of 8.0 mmol/L (309 mg/dL); (desirable levels are <4.0 mmol/L (≤155 mg/dL). See Chapter 18. He also smoked 15 cigarettes per day. He was given antismoking advice and was prescribed a statin. He tolerated the therapy well and 3 months later his cholesterol was 5.5 mmol/L 212 mg/dL. The dose of the statins was increased and after a further 3 months his cholesterol concentration was 4.1 mmol/L (158 mg/dL).

Comment. Partial inhibition of the HMG-CoA reductase brings about a lowering of total plasma cholesterol by 30–50% and LDL-cholesterol by 30–60%. A range of statins is now available: this follows the original discovery that compactin (later renamed mevastatin), a fungal metabolite isolated from *Penicillium citrinum*, had HMG-CoA reductase-inhibiting properties. The inhibition of HMG-CoA reductase activity leads to the lowering of intracellular cholesterol concentration, and to consequent increased expression of the apo B/E receptor (Chapter 17) and the lowering of the plasma LDL-cholesterol.

also explains why dietary restriction is only likely to achieve a moderate reduction in the plasma cholesterol concentration.

There are two sources of intracellular cholesterol: de novo synthesis and the external supply. The exogenous (dietary) cholesterol reaches cells predominantly as a component of VLDL remnants and LDL (see Chapter 18). These lipoproteins bind to the apoB/E receptor present on the plasma membranes and the lipoprotein/receptor complexes are internalized. In the cytoplasm, vesicles carrying the internalized complexes

are acted upon by lysosomal enzymes, which separate the LDL from the receptor molecule and hydrolyze cholesterol esters. Free cholesterol is released to the cytoplasm. The LDL apoprotein is hydrolyzed to its component amino acids.

Thus, the intracellular free cholesterol can either be derived from lipoproteins or be newly synthesized within the cell. These two sources of supply are reciprocally related. A key factor regulating cellular cholesterol synthesis is the intracellular cholesterol concentration. The rise in the intracellular free cholesterol concentration results in the following (Fig. 17.7):

- a reduction both in the activity and expression of HMG-CoA reductase, limiting further cholesterol synthesis
- downregulation of LDL receptors, limiting further cellular entry of cholesterol
- increase in cholesterol and phospholipid efflux from cell to apoproteins A
- increase in the rate of conversion of cholesterol to bile acids, and thus its excretion.

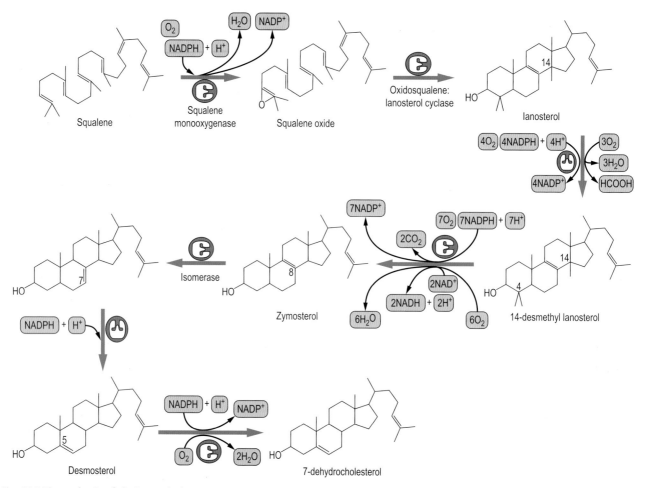

Fig. 17.6 **Biosynthesis of cholesterol**. These reactions occur while bound to a squalene- and sterol-binding protein. FAD, flavin adenine dinucleotide; NADH, reduced nicotinamide adenine dinucleotide.

Regulation of intracellular cholesterol concentration involves HMG-CoA reductase, LDL receptor, 7α-hydroxylase and a network of nuclear receptors

The liver X receptors (LXR) are ligand-activated transcription factors that are members of the nuclear receptor superfamily (see Chapter 40). They form heterodimers with other similar molecules, such as the retinoid X receptors (RXRs) and the farnesyl X receptors (FXR). The resultant complexes bind to the LXR response elements on the DNA, regulating gene expression.

LXR sense intracellular cholesterol concentration and regulate its synthesis and its efflux from cells. Interestingly, it is not the cholesterol itself that binds to the LXR but oxysterols, cholesterol metabolites such as 25-hydroxycholesterol or 27-hydroxycholesterol (see Fig. 17.1).

The ligand activation of LXR results in the upregulation of the synthesis of transcription factors known as the sterol regulatory element-binding proteins (SREBPs). SREBPs are synthesized as precursors integral to the endoplasmic reticulum membrane. They are cleaved by a protease to release the active transcription factors, which translocate to the nucleus and initiate transcription (see Fig. 17.7).

There is another intermediary molecule, the SREBP cleavage-activating protein (SCAP) which possesses a sterol-sensing domain and 'brings' the precursor SREBP to its active protease. This step is regulatory because it is blocked by sterols. Thus, when the intracellular cholesterol concentration is high, transcription of genes associated with cholesterol synthesis is repressed. On the other hand, when sterols are absent, SCAP/SREBP complex reaches the protease and the transcription begins. SREBPs act on the promoter regions of HMG-CoA reductase, HMG-CoA synthase and LDL receptor genes.

Apart from repressing intracellular cholesterol synthesis, the increased concentration of cholesterol in the hepatocyte induces, also through LXR, genes coding for cholesterol transporters that control its efflux from cells to HDL particles. This includes the expression of ABCA1 (a transporter that controls efflux of cholesterol from cells to nascent HDL) and ABCG1 (a transporter that stimulates efflux of cholesterol to more mature HDL 2 and HDL3; see Chapter 18). Note that the transcription factor PPARγ also acts through LXR regulating cholesterol efflux (see Chapter 18). Finally, high intracellular cholesterol concentration, also through one of the

Regulation of intracellular cholesterol

Factors increasing intracellular free cholesterol concentration

de novo biosynthesis

hydrolysis of intracellular cholesterol esters by the enzyme cholesterol ester hydrolase

dietary intake of cholesterol and uptake from chylomicrons

receptor-mediated uptake of cholesterol-containing lipoproteins (LDL)

Factors decreasing intracellular free cholesterol concentration

inhibition of cholesterol biosynthesis

downregulation of the LDL receptor

intracellular esterification of cholesterol by acyl-coenzyme A:cholesterol acyl transferase

release of cholesterol to high-density lipoproteins (HDL)

conversion of cholesterol to bile acids or steroid hormones

Factors influencing the activity of HMG-CoA reductase

intracellular concentration of HMG-CoA

intracellular concentration of cholesterol

hormones: insulin, tri-iodothyronine (+); glucagon, cortisol (−)

Table 17.1 Regulation of intracellular cholesterol (see also Fig. 17.1).

SREBPs, induces the enzymes catalyzing fatty acid synthesis, providing substrates for cholesterol esterification.

BILE ACIDS

The liver removes cholesterol either in a free form or as bile acids

Quantitatively, bile acids are the most important metabolic products of cholesterol. In man, there are four main bile acids (Fig. 17.8). They all have 24 carbon atoms with the terminal three carbon atoms of the cholesterol side chain being removed during synthesis. They also have a saturated steroid nucleus and differ only in the number and position of the additional hydroxyl groups. All these hydroxyl groups have the α-configuration (below the plane of the nucleus) and this means that isomerization of the 3β-hydroxyl group of cholesterol must occur.

Bile acids are synthesized in the liver

Biosynthesis of the bile acids occurs in liver parenchymal cells, where cholic and chenodeoxycholic acids are produced. They are known as the primary bile acids. The rate-limiting step in the biosynthesis is the microsomal 7α-hydroxylase enzyme (designated also CYP7A1), which introduces a hydroxyl group at 7α position of cholesterol ring. It is a microsomal monooxygenase which consists of cytochrome P-450 and requires NADPH and molecular oxygen.

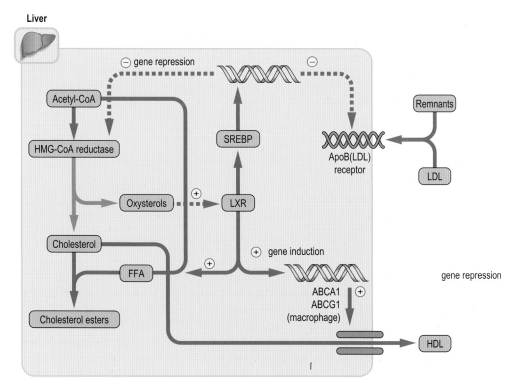

Fig. 17.7 **Regulation of intracellular cholesterol concentration.** Free cholesterol (and oxysterols) regulate intracellular cholesterol concentration by binding to nuclear receptors and inducing or suppressing gene expression. Note that increase in intracellular cholesterol concentration will suppress synthesis of HMG-CoA reductase and ApoB/E receptor and also increase cholesterol esterification and its transport from cells. FFA:free fatty acids, AcCoA: acetyl coenzyme A, LXR: liver X receptor, SREBP: sterol-regulatory-element binding protein.

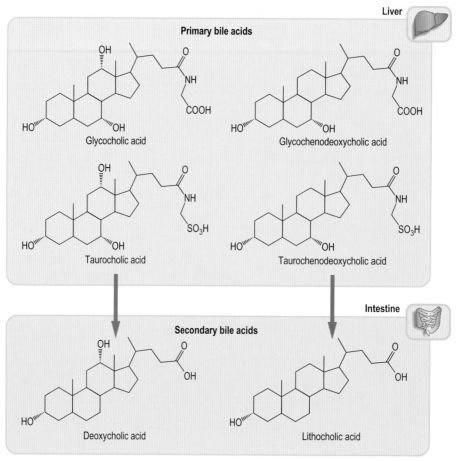

Fig. 17.8 **Structure of bile acids.** Primary bile acids are synthesized in the liver and secondary bile acids in the intestine.

GALL STONES

A 45-year-old woman complained of right upper quadrant abdominal pain and vomiting after fatty food. The only biochemical abnormality was a modestly raised alkaline phosphatase at 400 U/L (<260 U/L). However, an abdominal ultrasound showed that the gall bladder contained gall stones. She was referred to the surgeons.

Comment. Gall stones occur in up to 20% of the population of Western countries. The condition results from the formation of cholesterol-rich stones within the gall bladder. Cholesterol is present in high concentrations in bile, being solubilized in micelles that also contain phospholipids and bile acids. When the liver secretes bile with a cholesterol to phospholipid ratio greater than 1:1 it is difficult to solubilize all the cholesterol in micelles; thus there is a tendency for the excess to crystallize around any insoluble nuclei. This is compounded by further concentration of the bile in the gall bladder which occurs as a result of reabsorption of water and electrolytes. The condition may be managed conservatively by reducing dietary cholesterol and by increasing availability of bile acids that will assist with cholesterol solubilization in the bile and excretion via the gut. Alternative treatment includes disintegration of stones by shock waves (lithotripsy) and surgery. The elevated alkaline phosphatase is a marker of cholestasis (see Chapter 29).

Prior to their secretion, the primary bile acids are conjugated through the carboxyl group, forming amide linkages with either glycine or taurine (see Fig. 17.8). In man, there is a 3:1 ratio in favor of glycine conjugates. The secreted products are thus principally glycocholic, glycochenodeoxycholic, taurocholic and taurochenodeoxycholic acids. At physiologic pH, the bile acids are mainly ionized and so they occur as sodium or potassium salts. The terms 'bile acids' and 'bile salts' are used interchangeably. As their name suggests, these compounds are secreted from the liver via the bile canaliculi and larger bile ducts, either directly into the duodenum or for storage in the gall bladder. They are an important component of bile together with water, phospholipids, cholesterol and excretory products such as bilirubin. Cholesterol is pumped into bile by ABCG5 and ABCG8 proteins, the expression of which is regulated by the LXR (see above). Importantly, bile supersaturated with cholesterol facilitates formation of cholesterol gall stones.

The X receptors participate in bile synthesis and secretion

The X receptors coordinate expression of several genes relevant to cholesterol excretion including the expression of cholesterol 7α-hydroxylase. Cholesterol excretion into the bile is also regulated by other nuclear receptors. The farnesyl X receptor (FXR) heterodimerizes with retinoic X receptor and binds to bile acid response elements on the DNA. FXR acts as the cellular bile acid sensor by binding bile acids and suppressing their synthesis. FXR also induces bile acid export pump ABCBII which removes bile acids from the hepatocyte into the bile.

Secondary bile acids are formed in the intestine

Secondary bile acids form within the intestine through the action of the anaerobic bacteria (principally *Bacteroides*) on the primary bile acids. They are deoxycholic and lithocholic acids (see Fig. 17.8). Only a proportion of primary bile acids is converted into secondary bile acids. This requires hydrolysis of the amide link to glycine or taurine prior to removal of the 7α-hydroxyl group.

Bile acids assist the digestion of dietary fat

Secretion of bile from the liver and the emptying of the bile duct are controlled by the gastrointestinal hormones hepatocrinin and cholecystokinin, respectively. They are released when partially digested food passes from the stomach to the duodenum. Once secreted into the intestine, the bile acids act as detergents (they possess polar carboxyl and hydroxyl groups), assisting the emulsification of ingested lipids; this aids the enzymatic digestion and absorption of dietary fat (see Chapter 10).

Bile acids recirculate via the enterohepatic circulation

Up to 30g of bile acids pass from the bile duct into the intestine each day but only 2% of this (approximately 0.5 g) is lost through the feces. Most would be deconjugated and reabsorbed. Passive reabsorption of bile acids occurs in the jejunum and colon but the majority takes place in the ileum by active transport. Reabsorbed bile acids are transported in blood via the portal vein noncovalently bound to albumin, and are resecreted into the bile. The process is known as the enterohepatic circulation. The intestinal reabsorption explains why bile contains both primary and secondary bile acids. The total bile acid pool is only 3g and therefore they have to recirculate 5–10 times a day.

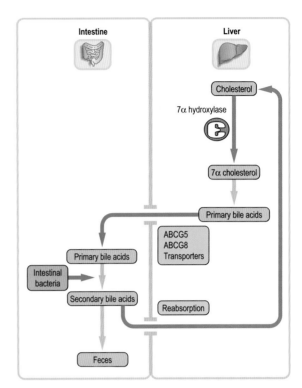

Fig. 17.9 **The enterohepatic circulation of bile acids**. For structures of the primary and secondary bile acids see Fig. 17.7.

This bile acid flux also contributes to the control of bile acid synthesis; 7α-hydroxylase is under feedback by the amount of bile acids returning to the liver through the portal vein. Dietary bile acids also decrease the expression of 7α-hydroxylase. Bile acid metabolism is summarized in Figure 17.9.

Cholesterol is excreted in the feces

Thus, there is a considerable flux of cholesterol from the liver into bile and then into the duodenum. About 1g of cholesterol is eliminated from the body each day through the feces. Approximately 50% of this is excreted as bile acids and the remainder as the isomeric saturated neutral sterols coprostanol (5β-) and cholestanol (5α-) produced by bacterial reduction of the cholesterol molecule.

Cholestyramine is a bile-acid binding resin which has been used to lower plasma cholesterol

Cholestyramine is a drug which interrupts enterohepatic circulation of the bile acids. It leads to an increase in 7α-hydroxylase activity, increased bile acid synthesis and increased bile acid excretion. Consequently, there is an increased cholesterol synthesis and increased expression of LDL receptor. Cholestyramine was one of the first effective cholesterol-lowering agents but now has been superseded by the statins. The newer lipid-lowering drug that acts on the intestine is the above-mentioned ezetimibe.

MEASUREMENT OF STEROIDS BY GAS CHROMATOGRAPHY-MASS SPECTROMETRY (GCMS)

In the clinical endocrinology laboratory, the measurement of urinary steroid metabolites aids the diagnosis of a number of inherited disorders of the synthesis and metabolism of adrenal steroids, and steroid-producing tumors. It is particularly valuable in identifying the site of the defect in congenital adrenal hyperplasia. These investigations are most often performed in neonates with ambiguous genitalia, children with precocious puberty and in patients with suspected Cushing's syndrome (see Chapter 40). The abnormalities in steroid synthesis are revealed by an alteration in the pattern of urinary steroid metabolites.

The procedure used is gas chromatography-mass spectrometry (GCMS); it is very similar to methods adopted for the identification of anabolic steroids in sport. Steroid metabolites are excreted in urine mostly as water-soluble sulfate or glucuronic acid conjugates. The first step in the analysis involves enzymatic release of the steroids from these conjugates; this is followed by chemical derivatization to increase their stability and improve separation, which is carried out by gas chromatography on capillary columns at high temperatures. Final detection is by mass fragmentation: for each steroid metabolite, a unique ion fragmentation 'fingerprint' is achieved, which allows positive identification and quantitation.

STEROID 21-HYDROXYLASE DEFICIENCY

A neonate is born with ambiguous genitalia. Within 48 hours the infant is hypotensive and distressed. Biochemical investigation reveals:

- Na^+ 115 mmol/L (135–145 mmol/L)
- K^+ 7.0 mmol/L (3.5–5.0 mmol/L)
- 17-hydroxyprogesterone 550 nmol/L (<50 nmol/L)

Comment. This baby has a severe form of steroid 21-hydroxylase deficiency, the commonest of a range of conditions characterized by defects in activity of one of the enzymes in the steroidogenic pathway, known as congenital adrenal hyperplasia. The condition has a genetic basis, and it leads to a failure to produce cortisol (and also possibly aldosterone). This results in reduced negative feedback inhibition of the pituitary production of ACTH. The ACTH continues to stimulate the adrenal gland to produce steroids upstream of the enzyme block. The steroids include 17-hydroxyprogesterone, which is further metabolized to testosterone (Fig. 17.10). This results in androgenization of a female neonate. Mineralocorticoid deficiency causes renal salt wasting and requires urgent treatment with steroids and fluids. Long-term maintenance therapy with hydrocortisone and a mineralocorticoid suppresses ACTH and androgen production. A less severe form of this condition, a partial enzyme deficiency, occurs in young women who present with menstrual irregularity and hirsutism as a consequence of excess of adrenal androgens.

STEROID HORMONES

Cholesterol is the precursor of all the steroid hormones

Mammals produce many steroid hormones, some of which differ only by a double bond or by the orientation of a hydroxyl group. Consequently, it has been necessary to employ systematic nomenclature to detail exact structures. There are three groups of steroid hormones (Fig. 17.10). The corticosteroids have 21 carbon atoms in the basic pregnane ring structure. Loss of the remaining two carbon atoms from the cholesterol side chain produces the androstane ring and the group of hormones known as the androgens. Finally, loss of the angular methyl group at carbon atom 19 as part of the aromatization of the A ring results in the estrane structure found in the estrogens. The presence and position of double bonds and the position and orientation of hydroxyl or other functional groups on the basic nucleus are particular characteristics of individual hormones.

Biosynthesis of the steroid hormones

Conversion of cholesterol into steroid hormones occurs in only three organs: the adrenal cortex, the testis in men and the ovary in women.

A simplification used in practice is to consider the corticosteroids as the products of the adrenal cortex, the androgens as the products of the testis and the estrogens as the products of the ovary. A simplified pathway of steroid synthesis is shown in Figure 17.11 (see also Chapter 39). The relative activity of the steroidogenic enzymes in each of the three organs determines the major secreted product; however, this is not absolute and all three organs are capable of secreting small amounts of steroids belonging to other groups. In pathologic situations, such as a defect in steroidogenesis or a steroid-secreting tumor, a very abnormal pattern of steroid secretion may occur.

Cytochrome P-450 monooxygenase enzymes control steroidogenesis

Most of the enzymes involved in converting cholesterol into steroid hormones are cytochrome P-450 proteins that require oxygen and NADPH. In its simplest form, this enzyme complex catalyzes the replacement of a carbon–hydrogen bond with a carbon–hydroxyl bond; hence, the collective term is monooxygenase. Hydroxylation of the adjacent carbon atoms is the forerunner to cleavage of the carbon–carbon bond. Comparison of the structure of cholesterol (see Fig. 17.2) with those of the steroid hormones (see Fig. 17.10) demonstrates that the biosynthetic pathway is largely made up of cleavage of carbon–carbon bonds and hydroxylation reactions. The enzymes involved have their own nomenclature in which the symbol CYP is followed by a specific suffix.

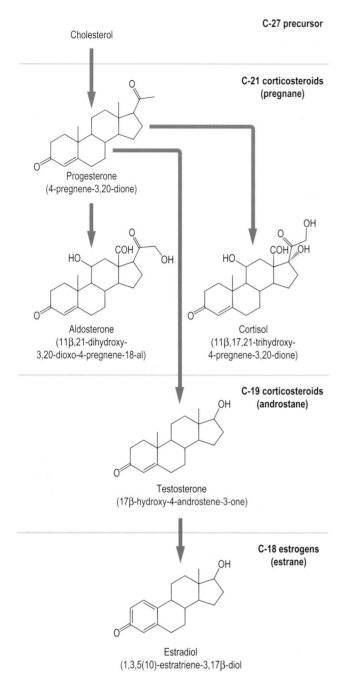

Fig. 17.10 **Structure and nomenclature of the most important human steroid hormones.** Their trivial and systematic names (in parentheses) are shown. For numbering of the atoms in a steroid molecule, see Fig. 17.1; see also Chapter 39.

Thus, CYP21A2 refers to the enzyme that hydroxylates carbon atom 21. (See also Chapter 29.)

Corticosteroids

The cellular substructure of the adrenal cortex is arranged in three layers. The inner two layers (*zona fasciculata* and *zona*

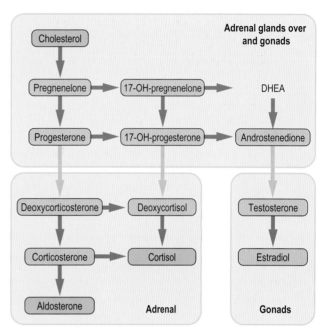

Fig. 17.11 **Steroid biosynthetic pathway.** Note how the pathway branches from cholesterol, eventually leading to synthesis of mineralo-corticoids (e.g. aldosterone), glucocorticoids (cortisol), androgens (testosterone) and estrogens (estradiol).

reticularis) are responsible for the synthesis of cortisol, the main glucocorticoid, and the adrenal androgens. The outer layer (*zona glomerulosa*) is responsible for the synthesis of aldosterone, the main mineralocorticoid (see Chapter 23). Although many of the steps are similar, they are controlled by very different mechanisms.

Biosynthesis of cortisol depends on stimulation by pituitary adrenocorticotropic hormone (ACTH) which binds to its plasma membrane receptor and triggers a range of intracellular events which cause hydrolysis of cholesterol esters stored in lipid droplets and activation of the cholesterol 20,22-desmolase enzyme which converts C-27 cholesterol into pregnenolone, the first of the C-21 pregnane family of corticosteroids. This is the rate-limiting step of steroidogenesis. Thereafter, conversion to cortisol requires a dehydrogenation-isomerization and three sequential hydroxylation reactions at C-17, -21 and -11, under the control of the CYP enzymes. Control of the rate of cortisol biosynthesis is achieved by negative feedback by cortisol on the secretion of ACTH (see Chapter 39).

The main stimulus to the synthesis of aldosterone is not ACTH but angiotensin II (see Chapter 23). Potassium is an important secondary stimulus. Angiotensin II, by binding to its receptor, and potassium, work cooperatively to activate the first step in the pathway: the conversion of cholesterol into pregnenolone. *Zona glomerulosa* lacks the 17α-hydroxylase but has abundant amounts of 18-hydroxylase which is the first of a two-stage reaction, forming the 18-aldehyde group found in aldosterone.

Androgens

Conversion of corticosteroids into androgens requires the 17-20 lyase/desmolase and a substrate that contains a 17α-hydroxyl group. This stimulates the addition of a 17α-hydroxyl group prior to breaking the C17–C20 bond to yield the androstane ring structure. This enzyme is abundant in the Leydig cells of the testis and in the granulosa cells of the ovary. In these cases, however, the rate-limiting cholesterol side chain cleavage step is stimulated by the luteinizing hormone (LH) in the testis and the follicle-stimulating hormone (FSH) in the ovary. Thus, in two different tissues the same biosynthetic step is controlled by two different hormones.

Estrogens

Conversion of androgens into estrogens involves removal of the methyl group at C-19 by the 19-aromatase (see Fig. 39.7). The A ring undergoes two dehydrogenations as part of the reaction, yielding the characteristic 1,3,5(10)-estratriene nucleus. This aromatase is most abundant in the granulosa cells of the ovary, although the enzyme in adipose tissue can also convert some testosterone into estradiol. Biological actions of the steroid hormones are diverse and are best considered as belonging to the trophic hormone system. This system is described in Chapter 39. Many genetic defects have been identified in the structure of the CYP enzymes –these defects lead to abnormal steroid biosynthesis and to clinical disorders such as congenital adrenal hyperplasia.

Mechanism of action and elimination of the steroid hormones

Steroid hormones act via nuclear receptors

All the steroid hormones act by binding to ligand-activated nuclear receptors. Steroid hormone receptors belong to a superfamily of hormone receptors, which include receptors for the thyroid hormone T3 and the active forms of vitamins A and D (see Chapter 40). The specificity of each receptor is being achieved through differing hydrophobic pockets in a small hormone-binding domain. Adjacent to the hormone-binding domain is a highly conserved DNA-binding domain, which is characterized by the presence of two zinc fingers (see Fig. 34.3). Binding of the steroid ligand facilitates translocation of the activated receptor to the nucleus and binding to a specific steroid response element in the promoter regions of target genes, leading to transcription (see Chapter 34). Genetic variability in the structure of steroid receptors may convey a variable degree of hormone resistance and diverse clinical presentations. Biological actions of the steroid hormones are best considered as part of the trophic hormone system described in Chapter 39.

Steroid hormones are excreted in the urine

Most steroid hormones are excreted via the kidney. There are two main steps in this process. First, the biological potency of the steroid must be removed and this is achieved by a series of reduction reactions. Second, the steroid structure must be rendered water soluble, achieved by conjugation to a glucuronide or sulfate moiety, usually through the hydroxyl group at C-3. As a result, many different steroid hormone conjugates are present in urine, some of them in high concentrations. Urinary steroid profiling by gas chromatography-mass spectrometry typically identifies more than 30 such steroids and their relative concentrations may be used to pinpoint specific defects in the steroidogenic pathway (Fig. 17.12).

VITAMIN D₃

Vitamin D_3 (cholecalciferol) is also derived from cholesterol and plays a key role in calcium metabolism. Vitamin D and its metabolites are described in Chapter 25.

A

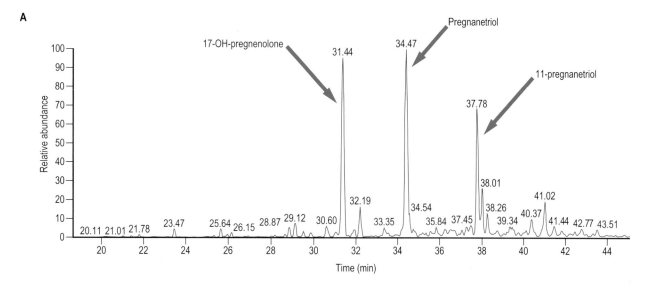

B

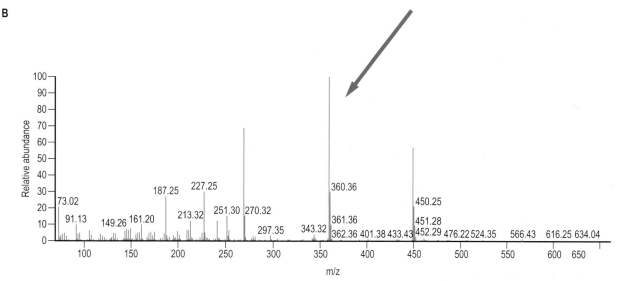

(A) Total ion chromatogram of a urinary steroid metabolite pattern from a patient with 21-hydroxylase deficiency variant of congenital adrenal hyperplasia. In this condition the most prominent steroid metabolites are 17-hydroxypregnanolone, pregnanetriol and 11-oxo-preganetriol.

   x-axis – time in minutes at which the chromatographically separated steroid metabolites are detected by the mass spectrometer. y-axis – relative abundance (quantity of ions)

(B) Complete pattern of ions produced from fragmentation of 11-oxo-pregnanetriol by the mass spectrometry detector.

   x-axis – m/z = mass to charge ratio

   y-axis – relative abundance (quantity of ions)

Fig. 17.12 **Separation of urinary steroids performed by mass spectrometry.** This clinical test box illustrates a urinary steroid metabolite pattern from a patient with 21-hydroxylase deficiency variant of congenital adrenal hyperplasia. In this condition the most prominent steroid metabolites are 17-hydroxypregnanolone, pregnanetriol and 11-oxo-pregnanetriol. x-axis, time in minutes at which the chromatographically separated steroid metabolites are detected by the mass spectrometer; y-axis, relative abundance (quantity of ions).

Summary

- Cholesterol is a vital constituent of cell membranes and the precursor molecule for bile acids, steroid hormones and vitamin D.
- Cholesterol is derived from the diet and is also synthesized de novo from acetyl-CoA. Cholesterol biosynthesis is strictly regulated. The rate-limiting enzyme is the HMG-CoA reductase.
- The metabolism of cholesterol into bile acids and steroid hormones involves several hydroxylation reactions catalyzed by cytochrome P-450 monooxygenase enzymes.
- Several clinical disorders are associated with abnormalities in the regulation of cholesterol homeostasis or metabolism.

ACTIVE LEARNING

1. Describe the regulation of intracellular cholesterol concentration.
2. What are the secondary bile acids and how are they produced?
3. Discuss the enterohepatic circulation of bile acids.
4. Discuss the role of monooxygenases in steroid synthesis.

Further reading

Charlton-Menys V, Durrington PN. Human cholesterol metabolism and therapeutic molecules. *Exp Physiol* 2007;**93**:27–42.

Janowski BA, Willy PJ, Devi TR, Falck JR, Mangelsdorf DJ. An oxysterol signaling pathway mediated by the nuclear receptor LXRa. *Nature* 1996;**383**:728–731.

Marcil M, Brooks-Wilson A, Clee SM et al. Mutations in the *ABC1* gene in familial HDL deficiency with defective cholesterol efflux. *Lancet* 1999; **354**:1341–1346.

Ory DS. Nuclear receptor signaling in the control of cholesterol homeostasis. *Circ Res* 2004;**95**:660–670.

Sakai J, Rawson RB. The sterol regulatory element-binding protein pathway: control of lipid homeostasis through regulated intracellular transport. *Curr Opin Lipidol* 2001;**12**:261–266.

Vegiopoulos A, Herzig S. Glucocorticoids, metabolism and metabolic diseases. *Mol Cell Endocrinol* 2007;**275**:43–61.

18. Lipoproteins and Lipid Transport

M H Dominiczak

LEARNING OBJECTIVES

After reading this chapter you should be able to:

- Describe the composition and functions of lipoproteins present in plasma: chylomicrons, very low-density lipoproteins, remnant particles, low-density lipoproteins and high-density lipoproteins.
- Describe the fuel transport pathway and the overflow pathway of lipoprotein metabolism.
- Describe the reverse cholesterol transport and its links with other pathways of lipoprotein metabolism.
- Outline mechanisms and regulation of intracellular cholesterol concentration, including the role of relevant transcription factors, receptors and enzymes.
- Comment on laboratory tests that assess lipid metabolism and cardiovascular risk.
- Discuss main component processes of atherogenesis: endothelial dysfunction, arterial deposition of lipids, chronic low-grade inflammation, and their relation to atherosclerotic plaque growth and rupture.

INTRODUCTION

Lipoprotein metabolism links closely with the metabolism of energy substrates. In health, lipoproteins transport triacylglycerols (synonymously called triglycerides; we use both terms) and cholesterol between organs and tissues. Abnormalities of lipoprotein metabolism are key factors in the development of atherosclerosis, a process affecting arterial walls and, consequently, blood supply and oxygen delivery to the heart (causing coronary heart disease), brain (causing stroke) and other large arteries (causing peripheral vascular disease). Atherosclerosis-related cardiovascular disease is presently the most frequent cause of death in the industrialized world.

Free fatty acids and triacylglycerols are transported between organs and tissues

Fatty acids are, together with glucose, the main compounds from which metabolism generates energy (energy substrates). Importantly, they can be stored to provide energy during periods of fasting. They are absorbed from the intestine as components of food but are also synthesized endogenously, primarily in the liver and intestine. Their main storage place is adipose tissue, where they are stored as esters of glycerol, triacylglycerols (Chapter 16). Fatty acids need to be transported from their places of absorption or synthesis to peripheral tissues. Free (nonesterified) short- and medium-chain fatty acids travel in plasma bound to albumin but long-chain fatty acids are too hydrophobic to be transported in this manner. Instead, they are transported as triacylglycerols packaged into particles known as lipoproteins. Thus, lipoproteins form a transport network which allows exchanges of triacylglycerols and cholesterol between organs and tissues.

LIPOPROTEINS

Plasma lipoproteins are particles of different size and density

Apart from triacylglycerols, lipoprotein particles contain cholesterol, phospholipids, and proteins (apolipoproteins). They also carry fat-soluble vitamins such as vitamin A and vitamin E. A lipoprotein particle contains a hydrophobic core of cholesterol esters and triacylglycerols (Fig. 18.1). Amphipathic phospholipids and free cholesterol, together with apolipoproteins, form its outer layer. Some proteins, such as apolipoprotein B (apoB), are embedded in the particle

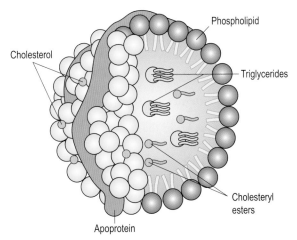

Fig. 18.1 **Lipoprotein particle.** A lipoprotein particle has a hydrophilic external surface and a hydrophobic interior. The external layer contains free cholesterol, phospholipids, and apolipoproteins. Cholesterol esters and triacylglycerols locate in the hydrophobic particle core.

Lipoprotein classes				
Particle	Density (kg/L)	Main component	Apoproteins*	Diameter (μm)
chylomicrons	<0.95	TG	B48 (A, C, E)	75–1200
VLDL	0.95–1.006	TG	B100 (A, C, E)	30–80
IDL	1.006–1.019	TG & cholesterol	B100, E	25–35
LDL	1.019–1.063	Cholesterol	B100	18–25
HDL	1.063–1.210	Protein	AI, AII (C, E)	5–12

*TG, triacylglycerol (triglyceride); VLDL, very low-density lipoproteins; IDL, intermediate-density lipoproteins; HDL, high-density lipoproteins. When separated by electrophoresis VLDL are called pre-β lipoproteins, LDL, β lipoproteins and HDL α lipoproteins. *Main apoproteins present in a given lipoprotein particle are indicated first, with those that are exchanged with other particles in brackets.*

Table 18.1 **Lipoprotein classes.**

surface while others, such as apoC, are only loosely bound and can be easily exchanged.

Lipoproteins present in plasma form a continuum of size and density (Table 18.1). They are classified on the basis of either their density or constituent apolipoproteins. Main lipoprotein classes are chylomicrons, very low-density lipoproteins (VLDL), remnant particles (which include intermediate-density lipoproteins, IDL), low-density lipoproteins (LDL), and high-density lipoproteins (HDL). VLDL and remnant particles are triacylglycerol rich, whereas LDL are triacylglycerol poor and cholesterol rich. Density of the particles increases, and size decreases, with decreasing triacylglycerol content, from chylomicrons (the lightest) through VLDL, IDL, LDL, to HDL (the heaviest). HDL contain different apolipoproteins, cholesterol and phospholipids, but relatively little triacylglycerol.

Apolipoproteins

Apolipoproteins, protein components of lipoprotein particles, play an active role in their metabolism. Also, during particle assembly, it is usually an apolipoprotein which forms a scaffolding for the addition of lipids (lipidation).

Apolipoproteins interact with cellular receptors

Apolipoproteins that sit on the surface of lipoprotein particles determine their metabolic fate through interactions with cellular receptors. They also serve as activators and inhibitors of enzymes participating in lipoprotein metabolism. Main apoproteins are listed in Table 18.2. The most important are apoA, apoB, apoC, apoE, and apo(a). Each class of lipoproteins contains a characteristic set of apoproteins. Apoproteins A (AI and AII) are present in HDL. Apoprotein B variant called apoB100 controls the metabolism of LDL, whereas its truncated form, apoB48 (an N-terminal 48% of apoB100; see Fig. 34.7), controls the chylomicrons.

 LIPOPROTEINS ARE SEPARATED BY ULTRACENTRIFUGATION

Every clinical laboratory uses simple centrifuges to separate red blood cells from serum or plasma. These machines develop a moderate centrifugal force, 2000–3000 g . However, in the specialist lipid, protein and nucleic acid biochemistry much larger centrifugal forces (40000–100000 g) are applied to plasma to separate particles and molecules. This technique is called ultracentrifugation and is extensively used in lipid research. When centrifugal force is applied to a solution, particles that are heavier than the surrounding solvent sediment, and those lighter than the solvent float to the surface at a rate proportional to the applied centrifugal force and to the particle size. The formula below shows factors that affect particle movement:

$$v = [d^2(P_p - P_s) - g]/18\mu$$

where v = sedimentation rate, d = diameter, P_p = particle density, P_s = solvent density, μ = viscosity of the solvent, and g = gravitational force.

In a technique known as flotation ultracentrifugation, plasma is overlayered with a solution of defined density, e.g. 1.063 kg/L, the density of VLDL. After several hours of centrifugation (with the rotor speeds around 40000 rev/min), the VLDL float to the surface, where they can be harvested. Other density solutions can be used to separate other lipoproteins. Modifications of the ultracentrifugation technique, such as density gradient centrifugation, can be applied to separate plasma into several 'bands' containing different lipoprotein fractions.

Apoprotein E controls the receptor binding of remnant particles. Apoproteins C act as enzyme activators and inhibitors and they are extensively exchanged between different lipoprotein classes. Apolipoprotein(a) is a component of lipoprotein(a) (Lp(a)) that may play a role in fibrinolysis.

Functions of apoproteins

Apoprotein	Structural function	Receptor	Effect on enzyme activity
AI	HDL	scavenger receptor	LCAT activator
		B1 (SRB1) putative	
		HDL receptor	
AII	HDL	HDL receptor?	LCAT cofactor
(a)	lp(a)	plasminogen receptor?	probably interferes with fibrinolysis
B48	chylomicrons	LRP	HTGL?
B100	VLDL, IDL, LDL	LDL receptor	–
CI, CII	–	–	LPL activation
CIII	–	–	LPL inhibition
E	remnant particles	LDL receptor	–

Note that apoE and apoB bind to the same cellular receptor: the apoB/E receptor. LCAT, lecithin:cholesterol acyltransferase; LRP, LDL receptor-related protein; HTGL, hepatic triglyceride lipase; LPL, lipoprotein lipase.

Table 18.2 **Functions of lipoproteins.**

LIPOPROTEIN RECEPTORS

LDL receptor is regulated by the intracellular cholesterol concentration

Lipoprotein receptors present on cell membranes mediate the uptake of these particles and thus allow cells to acquire cholesterol and other lipids. The main lipoprotein receptor is the apo B/E receptor also known as the LDL receptor. It was discovered by Joseph Goldstein and Michael Brown, who jointly received the Nobel Prize for this work in 1985. The receptor can bind *either apoB100 or apoE*. ApoE binds to the receptor with a higher affinity than apoB. The mature receptor protein contains 839 amino acids and spans the cell membrane (Fig. 18.2). The receptor gene is located on chromosome 19 and its expression is regulated by the intracellular cholesterol concentration. Importantly, the truncated form of apoB, apoB48, present in chylomicrons, cannot bind to the apoB/E receptor; however, the chylomicron remnants possess apoE that can bind to the apoB/E receptor and to another receptor called LDL receptor-related protein (LRP).

Scavenger receptors are nonspecific and nonregulated

While the apoB/E receptor has well-defined ligands, scavenger receptors are membrane receptors that can bind many

THERE ARE STRUCTURAL SIMILARITIES BETWEEN LIPOPROTEIN(a) AND PLASMINOGEN

Lipoprotein(a) is assembled in the liver and has a pre-β mobility on electrophoresis. Its density spans the LDL and HDL range (1.04–1.125 g/mL). It consists of an apoB100-containing LDL particle linked through a disulfide bond to another apoprotein, apo(a). Apo(a) is a glycoprotein characterized by considerable number of variants (isoforms) of different size. Molecular mass of these isoforms ranges between 200 and 800 kDa. Apo(a) possesses a protease domain and a number of repeating sequences of approximately 80–90 amino acids in length, stabilized by disulfide bonds into a triple-loop structure. These structures are called kringles (the name of Danish pastry of similar shape). One of the kringles, kringle IV, is repeated 35 times within the apo(a) sequence. The number of kringle IV repeats determines the size of the lipoprotein (a) isoforms. Interestingly, apo(a) exhibits a considerable sequence homology with plasminogen, a protein involved the clot resolution (fibrinolysis; see Chapter 6). Although it does not possess plasminogen's protease activity, it may impair the action of plasminogen.

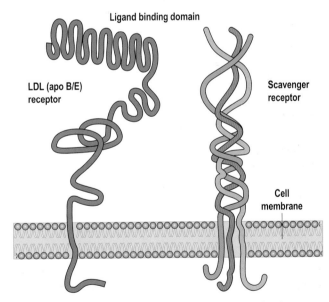

Fig.18.2 **Lipoprotein receptors.** The apoB/E receptor, also known as the LDL receptor, mediates the cellular uptake of intact LDL particles. The scavenger receptor internalizes chemically modified (e.g. oxidized) LDL. Both types of receptor span cell membranes. The expression of LDL receptor is regulated by the intracellular cholesterol concentration, while the scavenger receptor remains unregulated. The scavenger receptor type A, illustrated here, is present on macrophages and has a collagen-like structure. Scavenger receptor type BI participates in HDL metabolism (compare Fig. 26.5).

different molecules. They are present on phagocytic cells such as macrophages. They also differ from the LDL receptor in that they are not subject to feedback regulation, and therefore they may overload the cell with whatever ligand they bind. Scavenger receptors are designated as class A and class B and CD36. Class A receptors have a collagen-like triple helical structure. They do not bind intact LDL but readily bind chemically modified (e.g. oxidized) LDL (see Fig. 37.5). Class B receptor takes up HDL particles in the liver.

ENZYMES AND TRANSFER PROTEINS THAT PARTICIPATE IN LIPOPROTEIN METABOLISM

Two hydrolases, lipoprotein lipase (LPL) and hepatic triglyceride lipase (HTGL), remove triacylglycerols from lipoprotein particles. LPL is bound to heparan sulfate proteoglycans on the surface of the vascular endothelial cells, and HTGL is associated with plasma membranes in the liver. LPL digests triacylglycerols in the chylomicrons and VLDL, and releases fatty acids and glycerol to cells. HTGL acts on particles partially digested by LPL and facilitates the conversion of IDL into LDL (see below).

Lecithin:cholesterol acyltransferase (LCAT) is a glycoprotein enzyme synthesized in the liver, which is associated with HDL. LCAT esterifies cholesterol acquired by HDL from cells. LCAT is activated by apoAI. Note that within cells cholesterol is esterified by a different enzyme – acylCoA:acylcholesterol transferase (ACAT). There are two isoforms of ACAT: ACAT1 is the primary isoform in macrophages and ACAT2 is present in the intestine and liver. Another protein, the cholesterol ester transfer protein (CETP), facilitates the exchange of cholesterol esters for triacylglycerols between HDL and VLDL and IDL.

PATHWAYS OF LIPOPROTEIN METABOLISM

The main stages of lipoprotein metabolism are as follows:

- Assembly of lipoprotein particles. Chylomicrons are assembled in the intestine, and VLDL in the liver.
- Transfer of fatty acids from lipoproteins to cells. This is facilitated by LPL and HTGL and transforms chylomicrons and VLDL into remnant particles.
- Binding of the remnant particles to receptors and their cellular uptake.
- Transformation of some remnants into LDL, their subsequent binding to B/E receptor and uptake.
- Reverse cholesterol transport, i.e. removal of cholesterol from cells by the HDL particles.

The pathway involving the assembly of chylomicrons (after a meal) or the assembly of VLDL (in the fasting state), their transfer to peripheral tissues, their hydrolysis by lipoprotein lipase, and the cellular uptake of remnants is closely related to the feed–fast cycle (see Chapter 21) and, through this, to energy metabolism. Because the key process here is the transport of triacylglycerols, we will call it the *fuel transport pathway* (Fig. 18.3). The fuel transport pathway is closely linked to the reverse cholesterol transport through exchanges of lipoprotein components. It generates LDL as a byproduct of distribution of energy substrates. We will call the LDL metabolism, from the stage of hydrolysis of remnant particles by HTGL to LDL uptake by cells, *the overflow pathway*.

Fuel transport pathway of lipoprotein metabolism

Chylomicrons transport dietary lipids

Triacylglycerols present in food are acted upon by pancreatic lipases and are absorbed as monoacylglycerols, free fatty acids, and free glycerol (see Chapter 10). The intestinal cells (enterocytes) resynthesize triacylglycerols and, together with phospholipids, cholesterol and apoB48, assemble them into chylomicrons. These are secreted into the lymph and reach plasma through the thoracic duct.

Their main apoprotein is apoB48. Chylomicrons also contain apoproteins A, C, and E. Once the chylomicrons reach peripheral tissues, their triacylglycerols are hydrolyzed by the LPL, and the fatty acids enter cells. What is left of the chylomicrons are smaller particles called chylomicron remnants. Remnants acquire some cholesterol esters from the HDL (see below). The change in particle size uncovers apoE which mediates the remnant binding to the apoB/E receptor and to the LRP in the liver. The half-life of chylomicrons in plasma is less than 1 h. Chylomicrons normally appear in plasma only after fat-containing meals, giving plasma a milky appearance (see Fig. 18.3).

VLDL particles transport triacylglycerols synthesized in the liver

Triacylglycerols synthesized in the liver are transported by the VLDL. They are assembled in the liver around apoB100 molecules. The lipidation of apoB is facilitated by the microsomal triglyceride transfer protein (MTP). Unused apoB100 is degraded by ubiquitin-dependent protease (see Chapter 33, Fig. 33.10). After being secreted into plasma, VLDL acquire cholesteryl esters and apoproteins (apoC and apoE) from the HDL. In the peripheral tissues, their triacylglycerols are hydrolyzed by the LPL in a way analogous to chylomicrons; this yields VLDL remnants also called IDL. In the VLDL, the conformations of apoB100 and apoE do not allow

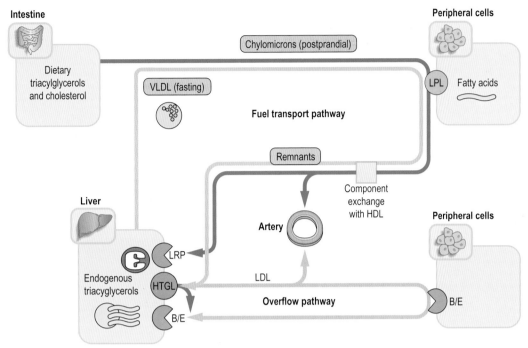

Fig.18.3 **Lipoprotein metabolism: the fuel transport pathway and the overflow pathway.** *The fuel transport pathway* is linked to energy metabolism and to the feed–fast cycle. In the fed state, chylomicrons transport triacylglycerols (triglycerides) to the periphery, where lipoprotein lipase hydrolyzes the triglycerides, liberating fatty acids into cells. Chylomicron remnants are metabolized in the liver. In the fasting state, VLDL transport fuel from the liver to peripheral tissues. Their remnants also return to the liver through the B/E receptor. Chylomicron remnants are also taken up by the LRP. Remnant particles acquire additional cholesteryl esters from the HDL in exchange for triglycerides. Remnants are short-lived and atherogenic. In clinical practice, the best indicator of the the activity of the fuel transport pathway is the measurement of plasma triglycerides. *The overflow pathway* is the pathway of LDL metabolism. LDL are generated from remnants in the fuel transport pathway, are cholesterol rich and atherogenic. Also their residence time in the circulation is longer than that of the remnants. They are taken up by the apoB/E receptor in response to decrease in intracellular cholesterol concentration. In clinical practice, the indicators of activity of the overflow pathway are the measurements of plasma total cholesterol and LDL-cholesterol. LPL, lipoprotein lipase; LRP, LDL receptor-related protein.

binding to the apoB/E receptor. However, in the remnant particles, apoE assumes a conformation that allows such binding. Thus, the remnants are either taken up by the liver or are further hydrolyzed by another enzyme, the hepatic triglyceride lipase, and transform into LDL.

Because of the loss of triglycerides, remnant particles are now relatively cholesterol rich. Also, their small size facilitates penetration of the endothelial layer – this makes them atherogenic.

Overflow pathway of lipid metabolism

LDL particles are taken up by cells by the same route as remnant particles

LDL is a small lipoprotein generated from the remnants by the hepatic triglyceride lipase. LDL are cholesterol rich and contain only one apolipoprotein: the apo B100. They are the main carrier of cholesterol in plasma. They remain in the circulation much longer than the remnants and are taken up through the apoB/E receptor (although they have lower

affinity for the receptor than apoE-containing remnants) either by the liver (approximately 80% of particles) or by the peripheral cells (see Fig. 18.3).

Intracellular cholesterol synthesis and uptake are interdependent

Most cells synthesize their own cholesterol. However, when the concentration of intracellular cholesterol decreases, cells can acquire it from the outside – and lipoproteins constitute a pool of extracellular cholesterol upon which the cells draw. After internalization, the LDL–receptor complex is digested by lysosomal enzymes and released cholesterol is esterified within the cell. The receptor protein recycles back to the membrane. Free cholesterol released within the cell is a feedback regulator of its own synthesis. This is mediated by a family of transcription factors called sterol regulatory element-binding proteins (SREBPs). SREBPs regulate transcription of genes coding for enzymes responsible for cholesterol synthesis: the 3-hydroxy-3-methylglutaryl coenzyme A synthase and HMG-CoA reductase, and also the gene

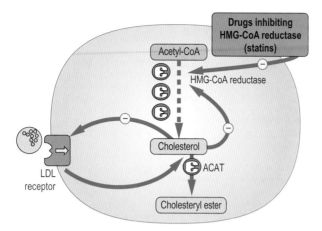

Fig. 18.4 **Regulation of the intracellular cholesterol concentration.** Intracellular cholesterol regulates the activity of the HMG-CoA reductase, the rate-limiting enzyme in cholesterol synthesis, and also the expression of LDL receptors on the cell membrane. The relevant gene expression is controlled by the SREBP transcription factors (see also Fig. 17.7). ACAT, acyl-CoA:acylcholesterol transferase; SREBP, sterol-regulatory-element binding protein.

coding for the apoB/E receptor (see also Chapter 17). Depletion of hepatic sterols increases the SREBP level and consequently cholesterol synthesis and the expression of the apoB/E receptor. On the other hand, increased intracellular cholesterol concentration inhibits the SREBP pathway, decreasing cholesterol synthesis and receptor expression (Fig. 18.4; see also Fig. 17.7).

Pathway of reverse cholesterol transport

Cholesterol is removed from cells to the HDL by specific transporter molecules

The function of HDL particles is to transport cholesterol in the 'reverse' direction: from peripheral tissues to the liver (Fig. 18.5). HDL are synthesized in the intestine and liver. Their main apolipoproteins are apoAI and apoAII but they also contain apoC and apoE. Importantly, HDL are able to exchange apoproteins, phospholipids, triacylglycerol and cholesteryl esters with chylomicrons, VLDL, and the remnants.

HDL are formed as discoid, lipid-poor particles (pre-β HDL) which contain mainly apoAI; they are partly constructed from the excess phospholipid shed from VLDL during their hydrolysis by LPL. These nascent HDL accept cholesterol from cells through the action of a membrane protein known as the ATP-binding cassette transporter A1 (ABCA1; see Chapter 8). ABCA1 uses ATP as a source of energy and is the rate-limiting controller of the efflux of free cholesterol to apoAI. Another ATP-binding cassette transporter, ABCG1, transfers cholesterol from cells to mature HDL particles. Others known as ABCG5 and ABCG8, reside in the apical

membranes of hepatocytes where they control the movement of cholesterol into bile. ABCA1 and ABCG1 genes are regulated by the liver X receptor (see Chapter 17).

After nascent HDL acquires the free cholesterol, it is esterified by LCAT and its cholesteryl esters move into the interior of the HDL particle. The particle, now known as HDL-3, enlarges, assuming a spherical shape. Aided by cholesterol ester transfer protein, it transfers some cholesteryl esters to triglyceride-rich lipoproteins (including VLDL and chylomicron remnants) in exchange for triglycerides; this allows cholesterol esters to reenter the VLDL-IDL-LDL pathway. The acquisition of triglycerides makes it still larger; it is now called HDL-2. HDL2 binds to the class B scavenger receptors in the liver and transfers cholesterol to the cell membrane. The particle is not taken up by cells but shrinks again, and its redundant parts become nascent HDL that participate in the next cycle of transport.

Apart from their participation in the reverse cholesterol transport, HDL have other atheroprotective properties. For instance, they activate the endothelial nitric oxide synthase, eNOS, promoting production of NO. They also have anti-inflammatory properties.

FAMILIAL HYPERCHOLESTEROLEMIA CAUSES EARLY HEART ATTACKS

A 32-year-old heavy smoker developed a sudden crushing chest pain. He was admitted to the casualty department. Myocardial infarction was confirmed by ECG changes and by high cardiac troponin concentration. On examination the patient had tendon xanthoma on hands and thickened Achilles tendons. There was a strong family history of coronary heart disease (his father had had a coronary bypass graft at the age of 40 and his paternal grandfather died of myocardial infarction in his early fifties). His cholesterol was 10.0 mmol/L (390 mg/dL), triglycerides 2 mmol/L (182 mg/dL) and HDL 1.0 mmol/L (38 mg/dL).

Comment. This patient has familial hypercholesterolemia (FH), an autosomal dominant disorder characterized by a decreased number of LDL receptors. FH carries a very high risk of premature coronary disease, and heterozygotic individuals may suffer heart attacks as early as the third or fourth decade of life. The frequency of FH homozygotes in Western populations is approximately 1:500. This patient was immediately treated with intravenous tissue plasminogen activator. Subsequently he underwent coronary artery bypass graft and was treated with lipid-lowering drugs (statins). His cholesterol concentration subsequently decreased to 4.8 mmol/L (185 mg/dL) and triglyceride (triacylglycerol) level to 1.7 mmol/L, with HDL-cholesterol increasing to 1.1 mmol/L (42 mg/dL).

PLASMA C-REACTIVE PROTEIN CONCENTRATION REFLECTS CHRONIC LOW-GRADE INFLAMMATION THAT CONTRIBUTES TO ATHEROGENESIS

Inflammatory reaction associated with infection can be detected by measuring the concentration of plasma C-reactive protein (CRP), a protein synthesized in the liver in response to stimulation by proinflammatory cytokines. Its name comes from its binding to the capsular (C) polysaccharide of bacteria such as *S. pneumoniae,* by which method it mediates their clearance. Very small increases in CRP concentration, which require a highly sensitive (hs) analytic method to detect, may reflect the chronic inflammatory processes in vascular walls. Epidemiologic studies demonstrated an association between the hsCRP concentration and cardiovascular events. Importantly, this association is independent of the link between plasma cholesterol and coronary disease. Increased plasma concentrations of other proinflammatory molecules, such as interleukin-6 (IL-6) and serum amyloid A, have also been linked to coronary heart disease (compare Fig. 26.9).

excess of lipoproteins, hypertension, diabetes or by components of cigarette smoke. Initially the damage is functional rather than structural. Endothelium loses its cell-repellent quality and admits inflammatory cells into the vascular wall. It also becomes more permeable to lipoproteins which deposit in the intima. Later, structural damage or a complete destruction of endothelial cells takes place.

Cell adhesion to the dysfunctional endothelium is mediated by the adhesion molecules present on its surface. Molecules called selectins mediate the initial interactions of cells with the endothelium. The key molecule that promotes adhesion of monocytes (white blood cells that are precursors of macrophages) and T lymphocytes is the vascular cell adhesion molecule-1 (VCAM-1). Adhering cells are stimulated by the monocyte chemoattractant protein-1 (MCP-1) to cross the endothelium and lodge in the intima. Animal experiments confirm that deficiency of VCAM-1 decreases the formation of atherosclerotic plaques.

Monocytes are also attracted to developing plaques by the chemoattractant cytokine CCL2 which binds to monocyte receptors. In the intima, under the influence of interferon-γ, tumor necrosis factor (TNF), granulocyte-macrophage colony-stimulating factor, and monocyte colony-stimulating factor secreted by the endothelial cells and VSMC, monocytes transform into macrophages. Some macrophages start to produce cytokines such as IL-1β, IL-6 and TNF-α. Other express scavenger receptors (such as the scavenger receptor class A, and CD36) become active in endocytosis. Importantly, macrophages produce reactive oxygen species, which oxidize LDL in the intima.

Production of NO in the damaged endothelium decreases. This promotes vasoconstriction. NO normally reduces monocyte adhesion and VSMC migration and proliferation, so these processes became disinhibited.

Activation of the renin-angiotensin-aldosterone system, apart from its effect on blood pressure, has proatherogenic effects. Angiotensin II (see Chapter 23) contributes to cell entry into the intima by increasing expression of VCAM-1 and MCP-1. Clinical studies show that drugs inhibiting that axis (ACE inhibitors) are beneficial in cardiovascular prevention.

Lipid entry into the arterial wall is a key factor in atherogenesis

Hypercholesterolemia contributes to induction of VCAM-1 and MCP-1. The intrusion of lipids into the vascular wall is a hallmark of atherosclerosis. The smaller lipoprotein particles, the remnants and the LDL, are most atherogenic because they enter the vascular wall more easily. Moreover, while in the plasma, LDL particles are protected against oxidation by antioxidants such as vitamin C and β-carotene. This protection is removed in the intima and phospholipids and fatty acids present in LDL became prone to oxidation mediated by enzymes such as lipoxygenases, myeloperoxidase, and NADPH oxidases that are present in the activated

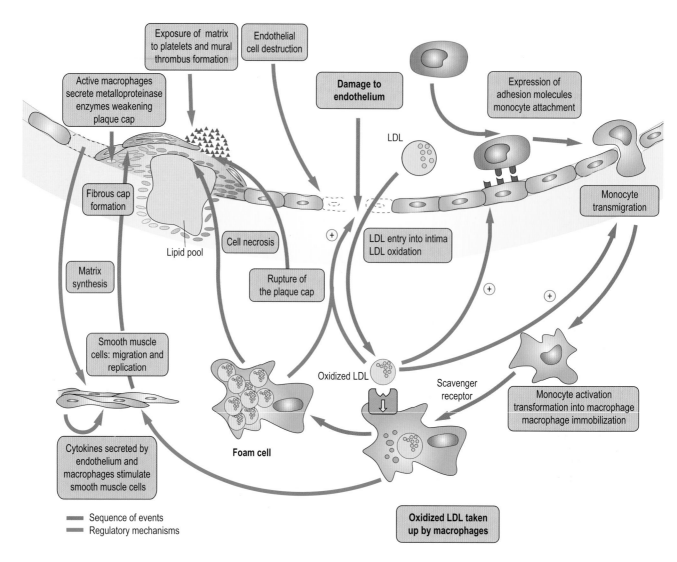

Fig. 18.7 Atherogenesis: the process. Atherogenesis is driven by signals mediated by cytokines and growth factors generated by endothelial cells, macrophages, T lymphocytes and vascular smooth muscle cells (VSMC). There are multiple activation paths: for instance, the expression of MCP-1 and VCAM-1 may be stimulated by signals generated by the macrophages as well as by the oxidized LDL. VSMC may be stimulated by the dysfunctional endothelial cells, by macrophages, and by T lymphocytes (note also the autocrine activation). Note that a hormone, angiotensin II, also participates in these processes. MCP-1, monocyte chemoattractant protein 1; VCAM-1, vascular cell adhesion molecule 1; ICAM-1, intracellular cell adhesion molecule 1; TNF-β, tumor necrosis factor β; TNF-α, tumor necrosis factor α; IFN-γ, interferon γ; NO, nitric oxide; PDGF, platelet-derived growth factor; bFGF, basic fibroblast growth factor; IGF-1, insulin-like growth factor 1; EGF, epidermal growth factor; TGF-β, transforming growth factor β; IL-1, interleukin-1.

macrophages. Oxidized LDL are quite toxic to their environment. They further stimulate expression of VCAM-1 and MCP-1. They damage the endothelial cells and are mitogenic for macrophages. The LDL apolipoprotein, apoB100, once oxidized, binds to the scavenger receptors rather than to the apoB/E receptor. Because scavenger receptors are not feed-back regulated by the intracellular cholesterol level, macrophages which take up oxidized LDL overload with lipids. As a result, their appearance changes into the so-called foam cells; conglomerates of such cells known as fatty streaks are visible in the arterial walls. Dying foam cells release the accumulated lipids, which form pools within the intima. These pools become centers of mature atherosclerotic plaques.

Migration and proliferation of the vascular smooth muscle cells change the structure of the vascular wall

All the above events take place in the arterial intima. However, secretion of growth factors such as the platelet-derived growth factor (PDGF), the epidermal growth factor (EGF) and the insulin-like growth factor-1 (IGF-1) by the endothelial cells and macrophages activates VSMC normally present in the media. VSMC proliferate and migrate into the intima. They also secrete a range of their own active molecules: the adhesion molecules, the MCP-1 as well as cytokines and growth factors such as interleukin-1 (IL-1), and TNF-α. Activated VSMC also synthesize extracellular matrix, in particular collagen, and deposit it in the growing

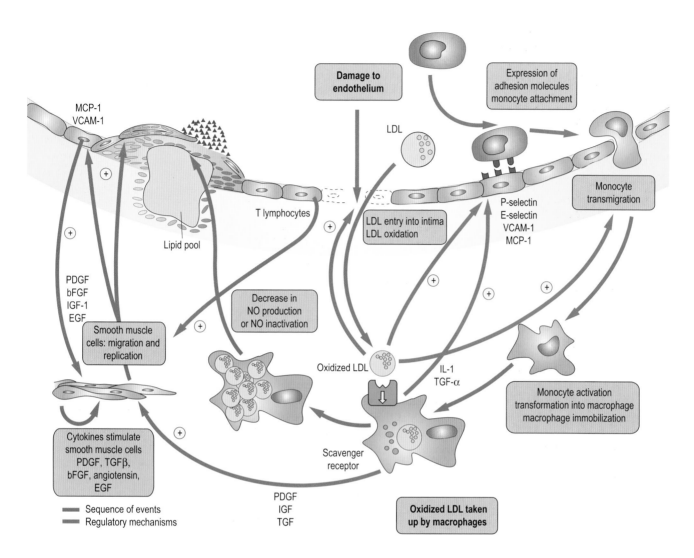

Fig.18.8 **Atherogenesis: the role of growth factors and cytokines.** Atherogenesis involves endothelial dysfunction, deposition of lipids in the arterial intima, inflammatory reaction, and the migration and proliferation of the vascular smooth muscle cells. Note the role of oxidized lipids in the formation of lipid-laden cells and the lipid center of the atherosclerotic plaque. The sequence of events is described in the text. (Compare Fig. 18.7.) Abbreviations are explained in Figure 18.7 on p. 230.

plaque. All this disrupts the normally ordered structure of the arterial wall. Newly formed plaques may protrude into the lumen of the artery, interfering with the blood flow.

Inflammation plays a fundamental role in atherogenesis

Exit of monocytes and T leukocytes from plasma and their activation in the intima are parts of the inflammatory response. Normally, such response is initiated by an antigen or trauma. Intriguingly, no specific antigen capable of initiating atherogenesis has been identified. There could be a molecular mimicry between such putative antigen(s) and the exogenous pathogens (Chapter 38). The antigen(s) might be infectious agents or modified molecules generated by reactive oxygen species. For instance, the phosphorylcholine group found in the oxidized LDL is also a component of the capsular polysaccharide of bacteria. Oxidized LDL remains a candidate

antigen that could be responsible for the stimulation of inflammatory reaction in atherogenesis.

Atherogenesis involves both innate and adaptive immunity. Innate immunity includes recognition of molecules by scavenger receptors A and CD36. When molecules that possess patterns encoded in immune memory bind to these receptors, they activate cells through, for instance, the pathway involving the transcription factor NFκB. T cells, involved in adaptive immunity, are also present in atherosclerotic lesions and circulating IgG and IgM-type antibodies against modified LDL have been identified in plasma (Chapter 38).

Prostaglandins and leukotrienes contribute to atherogenesis

One should mention here the role of active lipid molecules such as prostaglandins in atherogenesis. Prostaglandin synthesis from the arachidonic acid is catalyzed by the enzyme cyclooxygenase (COX). COX-1 in the platelets is inhibited by aspirin; this decreases production of prothrombotic thromboxane A_2 and is responsible for the cardioprotective effect of the drug. Proinflammatory prostaglandins such as prostaglandin E_2 (PGE_2) contribute to the inflammatory process. Leukotrienes (leukotriene A4 and B4), other lipids derived from the arachidonic acid, are generated by the enzyme 5-lipoxygenase and contribute to the recruitment of lymphocytes to atherosclerotic lesions.

Atherosclerotic plaques grow slowly, but the real danger is the possibility of sudden rupture

The foam cells and the lipid pool become centers of atherosclerotic plaques. VSMC which had migrated into the intima synthesize collagenous matrix which covers the lipid pool with a fibrous 'cap'. The cap also contains VSMC, active macrophages, and T lymphocytes. A mature plaque on the one hand penetrates the arterial wall, and on the other obstructs the arterial lumen (Fig. 18.9). Parts of advanced lesions may become calcified.

Importantly, growth of a plaque may be accelerated by a cycle of plaque rupture and thrombosis. In the plaque, active macrophages and T lymphocytes reside preferentially at its edges. Macrophages secrete enzymes which degrade extracellular matrix that belong to the metalloproteinase (MMP) family, which includes collagenases, gelatinases and stromyelysin. Lysosomal proteases (cathepsins) also contribute by degrading collagen and elastin. In addition, T cells activated by macrophages secrete interferon-γ (IFN-γ) and proinflammatory

cytokines IL-1, IL-2, and TNF-α. IFN-γ induces MMP expression and inhibits VSMC collagen synthesis, further weakening the cap. VSMC present in the most vulnerable edge regions of the plaque may undergo apoptosis. Such activity in the plaque makes it prone to rupture. When the plaque ruptures, it exposes its interior to the blood. Plaque interior is highly thrombogenic due to the presence of the tissue factor, a small-molecular-weight glycoprotein that initiates the extrinsic clotting cascade (see Chapter 7). Platelets also become activated and thrombus forms quickly on the ruptured surface. Such thrombus may completely occlude the lumen of the affected artery. This cuts off oxygen supply and causes tissue necrosis in the area supplied by the involved artery. Not all instances of plaque rupture result in complete lumen blockages and dramatic clinical events. However, even small hemorrhages and minute thrombi accelerate plaque growth.

ASSESSMENT OF CARDIOVASCULAR RISK

Cardiovascular risk is the probability that a person will suffer heart attack or stroke in a defined period in the future. The main cardiovascular risk factors are listed in Table 18.5. Knowledge of plasma concentrations of lipoproteins is essential for the assessment of cardiovascular risk.

Epidemiologic studies show that the risk of cardiovascular disease is primarily related to plasma concentrations of total cholesterol and LDL-cholesterol. It is also inversely related

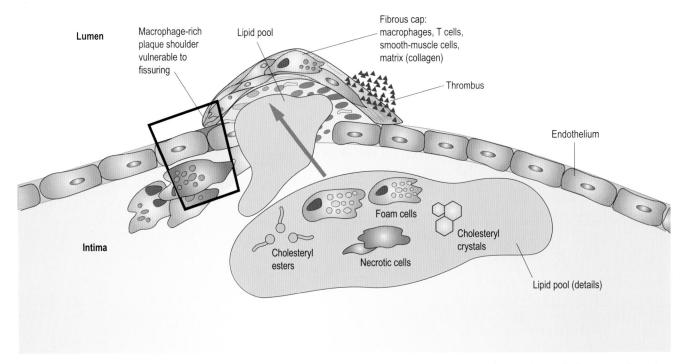

Fig. 18.9 **Atherosclerotic plaque.** The lipid center and fibrous cap are the main parts of a mature atherosclerotic plaque which emerges from the structurally remodeled vascular wall. A plaque that is rich in cells is unstable and may easily rupture. The key process leading to plaque rupture is digestion of the collagenous matrix of the plaque cap by metalloproteinase enzymes. The figure illustrates areas vulnerable to breakage and shows the obstructing thrombus that forms at the rupture site.

to the concentration of HDL-cholesterol. Inclusion of triglycerides (in clinical medicine the term triglyceride is used in preference to triacylglycerol) as determinants of risk has long been disputed. Recent research makes it quite clear that they contribute to risk. Particularly interesting are data which show an association between the postprandial (non-fasting) concentrations of triglycerides and the risk of future events.

As far as cholesterol concentrations are concerned, it seems that there is no lower threshold at which the risk

GENETICS OF ATHEROSCLEROSIS

Genes coding for LDL receptors, apolipoproteins and LRP6 are currently the only ones that have been directly linked with atherosclerotic disorders. However, the hope is that the new genome-wide association studies will identify more complex polygenic traits (Chapter 36). Particularly interesting recent data suggest that genes involved in the regulation of cell cycle may be linked to atherogenesis. The technical ability to perform genome-wide scans changed the way this type of research is conducted. Formerly, accumulation of results from many single studies would lead to elucidation of mechanisms and then perhaps a search for their role in disease. In contrast, genome-wide studies often provide evidence of association between a pathologic condition and a gene before anything is known about the underlying mechanisms. Only later would investigators search for processes that may underpin such association.

would plateau (in other words, the lower, the better). The risk clearly increases when total cholesterol concentration increases above 5.2 mmol/L (200 mg/dL). According to the US National Cholesterol Education Program Adult Treatment Panel III (ATPIII), the desirable level of total cholesterol is below 5.2 mmol/L (200 mg/dL) and the optimal level of LDL-cholesterol is below 2.6 mmol/L (100 mg/dL).

Importantly, the 'target' cholesterol concentration needs to be lower in people who are at increased risk of cardiovascular events, because they have several risk factors, and in those who already have atherosclerosis-related disease. In such persons the ATPIII recommends lowering LDL-cholesterol to below 2.6 mmol/L (100 mg/dL) and even 1.8 mmol/L (70 mg/dL).

The Joint British Societies' Guidelines (JBS2) published in 2005 recommend that the optimal total cholesterol concentration in persons who have an increased cardiovascular risk is 4 mmol/L (155 mg/dL) and optimal LDL-cholesterol concentration is 2.0 mmol/L (77 mg/dL). Triglyceride concentration should be no higher than 1.7 mmol/L.

In contrast to a high total cholesterol or LDL-cholesterol, it is the low concentration of HDL-cholesterol that signifies increased risk. HDL-cholesterol concentration below 1 mmol/L (40 g/dL) in men or 1.2 mmol/L (47 mg/dL) in women is regarded as undesirably low and a concentration above 1.6 mmol/L (60 mg/dL) provides some protection against coronary disease. The principles of lipid testing are summarized in Figure 18.10.

One should remember that the risk associated with plasma concentrations of the 'main' lipids can be modified by other

Cardiovascular risk factors and their management

Risk factor	Comment	Remedy
Male sex	the difference in cardiovascular risk between sexes equalizes in postmenopausal women	
Age		
Smoking		smoking cessation
High plasma cholesterol (high LDL-cholesterol)	2–3% decrease in risk for 1% decrease of total plasma cholesterol	diet low in saturated fats and, where appropriate, cholesterol-lowering drugs
Low plasma HDL		smoking cessation, regular exercise
Hypertension	major risk factor for stroke and a risk factor for CHD	control blood pressure: diet and drugs
Obesity		weight reduction
Sedentary lifestyle		regular exercise
Diabetes	cardiovascular disease is the main cause of death in diabetes	diet and drugs (insulin in type 1 diabetes) (see Chapter 21)

Table 18.5 **Cardiovascular risk factors and their management.** Plasma lipids are not the only factors that determine the risk of cardiovascular disease. This table lists the most important cardiovascular risk factors and the risk-reducing strategies used in cardiovascular prevention.

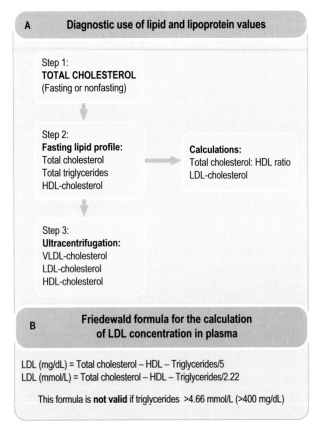

A   Diagnostic use of lipid and lipoprotein values

Step 1:
TOTAL CHOLESTEROL
(Fasting or nonfasting)

Step 2:
Fasting lipid profile:
Total cholesterol
Total triglycerides
HDL-cholesterol

Calculations:
Total cholesterol: HDL ratio
LDL-cholesterol

Step 3:
Ultracentrifugation:
VLDL-cholesterol
LDL-cholesterol
HDL-cholesterol

B   Friedewald formula for the calculation of LDL concentration in plasma

LDL (mg/dL) = Total cholesterol – HDL – Triglycerides/5
LDL (mmol/L) = Total cholesterol – HDL – Triglycerides/2.22

This formula is **not valid** if triglycerides >4.66 mmol/L (>400 mg/dL)

Fig.18.10 **Laboratory diagnosis of dyslipidemias.** (A) The initial screening test is the measurement of total cholesterol concentration in plasma. The next step, the fasting lipid profile, includes measurements of the total cholesterol, cholesterol present in the HDL fraction (HDL-cholesterol) and triacylglycerols (triglycerides). From these data, the cholesterol concentration in the LDL fraction (LDL-cholesterol) can be calculated. Analysis of lipoprotein subfractions using the ultracentrifugation method, and measurements of plasma apolipoproteins are specialist tests. Total cholesterol-to-HDL ratio is an important marker of cardiovascular risk: a ratio above 5 indicates increased risk. Note that the American ATPIII recommendations suggest performing a fasting lipid profile as the initial investigation, rather than screening for cholesterol only. (B) Calculation of plasma LDL-cholesterol concentration. LDL-cholesterol can be calculated from the values of total cholesterol, triglycerides, and HDL-cholesterol using the Friedewald formula.

factors, such as increased concentration of Lp(a), plasma homocysteine, fibrinogen or C-reactive protein (hsCRP). In fact, about 50% of persons who suffer from myocardial infarction have an 'average' cholesterol and LDL-cholesterol concentrations. The search for new biomarkers continues.

CLINICAL MANAGEMENT OF DYSLIPIDEMIAS

Since, as we discussed, arteriosclerosis is a multifactorial process, effective cardiovascular prevention needs an approach

 LIFESTYLE CHANGE IMPROVES PLASMA LIPID PROFILE

A 57-year-old man was referred to the lipid clinic because of hypertriglyceridemia (high triacylglycerol concentration). His triglycerides were 6 mmol/L (545 mg/dL), cholesterol was 5 mmol/L (192 mg/dL), and HDL was 1 mmol/L (39 mg/dL). He was obese, took 30 units of alcohol per week, and led a sedentary lifestyle. After initial difficulties, he eventually managed to lose 7 kg of weight over 6 months, cut drinking to below 20 units per week, and started to exercise regularly. Twelve months later, his triglycerides were 2.5 mmol/L (227 mg/dL), cholesterol 4.8 mmol/L (186 mg/dL), and HDL 1.2 mmol/L (46 mg/dL).

Comment. Lifestyle change may result in appreciable improvements in the lipid profile. To achieve this, individuals need to become committed to changing lifestyle and to maintaining the change over a prolonged period of time.
Note: 1 unit of alcohol is a one measure (60 mL) of liquor, one glass (170 mL) of wine or a half-pint (300 mL) of beer.

that combines lifestyle modification (smoking cessation, diet and regular exercise) with drug treatment of dyslipidemia, hypertension and diabetes (see Table 18.5). The concentration of plasma LDL (and consequently total plasma cholesterol) can decrease by approximately 15% when a person consistently follows a low-cholesterol diet. There are several classes of drugs that lower plasma cholesterol concentration.

Statins inhibit HMG-CoA reductase

Statins such as simvastatin, pravastatin, atorvastatin and rosuvastatin are competitive inhibitors of HMG-CoA reductase, the rate-limiting enzyme in cholesterol synthesis. They primarily lower plasma LDL-cholesterol. The inhibition of this enzyme results in a decrease in intracellular cholesterol concentration. This decrease, through SREBP transcription factors (see Fig. 17.7), increases expression of LDL receptors on the cell membrane. An increase in the number of cellular receptors leads to increased cellular uptake of LDL and, consequently, to a lower plasma cholesterol concentration. Treatment with statins decreases cholesterol concentration by 30–60% (depending on the preparation), and decreases future cardiovascular events by 20–30%.

Fibrates act through PPARα

Derivatives of fibric acid (fibrates) are agonists of PPARα transcription factor. They stimulate the LPL, decrease plasma triglyceride concentrations, and increase the concentration of HDL. Their effect on LDL and total cholesterol is less pronounced than that of the statins.

PRESENCE OF XANTHELASMA DOES NOT NECESSARILY INDICATE DYSLIPIDEMIA

A 28-year-old woman developed unsightly yellow marks around both eyes (xanthelasma). She was asymptomatic and had a good exercise tolerance. Her cholesterol was 5.0 mmol/L (192 mg/dL), triglycerides 0.7 mmol/L (64 mg/dL), and her HDL-cholesterol was 1.4 mmol/L (53 mg/dL). There was no family history of early coronary disease.

Comment. Xanthelasma may occur in individuals with completely normal lipid levels. On the other hand, lipid deposits in tendons (tendon xanthomata) are always diagnostic of familial lipid disorder. The patient was reassured and referred for cosmetic surgery.

Inhibitors of intestinal absorption bind bile acids and inhibit cholesterol transporter

Inhibitors of intestinal absorption of cholesterol include older drugs, the so-called bile acid-binding resins, that are now rarely used. They decreased plasma cholesterol concentration by interrupting the recirculation of cholesterol from the intestine and increasing its excretion. The newer drug ezetimibe inhibits the intestinal cholesterol transporter and lowers total cholesterol by approximately 20%. Longer-term studies of its clinical benefit are in progress.

Omega-3 fatty acids lower triglyceride concentration

A substantial decrease in plasma triglyceride concentration can be achieved by treatment with omega-3 fatty acids contained in fish oil.

Role of antioxidants continues to be studied

In animals, antioxidants such as probucol or vitamin E inhibit development of atherosclerosis. Epidemiologic studies have shown that those who take antioxidants such as vitamin E and C or β-carotene have a decreased risk of cardiovascular disease. However, prospective clinical trials of antioxidant treatment failed to confirm such preventive benefit. One tentative explanation is that it is the natural antioxidants (such as those contained in fruits) or their combinations that are protective, rather than single pure substances.

Summary

- Lipoproteins transport hydrophobic lipids between organs and tissues.
- Chylomicrons mediate the transport of dietary fat.
- VLDL mediate the transport of endogenously synthesized fat.

ACTIVE LEARNING

1. Compare the composition of VLDL and LDL.
2. What are the differences between the transport of dietary triacylglycerols and triacylglycerols synthesized in the liver?
3. Describe the transport pathway for dietary fatty acids.
4. Give examples of interactions between different cell types in atherogenesis.
5. How does atherosclerotic plaque rupture?
6. In what way does endothelial dysfunction contribute to atherosclerosis?

- Chylomicrons, VLDL and remnant lipoproteins are part of the organism's fuel distribution network: the fuel transport pathway.
- LDL are cholesterol-rich lipoproteins which emerge from the fuel transport pathway. When present in excess, they may enter the arterial wall.
- HDL mediate reverse cholesterol transport, e.g. removal of cholesterol from the peripheral cells to the liver.
- Atherogenesis involves endothelial dysfunction, lipid deposition, inflammatory reaction in the arterial wall, and activation and proliferation of the arterial smooth muscle cells.
- Interactions between different types of cells participating in atherogenesis are mediated by an array of cytokines, growth factors and adhesion molecules.
- Atherogenesis disrupts the structure of the arterial wall and results in the formation of atherosclerotic plaque, which narrows the lumen of the affected artery. However, the immediate cause of a heart attack is not the slow growth of the plaque, but its sudden rupture.
- Arteriosclerosis-related diseases are coronary heart disease, stroke and peripheral vascular disease.

Further reading

Dominiczak MH. Risk factors for coronary disease: the time for a paradigm shift? *Clin Chem Lab Med* 2001;**39**:907–919.

Durrington P. Dyslipidaemia. *Lancet* 2003;**362**:717–731.

Duval C, Muller M, Kersten S. PPAR alpha and dyslipidemia (review). *Biochim Biophys Acta Mol Biol Cell Biol Lipids* 2007;**1771**:961–971.

Expert Panel on Detection, Evaluation and Treatment of High Blood Cholesterol in Adults. Executive Summary of the Third Report of the National Cholesterol Education Program (NCEP) Expert Panel on Detection, Evaluation and Treatment of High Blood Cholesterol in Adults (Adult Treatment Panel III). *JAMA* 2001;**285**:2486–2497.

Grundy SM, Cleeman JI, Merz NB et al. Implications of recent clinical trials for the National Cholesterol Education Program Adult Treatment Panel III Guidelines. *Circulation* 2004;**110**:227–239.

Harrison GK. Inflammation, atherosclerosis and coronary artery disease. *N Engl J Med* 2005;**352**:1685–1695.

Joint British Societies' guidelines on prevention of cardiovascular disease in clinical practice. *Heart* 2005;**91(Suppl V)**:V1–V52.

LaRosa JC. Low-density lipoprotein cholesterol reduction: the end is more important than the means. *Am J Cardiol* 2007;**100**:240–242.

Libby P. Aikawa M. Stabilization of atherosclerotic plaques: new mechanisms and clinical targets. *Nature Med* 2002;**8**:1257–1262.

Rader DJ. Daugherty A. Translating molecular discoveries into new therapies for atherosclerosis. *Nature* 2008;**451**:904–913.

Websites

British Heart Foundation: www.bhf.org.uk/
American Heart Association: www.americanheart.org
National Heart, Lung and Blood Institute: www.nhlbi.nih.gov/nhlbi/nhlbi.htm/

19. Biosynthesis and Degradation of Amino Acids

Allen B Rawitch

LEARNING OBJECTIVES

After reading this chapter you should be able to:

- Describe the three mechanisms used by humans for removal of the nitrogen from amino acids prior to the metabolism of their carbon skeletons.
- Outline the sequence of reactions in the urea cycle and trace the flow of nitrogen from amino acids into and out of the cycle.
- Describe the role of vitamin B_6 in aminotransferase reactions.
- Define the terms and give examples of glucogenic and ketogenic amino acids.
- Summarize the factors that contribute to the input and the depletion of the pool of free amino acids in animals.
- Summarize the sources and use of ammonia in animals and explain the concept of nitrogen balance.
- Identify the essential amino acids and the metabolic sources of the nonessential amino acids.
- Explain the biochemical basis and the therapeutic rationale for treatment of phenylketonuria and maple syrup urine disease.

INTRODUCTION

In addition to their roles as building blocks for peptides and proteins, and as precursors of neurotransmitters and hormones, amino acids are a source of energy from the diet and during fasting. The carbon skeletons of some amino acids can be used to produce glucose through gluconeogenesis, thereby providing a metabolic fuel for tissues that require or prefer glucose; such amino acids are designated as glucogenic or glycogenic amino acids. The carbon skeletons of some amino acids can also produce the equivalent of acetyl-CoA or acetoacetate and are termed ketogenic, indicating that they can be metabolized to give immediate precursors of lipids or ketone bodies. In an individual consuming adequate amounts of protein, a significant quantity of amino acids may also be converted to carbohydrate (glycogen) or fat (triacylglycerol) for storage. Unlike carbohydrates and lipids, amino acids do not have a dedicated storage form equivalent to glycogen or fat.

When amino acids are metabolized, the resulting excess nitrogen must be excreted. Since the primary form in which the nitrogen is removed from amino acids is ammonia, and because free ammonia is quite toxic, humans and most higher animals rapidly convert the ammonia derived from amino acid catabolism to urea, which is neutral, less toxic, very soluble, and excreted in the urine. Thus the primary nitrogenous excretion product in humans is urea, produced by the urea cycle in liver. Animals that excrete urea are termed ureotelic. In an average individual, more than 80% of the excreted nitrogen is in the form of urea (25–30 g/24 h). Smaller amounts of nitrogen are also excreted in the form of uric acid, creatinine, and ammonium ion.

The carbon skeletons of many amino acids may be derived from metabolites in central pathways, allowing the biosynthesis of some, but not all, the amino acids in humans. Amino acids that can be synthesized in this way are therefore not required in the diet (nonessential amino acids), whereas amino acids having carbon skeletons that cannot be derived from normal human metabolism must be supplied in the diet (essential amino acids). For the biosynthesis of nonessential amino acids, amino groups must be added to the appropriate carbon skeletons. This generally occurs through the transamination of an α-keto acid corresponding to that specific amino acid.

METABOLISM OF DIETARY AND ENDOGENOUS PROTEINS

Relationship to central metabolism

Although body proteins represent a significant proportion of potential energy reserves (Table 19.1), under normal circumstances they are not used for energy production. In an extended fast, however, muscle protein is degraded to amino acids for the synthesis of essential proteins, and to keto acids for gluconeogenesis to maintain blood glucose concentration. This accounts for the loss of muscle mass during fasting.

In addition to its role as an important source of carbon skeletons for oxidative metabolism and energy production, dietary protein must provide adequate amounts of those amino acids that we cannot make, to support normal protein synthesis. The relationships of body protein and dietary protein to central amino acid pools and to central metabolism are illustrated in Figure 19.1.

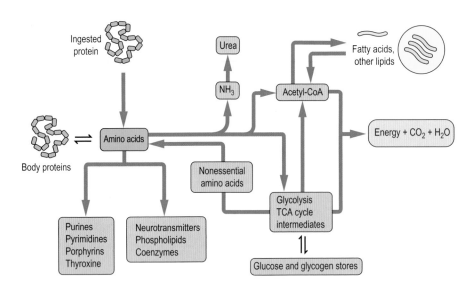

Fig. 19.1 **Metabolic relationships among amino acids.** The pool of free amino acids is derived from the degradation and turnover of body proteins and from the diet. The amino acids are precursors of important biomolecules, including hormones, neurotransmitters and proteins, and also serve as a carbon source for central metabolism, including gluconeogenesis, lipogenesis and energy production.

Storage forms of energy in the body

Stored fuel	Tissue	Amount (g)*	Energy (kj)	(kcal)
Glycogen	liver	70	1176	280
Glycogen	muscle	120	2016	480
Free glucose	body fluids	20	336	80
Triacylglycerol	adipose	15 000	567 000	135 000
Protein	muscle	6000	100 800	24 000

*in a 70-kg individual.

Table 19.1 **Storage forms of energy in the body.** Proteins represent a substantial energy reserve in the body. (Adapted with permission from Cahill GF Jr, *Clin Endocrinol Metab* 1976;**5**:398.)

Digestion and absorption of dietary protein

In order for dietary protein to contribute to either energy metabolism or pools of essential amino acids, the protein must be digested to the level of free amino acids or small peptides and absorbed across the gut. Digestion of protein begins in the stomach with the action of pepsin, a carboxyl protease that is active in the very low pH found in the gastric environment. Digestion continues as the stomach contents are emptied into the small intestine and mixed with pancreatic secretions. These pancreatic secretions are alkaline and contain the inactive precursors of several serine proteases including trypsin, chymotrypsin and elastase along with carboxypeptidases. The process is completed by enzymes in the small intestine (see Chapter 10). After any remaining di- and tripeptides are broken down in enterocytes, the free amino

 ALANINE AND INTERORGAN CARBON AND NITROGEN FLOW

Much of the carbon flow that occurs between peripheral tissues, such as skeletal muscle, and the liver is facilitated by the release of alanine into the blood by the peripheral tissues. The alanine is converted to pyruvate in the liver and the nitrogen component is incorporated into urea. The pyruvate can be used for gluconeogenesis to produce glucose, which is released into the blood for transport back to peripheral tissues. This 'glucose–alanine cycle' allows the net conversion of amino acid carbons to glucose, the elimination of amino acid nitrogen as urea, and the return of carbons to the peripheral tissues in the form of glucose (Chapter 21). This cycle works in a fashion similar to the Cori cycle (Chapter 21) in which lactate, released from skeletal muscle, is used for hepatic gluconeogenesis, the key difference being that alanine also carries a nitrogen atom to the liver. Alanine and glutamine are released in approximately equal quantities from skeletal muscle and represent almost 50% of the amino acids released by skeletal muscle into the blood – an amount that far exceeds the proportion of these amino acids in muscle proteins. Thus, there is substantial remodeling of protein-derived amino acids by transamination reactions, prior to their release from muscle.

acids are transported to the portal vein and carried to the liver for energy metabolism or biosynthesis, or distributed to other tissues to meet similar needs.

Turnover of endogenous proteins

In addition to the ingestion, digestion and absorption of amino acids from dietary protein, all the proteins in the body have a half-life or lifespan and are routinely degraded

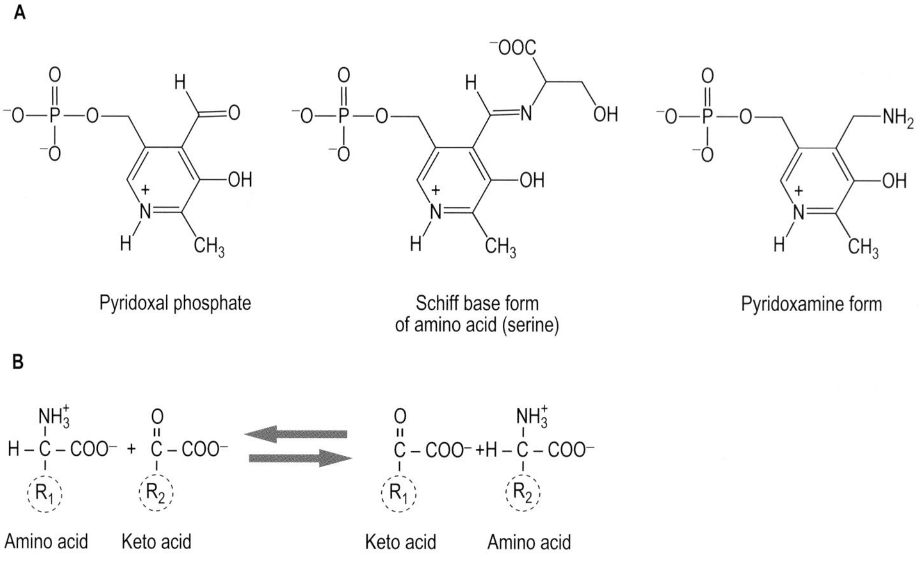

A

Pyridoxal phosphate

Schiff base form
of amino acid (serine)

Pyridoxamine form

B

Amino acid   Keto acid

Keto acid   Amino acid

Fig. 19.2 **The catalytic role of pyridoxal phosphate.** Aminotransferases or transaminases use pyridoxal phosphate as a cofactor. A pyridoxamine adduct acts as an intermediate in transfer of an amino group between an α-amino acid and an α-keto acid. (A) Structures of the components involved. The cofactor, pyridoxal phosphate, is used in a variety of enzyme-catalyzed reactions involving both amino and keto compounds, including transamination and decarboxylation reactions. (B) Transamination involves both a donor α-amino acid (R_1), and an acceptor α-keto acid (R_2). The products are an α-keto acid derived from the carbon skeleton of R_1 and an α-amino acid from the carbon skeleton of R_2.

to amino acids and replaced with newly synthesized protein. This process of protein turnover is carried out in the lysosome or by proteasomes. In the case of lysosomal digestion, protein turnover begins with engulfment of the protein or organelle in vesicles known as autophagosomes, by a process known as autophagy. The vesicles then fuse with lysosomes and the protein, lipid and glycans are degraded by lysosomal acid hydrolases. Cytosolic proteins are degraded primarily by proteasomes which are high molecular-weight complexes containing multiple proteolytic activities. There are both ubiquitin-dependent (Chapter 29) and ubiquitin-independent pathways for degradation of cytosolic proteins.

AMINO ACID DEGRADATION

Amino acids destined for energy metabolism must be deaminated to yield the carbon skeleton. There are three mechanisms for removal of the amino group from amino acids.

- **Transamination** – the transfer of the amino group to a suitable keto acid acceptor (Fig. 19.2)
- **Oxidative deamination** – the oxidative removal of the amino group, resulting in keto acids and ammonia (see Fig. 19.5)
- **Removal of a molecule of water by a dehydratase** – e.g. serine or threonine dehydratase; this reaction produces an unstable, imine intermediate that hydrolyzes spontaneously to yield an α-keto acid and ammonia (see Fig. 19.5).

Metabolism of the carbon skeleton and the amino group are coordinated

The principal mechanism for removal of amino groups from the common amino acids is via transamination, or the

MEASUREMENT OF BLOOD UREA NITROGEN

Serum urea measurements (also reported by laboratories as BUN or blood urea nitrogen) are critical in monitoring patients with a variety of metabolic diseases in which the metabolism of amino acids may be affected and in tracking the condition of individuals with renal problems. The traditional methodology used for measuring blood urea has relied on the action of the enzyme urease which converts urea to CO_2 and ammonia. The resulting ammonia can be detected spectrophotometrically by formation of a colored compound on reaction with phenol or a related compound (the Berthelot reaction).

REACTION TO MONOSODIUM GLUTAMATE

A healthy 30-year-old woman experienced the sudden onset of headache, sweating, and nausea after eating at an Oriental restaurant. She felt weak and experienced some tingling and a sensation of warmth in her face and upper torso. The symptoms passed after about 30 minutes and she experienced no further problems. Upon visiting her doctor the next day, she learned that some individuals react to foods containing high levels of the food additive monosodium glutamate, the sodium salt of glutamic acid.

Comment. The flu-like symptoms that develop, previously described as 'Chinese restaurant syndrome', have been attributed to central nervous system (CNS) effects of glutamate or its derivative, the inhibitory neurotransmitter γ-amino butyric acid (GABA). Interestingly, studies have shown that this phenomenon causes no permanent CNS damage and that, although bronchospasm may be triggered in individuals with severe asthma, the symptoms are generally brief and completely reversible.

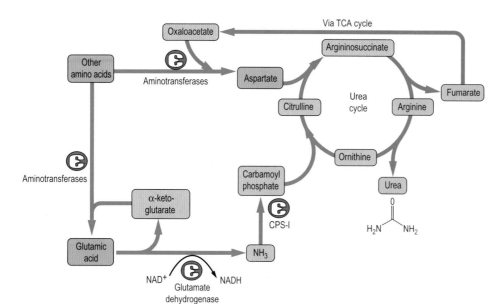

Fig. 19.3 **Sources of nitrogen atoms in the urea cycle.** Nitrogen enters the urea cycle from most amino acids via transfer of the α-amino group to either oxaloacetate or α-ketoglutarate, to form aspartate or glutamate, respectively. Glutamate releases ammonia in the liver through the action of GDH. The ammonia is incorporated into carbamoyl phosphate, and the aspartate combines with citrulline to provide the second nitrogen for urea synthesis. Oxaloacetate and α-ketoglutarate can be repeatedly recycled to channel nitrogen into this pathway. CPS-I, carbamoyl phosphate synthetase-I.

transfer of amino groups from the amino acid to a suitable α-keto acid acceptor, most commonly to α-ketoglutarate or oxaloacetate. Several enzymes, called aminotransferases (or transaminases), are capable of removing the amino group from most amino acids and producing the corresponding α-keto acid. Aminotransferase enzymes use pyridoxal phosphate, a cofactor derived from the vitamin B$_6$ (pyridoxine), as a key component in their catalytic mechanism; pyridoxamine is an intermediate in the reaction. The structures of the various forms of vitamin B$_6$ and the net reaction catalyzed by aminotransferases are shown in Figure 19.2.

Nitrogen atoms are incorporated into urea from two sources

The transfer of an amino group from one keto acid carbon skeleton to another may seem to be unproductive and not useful in itself; however, when one considers the nature of the primary keto acid acceptors that participate in these reactions (α-ketoglutarate and oxaloacetate) and their products (glutamate and aspartate), the logic of this metabolism becomes clear. The two nitrogen atoms in urea are derived exclusively from these two sources (Fig. 19.3), thereby linking amino acid catabolism to energy metabolism. Ammonia, which is produced primarily from glutamate via the glutamate dehydrogenase (GDH) reaction (Fig. 19.4B), enters the urea cycle as carbamoyl phosphate. The second nitrogen is contributed to urea by aspartic acid. Fumarate is formed in this process and may be recycled through the tricarboxylic acid (TCA) cycle to oxaloacetate, which can accept another amino group and reenter the urea cycle, or the fumarate may be used for energy metabolism or gluconeogenesis. Thus the funneling of amino groups from other amino acids into glutamate and aspartate provides the nitrogen for urea

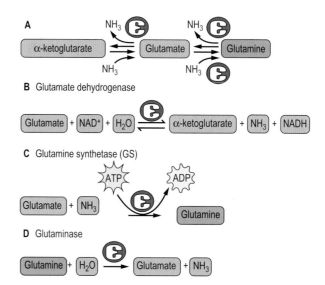

Fig. 19.4 **Relationships between glutamate, glutamine and α-ketoglutarate.** The several forms of the carbon skeleton of glutamic acid have key roles in the metabolism of amino groups. (A) Three forms of the same carbon skeleton. (B) The GDH reaction is a reversible reaction that can produce glutamate from α-ketoglutarate or convert glutamate to α-ketoglutarate and ammonia. The latter reaction is important in the synthesis of urea because amino groups are fed to α-ketoglutarate via transamination from other amino acids. (C) Glutamine synthetase catalyzes an energy-requiring reaction with a key role in transport of amino groups from one tissue to another; it also provides a buffer against high concentrations of free ammonia in tissues. (D) The second half of the glutamine transport system for nitrogen is the enzyme glutaminase, which hydrolyzes glutamine to glutamate and ammonia. This reaction is important in the kidney for management of proton transport and pH control. GDH, glutamate dehydrogenase.

synthesis in a form appropriate for the urea cycle (see Fig. 19.3). The other pathways that lead to the release of amino groups from some amino acids through the action of amino acid oxidase or dehydratases (Fig. 19.5) make

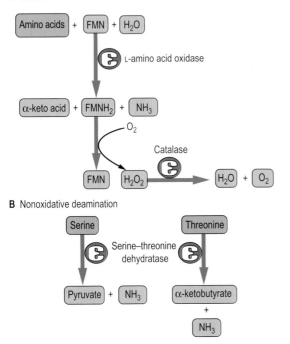

A Oxidative deamination

B Nonoxidative deamination

Fig. 19.5 **Deamination of amino acids.** The primary route for amino group removal is via transamination, but there are additional enzymes capable of removing the α-amino group. (A) L-amino acid oxidase produces ammonia and an α-keto acid directly, using flavin mononucleotide (FMN) as a cofactor. The reduced form of the flavin must be regenerated using molecular oxygen; this reaction is one of several that produce H_2O_2. The peroxide is decomposed by catalase. (B) A second means of deamination is possible only for hydroxyamino acids (serine and threonine), through a dehydratase mechanism; the Schiff base, imine intermediate hydrolyzes to form the keto acid and ammonia.

relatively minor contributions to the flow of amino groups from amino acids to urea.

The central role of glutamine

In addition to the role of glutamate as a carrier of amino groups to GDH, glutamate serves as a precursor of glutamine, a process that consumes a molecule of ammonia. This is important because glutamine, along with alanine, is a key transporter of amino groups between various tissues and the liver, and is present in greater concentrations than most other amino acids in blood. The three forms of the same carbon skeleton, α-ketoglutarate, glutamate, and glutamine, are interconverted via aminotransferases, glutamine synthetase, glutaminase, and GDH (see Fig. 19.4). Thus glutamine can serve as a buffer for ammonia utilization, as a source of ammonia, and as a carrier of amino groups. Because ammonia is quite toxic, a balance must be maintained between its production and utilization. A summary of the sources and pathways that use or produce ammonia is shown in Figure 19.6. It should be noted that the GDH reaction is reversible under physiologic conditions if amino groups are required for amino acid and other biosynthetic processes.

The urea cycle and its relationship to central metabolism

Urea is the principal nitrogenous excretion product in humans (Table 19.2). The urea cycle (see Fig. 19.3) was the first metabolic cycle to be well defined; its description

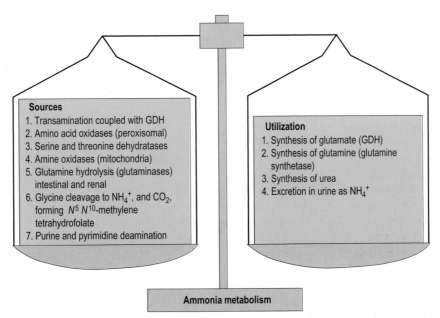

Fig. 19.6 **Balance in ammonia metabolism.** The balance between production and utilization of free ammonia is critical for maintenance of health. This figure summarizes the sources and pathways that use ammonia. Although most of these reactions occur in many tissues, urea synthesis is restricted to the liver. Glutamine and alanine function as the primary transporters of nitrogen from peripheral tissues to the liver.

preceded that of the TCA cycle. The start of the urea cycle may be considered the synthesis of carbamoyl phosphate from an ammonium ion, derived primarily from glutamate via GDH (see Fig. 19.3), and bicarbonate in liver mitochondria. This reaction requires two molecules of ATP and is catalyzed by the enzyme carbamoyl phosphate synthetase

I (CPS I) (Fig. 19.7), which is found at high concentration in the mitochondrial matrix.

The mitochondrial isozyme, CPS I, is unusual in that it requires *N*-acetylglutamate as a cofactor. It is one of two carbamoyl phosphate synthetase enzymes that have key roles in metabolism. The second, CPS II, is found in the cytosol, does not require *N*-acetylglutamate, and is involved in pyrimidine biosynthesis.

Ornithine transcarbamoylase catalyzes the condensation of carbamoyl phosphate with the amino acid ornithine, to form citrulline: see Figure 19.3 for pathway and Table 19.3

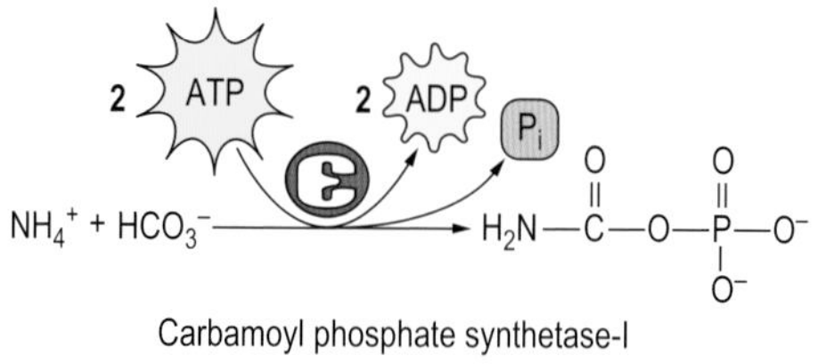

Urinary nitrogen excretion		
Urinary metabolite	**g excreted/24 h***	**% of total**
Urea	30	86
Ammonium ion	0.7	2.8
Creatinine	1.0–1.8	4–5
Uric acid	0.5–1.0	2–3

*Approximate values in an average adult male.

Table 19.2 **Urinary nitrogen excretion.**

Carbamoyl phosphate synthetase-I

Fig. 19.7 **Synthesis of carbamoyl phosphate.** The first nitrogen, derived from ammonia, enters the urea cycle as carbamoyl phosphate, synthesized by carbamoyl phosphate synthetase I in the liver.

Enzymes of the urea cycle			
Enzyme	**Reaction catalyzed**	**Remarks**	**Reaction product**
Carbamoyl phosphate synthetase	formation of carbamoyl phosphate from ammonia and CO_2	fixes ammonia released from amino acids, uses 2 ATP, located in the **mitochondrion,** deficiency leads to high blood concentrations of ammonia and related toxicity	Carbamoyl phosphate
Ornithine transcarbamoylase	formation of citrulline from ornithine and carbamoyl phosphate	releases P_i, an example of a transferase, located in the **mitochondrion,** deficiency leads to high blood concentrations of ammonia and orotic acid, as carbamoyl phosphate is shunted to pyrimidine biosynthesis	citrulline
Argininosuccinate synthetase	formation of arginino-succinate from citrulline and aspartate	requires ATP, which is cleaved to AMP + PP_i – an example of a ligase, located in the **cytosol,** deficiency leads to high blood concentrations of ammonia and citrulline	argininosuccinate
Argininosuccinase	cleavage of argininosuccinate to arginine and fumarate	an example of a lyase, located in **cytosol,** deficiency leads to high blood concentrations of ammonia and citrulline	fumarate + arginine
Arginase	cleavage of arginine to ornithine and urea	an example of a hydrolase, located in the **cytosol** and primarily in the liver, deficiency leads to moderately increased blood ammonia and high blood concentrations of arginine	urea + ornithine

Table 19.3 **Enzymes of the urea cycle.** Five enzymes catalyze the urea cycle in liver. The first enzyme, CPS-I, which fixes NH_4^+ as carbamoyl phosphate, is the regulatory enzyme and is sensitive to the allosteric effector, *N*-acetylglutamate.

for structures. In turn, the citrulline is condensed with aspartate to form argininosuccinate. This step is catalyzed by argininosuccinate synthetase and requires ATP; the reaction cleaves the ATP to adenosine monophosphate (AMP) and inorganic pyrophosphate (PPi) (2 ATP equivalents). The formation of argininosuccinate incorporates the second nitrogen atom destined for urea. Argininosuccinate is cleaved by argininosuccinase to arginine and fumarate, and the arginine is then cleaved by arginase to yield urea and ornithine. The ornithine can reenter the urea cycle, while the urea diffuses into the blood, is transported to the kidney and excreted in urine. The net process of ureogenesis is summarized in Table 19.4.

The urea cycle is split between the mitochondrial matrix and the cytosol

The first two steps in the urea cycle occur in the mitochondrion. The citrulline which is formed in the mitochondrion

Urea synthesis		
Component reactions in urea synthesis		
$CO_2 + NH_3 + 2\,ATP$	→	carbamoyl phosphate + 2 ADP + Pi
Carbamoyl phosphate + ornithine	→	citrulline + Pi
Citrulline + aspartate + ATP	→	argininosuccinate + AMP + PPi
Argininosuccinate	→	arginine + fumarate
Arginine	→	urea + ornithine
$CO_2 + NH_3 + 3\,ATP$ + aspartate	→	urea + 2 ADP + AMP + 2 Pi + PPi + fumarate

Table 19.4 **Urea synthesis.**

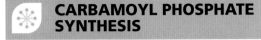

CARBAMOYL PHOSPHATE SYNTHESIS

The enzyme carbamoyl phosphate synthetase I (CPS I) is found in the mitochondrion and primarily in the liver; a second enzyme, CPS II, is found in the cytosol and in virtually all tissues. Although the product of both these enzymes is the same, namely carbamoyl phosphate, the enzymes are derived from different genes and function in ureogenesis (CPS I) or pyrimidine biosynthesis (CPS II), respectively. Additional differences between the two enzymes include their source of nitrogen (NH_3 for CPS I, and glutamine CPS II) and their requirement for *N*-acetylglutamate (required by CPS I but not by CPS II). Under normal circumstances, CPS I and II function independently and in different cellular compartments; however, when the urea cycle is blocked, e.g. as a result of a deficiency in ornithine transcarbamoylase, the accumulated mitochondrial carbamoyl phosphate spills over into the cytosolic compartment and may stimulate excess pyrimidine synthesis, resulting in a build-up of orotic acid in the blood and urine.

then moves into the cytosol by a specific passive transport system. The cycle is completed in the cytosol with the release of urea from arginine and the regeneration of ornithine. Ornithine is transported back across the mitochondrial

AMMONIA TOXICITY

Ammonia encephalopathy

The mechanisms involved in ammonia toxicity – the encephalopathy in particular – are not well defined. It is clear, however, that when its concentration builds up in the blood and other biologic fluids, ammonia diffuses into cells and across the blood–brain barrier. The increase in ammonia causes an increased synthesis of glutamate from α-ketoglutarate and increased synthesis of glutamine. Although this is a normal detoxifying reaction in cells, when concentrations of ammonia are significantly increased, supplies of α-ketoglutarate in cells of the CNS may be depleted, resulting in inhibition of the TCA cycle and a decrease in ATP production. There may be additional mechanisms accounting for the bizarre behavior observed in individuals with high blood concentrations of ammonia. Either glutamate, a major inhibitory neurotransmitter, or its derivative, γ-amino butyric acid (GABA), may also contribute to the CNS effects.

PARKINSON'S DISEASE

An otherwise healthy, 60-year-old man noticed an occasional tremor in his left arm when relaxing and watching television. He also noticed occasional muscle cramping in his left leg, and his spouse noticed that he would occasionally develop a trance-like stare. A complete physical examination and consultation with a neurologist confirmed a diagnosis of Parkinson's disease. He was prescribed a medication that contained L-dihydroxyphenylalanine (L-DOPA) and a monoamine oxidase inhibitor (MAOI). L-DOPA is a precursor of the neurotransmitter dopamine, while monoamine oxidase is the enzyme responsible for the oxidative deamination and degradation of dopamine. His symptoms improved immediately, but he gradually experienced significant side effects from the medication, especially the occurrence of involuntary movements.

Comment. Parkinson's disease is caused by the death of dopamine-producing cells in the substantia nigra and the locus ceruleus. Although medication can markedly reduce the symptoms, the disease is progressive and may result in severe disability. Dopaminergic agonists often have side effects and also have limited effect on tremor so that other treatments such as deep brain stimulation or ablation are used in selected cases. Monoamine oxidase is also involved in deamination of other amines in the brain, so that MAOIs have many undesirable side effects. Transplantation of dopaminergic fetal tissue is a controversial experimental treatment at present (see also Chapter 42).

HEREDITARY HYPERAMMONEMIA

An apparently healthy 5-month-old female infant was brought to a pediatrician's office by her mother, with a complaint of periodic bouts of vomiting and a failure to gain weight. The mother also reported that the child would oscillate between periods of irritability and lethargy. Subsequent examination and laboratory results revealed an abnormal electroencephalogram, a markedly increased concentration of plasma ammonia (323 mmol/L, 550 mg/dL; the normal range is 15–88 mmol/L, 25–150 mg/dL), and greater than normal concentrations of glutamine, but low concentrations of citrulline. Orotate, a pyrimidine nucleotide precursor, was found in her urine.

Comment. The infant was admitted to hospital and treated with intravenous phenylacetate and benzoate along with arginine. The benzoate and phenyllactate are metabolized to glycine and glutamate conjugates which are excreted, with their nitrogen content, into urine; arginine stimulates residual urea cycle activity. The infant improved rapidly and was discharged from hospital on a low-protein diet with arginine supplementation. Subsequent biopsy of the patient's liver indicated that her hepatic ornithine transcarbamoylase activity was about 10% of normal.

SCREENING FOR AMINO ACID METABOLIC DEFECTS IN THE NEWBORN

In most developed countries today, a spot of the blood of newborn infants is routinely collected on filter paper and tested for a series of compounds which are markers of inherited metabolic disease. The number of markers tested for may vary from state to state in the US, but generally ranges from 10 to 30. Because of the need for rapid screening, small sample size and reduced cost, older methodology is rapidly being replaced by technology which uses gas or liquid chromatography–mass spectrometry to measure the level of multiple markers simultaneously. The speed and high throughput capacity of this technology allow rapid screening of 20 or more markers from dried blood spots and the identification of infants who are potential victims of these inborn errors of metabolism. This technology is also applied to analysis of urine samples.

Regulation of the urea cycle

The urea cycle is regulated in part by control of the concentration of N-acetylglutamate, the essential allosteric activator of CPS I. Arginine is an allosteric activator of N-acetylglutamate synthase and also a source of ornithine (via arginase) for the urea cycle. Concentrations of urea cycle enzymes also increase or decrease in response to a high- or low-protein diet, and urea synthesis and excretion are decreased and NH_4^+ excretion is increased during acidosis as a mechanism to excrete protons into the urine. Lastly, it should be noted that during a fast, protein is broken down to free amino acids which are used for gluconeogenesis. The increase in protein degradation during fasting results in increased urea synthesis and excretion, a mechanism to dispose of the released nitrogen.

Defects in any of the enzymes of the urea cycle have serious consequences. Infants born with defects in any of the first four enzymes in this pathway may appear normal at birth, but rapidly become lethargic, lose body temperature, and may have difficulty breathing. Blood concentrations of ammonia increase quickly, followed by cerebral edema. The symptoms are most severe when early steps in the cycle are affected. However, a defect in any of the enzymes in this pathway is a serious issue and may cause hyperammonemia and lead rapidly to CNS edema, coma and death. Ornithine transcarbamoylase is the most common of these urea cycle defects and shows an X-linked inheritance pattern. The remainder of the known defects associated with the urea cycle are autosomal recessive. A deficiency of arginase, the last enzyme in the cycle, produces less severe symptoms but is nevertheless characterized by increased concentrations of blood arginine and at least a moderate increase in blood ammonia. In individuals

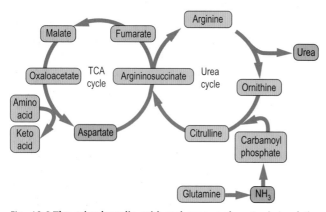

Fig. 19.8 **The tricarboxylic acid and urea cycles.** Analysis of the urea cycle reveals that it is really two cycles, with the carbon flow split between the primary urea synthetic process and the recycling of fumarate to aspartate; the latter cycle occurs in the mitochondrion and involves parts of the TCA cycle.

membrane to continue the cycle. Carbons from fumarate, released in the argininosuccinase step, may also reenter the mitochondrion after hydration to malate and be recycled by enzymes in the TCA cycle to oxaloacetate and ultimately to aspartate (Fig. 19.8), thus completing the second part of the urea cycle. Urea synthesis occurs virtually exclusively in the liver and the role of the enzyme, arginase, in other tissues is probably related more closely to ornithine requirements in those tissues than to the production of urea.

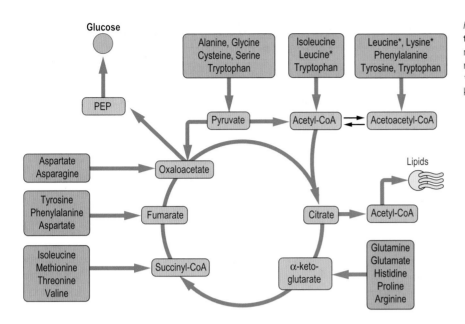

Fig. 19.9 **Amino acid metabolism and central metabolic pathways.** This figure summarizes the interactions between amino acid metabolism and central metabolic pathways. *The amino acids marked with an asterisk are ketogenic only. PEP, phosphoenolpyruvate.

with high blood concentrations of ammonia, hemodialysis must be used, often followed by intravenous administration of sodium benzoate and phenyllactate. These compounds are conjugated with glycine and glutamine, respectively, to form water-soluble adducts, trapping the ammonia in a nontoxic form that can be excreted in the urine.

The concept of nitrogen balance

Because there is no significant storage form of nitrogen or amino compounds in humans, nitrogen metabolism is quite dynamic. A careful balance is maintained between nitrogen ingestion and secretion. In an average, healthy diet, the protein content exceeds the amount required to supply essential and nonessential amino acids for protein synthesis, and the amount of nitrogen excreted is approximately equal to that taken in. Such a healthy adult would be said to be 'in neutral nitrogen balance'. When there is a need to increase protein synthesis, such as in recovering from trauma or in a rapidly growing child, the amount of nitrogen excreted is less than that consumed in the diet, and the individual would be in 'positive nitrogen balance'. The converse is true in protein malnutrition: because of the need to synthesize essential body proteins, other proteins, such as muscle protein or hemoglobin, are degraded and more nitrogen is lost than is consumed in the diet. Such an individual would be said to be in 'negative nitrogen balance'. Fasting, starvation and poorly controlled diabetes are also characterized by negative nitrogen balance, as body protein is degraded to amino acids and their carbon skeletons are used for gluconeogenesis. The concept of nitrogen balance is clinically important because it reminds us of the continuous turnover of amino acids and proteins in the body (see Chapter 22).

METABOLISM OF THE CARBON SKELETONS OF AMINO ACIDS

Metabolism of amino acids interfaces with carbohydrate and lipid metabolism

When one examines the metabolism of the carbon skeletons of the 20 common amino acids, there is an obvious interface with carbohydrate and lipid metabolism. Virtually all the carbons can be converted into intermediates in the glycolytic pathway, the TCA cycle or lipid metabolism. The first step in this process is the transfer of an α-amino group by transamination to α-ketoglutarate or oxaloacetate, providing glutamate and aspartate, the sources for the nitrogen atoms of the urea cycle (Fig. 19.9). The single exception to this is lysine, which does not undergo transamination. Although the details of pathways for the various amino acids vary, the general rule is that there is loss of the amino group, followed by either direct metabolism in a central pathway (glycolysis, the TCA cycle or ketone body metabolism), or one or more intermediate conversions to yield a metabolite in one of the central pathways. Examples of amino acids that follow the former scheme include alanine, glutamate and aspartate, which yield pyruvate, α-ketoglutarate and oxaloacetate, respectively. The branched-chain amino acids, leucine, valine and isoleucine, and the aromatic amino acids, tyrosine, tryptophan and phenylalanine, are examples of the latter, more complex pathways.

Amino acids may be either glucogenic or ketogenic

Depending on the point at which the carbons from an amino acid enter central metabolism, that amino acid

HOMOCYSTINURIA

A 21-year-old male was admitted to hospital following an episode of loss of speech and severe weakness on his right side. A diagnosis of ischemic stroke was made and the patient was treated with anticoagulant therapy and improved. Laboratory results indicated substantially elevated levels of blood homocysteine. The patient made a significant recovery and was discharged on a modified diet along with supplements of vitamin B_6, folic acid and vitamin B_{12}.

Comment. Homocystinuria is a relatively rare autosomal recessive condition (1 in 200 000 births) which results in a variety of symptoms including mental retardation, vision problems, and thrombotic strokes and coronary artery disease at a young age. The condition is caused by lack of an enzyme which catalyzes the transfer of sulfur from homocysteine to serine through the formation of a cystathionine intermediate. Some of these patients respond to vitamin supplementation. Moderately elevated levels of homocysteine in plasma are implicated in the development of cardiovascular disease and cerebrovascular ischemic episodes (stroke). Cross-sectional and retrospective studies suggest that even moderately elevated levels of homocysteine may be correlated with increased incidence of heart disease and stroke, but the jury is still out as to whether lowering homocysteine levels will reduce the development of these serious illnesses.

may be considered to be either glucogenic or ketogenic, i.e. possessing the ability to increase the concentrations of either glucose or ketone bodies, respectively, when fed to an animal. Those amino acids that feed carbons into the TCA cycle at the level of α-ketoglutarate, succinyl CoA, fumarate or oxaloacetate, and those that produce pyruvate can all give rise to the net synthesis of glucose via gluconeogenesis and are hence designated glucogenic. Those amino acids that feed carbons into central metabolism at the level of acetyl-CoA or acetoacetyl-CoA are considered ketogenic. Because of the nature of the TCA cycle, no net flow of carbons can occur between acetate or its equivalent to glucose via gluconeogenesis (see Chapter 13).

Several amino acids, primarily those with more complex or aromatic structures, can yield both glucogenic and ketogenic fragments (see Fig. 19.9). Only the amino acids, leucine and lysine, are regarded as being exclusively ketogenic and, because of its complex metabolism and lack of ability to undergo transamination, some authors do not consider lysine to be exclusively ketogenic. These classifications may be summarized as follows:

- **glucogenic amino acids**: alanine, arginine, asparagine, aspartic acid, cysteine, cystine, glutamine, glutamic acid, glycine, histidine, methionine, proline, serine, valine
- **ketogenic amino acids**: leucine, lysine
- **both glucogenic and ketogenic amino acids**: isoleucine, phenylalanine, threonine, tryptophan, tyrosine.

Metabolism of the carbon skeletons of selected amino acids

Alanine, aspartate and glutamate are examples of glucogenic amino acids. In each case, through either transamination or oxidative deamination, the resulting α-keto acid is a direct precursor of oxaloacetate via central metabolic pathways. Oxaloacetate can then be converted to PEP, and subsequently to glucose via gluconeogenesis. Other glucogenic amino acids reach the TCA cycle or related metabolic intermediates through several steps, after the removal of the amino group (see Fig. 19.9).

Leucine is an example of a ketogenic amino acid. Its catabolism begins with transamination to produce 2-ketoisocaproate. The metabolism of 2-ketoisocaproate requires oxidative decarboxylation by a dehydrogenase complex to produce isovaleryl CoA. Further metabolism of isovaleryl

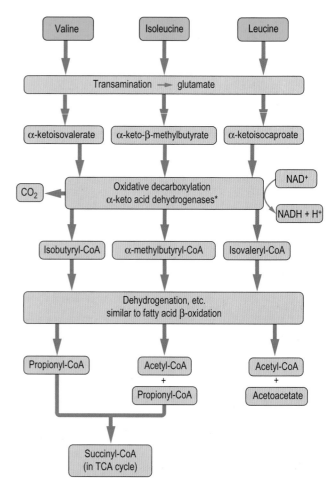

Fig. 19.10 **Degradation of branched-chain amino acids.** Metabolism of the branched-chain amino acids produces acetyl-CoA and acetoacetate. In the case of valine and isoleucine, propionyl-CoA is produced and metabolized, in two steps, to succinyl-CoA (Fig. 15.5). *The branched-chain amino acid dehydrogenases are structurally related to pyruvate dehydrogenase and α-ketoglutarate dehydrogenase, and use the cofactors thiamine pyrophosphate, lipoic acid, flavin adenine dinucleotide, NAD^+ and CoA.

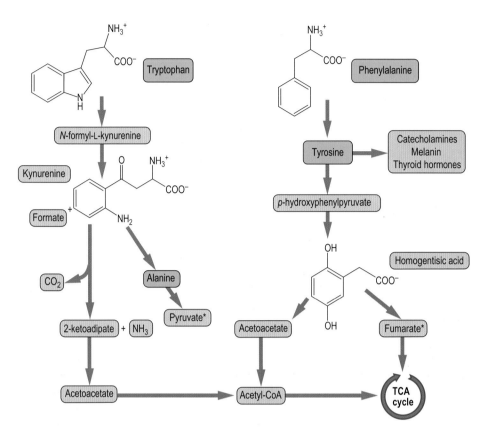

Fig. 19.11 **Catabolism of aromatic amino acids.** This figure summarizes the catabolism of the aromatic amino acids, illustrating the pathways that lead to ketogenic and glucogenic precursors derived from both tyrosine and tryptophan. *Both pyruvate and fumarate can lead to net glucose synthesis. They constitute the gluconeogenic portions of the metabolism of these amino acids.

CoA leads to formation of 3-hydroxy-3-methylglutaryl CoA, a precursor of both acetyl-CoA and the ketone bodies. The metabolism of leucine and the other branched-chain amino acids is summarized in Figure 19.10. Propionyl-CoA derived from either amino acid degradation or odd-chain fatty acid metabolism is converted to succinyl-CoA (see Fig. 15.5).

Tryptophan is a good example of an amino acid that yields both glucogenic and ketogenic precursors. After cleavage of its heterocyclic ring and a complex set of reactions, the core of the amino acid structure is released as alanine (a glucogenic precursor), while the balance of the carbons are ultimately converted to glutaryl-CoA (a ketogenic precursor). Figure 19.11 summarizes key points in the catabolism of the aromatic amino acids.

BIOSYNTHESIS OF AMINO ACIDS

Evolution has left our species without the ability to synthesize almost half the amino acids required for synthesis of proteins and other biomolecules

Humans use 20 amino acids to build peptides and proteins that are essential for the many functions of their cells. Biosynthesis of the amino acids involves synthesis of the carbon skeletons for the corresponding α-keto acids, followed by addition of the amino group via transamination. However, humans are capable of carrying out the biosynthesis of the carbon skeletons of only about half of those α-keto acids.

Origins of nonessential amino acids	
Amino acid	**Source in metabolism, etc.**
alanine	from pyruvate via transamination
aspartic acid, asparagine, arginine, glutamic acid, glutamine, proline	from intermediates in the citric acid cycle
serine	from 3-phosphoglycerate (glycolysis)
glycine	from serine
cysteine*	from serine; requires sulfur derived from methionline
tyrosine*	derived from phenylalanine via hydroxylation

These are examples of nonessential amino acids that depend on adequate amounts of an essential amino acid.

Table 19.5 **Origins of nonessential amino acids.**

Amino acids that we cannot synthesize are termed essential amino acids, and are required in the diet. While almost all the amino acids can be classified as clearly essential or nonessential, a few require further qualification. For example, although cysteine is not generally considered an essential

Essential amino acids		
Mnemonic	**Amino acid***	**Notes or comments**
P	phenylalanine	required in the diet also as a precursor of tyrosine
V	valine	one of three branched-chain amino acids
T	threonine	metabolized like a branched-chain amino acid
T	tryptophan	its complex heterocyclic side chain cannot be synthesized in humans
I	isoleucine	one of three branched-chain amino acids
M	methionine	provides the sulfur for cysteine and participates as a methyl donor in metabolism; the homocysteine is recycled
H	histidine	its heterocyclic side chain cannot be synthesized in humans
A	arginine	whereas arginine can be derived from ornithine in the urea cycle in amounts sufficient to support the needs of adults, growing animals require it in the diet
L	leucine	a pure ketogenic amino acid
L	lysine	does not undergo direct transamination

*The mnemonic PVT TIM HALL is useful for recalling the names of the essential amino acids.

Table 19.6 **Essential dietary amino acids.**

Examples of amino acids as effector molecules or precursors	
Amino acid	**Effector molecule or prosthetic group**
arginine	immediate precursor of urea, precursor of nitric oxide
aspartate	aspartate, an excitatory neurotransmitter
glycine	glycine, an inhibitory neurotransmitter; precursor of heme
glutamate	glutamate, excitatory neurotransmitter; precursor of γ-amino butyric (GABA), an inhibitory neurotransmitter
histidine	precursor of histamine, a mediator of inflammation and a neurotransmitter
tryptophan	precursor of serotonin, a potent smooth muscle contraction stimulation; precursor of melatonin, a regulator of circadian rhythm
tyrosine	precursor of the hormones and neurotransmitters, catecholamines, dopamine, epinephrine and norepinephrine, thyroxine

Table 19.7 **Examples of amino acids as effector molecules or precursors.**

whereas others may be converted to neurotransmitters or hormones through modification. Tyrosine is notable in that it serves as a precursor of several neurotransmitters, the catecholamines, and thyroid hormones.

INHERITED DISEASES OF AMINO ACID METABOLISM

In addition to deficiencies in the urea cycle, defects in the metabolism of the carbon skeletons of various amino acids were among the first disease states to be associated with simple inheritance patterns. These observations gave rise to the concept of the genetic basis of inherited metabolic disease states, also known as inborn errors of metabolism. Garrod considered a number of disease states that appeared to be inherited in a Mendelian pattern, and proposed a correlation between these abnormalities and specific genes, in which the disease state could be either dominant or recessive. Dozens of inborn errors of metabolism have now been described, and the molecular defect has been described for many of them. Three classic inborn errors of metabolism will be discussed in some detail here.

Phenylketonuria (PKU)

The common form of PKU results from a deficiency of the enzyme phenylalanine hydroxylase. The hydroxylation of

amino acid because it can be derived from the nonessential amino acid serine, its sulfur must come from the required or essential amino acid methionine. Similarly, the amino acid tyrosine is not required in the diet, but must be derived from the essential amino acid phenylalanine. This relationship between phenylalanine and tyrosine will be discussed further in considering the inherited disease phenylketonuria (PKU). Tables 19.5 and 19.6 list the nonessential and essential amino acids, and the source of the carbon skeleton in the case of those not required in the diet.

Amino acids are precursors of many essential compounds

In addition to their role as the building blocks for peptides and proteins, amino acids are essential precursors of a number of neurotransmitters, hormones, inflammatory mediators, and carrier and effector molecules (Table 19.7). Some of the amino acids may be used as neurotransmitters directly, for example glycine, aspartate and glutamate,

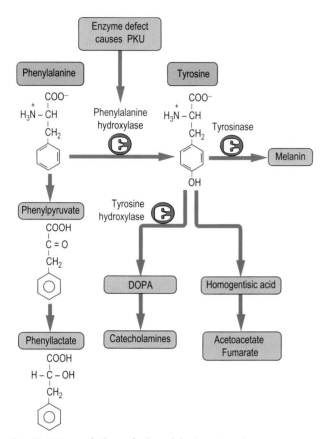

Fig. 19.12 **Degradation of phenylalanine.** In order to enter normal metabolism, phenylalanine must be hydroxylated by the enzyme phenylalanine hydroxylase. A defect in this enzyme leads to phenylketonuria (PKU). Tyrosine is a precursor of acetyl-CoA and fumarate, catecholamine hormones, the neurotransmitter dopamine, and the pigment melanin. DOPA, dihydroxyphenylalanine.

ALBINISM

A full-term infant, born to a normal and healthy mother and father, was observed to have a marked lack of pigmentation. The infant, who appeared to be otherwise normal, had blue eyes and very light blond, almost white, hair. This lack of pigmentation was confirmed as classic albinism on the basis of a family history and the establishment of a lack of the enzyme tyrosinase, which is responsible for a two-step hydroxylation of tyrosine to dihydroxyphenylalanine (DOPA) and a subsequent further oxidation to a quinone, a precursor of melanin in melanocytes (see Chapter 42).

Comment. A separate DOPA-producing enzyme, tyrosine hydroxylase, is involved in biosynthesis of the catecholamine neurotransmitters, so albinos do not appear to have neurologic deficits. As a result of their lack of pigmentation, however, they are quite sensitive to damage from sunlight and must take added precautions against ultraviolet radiation from the sun. Albinos have normal eyesight, in spite of the lack of pigmentation, but are generally very sensitive to bright light. (See Figure 19.15 for an outline of this pigment-forming pathway.)

PHENYLALANINE HYDROXYLASE

The hydroxylation of phenylalanine is a critical step in its catabolism and its conversion to tyrosine, thyroid hormone and the catecholamine hormones. Phenylalanine hydroxylase is an example of a mixed-function oxidase, an enzyme that uses a reduced cofactor and molecular oxygen to carry out a hydroxylation reaction. The cofactor is tetrahydrobiopterin, which is oxidized to dihydrobiopterin during the hydroxylation reaction. The residual hydrogens and oxygen are released as water. In order for this reaction to continue, the dihydrobiopterin must be reduced to its tetrahydro form and this requires a second enzyme, dihydrobiopterin reductase, which uses NADH to drive the reduction. The further hydroxylation of tyrosine, in the pathway that leads to catecholamines, requires a similar mixed-function oxidase, tyrosine hydroxylase. Phenylketonuria may develop as a result of mutations in either phenylalanine hydroxylase or enzymes involved in the synthesis or recycling of tetrahydrobiopterin.

phenylalanine is a required step in both the normal degradation of the carbon skeleton of this amino acid and the synthesis of tyrosine (Fig. 19.12). When untreated, this metabolic defect leads to excessive urinary excretion of phenylpyruvate and phenyllactate, and severe mental retardation. In addition, individuals with PKU tend to have very light skin pigmentation, unusual gait, stance, and sitting posture, and a high frequency of epilepsy. In the USA, this autosomal recessive defect occurs in about 1 in 30 000 live births. Because of its frequency, and the ability to prevent the most serious consequences of the defect by a low-phenylalanine diet, newborns in most developed countries are routinely tested for blood concentrations of phenylalanine. Fortunately, with early detection and the use of a diet restricted in phenylalanine but supplemented with tyrosine, most of the mental retardation can be avoided. Mothers who are homozygous for this defect have a very high probability of bearing children with congenital defects and mental retardation unless their blood phenylalanine concentrations can be controlled by diet. The developing fetus is very sensitive

to the toxic effects of high concentrations of phenylalanine and related phenylketones. Not all hyperphenylalaninemias are caused by a defect in phenylalanine hydroxylase. In some cases, there is a defect in biosynthesis or reduction of a required tetrahydrobiopterin cofactor.

SELENOCYSTEINE

In addition to the 20 common amino acids found in proteins, a 21st amino acid has been discovered and shown to be an active site amino acid in several enzymes, including the anti-oxidant enzyme glutathione peroxidase (Chapter 37) and 5'-deiodinases (Fig. 39.8). Selenocysteine is derived from serine and has unique chemical properties; substitution of seleno-cysteine with cysteine may have a pronounced inhibitory effect on enzyme activity. It is because of the need for selenocysteine that trace amounts of selenium are required in the diet.

Alkaptonuria (black urine disease)

A second inherited defect in the phenylalanine–tyrosine pathway involves a deficiency in the enzyme that catalyzes the oxidation of homogentisic acid, an intermediate in catabolism of tyrosine and phenylalanine. In this condition, which occurs in 1 in 1 000 000 live births, homogentisic acid accumulates and is excreted in urine. This compound oxidizes on standing or on treatment with alkali, and gives the urine a dark color. Individuals with alkaptonuria ultimately suffer from deposition of dark (ochre-colored) pigment in cartilage tissue, with subsequent tissue damage, including severe arthritis; the onset of these symptoms is generally in the third or fourth decade of life. This autosomal recessive disease was the first of several that Garrod considered in proposing his initial hypothesis for inborn errors of metabolism. Although alkaptonuria is relatively benign compared with PKU, little is available in the way of treatment, other than symptomatic relief.

Maple syrup urine disease (MSUD)

The normal metabolism of the branched-chain amino acids, leucine, isoleucine and valine, involves loss of the α-amino group, followed by oxidative decarboxylation of the resulting α-keto acid. This decarboxylation step is catalyzed by branched-chain keto acid decarboxylase, a multienzyme complex associated with the inner membrane of the mitochondrion. In approximately 1 in 300 000 live births, a defect in this enzyme leads to accumulation of the keto acids corresponding to these branched-chain amino acids in the blood, and then to branched-chain ketoaciduria. When untreated or unmanaged, this condition may lead to both physical and mental retardation of the newborn and a distinct maple syrup odor of the urine. This defect can be partially managed with a low-protein or modified diet, but not in all cases. In some instances, supplementation with high

CYSTINURIA

A 21-year-old man came to the emergency room with severe pain in his right side and back. Subsequent investigation indicated a kidney stone, and increased concentrations of cystine, arginine, and lysine in the urine. This patient exhibited the characteristic symptoms of cystinuria.

Comment. Cystinuria is an autosomal recessive disorder of intestinal absorption and proximal tubular reabsorption of dibasic amino acids; it does not result from a defect in cysteine metabolism per se. Because of the transport deficiency, cysteine, which is normally reabsorbed in the proximal renal tubule, remains in the urine. The cysteine spontaneously oxidizes to its disulfide form, cystine. Cystine is relatively insoluble and tends to precipitate in the urinary tract, forming kidney stones. The condition is generally treated by restricting the dietary intake of methionine (a biosynthetic precursor of cysteine), encouraging high fluid intake to keep the urine dilute and, more recently, with various drugs that may convert urinary cysteine to a more soluble compound that will not precipitate.

doses of thiamine pyrophosphate, a cofactor for this enzyme complex, has been helpful.

Summary

In this chapter, we have seen that the metabolism of amino acids is integrally related to the mainstream of metabolism. The catabolism of amino acids generally begins with the removal of the α-amino group, which is transferred to α-ketoglutarate and oxaloacetate, and ultimately excreted in the form of urea. The resulting carbon skeletons are converted to intermediates that enter central metabolism at various points. Because carbon skeletons corresponding to the various amino acids can be derived from or feed into the glycolytic pathway, the TCA cycle, fatty acid biosynthesis and gluconeogenesis, amino acid metabolism should not be considered as an isolated pathway. Although amino acids are not stored like glucose (glycogen) or fatty acids (triglycerides), they have an important and dynamic role, not only in providing the building blocks for the synthesis and turnover of protein, but also in normal energy metabolism, providing a carbon source for gluconeogenesis when needed and an energy source of last resort in starvation. In addition, amino acids provide precursors for the biosynthesis of a variety of small signaling molecules, including hormones and neurotransmitters. The severe consequences of inherited diseases such as phenylketonuria and maple syrup urine disease illustrate the effects of abnormal amino acid metabolism.

ACTIVE LEARNING

1. Tyrosine is included as a supplement in the diet plan for individuals with phenylketonuria. What is the rationale for this supplement? Compare the therapeutic approaches used for treatment of the various forms of PKU in which phenylalanine hydroxylase is not affected.

2. Review the rationale for the use of levodopa, catechol-O-methyltransferase inhibitors and monoamine oxidase inhibitors for treatment of Parkinson's disease.

3. Review the pathways for biosynthesis of the neurotransmitters serotonin, melatonin, dopamine, and the catecholamines. What enzymes are involved in the inactivation of these compounds?

Further reading

Cederbaum S. Phenylketonuria: an update. *Curr Opin Pediatr* 2002;**14**:702–706.

Gropman AL, Summar M, Leonard JV. Neurological implications of urea cycle disorders. *J Inherit Metab Dis* 2007;**30**:865–879.

Kuhara T. Noninvasive human metabolome analysis for differential diagnosis of inborn errors of metabolism. *J Chromatogr B Analyt Technol Biomed Life Sci* 2007;**855**:42–50.

Morris SM Jr. Regulation of enzymes of the urea cycle and arginine metabolism. *Annu Rev Nutr* 2002;**22**:87–105.

Ogier de Baulny H, Saudubray JM. Branched-chain organic acidurias. *Semin Neonatal* 2002;**7**:65–74.

Pitt JJ, Eggington M, Kahler SG. Comprehensive screening of urine samples for inborn errors of metabolism by electrospray tandem mass spectrometry. *Clin Chem* 2002;**48**:1970–1980.

Saudubray JM, Nassogne MC, de Lonlay P, Touati G. Clinical approach to inherited metabolic disorders in neonates: an overview. *Semin Neonatal* 2002;**7**:3–15.

Singh RH. Nutritional management of patients with urea cycle disorders. *J Inherit Metab Dis* 2007;**30**:880–887.

Steiner RD, Cederbaum SD. Laboratory evaluation of urea cycle disorders. *J Pediatr* 2001; **138**(Suppl 1): S21–S29.

Websites

Inborn errors of amino acid metabolism: www.gpnotebook.co.uk/simplepage. cfm?ID = -1811546080

Urea cycle disorders:
- www.nucdf.org
- www.ureacycle.com

Nitrogen metabolism: http://themedicalbiochemistrypage.org/nitrogen-metabolism.html

Maple syrup urine disease: www.msud-support.org/overview.htm

Parkinson's disease: www.enotes.com/nursing-encyclopedia/parkinson-s-disease

Phenylketonuria: http://www.nlm.nih.gov/medlineplus/phenylketonuria.html

20. Muscle: Energy Metabolism and Contraction

J A Carson and J W Baynes

LEARNING OBJECTIVES

After reading this chapter you should be able to:

- Describe muscle structure and its function in mechanical force production, including differences among skeletal, cardiac and smooth muscle types that are related to their physiologic functions.
- Describe the structure of the sarcomere and the mechanism of muscle contraction, including the composition of thick and thin filaments, the basis for banding patterns and the sliding filament model.
- Describe the sequence of events in excitation-contraction coupling, including the roles of membrane depolarization, the sarcoplasmic reticulum, and calcium triggering.
- Identify the key sites of energy utilization during muscle contraction, the relationship between force production and substrate utilization, the role of creatine phosphate in skeletal muscle, and the impact of skeletal muscle fiber type on substrate utilization and muscle function.
- Describe the changes in skeletal muscle mass and metabolism in diseases such as sarcopenia, metabolic syndrome, and wasting conditions.

INTRODUCTION

There are three types of muscle: skeletal, cardiac, and smooth muscle, each with a unique physiologic role. Their common function is the conversion of chemical energy to mechanical energy, but they differ in their mechanism of initiation of contraction, rate of force development, duration of contraction, and substrate utilization. Muscle accounts for about 40% of total body mass, and muscle activity is a major determinant of the overall metabolic rate in both the basal and active state. Changes in skeletal muscle metabolism occur with physical activity and are directly related to the required force output and duration of activity. These factors also affect the muscle's relative utilization of glucose and fatty acids for fuel. Besides locomotion, skeletal muscle is also a source of body heat, provides amino acids for hepatic gluconeogenesis during fasting, and is a major site of glucose and triglyceride disposal following a meal. Because of its critical role in the regulation of systemic fuel flux and metabolism, loss of muscle mass has a profound effect on overall metabolism. Advancing age and wasting diseases, such as AIDS and cancer, are conditions associated with loss of muscle mass, and this loss is associated with increased morbidity and mortality.

The primary focus of this chapter will be on skeletal muscle, supplemented by discussion of similarities and differences in skeletal, cardiac and smooth muscle structure, function and metabolism. The chapter will begin with a discussion of the mechanism of muscle contraction, proceed to the signaling that initiates the contractile process, and then examine energy metabolism essential for contraction.

 SARCOPENIA

Sarcopenia is defined as the loss of skeletal muscle mass with age. Sarcopenia is accelerated in humans after the fifth decade of life and can lead to frailty and loss of functional capacity. Besides the basic erosion of quality of life, loss of skeletal muscle mass also increases the risk of mortality and morbidity. The cause of sarcopenia appears to be related to both a biologic program of muscle fiber loss and decreased physical activity. Muscle fiber innervation by spinal motor neurones is critical to both development and maintenance of the mature muscle phenotype. Spinal motor neurones decrease in number with advancing age, possibly because of cumulative oxidative damage to these postmitotic cells. The decrease in muscle fiber number, accompanied by an increase in motor unit size, decreases fine motor skill. Sarcopenia has also been linked to age-induced systemic changes to the endocrine, cardiovascular, and immune systems, whose functions are all critical for the maintenance of skeletal muscle mass.

Comment. The scientific evidence is clear that most older individuals can increase muscle strength and mass with a regular resistance exercise program. Pharmaceutical treatments have also been examined for individuals who cannot regularly exercise. Currently there is no treatment for spinal motor neurone loss. Pharmaceutical treatments targeting muscle have had varying degrees of success, but are usually limited by side effects. The treatments include endocrine interventions with male or female sex hormone replacement therapy, and growth hormone therapy. Anti-inflammatory medication is also employed to allow individuals to participate in physical activity programs. One of the best defenses against sarcopenia may be regular exercise in order to maintain muscle mass during middle age.

MUSCLE STRUCTURE

The sarcomere: the functional contractile unit

A common characteristic of cardiac myocytes, smooth muscle cells and skeletal myofibers is that their cytoplasm is packed full of contractile protein. The contractile protein is arranged in linear arrays of sarcomere units in skeletal myofibers and cardiac myocytes, giving these muscles a striated appearance; thus, the term striated muscle. Contractile protein in smooth muscle cells is not organized into a sarcomeric structure, and this tissue is described as nonstriated muscle. Skeletal muscle's hierarchic structure (Fig. 20.1) consists of bundles (fasciculi) of elongated, multinucleated fiber cells (myofibers). The myofiber cells contain bundles of myofibrils which are, in turn, composed of myofilament proteins, primarily myosin and actin, that form the sarcomere (Table 20.1). Electron microscopic analysis of muscle reveals a repeating pattern of light- and dark-staining regions in the myofibril (Fig. 20.2). These regions are known as the I (isotropic)- and A (anisotropic)-bands, respectively. At the center of the I-band is a discrete, darker staining Z-line, while the center of the A-band has a lighter staining H-zone with a central M-line. The contractile unit, the sarcomere, is centered on the M-line, extending from one Z-line to the next. Smooth muscle lacks a defined Z-line.

Skeletal muscle structure	
Microscopic unit	fasciculus: bundle of muscle cells
Cellular unit	myofiber cell: long, multinucleated cell
Subcellular unit	myofibril: composed of myofilament proteins
Functional unit	sarcomere: contractile unit, repeating unit of the myofibril
Myofilament components	proteins: primarily actin and myosin

Table 20.1 **The structural elements of skeletal muscle arranged in descending order of size.**

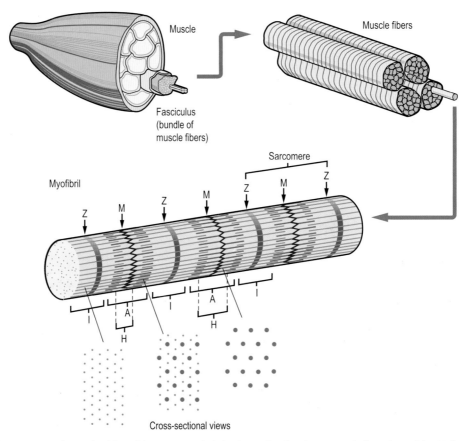

Fig. 20.1 **Hierarchic structure of muscle.** Hierarchic structure of skeletal muscle, showing an exploding view of fasciculi, myofibers, myofibrils and myofilament proteins. The location of the I-band (thin, actin filaments extending from the Z-line) and the A-band (thick, myosin filaments, extending from the M-line), with darker staining regions of the A-band corresponding to the region of overlap of actin and myosin filaments.

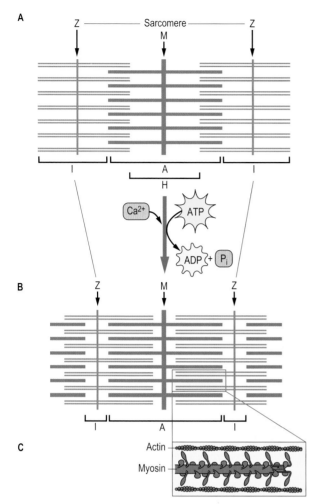

Muscle proteins and their functions	
Protein	**Function**
Myosin	Ca^{2+}-dependent ATPase activity
C-protein	assembly of myosin into thick filaments
M-protein	binding of myosin filaments to M-line
Actin	G-actin polymerizes to filamentous F-actin
tropomyosin	stabilization and propagation of conformational changes of F-actin
troponins-C, I and T	modulation of actin–myosin interactions
α- and β-actinins	stabilization of F-actin and anchoring to Z-line
nebulin	possible role in determining length of F-actin filaments
titin	control of resting tension and length of the sarcomere
desmin	organization of myofibrils in muscle cells
dystrophin	reinforcement of cytoskeleton and muscle cell plasma membrane

Table 20.2 **Muscle proteins and their functions.** Actin and myosin account for over 90% of muscle proteins, but several associated proteins are required for assembly and function of the actomyosin complex.

Fig. 20.2 **Schematic structure of the sarcomere, indicating the distribution of actin and myosin in the A- and I-bands.** (A) Relaxed sarcomere. (B) Contracted sarcomere. (C) Magnification of contracted sarcomere, illustrating the polarity of the arrays of myosin molecules. Increased overlap of actin and myosin filaments during contraction, accompanied by a decrease in the length of the H-zones and I-bands, illustrates the sliding filament model of muscle contraction.

The thick and thin filaments

The sarcomere may shorten by as much as 70% in length during muscle contraction (see Fig. 20.2). The components effecting the contraction are the thick and thin filaments. The thick filament is composed of myosin protein, and the thin filament is mainly made up of actin, with associated proteins, tropomyosin and troponins. Thick and thin filaments extend in opposite directions from both sides of the M- and Z-lines, respectively, and overlap and slide past one another during the contractile process (see Fig. 20.2). The M-and Z-lines are, in effect, base plates for anchoring the filaments. In striated muscle, increased thick–thin filament overlap during contraction causes the H-zone (myosin only) and I-bands (actin only) to shrink. In smooth muscle, thick and thin filaments are anchored at structures called dense

bodies that are further anchored by intermediate filaments. Although all three muscle types contain actin and myosin proteins, each muscle type expresses tissue-specific protein types or isoforms; the cardiac actin and troponins also differ slightly from those in skeletal muscle.

Sarcomere proteins

Myosin

Myosin is one of the largest proteins in the body, with a molecular mass of approximately 500 kDa, and accounts for more than half of muscle protein (Table 20.2). Under the electron microscope, myosin appears as an elongated protein with two globular heads. It is the primary component of the thick filament in muscle. Each myosin molecule is made up of two heavy chains (approx. 200 kDa) and four light chains (approx. 20 kDa). The heavy chain can be subdivided into the helical tail and globular head regions; the four light chains are bound to the globular heads. Structural analysis by limited proteolysis indicates that there are two flexible hinge regions in the myosin molecule (Fig. 20.3): one where the globular head attaches to the helical region and the other further into the helical region. The myosin filaments are

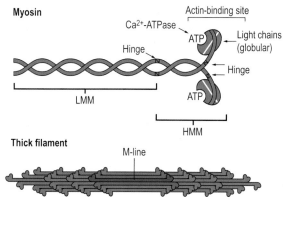

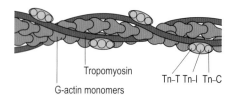

Fig. 20.3 **Polymerization of myosin and actin into thick and thin filaments.** Tn-C, calcium-binding troponin; Tn-I, troponin inhibitory subunit; Tn-T, tropomyosin-binding troponin. LMM: light meromyosin, HMM: heavy meromyosin.

associated through their helical regions and extend outward from the M-line toward the Z-line of each myofibril (see Figs 20.2 and 20.3). The hinge regions allow the myosin heads to interact with actin and provide the flexibility needed for reversible interactions and conformational changes during muscle contraction.

There are several features of myosin that are essential for muscle contraction.

- The myosin globular heads have binding sites for ATP and its hydrolysis products, ADP and phosphate (Pi).
- The myosin globular heads have a Ca^{2+}-dependent ATPase activity.
- Myosin binds reversibly to actin as a function of Ca^{2+}, ATP, and ADP + Pi concentrations.
- The binding of calcium and hydrolysis of ATP lead to major changes in the conformation of the myosin molecule and its interaction with actin.
- Myosin-ATPase activity, myosin–actin interactions and conformational changes are integrated into the sliding filament model of muscle contraction (below). They also explain the development of rigor mortis. The increase in Ca^{2+} in the muscle cytoplasm (sarcoplasm) and decrease in ATP after death lead to tight binding between myosin and actin, forming rigid muscle tissue.

Actin

Actin is composed of 42 kDa subunits, known as G-actin (globular), which polymerize into a filamentous array

(F-actin). Two polymer chains coil around one another to form the F-actin myofilament (see Fig. 20.3). F-actin is the major component of the thin filament and interacts with myosin in the actomyosin complex. The F-actin chains extend in opposite directions from the Z-line, overlapping with the myosin chains extending from the M-line. Each myosin-containing thick filament is surrounded by six actin molecule containing thin filaments. Each thin filament interacts with three myosin-containing thick filaments (see Fig. 20.1 for a cross-sectional view).

Tropomyosin and troponins

Calcium activation of muscle contraction in striated muscle involves thin filament-associated proteins, tropomyosin and the troponins. Tropomyosin is a fibrous protein that extends along the grooves of F-actin, each molecule contacting about seven G-actin subunits. Tropomyosin has a role in stabilizing F-actin and coordinating conformational changes among actin subunits during contraction. In the absence of Ca^{2+}, tropomyosin blocks the myosin-binding site on actin.

A complex of troponin proteins is bound to tropomyosin: Tn-T (tropomyosin-binding), Tn-C (calcium-binding) and Tn-I (inhibitory subunit). Troponins modulate the interaction between actin and myosin. Calcium binding to Tn-C, a calmodulin-like protein, induces changes in Tn-I which shift the interaction between tropomyosin and actin, exposing the myosin-binding site on F-actin and permitting actin–myosin interactions. For a description of the diagnostic use of cardiac troponin measurements see box on p. 262.

THE CONTRACTILE PROCESS

The sliding filament model of muscle contraction

The sliding filament model describes how a series of chemical and structural changes in the actomyosin complex can induce sarcomere shortening. The contractile response depends on a reversible, Ca^{2+}-dependent 'cross-bridge' formation between the myosin head and its binding site on actin. A conformational change in the hinge regions of myosin occurs after cross-bridge formation, providing the 'power stroke' for muscle contraction (Fig. 20.4). This conformational change, the relaxation of the high-energy form of myosin, is accompanied by dissociation of ADP and Pi. After the stroke is completed, the binding and hydrolysis

of ATP restore the high-energy conformation. The stability of the contracted state is maintained by multiple and continuous actin–myosin interactions, so that slippage is minimized until calcium is removed from the sarcoplasm, allowing dissociation of the actomyosin complex and muscle relaxation.

Higher myosin-ATPase activity increases cross-bridge cycling, which allows for increased rate of contraction. Different myosin isoforms have varying levels of ATPase activity, with fast muscles having higher myosin-ATPase activity. Isoforms of actin and myosin are also found in the cytoskeleton of nonmuscle cells, where they have roles in diverse processes such as cell migration, vesicle transport during endocytosis and exocytosis, maintenance or changing of cell shape, and anchorage of intracellular proteins to the plasma membrane.

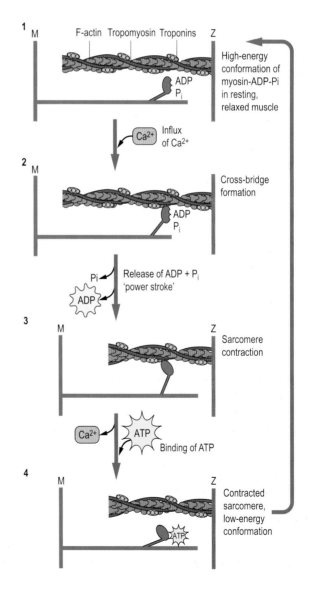

Fig. 20.4 **Proposed stages in muscle contraction, according to the sliding filament model.** (1) In resting, relaxed muscle, calcium concentration is $\sim 10^{-7}$ mol/L. The head group of myosin chains contains bound ADP and Pi, and is extended from the axis of the myosin helix in a high-energy conformation. Although the myosin-ADP-Pi complex has a high affinity for actin, binding of myosin to actin is inhibited by tropomyosin, which blocks the myosin-binding site on actin at low calcium concentration. (2) When muscle is stimulated, calcium enters the sarcoplasm through voltage-gated calcium channels (see Chapter 8). Calcium binding to Tn-C causes a conformational change in Tn-I, which is transmitted through Tn-T to tropomyosin. Movement of tropomyosin exposes the myosin-binding site on actin. Myosin-ADP-Pi binds to actin, forming a cross-bridge. (3) Release of Pi, then ADP, from myosin during the interaction with actin is accompanied by a major conformational change in myosin, producing the 'power stroke', which moves the actin chain about 10nm (100 Å) in the direction opposite the myosin chain, increasing their overlap and causing muscle contraction. (4) The uptake of calcium from the sarcoplasm and binding of ATP to myosin leads to dissociation of the actomyosin cross-bridge. The ATP is hydrolyzed, and the free energy of hydrolysis of ATP is conserved as the high-energy conformation of myosin, setting the stage for continued muscle contraction in response to the next surge in Ca^{2+} concentration in the sarcoplasm; compare Fig. 8.4.

Excitation-contraction coupling: muscle membrane depolarization

Skeletal muscle contraction is initiated by neuronal stimulation at the neuromuscular endplate. As described previously (see Fig. 8.4), this stimulus leads to depolarization of the electrochemical gradient across the muscle plasma membrane (sarcolemma). The depolarization, caused by an influx of Na^+, propagates rapidly along the sarcolemma membrane and signals a voltage-gated calcium release from the sarcoplasmic reticulum (SR), a membrane-bound, calcium-sequestering compartment within the muscle cell. The influx of Ca^{2+} from the SR to the sarcoplasm initiates cross-bridge formation and excitation-contraction coupling (see Fig. 20.4). In striated muscle, depolarization is transmitted into the muscle fiber by invaginations of the plasma membrane, called transverse tubules (T tubule) (Fig. 20.5). The transmission of depolarization through the highly branched T tubule network, which interacts closely with the SR, leads to rapid, concerted release of calcium from the SR into the sarcoplasm. In order for depolarization to occur again, sodium must be actively pumped out of the cytosol, by Na^+/K^+-ATPase pumps located in the sarcolemma. The rate of muscle repolarization is affected by both the rate and density of these pumps. Higher levels of Na^+/K^+-ATPase activity are found in fast contracting muscles, and increased Na^+/K^+-ATPase pump density is an important adaptation to exercise.

Skeletal, cardiac, and smooth muscle differ in their mechanism of neural stimulation, and have different structural adaptations for propagating the depolarization. Skeletal muscle contraction is volitional and fibers are innervated by motor nerve endplates that originate in the spinal cord; acetylcholine functions as the neurotransmitter (see Chapter 41). The neuromuscular junction is a special structural feature of skeletal muscle that is not found in cardiac or smooth muscle. Each individual fiber is innervated by only one motor nerve, and all the fibers innervated by one nerve are defined as a motor unit. Motor unit control and synchronization is the basis for coordinated whole-muscle contraction. Skeletal muscle cramping is nonvoluntary muscle contraction resulting from electrolyte imbalances after excessive fluid loss, often during exercise in hot, humid conditions.

Cardiac muscle is striated and contracts rhythmically under involuntary control. The general mechanism of contraction of heart muscle is similar to that in skeletal muscle; however, the sarcoplasmic reticulum is less developed and the transverse tubule network more developed in the heart. The heart is more dependent on, and actually requires, extracellular calcium for its contractile response (see Fig. 8.4); the influx of extracellular calcium enhances Ca^{2+} release from the SR. Lacking direct neural contact, cardiac myocytes propagate depolarization from a single node, the SA

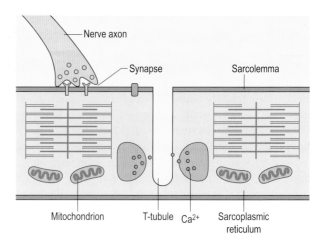

Fig. 20.5 **Side-view of the transverse tubular network in skeletal muscle cells.** Transverse tubules are invaginations of the sarcolemma, which are in close proximity to the sarcoplasmic reticulum (SR). The SR is a continuous, tubular compartment in close association with the myofibrils. The transverse tubules are extensions of the sarcolemma around the Z-line. They transmit the depolarizing nerve impulse to terminal regions of the SR, coordinating calcium release and contraction of the myofibril.

node, throughout the myocardium. The depolarization is passed cell to cell along specialized membrane structures called intercalated disks. Cardiac muscle is also more responsive to hormonal regulation. For example, cAMP-dependent protein kinases phosphorylate transport proteins and Tn-I, mediating changes in the force of contraction in response to epinephrine.

Smooth muscle can respond to both neural and circulating factors. Unlike skeletal muscle, neural input to smooth muscle innervates bundles of smooth muscle cells that cause both phasic (rhythmic) and tonic (sustained) contractions of the tissue. Smooth muscle can also be induced to depolarize by ligand–receptor interactions at the sarcolemma. This is called pharmacomechanical coupling, and is the basis for many drugs that target smooth muscle contraction or relaxation. Nitric oxide donors, such as amyl nitrite and nitroglycerine, used for treatment of angina, relax vascular smooth muscles, increasing the flow of blood to cardiac muscle.

Excitation-contraction coupling: the calcium trigger

The calcium content of the sarcoplasm is normally very low, 10^{-7} mol/L or less, but increases rapidly by over 100-fold in response to neural stimulation. The sarcoplasmic reticulum, a specialized organelle derived from the smooth endoplasmic reticulum, is rich in a Ca^{2+}-binding protein, calsequestrin, and serves as the site of calcium sequestration inside the cell. In striated muscle T tubule depolarization opens the Ca^{2+} channels in the SR (see Fig. 20.5). The influx of Ca^{2+}

into the sarcoplasm triggers both actin–myosin interactions and myosin-ATPase activity, leading to muscle contraction. Troponins are not expressed in smooth muscle. In this case, calcium triggers contraction by binding to calmodulin and activating myosin light chain kinase. Myosin phosphorylation enhances myosin–actin interaction.

Increased intracellular calcium activates more cross-bridges and causes sarcomere shortening through activation of myosin-ATPase. Thus, higher calcium levels increase muscle contractile force until saturation is reached. Calcium channel blockers used for treatment of hypertension, such as nifedipine (see Fig. 7.6), inhibit the flow of Ca^{2+} into the SR, thereby limiting the force of contraction of cardiac myocytes. While muscle contraction is triggered by increased calcium, muscle relaxation is dependent on calcium being actively pumped back into the SR. The rate of muscle relaxation is directly related to SR Ca^{2+}-ATPase activity. The SR is rich in Ca^{2+}-ATPase, which maintains cytosolic calcium in the sarcoplasm at submicromolar ($\sim 10^{-7}$ mol/L) concentrations. As intracellular calcium levels decrease, the number of active cross-bridges also decreases, and muscle contractile force declines.

MUSCLE ENERGY METABOLISM

ATP is used for muscle contraction

Three ATPases are required for muscle contraction: Na^+/K^+-ATPase, Ca^{2+}-ATPase and myosin-ATPase. Decreased ATP availability or inhibition of any of these ATPases will cause a decrease in muscle force production. However, the intracellular concentration of ATP does not change dramatically during exercise. Actively contracting muscle relies on the rapid resynthesis of ATP from ADP. Energy systems that synthesize ATP for muscle contraction include the creatine phosphate shuttle, anaerobic glycolysis, and aerobic metabolism via oxidative phosphorylation. The energy systems that synthesize ATP are not equivalent, and directly affect the amount and duration of power output from the contracting muscle.

Short-duration, high-power output contractions

A metabolic reality for skeletal muscle is that high force output can only be maintained for a short period of time. Contractions at or near maximal power levels depend on high myosin-ATPase and rapid ATP resynthesis by substrate-level phosphorylation using the high energy compound creatine phosphate (creatine-P). Creatine (see Table 9.2) is synthesized from arginine and glycine (Fig. 20.6) and is phosphorylated reversibly to creatine-P by the enzyme creatine (phospho)kinase (CK or CPK). CK is a dimeric protein and exists as three isozymes:

MALIGNANT HYPERTHERMIA

About 1 in 150 000 patients treated with halothane (gaseous halocarbon) anesthesia or muscle relaxants responds with excessive skeletal muscle rigidity and severe hyperthermia with a rapid onset, up to 2°C (4°F) within 1 hour. Unless treated rapidly, cardiac abnormalities may be life-threatening; mortality from this condition exceeds 10%. This genetic disease results from excessive or prolonged release of Ca^{2+} from the SR, most commonly the result of mutations in the Ca^{2+}-release channels within the SR. Excessive release of Ca^{2+} leads to a prolonged increase in sarcoplasmic Ca^{2+} concentration. Muscle rigidity results from Ca^{2+}-dependent consumption of ATP, and hyperthermia results from increased metabolism to replenish the ATP. As muscle metabolism becomes anaerobic, lacticacidemia and acidosis may develop. The cardiac abnormalities result from hyperkalemia, caused by release of potassium ions from muscle; as supplies of ATP are exhausted, muscle is unable to maintain ion gradients across its plasma membrane. Treatment of malignant hyperthermia includes use of muscle relaxants, e.g. dantrolene, an inhibitor of the ryanodine-sensitive Ca^{2+}-channel, to inhibit Ca^{2+} release from the SR. Supportive therapy involves cooling, administration of oxygen, correction of blood pH and electrolyte imbalances and also treatment of cardiac abnormalities.

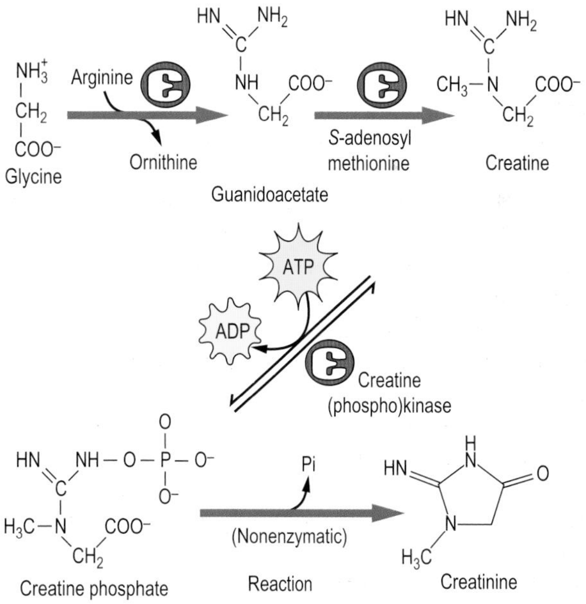

Fig. 20.6 Synthesis and degradation of creatine phosphate (creatine-P). Creatine is synthesized from glycine and arginine precursors. Creatine-P is unstable and undergoes slow, spontaneous degradation to Pi and creatinine, the cyclic anhydride form of creatine, which is excreted from the muscle cell into plasma and then into urine.

the MM (skeletal muscle), BB (brain) and MB isoforms. The MB isoform is enriched in cardiac tissue.

The level of creatine-P in resting muscle is several-fold higher than that of ATP (Table 20.3). Thus, ATP concentration

Metabolite	Metabolite concentration (mmol/kg dry weight)		
	Resting	3 minutes	8 minutes
ATP	27	26	19
Creatine-P	78	27	7
Creatine	37	88	115
Lactate	5	8	13
Glycogen	408	350	282

Changes in energy resources in working muscle

Table 20.3 **Changes in energy resources in working muscle.** Concentrations of energy metabolites in human leg muscle during bicycle exercise. These experiments were conducted during ischemic exercise, which exacerbates the decline in ATP concentration. They illustrate the rapid decline in creatine-P and the increase in lactate from anaerobic glycolysis of muscle glycogen. Data are adapted from Timmons JA *et al. J Clin Invest* 1998;**101**:79–85.

remains relatively constant during the initial stages of exercise. It is replenished not only by the action of CK, but also by adenylate kinase (myokinase) as follows:

$$\text{Creatine phosphokinase: creatine-P} + \text{ADP} \rightarrow \text{creatine} + \text{ATP}$$
$$\text{Adenylate kinase: 2 ADP} \rightleftharpoons \text{ATP} + \text{AMP}$$

Creatine phosphate stores decline rapidly during the first minute of high power output muscle contraction. As creatine phosphate stores are depleted, the muscle becomes unable to sustain the high force output, and contractile force rapidly declines. At this point, muscle glycogenolysis becomes a major source of energy. Calcium entry into muscle leads to formation of a Ca^{2+}–calmodulin complex, which activates phosphorylase kinase, catalyzing the conversion of phosphorylase b to phosphorylase a. AMP also allosterically activates muscle phosphorylase and phospho-fructokinase-1, accelerating glycolysis from muscle glycogen (see Chapter 12).

A further decline in force occurs as pyruvate and lactate gradually accumulate in the contracting muscle, resulting in a decrease in muscle pH. Force will then decline to a level that can be maintained by aerobic metabolism of fatty acids. Maximal aerobic power is about 20% of maximal power output, and about 50–60% of maximal aerobic power can be sustained for long periods of time.

Low-intensity, long-duration contractions

The availability and utilization of oxygen in working muscle are major limitations for maintaining continuous physical activity. Long-duration contractile activity requires adequate oxygen delivery and the capacity for the muscle to utilize the oxygen delivered. Oxygen delivery to muscle is affected by the red cell and hemoglobin concentrations in blood, the number of capillaries within the muscle and heart pump capacity. Highly oxidative muscle has a higher capillary density than glycolytic muscle, and muscle capillary density increases with endurance exercise training. Muscle oxygen utilization is also directly related to the number and size of muscle mitochondria. Muscles subjected to continual contractile activity, such as postural muscles, have more mitochondria than infrequently contracted muscle. A standard observation in muscle subjected to increased contractile demands is an elevation in oxidative enzyme activity.

At rest or at low intensities of physical work, oxygen is readily available and the aerobic oxidation of lipid predominates as the main source of ATP synthesis. However, at higher work intensities, oxygen availability and utilization lipid can become limiting, and subsequently the muscle work rate decreases. During the first 15–30 minutes of exercise, there is a gradual shift from glycogenolysis and aerobic glycolysis to aerobic metabolism of fatty acids. Perhaps this is an evolutionary response to deal with the fact that lactate, produced by glycolysis, is more acidic and less diffusible than CO_2. As exercise continues, epinephrine contributes to activation of hepatic gluconeogenesis, providing an exogenous source of glucose for muscle. Lipids gradually become the major source of energy in muscle during long-term, lower intensity exercise where oxygen is not limiting.

Long-term muscle performance (stamina) depends on levels of muscle glycogen

Marathon runners typically 'hit the wall' when muscle glycogen reaches a critically low level. Glycogen is the storage form of glucose in skeletal muscle and its muscle concentration can be manipulated by diet, e.g. by carbohydrate loading prior to a marathon run. Fatigue, which can be defined as an inability to maintain the desired power output, occurs when the rate of ATP utilization exceeds its rate of synthesis. For efficient ATP synthesis, there is a continuing requirement for a basal level of glycogen metabolism, even when glucose is available from plasma and when fats are the primary source of muscle energy. Glycogen metabolism is important as a source of pyruvate, which is converted to oxaloacetate by the anaplerotic, pyruvate carboxylase reaction. Oxaloacetate is required to maintain the activity of the TCA cycle, for condensation with acetyl-CoA derived from fats. To some extent, muscle glycogen can be spared and performance time increased during long-term vigorous physical activity by increasing the availability of circulating glucose, either by gluconeogenesis or by carbohydrate ingestion. Increased utilization of fatty acids during early stages of exercise is an important training adaptation to regular vigorous physical activity that can also serve to spare glycogen stores (see Chapter 21).

Muscle consists of two types of striated muscle cells: fast-glycolytic and slow-oxidative fibers

Striated muscle cells are generally classified by their physiologic contractile properties (fast versus slow) and primary type of metabolism (oxidative versus glycolytic). The muscle type is closely related to muscle function in skeletal muscle, and this comparison can easily be seen with muscles whose contraction is for infrequent-burst activities versus muscles used continuously for maintaining posture (antigravity). The coloring of the two striated muscle types readily distinguishes them. Fast-glycolytic muscle used for burst activity is white in appearance (like chicken breast – chickens cannot fly far!) because of less blood flow, lower mitochondrial density and decreased myoglobin content compared with slow-twitch oxidative muscle, which is red. Fast-glycolytic fibers also have increased glycogen stores and lower fat content; they rely on glycogen and anaerobic glycolysis for short bursts of contraction when additional muscle force is required such as in the 'fight or flight' stress response. These muscle fibers are not capable of sustaining contraction for long periods. In contrast, slow-oxidative fibers in postural muscles (and in goose breast – geese are migratory birds) are well perfused with blood, rich in mitochondria and myoglobin. This muscle type has the ability to sustain low-intensity contractions for long periods. Slow muscle uses fatty acid oxidation for ATP synthesis, which requires mitochondria. (Goose breast is a fairly fatty and dark meat, compared to chicken breast.) Cardiac muscle, which is continuously contracting, has many contractile and metabolic characteristics that are similar to slow-oxidative skeletal muscle. Cardiac muscle is well perfused with blood, rich in mitochondria, and relies largely on oxidative metabolism of circulating fatty acids.

DEVELOPMENT AND REGENERATION OF MUSCLE

To understand muscle regulation, it is helpful to understand its origin and development. Muscle is derived from proliferating cells that originate from the mesenchyme germ layer in the developing embryo. These cells are 'determined' into the muscle lineage and then become myoblasts. Myoblasts can leave the cell cycle and differentiate into a mature muscle cell phenotype. Differentiation involves the sequential activation of muscle-specific genes including contractile proteins by DNA-binding transcriptional regulator proteins from the family of myogenic regulatory factors (MRFs). Terminally

 MUSCLE WASTING SYNDROMES

Many patients with conditions that include HIV and many cancers experience severe body weight loss. Patients exhibiting wasting have an increased rate of morbidity and mortality. This loss of body weight is often independent of decreased caloric intake, and not just akin to starvation. Appetite stimulants alone are often not effective. The weight loss is associated with the loss of both muscle and adipose tissue. Health problems may be magnified in wasting individuals due to the metabolic dysregulation that can accompany the loss of adipose and muscle tissue. There also appears to be an effect of fiber type on muscle loss, which may be related to metabolism. Fast-glycolytic muscle fibers undergo more protein loss than slow-oxidative muscle fibers. This preferential loss of fast-glycolytic fibers with wasting is the opposite of what is seen in muscle with extended periods of disuse. Slow-oxidative fibers atrophy preferentially during muscle disuse. Although the exact mechanisms inducing wasting are not certain, prime candidates with many wasting syndromes involve systemic inflammatory signaling by cytokines, such as TNF-α and IL-6. Inflammatory signaling induced by the disease process can activate muscle protein degradation, inhibit muscle protein synthesis, and induce adipose tissue lipolysis. Maintaining or preventing severe body weight loss in many disease states can improve patient treatment options, survival and quality of life. Anabolic agents, like testosterone, have proven beneficial in maintaining muscle mass in AIDS patients and are widely used clinically. With other wasting diseases, research in animal models has demonstrated that inhibition of inflammatory signaling can inhibit wasting. Further research is necessary before this approach is widely applied to human populations.

 ASSAY OF CREATININE TO ASSESS RENAL FUNCTION AND URINE DILUTION

Since creatine phosphate concentration is relatively constant per unit muscle mass, the production of creatinine (see Fig. 20.6) is relatively constant during the day. Creatinine is eliminated in urine at a relatively constant amount per hour, primarily by glomerular filtration and to a lesser extent by tubular secretion. Since its concentration in urine varies with the dilution of the urine, levels of metabolites in random urine samples are often normalized to the urinary concentration of creatinine. Otherwise, a 24h collection would be required to assess daily excretion of a metabolite. Normal creatinine concentration in plasma is about 20–80mmol/L (0.23–0.90mg/dL). Increases in plasma creatinine concentration are commonly used as an indicator of renal failure. The albumin:creatinine ratio in a random urine sample, an indicator of protein filtration selectivity of the glomerulus, is used as a measure of the microalbuminuria to assess the progression of diabetic nephropathy (see also Chapter 23.).

MEASUREMENT OF CARDIAC TROPONIN IS ESSENTIAL FOR DIAGNOSIS OF MYOCARDIAL INFARCTION

Myocardial infarction (MI) is the result of blockage of blood flow to the heart (see Chapter 18). Tissue damage results in leakage of intracellular enzymes into blood (Fig. 20.7). Among these are glycolytic enzymes, such as LDH (Chapter 12); however, measurements of myoglobin, total plasma CK and CK-MB isozymes are more commonly used for diagnosis and management of MI. Myoglobin is a small protein (17 000 kDa) and rises most rapidly in plasma, within 2 hours following MI. Although it is sensitive, it lacks specificity for heart tissue. It is cleared rapidly by renal filtration and returns to normal within 1 day. Since plasma myoglobin also increases following skeletal muscle trauma, it would not be useful for diagnosis of MI, e.g. following an automobile accident. Total plasma CK and the CK-MB isozyme begin to rise within 3–10 hours following an MI, and reach a peak value of up to 25 times normal after 12–30 hours; they may remain elevated for 3–5 days. Total CK may also increase as a result of skeletal muscle damage but the measurement of CK-MB provides specificity for cardiac damage.

Comment. Enzyme-linked immunosorbent assays (ELISA) for the myocardial troponins are now recommended for the diagnosis and management of MI. These assays depend on the presence of unique isoforms of troponin subunits in the adult heart. Tn-T concentration in plasma increases within a few hours after a heart attack, peaks at up to 300 times normal plasma concentration, and may remain elevated for 1–2 weeks. An assay for a specific isoform in an adult heart, $Tn\text{-}T_2$, is essentially 100% sensitive for diagnosis of MI and yields fewer than 5% false-positive results. Significant increases in plasma Tn-T are detectable even in patients with unstable angina and transient episodes of ischemia in the heart. Troponins are commonly used as a component of an algorithm to differentiate high-risk from low-risk patients in terms of need for immediate invasive intervention. The recent definition of myocardial infarction is based on observed serum troponin concentrations.

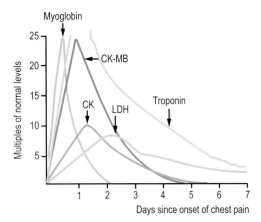

Fig. 20.7 **Serum enzyme changes after myocardial infarction (MI).** Various marker enzymes increase in plasma following MI. These are still used for the diagnosis of MI, but the currently recommended test is the measurement of serum troponin concentration. CK, creatine phosphokinase; CK-MB, cardiac isozyme of CK; LDH, lactate dehydrogenase. Adapted from Pettigrew AR, Pacanis A. Diagnosis of myocardial infarction. In: Dominiczak MH (ed) *Seminars in Clinical Biochemistry.* University of Glasgow Computer Publishing Unit, Glasgow, 1997.

differentiated myoblasts in the heart are called cardiac myocytes; these cells remain single or binucleated throughout life. To date, no myogenic stem cells have been found in cardiac muscle, which may explain the limited regenerative capacity of the heart after injury.

Smooth muscle myoblasts also differentiate into mature smooth muscle cells (SMC) but, unlike heart and skeletal muscle, they are not terminally differentiated. SMC phenotype also varies, based on its location and function. SMCs are found throughout the body in the vascular wall, and retain the ability to proliferate, e.g. in response to hypertension or during angiogenesis.

Skeletal muscle cells differ from the other muscle types in that they are multinucleated. Proliferating myoblasts fuse and terminally differentiate to form a multinucleated myotube. Innervation by a motor nerve endplate induces the myotube to take on mature muscle fiber characteristics. Satellite cells are undifferentiated muscle precursor cells, found only in skeletal muscle. Since muscle fiber nuclei are postmitotic, satellite cell proliferation and differentiation are critical events for postnatal muscle growth, e.g. in response to exercise, and for regeneration after damage. Alterations in satellite cell differentiation with advancing age or in wasting syndromes are thought to contribute to skeletal muscle loss under these conditions.

SUMMARY

Muscle is the major consumer of fuels and ATP in the body. Both glycolysis and lipid metabolism are essential for muscle activity. Reliance on these energy-producing pathways varies with muscle type and its prior contractile activity. The ATP produced in muscle drives the maintenance of ion gradients, restoration of intracellular calcium levels, and the contractile process. Fast, glycolytic muscle relies largely on glycogen and anaerobic glycolysis for short, high-intensity bursts of muscle activity. Slow, oxidative muscle is an aerobic tissue; at rest, it uses fats as its primary source of energy. During the initial phases of exercise, it relies on glycogenolysis and glycolysis but then gradually converts to fat metabolism for long-term energy production.

ACTIVE LEARNING

1. When chickens are frightened, they squawk a lot, may jump high and fly for short distances, but are unable to take flight and fly for great distances, either normally or to escape danger. In contrast, geese have the ability to fly for great distances, e.g. during semi-annual migrations. Compare the types of muscle fibers and energy resources in the breast of chicken and geese and explain how the differences in fiber type are compatible with the flying capacity of these birds.
2. Discuss the impact of muscle glycogen phosphorylase deficiency (McArdle's disease) and carnitine or carnitine palmitoyl transferase I deficiency on muscle performance during short- and long-duration exercise.
3. Review the merits of blood doping, carbohydrate loading and creatine supplementation to enhance performance during marathon events.

Skeletal, cardiac, and smooth muscle have a common actomyosin contractile complex, but differ in innervation, contractile protein arrangement, calcium regulation of contraction, and propagation of depolarization from cell to cell. The sarcomere is the fundamental contraction unit of striated muscle and is defined by Z-lines and thick and thin filament overlap. Contraction is described by a 'sliding filament' model in which hydrolysis of ATP is catalyzed by an influx of Ca^{2+} into the sarcoplasm and is coupled to changes in the conformation of myosin. Relaxation of the high-energy conformation of myosin during interaction with actin produces a 'power stroke', resulting in increased overlap of the actin–myosin filaments and shortening of the sarcomere. Measurements of CK activity are used as a marker of skeletal muscle damage. Troponin measurements are now essential investigations in the diagnosis of myocardial infarction.

Further reading

Coffey VG, Hawley JA. The molecular bases of training adaptation. *Sports Med* 2007;**37**: 737–763.

Joseph AM, Pilegaard H, Litvintsev A, Leick L, Hood DA. Control of gene expression and mitochondrial biogenesis in the muscular adaptation to endurance exercise. *Essays Biochem* 2006;**42**:13–29.

Nistasla R, Stump CS. Skeletal muscle insulin resistance is fundamental to the cardiometabolic syndrome. *J Cardiometab Syndr* 2006;**1**:47–52.

Thomas DR. Loss of skeletal muscle mass in aging: examining the relationships of starvation, sarcopenia and cachexia. *Clin Nutr* 2007;**4**:389–399.

Yudkin JS. Inflammation, obesity, and the metabolic syndrome. *Horm Metab Res* 2007;**39**:707–709.

Websites

Carnitine deficiency: www.emedicine.com/ped/topic321.htm

McArdle's disease: www.muscular-dystrophy.org/information_resources/factsheets/medical_conditions_factsheets/mcardles.html

Muscular dystrophy: www.ninds.nih.gov/health_and_medical/disorders/md.htm; www.nlm.nih.gov/medlineplus/musculardystrophy.html

Animations:

http://trc.ucdavis.edu/biosci10v/bis10v/week10/08muscularsystem.html

http://entochem.tamu.edu/MuscleStrucContractswf/index.html

21. Glucose Homeostasis and Fuel Metabolism

M H Dominiczak

LEARNING OBJECTIVES

After reading this chapter you should be able to:

■ Characterize the main energy substrates (metabolic fuels).
■ Outline the actions of insulin and glucagon.
■ Compare and contrast metabolism in the fasting and postprandial states.
■ Describe the metabolic response to injury and compare it with metabolism in diabetes.
■ Characterize type 1 and type 2 diabetes.
■ Explain the basis of laboratory tests relevant to fuel metabolism and monitoring of diabetes.

Continuous provision of energy is essential to maintain life. This chapter describes the metabolism of compounds known as energy substrates (metabolic fuels). It also discusses the most common metabolic disease, diabetes mellitus.

Most important energy substrates are glucose and fatty acids: both can be stored in the body

The most important energy substrates in mammals are glucose and fatty acids. After ingestion of food, their excess is stored to be released again in case of need. This safeguards energy supply between meals and in extreme circumstances can ensure an organism's survival for weeks and months. The main pathways of fuel metabolism and key metabolites are listed in Table 21.1.

Glucose is stored as glycogen and can be synthesized from noncarbohydrate compounds

In normal circumstances glucose is the only fuel used by the brain; therefore its continuous supply is essential for survival. Glucose is also preferentially used by muscle during initial stages of exercise. In spite of occasional large demand, the amount of free glucose present in the extracellular fluid is small – only about 20 g (<1 oz), the equivalent of 80 kcal (335 kJ). To safeguard continuous supply, glucose can be released into the circulation from the 'emergency store' of its polymer, glycogen. Glycogen is stored in the liver (approximately 75 g (2.5 oz)) and in muscle (400 g (<1 lb)). This is equivalent to about 1900 kcal (7955 kJ) and can provide a supply of glucose for approximately 16 h of fasting (compare Table 19.1 and Table 20.3). If the fast lasts longer, another mechanism of glucose supply comes into play: its synthesis from noncarbohydrate compounds (gluconeogenesis).

Principal anabolic and catabolic pathways, and their main substrates and products

Pathway	Main substrates	End products
Anabolic		
gluconeogenesis	lactate, alanine, glycerol	glucose
glycogen synthesis	G-1-P	glycogen
protein synthesis	amino acids	proteins
fatty acid synthesis	acetyl-CoA	fatty acid
lipogenesis	glycerol, fatty acids	triacylglycerols (triglycerides)
Catabolic		
glycolysis	glucose	pyruvate, ATP
tricarboxylic acid cycle	pyruvate	$NADH + H^+$, $FADH_2$
		acetyl-CoA, pyruvate CO_2, H_2O, ATP
glycogenolysis	glycogen	G-1-P, glucose
pentose phosphate pathway	G-6-P	$NADH + H^+$, pentoses, CO_2
fatty acid oxidation	fatty acids	CO_2, H_2O, ATP (ketones)
lipolysis	triglycerides	glycerol, fatty acids
proteolysis	proteins	amino acids, glucose

Note that metabolites such as pyruvate and acetyl-CoA are common to several different pathways. This enables their integrated regulation. Note also which pathways generate reducing equivalents (NADH, NADPH and FADH$_2$) serving as substrates for the mitochondrial respiratory chain.

Table 21.1 **Principal anabolic and catabolic pathways, and their main substrates and products.**

Safeguarding a constant glucose supply is one of the main functions of energy metabolism.

Fatty acids are stored as esters of glycerol (triacylglycerols or triglycerides) and cannot be converted into carbohydrates

The body has virtually unlimited capacity for the accumulation of fat in the adipose tissue as esters of glycerol (triacylglycerols). The caloric value of fat (9 kcal/g, 37 kJ/g) is higher than that of either carbohydrates (4 kcal/g, 17 kJ/g) or proteins (4 kcal/g) (see Table 22.3). A 70 kg (154 lb) man will have approximately 15 kg (33 lb) of fat stored. This is equivalent to over 130 000 kcal (544 300 kJ; compare the caloric value of glycogen above). Fatty acids support body energy needs during prolonged periods of fasting. In extreme circumstances, people can fast for as long as 60–90 days and obese persons may survive for over a year without food.

Amino acids can be used as a fuel after conversion to glucose

Amino acids normally are not a source of energy but are substrates for synthesis of the body's proteins. However, in certain situations they become energy substrates. First, during a prolonged fast or during metabolic stress induced by illness or injury, body proteins are degraded and the constituent amino acids are converted into glucose during gluconeogenesis. Second, when an excessive amount of amino acids is taken as food, they are converted to carbohydrates and are either stored or metabolized (see Chapter 19).

Various organs and tissues handle fuels differently

At rest, the brain uses approximately 20% of all oxygen (O_2) consumed by the body. Glucose is normally the brain's only fuel: during starvation, however, the brain can use ketones as an alternative energy source.

The two endogenous pathways that provide glucose are glycogenolysis and gluconeogenesis. When glucose concentration in the extracellular fluid decreases, it is quickly replenished through the degradation of liver glycogen. However, when fasting extends, more glucose starts to be formed by gluconeogenesis. Gluconeogenesis takes place primarily in the liver but the kidneys contribute during prolonged fast. The main substrates for gluconeogenesis are lactate (from anaerobic glycolysis), alanine (from the breakdown of muscle protein) and glycerol (from the breakdown of adipose tissue triacylglycerols (triglycerides);(see Chapter 13).

Muscle uses both glucose and fatty acids as energy sources. During short-term exercise, glucose is the preferred substrate but at rest and during prolonged exercise, fatty acids are the main energy source (see Chapter 20). Muscle handles carbohydrates differently from the liver. It cannot release glucose directly into the circulation because, in contrast to the liver, it does not possess glucose-6-phosphatase (Glc-6-Pase) enzyme. Therefore, it can only use glycogen for its own energy needs. However, it contributes to liver gluconeogenesis by releasing lactate, which is transported to the liver.

GLUCOSE HOMEOSTASIS

In the fasting state, a person weighing 70 kg (154 lb) metabolizes glucose at a rate of approximately 2 mg/kg/min (200 g/24 h). Glucose concentration in plasma reflects the balance between

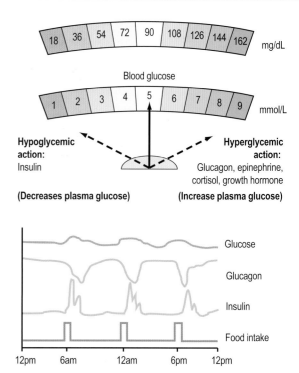

Fig. 21.1 **Hormonal control of glucose homeostasis.** Plasma glucose concentration reflects the balance between the hypoglycemic (glucose-decreasing) action of insulin and the hyperglycemic (glucose-increasing) action of anti-insulin hormones. The lower panel illustrates daily patterns of insulin and glucagon secretion, and corresponding pattern of plasma glucose concentration. Glucose concentration is maintained within a relatively narrow range throughout the day. To obtain glucose concentrations in mg/dL, multiply by 18.

its intake (glucose absorption from the gut) or its endogenous production (glycogenolysis and gluconeogenesis) and its tissue utilization (glycolysis, pentose phosphate pathway, tricarboxylic acid (TCA) cycle and glycogen synthesis) (see Fig. 13.2).

Insulin and glucagon are the main hormones responsible for controlling plasma glucose concentration

Glucose homeostasis is controlled by, on the one hand, anabolic hormone insulin and on the other, catabolic hormones (glucagon, catecholamines, cortisol, and growth hormone) known also as antiinsulin or counterregulatory hormones (Fig. 21.1).

Insulin and glucagon are both secreted from the same anatomic location – the pancreatic islets of Langerhans. Insulin is secreted by β-cells (approximately 70% of all islet cells) and glucagon by the α-cells. The molar ratio of insulin to glucagon at any given time is the key determinant of fuel metabolism.

INSULIN

Insulin molecule

The insulin molecule consists of two peptide chains linked by two disulfide bonds. The α-chain contains 21 amino acids

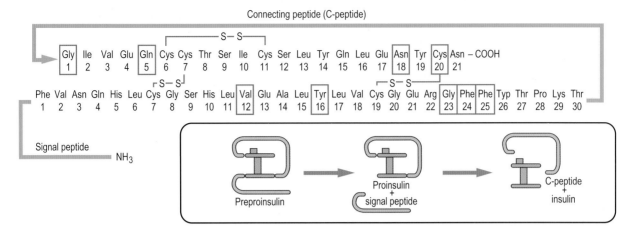

Fig. 21.2 **Insulin.** The insulin molecule consists of two polypeptide chains joined by two disulfide bonds. The third bond is internal to the β-chain. Insulin is synthesized as a longer peptide, preproinsulin, which is split into the signal peptide and proinsulin. Before secretion from the β-cell, proinsulin is split further into the C-peptide and insulin. Boxes drawn around amino acid residues indicate amino acids participating in the binding to the insulin receptor.

and the β-chain 30 amino acids. Its molecular weight is 5500 Da. Insulin is synthesized in the rough endoplasmic reticulum of the pancreatic β-cells and is packaged into the secretory vesicles in the Golgi apparatus. The precursor of insulin is the single chain molecule, preproinsulin. First, a 24-amino acid signal sequence is cleaved from preproinsulin by a peptidase, yielding proinsulin. Proinsulin is then split by endopeptidases into insulin and C-peptide (Fig. 21.2; see also box on p. 94), both of which are released from the cell in equimolar amounts. This is exploited for the assessment of β-cell function in patients treated with insulin injections. In such persons endogenous insulin cannot be measured directly, because the administered insulin would interfere in the assay. However, since C-peptide is present in the same molar concentration as native insulin, it serves as a marker of β-cell function.

Insulin secretion is determined by glucose metabolism in the β cell

During a meal containing carbohydrate, glucose concentration is sensed by the pancreatic β-cells. As glucose enters the β-cell, the increased rate of its metabolism triggers insulin secretion (this is known as the metabolism-secretion coupling). In parallel to stimulating insulin secretion, glucose suppresses secretion of glucagon.

The β-cell takes up glucose through the membrane transporter GLUT-2 (see Chapter 8 and Table 8.2). On entering the cell, glucose is phosphorylated by glucokinase. As glucose metabolism is stimulated, the ATP/ADP ratio in the cell increases. This closes the ATP-sensitive potassium channels in the cell membrane and depolarizes the cell, opening the calcium channel. Calcium ions enter the cell (see Chapter 40) and stimulate the release of secretory granules containing preformed insulin. This is known as the first phase of insulin secretion (compare this with the neurosecretory granules, Chapter 41) (Fig. 21.3). Loss of this phase is the early functional

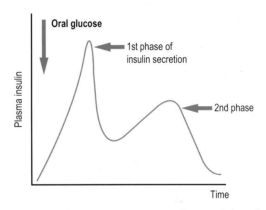

Fig. 21.3 **Phases of insulin secretion.** Note the two phases of insulin secretion. Glucose is the most important stimulator of insulin secretion, but secretion is also stimulated by some amino acids (branched-chain amino acids), by the stimulation of the vagus nerve and by the hormones secreted by the gut.

sign of islet cell damage. The second phase of insulin secretion involves synthesis of new insulin and responds to signals such as an increase in the concentration of the cytosolic long-chain acetyl-CoA.

Gut hormones potentiate insulin secretion

Insulin secretion is also stimulated by amino acids, such as leucine, arginine, and lysine. Gastrointestinal hormones, such as glucose-dependent insulinotropic peptide (GIP), cholecystokinin, glucagon-like peptide-1 (GLP-1) and vasoactive intestinal peptide (VIP), secreted following ingestion of foods, potentiate insulin secretion. This explains why insulin response to orally administered glucose is greater than to its intravenous infusion. GLP-1 and GIP are degraded by the enzyme dipeptidyl peptidase-4 (DPP-4).

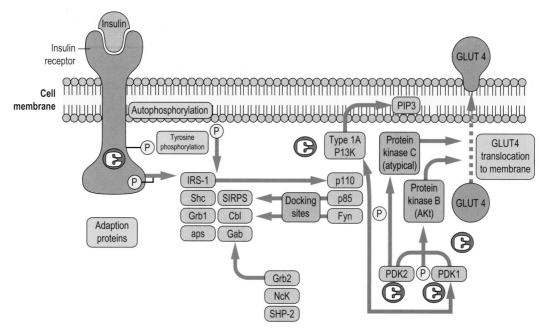

Fig. 21.4 **Insulin signaling.** Insulin signaling cascades transfer the signal from the insulin molecule to target molecules such as regulatory enzymes in key pathways or the membrane glucose transporter GLUT-4. One signaling pathway leads from the insulin receptor, through receptor phosphorylation to the phosphorylation of IRS-1, the phosphoinositol (PI3) kinase, then PDKs and two downstream kinases Akt/PKB and PKC. There are also other mediators of Akt and PKC action (not shown here) which determine GLUT-4 cycling between endoplasmic reticulum and cell membrane (compare Fig 13.7). PDK, phosphoinositide-dependent kinase; PKB, protein kinase B; PKC, protein kinase C.

Insulin action

Insulin signaling within cells involves a membrane receptor and multistep phosphorylation cascades

Much progress has been made in recent years in our understanding of how the insulin molecule conveys its metabolic message (Fig. 21.4; compare Fig. 13.7).

Cellular propagation of insulin signal includes multiple phosphorylations at different sites (tyrosine phosphorylation sends signals differently from serine-threonine phosphorylation). These phosphorylations help create conformational changes that enable binding (docking) of other proteins that transfer the signal downstream.

First, insulin binds to its receptor, a four-subunit protein, which spans membranes of the target cells. The β-subunit of the receptor contains an ATP-binding site and has tyrosine kinase activity. Binding of insulin causes the receptor to autophosphorylate. The receptor also recruits and phosphorylates several other proteins: insulin receptor substrates, designated IRS1–4, and adaptor proteins Gab1, Shc, Grb1, SIRPS and others. These in turn generate docking sites for other proteins such as the 1 A phosphatidylinositol 3-kinase (PI3K), protein tyrosine phosphatase (SHP2) and Fyn kinase.

PI3K generates lipid-based messengers, the phosphoinositol phosphates: PI-3,4-P2 and PI-3,4,5-P3 (see Chapter 40). They in turn recruit the serine-threonine kinase (protein kinase B, PKB, also called Akt) and the 3'-phosphoinositide-dependent kinases 1 and 2 (PDK1 and 2). PDK1 phosphorylates PKB and

PKC (see below). A form of PKB known as PKB β is involved in glucose transport and translocation in adipocytes. Several isoforms of another kinase, atypical protein kinase C (PKC), are involved in glucose transport in adipocytes and skeletal muscle. It becomes activated when its regulatory domain binds lipid messengers such as inositol trisphosphate, and after phosphorylation by PDK-1.

Serine-threonine kinases can also phosphorylate IRS1; this decreases its susceptibility to phosphorylation by the insulin receptor, introducing a further regulatory loop. In addition, phosphatases such as the phosphotyrosine phosphatase 1B contribute to the termination of insulin signal.

Finally, there is the PI3K-independent pathway of insulin signaling that also activates glucose transport; the insulin receptor phosphorylates a protein called Cbl, using associated protein substrate (APS) as an adaptor. Phosphorylated Cbl binds to Cbl-associated protein (CAP). CAP in turn binds to flotillin, a protein associated with lipid rafts in the membrane. Flotillin docks guanyl nucleotide exchange factor (C3G) with mediation of another adaptor molecule, CrkII. This activates a G-protein called TC-10 which participates in GLUT-4 translocation in adipocytes.

Metabolic effects of insulin

Insulin promotes the anabolic state by channeling metabolism towards the storage of carbohydrates and lipids, and towards protein synthesis. It also suppresses the relevant

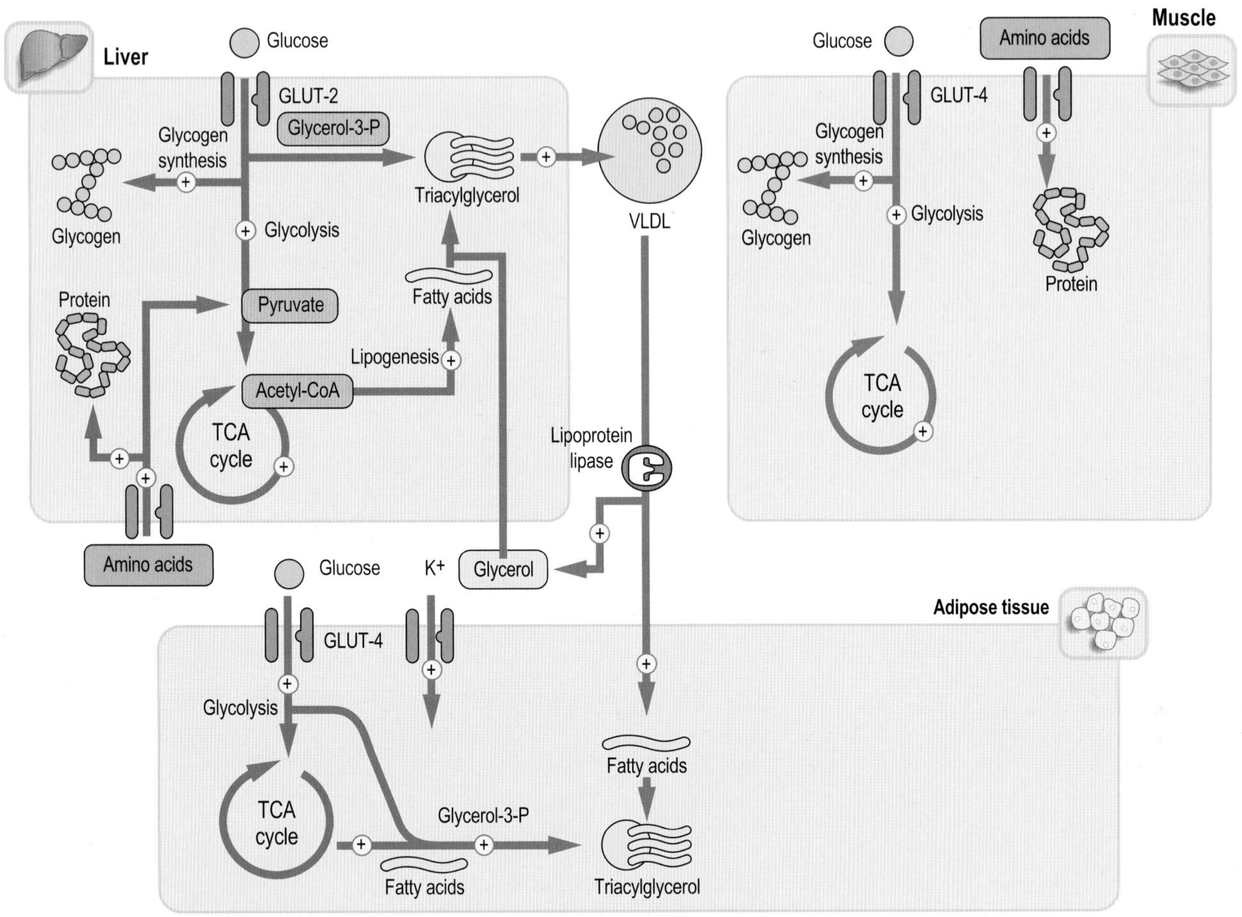

Fig. 21.5 **Metabolic effects of insulin.** The main insulin target tissues are liver, muscle, and adipose tissue. Insulin affects carbohydrate, lipid, and protein metabolism, and also promotes cellular potassium uptake. Glucose transport in muscle and adipose tissue is mediated by the GLUT-4 transporter and is insulin dependent. However, the glucose transporter in liver (GLUT-2) is insulin independent (compare Fig. 13.7).

catabolic pathways. Insulin acts on three main target tissues: liver, adipose tissue and skeletal muscle (Fig. 21.5).

In the liver, insulin stimulates glycolysis and glycogen synthesis. At the same time, it suppresses lipolysis and gluconeogenesis. It stimulates synthesis of long-chain fatty acids and triacylglycerols (the latter is known as lipogenesis). It promotes lipid transport from the liver to the peripheral cells involving particles of very low-density lipoproteins (VLDL). In the peripheral tissues, insulin induces endothelial lipoprotein lipase, an enzyme that liberates triacylglycerol from chylomicrons and VLDL (see Chapter 18).

In the adipose tissue, insulin stimulates triglyceride synthesis from glycerol-3-phosphate and fatty acids.

In muscle, it stimulates glucose transport, glucose metabolism, and glycogen synthesis. It increases cellular uptake of amino acids and stimulates protein synthesis.

Insulin-dependent glucose transport across cell membrane

Insulin-dependent glucose entry into cells is mediated by glucose transporters (see Table 8.2). The GLUT-4 transporter controls glucose uptake in skeletal muscle and adipocytes.

GLUT-4 cycles between the endosomal compartment and membrane. In an unstimulated cell, most of the GLUT-4 molecules reside intracellularly and no more than 10% are present in the plasma membrane. In humans, insulin doubles recruitment of the transporter to cell membrane. GLUT-4 translocation is affected by insulin signals transmitted through IRS1, the phosphatidylinositol 3-kinase (PI3K), PKB/Akt and the atypical PKC. Importantly, muscular contraction increases the expression of GLUT-4 independently of insulin. On the other hand, fatty acids decrease the expression of GLUT-4 in muscle.

Insulin resistance is a major factor in the development of type 2 diabetes

Insulin resistance is a condition in which insulin produces a less than expected response. This may be due either to its inadequate synthesis or secretion or, most often, to inability of the insulin molecule to exert its normal effect in a cell. Mildly insulin-resistant individuals have normal plasma glucose concentration but have hyperinsulinemia. This indicates that more insulin is required to produce a 'normal' effect. When resistance becomes more severe, plasma glucose

Sites of insulin resistance

Site of resistance	Possible defect	Role in diabetes
Prereceptor	insulin receptor antibodies, abnormal molecule	rare
Receptor	decreased number or affinity of insulin receptors	not significant in diabetes
Postreceptor	defects in signal transduction: defective tyrosine phosphylation, mutations in genes coding for IRS-1, phosphatidylinositol-3' kinase defective translocation of GLUT-2 to cell membrane	postreceptor resistance is the most common type of insulin resistance
	elevated concentration of fatty acids	

Table 21.2 **Sites of insulin resistance.**

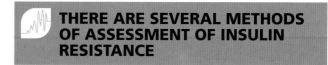

THERE ARE SEVERAL METHODS OF ASSESSMENT OF INSULIN RESISTANCE

Insulin resistance can be assessed by function tests, which are used mostly for research purposes. One such test is the hyper-insulinemic euglycemic clamp: insulin is infused at a constant rate together with variable amounts of glucose. The rate of glucose infusion is adjusted to keep plasma glucose concentration at 5–5.5 mmol/L (90–99 mg/dL). When a steady state is attained, the rate of glucose infusion is equal to the peripheral glucose uptake and is a measure of insulin sensitivity/resistance. Other tests of insulin resistance are based on the oral glucose tolerance test (see below) and involve frequent measurements of plasma glucose and insulin concentrations after glucose load.

concentration increases. Clinically, it is seen first as impaired glucose tolerance and subsequently as type 2 diabetes. Insulin resistance is common in obesity, which is a major risk factor for the development of type 2 diabetes.

The most important cause of insulin resistance is defective insulin signaling

Within a cell, insulin resistance may be caused by defects at several levels (Table 21.2). It could be a compromised insulin binding to its receptor, for instance due to a very rare mutation in the insulin receptor gene. Resistance can also be caused by antireceptor autoantibodies. The most important causes, however, are defects in the insulin signaling pathways. In type 2 diabetes and in persons with a strong family history of diabetes, the IRS-phosphoinositol kinase pathway may not operate normally. This impairs cellular translocation of the GLUT-4 transporter, and consequently glucose uptake in the adipose tissue. Reduced expression and impaired translocation of GLUT-4 in adipocytes (but not in skeletal muscle) have been observed in obesity and diabetes. Interestingly, adipocytes of GLUT-4 deficient (GLUT-4 knock-out) mice also show overexpression of a gene for another protein, the retinol-binding protein (RBP). Although RBP originates in adipocytes, it was found to impair insulin signaling in muscle; thus it serves as an inter-tissue messenger that propagates insulin resistance.

Other causes of insulin resistance include variants of genes coding for IRS1 and phosphatidylinositol 3-kinase. Elevated fatty acids also contribute to insulin resistance by

inhibiting peripheral glucose disposal, enhancing hepatic glucose output and damaging β-cell function. Steatosis (accumulation of triacylglycerols in liver and muscle), seen in patients with dyslipidemia and high plasma triacylglycerol concentration, also contributes to insulin resistance.

Effects of glucagon and anti-insulin hormones

Anti-insulin hormones antagonize the effect of insulin, promoting hyperglycemia

Antiinsulin hormones mobilize glucose through stimulation of glycogenolysis and gluconeogenesis. This causes an increase in plasma glucose concentration (hyperglycemia).

Glucagon acts on the liver

Glucagon is a small, single-chain, 29-amino acid peptide, with a molecular weight of 3485 Da. It acts on the liver and its function is to mobilize fuel reserves to maintain blood glucose concentration between meals. It directs metabolism towards catabolism and inhibits anabolism. It stimulates glycogenolysis, gluconeogenesis (Table 21.3), oxidation of fatty acids and ketogenesis, and inhibits glycolysis, glycogen synthesis and the synthesis of triacylglycerols (lipogenesis) (Fig. 21.6).

Glucagon binds to its own membrane receptor (see Chapter 13, Fig. 13.4), which signals through the membrane-associated G-proteins and the cyclic AMP cascade. First, the glucagon–receptor complex causes binding of guanosine 5'-triphosphate (GTP) to a G-protein complex (see Chapter 40 for details). This leads to the dissociation of G-protein subunits. One of the subunits (Gα) activates the adenylate cyclase, which converts ATP into cyclic AMP (cAMP). cAMP in turn activates cAMP-dependent protein kinase which, through phosphorylation of several regulatory enzymes, controls the

Reciprocal effects of insulin and glucagon on the key enzymes of gluconeogenesis

Enzyme	Effect of glucagon	Effect of insulin
Glc-6-Pase	+	−
Fru-1,6-BPase	+	−
PEPCK	+	−

On a high-carbohydrate diet, insulin induces gene transcription of the glycolytic enzymes glucokinase, PFK, pyruvate kinase, and glycogen synthase. At the same time, it represses the key enzymes of gluconeogenesis, pyruvate carboxylase (PC), phosphoenolpyruvate carboxykinase (PEPCK), Fru-1,6-BPase, and Glc-6-Pase. Glucagon effects oppose those of insulin. On a high-fat diet, glucagon represses the synthesis of glucokinase, PFK-1, and pyruvate kinase, and induces the transcription of PEPCK, Fru-6-Pase, and Glc-6-Pase.

Table 21.3 **Reciprocal effects of insulin and glucagon on the key enzymes of gluconeogenesis.**

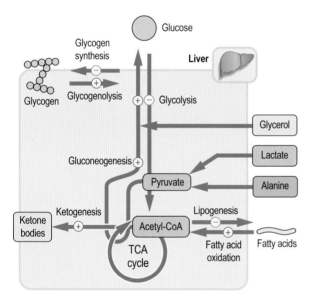

Fig. 21.6 **Metabolic effects of glucagon.** Glucagon mobilizes glucose from every available source; it also increases lipolysis, and ketogenesis from acetyl-CoA. Glucagon action is confined to the liver (compare Fig 13.4).

activity of key enzymes in carbohydrate and lipid metabolism (Figs 21.6 and 21.7).

Importantly, there are no glucagon receptors on muscle cells; muscle glycogenolysis is stimulated by another anti-insulin hormone, epinephrine.

The action of epinephrine

The metabolic effects of epinephrine (adrenaline) are similar to glucagon. It inhibits glycolysis and lipogenesis, and stimulates

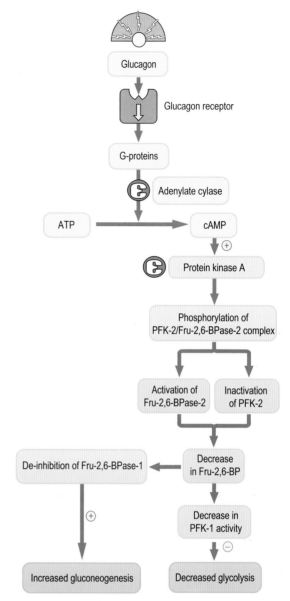

Fig. 21.7 **Regulation of glycolysis and gluconeogenesis by phosphofructokinase.** Glucagon regulates gluconeogenesis by controlling the bifunctional enzyme complex that contains activities of both phosphofructokinase-2 (PFK-2) and fructose 2,6-biphosphatase-2 (Fru-2,6-BPase-2). Glucagon binds to its membrane receptor and signals through G-proteins, and adenylate cyclase, generating cyclic AMP. cAMP activates protein kinase A. This kinase in turn phosphorylates the PFK-2:Fru-2,6-BPase complex. Phosphorylation activates the bisphosphatase which degrades Fru-2,6-BP. Lowering of Fru-2,6-BP dis-inhibits another enzyme, Fru-2,6-BPase-1, in the main gluconeogenic pathway. Gluconeogenesis is stimulated. Ingeniously, the decrease in Fru-2,6-BP has a reciprocal inhibitory effect on mainline phosphofructokinase (PFK-1). This inhibits glycolysis. Overall, glucagon action results in stimulation of gluconeogenesis and inhibition of glycolysis.

gluconeogenesis. Its receptors are the α- and β-adrenergic receptors (mainly the β_2 receptor; see Fig 13.5) and they link to the cAMP signaling cascade. Epinephrine is a key hormone responsible for hyperglycemia in response to stress.

Hormones regulate key enzymes in metabolic pathways by different mechanisms

The way to change the rate and direction of metabolic pathways is to control the activity of key (regulatory) enzymes. Hormones target regulatory enzymes. Regulation of enzyme activity can be exerted through several mechanisms: induction or repression of genes that code for these enzymes, phosphorylation and dephosphorylation of enzyme molecules, and other mechanisms such as substrate interactions and allosteric changes. Cell energy level and the redox state of the cell also control their activity (see Chapter 6).

Transcription factors directly control gene induction

Induction or repression of genes (see Table 21.3) takes days or weeks to take effect, and may occur in response to diet, chronic stress or illness. For example, activities of several hepatic enzymes are different in people on a high-fat diet compared to those on a high-carbohydrate diet.

Gene induction is controlled by proteins known as transcription factors that bind to the response elements in gene promoters (see Chapter 34, Fig. 34.2). Transcription factors act within translational complexes that include more than one transcription factor and also other molecules called coactivators and corepressors. This complexity allows for different transcriptional responses in different tissues, and also for interactions between different genes. Transcription factors themselves are often targets of the hormonal signaling cascades.

Phosphorylation is a key regulatory mechanism in metabolic pathways and signaling cascades

Short-term regulation involves phosphorylation and dephosphorylation of key molecules. Enzymes are commonly controlled by this mechanism. Signaling cascades often involve several levels of kinases and phosphatases. Phosphorylation/dephosphorylation is also a mechanism which can regulate transcription factors. Figures 21.7 and 21.8 illustrate how this mechanism controls enzymes that regulate glycogenolysis, gluconeogenesis and lipolysis.

Insulin and glucagon switch genes on and off during feed-fast cycle

Insulin regulates synthesis of key enzymes by controlling the activity of so-called forkhead transcription factors (they have a helix-turn-helix structure with two additional loops or wings). Two such transcription factors, Foxo1 and Foxa2, are essential for switching metabolism from anabolism to catabolism. The transcription factor Foxo1 promotes gluconeogenesis in the liver in the fasted state, and Foxa2 regulates fatty acid oxidation. They are both inactivated by phosphorylation by kinases in the IRS-PKB/Akt pathway.

Foxo1 and its coactivators Pgc-1 and TORC2 (the latter being cAMP responsive) stimulate gluconeogenesis by activating genes that code for rate-limiting enzymes PEPCK and G-6-Pase. During feeding, insulin, again through the IRS-PKB/Akt pathway, phosphorylates Foxo1, inactivating it. This inhibits hepatic gluconeogenesis. Insulin also deactivates TORC2. Glucagon, on the other hand, dephosphorylates TORC2, activating it and facilitating induction of gluconeogenic enzymes.

Foxa2 regulates fat breakdown in the fasted state by inducing genes encoding enzymes of glycolysis, fatty acid

SENSITIVITY OF TRANSCRIPTION FACTORS TO INSULIN MAY VARY

The transcription factor Foxa 2 is more sensitive to being switched off by insulin than Foxo 1. This creates a situation where insulin may stimulate lipogenesis and inhibit Foxa 2-controlled fatty acid oxidation, but fail to suppress Foxo 1-controlled gluconeogenesis. This leads to parallel uninhibited gluconeogenesis and lipogenesis and results in accumulation of triacylglycerols in the liver (hepatic steatosis). Steatosis aggravates insulin resistance (see Fig. 34.2).

REGULATORY ROLE OF THE TRANSCRIPTION FACTOR PPARγ

Peroxisome proliferator activator receptors (PPARs) are ligand-activated nuclear receptors belonging to the steroid receptor family. Binding of a ligand induces conformational change which allows a PPAR to form a heterodimer with another receptor, retinoid X receptor (RXR). PPAR may also bind or release small molecules, coactivators or corepressors. The complex binds to response elements in gene promoters (Fig. 21.9).

There are three types of PPAR: PPARα which is discussed in Chapter 18, PPARγ and PPARβ. PPARγ is predominantly expressed in adipose tissue but also in muscle, liver, intestine and heart. It is activated by polyunsaturated fatty acids and by components of oxidized LDL. It regulates carbohydrate and fatty acid metabolism inducing, among others, genes coding for lipoprotein lipase (LPL), GLUT-4 glucose transporter and glucokinase. It also induces the ABCA1 transporter, increasing transfer of cholesterol from cells to the HDL (Chapter 18). It also inhibits macrophage activation and the production of cytokines such as tumor necrosis factor (TNF-α), interferon-γ and interleukin-1 (IL-1). PPAR-α is a target of thiazolidine diones, drugs used in the treatment of type 2 diabetes.

oxidation, and ketogenesis. This leads to an increase in the concentrations of free fatty acids, ketone bodies and triglycerides, and to a decrease in liver triglyceride content. Insulin phosphorylates and inhibits Foxa2 through the IRS-PKB/Akt pathway.

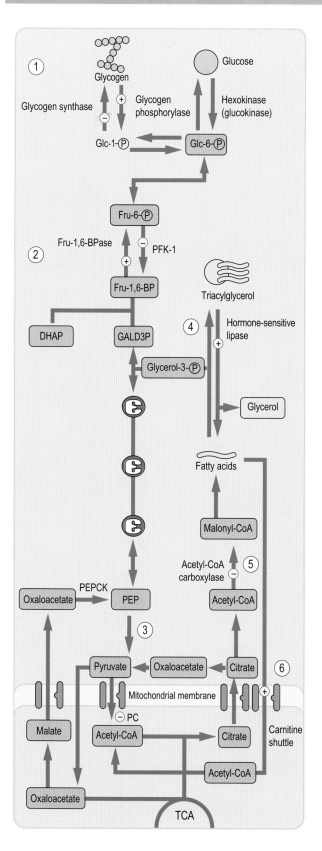

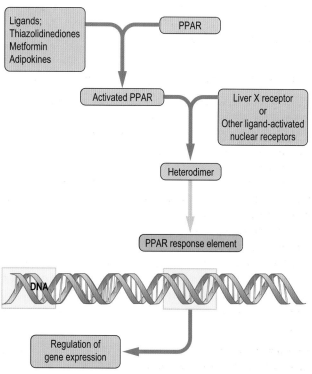

Fig. 21.9 **Transcriptional regulation by peroxisome proliferator-activator receptors (PPARs).** PPARs are activated by ligands that may be metabolites or drugs. They form heterodimer complexes with a range of other nuclear receptors. Resulting complexes bind to the PPAR response elements located in gene promoters, regulating gene expression.

Fig. 21.8 **Regulatory role of enzyme phosphorylation.** Carbohydrate and lipid metabolism is regulated by the phosphorylation of key enzymes, controlled by glucagon and epinephrine. Note that phosphorylation usually stimulates enzymes in catabolic pathways and inhibits these in anabolic ones. Thus:
In glycogen metabolism: glycogen phosphorylase is activated and glycogen synthase is inactivated. This promotes glycogen breakdown (1). **In gluconeogenesis:** Fru-2,6-BPase-2 is activated and PFK-2 is inhibited. This decreases Fru-2,6-BP formation which inhibits PFK-1 (glycolysis) and stimulates FBPase (gluconeogenesis) (2). **In glycolysis:** Fru-1,6-BP also allosterically activates pyruvate kinase downstream in the glycolytic pathway. Because its formation is decreased, glycolysis slows down (3). **In lipolysis:** phosphorylation stimulates hormone-sensitive lipase-stimulating lipolysis (the release of fatty acids from triglycerides) (4). **In fatty acid oxidation:** phosphorylation inhibits acetyl-CoA carboxylase, inhibiting generation of malonyl-CoA (5). Malonyl-CoA normally inhibits carnitine-palmitoyl transferase-1. Lack of malonyl-CoA disinhibits it (6), facilitating the entry of fatty acids into mitochondria. This stimulates lipid oxidation. DHAP, dihydroxyacetone phosphate; GALD3P, glyceraldehyde-3-phosphate; PEP, phosphoenolpyruvate.

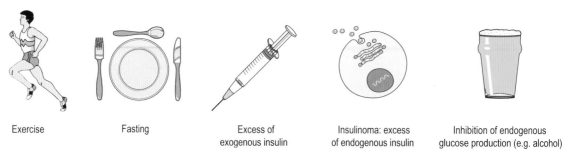

Exercise   Fasting   Excess of exogenous insulin   Insulinoma: excess of endogenous insulin   Inhibition of endogenous glucose production (e.g. alcohol)

Fig. 21.10 **Causes of hypoglycemia.** Hypoglycemia is plasma glucose concentration below 4 mmol/L (72 mg/dL). Severe hypoglycemia is glucose concentration below 2.5 mmol/L (45 mg/dL). Hypoglycemia may result from decreased supply of glucose or from an increased concentration of insulin. It also results from increased utilization of glucose by tissues (exercise).

HYPOGLYCEMIA

We define hypoglycemia (low blood glucose) as blood glucose concentration below 4 mmol/L (72 mg/dL). Low plasma glucose stimulates the sympathetic nervous system. Epinephrine and glucagon are released, initiating the stress response, manifested as sweating, tremor, increased heart rate, and a feeling of hunger. If glucose continues to fall, brain function becomes compromised because of lack of glucose (neuroglycopenia: this usually happens when glucose concentration falls below 2.5 mmol/L (45 mg/dL)). The person becomes confused and may lose consciousness. Profound hypoglycemia can be fatal.

Hypoglycemia in healthy individuals is usually mild and may occur during exercise, after a period of fasting or as a result of drinking alcohol. Alcohol increases the intracellular $NADH + H^+/NAD^+$ ratio, which favors conversion of pyruvate to lactate and reduces the amount of pyruvate available for gluconeogenesis (see Clinical Box on p. 168). Hypoglycemia may also occur when there is an insufficient amount of counterregulatory hormones to balance the effects of insulin; this happens in adrenal or pituitary insufficiency when cortisol concentration is low (in the latter there is an insufficient amount of adrenocorticotrophic hormone (ACTH; see Chapter 39). Another endocrine cause of hypoglycemia is a rare tumor of β-cells, insulinoma, which secretes large amounts of insulin. Glycogen storage diseases are rare causes of hypoglycemia in childhood (see Chapter 13 and Clinical Boxes on pp. 158 and 163). The causes of hypoglycemia are summarized in Fig. 21.10.

FEED–FAST CYCLE

Human metabolism oscillates between fed and fasting states. The key switch which determines metabolic changes is the molar ratio of insulin to glucagon in plasma. A high-insulin/low-glucagon state occurs during a meal and for several hours after (this is called the absorptive, postprandial or fed state), and a low-insulin/high-glucagon state occurs on fasting. Fasting for 6–12 h is called the postabsorptive state.

Fasting that lasts longer than 12 h is 'prolonged fasting' or 'starvation'.

Fed (absorptive) state

Meal stimulates insulin release and inhibits glucagon secretion

Nutrients in a meal stimulate insulin release and suppress the secretion of glucagon. This affects metabolism of the liver, adipose tissue, and muscle (Fig. 21.11). Glucose utilization by the brain remains unchanged.

There is an increase in glucose uptake in the insulin-dependent tissues, principally in the skeletal muscle. Glucose oxidation and glycogen synthesis are stimulated, and lipid oxidation is inhibited. Glucose taken up by the liver is phosphorylated by glucokinase, yielding Glc-6-P. Excess glucose is directed into the pentose phosphate pathway, generating $NADPH + H^+$ that is used in biosyntheses that require reductions, such as synthesis of fatty acids and cholesterol.

Fat (triacylglycerols) absorbed in the intestine is transported in chylomicrons to peripheral tissues, where it is hydrolyzed to glycerol and free fatty acids by lipoprotein lipase (see Chapter 18). Fatty acids are taken up by cells. They are reassembled into triacylglycerols and stored; in muscle they are used as a fuel. Synthesis of triacylglycerols from fatty acids requires glycerol, which is provided from glycolysis (triose phosphate being reduced to glycerol-3-phosphate). Insulin stimulates synthesis of fatty acids in the liver and adipose tissue. It also stimulates amino acid uptake and protein synthesis, and decreases protein degradation in liver, muscle, and adipose tissue.

Fasting (postabsorptive) state

During fasting the liver switches from a glucose-utilizing to a glucose-producing organ

During fasting, insulin secretion decreases and glucagon secretion increases (Fig. 21.12). As a consequence, there is

Postprandial metabolism

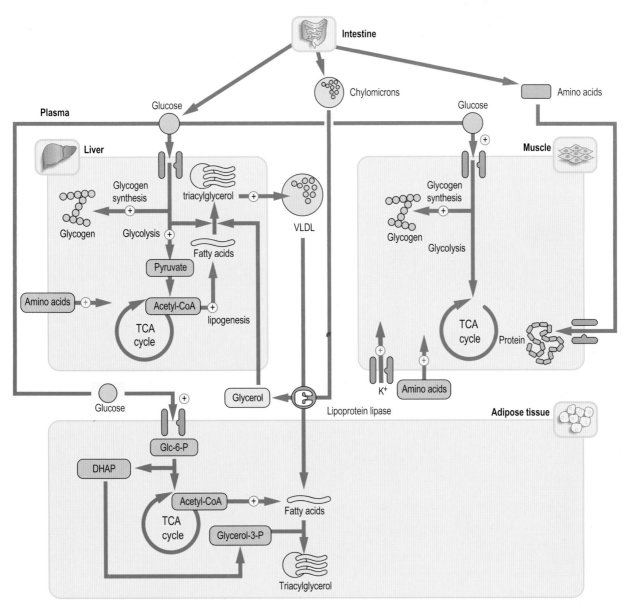

Fig. 21.11 **Metabolism in the fed (postprandial) state.** Carbohydrates, amino acids and fats are absorbed in the intestine and insulin secretion is stimulated. Insulin directs metabolism towards storage and synthesis (anabolism). In the liver, glucose is taken up by the GLUT-2 transporter and is channeled into glycolysis, glycogen synthesis. Aerobic glycolysis supplies the acetyl-CoA which is a substrate for lipogenesis. The synthesized fatty acids are esterified by glycolysis-derived glycerol, forming triacylglycerols. These are packaged into VLDL for transport to peripheral tissues. Muscle glycogen synthesis, amino acid uptake and protein synthesis are stimulated. In the adipose tissue, VLDL triacylglycerols are hydrolyzed and fatty acids are taken up by cells. Triacylglycerols are resynthesized intracellularly as adipocyte storage material. DHAP, dihydroxyacetone phosphate; Glc-6-P, glucose-6-phosphate (compare Fig. 16.8).

a decrease in glycogen synthesis and an increase in glycogenolysis. This transforms the liver from a glucose-utilizing to a glucose-producing organ. A steady state, with hepatic glucose production equal to its peripheral uptake, is achieved after an overnight fast.

Three key substrates for gluconeogenesis are lactate, alanine and glycerol

In the fasting state, as much as 80% of all glucose is taken up by insulin-independent tissues. Of this, 50% goes to the brain and 20% to the erythrocytes. Insulin-dependent tissues use relatively little glucose – the muscle and adipose tissue together use only 20% of all available glucose. After a 12 h fast, 65–75% of synthesized glucose is still derived from glycogen; the rest comes from gluconeogenesis. If fasting lasts longer, the contribution of gluconeogenesis steadily increases. Muscle helps gluconeogenesis by releasing lactate, which is taken up by the liver and oxidized to pyruvate before it enters gluconeogenesis. Glucose released from the liver returns to the skeletal muscle, closing the loop known as the Cori cycle (Fig. 21.13).

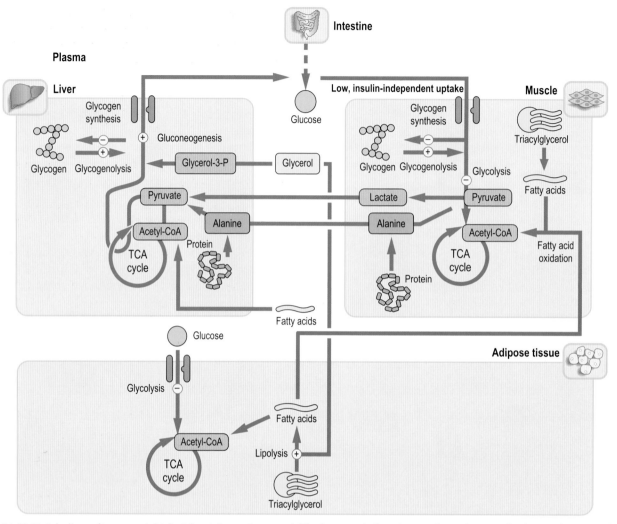

Fig. 21.12 **Metabolism after overnight fast (postabsorptive state).** The liver metabolism changes from glucose utilization to glucose production (gluconeogenesis stimulated by glucagon). Glucagon also stimulates glycogenolysis and inhibits glycolysis. Note the substrates for gluconeogenesis: alanine, lactate and glycerol. Alanine and lactate are transported to the liver from muscle (see Fig. 21.13). Glucose uptake by the muscle and adipose tissue decreases. Lipolysis and fatty acid oxidation are stimulated, providing energy.

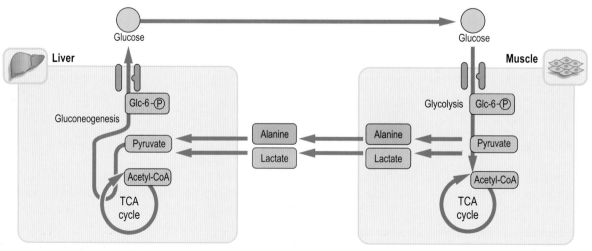

Fig. 21.13 **Cori cycle and glucose–alanine cycle.** The Cori (glucose–lactate) cycle allows recycling of lactate back to glucose, but does not contribute to the de novo synthesis of glucose. Alanine is derived mostly from muscle proteolysis.

Low insulin concentration stimulates proteolysis and leads to the release of amino acids (primarily alanine and glutamine) from muscle. Released alanine is taken up by the liver, and converted to pyruvate that enters gluconeogenesis. This glucose–alanine cycle parallels the Cori cycle.

Glucagon stimulates hydrolysis of triacylglycerols (lipolysis) by the hormone-sensitive lipase. This releases glycerol, which is the third (after lactate and alanine) gluconeogenic substrate, and generates free fatty acids. Fatty acid metabolism in turn stimulates ketogenesis from acetyl-CoA. Ketogenesis yields ketone bodies: acetoacetate, hydroxybutyrate, and the product of spontaneous decarboxylation of acetoacetate, acetone. During prolonged fasting, ketone bodies can be used as energy substrates in the heart and skeletal muscle.

Prolonged fasting (starvation)

Starvation is a chronic low-insulin, high-glucagon state. There is also a decrease in thyroid hormone concentration which decreases the metabolic rate. Free fatty acids are now the major energy substrate. Because gluconeogenesis uses oxaloacetate, the TCA cycle metabolite, its concentration in the mitochondria falls; this limits activity of the TCA cycle (see Chapter 14). Slowing down of the cycle leads to accumulation of acetyl-CoA from the β-oxidation of fatty acids. Acetyl-CoA is channeled into ketogenesis and the concentration of ketone bodies in plasma increases.

Several mechanisms during starvation minimize the need for synthesis of glucose from body proteins

During starvation gluconeogenesis takes place in both the liver and the kidneys. Muscle proteolysis increases, leading to a release of alanine and glutamine. However, the use of body proteins as substrates for gluconeogenesis is minimized by almost total dependence on fat as energy source (Fig. 21.14). Also, the Cori cycle decreases the requirement for endogenous glucose production and the amount of the GLUT-4 transporter in adipose tissue and muscle decreases, 'saving'

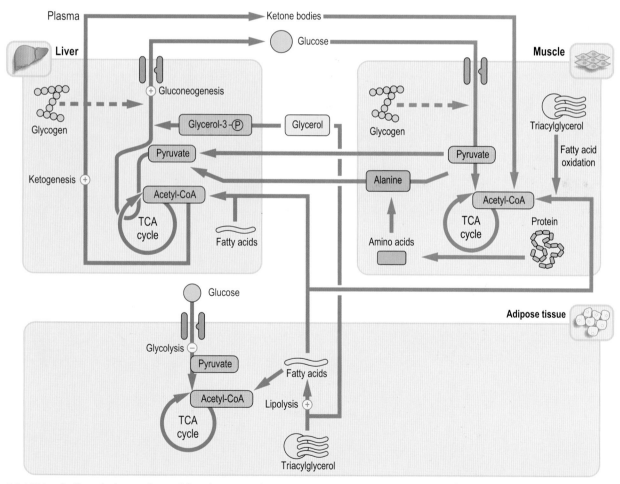

Fig. 21.14 **Metabolism during prolonged fast (starvation).** The direction of metabolism is similar to that during short-term fasting, but adaptive responses are in operation. Glycogen stores are depleted. The supply of metabolic fuels depends on gluconeogenesis and lipolysis. Ketone bodies produced from acetyl-CoA are becoming an important energy source for the muscle, and the brain also adapts to their use. Importantly, a decrease in the demand for glucose (and thus gluconeogenesis) spares muscle proteins.

more glucose. Eventually, the brain also adapts to the use of ketone bodies as fuel. Some brain tissue actually switches from the complete oxidation of glucose to glycolysis.

METABOLISM DURING STRESS

Response to stress is driven by the antiinsulin hormones

This type of metabolic response not only occurs during 'fight and flight' reactions but is also triggered by trauma, burns, surgery and infection. It is associated with hypermetabolism. The sympathetic nervous system plays a major role in its development. The metabolic response is driven by the anti-insulin hormones: catecholamines, primarily epinephrine (see Fig 13.5), glucagon and cortisol. Metabolic response to stress includes suppression of anabolic pathways (glycogen synthesis, lipogenesis), increased catabolism (glycogenolysis, lipolysis, and proteolysis) and increased insulin-independent peripheral glucose uptake (Fig. 21.15). Clinically, there is early vasoconstriction, which aims to limit

possible blood loss. There is also fever, tachycardia, tachypnea (increased respiratory rate), and leukocytosis (increased number of white blood cells).

Stress response safeguards glucose supply through glycogenolysis and gluconeogenesis

During stress response, energy substrates are mobilized from all available sources. The priority is to provide glucose for the brain: epinephrine and glucagon stimulate glycogenolysis and gluconeogenesis. In addition, decreased peripheral uptake of glucose makes more glucose available to the brain. Later, metabolic rate increases and fatty acids become the major source of energy. Muscle proteins supply amino acids for gluconeogenesis; this leads to the negative nitrogen balance within 2–3 days after injury.

Stress induces insulin resistance

Insulin-dependent transport of glucose into cells, mediated by GLUT-4, decreases. Glucocorticoid hormones contribute to this. They also facilitate stimulation of gluconeogenesis by glucagon and catecholamines by inducing genes coding for Glc-6-Pase

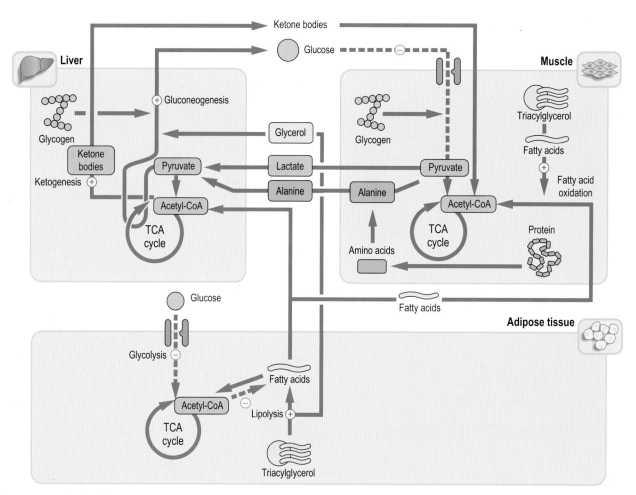

Fig. 21.15 **Metabolism during stress and injury.** The response to stress is catabolic and is broadly analogous to fasting. Glucose is mobilized from all available sources. Epinephrine plays a key role and, together with glucagon, inhibits insulin secretion. The effect of antiinsulin hormones prevails. Stress also induces peripheral insulin resistance, further sparing glucose. Energy is provided from glucose, fatty acids and from protein catabolism.

and phosphoenolpyruvate carboxykinase (PEPCK) (see Table 21.2). At the same time, insulin-independent glucose uptake increases, particularly in muscle. This is mediated by tumor necrosis factor α (TNF-α) and other cytokines such as interleukin-1 (IL-1) (see Chapter 43). TNF-α also stimulates muscle glycogen breakdown. Cytokines, such as IL-6, help induce PEPCK, stimulate lipolysis in the adipose tissue and contribute to muscle proteolysis. There is an increase in lactate production.

Stress response affects results of laboratory tests

Metabolic response to stress affects the results of common laboratory tests. A key finding is hyperglycemia; during stress it should not be confused with diabetes mellitus. Also, injury, infection, and trauma are associated with the so-called acute phase response, during which synthesis of a range of proteins, such as α_1-antitrypsin, C-reactive protein (CRP), haptoglobin, α_1-acid glycoprotein, complement proteins and others, increases. Measurements of CRP are important in monitoring the progress of treatment in patients with severe infections (see Chapter 4).

DIABETES MELLITUS

Diabetes is a disorder of fuel metabolism characterized by hyperglycemia and vascular damage

There are two major components to the syndrome of diabetes mellitus: hyperglycemia and vascular complications. Diabetes is increasingly common; the number of people with diabetes worldwide increased from 30 million in 1985 to over 170 million, and the WHO predicts that it will reach 300 million in 2025. The International Diabetes Federation's estimate is even higher at 380 million. There are approximately 440 000 children with type 1 diabetes worldwide and type 2 diabetes affects approximately 5% of the populations in developed countries (Table 21.4).

There are several forms of diabetes mellitus

There are four main forms of diabetes mellitus: type 1 diabetes, type 2 diabetes, secondary diabetes, and gestational diabetes (GDM, diabetes of pregnancy). The most common is type 2 diabetes; 90% of all diabetic patients have type 2 diabetes, and 5–10% have type 1. The other two forms are, in comparison, rare (see Table 21.4). Diabetes has a strong genetic component but is often unmasked by lifestyle factors. Importantly, some diabetic patients have no clinical symptoms at all. In these individuals the diagnosis is made solely on the basis of laboratory results.

Diabetes leads to changes in the walls of small (microangiopathy) and large (macroangiopathy) arteries, induced by a combination of oxidative stress, excessive formation of advanced glycation (glycoxidation) endproducts (AGE) and increased substrate flux through the polyol pathway (see below). Microangiopathy occurring in the kidney (diabetic nephropathy) leads to kidney failure (see box on p. 317), microangiopathy developing in the retina (diabetic retinopathy) may cause blindness, and that occurring in the nervous system (diabetic neuropathy) leads to impairment of the autonomic nerve function. Diabetic patients also develop lens opacities (cataracts). Diabetes is the main cause of blindness in the Western world and one of the main causes of kidney failure.

Diabetic macroangiopathy is associated with a 2–3 times greater risk of myocardial infarction than in nondiabetic persons of similar age. Macroangiopathy affecting peripheral arteries leads to diabetic peripheral vascular disease, and to foot ulceration: diabetes is a major cause of lower limb amputations. However, the most prevalent complication of diabetes is cardiovascular disease. It is also the main cause of death among people with type 2 diabetes.

Type 1 diabetes

Type 1 diabetes usually develops in people below 35 years of age, with the peak incidence at approximately 12 years. It is caused by autoimmune destruction of the pancreatic β-cells. Its precipitating cause is still unclear; it could be a viral infection, environmental toxins or foods. The autoimmune reaction could be initiated by the cytokine response to infection. In addition to the inflammatory infiltration of the

Classification of diabetes	
Syndrome	**Comments**
Type 1	autoimmune destruction of β-cells
Type 2	insulin resistance and β-cell failure
Other types	genetic defects of β-cells (e.g. mutations of glucokinase gene). Rare insulin resistance syndromes
	diseases of exocrine pancreas. Endocrine diseases (acromegaly, Cushing's syndrome). Drugs and chemical-induced diabetes, infections (e.g. mumps)
	rare syndromes with the presence of antireceptor antibodies Diabetes accompanying other genetic diseases (e.g. Down syndrome)
Gestational diabetes	any degree of glucose intolerance diagnosed in pregnancy

Type 1 diabetes was in older literature described as insulin-dependent diabetes (IDDM) and type 2 as noninsulin-dependent diabetes (NIDDM) or maturity-onset diabetes. Approximately 90% of all diabetic patients have type 2 diabetes.

Table 21.4 **Classification of diabetes.**

PLASMA GLUCOSE AFTER MYOCARDIAL INFARCTION

A 66-year-old woman was admitted to the cardiology ward with chest pain. Myocardial infarction was diagnosed on the basis of ECG and increased plasma troponin concentration. She was successfully treated with thrombolysis. At that time her random plasma glucose concentration was 10.5 mmol/L (189 mg/dL). Next day the fasting blood glucose was only slightly raised at 7.5 mmol/L (117 mg/dL). Normal fasting plasma glucose is <6.1 mmol/L.

Comment. Major stress associated with myocardial infarction is associated with the counterregulatory hormone response and this leads to the elevation of blood glucose concentration. Care is needed in the interpretation of raised fasting glucose levels in the context of acute illness. Glucose tolerance test should not be performed during acute illness.

MAJOR STRESS AFFECTS WATER AND ELECTROLYTE METABOLISM

A 65-year-old woman underwent partial gastrectomy. After surgery she was given a standard intravenous fluid replacement. The volume of fluids to be replaced was calculated on the basis of fluid lost in urine, through gastric drainage, and included an allowance for an insensible loss (water loss with breath and sweat). In spite of this carefully calculated volume of administered fluid, and a normal renal function, the patient developed hyponatremia and became clinically overloaded with fluid.

Comment. Response to stress, such as major surgery, includes stimulation of vasopressin secretion from the posterior pituitary. This increases water reabsorption by the kidney and causes water retention, which needs to be taken into account when prescribing postoperative fluid therapy (see also Chapters 22 and 23). Rapid onset of hyponatremia may cause convulsions or coma due to cerebral edema.

islets, a proportion of patients have circulating antibodies against various β-cell proteins, which may appear years before diagnosis. Autoantibodies to insulin, to glutamic acid decarboxylase and to protein tyrosine phosphatase have also been observed.

Susceptibility to type 1 diabetes is inherited. A sibling of a type 1 diabetic patient has a 10% chance of developing diabetes by the age of 50. Susceptibility genes are located on chromosome 6 in the major histocompatibility complex (MHC; Chapter 38). Approximately 50% of the genetic susceptibility to diabetes resides in the HLA genes: HLA genotypes DR and DQ, and to a lesser extent in other loci known as IDDM2 (insulin-VNTR) and IDDM12 (CTLA-4) are linked to diabetes. Both genes imparting risk and genes imparting protection have been identified within the HLA complex. Interestingly, this region also contains susceptibility genes associated with other autoimmune diseases; this means that patients with type 1 diabetes are more susceptible to other autoimmune disorders such as Graves' disease, Addison's disease and celiac disease. Persons with type 1 diabetes are prone to the development of ketoacidosis and are dependent on the insulin treatment.

Type 2 diabetes

Type 2 diabetes usually develops in obese patients who are over 40 years old. Its pathogenesis involves a combination of insulin resistance and impairment of insulin secretion.

There is a strong hereditary component to type 2 diabetes. Monozygotic twins are 90–95% concordant for diabetes, and first-degree relatives of diabetic persons have a 40% chance of developing the disease. By contrast, in people with no diabetic relatives such risk is only 10%. In 2007, a genome-wide study defined approximately 70% of the genetic risk for type 2 diabetes. The identified genes include previously known gene TCF7L2 and four others, the most important being SLC30A8, a gene, somewhat surprisingly, coding for a zinc transporter.

There is also a rare autosomal dominant form of type 2 diabetes known as maturity-onset diabetes of the young (MODY). MODY results from mutations of at least six different genes; among them are enzyme glucokinase (MODY2) and several transcription factors (e.g. hepatocyte nuclear factor HNF-4α (MODY1) and HNF-α$_1$ (MODY3)). There is also a mitochondrial DNA mutation that leads to impaired oxidative phosphorylation and to the so-called mitochondrial diabetes. To complicate things further, approximately 10% of patients diagnosed with type 2 diabetes also have autoantibodies to glutamic acid decarboxylase; these are actually individuals who are developing a form of type 1 diabetes, sometimes called latent autoimmune diabetes in adults (LADA).

In type 2 diabetes, ketoacidosis is rare. Patients may develop microvascular complications as in type 1 but the main problem is macrovascular complications, which eventually lead to coronary heart disease, peripheral vascular disease and stroke. Obesity is a major factor for the development of type 2 diabetes. Type 1 and type 2 diabetes are compared in Table 21.5.

Metabolism in diabetes

In type 1 diabetes, glucose cannot enter insulin-dependent cells such as adipocytes and myocytes because of the lack of

Comparison of type 1 and type 2 diabetes

	Type 1	Type 2
Onset	usually under 20 years of age	usually over 40 years of age
Insulin synthesis	absent: immune destruction of β-cells	preserved: combination of insulin resistance and impaired β-cell function
Plasma insulin concentration	low or absent	low, normal or high
Genetic susceptibility	yes	yes
Islet cell antibodies at diagnosis	yes	no
Obesity	uncommon	common
Ketoacidosis	yes	rare – can be precipitated by major metabolic stress
Treatment	insulin	hypoglycemic drugs and insulin

Table 21.5 **Comparison of type 1 and type 2 diabetes.**

insulin. Glycolysis and lipogenesis are inhibited, whereas glycogenolysis, lipolysis, ketogenesis, and gluconeogenesis are stimulated by glucagon (Fig. 21.16). The liver turns into a glucose-producing organ. This, combined with impaired glucose transport, leads to fasting hyperglycemia. When plasma glucose concentration exceeds renal capacity for reabsorption, glucose appears in the urine. Because glucose is osmotically active, its excretion is accompanied by increased water loss (osmotic diuresis). Poorly controlled diabetic patients pass large volumes of urine (polyuria) and drink a lot of fluids (polydypsia). The fluid loss eventually leads to dehydration (see Chapter 23).

In parallel to the disturbed water balance, lipolysis generates an excess of acetyl-CoA, which enters ketogenesis. Concentration of ketone bodies in plasma increases (ketonemia) and they are excreted in the urine (ketonuria). Overproduction of acetoacetic and β-hydroxybutyric acids increases the blood hydrogen ion concentration (pH decreases). This is a metabolic acidosis (see Chapter 24) known as diabetic ketoacidosis (Fig. 21.17). In some patients, acetone can be smelled on the breath.

Ketoacidosis is a major acute complication of poorly controled diabetes

Key features of diabetic ketoacidosis are hyperglycemia, ketonuria, dehydration and metabolic acidosis. Diabetic ketoacidosis may develop quickly, sometimes after a person misses just a single dose of insulin. Ketoacidosis develops predominantly in persons with type 1 diabetes who have no, or very little, insulin in plasma and, consequently, a very low insulin-to-glucagon concentration ratio. It is rare in type 2 diabetes but may occur after a major stress, such as myocardial infarction. Ketoacidosis, if untreated, becomes life threatening.

Note that there are substantial similarities between metabolism in the fasting state and in diabetes; this is why it was once described as 'starvation in the midst of plenty'. However, whereas fasting leads just to moderate ketonemia, in diabetes accumulation of large amounts of ketone bodies eventually causes diabetic ketoacidosis.

Hypoglycemia is the most common complication of diabetes

It is worth remembering that the most common acute complication of diabetes is not ketoacidosis but hypoglycemia. It occurs in both type 1 and type 2 diabetes. It develops as a result of imbalance between insulin dose, carbohydrate supply, and physical activity. Thus, it may occur after taking too much insulin or missing a meal. Importantly, because exercise increases insulin-independent tissue glucose uptake, diabetic patients need to decrease their insulin dose before strenuous exercise to avoid hypoglycemia. Mild hypoglycemia can be controlled by taking a sweet drink or eating a few lumps of sugar. Severe hypoglycemia, however, is a medical emergency that requires treatment with intravenous glucose or intramuscular injection of glucagon.

The path from obesity to type 2 diabetes

In type 1 diabetes, the development of clinical disease may happen fast and diabetic ketoacidosis may be its first presentation. The development of type 2 diabetes is slower and forms a continuum which includes obesity and insulin resistance.

The two most important risk factors for type 2 diabetes are family history and obesity. Family history reflects the genetic background. Obesity is often closely linked to insulin resistance. Insulin resistance first presents as hyperinsulinemia with normal glucose concentration. When increased concentrations of insulin are insufficient to compensate for tissue resistance, plasma glucose concentration may increase slightly on fasting (this condition is known as impaired fasting glucose) or in response to glucose load (impaired glucose tolerance, IGT). Both IFG and IGT are predictors of diabetes and IGT is associated with an increased risk of macrovascular complications. Further increase in insulin resistance and the consequent impairment of insulin secretion lead to overt type 2 diabetes. The importance of being aware of the described continuum is that the entire process can be slowed down or, occasionally, reversed by weight reduction and exercise. Thus, emergence of IFG or IGT should be a strong signal to change the lifestyle to minimize the chance of overt diabetes later.

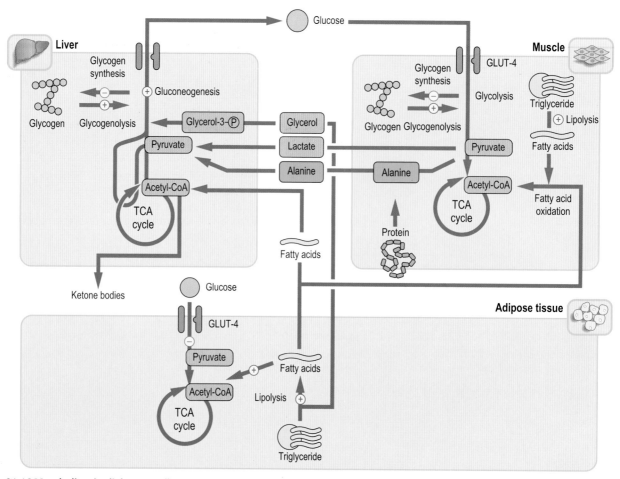

Fig. 21.16 **Metabolism in diabetes mellitus.** There is a decreased ability of tissues to use glucose because of either insulin lack or defective insulin action. Hyperglycemia is caused by the combined effect of the impaired peripheral glucose uptake and increased liver gluconeogenesis. Note that the excess of fatty acids available to the liver, together with the less efficient TCA cycle due to oxaloacetate being used for gluconeogenesis, results in the accumulation of acetyl-CoA and its conversion into ketone bodies.

UNEXPECTED DIABETIC KETOACIDOSIS

A 15-year-old girl, never known to have diabetes, was admitted to the accident and emergency department. She was confused and her breath had a smell of acetone. She had signs of dehydration with reduced tissue turgor and dry tongue. She also had rapid pauseless respirations. Her blood glucose was 18.0 mmol/L (324 mg/dL) and ketones were present in the urine. Her serum potassium concentration was 4.9 mmol/L (normal 3.5–5.0 mmol/L) and her arterial blood pH was 7.20 (normal 7.37–7.44).

Comment. This is a typical presentation of diabetic ketoacidosis. Hyperventilation is a compensatory response to acidosis (see Chapter 24). Diabetic ketoacidosis is a medical emergency. The patient received an intravenous infusion containing physiologic saline with potassium supplements to replace lost fluid and an infusion of insulin. Note that a substantial proportion of children present with ketoacidosis at the time of diagnosis.

Obesity, diabetes and hypertension are linked with cardiovascular disease

Obesity, insulin resistance and glucose intolerance may be accompanied by dyslipidemia (see Chapter 18) and by increased arterial blood pressure (arterial hypertension). This cluster has been described as the metabolic syndrome. It is associated (as is obesity) with low-grade inflammation affecting the vasculature (Chapter 18), and with an increased tendency to thrombosis (hypercoagulable state; Chapter 7). Importantly, it is also characterized by an increased risk of cardiovascular disease.

Metabolic syndrome is not a clinical condition – it is a concept formulated to increase clinicians' awareness of multiple cardiovascular risk factors. The search for a possible common denominator for all involved risk factors continues; increasingly there is realization that diabetes mellitus and cardiovascular disease may have what some researchers call 'common soil'. Relationships between obesity, diabetes and atherosclerosis are illustrated in Figure 21.18.

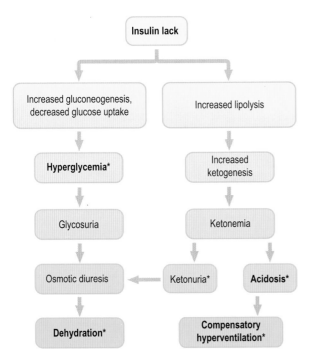

Fig. 21.17 Diabetic ketoacidosis. The clinical picture of ketoacidosis is a consequence of insulin lack and resulting hyperglycemia and its complications (osmotic diuresis, dehydration), increased lipolysis and ketogenesis (ketonemia and acidosis). Treatment of ketoacidosis is devised to combat these problems and includes insulin infusion, rehydration and potassium supplementation. *Indicates the most important clinical and laboratory findings.

Oxidative stress, advanced glycation (glycoxidation) endproducts and activity of the polyol pathway contribute to the development of vascular complications of diabetes

The toxicity of glucose in diabetes is due in particular to its involvement in reactions that generate reactive oxygen species (ROS; see Chapter 37). In the presence of transition metals such as copper, glucose undergoes autooxidation. This generates ROS. Glucose also attaches nonenzymatically to lysine and valine residues on tissue and plasma proteins in a process known as protein glycation (Fig. 21.19). When glucose interacts with a protein, first it forms a labile compound known as a Schiff base. This, through the so-called Amadori rearrangement, transforms spontaneously to ketoamine. The most widely studied Amadori product is glycated hemoglobin (hemoglobin A_{1c}, HbA_{1c}). Other proteins such as albumin, collagen and apolipoprotein B also undergo glycation. Glycation affects the function of proteins, for instance their binding to membrane receptors. For example, glycation of apolipoprotein B inhibits cellular uptake of the LDL particles (see Chapter 18).

Further oxidation, rearrangement, dehydration and fragmentation of the Amadori products lead to the formation of a family of compounds known as advanced glycation (glycoxidation) endproducts (AGE). It also generates compounds with chemically active carbonyl groups, such as 3-deoxyglucosone, glyoxal and methylglyoxal (see Fig. 21.19 and Fig. 44.6). Some of the AGEs are in fact protein crosslinks, which form, for instance, on collagen or myelin, decreasing the elasticity of these proteins. AGE concentration normally increases with aging but in diabetes their accumulation is faster at any given age. AGE bind to their membrane receptors on the endothelial cells and this generates oxidative stress. This damages endothelial cells and stimulates the proinflammatory pathway involving the transcription factor NFκB. NFκB in turn controls the expression of a range of inflammatory cytokines such as TNF-α, and IL-1β and IL-6. The result is chronic low-grade inflammation, known to harm vascular endothelium further. Formation of AGE seems important in the development of the microvascular complications of diabetes. AGE accumulation also contributes to atherosclerosis. They may be involved in the pathogenesis of other age-related diseases such as Alzheimer's disease.

ROS generated during hyperglycemia impair endothelium-dependent relaxation of the vascular smooth muscle cells. The vasodilatory nitric oxide (NO) is generated by the endothelial cells from arginine in a reaction that utilizes NADPH. It is rapidly deactivated by superoxide, forming peroxynitrite radical, which itself is an oxidant. ROS also interfere with signaling cascades, affecting, for instance, activation of protein kinase C. Hyperglycemia aslo increases the amount of proton donors within mitochondria. This leads to increased electrochemical potential difference across the inner mitochondrial membrane and consequently the production of ROS by the respiratory chain (see Fig. 37.4). It has been suggested that the increased mitochondrial ROS production is the primary cause of long-term diabetic complications.

Increased activity of the polyol pathway is associated with diabetic neuropathy and ocular cataracts

Hyperglycemia alters cellular redox state by increasing the $NADH/NAD^+$ ratio and decreasing $NADPH/NADP^+$. This increases substrate flux into the polyol pathway where glucose is reduced to sorbitol by aldose reductase (AR; Fig. 21.20). Importantly, AR and nitric oxide synthase compete for NADPH (see above). Sorbitol is further oxidized to fructose by sorbitol dehydrogenase. Because aldose reductase has a high K_m for glucose, the polyol pathway is not very active at normal glucose concentrations. However, during hyperglycemia, glucose concentration in insulin-independent tissues (red blood cells, nerve, and lens) increases, and this activates the pathway. Sorbitol, similarly to glucose, is osmotically active. Its accumulation in the ocular tissue contributes to the development of diabetic cataracts. In the nerve tissue, high concentration of sorbitol decreases cellular uptake of another alcohol, myoinositol: this decreases the activity of the membrane Na^+/K^+-ATPase, and affects nerve function. Sorbitol accumulation, along with hypoxia and reduced nerve blood flow, contributes to the development of diabetic neuropathy. Processes that contribute to the long-term diabetic complications are summarized in Fig. 21.21.

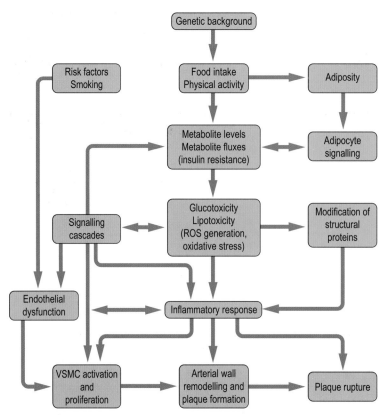

Fig. 21.18 Relationships between obesity, glucose intolerance, diabetes and atherosclerosis. In obesity the endocrine activity of the enlarging adipose tissue is important in the development of insulin resistance, glucose intolerance and type 2 diabetes. Low-grade inflammation and increased oxidative stress can be induced by obesity and also by the classic cardiovascular risk factors. This results in endothelial damage and the initiation of atherosclerosis. Once diabetes is present, protein glycation and formation of the advanced glycation (glycoxidation) endproducts further contribute to vascular damage.

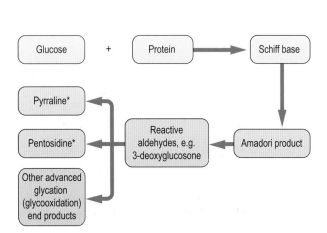

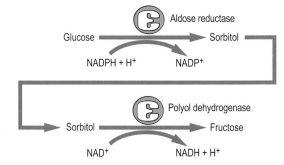

Fig. 21.20 The polyol pathway. The polyol pathway contributes to the development of diabetic neuropathy which results from a combination of vascular and structural tissue changes. This pathway may be inhibited by inhibitors of its rate-limiting enzyme, aldose reductase.

Fig. 21.19 Modification of proteins by glucose: the Maillard reaction. Nonenzymatic, concentration-dependent, glycation reaction between glucose and protein modifies structure and function of affected proteins. Glycated proteins (Amadori products) are substrates for the formation of the advanced glycation (glycoxidation) end products (AGE). Also, glucose metabolism through glycolysis to triose phosphates and through the polyol pathway can generate reactive compounds such as methylglyoxal and 3-deoxyglucosone which also are precursors of AGE. Excess production of these compounds is to a large extent responsible for the toxicity of glucose observed in diabetes. (Compare Fig. 44.6)

LABORATORY ASSESSMENT OF FUEL METABOLISM AND DIABETES MELLITUS

Results of laboratory tests need to be related to the feed–fast cycle described above. The best time to assess metabolism is after an 8–12 h fast (in the postabsorptive state Fig. 21.12).

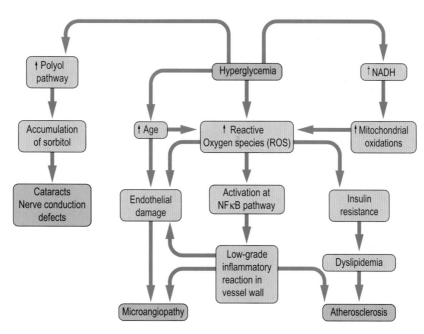

Fig. 21.21 **Mechanism of development of microvascular and macrovascular complications of diabetes mellitus.** Glycemic control is associated with the development of microvascular complications in type 1 and type 2 diabetes and with increased cardiovascular risk, particularly in type 2 diabetes. Oxidative stress, protein glycation and formation of advanced glycation (glycoxidation) endproducts are the most important candidate mechanisms of the development of microvascular complications. Hyperglycemia stimulates generation of the reactive oxygen species (ROS) through increase in the flow of reductive equivalents through the respiratory chain and the formation of AGE, which generate ROS at different stages of their metabolism. ROS toxicity is associated with structural and functional damage to proteins and with inflammatory phenomena induced through, for instance, the proinflammatory NFκB pathway. Endothelial damage is particularly important. ROS also interfere with insulin signaling, contributing to insulin resistance. Inflammation and insulin resistance are important in the development of atherosclerosis causing macrovascular disease (see Chapter 18). Importantly, increased oxidative stress and low-grade chronic inflammation have also been observed in obesity before diabetes develops.

Plasma glucose is the key test for the diagnosis of diabetes

Measurement of plasma glucose concentration is the most important test of fuel metabolism. The clinician wants to know whether a patient's glucose concentration is normal (normoglycemia), too high (hyperglycemia) or too low (hypoglycemia). Glucose concentration increases after food, so it is important to relate the time of blood sampling to the time of the last meal. Glucose concentration measured irrespective of the meal times is known as the random plasma glucose. It helps diagnose hypoglycemia or severe hyperglycemia, but is less useful in mild hyperglycemia. Two types of measurement that are used as diagnostic criteria for diabetes are fasting glucose concentration (no caloric intake for approx 10 h) and the concentration measured 2 h after oral ingestion of a standard amount of glucose.

Fasting plasma glucose is remarkably stable. Normally, it should remain below 6.1 mmol/L (<110 mg/dL). The prediabetic abnormalities of carbohydrate metabolism are defined as either impaired fasting glucose (IFG) or impaired glucose tolerance (IGT). The diagnosis of IFG is recommended by the American Diabetes Association. The diagnosis of IGT is recommended by the World Health Organization (WHO) and is accepted in Europe. The main principle behind

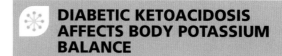

DIABETIC KETOACIDOSIS AFFECTS BODY POTASSIUM BALANCE

Insulin increases cellular potassium uptake and lack of insulin leads to the release of potassium from cells. Since uncontrolled diabetes is accompanied by osmotic diuresis, the released potassium is excreted in urine. As a result, most patients admitted with ketoacidosis are potassium depleted but, paradoxically, often have normal or raised levels of plasma potassium concentration. When exogenous insulin is given to such patients, it stimulates entry of potassium into cells and can lead to very low plasma potassium levels (hypokalemia). Hypokalemia is dangerous, owing to its effects on cardiac muscle. Thus, except for patients with very high plasma concentrations, potassium needs to be given during treatment of diabetic ketoacidosis. (See also Chapters 22 and 23.)

the diagnostic criteria for diabetes mellitus is evidence that higher fasting glucose concentrations constitute a risk for the development of microvascular complications. These criteria are not absolute – they are likely to be modified in the light of future research.

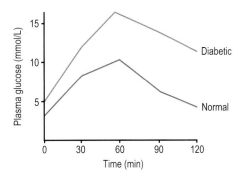

Fig. 21.22 **Oral glucose tolerance test (OGTT).** The principle of the test is the measurement of plasma glucose concentration before and after a standard (75 g) oral glucose load. Glucose concentration increases, achieving a peak between 30 and 60 min after the load. It should return to near-fasting values after 2 h. Note higher plasma glucose values at all time points in a diabetic patient.

IGT is associated with cardiovascular risk (the role of postprandial phenomena in atherogenesis is increasingly recognized), whereas IFG is simply a risk factor for the future development of diabetes. IGT is diagnosed when fasting plasma glucose is normal but there is an elevated postload concentration. IFG is defined as plasma glucose concentration higher than 6.0 mmol/L but lower than 7.0 mmol/L (126 mg/dL). Fasting plasma glucose of 7.0 mmol/L (126 mg/dL) or above, if confirmed, indicates diabetes. Laboratory diagnosis of diabetes is summarized in Table 21.6.

Oral glucose tolerance test (OGTT) tests blood glucose response to a carbohydrate load

The WHO recommends that the OGTT is performed in all individuals whose fasting plasma glucose falls into the IFG category.

It is essential that the test is performed under standard conditions. The patient should attend in the morning, after an approximately 10 h fast. To avoid stress- or exercise-related change in plasma glucose, the person should sit throughout the test. The test should not be performed during or immediately after an acute illness. Fasting plasma glucose is measured first. Next, the patient is given a standard quantity of glucose to drink (75 g in 300 mL of water) and glucose is measured again after 120 min (Fig. 21.22). In some procedures glucose is measured more often, e.g. after 20, 60 and 120 min. Normally, plasma glucose rises to a peak concentration after approximately 60 min and returns to a near-fasting state within 120 min. If it remains above 11.1 mmol/L (200 mg/dL/min) in the 120 min sample, the patient has diabetes, even if the fasting blood glucose is normal. Nondiabetic fasting blood glucose with postload concentration between 6.1 and 7.8 mmol/L (100–140 mg/dL) signifies IGT. Interpretation of the OGTT is summarized in Table 21.6.

Urine glucose measurement is not a diagnostic test for diabetes

Diagnostic criteria for diabetes mellitus and glucose intolerance		
Condition	**Diagnostic criteria (mmol/L)**	**Diagnostic criteria (mg/dL) Comments**
normal fasting plasma glucose	below 6.1	below 110
impaired fasting glucose (IFG)	equal or above 6.1 but below 7.0	equal or above 110 but below
impaired glucose tolerance (IGT)	plasma glucose 2 h after 75 g load 7.8 or above, but below 11.1	plasma glucose 2 h after 75 g load 140 or above, diagnosed during OGIT but below 200
Diabetes mellitus*		
criterion 1	random plasma glucose 11.1 or above†	random plasma glucose 200 or above†
criterion 2	fasting plasma glucose 7.0 or above	fasting plasma glucose 126 or above
criterion 3	2 h value during OGTT 11.1 or above	2 h value during OGTT 200 or above

*If one of the criteria is fulfilled, diagnosis is provisional. Diagnosis needs to be confirmed next day using a different criterion.
†If accompanied by symptoms (polyuria, polydypsia, unexplained weight loss). These are the criteria proposed by the American Diabetes Association in 1997 (see Further Reading).

Table 21.6 **Diagnostic criteria for diabetes mellitus and glucose intolerance.**

At normal plasma concentration, glucose filtered through the renal glomeruli is reabsorbed in the proximal kidney tubules, and none appears in the urine (Chapter 23). The urinary threshold for glucose reabsorption is approximately 10.0 mmol/L (180 mg/dL). At higher plasma glucose concentrations, the capacity of the renal tubular transport system is exceeded, and glucose appears in the urine (glucosuria). Note that healthy persons may have a low renal glucose threshold and may show glucosuria at nondiabetic blood glucose levels. Therefore, diabetes cannot be diagnosed on the basis of urine glucose testing alone.

Ketone bodies in urine of a diabetic person signify metabolic decompensation

High concentration of ketones in urine (ketonuria) signifies a high rate of lipolysis. Mild ketonuria occurs in healthy individuals during prolonged fasting or on a high-fat diet (see box in Chapter 15, p. 191). However, in a diabetic patient, ketonuria is an important sign of metabolic decompensation, which requires adjustment of treatment regimen.

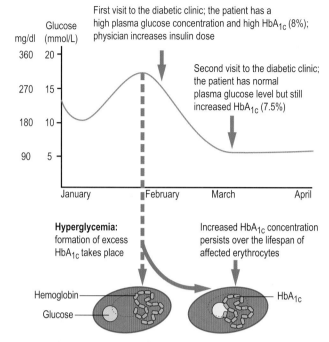

First visit to the diabetic clinic; the patient has a high plasma glucose concentration and high HbA$_{1c}$ (8%); physician increases insulin dose

Second visit to the diabetic clinic; the patient has normal plasma glucose level but still increased HbA$_{1c}$ (7.5%)

Hyperglycemia: formation of excess HbA$_{1c}$ takes place

Increased HbA$_{1c}$ concentration persists over the lifespan of affected erythrocytes

Hemoglobin

Glucose

HbA$_{1c}$

Fig. 21.23 **Hemoglobin A$_{1c}$ measurement reflects the time-averaged control of glycemia.** Hemoglobin A$_{1c}$ is hemoglobin A posttranslationally modified by a nonenzymatic glycation. The degree of glycation is proportional to hemoglobin's exposure to glucose during the lifespan of an erythrocyte. Hemoglobin A$_{1c}$ concentration below 7% is regarded as adequate glycemic control (American Diabetes Association 2008) although this may vary with the type of patient and their tendency to hypoglycemia. To obtain glucose concentrations in mg/dL, multiply by 18 (see boxes on pp. 54 and 289).

Increased plasma lactate indicates inadequate oxygenation

High plasma lactate level indicates increased anaerobic metabolism, and is a marker of inadequate tissue oxygenation (hypoxia; see also Chapter 5). In extreme cases, such as cardiac arrest, this causes severe acidosis (lactic acidosis). In diabetes, measurements of plasma lactate are important in rare instances of hyperglycemic nonketotic coma, a life-threatening condition where very high plasma glucose levels and extreme dehydration occur in the absence of ketoacidosis.

Average concentration of plasma glucose in a diabetic patient can be assessed by measuring the concentration of glycated hemoglobin

One can assess average glycemia in a patient by performing multiple plasma glucose measurements but this is cumbersome. The measurement of glycated hemoglobin (hemoglobin A$_{1c}$, HbA$_{1c}$) makes this much easier. Glycation reaction is irreversible, therefore glycated hemoglobin remains in the circulation for the entire life of the erythrocyte. The extent of hemoglobin glycation is proportional to plasma glucose concentration. The amount of glycated hemoglobin (measured as a percentage of total hemoglobin) reflects the

average concentration of plasma glucose (Fig. 21.23) over approximately 3–6 weeks preceding its measurement. This is difficult to calculate precisely because at any time populations of erythrocytes of different ages are present in plasma. Values such as 4–8 weeks and 3–4 months have also been reported in the literature. The exposure to glucose over 30 days before measurement contributes approximately 50% to observed changes in HbA$_{1c}$. The value of HbA$_{1c}$ is used as a target for therapy. Normal concentration of HbA$_{1c}$ is 4–6%. The current recommendations are that in diabetic patients one should aim to achieve a HbA$_{1c}$ concentration below 7% (American Diabetes Association 2008) or below 6.5% (Joint British Societies, JBS2, 2005). In some patients, particularly the elderly, this may be difficult to achieve because of the risk of hypoglycemia. There is ongoing discussion among experts over whether HbA$_{1c}$ should be used as a screening test for diabetes.

Urinary albumin excretion is important in the assessment of diabetic nephropathy

Development of diabetic nephropathy can be predicted by detecting small amounts of albumin in urine (microalbuminuria). To do this, laboratories employ a method that is more sensitive than the conventional one used for the measurement of albumin. The test is positive if more than 200 mg of albumin is excreted over 24 h. Urine protein above 300 mg/day signifies overt proteinuria. In diabetic patients plasma urea and creatinine concentrations are also routinely checked (see Chapter 23).

Periodic assessment of a diabetic patient

To summarize, during a periodic assessment of a diabetic patient, the physician would first of all check blood glucose and HbA$_{1c}$ concentration to assess glycemic control. She would perform an eye examination (looking for signs of retinopathy), neurologic examination (neuropathy) and arrange an ECG (coronary heart disease). She would also measure urea and creatinine in plasma and microalbumin/protein in urine (nephropathy), and measure plasma lipids (risk of coronary heart disease, see Chapter 18).

TREATING DIABETES

The goal of treatment in diabetes is prevention of acute and chronic complications.

Lifestyle change is the mainstay of diabetes prevention and a key element of its treatment

Diet and exercise are the key lifestyle factors in the management of diabetes mellitus, and they must underpin all drug treatments. They are also essential preventive measures to avoid or delay the development of diabetes. The Diabetes Prevention Program demonstrated a 58% decrease in development of type 2 diabetes after lifestyle interventions involving diet and exercise (see Further reading). Unfortunately, less than 20% of patients who have diabetes can be controlled by lifestyle measures alone.

Good glycemic control prevents complications of diabetes

Maintenance of good glycemic control is fundamental for diabetes care. Two major clinical trials, the Diabetic Control and Complications Trial (DCCT) in type 1 diabetes and the UK Prospective Diabetes Study (UKPDS) in type 2 patients, confirmed that microvascular complications are associated with the level of glycemia (see Further Reading). There is increasing evidence that therapeutic intervention that includes both glycemic control and the management of cardiovascular risk is optimal for the prevention of long-term complications. Thus, in addition to striving to maintain the concentration of plasma glucose close to normal, intensive management of cardiovascular risk factors such as hypertension and dyslipidemia is necessary.

Patients with type 1 diabetes are treated with insulin

Insulin was first isolated in 1921–22 by Frederick Banting and Charles Best working in Toronto (see Further Reading). In 1979, human insulin became the first recombinant protein to be produced commercially. Insulin remains absolutely necessary for the treatment of type 1 diabetes. The treatment involves daily subcutaneous injections throughout life. Different types of insulin are available and they differ in the duration of their action. Newer analogs of human insulin are insulin-lispro and insulin-aspart (short-acting) and insulin-glargine (long-acting). Patients usually take two subcutaneous injections of intermediate-acting insulin per day or a mixture of a short-acting and intermediate-acting insulin. The greatest challenge of insulin treatment is replicating normal daily patterns of insulin secretion with insulin injections. Multiple injections of short-acting insulin are used in more difficult cases. Rarely, patients need a constant insulin infusion, delivered by a portable pump programmed to increase the rate of delivery at meal times.

Emergency treatment of diabetic ketoacidosis includes insulin, rehydration and potassium supplementation

Emergency treatment of diabetic ketoacidosis addresses four issues: insulin lack, dehydration, potassium depletion, and acidosis. Insulin infusion is required to reverse the metabolic effect of the excess of anti-insulin hormones, and the infusion of fluids to treat dehydration. Administered fluids normally contain potassium to prevent hypokalemia. Such treatment is usually sufficient to control the metabolic acidosis; however, in severe acidosis, infusion of an alkaline solution (sodium bicarbonate) may also be required (see case described on p. 282).

Patients with type 2 diabetes are treated with oral hypoglycemic drugs but may require insulin

Type 2 diabetic patients may not require insulin treatment because their insulin synthesis is at least partly preserved; they can usually be treated with oral hypoglycemic drugs. However, they do require insulin if adequate control cannot be achieved with oral hypoglycemic drugs; each year 5–10% of patients treated with hypoglycemic drugs need to commence treatment with insulin. Currently used oral hypoglycemic drugs target two main mechanisms of development of type 2 diabetes: insulin resistance and insulin secretion.

Sulfonylureas are drugs that increase insulin secretion

Sulfonylureas bind to a receptor in the plasma membrane of the pancreatic β-cells. The receptor contains the ATP-sensitive potassium channel. Binding of the drug closes the channel, depolarizes the membrane and opens the calcium channel. Increasing intracellular cytoplasmic calcium concentration stimulates exocytosis of insulin.

Metformin decreases insulin resistance

Metformin, a biguanide, is currently the preparation most commonly used in the treatment of type 2 diabetes. It reduces hepatic gluconeogenesis, suppresses the effects of glucagon and increases peripheral insulin sensitivity. It also inhibits glycogenolysis by inhibiting the activity of glucose-6-phosphatase. Metformin increases insulin-dependent glucose uptake in the skeletal muscle, and reduces fatty acid oxidation.

Thiazolidinediones act on the transcriptional level and decrease insulin resistance

Thiazolidinediones improve peripheral glucose utilization and insulin sensitivity. They are ligands of the PPARγ in the adipose tissue and, to a lesser extent, in muscle. PPARγ activation increases transcription of a range of genes responsible for glucose and lipid metabolism such as the ones coding for the fatty acid transporter aP2 (this increases the uptake of fatty acids and lipogenesis), the lipoprotein lipase, acyl-CoA synthase and GLUT-4. Thiazolidinediones also activate the IRSphosphoinositol kinase signaling pathway.

The glitazar group of drugs is currently being tested; these are agents that stimulate both PPARγ and PPARα and therefore, apart from thiazolidinedione-like action, they may influence lipid metabolism by raising HDL and decreasing plasma triglyceride concentration (see Chapter 18).

Intestinal hormones and intestinal absorption of carbohydrates are also targets for antidiabetic drugs

Other drugs that promote insulin secretion include a glucagon-like peptide-1 (GLP-1) receptor agonist, exenatide. GLP1 and GIP are incretin hormones that stimulate glucose-dependent insulin release. GLP-1 inhibits glucagon release and is decreased in diabetes. The enzyme dipeptidyl peptidase IV (DPP-IV) cleaves and inactivates incretin hormones. DPP-IV inhibitors such as sitaglyptin increase insulin secretion.

Finally, acarbose is an inhibitor of intestinal α-glucosidase, which digests complex sugars. It delays intestinal absorption of glucose.

SEVERE HYPOGLYCEMIA IS A MEDICAL EMERGENCY

A 12-year-old diabetic boy was playing with his friends. He received his normal insulin injection in the morning but continued playing through the lunch time without a meal. He became increasingly confused and finally lost consciousness. He was given an injection of glucagon from the emergency kit his father carried, and recovered within minutes.

Comment. An immediate improvement after glucagon injection confirms that this boy's symptoms were caused by hypoglycemia, caused by the combination of the administration of exogenous insulin and insufficient food intake. Recovery from hypoglycemia was due to the action of glucagon. In the hospital, hypoglycemic patients who cannot eat or drink are usually treated with intravenous glucose. An intramuscular glucagon injection is an emergency measure that can be applied at home.

INSULIN RESISTANCE INCREASES THE RISK OF HEART ATTACK

A 45-year-old man was referred to the cardiology outpatient clinic for investigation of chest discomfort which he felt when climbing steep hills and when he was stressed or excited. The patient was 170 cm tall and weighed 102 kg (224 lb). His blood pressure was 160/98 mmHg (upper limit of normal 140/90 mmHg), triglyceride concentration was 4 mmol/L (364 mg/dL) (desirable level <1.7 mmol/L, 148 mg/dL), and fasting plasma glucose was 6.5 mmol/L (117 mg/dL). His resting ECG was normal but an ischemic pattern was observed during exercise testing.

Comment. This obese man presented with arterial hypertension, hypertriglyceridemia, and impaired fasting glucose. The impaired fasting of glucose in this case was due to peripheral insulin resistance. Such cluster of abnormalities is known as metabolic syndrome and carries an increased risk of coronary heart disease.

MEASUREMENT OF HbA₁c IDENTIFIES DIABETIC PATIENTS WHO DO NOT COMPLY WITH TREATMENT

A 15-year-old insulin-dependent boy visited a diabetic clinic for a routine check-up. He told the doctor that he followed all the dietary advice and never missed insulin injections. Although his random blood glucose was 6 mmol/L (108 mg/dL), HbA₁c concentration was 11% (adequate control: below 7%). He had no glycosuria or ketonuria.

Comment. Blood and urine glucose results indicate good control of this boy's diabetes at the time of measurement, but the HbA₁c level suggests poor control over the last 3–6 weeks. The probability is that he only complied with treatment days before he was due to come to the clinic. This is not uncommon in adolescents, who find it hard to accept the necessity to adjust their lifestyle to, sometimes demanding, diabetes treatment.

Summary

- Glucose homeostasis involves interactions between key tissues and organs – liver, adipose tissue, skeletal muscle and pancreas.
- Disruption of this homeostatic system results in potentially life-threatening conditions – hypoglycemia and diabetes mellitus.
- Organism alternates between the fed and fasting state. Metabolite concentrations in blood change during the feed–fast cycle, and are influenced by stress and disease.
- Measurement of plasma glucose concentration is part of a routine assessment of every patient admitted to hospital. In diabetic patients, measurements of glucose, ketones, HbA₁c, and tests of renal function, including microalbuminuria, are performed.

ACTIVE LEARNING

1. Describe how insulin causes an increase in cellular glucose uptake.
2. What are antiinsulin hormones?
3. Why would a nondiabetic patient brought to the emergency unit with extensive burns have an increased plasma glucose concentration? Describe her metabolic state.
4. You have asked a patient to come to the outpatient clinic to have plasma triglycerides tested. The patient asks whether he needs to be fasting that day. Please provide an answer and explain your reasons.
5. Do people with impaired glucose tolerance develop long-term vascular complications?
6. What do obesity and diabetes mellitus have in common?

Further reading

Ahmed W, Ziouzenkova O, Brown J et al. PPARs and their metabolic modulation: new mechanisms for transcriptional regulation? *J Intern Med* 2007; **262**: 184–198.

Bliss M. *The Discovery of Insulin.* Paul Haris Edinburgh Publishing, 1983:304 pp.

Daneman D. Type 1 diabetes. *Lancet* 2006; **367**: 847–858.

Diabetes Control and Complications Trial (DCCT) Research Group. The effect of intensive treatment of diabetes on the development and progression of long-term complications in insulin-dependent diabetes mellitus. *N Engl J Med* 1993; **329**: 977–986.

Diabetes Prevention Program Research Group. Reduction in the incidence of type 2 diabetes with lifestyle intervention or metformin. *N Engl J Med* 2002; **24**: 387–388.

Dominiczak MH. Obesity, glucose intolerance and diabetes and their links to cardiovascular disease. Implications for laboratory medicine. *CCLM* 2003; **41**: 1266–1278.

Expert Committee on the Diagnosis and Classification of Diabetes Mellitus. Report of the Expert Committee on the Diagnosis and Classification of Diabetes Mellitus. *Diabetes Care* 2003; **26**: S4–S20.

Jeffcoate SL. Diabetes control and complications: the role of glycated hemoglobin, 25 years on. *Diabetic Med* 2004; **21**: 6576–6665.

Sheen AJ. Exenatide once weekly in type 2 diabetes. *Lancet* 2008;**372**:1197–8.

Sladek R, Rocheleau G, Rung J et al. A genome-wide association study identifies novel risk loci for type 2 diabetes. *Nature* 2007; **445**: 881–885.

Stern MP. Diabetes and cardiovascular disease. The 'common soil' hypothesis. *Diabetes* 1995; **44**: 369–374.

Stumvoll M, Goldstein BJ, von Haeften TW. Type 2 diabetes: principles of pathogenesis and therapy. *Lancet* 2005; **365**: 1333–1346.

UK Prospective Diabetes Study (UKPDS) Group. Intensive blood-glucose control with sulphonylureas or insulin compared with conventional treatment and risk of complications in patients with type 2 diabetes (UKPDS 33). *Lancet* 1998; **352**: 837–853.

Wong TY, Liew G, Tapp RJ et al. Relation between fasting glucose and retinopathy for diagnosis of diabetes: three population-based cross-sectional studies. *Lancet* 2008; **371**: 736–743.

Zimmet P, Alberti KGMM, Shaw J. Global and societal implications of the diabetes epidemic. *Nature* 2001; **414**: 782–787.

Zorzano A, Palacin M, Gumà A. Mechanisms regulating GLUT4 glucose transporter expression and glucose transport in skeletal muscle. *Acta Physiol Scand* 2005; **183**: 44–48.

22. Nutrition and Energy Balance

M H Dominiczak

LEARNING OBJECTIVES

After reading this chapter you should be able to:

- Describe mechanisms controlling food intake.
- Describe the role of AMPK-activated kinase in maintaining cellular energy balance.
- Identify the main categories of nutrients, and essential nutrients within these categories.
- Relate your knowledge of energy metabolism to current nutritional recommendations.
- Characterize malnutrition and obesity.
- Discuss nutritional assessment.

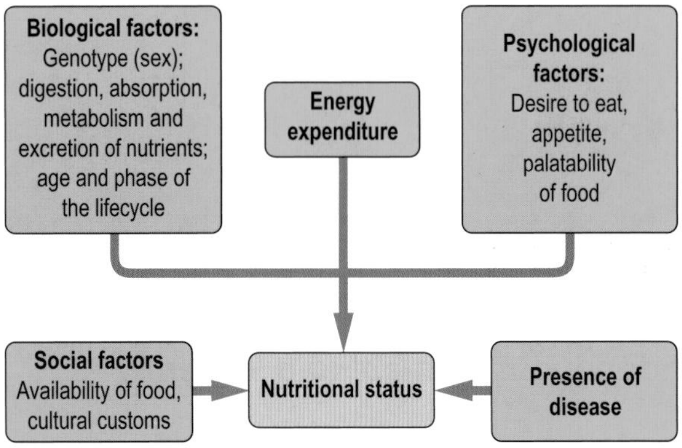

Fig. 22.1 **Factors that determine the state of nutrition.**

INTRODUCTION

From the biochemistry point of view, nutrition is an essential interaction of an organism with the environment. Nutrients, apart from providing energy for survival, signal the organism in diverse ways, and this in turn affects their use and storage. Nutrition underpins health and affects susceptibility to disease; both malnutrition and obesity put an organism at risk.

Nutritional status is determined by biologic, psychologic and social factors

The factors that determine nutritional status of an individual are the genetic background, the environment, the phase of the life cycle, the level of physical activity and the presence of disease (Fig. 22.1). Nutritional status is influenced by the availability of food, its palatability and variety, and the absence or presence of illness. Nutritional deficiencies may result from dietary inadequacies or from genetically determined metabolic errors.

REGULATION OF FOOD INTAKE

Food intake is controlled by hunger (a desire to eat) and appetite (a desire for a particular food).

The main centers regulating appetite are located in the hypothalamus in the central nervous system (CNS). The appetite is regulated by the hypothalamic arcuate and paraventricular nuclei.

The brain regulates energy homeostasis and is also the primary regulator of body weight (Fig. 22.2). According to the lipostatic model of energy homeostasis, signals controlling energy intake originate from the adipose tissue and are sent to the central nervous system. These signals are mediated by the adipokine leptin and by insulin. In response, the brain sends efferent signals through the complex network of neuropeptides. These signals regulate appetite and hunger. The neurones in the arcuate nucleus express two neuropeptides: catabolic proopiomelanocortin (POMC), and anabolic neuropeptide Y/agouti-related protein (NPY/AgRP). POMC is cleaved yielding melanocortins, such as α-MSH, that decrease food intake. NPY/AgRP links to neurones expressing melanin-concentrating hormone (MCH) and orexins A and B. They, in turn, are involved in the control of food intake by acting on brainstem neurones. These neurones connect with the brain cortex (the satiety center) to promote hunger and to stimulate yet another set of hormones such as thyreoliberin (TRH), corticoliberin (CRH) and oxytocin. Thyreoliberin increases thermogenesis and food intake, whereas corticoliberin decreases food intake and, through the sympathetic activity, increases energy expenditure. Further signals that control food intake are conveyed by gastrointestinal peptides such as glucagon, cholecystokinin, glucagon-like peptide, amylin and bombesin-like peptide. Ghrelin, secreted by the stomach, stimulates NPY/AgRP-expressing neurones. It is the only known appetite-stimulating peptide. Gastric stretch also affects food intake. Finally, hypoglycemia decreases the activity of the satiety center.

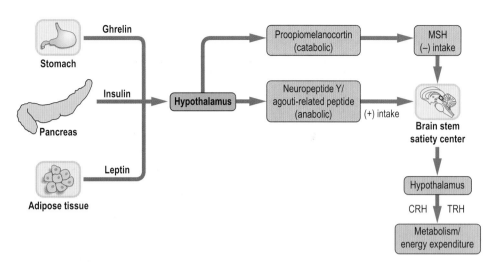

Fig. 22.2 **Regulation of food intake.** Regulation of food intake is accomplished by signals generated in the adipose tissue, pancreas, stomach and brain. The hypothalamus translates signals related to the energy balance into eating behavior through secretion of a range of neuropeptides. The (+) sign means action leading to increase of appetite and food intake, and the sign (−) to a decrease. CRH, corticoliberin; TRH, thyreoliberin; MSH, melanocyte-stimulating hormone.

Endogenous cannabinoid system

The hypothalamus and brainstem translate the information about energy balance into eating behavior. This involves the endogenous cannabinoid system. Endocannabinoids are compounds synthesized from membrane phospholipids. They include Δ^9-tetrahydrocannabinol and anandamide formed as a result of hydrolysis of *N*-arachidonyl phosphatidyl ethanolamine by phospholipase D. Endocannabinoids are released at the synapses and bind to the synaptic receptors called CB1. The receptors are present in the central nervous system and also in gut, adipose tissue, liver, muscle and pancreas. They are coupled to G-proteins and adenylate cyclase and they also regulate potassium and calcium channels. The binding of endocannabinoids to the receptors modulates release of neurotransmitters such as GABA, noradrenaline, glutamate and serotonin. Hypothalamic levels of endocannabinoids increase during food deprivation. A CB1 receptor antagonist, rimonabant, is now used in the treatment of obesity.

REGULATION OF ENERGY BALANCE

Adipose tissue is an active endocrine organ

Adipose tissue, far from being an inert depot of storage fat, is an active endocrine organ (Fig. 22.3). Its products are known as adipokines. This endocrine activity influences development of obesity and conditions such as insulin resistance and type 2 diabetes. The two major adipokines secreted by the adipose tissue are leptin and adiponectin.

Leptin regulates adipose tissue mass and responds to the energy status

Leptin is a 16 kDa protein. Its secretion is linked to the adipose tissue mass and the size of adipocytes. In the central

nervous system it decreases food intake. It also acts on the skeletal muscle, liver, adipose tissue and pancreas. Leptin gene expression is regulated by food intake, energy status, hormones and inflammatory state. It affects metabolism by stimulating fatty acid oxidation and by decreasing lipogenesis. Importantly, it also decreases ectopic deposition of fat in liver or muscle.

Leptin signals through a membrane receptor that has an extracellular binding domain and intracellular tail. Its signaling pathways involve Janus kinase and signal transducer and activator of transcription (JAK/STAT; see Chapter 40). Mitogen-activated protein kinase and phosphatidyl-inositol 3' kinase are also involved. Its signaling involves the AMP-activated kinase (AMPK) (see below).

Adiponectin increases insulin sensitivity and its lack leads to insulin resistance

Adiponectin is a 244 amino acid protein with a structural homology with collagens type VIII and X and with complement factor C1q. Several forms exist in the circulation: globular, trimeric and high molecular weight. Adiponectin stimulates glucose utilization in muscle and increases fatty acid oxidation in muscle and liver, thus increasing insulin sensitivity. It also decreases hepatic glucose production. Low adiponectin levels are linked with insulin resistance and with hepatic steatosis. Adiponectin downregulates the secretion of proinflammatory cytokines interleukins 6 and 8 (IL-6 and IL-8) and monocyte chemoattractant protein-1 (MCP-1).

Physical training increases adiponectin expression and upregulates its receptors in the skeletal muscle. On the other hand, its concentration decreases in obesity and in type 2 diabetes. Low levels of adiponectin are also associated with low-grade inflammation, oxidative stress and endothelial dysfunction. Adiponectin receptors activate AMPK, p38 mitogen-activated protein kinase, and PPARα, which in turn regulates fatty acid metabolism (see Chapter 18).

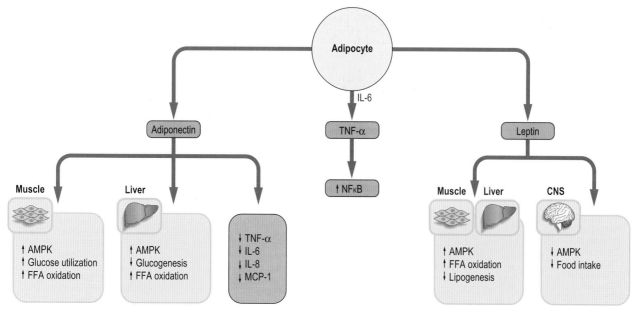

Fig. 22.3 **Endocrine activity of adipose tissue.** Adipose tissue is an endocrine organ and its products are known as adipokines. Leptin and adiponectin play an essential role in adjusting metabolism to body energy needs. They activate the 'energy sensor enzyme', AMP-activated kinase (AMPK). Adipocytes also secrete a range of proinflammatory cytokines (among others TNF-α, IL-6) . TNF-α is known to stimulate the transcription factor NFκB, a key factor in the induction of genes involved in the inflammatory response. AMPK, AMP-activated kinase; FFA, free fatty acids; CNS, central nervous system. IL, interleukin; TNF-α, tumor necrosis factor α .

Adipose tissue secretes proinflammatory cytokines

Adipose tissue secretes the proinflammatory cytokines tumor necrosis factor α (TNF-α) and IL-6. TNF-α is highly expressed in obese animals and humans, and it also induces insulin resistance and type 2 diabetes. TNF-α activates the proinflammatory NFκb pathway (see Chapter 38).

AMP-stimulated kinase (AMPK) responds to cellular energy levels

AMPK is a serine-threonine kinase. It is a heterotrimer encoded by three genes: it has a catalytic subunit a and two regulatory subunits, β and γ. It is activated by phosphorylation by a kinase known as LKB1, which is a tumor suppressor molecule. The key activator of the AMPK is cellular accumulation of 5′-AMP and the increase the ratio of 5′-AMP/ATP. A low creatine/phosphocreatine ratio also activates the enzyme. High 5′-AMP concentration induces allosteric changes and the phosphorylation of the AMPK catalytic subunit.

AMPK stimulates energy-producing pathways and suppresses energy-utilizing ones

In the skeletal muscle, AMPK activation promotes glucose transport, glycolysis and fatty acid oxidation. It inhibits fatty acid synthesis by phosphorylating acetyl-CoA carboxylase. This leads to a decrease in malonyl-CoA, and to disinhibition of carnitine palmitoyl transferase 1 and consequent facilitation of fatty acid transport into mitochondria. Increased

fatty acid oxidation prevents tissue lipid accumulation. In the liver, AMPK inhibits lipogenesis and cholesterol synthesis; its activation suppresses the sterol regulatory element-binding protein 1c (SREBP1c) (see Chapter 18).

In the skeletal muscle, AMPK is activated during exercise and is involved in contraction-stimulated glucose transport and fatty acid oxidation (it is known that exercise enhances insulin sensitivity). In the heart it is activated by ischemia.

AMPK also acts at the hypothalamic level. Expression of AMPK in the hypothalamus reduces food intake. Leptin and adiponectin stimulate AMPK in the skeletal muscle, liver and adipose tissue. Insulin and leptin inhibit it in the hypothalamus. Drugs such as thiazolidinediones and biguanides act in part through AMPK (Chapter 21). Effects of AMPK activation are summarized in Figure 22.4 (see also box on p. 100).

Energy expenditure

Total daily energy expenditure is a sum of basal metabolic rate, the thermic effect of food and the energy used up in physical activity.

Energy expenditure can be measured by direct calorimetry, which relies on measurements of heat production. Indirect calorimetry is based on measurement of the oxygen consumption rate (VO_2). The ratio of VCO_2 to VO_2 is known as the respiratory exchange rate (RER) or respiratory quotient. For carbohydrates, RER = 1; for fat, RER = 0.7.

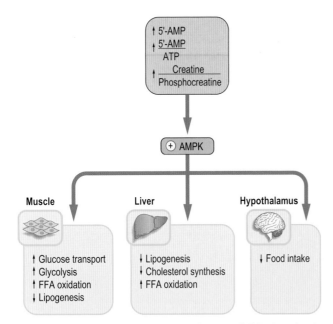

Fig. 22.4 **AMP-activated kinase (AMPK).** AMPK fulfills the role of a sensor of cellular energy levels. Its main stimulator is the increase in 5'-AMP, a product of ATP conversion. Increased 5'-AMP-to-ATP ratio signals low cellular energy level. Activated AMPK phosphorylates rate-limiting enzymes in energy-producing and energy-using pathways. The final effect is inhibition of energy-utilizing pathways such as lipogenesis or cholesterol synthesis, and stimulation of pathways that generate energy: glycolysis and FFA oxidation. FFA, free fatty acids.

Energy expenditure required to maintain body function at complete rest is called the basal metabolic rate (BMR). The BMR is dependent on sex, age and body weight. At rest, energy is required for membrane transport (30% of the total), protein synthesis and degradation (30%), and for maintaining temperature, physical activity and growth. Certain organs use particularly high amounts of energy: in a 70 kg person brain metabolism constitutes approximately 20% of basal metabolic demand, liver 25% and muscle 25%. On the other hand, in very low birth weight babies, the brain is responsible for as much as 60% of the BMR, liver for 20% and muscle for only 5%.

In health, physical activity is the most important change-able component of energy expenditure. It is normally expressed as multiplies of the BMR. Examples of energy expenditure associated with different activities are given in Table 22.1. Energy requirement also depends on sex and age (Table 22.2).

DEFINITIONS IN NUTRITION SCIENCE

Diet is the total of all the foods and drinks ingested by an individual. The food or foodstuff is the particular food that is ingested and nutrients are chemically defined components of food required by the body.

Energy expenditure during physical activity

Physical activity ratio	Activity
1.0–1.4	Watching TV, reading, writing
1.5–1.8	Washing dishes, ironing
1.9–2.4	Dusting and cleaning, cooking
2..5–3.3	Dressing and undressing, making beds, walking slowly
3.4–4.4	Cleaning windows, golf, carpentry
4.5–5.9	Volley ball, fast walk, dancing, slow jogging, digging and shoveling
6.0–7.9	Climbing stairs, cycling, football, skiing

Table 22.1 **Energy expenditure during physical activity.** Energy expenditure is expressed as physical activity ratios (multiples of the basal metabolic rate, BMR) for different types of activities. Data from Dietary Reference Values for Food Energy and Nutrients for the United Kingdom; Report of the Panel on Dietary Reference Values of the Committee on Medical Aspects of Food Policy, London: TSO 2003.

Daily energy requirements

	EAR kcal/day (mJ)	
Age	**Males**	**Females**
0–3 months	545 (2.28)	515 (2.16)
4–6 months	690 (2.89)	645 (2.69)
4–6 years	1715 (7.16)	1545 (6.46)
15–18 years	2755 (11.51)	2110 (8.83)
19–50 years	2550 (10.60)	1940 (8.10)
75+ years	2100 (8.77)	1810 (7.61)

Table 22.2 **Daily energy requirements.** Estimated average requirements (EAR) for energy for selected age and sex groups. Data from Dietary Reference Values for Food Energy and Nutrients for the United Kingdom; Report of the Panel on Dietary Reference Values of the Committee on Medical Aspects of Food Policy, London: TSO 2003.

Recommendations on nutrient intake are based on dietary reference intakes (DRI)

Dietary intake is not easy to assess. Available data are based on (sometimes incomplete) population surveys. Sets of values derived from these describe suggested minimal, average, and adequate intakes of particular nutrients. Different values are used in different countries, and there has been a degree of confusion and overlap between various definitions (see box). Currently the estimates of nutrient intake are based

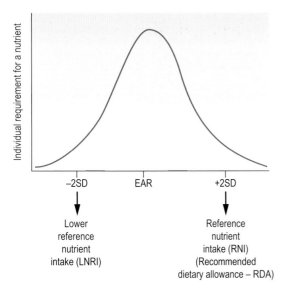

Fig. 22.5 **Dietary reference intakes (RDA): the component values.** While the estimated average requirement (EAR) reflects the intake adequate for half of a population, the RNI (or RDA) are values representing intake adequate for the great majority of individuals SD: standard deviation.

✦ DEFINITIONS IN NUTRITION SCIENCE

The definitions below are used by the Food and Nutrition Board, Institute of Medicine (IOM) of the National Academies in the United States.

Estimated Average Requirement (EAR): average daily nutrient intake estimated to meet the requirement of half of the healthy individuals in a particular gender group at a particular stage of life. The EAR is complemented by two other values:

(1) Recommended Daily Allowance (RDA; in the UK the Reference Nutrient Intake, RNI). It describes the average daily nutrient intake level sufficient to meet the nutrient requirement of nearly all (97–98%) healthy individuals.
(2) The Lower Reference Nutrient Intake (LNRI) used in the UK: the daily intake observed at the low end of intake distribution in a population (about 2%). If intake falls below this, a deficiency may occur.

Adequate Intake (AI): recommended average daily nutrient intake based on estimates of nutrient intake by a group of healthy people that are assumed to be adequate – used when an RDA cannot be determined.

Tolerable Upper Intake Level (UL): highest average daily intake likely to pose no health risk to almost all individuals in a particular gender group at a particular stage of life. As intake increases above the UL, the risk of adverse effects increases.

Note that the Dietary Reference Intakes have replaced the Dietary Reference Values (DRVs) used previously in the UK, and the Recommended Dietary Allowances (RDAs) used in the USA. Refer to Further Reading for details.

on the dietary reference intakes (DRI), the sets of values that describe the intake of a given nutrient in a population (Fig. 22.5). The DRI include:

- estimated average requirement (EAR)
- recommended daily allowance (RDA)
- adequate intake (AI)
- tolerable upper intake (UL).

The EAR and RDA values are given for a nutrient or, if these cannot be determined, AI is used. See the box for relevant definitions. Bear in mind that DRI are intended for healthy people. Also, a DRI established for any one nutrient presupposes that requirements for other ones are being met.

NUTRIGENOMICS

The variable individual response to nutrients is to a substantial extent determined by genetics. Genes influence digestion and absorption of nutrients, their metabolism and excretion. Perceptions such as taste or satiety are also, to an extent, genetically determined. This has consequences for nutritional guidelines: because the gene pool varies between populations, optimal nutritional guidelines should be population specific, rather than general. Nutrigenomics has huge potential implications for future nutritional interventions. It is analogous to pharmacogenomics: it aims to exploit the knowledge accumulated by the Human Genome Project, and the ability to monitor the expression of a large number of genes, to devise individual dietary treatments customized to a genetic background. Metabolomics, the monitoring of metabolic response patterns to nutrients, offers further opportunities to determine individual nutrition profiles (see Chapter 36).

Genotype influences plasma concentrations of nutrients

An example of the genotype effect on nutrient intake is the response of plasma cholesterol concentration to its dietary content. Approximately 50% of individual variation in plasma cholesterol is genetically determined. Response to a cholesterol-containing diet is associated with the apoprotein E (apoE) genotype. ApoE is a protein synthesized in the liver, and is the main metabolic driver of the remnant particles (Chapter 18). It occurs in several isoforms coded by alleles designated e2, e3 and e4. It has been demonstrated that plasma cholesterol concentration increases on low-fat/high-cholesterol diet in people with the E4/4 but not E2/2 phenotype.

There are many examples of nutrients affecting gene expression. For instance, the activities of key hepatic enzymes differ in persons on a long-term high-fat diet compared to a high-carbohydrate diet. The amount of dietary cholesterol affects the activity of HMG-CoA reductase. Polyunsaturated fatty acids inhibit the expression of fatty acid synthase and the ω-3 fatty acids (see below) reduce the synthesis of RNA for the platelet-derived growth factor (PDGF) and inflammatory cytokine interleukin 1 (IL-1). In essential hypertension, sensitivity to dietary salt is controlled, at least to an extent, by the angiotensinogen gene variants. Only 50% of patients are sensitive to salt intake: 30–60% of blood pressure variation is genotype related. Genetic factors are also fundamental in obesity: more than 50% of variation in weight is associated with the genetic background. Obesity is concordant in 74% between monozygotic and 32% between dizygotic twins.

Nutrition, life cycle and metabolic adaptation

Demand for nutrients is affected by both physiology and disease. Pregnancy, lactation, and growth (in particular the intensive growth in utero, growth during infancy and the adolescent growth spurt) are the three most important physiologic states associated with increased demand for nutrients.

Pregnancy is an example of metabolic adaptation termed expansive adaptation. Here the body of the mother adapts to carrying the fetus and supplying it with nutrients. Around the time of conception the mother's body prepares for the metabolic demands of the fetus. In early pregnancy the mother sets up the 'supply capacity' and later in pregnancy such supply takes place. Ninety percent of fetal weight is gained between the 20th and 40th weeks of pregnancy and the steepest growth is established between the 24th and 36th weeks. The total amount of energy stored during pregnancy is about 70 000 kcal (293 090 kJ), amounting to approx 10 kg of weight.

Nutrient intake changes during the life cycle. After delivery there is a transition from feeding through the placenta to breastfeeding and then, gradually, the baby adapts to a free diet. Up to the breastfeeding stage, nutrition is controled by substrates and the infant is entirely dependent on the mother for nutrition. Later, the growth hormone assumes a major role in directing development. At school age, new eating and activity patterns emerge as a child learns to be independent from its parents. This continues during adolescence. At this stage, sex hormones begin to play a prominent developmental role. In adulthood, muscle mass increases between 20 and 30 years of age and at that point the level of physical activity stabilizes. Thereafter, muscle mass starts to decline and the fat mass starts to increase. This accelerates after the age of 60. The bone mass also declines with age.

When nutrients are in short supply, either because of increased nutritional need or reduced availability of food, the so-called reductive adaptation takes place: the metabolic rate falls and the desire to eat decreases. This limits weight loss.

MAIN CLASSES OF NUTRIENTS

The main nutrients are carbohydrates (including fiber), fats, proteins, minerals and vitamins. Carbohydrates, proteins, fat, fiber and some minerals are macronutrients. Vitamins and

Caloric content of nutrients		
	Energy	
Nutrient	**kJ**	**kcal/g**
Starch	17	4
Glucose	17	4
Fat	37	9
Protein	17	4
Alcohol	30	7

Table 22.3 **Caloric content of nutrients** (1 kJ = 239 cal; 1 kcal = 4.184 kJ).

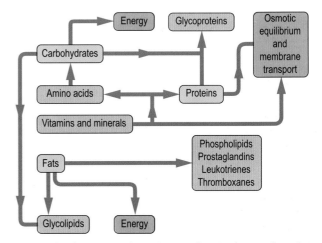

Fig. 22.6 **The functions of nutrients.** All main classes of nutrients can be used to produce energy, and all contribute to the synthesis of more complex compounds. The main role of vitamins and minerals is participation in enzymatic reactions. Prostaglandins, thromboxanes and leukotrienes, refer to Chapter 40; Glycoproteins, Chapter 26; Glycolipids, Chapter 27.

trace metals are micronutrients (see Chapter 11). The caloric value of the main nutrients is given in Table 22.3. The functions of nutrients are summarized in Figure 22.6.

Carbohydrates

Carbohydrates and fats are the most important energy sources. They also are precursors of glycoproteins, glycolipids, and mucopolysaccharides. Dietary carbohydrates include refined carbohydrates such as sucrose in sweets, drinks and fruit juices, and complex carbohydrates such as starch, present in grains and potatoes. Fiber is carbohydrate which is indigestible by the human gut such as cellulose, hemicellulose, lignin, pectin, and β-glucan. Fiber is present in unprocessed cereals, legumes, vegetables, and fruits. Its main role is to regulate gut motiity and transit.

Daily protein requirements		
Age	g/day males	g/day females
0–3 months	12.5	12.5
10–12 months	14.9	14.9
4–6 years	19.7	19.7
15–18 years	55.2	45
19–50 years	55.5	45
50+ years	53.3	46.5

Table 22.4 **Daily protein requirements.** Protein requirements are age and sex dependent. Here reference nutrient intakes (RNI) for selected age groups are shown. Data from Dietary Reference Values for Food Energy and Nutrients for the United Kingdom; Report of the Panel on Dietary Reference Values of the Committee on Medical Aspects of Food Policy, London: TSO 2003.

Proteins

Dietary proteins are digested to their component amino acids. Amino acids are used as a material to build the host's own proteins. They also serve as the 'last resort' energy substrate (see Chapter 19). Due to the different composition of animal and plant proteins, eating no animal products at all may lead to nutrient deficiencies such as those of vitamin B_{12}, calcium, iron, and zinc. Similarly to energy requirements, protein requirements change during the life cycle (Table 22.4). Increased demand for dietary protein is associated with pregnancy, lactation and the adolescent growth spurt.

Fats

Fats are the most important nutrients used for energy storage. Lipids also provide thermal insulation for the organism. They are essential components of biologic membranes and serve as substrates for synthesis of glycolipids and glycoproteins, and also phospholipids, prostaglandins, leukotrienes, and thromboxane. They are particularly important for the development of brain and retina (see also Table 3.2).

Fatty acids are signaling molecules

Lipid-derived molecules have many signaling functions and are activating ligands for transcription factors. Fatty acids, for instance, stimulate accumulation of diacylglycerol (DAG), activate the δ isoform of protein kinase C (PKC) in the liver, and decrease tyrosine phosphorylation of insulin receptor substrate proteins 1 and 2 (IRS1 and 2). PKC in turn activates NADPH oxidase and increases generation of reactive oxygen species, increasing oxidative stress. Free fatty acids (FFA) also stimulate the NFκB pathway.

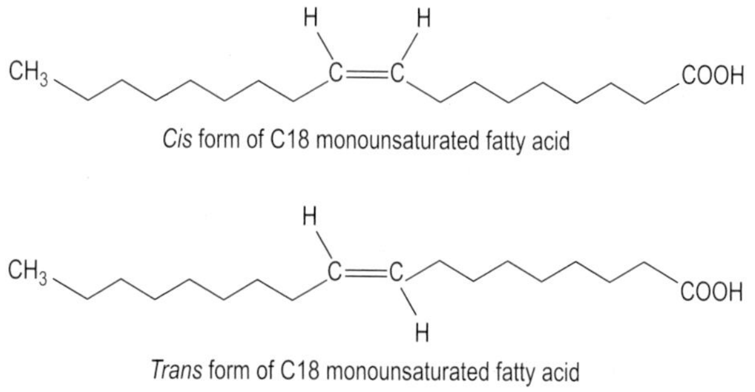

Fig. 22.7 **The example of *cis*- and *trans*-monounsaturated fatty acid (18-carbon oleic acid).** *Trans* fatty acids are produced during hydrogenation of liquid vegetable oils.

Fats are classified into saturated and unsaturated (and within the latter category there is a subdivision into mono- and polyunsaturated).

Saturated fats

Long-chain fatty acids are not soluble in water but short- (C4–6) and medium-chain fatty acids (C8–10) are. Short- and medium-chain fatty acids are transported in plasma rather than in chylomicrons. The most common saturated fatty acid is palmitic acid (C16). Others are stearic (C18), myristic (C14), and lauric (C12). All animal fats (beef fat, butterfat, lard) are highly saturated. Saturated fats are also present in palm oil, cocoa butter and coconut oil.

Monounsaturated fats

Oleic acid (ω-9) is the only significant dietary monounsaturated fatty acid

Monounsaturated fatty acids are present in all animal and vegetable fats. Olive oil is a particularly rich source of monounsaturated fats. Monounsaturated *trans* fatty acids (Fig. 22.7), the isomers of *cis*-oleic acid, are byproducts of the hydrogenation process of liquid vegetable oils. *Trans* fatty acids arising from hydrogenation of fats are associated with an increased risk of coronary disease.

Polyunsaturated fats

Polyunsaturated fatty acids include ω-6 and ω-3 acids

The ω-6 acids are arachidonic acid (ω-6, C-20:4, $\Delta^{5,8,11,14}$) and its precursor linoleic acid (ω-6, C-18:2, $\Delta^{9,12}$). They are present in vegetable seed oils. The ω-6 fatty acids are present in soybean and canola oils and in fish oils (particularly in fatty fish such as salmon, sardines, and pilchards).

The ω-3 fatty acids are α-linolenic (ω-3, C-18:3, $\Delta^{9,12,15}$), eicosapentaenoic (ω-3, C-20:5, $\Delta^{5,8,11,14,17}$), and docosahexaenoic (ω-3, C-22:6, $\Delta^{4,7,10,13,16,19}$) acids. They are present primarily in fish, shellfish, and phytoplankton and also in some vegetable oils such as olive, safflower, corn, sunflower, and soybean and leafy vegetables.

ESSENTIAL (LIMITING) NUTRIENTS

Essential nutrients cannot be synthesized in the human body and therefore need to be supplied from outside. They include essential amino acids, essential fatty acids (EFA), and some vitamins and trace elements. Carbohydrates (glucose and starches) are not essential nutrients.

Essential amino acids

Essential amino acids are phenylalanine (tyrosine can be synthesized from phenylalanine), the branched-chain amino acids valine, leucine, isoleucine, threonine, and methionine and lysine. Some plant proteins are relatively deficient in essential amino acids, whereas animal proteins usually contain a balanced mixture (see Chapter 19).

Essential lipids

The essential fatty acids (EFA) are linoleic acid and α-linolenic acid. Arachidonic acid, eicosapentaenoic acid, and docosahexaenoic acid can be made in limited amounts from EFA; however, they become essential nutrients when EFA are deficient.

MINERALS

Major minerals are sodium, potassium, chloride, calcium, phosphate, and magnesium

Sodium is important in the maintenance of extracellular fluid volume (Chapter 23). It participates in electrophysiologic phenomena and, together with potassium, is essential in maintaining transmembrane potential (Chapter 8). Potassium is the main intracellular cation. Importantly, hyperkalemia and hypokalemia lead to arrhythmias and may be life-threatening. Potassium is contained in vegetables and fruit, particularly bananas, and in fruit juices. Dietary potassium intake needs to be limited in renal disease because of its impaired excretion and a tendency to hyperkalemia (Chapter 23).

Calcium and phosphate balance is important for maintaining bone structure (Chapter 25). Calcium is present in milk and milk products, and in some vegetables. Phosphates are present in plant and animal cells.

Magnesium is important for skeletal development and for the maintenance of electrical potential in nerve and muscle membranes. It is also a co-factor for ATP-requiring enzymes, and is important for the replication of DNA and for RNA synthesis. Magnesium deficiency develops in starvation and malabsorption, may be due to the loss from the gastrointestinal tract in diarrhea and vomiting, and sometimes occurs as a result of diuretic treatment and surgical procedures on the gastrointestinal tract. It is also associated with acute pancreatitis and alcoholism. Hypomagnesemia is often accompanied by hypocalcemia. Magnesium deficiency leads to muscle weakness and cardiac arrhythmias.

Iron

Iron is important in the transfer of molecular oxygen and is a component of heme in hemoglobin and myoglobin (Chapter 5). Cytochromes a, b, and c also contain iron (Chapter 9). Altogether, there are 3–4 g of iron in the body. Seventy-five percent of body iron is in hemoglobin and myoglobin, and 25% is stored in tissues such as bone marrow, liver, and reticuloendothelial system.

Iron is absorbed in the upper small intestine. Meat and ascorbic acid increase its absorption, and vegetable fiber inhibits it. It is transported in blood bound to transferrin and is stored as ferritin and hemosiderin. Transferrin is normally about 30% saturated with iron. Iron is lost through the skin and through the gastrointestinal tract. Humans do not have a mechanism to excrete iron and free iron is toxic.

Dietary iron is in the ferric Fe^{3+} form. It is reduced in the gastrointestinal tract to divalent Fe^{2+} by ascorbate and a ferrireductase enzyme located in the intestinal brush border. Fe^{2+} is transported into the cells by a divalent metal transporter (which also transports most trace metals). The iron pool within the enterocyte is controlled by the iron regulatory proteins. The erythrocyte content of iron affects iron absorption from the intestine. If erythrocytes are iron rich, the iron is stored in the enterocytes incorporated into ferritin. Otherwise, it is transported through the basolateral membrane, where one of the transport-facilitating proteins, ferroxidase, also called hephaestin, oxidizes Fe^{2+} to Fe^{3+}, which is then bound to transferrin in plasma. Transferrin is taken up in the bone marrow by erythrocyte precursors cells in a receptor-dependent process. Within the cells, iron is released, reduced to Fe^{2+}, and transported to the mitochondria for incorporation into the heme molecule in the Fe^{2+} form. After destruction of the old erythrocytes by macrophages in the reticuloendothelial system, the iron is released as Fe^{2+}, oxidized to Fe^{3+} again, and loaded back onto transferrin. The outline of iron metabolism is shown in Figure 22.8.

The requirement for iron increases during growth and pregnancy. Iron deficiency results in defective erythropoiesis and in normocytic or microcytic (small erythrocytes) hypochromic anemia. This is most likely to develop in infants and adolescents, in pregnant and menstruating women, and also in the elderly. Iron deficiency most often develops as a result of abnormal blood loss, and therefore persons who present with iron deficiency anemia always need to be investigated for causes of bleeding, particularly from the gastrointestinal tract.

Dietary sources of iron include organ meats, poultry and fish and oysters, and also egg yolks, dried beans, dried figs and dates, and some green vegetables. Assessment of iron status includes the measurements of transferrin and ferritin

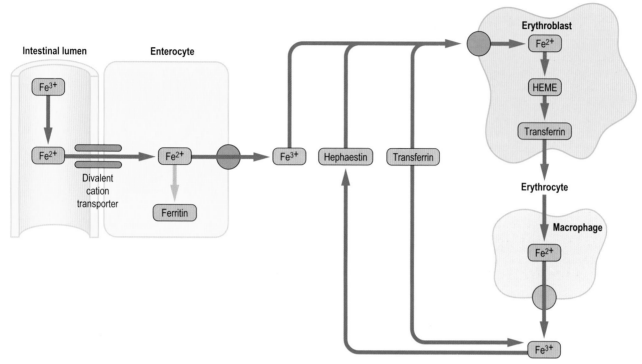

Fig. 22.8 **Iron metabolism.** Dietary iron is absorbed in the intestine and either stored in enterocytes as ferritin or transported out to plasma. In plasma, iron remains bound to transferrin. It is taken up by other cells, e.g. erythroblasts, through the mediation of the membrane transferrin receptor. In erythroblasts, iron is incorporated into heme, and then hemoglobin. Old erythrocytes are degraded by macrophages in the reticuloendothelial system. Liberated iron is released from cells and recycled bound to transferrin. Note that the dietary iron is in the ferric (Fe^{3+}) form. This is reduced to ferrous ion (Fe^{2+}) at the intestinal brush border. The transported form of iron is ferric again, but the form incorporated into heme is ferrous (see also Fig. 34.8).

HEMOCHROMATOSIS

Hemochromatosis is an autosomal recessive disorder resulting from the increased absorption of iron. It is the most common inherited disorder in persons of North European ancestry. Iron accumulates in heart, liver and pancreas and can cause liver cirrhosis, hepatocellular carcinoma, diabetes, arthritis and heart failure. In the classic form of hemochromatosis, the mutated gene encodes the protein known as hereditary hemochromatosis protein (HFE), which is structurally similar to class I major histocompatibility antigens (see Chapter 38). It is now known that mutations of other proteins can lead to a very similar clinical picture.

in plasma, hematologic variables, and the bone marrow smear.

Trace metals and vitamins

Vitamins and trace metals are important for the catalysis of chemical reactions. They act as coenzymes and form functionally important prosthetic groups of enzymes. They are discussed in detail in Chapter 11.

NUTRITIONAL ASSESSMENT

Nutritional assessment includes clinical assessment of the state of nutrition, the assessment of dietary habits and dietary history, a range of body (anthropometric) measurements, and biochemical and hematologic laboratory tests. Since there is no single definitive marker of nutritional status, assessment relies on the interpretation of a range of variables.

Body weight and the body mass index

Body weight in relation to height is the most commonly used measurement in nutritional assessment. Relationship between the two is expressed as the body mass index (BMI) calculated according to the formula:

$$BMI = weight\ (kg)/height\ (cm)^2$$

The BMI is used to categorize the nutritional status as shown in Table 22.5. As mentioned above, the BMI alone should not be used as a sole/definitive indication of the nutritional status.

Other measurements used in nutritional assessment are the waist-to-hip ratio, the mid-arm circumference and the

THE ABC OF EMERGENCY TREATMENT

Eating and drinking, like breathing, connect living organisms with the environment. To survive we need oxygen, water and nutrients. One can exist without oxygen for minutes only. Without water the survival time is days. With these two supplied, a human can survive without food for between 60 and 90 days.

These considerations determine the urgency of treatment when things go wrong. Reestablishment of oxygen supply and circulating volume is the first priority (ABC of resuscitation: Airway, Breathing, Circulation). Repletion of lost fluid and electrolytes is also necessary within hours to days, depending on the state of the patient. Provision of other nutrients becomes important as soon as the life-saving measures have been taken. The rule of thumb is that patients unable to eat would need nutritional support if they have been (or will be) unable to take food for 5–7 days. This period is shorter in hypercatabolic persons.

skinfold thickness measured with carefully calibrated calipers. The simple measurement of waist circumference correlates with the amount of visceral fat and is used in the diagnosis of the metabolic syndrome (Chapter 21). More detailed analysis includes assessment of total body water, analysis of body bioelectrical impedance and the measurements of lean body mass using dual-energy X-ray absorptiometry (DEXA). Some of these measurements allow calculation of variables such as body fat content and composition. Functional measurements such as grip strength or peak expiratory flow are also relevant to nutritional assessment. Full assessment involves measurements of vitamins and trace metals. This is particularly important in patients who remain on long-term parenteral nutrition.

Biochemical markers of nutritional status

Urinary nitrogen excretion helps to assess nitrogen balance

Nitrogen balance relates to body protein requirements. It is the difference between the intake of nitrogen and its excretion. Positive nitrogen balance means that the intake exceeds loss. Negative nitrogen balance signifies that the loss exceeds intake. The 24 h urinary nitrogen excretion is an estimate of the quantity of proteins metabolized by the body. Ninety percent of the excreted nitrogen appears in the urine (80% of this as urea). The rest is excreted in the stool, hair, and sweat. Nitrogen excretion adjusts to protein intake over 2–4 days. Measurement of urinary nitrogen (or urea) excretion is the most reliable way of assessing daily protein requirements. Currently, it is rarely used outside the research setting. As a guide, most people require 1–1.2 g protein/kg body weight/day. Age-related protein requirements are listed in Table 22.4 (see also Chapter 19).

Body mass index (BMI) and nutritional status	
BMI	**Interpretation**
<18.5	malnourished
18.5–20	underweight
21–25	desirable
26–30	overweight
>30	obese

Table 22.5 **Body mass index (BMI) and nutritional status.**

 A WOMAN WITH RENAL FAILURE AND WEIGHT LOSS

A 59-year-old woman was admitted to the renal unit with recurrent infections and recurrent endocarditis. She had been treated with hemodialysis for 5 years and over a period of 2 years had lost 33% of her body weight. She had a very poor appetite and had been taking two cartons (1.5 kcal/ml) of milkshake sip feeds daily. She was anuric and her fluid intake was restricted to 1000 ml daily. Her height was 1.68 m and she weighted 52.7 kg; BMI was 18. Her most recent biochemistry results revealed persistent hyperkalemia between 5.7 and 6.2 mmol/L.

Comment. Because of her poor nutritional status and continuous weight loss she needs to continue taking nutritional supplements to minimize further weight loss. However, due to the hyperkalemia, a low-electrolyte sip feed should be considered. She was initially taking 22 mmol of potassium from the 1.5 kcal/ml milkshake. Subsequently this was changed to a low electrolyte sip feed, which provided 12 mmol in total. The UK Renal Nutrition Group Standards recommend that daily potassium intake in this type of patient should be less than 1 mmol/kg body weight. Low-electrolyte/volume sip feeds should always be considered for renal patients and the serum electrolyte concentrations need to be closely monitored. (See Chapter 23.)

Different plasma proteins have been used as markers of nutritional status

Concentration of a protein in plasma may reflect the nutritional status over the time-period related to its half-life. Proteins most commonly used for this purpose are albumin and transthyretin (prealbumin). Many studies confirm the link between liver albumin synthesis (albumin half-life is approximately 20 days; see Chapter 4) and nutritional status. Transthyretin, which has a half-life of 2 days, has also been used in nutritional assessment. It is synthesized in the liver and forms a complex with retinal-binding protein in plasma. Unfortunately, interpretation of plasma concentrations of nutritionally relevant proteins is often difficult, because they are not exclusively determined by the state of nutrition. For instance, albumin concentration in plasma also depends on the state of hydration; it decreases in overhydrated patients. In addition, albumin and transthyretin are affected by the acute phase response (transthyretin concentration increases during the acute phase reaction and albumin concentration decreases). All this means that they cannot be interpreted in isolation but are helpful when seen as part of the entire clinical picture.

General laboratory tests provide information supplementing nutritional assessment

Measurement of hemoglobin may uncover iron deficiency. Checking the liver (Chapter 29) and kidney (Chapter 23) function, the measurements of serum sodium, potassium, chloride, bicarbonate, calcium, phosphate and magnesium, and the assessment of iron metabolism, all provide useful additional information. Assessing daily fluid intake and loss is essential in patients who are being considered for nutritional support.

MALNUTRITION

Malnutrition is a gradual decline in nutritional status, which in its more advanced stages leads to a decrease in functional capacity and other complications. Protein energy malnutrition (PEM) is defined as poor nutritional status due to inadequate nutrient intake.

Reduced food intake leads to reductive adaptation which includes a decrease in nutrient stores, changes in body composition and the more efficient use of fuels such as the use of ketone bodies by the brain (metabolic changes that accompany starvation are described in Chapter 21).

Malnutrition is one of the key issues faced by public health in the developing world and needs to be viewed from not only medical, but also social and economic perspectives. Mortality in malnourished patients (BMI between 10 and 13) is four times higher compared to well-nourished people. The effects of malnutrition are summarized in Table 22.6. Worldwide, malnutrition contributes to 54% of the 11.6 million deaths annually among children below 5 years of age.

In the developed world, malnutrition is a problem in hospitalized patients who are unable to eat because of their primary problem, for instance, stroke or cancer. Gastrointestinal problems, particularly colon pathology and celiac disease (see case, Chapter 10), or postoperative conditions are associated with specific nutritional problems. Malnutrition also affects a large group of older individuals. In the UK, up to 40% of patients admitted to hospitals are undernourished. In addition to malnutrition, specific deficiencies such as those of vitamin D, iron, and vitamin C may occur.

There are two types of protein-calorie malnutrition: marasmus and kwashiorkor

Marasmus results from a prolonged inadequate intake of calories and protein. It is a chronic condition, which develops over months or years. It is characterized by loss of muscle tissue and subcutaneous fat with the preservation of the synthesis of visceral proteins such as albumin. There is a clear loss of weight.

Kwashiorkor is a more acute form of undernutrition, which may also occur on the background of marasmus. It also develops because of inadequate nutrient intake after trauma or infection. In kwashiorkor, in contrast to marasmus, visceral tissues are not spared: the hallmark of kwashiorkor is edema due to the low concentration of plasma albumin and the loss of oncotic pressure (Chapter 23). The edema may mask the weight loss. Complications of kwashiorkor are dehydration, hypoglycemia, hypothermia, electrolyte disturbances and septicemia. These patients have impaired immunity and wound healing, and are prone to infection.

The WHO classification of malnutrition is based on anthropometry and the presence of bilateral pitting edema. Another classification has been proposed which distinguishes complicated from uncomplicated malnutrition (Table 22.7). Marasmus and kwashiorkor are terms rarely used in the hospital practice in developed countries; malnutrition and complicated malnutrition are probably more appropriate.

Inappropriate treatment of a malnourished person may lead to refeeding syndrome

The inpatient treatment of malnutrition in famine areas includes standard preparations such as Formula 100 therapeutic milk (F100). F100 is a liquid diet with an energy content of 100 kcal/100 ml. It includes dried skimmed milk, oil,

Consequences of protein-calorie malnutrition
Decreased protein synthesis
Decreased activity of Na$^+$/K$^+$-ATPase
Decreased glucose transport
Fatty liver, liver necrosis, liver fibrosis
Depression, apathy, mood changes
Hypothermia
Compromised ventilation
Compromised immune system: impaired wound healing
Risk of wound breakdown
Decreased cardiac output
Decreased renal function
Loss of muscle strength
Anorexia
Decreased mobility

Table 22.6 **Consequences of protein-calorie malnutrition.**

Classification of malnutrition

	Moderate	Severe	Complicated
Weight for height (% of median)	70–80	<70	<80
– or pitting edema	no	yes	yes
– or mid upper arm circumference	110–125	<110 mm	<110 mm
Appetite, clinically well, alert	yes	yes	no*

Note that, in the classic classification of malnutrition, the presence of edema is also the main differentiating feature between marasmus and kwashiorkor.

Patients with complicated malnutrition may develop anorexia, high fever, anemia and dehydration. After Collins S, Yates R. The need to update the classification of acute malnutrition. Lancet 2003;362**:249.*

Table 22.7 **Classification of malnutrition.**

OBESE MAN WITH TYPE 2 DIABETES, CORONARY DISEASE, AND ARTHRITIS

Mr K is a 55-year-old man with type 2 diabetes and coronary disease. He gets angina on effort and also suffers from severe arthritic knee pain. When he initially presented to the outpatient clinic his weight was 140 kg and his height 1.80 m (BMI 43). Within a year he managed to lose 12 kg by dieting. He was prescribed a lipase inhibitor, which he tolerated well. However, his arthritis worsened and he was increasingly less able to exercise. As a result his weight increased again to 137 kg. He was referred to the surgeons and is now being considered for gastric banding surgery.

Comment. This patient illustrates multiple problems associated with obesity and in particular the way a concomitant disease may interfere with weight reduction programs. Weight loss is, to a substantial extent, dependent on the level of exercise. This patient lost weight initially but the maintenance of lower body weight was compromised by decreased mobility caused by arthritis.

---

sugar and a mix of vitamins and minerals (without iron). In the areas of famine, community feeding programs use the so-called life-sustaining general rations (at least 2100 kcal; 8786 kJ/day) containing grains, legumes, and vegetable oil. During the treatment of malnutrition, this needs to be combined with providing adequate water, sanitation, and basic health care.

It is important to take time to replete a starved person nutritionally. Too quick a replacement may be dangerous due to a major shift between intracellular and extracellular fluid. This is known as the refeeding syndrome, and is characterized

Obesity is associated with an increased risk for a range of conditions

Type 2 diabetes
Hypertension and stroke
Dyslipidemia
Gall stones, particularly in women
Some cancers: breast, endometrial, ovarian, gall bladder, colon
Respiratory disorders
Musculoskeletal disorders (however, reduction of risk of osteoporosis)
Psychologic problems

Table 22.8 **Obesity is associated with an increased risk for a range of conditions.**

by a severe decrease in concentrations of serum magnesium, phosphate and potassium (the latter because of the stimulation of insulin secretion). Also, if thiamin deficiency is present, carbohydrate feeding can precipitate the Wernicke-Korsakoff syndrome (see Chapter 11). Frequent simple meals at short intervals are recommended during famine relief and, in a hospital setting, gradual introduction of nutritional support and close monitoring are required.

OBESITY

Obesity has emerged as a major health problem worldwide

Worldwide obesity has increased by more than 70% since 1980. In the USA, 61% of adults are overweight and 26% are obese (USA National Center for Health Statistics Report 2002). Main causes of this seem to be the wide availability of highly caloric food, and the significant recent decrease in physical activity both at work and during leisure time. There is also a genetic predisposition to obesity: in a great majority of cases it appears to be polygenic. Over 50 chromosomal regions were quoted to contain obesity-related genes. Rare mutations in at least six human genes, including leptin, have been linked to morbid obesity.

Obesity is associated with an increased risk of medical and surgical problems

Obesity is associated with an increased risk of several diseases (Table 22.8). In particular, it is a risk factor for type 2 diabetes mellitus (see Chapter 21); the increased incidence of diabetes worldwide parallels that of obesity. Insulin resistance, which develops in obesity, is an important common denominator between obesity and diabetes. The metabolic syndrome, closely associated with obesity (Chapter 21), carries an increased risk of cardiovascular disease.

DIET IN HEALTH AND DISEASE

Dietary history should include more than the details of food intake

Dietary habits include meal patterns and the amount and composition of food. Individual diet is determined by biologic, psychologic, sociologic and cultural factors. Biologic factors involved are the state of the systems responsible for the intake, digestion, absorption and metabolism of nutrients. Enzyme deficiencies, such as, for instance, that of lactase (Chapter 10), cause impaired absorption of foodstuffs (in this case, milk).

Psychologic factors play an important role in determining food intake; eating disorders such as anorexia nervosa and bulimia nervosa may lead to severe malnutrition. Sociologic factors include availability and price of food, and measures taken by society to improve diets such as, for instance, school meals or subsidized meals for the elderly or disabled persons. Cultural factors also determine eating patterns and the type of preferred foodstuffs. All the above are important when taking the nutritional/dietary history. Individual food intake can be assessed by food frequency questionnaires, 24-h dietary recalls, food records, and also by direct analysis of foods and by metabolic balance studies. The newer method of diet research is the so-called structured assessment of dietary patterns.

Diets in health

Current dietary recommendations for general population focus on balanced eating

An example of dietary recommendations for a healthy population is the Food Pyramid developed by the US Department of Agriculture (Fig. 22.9). These recommendations suggest eating a wide variety of foods. They stress the balance between food intake and physical activity. They recommend a

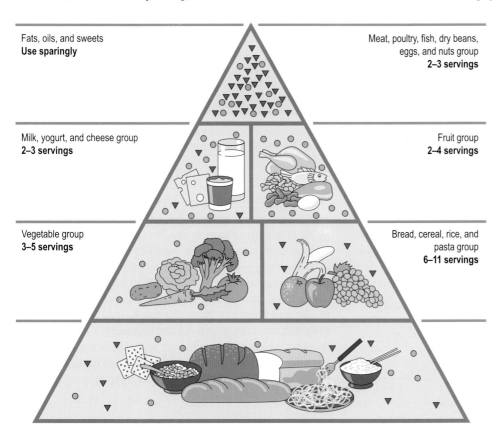

Fig. 22.9 **The Food Pyramid.** This illustrates current recommendations on healthy eating (US Department of Agriculture).

Fats, oils, and sweets
Use sparingly

Meat, poultry, fish, dry beans, eggs, and nuts group
2–3 servings

Milk, yogurt, and cheese group
2–3 servings

Fruit group
2–4 servings

Vegetable group
3–5 servings

Bread, cereal, rice, and pasta group
6–11 servings

What is the food guide pyramid?
The pyramid is an outline of what to eat each day. It's not a rigid prescription, but a general guide that lets you choose a healthful diet that's right for you.
The pyramid calls for eating a variety of foods to get the nutrients you need and at the same time the right amount of calories to maintain or improve your weight.
The pyramid also focuses on fat because most American diets are too high in fat, especially saturated fat.

⊙ Fat (naturally occurring and added)
▼ Sugars (added)

These symbols show fat and added sugars in food

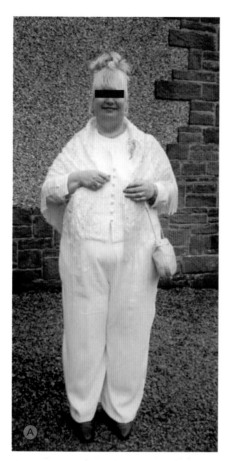
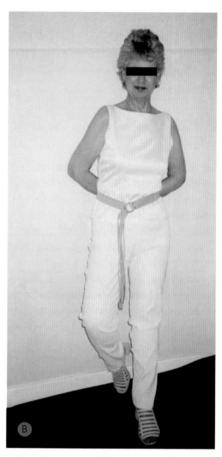

Fig. 22.10 **Surgical treatment of severe obesity.** These photographs show the same patient before and after gastric banding surgery. Her weight before surgery was 136.1 kg; within 3 years it decreased to 63 kg. Courtesy of the patient and Mr D Galloway, Consultant Surgeon, Glasgow.

diet containing plenty of complex carbohydrates in the form of grain products, vegetables and fruits. Diet should be low in saturated fat and cholesterol and moderate in sugars, salt and sodium. Alcohol should be taken in moderation. The Food Pyramid consists of several groups of foodstuffs which need to be taken daily in a decreasing number of daily servings.

- The bread, pasta, and cereal group forms the basis of nutrition with 6–11 recommended servings
- Fruit (2–4 servings) and vegetable (3–5 servings)
- Milk, yoghurt, cheese (2–3 servings)
- Meat, poultry, fish, dry beans, eggs, and nuts (2–3 servings)
- Fats, oils, and sweets (to be used sparingly).

Weight reduction

Losing weight increases life expectancy, decreases blood pressure, decreases visceral fat deposition, improves plasma lipid concentrations, increases insulin sensitivity and normalizes glycemia, improves clotting and platelet function, and enhances the quality of life.

To lose weight, one needs to change the balance between energy intake and expenditure, i.e between food intake and physical activity. However, the process involves many other factors, such as motivation, available time, cost, and access to appropriate weight reduction programs. Low-calorie diets contain approximately 1200–1300 kcal/day and very low-calorie diets around 800 kcal/day. Generally, a combination of diet and exercise is more effective in inducing weight loss than diet alone. In severe obesity, treatment with fat absorption inhibitors and antagonists of endocannabinoid receptors have been used. Surgical treatments such as gastric plication (banding) and jejuno-ileal bypass surgery can be considered in extreme cases (Fig. 22.10).

Low-carbohydrate diets for weight reduction

Low-carbohydrate, high-fat diets appear to be effective in weight reduction (see box on p. 191), at least in the short term, and they consistently lower plasma glucose concentration. As with many other aspects of dietary management, they are not completely evidence based. There are persisting concerns that include potential risk of abnormalities of liver and kidney function, and the long-term effects of higher fat intake on cardiovascular risk. Research in the field continues.

Diet is important in the prevention of coronary disease

Nutrients which affect atherosclerosis are dietary cholesterol, saturated fat and *trans* fatty acids. Excessive caloric intake and consequent obesity also facilitate atherosclerosis. High dietary cholesterol and high saturated fat decrease the LDL receptor expression mediated through an increase in the intracellular cholesterol content in the hepatocytes: this leads to an increase in plasma cholesterol concentration (Chapter 17). Foods containing saturated fatty acids (full-fat milk, cheese, butter, and red meats) are atherogenic in excess. The rationale behind low-cholesterol diets is that LDL receptor expression can be increased if dietary cholesterol content is sufficiently low. The typical Western diet contains approximately 400–500 mg of cholesterol daily. The intake required to achieve reduction in plasma cholesterol is much lower – below 200 mg or even below 100 mg daily.

Nutrients that seem to be protective against atherosclerosis include polyunsaturated ω-6-rich fatty acids (contained in vegetable oils) and ω-3-rich fish and fish oils, monounsaturated fat, and soluble fiber such as β-pectin. Polyunsaturates reduce plasma cholesterol concentration. The ω-3 fatty acids reduce triglycerides by decreasing VLDL synthesis and increasing its catabolism. They are also antithrombotic: fish oil inhibits thromboxane and PDGF synthesis, reduces blood viscosity and enhances fibrinolysis. Interestingly, it seems to electrically stabilize the heart muscle, preventing arrhythmias and decreasing the incidence of sudden death in people who have suffered myocardial infarction. Monounsaturated fats increase the HDL concentration, increase insulin sensitivity and decrease plasma triglyceride concentration.

Diets low in fat and cholesterol have been a hallmark of cardiovascular prevention

These diets normally result in an approximately 10% decrease in serum cholesterol if applied during clinical trials and a lesser decrease (usually below 5%) when applied to the general population. Alcohol seems to be protective against coronary disease but taken in excess it carries many other risks, obesity included. Unfortunately, low-fat diets, if the protein content is kept constant, tend to be high in carbohydrates. In spite of recommendations to use predominantly complex carbohydrates, in many populations refined sugars constitute too high a proportion of carbohydrate intake, and this promotes obesity. High-carbohydrate diets may also lead to hypertriglyceridemia. Unfortunately, low-fat diets seem to decrease HDL-cholesterol by 10–20%.

NUTRITION AND CHRONIC DISEASE

Diabetes mellitus

The management of diabetes is closely linked to nutrition

To ensure optimal glycemic control, not only the quality and quantity of food, but also timing and regularity of meals are important. Importantly, in persons with glucose intolerance, a comprehensive approach including weight reduction, reduction of sugar and fat intake, increase in fiber intake, and increase in physical activity decreases the risk of developing diabetes.

Cancer

Lifestyle and diet may influence the incidence of cancer

High intake of fruit and vegetables seems to be protective against cancer, possibly due to the presence of antioxidants and fiber. Dairy products seem also to be protective. There were suggestions that high-fat diets may increase cancer risk, but epidemiologic evidence for this is weak. In clinical studies β-carotene, retinoids (see Chapter 11), fiber, and calcium were not found to be effective in cancer prevention. However, coincidental findings suggest that vitamin E prevents development of prostate cancer, and selenium is beneficial in prostate and colorectal cancers.

Renal disease

Factors contributing to the development of malnutrition in renal failure (uremia, see Chapter 23) include, in addition to poor nutrient intake, increased catabolism, chronic inflammation, and endocrine changes. Maintaining adequate protein and energy intake is important and a low-potassium, low-phosphate diet is recommended due to the tendency to retain potassium and phosphate when renal function deteriorates.

Nutritional support

Nutritional support is required for a substantial number of hospitalized patients and ranges from simple assistance with meals, through enriched or special-consistency diets, to enteral nutrition and total parenteral nutrition (Table 22.9).

Enteral nutrition entails feeding a person through special tubes placed in the stomach or jejunum, and parenteral nutrition is essentially intravenous feeding. Enteral nutrition is appropriate when there are difficulties with taking food orally but the gastrointestinal tract functions properly.

Table 22.9 The levels of nutritional support.

Special diets

Assistance with eating

Enteral nutrition (feeding through different feeding tubes: nasogastric, nasoduodenal; gastrostomy and jejunostomy)

Parenteral (intravenous) nutrition

A comprehensive guide to nutritional support can be consulted at http://www.nhsggc.org.uk/nutritionteam.

When the gastrointestinal tract does not function because of, for instance, intestinal obstruction, or when large parts of it have been surgically removed, total parenteral nutrition is appropriate.

Total parenteral nutrition, while in many instances life-saving, is a treatment potentially associated with complications caused by intravenous line infections (it requires strictly sterile procedures) as well as metabolic problems. For this reason, parenteral nutrition treatment in hospitals is managed by multidisciplinary teams that include specialist nurses, surgeons, gastroenterologists, dieticians, pharmacists, and laboratory medicine physicians.

Summary

- Appropriate nutrition underpins health and well-being, and poor nutrition increases susceptibility to disease.
- Food intake is controlled by a neuroendocrine system responding to signals generated in adipose tissue.
- Genotype, food availability, state of health, and physical activity are factors which determine nutritional status.
- Nutritional needs change during the life cycle.
- Main categories of nutrients are carbohydrates, fats, proteins, and vitamins and minerals. Water balance is closely associated with nutrition.
- Assessment of nutritional status is an important part of general clinical assessment. It includes the assessment of current diet, dietary history, clinical examination and a range of biochemical and hematologic tests.
- Malnutrition affects large areas of the developing world, and in the developed world is an issue among disadvantaged social groups and also in hospitalized persons.
- Obesity has become a major health problem worldwide.
- Nutritional support includes graded assistance with nutrient intake, ranging from assistance with meals to total parenteral nutrition.

ACTIVE LEARNING

1. Outline the processes that maintain energy homeostasis.
2. Describe the role of different classes of fatty acids in nutrition.
3. List the principles of a weight reduction program.
4. Discuss instances when increased nutritional demand can precipitate malnutrition.
5. What diet would you recommend for a diabetic patient?

Further reading

Collins S, Yates R. The need to update the classification of acute malnutrition. *Lancet* 2003;**362**:249.

Cota D. CXB1 receptors: emerging evidence for central and peripheral mechanisms that regulate energy balance, metabolism, and cardiovascular health. *Diabetes/Metabol Res Rev* 2007;**23**:507–517.

Crowley VEF. Overview of human obesity and central mechanisms regulating energy homeostasis. *Ann Clin Biochem* 2008;**45**:245–255.

Dietary Reference Values for Food Energy and Nutrients for the United Kingdom. *Report of the Panel on Dietary Reference Values of the Committee on Medical Aspects of Food Policy Department of Health* London: TSO, 2003.

Eckel RH. Nonsurgical management of obesity. *N Engl J Med* 2008;**358**: 1941–1950.

Gidden F, Shenkin A. Laboratory support of the clinical nutrition service. *Clin Chem Lab Med* 2000;**38**:693–714.

James WPT. The fundamental drivers of the obesity epidemics. *Obesity Rev* 2008; **9** (suppl 1): 6–13.

Kopelman PG. Obesity as a medical problem. *Nature* 2000;**404**:635–643.

Mann J, McAuley K. Carbohydrates: is the advice to eat less justified for diabetes and cardiovascular health?. *Curr Opin Lipidol* 2007;**18**:9–12.

Munoz M, Breymann C, Garcia-Erce JA et al. Efficacy and safety of intravenous iron therapy as an alternative/adjunct to allogeneic blood transfusion. *Vox Sang* 2008;**94**:172–183.

Schneider BD, Leibold EA. Regulation of mammalian iron homeostasis. *Curr Opin Clin Nutr Metab Care* 2000;**3**:267–273.

Vincent HK, Innes KE, Vincent KR. Oxidative stress and potential interventions to reduce oxidative stress in overweight and obesity. *Diabetes Obesity Metabol* 2007; **9**:813–839.

World Health Organization. *Management of Severe Malnutrition: A Manual for Physicians and Other Senior Health Workers* Geneva: World Health Organization, 1999; Available online at: www.who.int/nut/documents/manage_severe_malnutrition_eng.pdf.

Websites

Dietary Reference Intakes: Applications in Dietary Planning (2003). Food and Nutrition Board, Institute of Medicine (IOM) of the National Academies: www.iom.edu

UK Food Standards Agency: http://www.Foodstandards.gov.uk

American Dietetic Association: http://www.eatright.org

The Food Pyramid: http://www.nal.usda.gov

Nutrition Team: http://www.nhsggc.org.uk/nutritionteam

23. Water and Electrolyte Homeostasis

M H Dominiczak and M Szczepanska-Konkel

LEARNING OBJECTIVES

After reading this chapter you should be able to:

- Describe the body water compartments in the adult and the composition of the main body fluids.
- Explain the role of albumin in movement of water between plasma and interstitial space, including the consequences of proteinuria.
- Describe how sodium influences the movement of water between the extracellular and intracellular space.
- Explain why sodium-potassium ATPase is essential for normal cell hydration, and comment on the consequences of its inhibition.
- Describe factors affecting plasma potassium concentration.
- Discuss links between sodium and water homeostasis.
- Describe clinical assessment of water and electrolyte status.

INTRODUCTION

Water and electrolytes are constantly exchanged with the environment and their body content depends on the balance between intake and loss.

Water is essential for survival and accounts for approximately 60% of the body weight in an adult person. This changes with age: it is about 75% in the newborn and decreases to below 50% in older individuals. Water content is greatest in brain tissue (about 90%) and least in adipose tissue (10%).

The stability of subcellular structures and activities of numerous enzymes are dependent on adequate cell hydration. Both a deficiency of water and its excess impair function of tissues and organs. Water balance and water distribution between cells and surrounding fluid are subject to complex regulation.

Maintenance of ion gradients and electrical potential across membranes is also crucial for survival and underlies muscle contraction, nerve conduction and secretory processes (Chapter 8). The kidneys play a major role in the regulation of water and electrolyte homeostasis. Water and electrolyte disorders are common in clinical practice.

WATER

Body water compartments

Approximately two-thirds of total body water is in the intracellular fluid (ICF), and one-third remains in the extracellular fluid (ECF). ECF consists of interstitial fluid and lymph (15% body weight), plasma (3% body weight), and the so-called transcellular fluids, which include gastrointestinal fluid, urine and cerebrospinal fluid (CSF) (Fig. 23.1). Two 'barriers' are important for the understanding of exchanges taking place between different compartments: the cell membrane and the wall of a capillary vessel.

Capillary vessel wall separates plasma from the surrounding interstitial fluid

The capillary wall separates plasma from the interstitial fluid and is freely permeable to water and electrolytes but

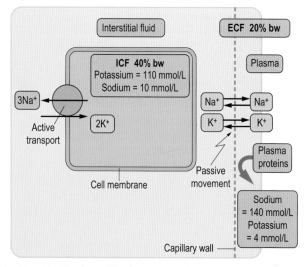

Fig. 23.1 **Distribution of body water, sodium and potassium.** Main body water compartments are the intracellular fluid (ICF) and the extracellular fluid (ECF). ECF includes interstitial fluid and plasma. The gradient of sodium and potassium concentration is maintained across cell membranes by Na⁺/K⁺-ATPase. Sodium is a major contributor to the osmolality of the ECF, and a determinant of the distribution of water between ECF and ICF. Distribution of water between plasma and interstitial fluid is determined by the oncotic pressure exerted by plasma proteins. bw, body weight.

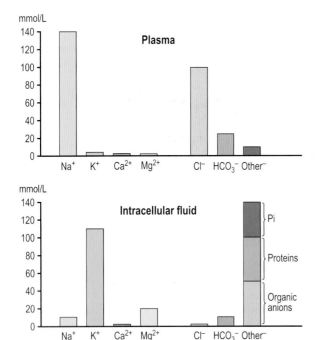

Fig. 23.2 **Ions present in the plasma and in the intracellular fluid.** The most important ions in plasma are sodium, potassium, calcium, chloride, phosphate, and bicarbonate. Sodium chloride, in a concentration close to 0.9% (thus 'physiologic saline'), is the main ionic component of the extracellular fluid. Potassium is the main intracellular cation. Glucose and urea also contribute to plasma osmolality. Their contribution is normally small, because they are present in plasma in relatively low molar concentrations (about 5 mmol/L each). However, when glucose concentration increases in diabetes, its contribution to osmolality becomes significant. Plasma urea increases in renal failure but it does not contribute to water movement between ECF and ICF because it freely crosses cell membranes. The main intracellular cation is potassium and the main anions are phosphates and proteins. There is also a substantial amount of magnesium in cells.

not to proteins. Ions and low molecular-weight molecules are present in similar concentrations in the ECF and plasma but protein concentration is 4–5 times greater in plasma than it is in the interstitial fluid. The total plasma concentration of cations is about 150 mmol/L, of which sodium is approximately 140 mmol/L and potassium 4 mmol/L. The most abundant plasma anions are chloride and bicarbonate, with average concentrations of 100 mmol/L and 25 mmol/L, respectively (Fig. 23.2). The rest of the anions are, for the purposes of electrolyte balance, considered together, constituting the so-called anion gap which is calculated as follows:

$$Anion\,gap = \{[Na^+] + [K^+]\} - \{[Cl^-] + [HCO_3^-]\}$$

The 'anion gap' includes phosphate, sulfate, protein, and organic anions such as lactate, citrate, pyruvate, acetoacetate, and 3-hydroxybutyrate. In a healthy person, the anion gap is approximately 10 mmol/L. However, it may increase several-fold in conditions where inorganic and organic anions accumulate, e.g. in renal failure or diabetic ketoacidosis. For this reason it is clinically important.

Plasma membrane separates intracellular and extra-cellular fluid

In the ICF, the main cation is potassium, present in a concentration of about 110 mmol/L. This is almost 30-fold greater than its concentration in the ECF and in plasma (4 mmol/L). The main anions in the ICF are proteins and phosphate.

In the ECF, the situation is reversed: the main cation is sodium, present in a concentration of about 145 mmol/L. In the ICF the concentration of sodium (and chloride) is only 10 mmol/L.

Water diffuses freely across most cell membranes but the movement of ions and neutral molecules is restricted

Small molecules are transported across cell membranes by specific transport proteins, the ion pumps. The most important is the sodium/potassium ATPase (Na^+/K^+-ATPase), also referred to as the sodium–potassium pump.

Na^+/K^+-ATPase maintains the sodium and potassium gradients across the cell membrane

Na^+/K^+-ATPase is a major determinant of cytoplasmic sodium concentration (see also Chapter 8). It also has an important role in regulating cell volume, cytoplasmic pH and calcium levels through the $Na^+–H^+$ and $Na^+–Ca^{2+}$ exchangers. One of the primary requirements for sodium pump-driven adaptation comes from changes in dietary sodium and potassium. Hormones that control the volume and ionic composition of ECF often act directly on the sodium pump in the kidney and intestine. Also, because water and sodium transport across epithelia is invariably linked, the work of the sodium pump is also critical to water absorption in the intestine and reabsorption in the kidney. Impairment of the sodium pump in kidney and small intestine is linked to pathophysiology of hypertension and chronic diarrhea, respectively.

Na^+/K^+-ATPase can be considered either as an ion transporter (sodium pump) or as an enzyme (ATPase). It maintains chemical and electrical potential gradients (it is electrogenic) across the cell membrane (Fig. 23.3). It hydrolyzes one ATP molecule, and the released energy drives the transfer of three sodium ions from the cell to the outside, and two potassium ions from the outside into the cell (Fig. 23.4). It is activated by sodium and ATP at cytoplasmic sites. The structure of the catalytic subunit of the enzyme and its phosphorylation sites are shown in Figure 23.5. Half-maximal activation of the enzyme by intracellular sodium occurs at sodium concentration of 10–40 mM, which is often above the steady-state concentration. Accordingly, small changes in the cytoplasmic sodium can have dramatic effects on the Na^+/K^+-ATPase activity. Some hormones appear

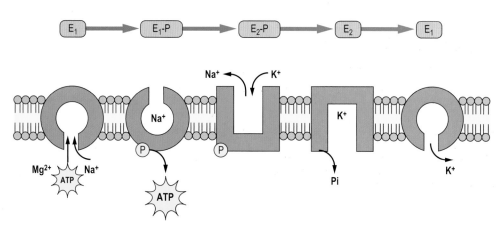

Fig. 23.3 Na⁺/K⁺-ATPase (the sodium–potassium pump) generates transmembrane potential and ion concentration gradients across the cell membrane. For each molecule of hydrolyzed ATP, it moves two potassium ions into the cell and three sodium ions out of the cell. Na⁺/K⁺-ATPase consists of two main subunits – catalytic subunit (α) and structural subunit (β).

Fig. 23.4 Catalytic function of the Na⁺/K⁺-ATPase. The Na⁺/K⁺-ATPase catalytic subunit can be either phosphorylated (E1-P and E2-P) or dephosphorylated (E1 and E2) and this changes its conformation and affinity towards substrates. The E1 form exhibits high affinity towards ATP, magnesium and sodium and low affinity towards potassium, whereas the E2 form exhibits high affinity for potassium and low for sodium. After the release of ADP, there is conformational change from E1-P to E2-P. This promotes extracellular delivery of sodium and the binding of extracellular potassium. The latter process induces dephosphorylation of E2-P and potassium release into the intracellular compartment.

to alter it by changing its apparent affinity for sodium (for instance, the affinity is increased by angiotensin II and insulin).

Passive movement of electrolytes through ion channels is driven by electrochemical gradient

For most cells, the membrane potential ranges from 50 to 90 mV, being negative inside the cell. The electrochemical gradient is a source of energy for transport of many substances such as the cotransport of sodium ions with glucose, amino acids, and phosphate. Membrane depolarization promotes an increase in intracellular calcium by activating voltage-dependent Ca channels (see also Chapter 8). The role of ion gradients in nerve transmission is described in Chapter 42.

🐾 BODY FLUIDS DIFFER IN IONIC COMPOSITION

Clinical abnormalities that may develop after fluid loss depend on the composition of what is lost. For instance, sweat contains less sodium than extracellular fluid: therefore excessive sweating leads to a predominant loss of water and 'concentrates' sodium in the extracellular fluid, causing hypernatremia. On the other hand, sodium content of the intestinal fluid is similar to that of plasma but contains considerable amounts of potassium. Thus its loss (for instance, in severe diarrhea) would result in dehydration and hypokalemia, but may not change plasma sodium concentration (Table 23.1).

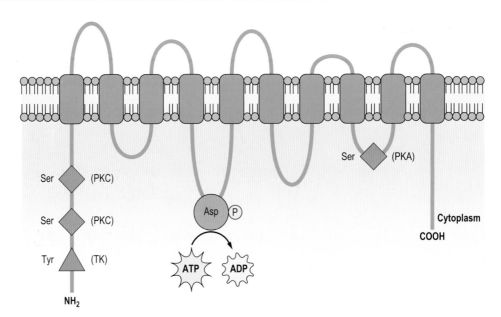

Fig. 23.5 **Structure of the α subunit of the Na+/K+-ATPase.** The α subunit consists of 10 membrane-spanning domains (M1–M10) with intracellular amino- and carboxy-terminal domains. The ATP-binding domain and the phosphorylation site are located in the long M4–M5 cytoplasmic loop (where Asp residue undergoes phosphorylation). Other phosphorylation sites on serine and tyrosine residues are mediated by protein kinase A (PKA), protein kinase C (PKC) and tyrosine kinase (TK).

Electrolyte content of body fluids				
	Sodium (mmol/L)	Potassium (mmol/L)	Bicarbonate (mmol/L)	Chloride (mmol/L)
Plasma	140	4	25	100
Gastric juice	50	15	0–15	140
Small intestinal fluid	140	10	variable	70
Feces in diarrhea	50–140	30–70	20–80	variable
Bile, pleural, and peritoneal fluids	140	5	40	100
Sweat	12	10	–	12

Table 23.1 **Ionic composition of body fluids.** Loss of fluid that has an electrolyte content similar to that of plasma leads to dehydration with normal plasma electrolyte concentrations. On the other hand, when the sodium content of the lost fluid is less than that of plasma (e.g. sweat), dehydration may be accompanied by hypernatremia. Overhydration is usually accompanied by hyponatremia. (Adapted with permission from Dominiczak MH (ed). Seminars in Clinical biochemistry, 2nd edn. Glasgow: Glasgow University, 1997.) Electrolyte content of body fluids

OSMOLALITY

Osmolality depends on the concentration of molecules in water. All molecules dissolved in the body water contribute to the osmotic pressure, which is proportional to the molal concentration of a solution. One millimole of a substance dissolved in 1 kg H_2O at 37°C exerts an osmotic pressure of approximately 19 mmHg. Under physiologic conditions, the average concentration of all osmotically active substances in the ECF is 290 mmol/kg H_2O. Normally, the ICF osmolality is identical.

Movement of water between intracellular and extracellular fluid is caused by differences in osmolality

A change in the concentration of osmotically active ions in one of the two compartments creates a gradient of osmotic pressure and, consequently, causes movement of water. Water always diffuses from lower osmolality to higher to equalize osmotic pressures.

Because sodium is the most abundant ion in the ECF, it is the most important determinant of its osmolality. Glucose is normally present in plasma in a concentration too low to contribute significantly to osmolality (5 mmol/L; 90 mg/dL) but it may become a major determinant of osmolality when its concentration increases in diabetes (see Chapter 21) (Fig. 23.6).

Movement of water between the plasma and interstitial fluid depends on plasma protein concentration

Proteins, particularly albumin, exert osmotic pressure in the plasma, (about 3.32 kPa; 25 mmHg). This is known as the oncotic pressure and it retains water in the vascular bed. It is balanced by the hydrostatic pressure, which forces fluid out of the capillaries. In the arterial part of capillaries, the hydrostatic pressure prevails over the oncotic pressure and water and low molecular-weight compounds filter out into the extravascular space. In contrast, in the venous part of

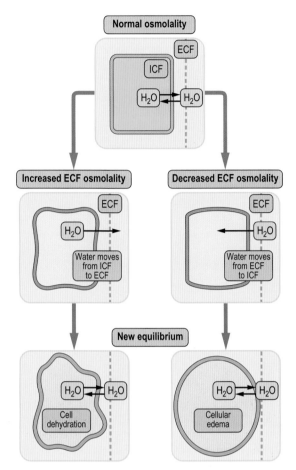

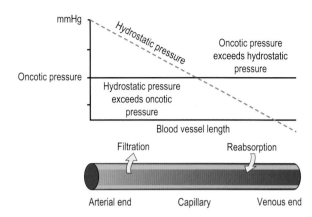

Fig. *23.7* **Oncotic and hydrostatic pressures determine movement of fluid between plasma and interstitial fluid.**

Fig. *23.6* **Water redistribution caused by changes in osmolality.** Osmotic pressure controls the movement of water between compartments. An increase in ECF osmolality draws water from the cells, and leads to cellular dehydration. On the other hand, when ECF osmolality decreases, water moves into the cells and this may cause cell edema. The arrows indicate direction of water movement.

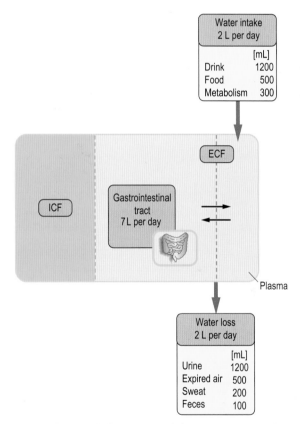

Fig. *23.8* **Daily water balance in an adult person.** Water is obtained from the diet and from oxidative metabolism, and is lost through the kidneys, skin, lungs, and intestine. Note how much water enters and leaves the gastrointestinal tract daily; this explains why severe diarrhea quickly leads to dehydration.

capillaries, oncotic pressure prevails over hydrostatic pressure, and fluid is drawn into the vascular lumen (Fig. 23.7). A reduction in plasma oncotic pressure, which occurs, for instance, as a consequence of a decrease in the plasma albumin concentration, results in the movement of fluid into the extravascular space and in edema.

Cells protect themselves against changes of osmolality and volume

An increase in intracellular concentration of sodium stimulates the Na^+/K^+ ATPase, which extrudes sodium from the cell. This protects the cell from volume changes. Another protective mechanism is intracellular generation of osmotically active substances. For instance, the brain cells adapt to increased ECF osmolality by increasing their amino acid concentration, and cells in the renal medulla exposed to a hyperosmotic environment produce an osmotically active alcohol, sorbitol, and increase the concentration of an amino acid taurine.

The body constantly exchanges water with the environment

In a steady state, the intake of water equals its loss. The main source of water is oral intake and the main source of loss is urine excretion. We also lose water through the lungs, sweat and feces: this is called the 'insensible' loss and amounts to approximately 500 mL daily (Fig. 23.8). The insensible

EDEMA RESULTS FROM A LOSS OF PROTEIN

An 8-year-old girl was referred to a nephrologist after it had been noticed that her face was puffy and her ankles swollen over a period of about 2 weeks. Dipstick test for urine protein yielded a strongly positive (++++) result and measurement in a 24-hour collection showed protein excretion of 7 g/day. The reference value for urinary protein excretion is less than 0.15 g/day.

Comment. Renal biopsy showed the so-called minimal change disease. The cause of the proteinuria was damage to the renal filtration barrier, with the urinary protein loss causing in turn a decrease in the plasma oncotic pressure and retention of water in the ECF. This led to edema. The condition went into remission after treatment with a glucocorticoid.

loss can increase substantially in high temperatures, during intensive exercise, and also as a result of diarrhea or fever.

KIDNEYS

Kidneys maintain the composition, osmolality, and volume of the ECF and also control the acid–base balance

The kidneys remove products of metabolism such as urea, uric acid, and creatinine in urine, and retain substances such as glucose, amino acids, and proteins. They also metabolize and remove drugs and toxins. Kidney function is regulated hormonally by vasopressin (antidiuretic hormone, ADH) produced in the posterior pituitary and by the renin-angiotensin system. The kidneys produce calcitriol (1α,25-dihydroxycholecalciferol, $1,25(OH)_2D_3$) involved in calcium homeostasis (see Chapter 25), and erythropoietin which controls the production of erythrocytes.

Kidneys consume large amounts of oxygen, mainly to support active sodium transport

Most of the metabolic processes in the kidneys are aerobic, and consequently oxygen consumption in the kidneys is high: it approximately equals that of the cardiac muscle, and is three times greater than that of the brain. Such high metabolic activity is required to maintain tubular reabsorption; about 70% of the consumed oxygen is used to support active sodium transport, which determines reabsorption of glucose and amino acids. The main energy substrates in the renal cortex are fatty acids, lactate, glutamate, citrate, and ketone bodies. Renal tubular cells with a high Na^+/K^+-ATPase activity possess multiple mitochondria close to the

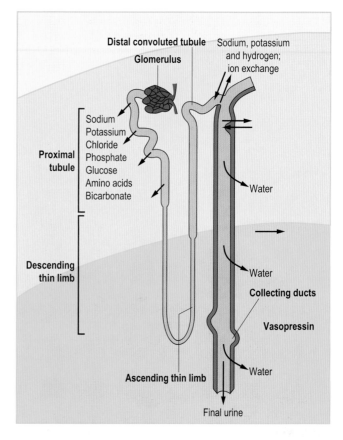

Fig. 23.9 **The nephron and its major transport sites.**

plasma membrane, so that the ATP released into the cytosol is easily accessible.

The functional unit of the kidney is the nephron

Each kidney consists of approximately 1 million tiny structures called nephrons (Fig. 23.9). Glomeruli located in the kidney cortex are biologic filters connecting the plasma to the excretory tubules. The renal tubules are divided into proximal tubules, the so-called loop of Henle and distal tubules, and the collecting duct.

Plasma filtration takes place in the kidney glomeruli

The excretory function of the kidneys involves filtration of the plasma in the glomeruli, transport of water and solutes from the tubular lumen back to the blood (tubular reabsorption), and secretion of different substances from the tubular cells into the lumen.

Plasma from the glomerular capillaries is filtered into the interior of the glomerulus, the Bowman's space. Glomerular filtration depends on the filtration surface and on the permeability of the filtration barrier, which includes the layer of endothelial cells that line glomerular blood vessels, the basement membrane, and epithelial cells (podocytes) with characteristic foot processes (Fig. 23.10).

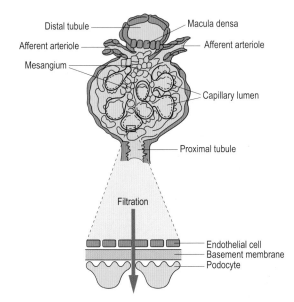

Distal tubule
Macula densa
Afferent arteriole
Afferent arteriole
Mesangium
Capillary lumen
Proximal tubule
Filtration
Endothelial cell
Basement membrane
Podocyte

Fig. 23.10 **Glomerular filtration barrier.** This consists of endothelial cells, the basement membrane, and the podocytes. Macula densa cells are part of the juxtaglomerular apparatus: they sense chloride concentration in the distal tubule and adjust the diameter of afferent arterioles, regulating the glomerular blood flow.

The main component of the glomerular basement membrane is type IV collagen which forms a network of filaments which provide elasticity and resistance to hydrostatic pressure. The membrane also contains laminin, fibronectin and proteoglycans with negatively charged heparan sulfate groups, which form an electrostatic barrier for proteins filtered from plasma.

Podocytes and mesangial cells possess receptors for a range of vasoactive substances such as angiotensin II, vasopressin, bradykinin, ATP, endothelin, prostaglandins, dopamine, natriuretic peptides and adenine nucleotides.

The fenestrations in the endothelial layer and the spaces between foot processes of the podocytes form a sieve that filters water and small molecules. Filtration of larger molecules is limited by their size, shape, and electric charge. For instance, at pH 7.4, most plasma proteins are negatively charged, and so is the filtration barrier; this hinders filtration of even the smallest proteins, such as myoglobin (molecular mass 17 kDa), and almost completely prevents filtration of the larger (69 kDa) albumin.

Glomerular filtration is driven by the hydrostatic pressure in the glomerular capillaries, which is approximately 50 mmHg. The hydrostatic pressure is counteracted by the oncotic pressure of the plasma and the back-pressure (approximately 10 mmHg) of the filtrate in the glomerular capsule. Changes in glomerular filtration rate alter the total amount of filtered water and solute, but not the composition of the filtrate. A decrease in the blood pressure in the afferent arteriole of the glomerulus is sensed by the group of cells known as the juxtaglomerular apparatus. This stimulates renin secretion and activates the renin–angiotensin system.

Glomerular filtrate: urine formation

The volume, composition, and osmolality of the glomerular filtrate change as it flows through renal tubules. Approximately 80% of the filtrate is reabsorbed in the proximal tubule. Sodium is reabsorbed by several mechanisms: through specific ion channels, in exchange for the hydrogen ion, and in cotransport with glucose, amino acids, phosphate, and other anions. The movement of sodium causes reabsorption of water. Entry of sodium into the proximal tubular cells is passive. This is possible because the Na^+/K^+ ATPase maintains low sodium concentration in the cytoplasm of tubular cells.

The fluid leaving the proximal tubule is isotonic. Different permeability of the ascending and descending limbs of the loop of Henle maintains the high osmolality of the medulla. This is essential for the efficient reabsorption of water (Fig. 23.11). The fluid that leaves the loop of Henle is diluted (hypotonic). More sodium is reabsorbed in the distal tubule and in the collecting duct in exchange for potassium or hydrogen ion. This process controlled by the hormone aldosterone (Fig. 23.12). Water reabsorption in the collecting duct is controlled by vasopressin (see below).

Na^+/K^+-ATPase in the kidney

Na^+/K^+-ATPase activity in the kidney is a few thousand times higher than in other tissues. In the kidney, its major function is sodium reabsorption by catalyzing extrusion of sodium to the interstitial fluid. There is a close relationship between the amount of Na^+/K^+-ATPase and sodium reabsorptive capacity of different segments of the nephron. In renal tubular cells, as in all sodium-reabsorbing epithelial cells, Na^+/K^+ ATPase is present in the basolateral membrane.

In humans, the kidney reabsorbs about 18 moles of sodium per day and utilizes about 6 moles of ATP for this process. Thus, Na^+/K^+-ATPase is an energy transducer that converts metabolic energy into ionic gradients.

Regulation of Na^+/K^+-ATPase activity

Na^+/K^+-ATPase is subject to both short- and long-term regulation by a number of hormones, including aldosterone (see below). Short-term regulation involves either direct effects on the kinetic properties of the enzyme or its translocation between the plasma membrane and intracellular stores. Long-term regulatory mechanisms affect enzyme synthesis or degradation.

Peptide hormones such as vasopressin and PTH that act through G-protein coupled receptors can also affect the activity of Na^+/K^+-ATPase. The G-proteins activate adenylyl cyclase, which generates cAMP. cAMP activates protein kinase A (PKA). PTH, angiotensin II, norepinephrine and dopamine also trigger G-protein mediated activation of phospholipase C,

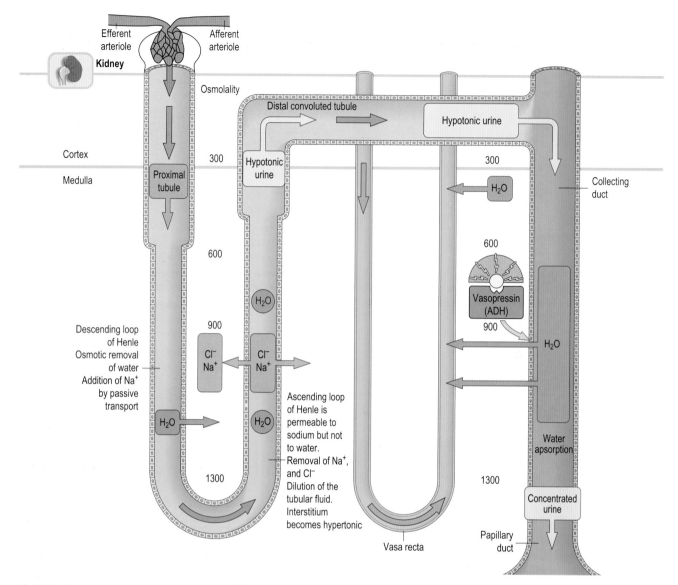

Efferent arteriole

Afferent arteriole

Kidney

Osmolality

Distal convoluted tubule

Hypotonic urine

Cortex — 300

Hypotonic urine

H_2O — 300

Collecting duct

Medulla

Proximal tubule

600

H_2O

600

900

Vasopressin (ADH)

H_2O

Descending loop of Henle Osmotic removal of water Addition of Na^+ by passive transport

900

Cl^- Na^+

Cl^- Na^+

H_2O

H_2O

H_2O

1300

1300

Concentrated urine

Ascending loop of Henle is permeable to sodium but not to water. Removal of Na^+, and Cl^- Dilution of the tubular fluid. Interstitium becomes hypertonic

Water apsorption

Vasa recta

Papillary duct

Fig. 23.11 **Counter-current exchange and multiplication in the renal tubules.** The counter-current mechanism is essential for the formation of urine, and for reabsorption of water in the distal tubule. In the ascending arm of the loop of Henle, sodium and chloride ions are pumped into the interstitial fluid. They then diffuse freely into the lumen of the descending limb, creating a functional loop, which perpetuates the increase in osmolality of the filtrate reaching the ascending limb. This is known as counter-current multiplication. As a result of this, the osmolality of the renal cortex is similar to that of plasma (300 mmol/L), whereas in the medulla it might reach 1300 mmol/L. High osmolality of the medulla later facilitates reabsorption of water in the collecting ducts. This is known as counter-current exchange. The amount of reabsorbed water is controlled by vasopressin.

which activates protein kinase C (PKC). Both PKA and PKC affect Na^+/K^+-ATPase by serine phosphorylation of its subunit a (see Fig 23.5).

Urine

The kidneys excrete from 0.5 L to more than 10 L of urine daily; the average daily volume is 1–2 L. The minimum volume necessary to remove the products of metabolism (mainly nitrogen excreted as urea) is approximately 0.5 L/24 h. The osmolality of the glomerular filtrate is about 300 mmol/L and the osmolality of urine varies from about 80 to 1200 mmol/L. Thus the maximal urine concentration is approximately fourfold, and to excrete excess water it may be diluted below the osmolality of plasma.

Only small amounts of amino acids (0.7 g/24 h), and almost no glucose, are normally present in the urine. Each substance reabsorbed in the renal tubules has its own renal transport maximum (T_{max}). T_{max} can be exceeded either

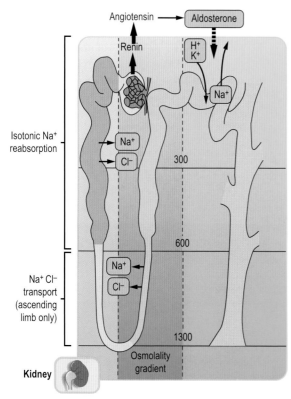

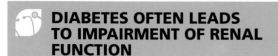

Fig. 23.12 **Sodium reabsorption in the renal tubules.** More than 80% of filtered sodium is actively reabsorbed in the proximal tubule. Sodium and chloride ions are also reabsorbed in the ascending limb of the loop of Henle. A different mechanism operates in the distal tubule, where sodium reabsorption is stimulated by aldosterone and is coupled with the secretion of hydrogen and potassium ions. Aldosterone causes sodium retention and an increase in potassium excretion.

DIABETES OFTEN LEADS TO IMPAIRMENT OF RENAL FUNCTION

A 37-year-old woman with a 12-year history of type 1 diabetes came for a routine visit to the diabetic clinic. Her glycemic control was poor and glycated hemoglobin (HbA$_{1c}$) was 8%. Blood pressure was mildly raised at 145/88 mmHg. A quantitative measurement of albumin in urine revealed protein concentration of 5 mg/mmol creatinine, indicating microalbuminuria. Reference values are:

- **HbA$_{1c}$:** desirable value below 7%
- **urine microalbumin:** less than 3.5 mg/mmol creatinine.

Comment. This patient had mildly impaired renal function and raised blood pressure as a result of glomerular damage from diabetes. The presence of microalbuminuria predicts future overt diabetic nephropathy. Blood pressure should be maintained at <130/80 mmHg preferably with an ACE inhibitor drug.

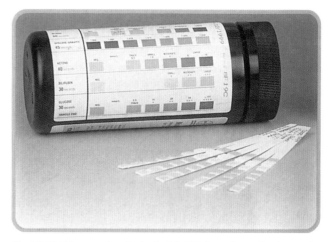

Fig. 23.13 **Urine testing (urinalysis).** This is performed using ready-made dry tests, strips coated with reagents immobilized on a plastic support. Dipping the strip in the urine initiates a reaction that yields a colored product. The readout is against a standardized color scale.

when the amount of filtered substance becomes too large to handle or when the tubular cells do not function properly. Thus, aminoaciduria may result from an impaired tubular function or from the accumulation of amino acids such as phenylalanine, leucine, isoleucine, and valine in the plasma.

Urine analysis can provide a lot of clinically important information

Analysis of urine (urinalysis) in clinical laboratories includes testing for the presence of protein, glucose, ketone bodies, bilirubin, and urobilinogen, and for traces of blood. Measuring urinary osmolality assesses the concentrating capacity of the kidney. The urine is also tested for the presence of leukocytes and various crystals and deposits (Fig. 23.13). Specialist investigations include analysis of urinary amino acids, hormones and other metabolites.

Only traces of protein are normally detectable in the urine. This increases when the glomeruli are damaged; presence of significant amounts of protein in urine is an important sign of renal disease. Even a minimal amount of albumin in the urine (microalbuminuria) predicts the development of diabetic nephropathy (see Chapter 21). Larger proteins such as immunoglobulins appear in the urine when the damage is more extensive: the immunoglobulin light chains (Bence-Jones protein) are present in urine in multiple myeloma (see Chapter 4). In hemolytic anemia, urine may contain free hemoglobin and urobilinogen. The presence of myoglobin is a marker of muscle damage (rhabdomyolysis). The measurement of urine glucose and ketones is important in the assessment of glycemic control in diabetic patients (see Chapter 21). Measurements of urobilinogen and bilirubin help to assess liver function (see Chapter 29).

ASSESSMENT OF RENAL FUNCTION

Glomerular filtration rate is the most important characteristic describing kidney function

The renal clearance is the volume of plasma (in milliliters) that the kidney clears of a given substance every minute. The glomerular filtration rate (GFR) is the most important characteristic describing kidney function. GFR could be estimated by measuring the clearance of a substance, such as the polysaccharide inulin, that is neither secreted nor reabsorbed in the renal tubules. The amount of inulin filtered from plasma (i.e. its plasma concentration, P_{in}, multiplied by GFR) equals the amount recovered in urine (i.e. its urinary concentration, U_{in}, multiplied by the urine formation rate, V):

$$P_{in} \times GFR = U_{in} \times V$$

From this we calculate the GFR:

$$GFR = U_{in} \times V/P_{in}$$

The average GFR is 120 mL/min for men and 100 mL/min for women. The renal clearance of inulin equals the GFR.

Serum urea and creatinine are first-line tests in the diagnosis of renal disease

To administer inulin intravenously every time one would want to assess the GFR is impractical. In clinical practice, we use creatinine clearance instead. Creatinine is derived from skeletal muscle phosphocreatine. Its clearance is similar to that of inulin. Although some creatinine is reabsorbed in the renal tubules, this is compensated by an equivalent tubular secretion. To calculate creatinine clearance, one needs a sample of blood, and urine collected over 24 hours. The concentrations of creatinine in serum and urine are measured first. Urine excretion rate is calculated by dividing the urine volume by the collection time (V, above). The creatinine clearance is then calculated according to the formula:

$$Creatinine\ clearance = U_{in} \times V/P_{in}$$

Serum concentration of creatinine is 20–80 mmol/L (0.28–0.90 mg/dL). An increase in serum creatinine concentration reflects the decrease in GFR: serum creatinine concentration doubles when the GFR decreases by 50%. Another test used to assess kidney function is measurement of serum urea. However, because urea is an endproduct of protein catabolism, its level in plasma is also dependent on factors such as the dietary protein intake (Chapter 22) and the rate of tissue breakdown.

In clinical practice, serum urea and creatinine are first-line tests in the diagnosis of renal failure (Fig. 23.14). Renal failure leads to a decrease in urine volume and creatinine clearance, and to an increase in serum urea and creatinine. Recent refinements in laboratory testing include standardization of creatinine measurements by making methods used in clinical laboratories traceable to the reference method which is isotope dilution mass spectroscopy.

Cystatin C concentration is another marker of the GFR

Cystatin C is a 122-amino acid, 13 kDa protein belonging to the family of cysteine proteinase inhibitors. It is a product of

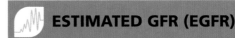

ESTIMATED GFR (EGFR)

Creatinine clearance changes with age, body surface, gender and race. Also, the relationship between GFR and creatinine concentration may differ between healthy populations and patients with renal disease. Currently, GFR values are being fine-tuned using calculation formulas that include serum creatinine concentrations together with factors such as age, gender and weight. There is currently no evidence that such estimated GFR (eGFR) identifies the risk of decline in renal function better than serum measurements. However, it might be helpful in staging renal disease once it has been diagnosed.

Serum creatinine values need to be interpreted in the context of clinical history, patient examination and results of other laboratory tests.

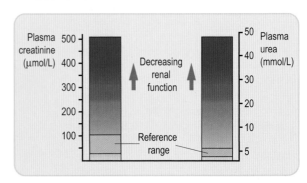

Fig. 23.14 **Serum urea and creatinine concentrations are important markers of renal function.** The upper panel shows the conversion of muscle phosphocreatine to creatinine. Loss of 50% of nephrons results in approximate doubling of serum creatinine concentration.

the housekeeping gene expressed in all nucleated cells, and is produced at a constant rate. Because of its small size and basic isoelectric point, cystatin C is freely filtered through the glomerulus. It is not secreted by the tubules and although it is reabsorbed, it is subsequently catabolized and therefore does not return to plasma. Its concentration is affected by age. Other factors, independent of the GFR, such as the inflammatory phenomena may affect cystatin C concentration.

POTASSIUM

Monitoring potassium concentration in persons with fluid and electrolyte disorders is fundamentally important.

Measurement of serum potassium concentration is clinically very important (Fig. 23.15). Normal serum concentration of potassium is 3.5–5 mmol/L. Because its intracellular concentration is much higher than concentration in plasma, a relatively minor shift of potassium between the ECF and ICF may result in major changes in its serum concentration. Both high and low concentrations of potassium (hyperkalemia and hypokalemia, respectively) can be life threatening. A potassium concentration below 2.5 mmol/L or above

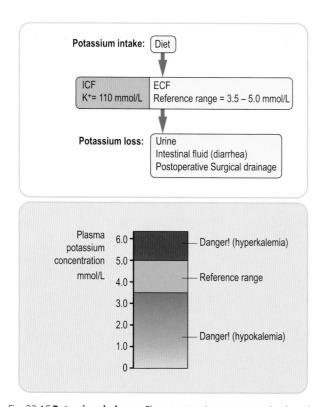

Fig. 23.15 **Potassium balance.** Plasma potassium concentration is maintained within narrow limits. Both low (hypokalemia) and high (hyperkalemia) concentrations may be dangerous, as potassium affects the contractility of heart muscle. The upper panel shows the main sources of potassium loss.

6.0 mmol/L is dangerous. Monitoring potassium concentration in persons with fluid and electrolyte disorders is fundamentally important. The most common cause of severe hyperkalemia is renal failure: in this condition potassium cannot be adequately excreted in the urine. On the other hand, low serum potassium usually results from excessive losses, either in urine or through the gastrointestinal tract. Kidneys account for more than 90% of the body potassium loss. Changes in serum potassium concentration are also associated with acid–base disorders (see Chapter 24).

RENIN-ANGIOTENSIN SYSTEM

Renin-angiotensin system controls blood pressure and vascular tone

Renin is produced principally in the juxtaglomerular apparatus of the kidney; it is stored in secretory granules and released in response to decreased renal perfusion pressure. Renin is a protease that uses angiotensinogen as its substrate. Angiotensinogen is a glycoprotein of more than 400 amino acids, is synthesized in the liver, and its different forms have a variable structure and molecular weight. Renin cleaves the angiotensin I from angiotensinogen. Angiotensin I is a 10-amino acid peptide. It becomes a substrate for peptidyl-dipeptidase A (angiotensin-converting enzyme; ACE). ACE removes two amino acids from angiotensin I, producing angiotensin II. This reaction can also be catalyzed by enzymes such as chymase and cathepsin. Another form of angiotensin, angiotensin 1-9, is formed by the isoform of ACE (ACE2) and is subsequently degraded to angiotensin 1-7. The latter can also be formed from angiotensin II by endopeptidases. The renin-angiotensin system is illustrated in Figure 23.16.

Angiotensin receptors are important in the pathogenesis of cardiovascular disease

Angiotensin II constricts vascular smooth muscle, thereby increasing blood pressure and reducing renal blood flow and glomerular filtration rate. It also promotes aldosterone release and vascular smooth muscle proliferation through the activation of AT1 receptors which signal through G-proteins and phospholipase C (Fig. 23.17). Generally, AT1 receptor activation has effects that promote cardiovascular disease: stimulation of inflammatory phenomena, extracellular matrix deposition and generation of reactive oxygen species (ROS). It is also prothrombotic. These actions are counteracted by the stimulation of the AT2 receptor, which leads to vasodilatation through stimulation of the NO production, promotes sodium loss and inhibits vascular smooth muscle cell proliferation. The actions of angiotensin (1-7) which acts through the so-called Mas receptor (it may also bind to AT1 and AT2) also seem to be cardioprotective.

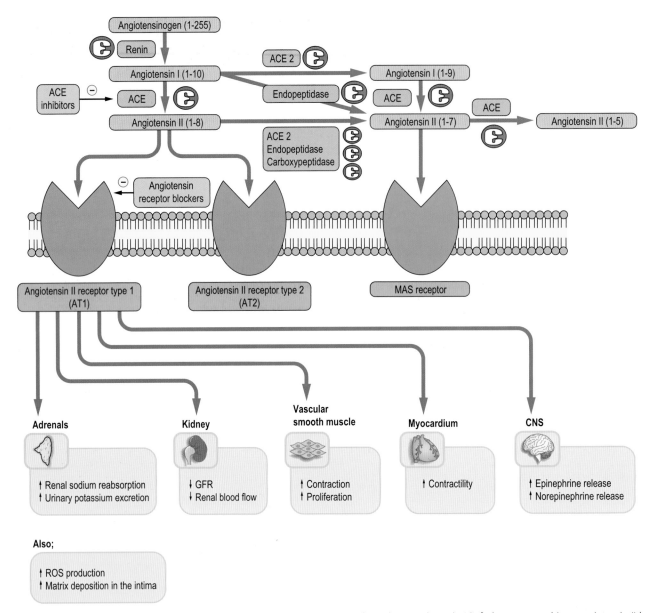

Fig. 23.16 **Renin-angiotensin system.** Renin converts angiotensinogen into angiotensin I. Angiotensin I is futher converted into angiotensin II by the angiotensin-converting enzyme (ACE). It also yields other angiotensin peptides. Cellular actions of angiotensins are mediated by angiotensin receptors type 1 (AT1), type 2 (AT2) and Mas receptors that bind angiotensin (1-7). The renin-angiotensin system is a target for two major classes of hypotensive drugs: ACE blockers (e.g. ramipril, enalapril) and AT1 receptor antagonists (e.g. losartan). ACE blockers are also extensively used in the treatment of heart failure. VSMC, vascular smooth muscle cells; CNS, central nervous system. *AT1 receptor blocked by, e.g., losartan. **AT2 receptor blocked by saralasin. ROS: reactive oxygen species.

Drugs that inhibit ACE are now extensively used in the treatment of hypertension and heart failure (see Fig. 23.17 and box on p. 66).

Substantial amounts of angiotensin II are formed in the kidney. Juxtaglomerular cells contain ACE, angiotensin I and angiotensin II. Angiotensin II is also synthesized in the glomerular and tubular cells and is secreted into the tubular fluid and interstitial space. Angiotensin II receptors are present on the tubular and renal vascular cells: therefore, locally produced angiotensin II probably influences tubular

reabsorption and renal vascular tone through autocrine and paracrine action.

Aldosterone

Aldosterone regulates sodium and potassium homeostasis

Aldosterone is a major mineralocorticosteroid hormone in man, and is produced in the adrenal cortex. It regulates the

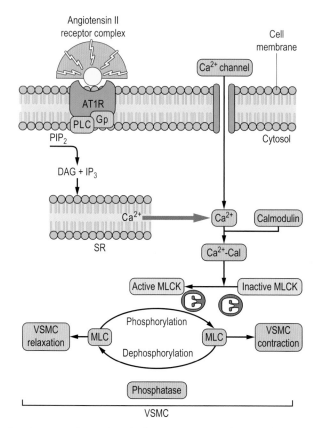

Fig. 23.17 **Angiotensin II-induced vasoconstriction.** The angiotensin receptor (AT1R) is coupled to G-proteins. The binding of angiotensin II leads to phospholipase C-mediated formation of inositol 1,4,5-trisphosphate (IP_3) and 1,2-diacylglycerol. This mobilizes Ca^{2+} from the sarcoplasmic reticulum (SR), and causes entry of the extracellular Ca^{2+} through activated calcium channels. An increase in the cytosolic Ca^{2+} initiates contractile response of the vascular smooth muscle cells. Ca^{2+} subsequently binds to calmodulin (Cal). The Ca^{2+}–calmodulin complex activates myosin light-chain kinase. The kinase phosphorylates myosin light chains and elicits muscular tension. This effect is terminated by the dephosphorylation of myosin (see also Chapter 20). AT1 receptor antagonists, such as losartan, inhibit vasoconstrictor effects of angiotensin II and are used in the treatment of hypertension. AT1R: Angiotensin AT1 receptor; DAG: 1,2,diacylglycerol; VSMC: vascular smooth muscle cell, MLCK: myosin light-chain kinase; Cal: calmodulin.

extracellular volume and vascular tone and controls renal sodium and potassium transport. It binds to the cytosolic mineralocorticoid receptor in the epithelial cells, principally in the renal collecting duct. The receptor moves to the nucleus and binds to specific domains on targeted genes, altering gene expression.

Aldosterone regulates the Na^+/K^+-ATPase in both the long and short term and also regulates transporters such as the Na^+/H^+ exchanger type 3 in the proximal tubule, the Na^+/Cl^- cotransporter in the distal tubule, and the epithelial sodium channel in the collecting duct. The overall result is an increased sodium reabsorption, and increased potassium and hydrogen ion secretion.

 ### DIAGNOSTIC USE OF THE BRAIN NATRIURETIC PEPTIDE (BNP) PROPEPTIDES

Instead of measuring the active forms of natriuretic peptides in plasma, it is more convenient to measure the propeptides present in plasma in equimolar amounts to the active species. Thus proBNP (1-76) reaches higher levels in cardiac failure than BNP 32. Similarly, proANP (1-98) has a longer half-life in plasma than biologically active 1-28 ANP and therefore is present in the circulation in higher concentrations.

 ### ACUTE RENAL FAILURE LEADS TO A STEEP FALL IN OUTPUT OF URINE, AND CAUSES HIGH SERUM UREA AND CREATININE CONCENTRATIONS

A 25-year-old man was admitted to hospital unconscious after a motorcycle accident. He had evidence of shock with hypotension and tachycardia, a fractured skull and multiple injuries to his limbs. Despite treatment with intravenous colloid and blood he showed persistent oliguria (urine output 5–10 ml/h: oliguria is <20 ml/h). Oliguria due to acute tubular necrosis can be distinguished from prerenal uremia by measuring urine osmolality (>500 mOsm/kg in prerenal uremia and <350 mOsm/kg in acute renal failure) and urine sodium concentration (<20 mmol/L in prerenal azotemia and >40 mmol/L in acute renal failure). On the third day, his serum creatinine concentration had risen to 300 μmol/L (3.9 mg/dL) and his urea concentration to mmol/L (132 mg/dL). Reference values are:

- **creatinine:** 20–80 μmol/L (0.23–0.90 mg/dL)
- **urea:** 2.5–6.5 mmol/L (16.2–39 mg/dL).

Comment. This young man has developed acute renal failure due to acute tubular necrosis as a consequence of hypovolemic shock. He subsequently underwent emergency hemofiltration. Renal function started to recover after 2 weeks with an initial increase in urine volume, the so-called 'diuretic phase'.

- **urea** mg/dL = mmol/L × 6.02
- **creatinine** mg/dL = μmol/L × 0.0113

Hyperaldosteronism is a common finding in hypertension

Primary hyperaldosteronism occurs as a result of abnormal adrenal activity and is rare. It may be a result of a single adrenal tumor, an adenoma (Conn's syndrome). The more common secondary hyperaldosteronism is due to an increased secretion of renin. Pheochromocytomas are catecholamine-secreting tumors that cause hypertension in about 0.1% of hypertensive patients. It is important to correctly diagnose

RENIN-ANGIOTENSIN-ALDOSTERONE SYSTEM AND CARDIAC FAILURE

A 65-year-old man with a previous anterior myocardial infarction presented with increasing fatigue, shortness of breath and ankle edema. Physical examination showed mild tachycardia, and a raised jugular venous pressure. An echocardiogram showed that the function of the left ventricle during systole was poor. The patient's serum measurements revealed: sodium 140 mmol/L, potassium 3.5 mmol/L, protein 34 (normal 35–45) g/dL, creatinine 80 μmol/L (0.90 mg/dL), and urea 7.5 mmol/L (45 mg/dL).

Comment. This man presents with symptoms and signs of cardiac failure. The impaired function of the heart leads to a decreased blood flow through the kidney, activation of the renin-angiotensin system and stimulation of aldosterone secretion. Aldosterone causes an increased renal reabsorption of sodium and water retention, thereby increasing extracellular fluid volume and edema.

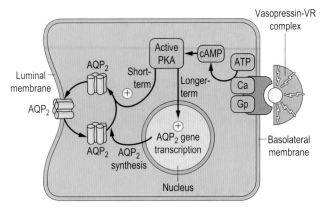

Fig. 23.18 **Vasopressin regulates water reabsorption in the collecting duct.** Vasopressin controls the aquaporin 2 (AQP2) water channel. Vasopressin binds to its receptor (VR) and through G-proteins stimulates production of cAMP, which in turn activates protein kinase A (PKA). PKA phosphorylates cytoplasmic AQP2 and induces its translocation to the cell membrane, increasing capacity for water transport. Vasopressin also regulates expression of the AQP2 gene.

pheochromocytoma, because it can be surgically removed (see Chapter 43 and box on p. 588).

Natriuretic peptides

Natriuretic peptides are important markers of heart failure

A family of peptides known as the natriuretic peptides is involved in the regulation of fluid volume. The two main peptides are atrial natriuretic peptide (ANP) and brain natriuretic peptide (BNP). ANP is synthesized predominantly in the cardiac atria as a 126-amino acid propeptide (pro-ANP). It is then cleaved into a smaller 98-amino acid propeptide and the biologically active 28-amino acid ANP. BNP is synthesized in the cardiac ventricles as a 108-amino acid propeptide, and is cleaved into a 76-amino acid propeptide and a biologically active 32-amino acid BNP. BNP 32 and another peptide, CNP (23 amino acids long), were isolated from the porcine brain, thus the name. All natriuretic peptides possess a ring-type structure due to the presence of a disulfide bond.

Natriuretic peptides promote sodium excretion and decrease blood pressure. ANP and BNP are secreted in response to atrial stretch and to ventricular volume overload. They bind to G-protein linked receptors: the A-type receptors are located predominantly in the endothelial cells and the B-type receptors in the brain. There is cross-reactivity between different natriuretic receptors with regard to these peptides. Importantly, the levels of ANP and BNP are increased in heart failure and therefore their measurements are used as

early biochemical markers of this condition. These measurements are particularly useful for excluding heart failure in patients who present with nonspecific symptoms such as shortness of breath.

Vasopressin and aquaporins

Reabsorption of water in the collecting ducts of the kidney is controlled by the posterior pituitary hormone vasopressin which controls the activity of membrane water channels, aquaporins.

Vasopressin determines the final volume and concentration of the urine

Vasopressin (also known as the antidiuretic hormone, ADH) controls water reabsorption in the collecting ducts of the kidney (Fig. 23.18). Vasopressin is synthesized in the supraoptic and paraventricular nuclei of the hypothalamus and is transported along axons to the posterior pituitary where it is stored before being further processed and released. It binds to a receptor located on the membranes of tubular cells in the collecting ducts. The receptor is coupled to G-proteins and activates protein kinase A (PKA). PKA phosphorylates aquaporin 2 (AQP2), which stimulates its translocation to the cell membrane, increasing water reabsorption in the collecting duct. Vasopressin secretion needs to be suppressed to allow urine dilution. Failure to maximally suppress AVP results in the inability to dilute urine below the osmolality of plasma.

Other hormones affect vasopressin secretion. Glucocorticoids stimulate it primarily through their hemodymamic

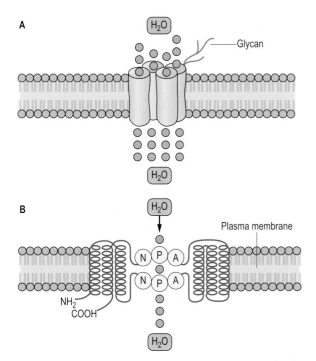

A

B

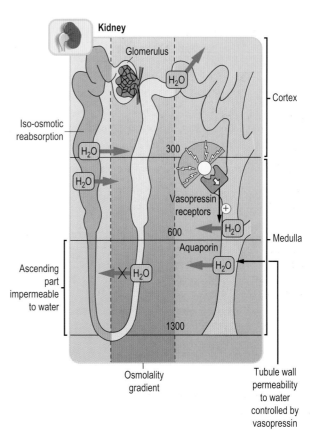

Fig. 23.19 **Aquaporin water channel.** Aquaporin 1 is a multisubunit water channel with a glycan unit attached to one of the subunits (A). Each of the two monomers has two tandem repeat structures, each consisting of three membrane-spanning regions (B) and connecting loops embedded in the membrane.

Fig. 23.20 **Renal handling of water.** Permeability of the tubular walls to water differs along the nephron. About 80% of filtered water is reabsorbed in the proximal tubule, by isoosmotic reabsorption. The ascending loop of Henle is impermeable to water. In the collecting duct, vasopressin controls the water reabsorption through aquaporin water channels.

effects which decrease arterial pressure. Incidentally, AVP is also stimulated by nicotine.

Aquaporins are membrane channel proteins which transport water

The aquaporin water channel is illustrated in Figure 23.19. Aquaporin 1 (AQP1) is expressed on the apical and basolateral membranes of the proximal tubule and in the descending loop of Henle and is not under vasopressin control. It is also present in erythrocytes, renal proximal tubular cells, and in the capillary endothelium. AQP2 and 3 are present in the collecting duct and are regulated by vasopressin.

Defects in vasopressin secretion and mutations of genes coding for aquaporins cause clinical conditions

Vasopressin deficiency causes the condition known as diabetes insipidus, in which large amounts of dilute urine are lost. On the other hand, an excessive secretion of vasopressin may occur following major trauma or surgery. This is known as the syndrome of inappropriate antidiuretic hormone secretion (SIADH), and leads to water retention.

Mutations in the vasopressin receptor gene and also in the AQP2 gene lead to different types of the so-called nephrogenic diabetes insipidus, a condition associated with passing large amounts of urine and dehydration. Figure 23.20 summarizes the renal handling of water.

DIURETICS ARE USED FOR TREATMENT OF EDEMA, CARDIAC FAILURE AND HYPERTENSION

Diuretics are drugs that stimulate water and sodium excretion. Thiazide diuretics, e.g. bendrofluazide, decrease sodium reabsorption in the distal tubules by blocking sodium and chloride cotransport. Loop diuretics, such as frusemide, inhibit sodium reabsorption in the ascending loop of Henle. Spironolactone, a potassium-sparing diuretic, is a competitive inhibitor of aldosterone: it inhibits sodium–potassium exchange in the distal tubules, and decreases potassium excretion.

An osmotic diuresis may be induced by the administration of the sugar alcohol, mannitol. The net effect of treatment with diuretics is increased urine volume and loss of sodium and water. Diuretics are important in the treatment of edema associated with circulatory problems such as heart failure, in which impaired cardiac function may lead to a severe breathlessness caused by pulmonary edema. They are also essential in the treatment of hypertension.

POOR FLUID INTAKE LEADS TO DEHYDRATION

An 80-year-old man had been admitted to hospital after lying for a prolonged period on the floor at home as a result of an acute stroke. He had poor tissue turgor, dry mouth, tachycardia and hypotension. Serum measurements revealed: sodium 150 mmol/L, potassium 5.2 mmol/L, bicarbonate 35 mmol/L, creatinine 110 μmol/L (1.13 mg/dL), and urea 19 mmol/L (90.3 mg/dL).
Reference values are:

- **sodium:** 135–145 mmol/L
- **potassium:** 3.5–5.0 mmol/L
- **bicarbonate:** 20–25 mmol/L
- **creatinine:** 20–80 μmol/L (0.28–0.90 mg/dL)
- **urea:** 2.5–6.5 mmol/L (16.2–39 mg/dL)

Comment. This patient presents with dehydration, indicated by the high sodium and urea values. He was treated with intravenous fluid predominantly in the form of 5% dextrose to replace the water deficit.

ARTERIAL HYPERTENSION IS A COMMON DISEASE

Hypertension is inappropriately increased arterial blood pressure. The desirable level of systolic blood pressure is below 140 mmHg and diastolic pressure 90 mmHg (optimal values are still lower, below 120/80 mmHg). According to the World Health Organization, up to 20% of the population of the developed world may suffer from the condition. Arterial hypertension has been classified as 'essential' (primary) or 'secondary'. A cause of essential hypertension has not yet been identified, although it is known to involve multiple genetic and environmental factors including neural, endocrine, and metabolic components. A sodium-rich diet is a recognized factor in the development of hypertension.

Hypertension is associated with an increased risk of stroke and myocardial infarction and causes one in every eight deaths worldwide. A range of drugs is used in the modern treatment of hypertension. These include diuretics such as bendrofluazide, drugs blocking adrenoreceptors, inhibitors of the angiotensin converting enzyme and the antagonists of angiotensin receptors AT1 (see box p. 323 and box on p. 66; pheochromocytoma is described on p. 588).

INTEGRATION OF WATER AND SODIUM HOMEOSTASIS

Aldosterone and vasopressin together control the handling of sodium and water

Normally, despite variations in fluid intake, plasma osmolality is maintained within narrow limits (280–295 mmol/kg H$_2$O). Vasopressin contributes to the control of plasma osmolality by regulating water metabolism. It responds to both osmotic and volume signals. On the one hand, its secretion, and thirst, are stimulated by signals from osmoreceptors which respond to very small (about 1%) increases in plasma osmolality. On the other, vasopressin release is stimulated by a decrease (more than 10%) in circulating volume.

Water excess increases plasma volume, renal blood flow, and GFR

When there is water excess, production of renin is suppressed. Low concentration of aldosterone allows urinary sodium loss. Because excess water 'dilutes' plasma, plasma osmolality decreases. The decrease in osmolality, sensed by the hypothalamic osmoreceptors, suppresses thirst and the secretion of vasopressin. Suppression of vasopressin leads to urinary loss of water. Thus, the overall response to water excess is increased excretion of sodium and water.

Water deficit (dehydration) decreases plasma volume, renal blood flow and GFR

When there is dehydration, the decrease in renal blood flow stimulates the renin-angiotensin-aldosterone system.

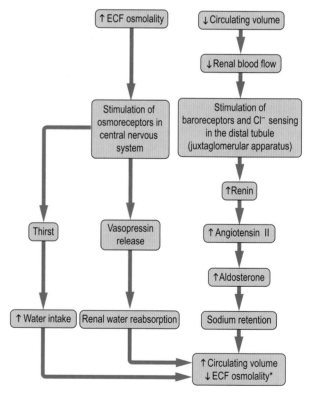

Fig. 23.21 **Links between water and sodium metabolism.** Water and sodium metabolism are closely interrelated. An increase in ECF osmolality stimulates secretion of vasopressin and leads to increased renal water reabsorption. This 'dilutes' the ECF and the osmolality decreases. This response is reinforced by the stimulation of thirst. A decrease in the plasma volume also stimulates water retention through stimulation of the pressure-sensitive receptors (baroreceptors) in the juxtaglomerular apparatus. *Osmolality will decrease if the degree of water retention is relatively greater than that of sodium retention.

Aldosterone inhibits urinary sodium excretion. In addition, because of loss of water, the plasma osmolality increases. This stimulates vasopressin secretion, with a consequent decrease in the urine volume. Thus, the response to water deficit is sodium and water retention (Fig. 23.21).

Serum sodium concentration is a marker of fluid and electrolyte disorders

Water and electrolyte disturbances result from an imbalance between the intake of fluids and electrolytes and their loss and from a movement of water and electrolytes between body compartments. A decreased sodium concentration (hyponatremia) usually indicates that the extracellular fluid is being 'diluted' (excess water is present), whereas an increasing sodium concentration means that the extracellular fluid is being 'concentrated' (water has been lost). Hyponatremia may also result from the loss of sodium but this is rare.

Assessment of water and electrolyte status is an important part of clinical practice

The assessment of water and electrolyte balance is an important part of clinical examination. In addition to the physical examination and medical history, the following measurements are required:

- serum electrolyte concentrations: the profile commonly requested by a physician includes sodium, potassium, chloride and bicarbonate concentrations
- serum urea (blood urea nitrogen) and creatinine
- urine volume, osmolality and sodium concentration
- serum osmolality.

Patients who have or who are at risk of developing abnormalities of water or electrolyte balance need a daily record of fluid intake and loss (a fluid chart).

Summary

- Both deficit of body water (dehydration) and its excess (overhydration) cause potentially serious clinical problems. Therefore, assessment of water and electrolyte balance is an important part of clinical examination.

ACTIVE LEARNING

1. Comment on the role of Na^+/K^+-ATPase in maintaining the ion gradients across cell membrane.
2. Explain the role of renin-angiotensin system in the maintenance of blood pressure.
3. Describe water movements between ECF and ICF which take place in water deprivation.
4. Why does the low concentration of albumin in plasma lead to edema?

- Body water balance is closely linked to the balance of dissolved ions (electrolytes), the most important of which are sodium and potassium.
- Movement of water between ECF and ICF is controlled by osmotic gradients.
- Movement of water between the lumen of a blood vessel and the interstitial fluid is controlled by the osmotic and hydrostatic pressures.
- The main regulators of water and electrolyte balance are vasopressin (water) and aldosterone (sodium and potassium).
- The renin-angiotensin-aldosterone system is the principal regulator of blood pressure and vascular tone.
- Measurements of natriuretic peptides help to diagnose cardiac failure.
- Serum concentrations of urea and creatinine are key tests in the assessment of renal function.

Further reading

Androgue HJ, Madias NE. Mechanisms of disease: sodium and potassium in the pathogenesis of hypertension. *N Engl J Med* 2007;**356**:1966–1978.

Bekheirnia R, Schrier RW. Pathophysiology of water and sodium retention: edematous states with normal kidney function. *Curr Opin Pharmacol* 2006;**6**:202–207.

Chobanian A, Bakris GL, Black HR et al. The Seventh Report of the Joint National Committee on Prevention, Detection, Evaluation and Treatment of High Blood Pressure. *JAMA* 2003;**289**:2560–2572.

Li J, Gobe G. Protein kinase C activation and its role in kidney disease. *Nephrology* 2006;**11**:428–434.

Moro C, Berlan M. Cardiovascular and metabolic effects of natriuretic peptides. *Fund Clin Pharmacol* 2006;**20**:41–49.

Schrier RW. Body water homeostasis: clinical disorders of urinary dilution and concentration. *J Am Soc Nephrol* 2006;**17**:1820–1832.

24. Regulation of Hydrogen Ion Concentration (Acid–Base Balance)

M H Dominiczak and M Szczepanska-Konkel

LEARNING OBJECTIVES

After reading this chapter you should be able to:

- Explain the nature of the bicarbonate buffer.
- Describe the gas exchange occurring in the lungs.
- Describe the respiratory and metabolic components of the acid–base balance.
- Define and classify acidosis and alkalosis.
- Comment on clinical conditions associated with disturbances of the acid–base balance.

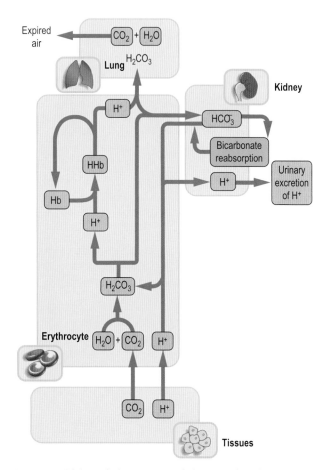

Fig. 24.1 **Acid–base balance.** Lungs, kidneys, and erythrocytes contribute to the maintenance of acid–base balance. The lungs control gas exchange with the atmospheric air. Carbon dioxide generated in tissues is transported in plasma as bicarbonate; the erythrocyte hemoglobin (Hb) also contributes to CO_2 transport. Hemoglobin buffers hydrogen ion derived from carbonic acid. The kidneys reabsorb filtered bicarbonate in the proximal tubules and generate new bicarbonate in the distal tubules, where there is a net secretion of hydrogen ion.

Metabolism generates carbon dioxide. Carbon dioxide generated in tissues dissolves in H_2O, forming carbonic acid, which in turn dissociates, releasing hydrogen ion. In addition, metabolism generates strong acids such as sulfuric acid, and organic acids such as uric acid, lactic acid and others; all become sources of hydrogen ion in the extracellular fluid. In spite of this, the blood concentration of hydrogen ion (or its negative logarithm, the pH) is surprisingly constant: it remains between 36 and 46 nmol/L (pH 7.36–7.46). Changes in pH affect the ionization of protein molecules (Chapter 2) and, consequently, activity of many enzymes. Importantly, changes in pH together with the partial pressure of carbon dioxide (pCO_2) change the shape of the hemoglobin saturation curve, affecting tissue oxygenation (see Chapter 5). A decrease in pH increases sympathetic tone and may lead to cardiac dysrhythmias.

Maintaining the acid–base balance involves lungs, erythrocytes and kidneys

The maintenance of the acid–base balance involves the lungs, the erythrocytes, and the kidneys (Fig. 24.1). The lungs control the exchange of carbon dioxide and oxygen between the blood and the external atmosphere; erythrocytes transport gases between lungs and tissues; and the kidneys control plasma bicarbonate synthesis and the excretion of hydrogen ion.

Clinically, the understanding of the acid–base balance is important in many subspecialties of medicine and surgery, and particularly in critical care medicine.

THE BODY BUFFER SYSTEMS

Metabolic production of CO_2, the metabolism of sulfur-containing amino acids and phosphorus-containing compounds all generate substantial quantities of inorganic and organic acids. Metabolism also generates lactic acid and ketoacids (acetoacetate and β-hydroxybutyrate).

Buffers in the human body			
Buffer	Acid	Conjugate base	Main buffering action
Hemoglobin	HHb	Hb⁻	erythrocytes
Proteins	HProt	Prot⁻	intracellular
Phosphate buffer	$H_2PO_4^-$	HPO_4^{2-}	intracellular
Bicarbonate	$CO_2 \rightarrow H_2CO_3$	HCO_3^-	extracellular

Table 24.1 **Main buffers in the human body.** See Chapter 2 for the principles of buffering action.

Accumulation of lactic acid is the hallmark of hypoxia and ketoacid excess is important in diabetes (see Chapter 21). Acids derived from sources other than CO_2 are known as nonvolatile; by definition, they cannot be removed through the lungs, and must be excreted via the kidney. The net production of nonvolatile acids is of the order of 50 mmol/24 h.

Blood and tissues contain buffer systems that minimize changes in hydrogen ion concentration

The main buffer that neutralizes hydrogen ions released from cells is the bicarbonate buffer. Hemoglobin buffers hydrogen generated from the carbonic anhydrase reaction (see below). Hydrogen ion is neutralized by intracellular buffers, mainly proteins and phosphates (see Table 24.1 and also Chapter 2).

The bicarbonate buffer

The bicarbonate buffer remains in equilibrium with atmospheric air, creating an open system the capacity of which exceeds all the 'closed' buffer systems. The metabolically produced carbon dioxide diffuses through cell membranes and dissolves in plasma. The plasma solubility coefficient of CO_2 is 0.23 if pCO_2 is measured in kPa (0.03 if pCO_2 is measured in mmHg; 1 kPa = 7.5 mmHg or 1 mmHg = 0.133 kPa). Thus, at the normal pCO_2 of 5.3 kPa (40 mmHg), the concentration of dissolved CO_2 (dCO_2) is:

$$dCO_2 \text{ (mmol/L)} = 5.3 \text{ kPa} \times 0.23 = 1.2 \text{ mmol/L}$$

CO_2 equilibrates with H_2CO_3 in plasma in the course of a slow, nonenzymatic reaction. Normally plasma H_2CO_3 concentration is very low, about 0.0017 mmol/L. However, because of the equilibrium between H_2CO_3 and dissolved CO_2 (theoretically all dissolved CO_2 could eventually convert into

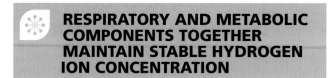

RESPIRATORY AND METABOLIC COMPONENTS TOGETHER MAINTAIN STABLE HYDROGEN ION CONCENTRATION

Both lungs and kidney contribute to maintenance of the blood pH. They are called the respiratory and metabolic components of the acid–base balance, respectively. The two components are closely interrelated. When the primary disorder is respiratory and causes accumulation of CO_2, a compensatory increase in bicarbonate reabsorption by the kidney takes place. Conversely, a decrease in pCO_2 decreases bicarbonate reabsorption. When the primary problem is metabolic, a decrease in bicarbonate concentration (and the resulting decrease in pH) stimulate the respiratory center to increase the ventilation rate. CO_2 is blown off and plasma pCO_2 decreases. This is why patients with metabolic acidosis hyperventilate. On the other hand, an increase in plasma bicarbonate (causing an increase in pH) leads to a decrease in the ventilation rate, and CO_2 retention. *The compensatory change always helps to return the pH to normal.*

H_2CO_3), this component of the bicarbonate buffer is equal to the sum of H_2CO_3 and dissolved CO_2 (in practice it equals the dissolved CO_2).

The key equation describing the behavior of the bicarbonate buffer is the Henderson–Hasselbalch equation (see Chapter 2). It expresses the relationship between pH and the components of the buffer:

$$pH = pK + \log[\text{bicarbonate}]/pCO_2 \times 0.23$$

It demonstrates that the plasma pH is determined by the ratio between the concentrations of plasma bicarbonate (the 'base' component of the buffer) and the dissolved CO_2 (the 'acid' component). Normally, at a plasma pCO_2 of 5.3 kPa (dCO_2 concentration 1.2 mmol/L), the plasma bicarbonate concentration is about 24 mmol/L. The pK of the bicarbonate buffer is 6.1. Let's insert the concentrations of buffer components into the above equation:

$$pH = 6.1 + \log(24/1.2) = 7.40$$

Thus, pH 7.40 (hydrogen ion concentration 40 nmol/L) is the pH of the extracellular fluid corresponding to normal concentration of bicarbonate and normal partial pressure of CO_2.

The bicarbonate buffer minimizes changes in hydrogen ion concentration when either acid or alkali is added to blood. When an acid (H^+) is added, it reacts with bicarbonate; this forms carbonic acid which on dissociation releases

CO_2. The blood pCO_2 increases slightly and the CO_2 is eliminated through the lungs. The excess hydrogen ion has been neutralized.

$$H^+ + HCO_3^- \rightleftharpoons H_2CO_3 \rightleftharpoons CO_2 + H_2O$$

When alkali (OH^-) is added, it reacts with the carbonic acid, yielding water. The bicarbonate concentration increases slightly.

$$OH^- + H_2CO_3 \rightleftharpoons H_2O + HCO_3^-$$

as a consequence of a decrease in the H_2CO_3 concentration; the reaction

$$CO_2 + H_2O \rightleftharpoons H_2CO_3$$

proceeds to the right, supplementing the used H_2CO_3. The excess of OH^- has been neutralized. Depletion of CO_2 is subsequently compensated by a decreased ventilation rate.

The above illustrates that the denominator in the Henderson–Hasselbalch equation (the pCO_2) is controlled by the lungs. It is called 'the respiratory component of the acid–base balance'. On the other hand, plasma bicarbonate concentration is controlled by the kidneys and erythrocytes and is called 'the metabolic component of the acid–base balance'.

Erythrocytes and renal tubular cells contain a zinc-containing enzyme, carbonic anhydrase (CA), which converts dissolved CO_2 into carbonic acid. Carbonic acid dissociates, yielding the hydrogen and bicarbonate ions:

$$CO_2 + H_2O \rightleftharpoons H_2CO_3 \rightleftharpoons H^+ + HCO_3^-$$

This is how renal tubular cells and erythrocytes produce bicarbonate. The kidneys regulate bicarbonate reabsorption and synthesis, and the erythrocytes adjust its concentration in response to changes in pCO_2.

Intracellular buffering

Intracellular buffers are proteins and phosphates

Hydrogen ion enters cells in exchange for potassium (this may result in an increase in plasma potassium concentration). Conversely, decrease in plasma hydrogen ion, or bicarbonate excess, would be buffered by cell-derived hydrogen ion. Hydrogen ion would enter plasma in exchange for potassium, decreasing plasma potassium.

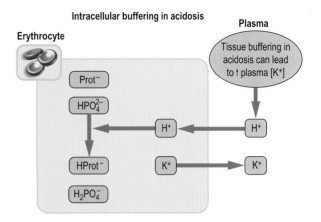

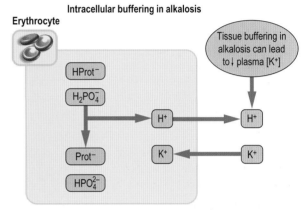

Fig. 24.2 **Intracellular buffers: proteins, phosphates, and potassium exchange.** Intracellular buffers are primarily proteins and phosphates. Hydrogen ion from the plasma enters cells in exchange for potassium. Therefore, an accumulation of the hydrogen ion in the plasma (acidemia) and the consequent entry of hydrogen ion into cells increase plasma potassium concentration. Conversely, a deficit of hydrogen ion in plasma (alkalemia) may lead to a low plasma potassium concentration. Prot, protein.

Thus acidemia (low plasma pH) may be associated with hyperkalemia and alkalemia (high blood pH) with hypokalemia (Fig. 24.2).

Classification of the acid–base disorders

The concept of respiratory and metabolic components of acid–base balance is a basis for the classification of the disorders of acid–base balance (Fig. 24.3). They are divided into acidosis or alkalosis. Acidosis is a process that leads to the accumulation of hydrogen ion. Alkalosis causes a decrease in hydrogen ion concentration (acidemia and alkalemia are terms that simply describe blood pH; thus, acidosis and alkalosis result in acidemia and alkalemia, respectively).

Depending on the primary cause, acidosis or alkalosis can be either respiratory or metabolic. Thus there are four main disorders of acid–base balance: respiratory acidosis, metabolic acidosis, respiratory alkalosis, and metabolic alkalosis

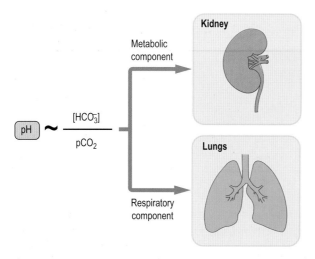

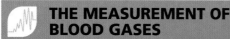

$$pH \sim \frac{[HCO_3^-]}{pCO_2}$$

Fig. 24.3 Components of the bicarbonate buffer. Blood pH is proportional to the ratio of plasma bicarbonate to the partial pressure of carbon dioxide in blood (pCO$_2$). The components of the bicarbonate buffer are carbon dioxide and bicarbonate. The pCO$_2$ is called 'the respiratory component of the acid–base balance' and bicarbonate is the 'metabolic component'.

(Fig. 24.4). However, mixed disorders can also develop; we consider them later in the chapter.

LUNGS: THE GAS EXCHANGE

Lungs supply oxygen necessary for tissue metabolism and remove CO$_2$ produced by metabolism

Approximately 10 000 L of air pass through the lungs of an average person each day. The lungs lie in the thoracic cavity

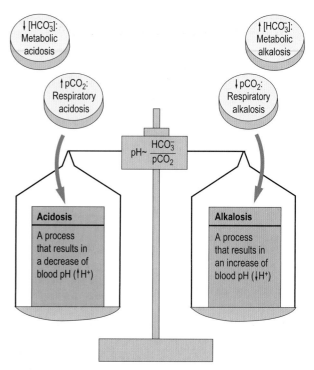

Fig. 24.4 The acid–base disorders. Primary increase in pCO$_2$, or a decrease in plasma bicarbonate concentration, lead to acidosis. A decrease in pCO$_2$, or an increase in plasma bicarbonate, lead to alkalosis. If the primary change is in pCO$_2$, the disorder is called respiratory, and if the primary change is in plasma bicarbonate it is called metabolic.

surrounded by the pleural sac, a thin 'bag' of tissue that lines the thoracic cage at one end and attaches to the external surface of the lungs at the other. When the thoracic cage expands during inspiration, negative pressure created in the expanding pleural sac inflates the lung.

The airways are a set of tubes of progressively decreasing diameter. They consist of the trachea, large and small bronchi,

THE MEASUREMENT OF BLOOD GASES

The so-called 'blood gas measurement' is an important first-line laboratory investigation. In respiratory failure, the results of such measurements are also an essential guide to oxygen therapy and assisted ventilation.

The measurements are performed on a sample of arterial blood, taken usually from the radial artery in the forearm. The jargon term 'blood gases' means the measurements of pO$_2$, pCO$_2$, and pH (or hydrogen ion concentration) from which the concentration of bicarbonate is calculated using the Henderson–Hasselbalch equation. Several other indices are also computed: they include the total amount of buffers in the blood (so-called buffer base) and the difference between the desired (normal) amount of buffers in the blood and the actual amount (base excess). The reference values for pH, pCO$_2$, and O$_2$ are given in Table 24.2.

RESPIRATORY ALKALOSIS IS CAUSED BY HYPERVENTILATION

A 25-year-old man was admitted to hospital with an asthmatic attack. Peak expiratory flow rate was 75% of his best. His blood gas values were pO$_2$ 9.3 kPa (70 mmHg) and pCO$_2$ 4.0 kPa (30 mmHg), with pH 7.50 (hydrogen ion concentration 42 nmol/L). He was treated with nebulized salbutamol, a β$_2$-adrenergic stimulant (see Chapter 41) which is a bronchodilator, and made a good recovery.

Comment. This man's blood gases show a mild degree of respiratory alkalosis caused by hyperventilation and 'blowing off' the CO$_2$. Respiratory alkalosis causes reduction in serum levels of ionized calcium, leading to neuromuscular irritability. Ventilatory impairment that leads to CO$_2$ retention and respiratory acidosis is characteristic of a severe asthma. Reference ranges are given in Table 24.2.

Reference ranges for blood gas results		
	Arterial	**Venous**
[H$^+$]	36–43 mmol/L	35–45 mmol/L
pH	7.37–7.44	7.35–7.45
pCO$_2$	4.6–6.0 kPa	4.8–6.7 kPa
pO$_2$	10.5–13.5 kPa	4.0–6.7 kPa
bicarbonate	19–24 mmol/L	

Table 24.2 **The reference values for blood gases.** The primary values are the pH, pCO$_2$ and pO$_2$; bicarbonate concentration is calculated from pH and pCO$_2$ values; pH below 7.0 or above 7.7 is life threatening.

and even smaller bronchioles (Fig. 24.5). At the end of the bronchioles, there are pulmonary alveoli – structures lined with endothelium and covered with a film of surfactant – the main component of which is dipalmitoylphosphatidylcholine (see Chapter 27). Surfactant decreases the surface tension of the alveoli. The gas exchange takes place in the alveoli.

Respiration rate is controlled by the respiratory center located in the brainstem. Both pO$_2$ and pCO$_2$ affect the

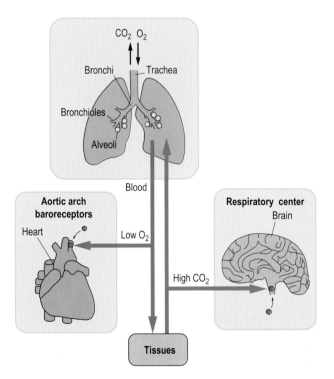

Fig. 24.5 **Lungs and the regulation of the respiratory rate by pCO$_2$ and pO$_2$.** Lung ventilation and perfusion are the main factors controlling gas exchange. The pCO$_2$ regulates the ventilation rate through the central chemoreceptors in the brainstem. When pO$_2$ decreases, this control switches to pO$_2$-sensitive peripheral receptors in the carotid bodies and in the aortic arch.

RESPIRATORY ACIDOSIS OCCURS IN CHRONIC LUNG DISEASES

A 56-year-old woman was admitted to a general ward with increasing breathlessness. She had smoked 20 cigarettes a day for the previous 25 years and reported frequent attacks of 'winter bronchitis'. Blood gas measurements revealed a pO$_2$ of 6 kPa (45 mmHg), pCO$_2$ of 8.4 kPa (53 mmHg), and pH 7.35 (hydrogen ion concentration 51 nmol/L); bicarbonate concentration was 35 mmol/L (for reference ranges, refer to Table 24.2).

Comment. This patient suffered from an exacerbation of chronic obstructive pulmonary disease and a respiratory acidosis. Her pCO$_2$ was high, and her ventilation was probably dependent on the hypoxic drive. Her bicarbonate was also increased, as a result of metabolic compensation of respiratory acidosis. One must be careful when treating such patients with high concentrations of oxygen, because the increased pO$_2$ may remove hypoxic drive and cause respiratory depression. Monitoring of arterial pO$_2$ and pCO$_2$ on oxygen treatment is mandatory. This patient was successfully treated with a 28% concentration of oxygen.

ventilation rate: the respiratory center has chemoreceptors sensitive to pCO$_2$ and to pH. Under normal circumstances it is not the pO$_2$ that stimulates ventilation but an increase in pCO$_2$ or a decrease in pH. However, when the pO$_2$ falls and hypoxia develops, it begins the control of ventilation through a set of receptors located in the carotid bodies in the aortic arch. When arterial pO$_2$ decreases to less than 8 kPa (60 mmHg), this 'hypoxic drive' becomes the main controller of ventilatory rate. People who suffer from hypoxia due to chronic lung disease depend on hypoxic drive to maintain their ventilation rate (see clinical box).

Ventilation and lung perfusion determine gas exchange

Blood supply to the pulmonary alveoli is provided by the pulmonary arteries that carry deoxygenated blood from the periphery through the right ventricle. After oxygenation in the lungs, blood flows through pulmonary veins to the left atrium. In the alveolar capillaries of the lungs, it accepts oxygen which diffuses through the alveolar wall from the inspired air; at the same time the CO$_2$ diffuses from the blood into the alveoli (see Fig. 24.5) and is removed with the expired air.

The rate of diffusion of gases in and out of the blood is determined by the difference in partial pressures between alveolar air and blood. Table 24.3 shows the partial pressures of oxygen (pO$_2$) and carbon dioxide (pCO$_2$) in the lungs. Compared with the atmospheric air, the pCO$_2$ in the alveolar air is slightly higher and pO$_2$ slightly lower (this is due to the water vapor pressure). Carbon dioxide is much more soluble in water than oxygen, and equilibrates with blood more rapidly. Therefore, when problems develop, one first notices a decrease in blood pO_2 (hypoxia). An increase in pCO_2 (hypercapnia) occurs later and usually indicates a more severe disease.

The other major factor determining gas exchange is the rate at which the blood flows through the lungs (the perfusion rate). Normally, the alveolar ventilation rate is approximately 4 L/min and the perfusion 5 L/min (the ratio of ventilation to perfusion (Va/Q) is 0.8). In pathologic conditions, some parts of the lung may be well perfused but poorly ventilated. This occurs when some alveoli collapse and are unable to exchange gases. As a result, the blood pO_2 decreases because there is no diffusion of oxygen from the alveolar air. The presence of oxygen-poor blood in the arterial circulation is known as a 'shunt' condition. On the other hand, when ventilation is adequate but perfusion poor, gas exchange cannot take place; in such cases, part of the lung behaves as if it had no alveoli at all, forming the 'physiologic dead space' (Table 24.4). Examples of conditions related to poor ventilation, poor perfusion, or the combination of both, are given below:

- rib cage deformities impair ventilation by limiting lung movement
- chest trauma may decrease ventilation as a result of lung collapse; alveoli may be actually destroyed in pulmonary emphysema; inadequate synthesis of surfactant leads to the collapse of alveoli and to the respiratory distress syndrome

- the bronchial tree may be mechanically obstructed by inhaled objects or narrowed by a growing tumor: this impairs ventilation
- constriction of the bronchi occurs in asthma
- ventilatory efficiency may be reduced by impaired elasticity of the lung or dysfunction of relevant muscles (the diaphragm and intercostal muscles of the chest wall)
- diffusion of gases is impaired when fluid is present in the alveoli (pulmonary edema)
- lung movement is affected by defects in neural control
- lung perfusion is compromised in circulatory problems such as shock and heart failure.

Handling of carbon dioxide by erythrocytes

The body produces CO_2 at a rate of 200–800 mL/min. The CO_2 dissolves in water and generates carbonic acid, which in turn dissociates into hydrogen and bicarbonate ions. Thus, CO_2 generates large amounts of hydrogen ion:

$$CO_2 + H_2O \rightleftharpoons H_2CO_3 \rightleftharpoons H^+ + HCO_3^-$$

Erythrocytes transport CO_2 to the lungs

We already know that in plasma, the above reaction is nonenzymatic and proceeds slowly, generating only minute amounts of carbonic acid, which remain in equilibrium with a large amount of dissolved CO_2. The same reaction in the erythrocytes is catalyzed by carbonic anhydrase, which 'fixes' CO_2 as bicarbonate. The generated hydrogen ion is buffered by hemoglobin.

Bicarbonate produced by erythrocyte carbonic anhydrase moves to plasma in exchange for the chloride ion (the 'chloride shift') (Fig. 24.6). As much as 70% of all CO_2 produced in tissues becomes bicarbonate; approximately 20% is carried 'fixed' to hemoglobin as carbamino groups (see Chapter 5), and only 10% remains dissolved in plasma.

In the lungs, higher pO_2 facilitates dissociation of CO_2 from hemoglobin. This is known as the Haldane effect. The

Partial pressures of oxygen and carbon dioxide in air, alveoli, and blood.				
	Dry air	**Alveoli**	**Systemic arteries**	**Tissue**
pO_2	21.2 kPa	13.7 kPa	12 kPa	5.3 kPa
pCO_2	<0.13 kPa	5.3 kPa	5.3 kPa	6 kPa
Water vapor		6.3 kPa		

Table 24.3 **Partial pressures of oxygen and carbon dioxide in atmospheric air, lung alveoli, and the blood.** Partial pressure gradients determine diffusion of gases through the alveolar/blood barrier (1 kPa = 7.5 mmHg).

Blood pCO_2 and pO_2 are affected by the perfusion and ventilation of the lungs					
	Alveolar pO_2	**Alveolar pCO_2**	**Arterial pO_2**	**Arterial pCO_2**	**Comment**
Poor ventilation, adequate perfusion	decreased	increased	decreased	normal	physiologic shunt
Adequate ventilation, poor perfusion	increased	decreased	decreased*	increased*	physiologic dead space

Table 24.4 **Blood partial pressures of oxygen and carbon dioxide depend on lung perfusion and ventilation.** *Depending on the degree of shunt.

ANEMIA CAUSES TIREDNESS AND SHORTNESS OF BREATH

A 35-year-old man complained of shortness of breath after climbing two flights of stairs. His chest radiograph was normal, as were examination of the heart and the electrocardiogram; blood gases were normal. He was taking a nonsteroidal anti-inflammatory agent (NSAID) for joint pain. His blood cell count revealed a hemoglobin value of 10 g/dL (reference range for men 13–18 g/dL) and a reduced mean corpuscular volume of 72 dL (reference range 80–96). Seru m ferritin concentration was low at 10 µg/L (reference range 14–200).

Comment. This man had chronic iron deficiency anemia. Anemia can present with general symptoms such as tiredness or breathlessness. The patient had a gastric ulcer caused by the NSAID with loss of blood from the gastrointestinal tract.

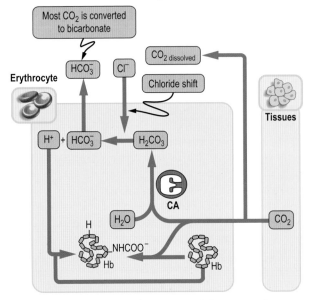

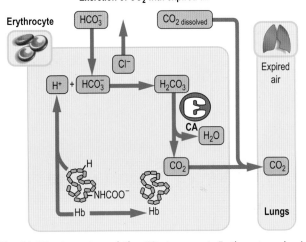

Fig. 24.6 **Erythrocyte and the CO_2 transport.** Erythrocyte carbonic anhydrase converts most of the CO_2 produced in tissues into bicarbonate for transport to the lungs; approximately 20% of the total amount is transported bound to hemoglobin, and the rest as dissolved gas in plasma.

hemoglobin releases its hydrogen ion, which reacts with bicarbonate and forms carbonic acid which releases CO_2.

HANDLING OF BICARBONATE BY THE KIDNEYS

The kidneys play an essential role in the control of plasma bicarbonate concentration and in the removal of hydrogen ion. In common with erythrocytes, the renal (proximal and distal) tubular cells contain carbonic anhydrase.

Proximal tubules reabsorb bicarbonate

Bicarbonate is reabsorbed in the proximal tubule and the urine is almost bicarbonate free. The surfaces of the renal tubular cells facing the lumen are impermeable to bicarbonate. Filtered bicarbonate combines with hydrogen ion secreted by the cells, and forms carbonic acid that is converted into CO_2 by carbonic anhydrase located on the luminal membrane. The CO_2 diffuses into cells where intracellular carbonic anhydrase converts it back into carbonic acid, dissociating into hydrogen and bicarbonate ions. Bicarbonate is returned to the plasma and the hydrogen ion is secreted into the lumen of the tubule, to trap more of the filtered bicarbonate. Note that in this process hydrogen ion is used exclusively to aid bicarbonate reabsorption – no net excretion takes place (Fig. 24.7).

Distal tubules generate new bicarbonate and excrete hydrogen

In the distal tubule bicarbonate generation takes place. The mechanism is identical to that of bicarbonate reabsorption but this time there is both a net loss of hydrogen ions

from the body and a net gain of bicarbonate. CO_2 diffuses into cells. The distal tubule carbonic anhydrase converts it into carbonic acid which dissociates into hydrogen ion and bicarbonate. Bicarbonate is transported to the plasma and hydrogen ion is secreted into the tubule lumen. However, no bicarbonate is present in the lumen of the distal tubule (all has been reabsorbed earlier) and the hydrogen ion is trapped (buffered) by the phosphate ions present in the filtrate, and by ammonia synthesized by the proximal tubules. It is subsequently excreted in the urine (Fig. 24.8).

The ammonia is generated during the transformation of glutamine into glutamic acid in a reaction catalyzed by

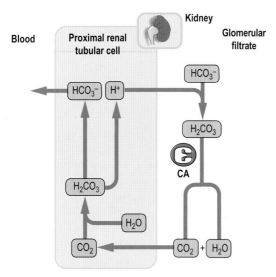

Fig. 24.7 **Bicarbonate reabsorption in the kidney.** Bicarbonate reabsorption takes place in the proximal tubule. There is no net excretion of hydrogen ion.

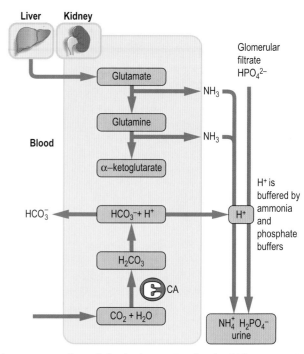

Fig. 24.8 **Excretion of the hydrogen ion by the kidney.** Excretion of the hydrogen ion takes place in the distal tubules. Hydrogen ion reacts with ammonia, forming the ammonium ion. Hydrogen ion is also buffered by phosphate. The daily excretion of hydrogen ion is approximately 50 mmol. CA, carbonic anhydrase.

glutaminase. Ammonia diffuses through the luminal membrane and the hydrogen ion is trapped inside the tubule as the ammonium ion (NH_4^+) to which the membrane is impermeable.

Defects in renal handling of bicarbonate and hydrogen ion lead to a group of relatively rare disorders known as renal tubular acidoses (RTA). The distal RTA is due to the impairment of hydrogen ion excretion in the distal tubule, and the proximal RTA to the impaired reabsorption of bicarbonate. Proximal RTA is usually accompanied by other defects in proximal transport mechanisms (this is known as the Fanconi syndrome).

RESPIRATORY AND METABOLIC DISORDERS OF ACID–BASE BALANCE CAN OCCUR TOGETHER

During resuscitation of a 60-year-old man from a cardiorespiratory arrest, blood gas analysis revealed pH 7.00 (hydrogen ion concentration 100 nmol/L) and pCO_2 7.5 kPa (52 mmHg). His bicarbonate concentration was 11 mmol/L. pO_2 was 12.1 kPa (91 mmHg) during treatment with 48% oxygen.

Comment. This patient had a mixed disorder: a respiratory acidosis caused by lack of ventilation, and metabolic acidosis caused by the hypoxia that had occurred before oxygen treatment was instituted. The acidosis was caused by an accumulation of lactic acid: the measured lactate concentration was 7 mmol/L (reference range is 0.7–1.8 mmol/L, 6–16 mg/dL). The terms acidosis and alkalosis do not just describe blood pH changes: they relate to the processes that result in these changes. Therefore, in some instances, two independent processes may occur: for example, a patient may be admitted to hospital with diabetic ketoacidosis and coexisting emphysema causing respiratory acidosis. The final result could be a more severe change in pH than would have resulted from a simple disorder (Table 24.5). Any combination of disorders can occur; the skills of an experienced physician are usually required to diagnose this.

DISORDERS OF THE ACID–BASE BALANCE

The lung and the kidney work in a concerted way to minimize changes in plasma pH, and can compensate for each other when problems occur

Disturbances of acid–base balance may be caused by primary problems affecting the respiratory component or bicarbonate concentration (the metabolic component). The Henderson–Hasselbalch equation shows that acidosis is accompanied by an increased ratio of plasma bicarbonate to pCO_2, and alkalosis by a decreased ratio.

Acidosis

Clinically, acidosis is much more common than alkalosis (Table 24.5) and it can be either respiratory or metabolic.

Metabolic, respiratory and mixed acidosis			
Disorder	pH	pCO$_2$	Bicarbonate
metabolic acidosis	decrease	decrease (respiratory compensation)	decrease (primary change)
respiratory acidosis	decrease	increase (primary change)	increase (metabolic compensation)
mixed respiratory and metabolic acidosis	large decrease	increase (respiratory acidosis)	decrease (metabolic acidosis)

Metabolic, respiratory and mixed alkalosis			
Disorder	pH	pCO$_2$	Bicarbonate
metabolic alkalosis	increase	increase (respiratory compensation)	increase (primary change)
respiratory alkalosis	increase	decrease (primary change)	decrease (metabolic compensation)
mixed respiratory and metabolic alkalosis	large increase	decrease (respiratory alkalosis)	increase (metabolic acidosis)

Table 24.5 **Simple and mixed acid–base disorders.** Mixed acid–base disorders result in a greater change in blood pH than simple disorders; they may pose diagnostic difficulties.

ACID–BASE DISORDERS AFFECT PLASMA POTASSIUM CONCENTRATION

Potassium affects the contractility of the heart and either a too high or too low plasma concentration (hyperkalemia and hypokalemia, respectively) can be life threatening. The effects of potassium on heart function can be observed on the electrocardiogram. Hypokalemia leads to an increased excretion of hydrogen ion and, consequently, to metabolic alkalosis. The converse is also true: metabolic alkalosis leads to an increased renal excretion of potassium, and hypokalemia. Plasma potassium concentration needs to be checked whenever a disorder of acid–base balance is suspected (see Fig. 23.15).

Respiratory acidosis occurs most often in lung disease and results from decreased ventilation

The most common cause is chronic obstructive airways disease (COAD). Severe asthmatic attack can result in respiratory acidosis because of bronchial constriction. Respiratory acidosis often accompanies hypoxia (respiratory failure); in such a case, an increase in pCO$_2$ often parallels the decrease in pO$_2$.

Metabolic acidosis results from the excessive production, inefficient metabolism or impaired excretion of nonvolatile acids

A classic example of metabolic acidosis is diabetic ketoacidosis, when ketoacids, acetoacetic acid, and β-hydroxybutyric acid accumulate in the plasma (see Chapter 21). Acidosis may also occur during extreme physical exertion, when there

VOMITING MAY LEAD TO METABOLIC ALKALOSIS

A 47-year-old man came to the outpatient clinic with a history of intermittent profuse vomiting and loss of weight. He had tachycardia, reduced tissue turgor, hypotension and an abdominal succussion splash. His blood pH was 7.55 (hydrogen ion concentration 28 nmol/L) and pCO$_2$ was 6.4 kPa (48 mmHg). His bicarbonate concentration was 35 mmol/L and there was also hyponatremia and hypokalemia. Despite the systemic alkalosis, urine pH was only 3.5.

Comment. This patient presents with metabolic alkalosis caused by the loss of hydrogen ion through vomiting. Investigations showed gastric outlet obstruction of the stomach entrance due to scarring from chronic peptic ulceration. He subsequently underwent surgery for pyloric stenosis, with a good outcome. Note the increased pCO$_2$ as a result of respiratory compensation of metabolic alkalosis. The paradoxically acid urine is probably due to depletion of chloride which then limits reabsorption of sodium in the thick ascending limb of the loop of Henle of the kidney, so that sodium is then exchanged for hydrogen ions and potassium in the distal nephron.

is accumulation of lactate generated from muscle metabolism; in normal circumstances, lactate is quickly metabolized on cessation of exercise. However, when large amounts of lactate are generated as a consequence of hypoxia, lactic acidosis may become life-threatening, as happens, for instance, in shock.

Excretion of nonvolatile acids is also impaired in renal failure and this also causes metabolic acidosis. Renal failure

Respiratory and metabolic compensation of acid–base disorders

Acid–base disorder	Primary change	Compensatory change	Timescale of compensatory change
metabolic acidosis	decrease in plasma bicarbonate concentration	decrease in pCO_2 (hyperventilation)	minutes/hours
metabolic alkalosis	increase in plasma bicarbonate concentration	increase in pCO_2 (hypoventilation)	minutes/hours
respiratory acidosis	increase in pCO_2	increase in renal bicarbonate reabsorption increase in plasma bicarbonate concentration	days
respiratory alkalosis	decrease in pCO_2	decrease in renal bicarbonate reabsorption decrease in plasma bicarbonate concentration	days

Table 24.6 **Respiratory and metabolic compensation in the acid–base disorders minimizes changes in the blood pH.** A change in the respiratory component leads to metabolic compensation, and a change in the metabolic component stimulates respiratory compensation. Metabolic compensation involves a change in renal bicarbonate handling, and respiratory compensation means changes in the ventilation rate. A compensatory increase or decrease in the rate of ventilation (hyper- or hypoventilation) is seen within minutes; however, an adjustment of the rate of bicarbonate reabsorption may take days.

Clinical causes of acid–base disorders

Metabolic acidosis	Respiratory acidosis	Metabolic alkalosis	Respiratory alkalosis
diabetes mellitus (ketoacidosis)	chronic obstructive airways disease	vomiting (loss of hydrogen ion)	hyperventilation (anxiety, fever)
lactic acidosis (lactic acid)	severe asthma	nasogastric suction (loss of hydrogen ion)	lung diseases associated with hyperventilation
renal failure (inorganic acids)	cardiac arrest	hypokalemia	anemia
severe diarrhea (loss of bicarbonate)	depression of respiratory center (drugs, e.g. opiates)	intravenous administration of bicarbonate (e.g. after cardiac arrest)	salicylate poisoning
surgical drainage of intestine (loss of bicarbonate)	weakness of respiratory muscles (e.g. poliomyelitis, multiple sclerosis)		
renal loss of bicarbonate (renal tubular acidosis type 2 – rare)	chest deformities		
impairment of renal H^+ excretion (renal tubular acidosis type 1 – rare)	airway obstruction		

Table 24.7 **The clinical causes of acid–base disorders.** Disorders of the acid–base balance are acidosis and alkalosis: each of them can be either respiratory or metabolic. Respiratory acidosis is common and is caused primarily by diseases of the lung that affect gas exchange. Respiratory alkalosis is rarer and is caused by hyperventilation, which decreases pCO_2. Metabolic acidosis is common and results from either overproduction or retention of nonvolatile acids in the circulation. Metabolic alkalosis is rarer: its most common causes are vomiting and gastric suction, both causing loss of hydrogen ion from the stomach.

develops when the perfusion of the kidneys is inadequate (e.g. in trauma, shock or dehydration) or if there is an intrinsic kidney disease such as glomerulonephritis (inflammatory reaction in the renal tubular tissue; see Chapter 23 and box on p. 321).

Excessive loss of bicarbonate can also be a cause of metabolic acidosis. This may occur when the renal reabsorption mechanism is defective but is more common when bicarbonate present in the intestinal fluid is lost as a result of severe diarrhea or surgical drainage after bowel surgery.

Alkalosis

Alkalosis is rarer than acidosis (see Tables 24.6 and 24.7)

A mild respiratory alkalosis may be a consequence of hyperventilation during exercise, anxiety attack or fever. It also occurs in pregnancy. Metabolic alkalosis is often associated with abnormally low potassium concentration in plasma, as a result of cellular buffering. Cellular entry or exit of potassium ion is associated with the movement of hydrogen ion in an opposite direction. Thus, alkalosis can cause hypokalemia while hypokalemia (see Chapter 23) may lead to alkalosis. Severe metabolic alkalosis may also occur as a result of the massive loss of hydrogen ion from the stomach during vomiting (see box on p. 335), or as a result of nasogastric suction after surgery. Lastly, it may occur when too much bicarbonate is given intravenously, for instance during resuscitation from the cardiac arrest.

SUMMARY

■ Maintenance of the hydrogen ion concentration within a narrow range is vital for cell survival.

■ Acid–base balance is regulated by the concerted action of lungs and kidneys. The erythrocytes play a key role in the transport of carbon dioxide in blood.

■ The main buffers in blood are hemoglobin and bicarbonate, whereas in the cells they include proteins and phosphate. The bicarbonate buffer system communicates with atmospheric air.

■ Acid–base disorders are acidosis and alkalosis and each of them can be either metabolic or respiratory.

■ Determination of pH, pCO_2 and bicarbonate, and pO_2 is a first-line investigation and is frequently required in emergencies.

ACTIVE LEARNING

1. Describe how the bicarbonate buffer copes with an addition of acid to the system.
2. Compare bicarbonate handling by the proximal and distal tubules of the kidney.
3. Outline the role of ventilation in acid–base disorders.
4. Which disorders of the acid–base balance may be associated with gastrointestinal surgery?
5. Discuss the association between acid–base disorders and plasma potassium concentration.

Further reading

Corey HE. Bench-to-bedside review: fundamental principles of acid–base balance. *Crit Care* 2005;**9**:184–192.

Kellum JA. Disorders of acid–base balance. *Crit Care Med* 2007;**35**:2630–2636.

25. Calcium and Bone Metabolism

W D Fraser and M H Dominiczak

LEARNING OBJECTIVES

After reading this chapter you should be able to:

- Describe the chemical composition of bone, and the process of mineralization.
- Recognize the major cells in bone and their interactions in the bone remodeling cycle.
- Understand the role of major factors contributing to the regulation of serum calcium concentration.
- Know the causes of hypercalcemia and hypocalcemia.
- Explain the pivotal role of parathyroid hormone related protein in hypercalcemia of malignancy.
- Understand the role of vitamin D and its metabolism in health and disease.
- Define osteoporosis, its causes and treatment.
- Recognize the causes of osteomalacia and its presentation in adults.

BONE STRUCTURE AND BONE REMODELLING

Bone is a specialized connective tissue that, along with cartilage, forms the skeletal system. In addition to serving a supportive and protective role, it is the site of substantial metabolic activity. Two types of bone are recognized: the thick, densely calcified external bone (cortical or compact bone), and a thinner, honeycomb network of calcified tissue on the inner aspect of bone (trabecular bone).

Collagen and hydroxyapatite are the main components of the bone matrix

Within the bone matrix, type 1 collagen is the major protein (90%; see box on p. 12) and calcium-rich crystals of hydroxyapatite ($Ca_{10}[PO_4]_6[OH]_2$) are found on, within, and between the collagen fibers. The attachment of hydroxyapatite to collagen and the calcification of bone are, in part, controlled by the presence of glycoproteins and proteoglycans with a high ion-binding capacity. Collagen fibers orientate so that they have the greatest density per unit volume and are packed in layers, giving the lamellar structure observed on microscopy. Posttranslational modifications of collagen occur that result in the formation of intra- and intermol-ecular pyridinoline and pyrrole crosslinks, which have an important role in fibril strength and matrix mineralization. This microarchitecture allows bone to function as the major reservoir of calcium for the body. The noncalcified organic matrix within bone, known as osteoid, becomes mineralized through two mechanisms.

Within the bone extracellular space, plasma membrane-derived matrix vesicles act as a focus for deposition of calcium phosphate, the lipid-rich inner membrane of these vesicles being the nidus for the formation of hydroxyapatite crystals. Crystallization proceeds rapidly, eventually obliterating the vesicle membrane and leaving a collection of clustered hydroxyapatite crystals. Within this environment, osteoblasts (bone-forming cells) can also secrete preorganized packets of matrix proteins that rapidly mineralize, and these combine with matrix vesicle-derived crystals to form a mineralized tissue within the matrix space. Molecules that inhibit this process, for example pyrophosphate, exist within the matrix environment. The secretion of alkaline phosphatase by osteoblasts destroys pyrophosphate, allowing mineralization to occur.

Mineralization is highly dependent on an adequate supply of calcium and phosphate. When mineral deprivation exists, there is an increase in the percentage of osteoid (the nonmineralized organic matrix) within bone, resulting in the clinical condition of osteomalacia.

Small amounts of calcium are exchanged daily between bone and the extracellular fluid (ECF) as a result of constant bone remodeling, i.e. coupled processes of resorption by osteoclasts (bone-resorbing cells) and formation by osteoblasts (Fig. 25.1). This exchange maintains a relative calcium balance between newly formed bone and older resorbed bone. Bone remodeling is a coupled process of resorption by osteoclasts and formation by osteoblasts.

Bone constantly changes its structure through remodeling

Bone is a dynamic structure. It undergoes constant mechanical adaptation. The process is known as remodeling and is a result of concerted action of two types of cells: osteoblasts and osteoclasts. Increased mechanical load stimulates bone formation and excess osteoclastic activity underpins several diseases, in particular osteoporosis, rheumatoid arthritis, and metastatic cancers.

Factors affecting bone resorption are listed in Table 25.1.

Osteoclasts

Osteoclasts are bone-resorbing cells

Osteoclasts are multinucleated giant cells (tissue-specific macrophages). They remain in contact with a calcified surface generated by their resorptive activity. Osteoclasts are

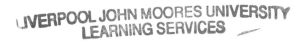

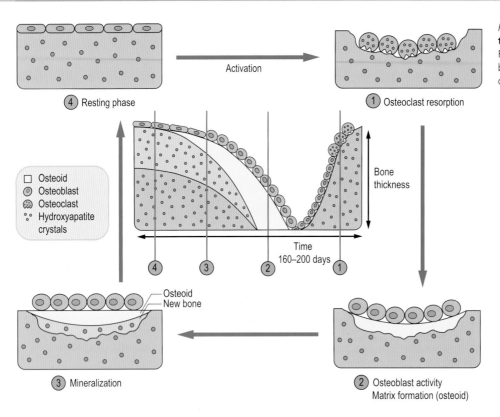

Fig. 25.1 **Maintaining bone mass: the bone remodeling cycle.** Resorption and formation of bone by osteoclasts and osteoblasts is coupled.

① Osteoclast resorption

② Osteoblast activity Matrix formation (osteoid)

③ Mineralization

④ Resting phase

Bone thickness

Time 160–200 days

Osteoid
Osteoblast
Osteoclast
Hydroxyapatite crystals

Osteoid
New bone

Factors affecting bone resorption	
Factors stimulating bone resorption	**Factors inhibiting bone resorption**
1,25-OH$_2$D$_3$	Calcium
PTH	Estrogens
PTHrP	Calcitonin
PGE$_2$	TGF-β
IL-1	IL-17
IL-6	
TNF	
Prolactin	
Corticosteroids	

PGE$_2$, prostaglandin E2; IL, interleukin; TNF, tumor necrosis factor; TGF, tumor growth factor; PTH, parathyroid hormone; PTHrP, parathyroid hormone-related protein.

Table 25.1 **Factors affecting bone resorption.**

derived from pluripotent hematopoietic mononuclear cells in the bone marrow.

RANK receptor and its ligand RANKL are essential for the differentiation, maturation, and regulation of osteoclasts

The maturation of osteoclasts from their progenitor cells is directed by growth factors, particularly colony-stimulating factor 1 (CSF1). Another essential factor is the receptor protein structurally related to the tumor necrosis factor receptor, called receptor activator of nuclear factor NFκB (RANK). It binds the TNF-related cytokine called RANK ligand (RANKL). The binding of RANKL to RANK can be blocked by osteoprogenerin (OPG) which is also a protein structurally related to the TNF receptor. RANKL and OPG control the differentiation and activation of osteoclasts. RANKL stimulates and OPG inhibits bone resorption. Importantly, estrogens induce OPG synthesis.

Genetic manipulation of animals, producing targeted disruption of the OPG gene, results in profound osteoporosis. RANKL knockout mice lack osteoclasts and suffer osteopetrosis with excessively thickened bone.

RANK controls the osteoclast through intracellular signaling cascades and transcription factors

Essentially, RANK prepares the osteoclast to resorb bone. As with other membrane receptors (see Chapter 40), it stimulates intracellular signaling cascades, which in turn activate transcription factors that control genes. Intracellular signaling pathways of the RANK involve proteins known as adaptor molecules (TNFR-associated cytoplasmic factors; TRAFs). TRAFs in turn assemble further signaling proteins and activate pathways involving NFκB and activator protein-1 (AP-1). Other pathways involve C-Jun terminal kinase (JNK), p38 stress-activated protein kinase, extracellular signal-regulated kinase (ERK) and the src pathway which involves PI3K and Akt kinase (for more details on these see Chapter 40). The end result of osteoclast activation is the induction of genes coding for tartrate-resistant acid phosphatase, cathepsin K′ calcitonin and the β2 integrin which directly control bone resorption. Osteoclast resorption of bone releases collagen peptides, pyridinoline crosslink fragments, and calcium from the bone matrix through the production, secretion, and action of lysosomal enzymes, collagenases, and cathepsins at an acidic pH. Collagen breakdown products in serum and urine (e.g. hydroxyproline) and collagen fragments (amino or carboxy telopeptides NTX and CTX, respectively) can be measured.

Parathyroid hormone contributes to osteoclast activation

Parathyroid hormone (PTH) activates osteoclasts indirectly via osteoblasts and calcitonin. Local factors such as the cytokines interleukin-1 (IL-1), tumor necrosis factor (TNF), transforming growth factor-β (TGF-β) and interferon-γ (INF-γ) are also important regulators of osteoclasts and act through RANKL and OPG.

Osteoblasts

Osteoblasts are bone-forming cells

The osteoblast progenitor cell is derived from mesenchyme. Mature osteoblasts synthesize type 1 collagen, osteocalcin (also known as bone Gla protein), cell attachment proteins (thrombospondin, fibronectin, bone sialoprotein, osteopontin), proteoglycans, and growth-related proteins, and they control bone mineralization. Osteoblast function and activity are altered by several hormones and growth factors.

PTH binds to a specific receptor, stimulating production of cyclic adenosine monophosphate (cAMP), ion and amino acid transport, and collagen synthesis. 1,25-Dihydroxycholecalciferol $(1,25(OH)_2D_3;$ calcitriol) stimulates synthesis of alkaline phosphatase, matrix, and bone-specific proteins and can decrease osteocalcin secretion. Growth factors TGF-β, insulin-like growth factors (IGFs)-1 and -2, and platelet-derived growth factor (PDGF) serve as autocrine regulators of osteoblast function. Serum biochemical markers reflecting osteoblast function are bone-specific alkaline phosphatase, osteocalcin, and markers of collagen formation: carboxy-terminal procollagen extension peptide (ICTP) and amino or carboxy-terminal procollagen extension peptides (PINP, P1CP).

The functions of osteoblasts and osteoclasts are connected by a process called coupling. For instance, osteoblasts express RANKL on their surface and it interacts with RANK expressed on osteoclast progenitor cells. This increases osteoclast differentiation and activates mature osteoclasts, providing a link between bone formation and resorption.

A protein that plays an important role in osteoblast differentiation is a member of the LDL-receptor family (see Chapter 18) known as the LDL-receptor protein 5 (LRP5). LRP5 together with another receptor activates the so-called Wnt signaling pathway leading to cell differentiation. This pathway is important in controling the formation of new bone.

Mutation of the gene encoding for LRP5 was shown to cause high bone mass and formation of dense bone. On the other hand, the loss-of-function mutation caused osteoporosis.

CALCIUM METABOLISM

Bone serves as a store of calcium

In calcium homeostasis, bone serves as the reservoir of calcium when deficiency exists, and as its store when the body is replete.

The skeleton contains 99% of the calcium present in the body in the form of hydroxyapatite; the remainder is distributed in the soft tissues, teeth, and ECF. Many cell and organ functions are dependent on the tight control of extracellular calcium concentration; these include neural transmission, cellular secretion, contraction of muscle cells, cell proliferation, the stability and permeability of cell membranes, blood clotting, and the mineralization of bone. Total serum calcium is maintained between 2.2 and 2.60 mmol/L (8.8–10.4 mg/dL). Calcium exists in the circulation in three forms (Fig. 25.2):

- **ionized Ca²⁺**: the most important, physiologically active form (50% of total calcium)
- **protein bound Ca²⁺**: the majority of the remaining calcium, mainly bound to negatively charged albumin (40%)
- **Ca²⁺ complexed to substances such as citrate and phosphate**: a smaller fraction (10%).

If serum protein concentration increases (as in dehydration and after prolonged venous stasis), protein-bound calcium and total serum calcium increase. In conditions of reduced serum proteins (e.g. liver disease, nephrotic syndrome, malnutrition), the protein-bound calcium concentration is reduced, decreasing the total calcium, although ionized calcium is maintained within the reference range 1.1–1.3 mmol/L (4.4–5.2 mg/dL). Many acute and chronic illnesses decrease serum albumin concentration, which consequently decreases serum total calcium. Because of this, in

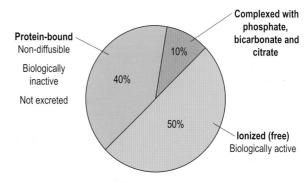

Total Ca²⁺ = Ionized Ca²⁺ + Protein bound Ca²⁺ + Complexed Ca²⁺
(2.2–2.6 mmol/L) (1.1–1.3 mmol/L) (0.9–1.0 mmol/L) (0.2–0.3 mmol/L)

Fig. 25.2 **Circulating calcium fractions.** The three forms of circulating calcium.

clinical situations it is important to calculate the 'adjusted calcium' – total serum calcium, adjusted for the patient's prevailing albumin concentration. This is achieved by means of a formula utilizing the population mean albumin concentration of 40 g/L (4 g/dL):

$$\text{Adjusted Ca}^{2+} = \text{measured Ca (mmol/L)} \\ + 0.02(40 - \text{albumin [g/L]})$$

Hormonal control of calcium homeostasis

Parathyroid hormone

Parathyroid hormone responds to changes in ionized calcium and phosphate

When plasma calcium decreases, PTH is released from the parathyroid glands, stimulating osteoclast-mediated bone resorption, reabsorption of calcium at the kidney, and absorption of calcium at the small intestine (mediated by $1,25(OH)_2D_3$). PTH secretion is in turn regulated by calcium, completing the homeostatic loop: an increase in calcium decreases PTH secretion. It also stimulates calcitonin release from the thyroid, which inhibits resorption of bone (Fig. 25.3).

PTH is an 84-amino acid, single-chain peptide hormone secreted by the chief cells of the parathyroid glands. A decrease in extracellular ionized calcium or an increase in serum phosphate concentration stimulates its secretion, chronic severe magnesium deficiency can inhibit its release from secretory vesicles, and low concentrations of $1,25(OH)_2D_3$ interfere with its synthesis. $PTH_{(1-84)}$ is mainly metabolized into a biologically active $PTH_{(1-34)}$ amino-terminal fragment and an inactive carboxy-terminal fragment, $PTH_{(35-84)}$ (Fig. 25.4). Most of the classic cellular actions of PTH are mediated by cAMP, which is generated through G-protein stimulated adenylyl cyclase.

Calcium-sensing receptor is a cell-surface G-protein receptor

Ionized calcium is maintained within a narrow range through an extracellular calcium-sensing receptor (CaSR) that is a cell surface G-protein (see box on p. 160 and Fig. 40.2) coupled receptor present in the chief cells of the parathyroid gland, the thyroidal C-cells and along the kidney tubules. Minute changes in ionized calcium modulate cellular function to maintain normocalcemia.

Vitamin D

Vitamin D is synthesized in the skin by UV radiation

The synthesis and metabolism of vitamin D are illustrated in Figure 25.5. Vitamin D_2 (ergocalciferol) is synthesized in the skin by UV radiation of ergosterol. Vitamin D_3 (cholecalciferol) is derived also by UV irradiation from 7-dehydrocholesterol in the skin of animals. Vitamin D_3 and its hydroxylated metabolites are transported in the plasma bound to a specific globulin, vitamin D-binding protein (DBP). The affinity of cholecalciferol for DBP is low but that for D_3 is high, thus ensuring the movement of D_3 from the skin to the circulation. Vitamin D_3 is also found in the diet where its absorption is associated with other fats, and it is transported to the liver in chylomicrons. It is released from chylomicrons in the liver by DBP and hydroxylated at the 25-position forming 25-hydroxycholecalciferol (($25(OH)D_3$, calcidiol).

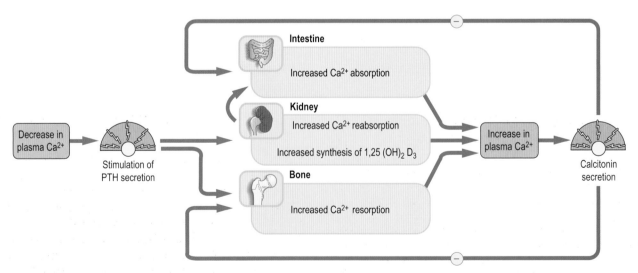

Fig. 25.3 **Major hormones influencing calcium homeostasis.** A decrease in plasma ionized calcium stimulates release of PTH; this promotes Ca^{2+} reabsorption from the kidney, resorption from bone, and absorption by the gut via increased production of $1,25(OH)_2D_3$. As a result, plasma calcium increases. Conversely, an increase in plasma ionized calcium stimulates release of calcitonin, which inhibits reabsorption of calcium by the kidney and osteoclast-mediated bone resorption.

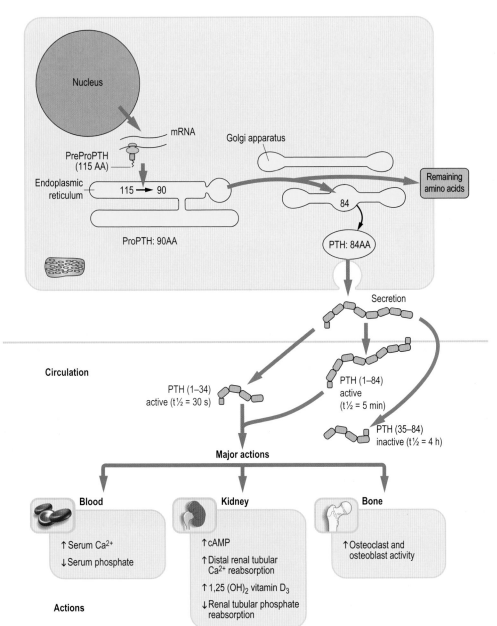

Fig. 25.4 **Synthesis and major actions of the parathyroid hormone (PTH)**. PTH mobilizes calcium from all available sources and decreases its renal excretion. AA: amino acids.

MEASUREMENT OF PARATHYROID HORMONE

Intact $PTH_{(1-84)}$ is the most important biologically active form of PTH, and can be measured by specific immunoradiometric assays (IRMAs) without interference from its amino- or carboxy-terminal fragments. These assays utilize a double-antibody technique, with a capture antibody directed against one end of the intact molecule, and the labeled detection antibody directed against the opposite end of the molecule. Only the full-length, 1-84 amino acid molecule can bind to the two antibodies, which means that fragments of PTH produced during its metabolism (Fig. 25.2) are not measured by these assays.

25-hydroxycholecalciferol (25(OH)D₃) is the main liver storage form of vitamin D

The 25-hydroxylation step is carried out by a hepatic microsomal enzyme and is the rate-limiting step in conversion of vitamin D_3 to its active metabolite. The hepatic content of $25(OH)D_3$ regulates the rate of 25-hydroxylation. $25(OH)D_3$ is the major form of the vitamin found in both the liver and the circulation, in each case bound to DBP, and its levels in the circulation reflect hepatic stores of the vitamin. A significant proportion of $25(OH)D_3$ is subject to enterohepatic circulation, being excreted in the bile and reabsorbed in the small bowel. Disturbance in the enterohepatic circulation can lead to deficiency of this vitamin.

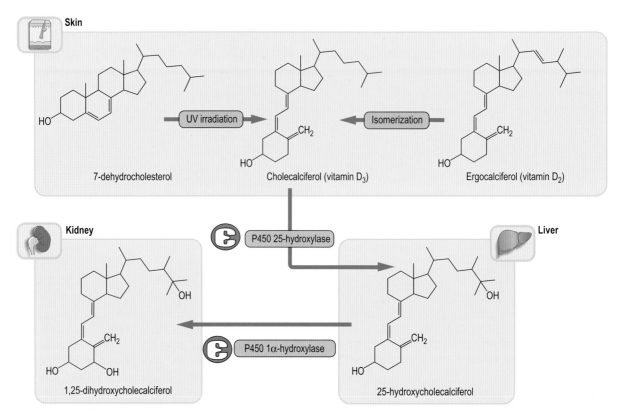

Fig. 25.5 **Vitamin D metabolism.** Vitamin D is mainly synthesized in response to the action of sunlight on the skin; a smaller component comes from the diet. Normal liver and kidney function are essential to the formation of the active form $1,25(OH)_2D_3$. Plasma calcium concentration controls the level of $1,25(OH)_2D_3$ through the parathyroid hormone. $1,25(OH)_2D_3$, 1,25-dihydroxycholecalciferol, calcitriol.

The active metabolite of vitamin D is 1α,25-dihydroxy-cholecalciferol $(1,25(OH)_2D_3)$

The main site for further hydroxylation of the $25(OH)D_3$ at the 1-position are the renal tubules, although bone and the placenta can also carry out this reaction. The $25(OH)D_3$ 1α-hydroxylase is a mitochondrial enzyme. The product, $1,25(OH)_2D_3$ (calcitriol) is the most potent of the vitamin D metabolites and the only naturally occurring form of vitamin D that is active at physiologic concentrations. The 1α-hydroxylase activity is stimulated by PTH, low serum concentrations of phosphate or calcium, vitamin D deficiency, calcitonin, growth hormone, prolactin, and estrogen. Conversely, the activity of 1α-hydroxylase is feedback inhibited by $1,25(OH)_2D_3$, hypercalcemia, high phosphate and hypoparathyroidism.

The renal tubules, cartilage, intestine, and placenta also contain a 24-hydroxylase, producing the inactive 24,25-dihydroxycholecalciferol $(24,25[OH]_2D_3$; 24(R)-hydroxycalcidiol). The level of the $24,25[OH]_2D_3$ in the circulation is reciprocally related to the level of the $1,25(OH)_2D_3$.

$1,25(OH)_2D_3$ is transported in plasma, also bound to DBP. Since it affects Ca^{2+} transport and metabolism at a distance, vitamin D may be described as a hormone. In the intestinal epithelial cells it binds to a cytoplasmic receptor like other steroid hormones (see Chapter 17 and Chapter 34) and this

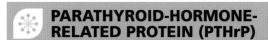

PARATHYROID-HORMONE-RELATED PROTEIN (PTHrP)

PTHrP is synthesized as three isoforms containing 139, 141, and 173 amino acids, as a result of alternative differential splicing of RNA. There is amino-terminal sequence homology with PTH: eight of the first 13 amino acids are identical in PTHrP and PTH, three are identical within residues 14-34, and a further three are identical within residues 35-84. Activation of the classic PTH receptor is by the amino-terminal portion of both PTH and PTHrP, and there is a common α-helical secondary structure in the binding domain of both peptides. As a result of this structural similarity, PTHrP possesses many of the biologic actions of PTH.

There is, to date, little evidence to suggest that PTHrP has a role in normal adult calcium homeostasis, but evidence from animal models indicates that it is important in regulating fetal calcium homeostasis and skeletal development. Deletion of the PTHrP gene results in either severe skeletal abnormalities (heterozygotes) or a lethal mutation (homozygotes). PTHrP has an important role in the etiology of hypercalcemia associated with malignancy (HCM) (see below). PTHrP is subject to posttranslational processing, producing fragments with biologic activities that have yet to be characterized. The structural and functional relationships of PTHrP as they are currently understood are summarized in Figure 25.7.

ligand–protein complex is transported to the nucleus where $1,25(OH)_2D_3$ induces gene expression affecting calcium metabolism.

$1,25(OH)_2D_3$ increases serum concentrations of calcium and phosphate

$1,25(OH)_2D_3$ increases the absorption of calcium and phosphate from the gut via active transport by calcium-binding proteins. Together with PTH, it stimulates bone resorption by osteoclasts. These effects increase serum calcium and phosphate concentrations. Low $1,25(OH)_2D_3$ causes abnormal mineralization of newly formed osteoid. This is a result of low calcium and phosphate availability and reduced osteoblast function, which result in rickets (in infants and children) or osteomalacia (in adults).

Calcitonin inhibits osteoclastic bone resorption

Calcitonin is a 32-amino acid peptide synthesized and secreted primarily by the parafollicular cells of the thyroid gland (C-cells). Its secretion is regulated acutely by serum calcium through the calcium-sensing receptor (CaSR): an increase in serum calcium results in a proportional increase in calcitonin, and a decrease elicits a corresponding reduction in calcitonin. Chronic stimulation results in exhaustion of the secretory reserve of the C-cells. The precise biologic role of calcitonin is not known, but the main effect is inhibition of osteoclastic bone resorption. There is significant species homology for calcitonin, with a 1-7 amino-terminal disulfide bridge, a glycine residue at position 28, and a carboxy-terminal proline amide residue. Basic amino acid substitutions enhance potency; because of this, salmon and eel calcitonins have increased biologic activity in mammalian systems, compared with that of endogenous calcitonin.

Calcium is absorbed in the small intestine and is excreted in urine and feces

Calcium is absorbed predominantly in the proximal small intestine; this is regulated through the quantity of calcium ingested in the diet, and two cellular calcium transport processes:

- active saturable transcellular absorption which is stimulated by $1,25(OH)_2D_3$
- nonsaturable paracellular absorption which is controlled by the concentration of calcium in the intestinal lumen relative to the serum concentration.

In a normal adult taking a Western diet, calcium balance is maintained: the amount of calcium intake and its deposition in bone are exactly matched by the excretion in urine and feces. During growth, a child will be in positive calcium balance, whereas elderly and individuals suffering from several diseases may be in negative calcium balance. Reduced or increased calcium absorption reflects alterations in dietary calcium intake, intestinal calcium solubility, and vitamin D metabolism.

Generally, as serum calcium increases, calcium excretion increases. When hypercalcemia is caused by hyperparathyroidism (HPT), PTH will act on the renal tubule, promoting reabsorption of filtered calcium and thus diminishing the effects of the increased filtration of calcium and inhibition of renal tubular reabsorption that are caused by increased serum calcium. Decreasing serum calcium is associated with a reduction in urinary excretion of calcium, mainly as a result of decreased amounts of filtered calcium. In hypoparathyroid patients, who lack PTH secretion, renal tubular reabsorption of calcium is reduced.

Other hormones also affect calcium homeostasis

Several hormones directly or indirectly affect calcium homeostasis and skeletal metabolism.

Thyroid hormone stimulates osteoclast-mediated resorption of bone. Adrenal and gonadal steroids, particularly estrogen in women and testosterone in men, have important regulatory effects, increasing osteoblast and decreasing osteoclast function. They also decrease renal calcium and phosphate excretion and intestinal calcium excretion.

Growth hormone has anabolic effects on bone, promoting the growth of the skeleton. These effects are believed to be mediated by insulin-like growth factors (IGF-1 and IGF-2) acting on cells of the osteoblast lineage. Growth hormone increases the urinary excretion of calcium and hydroxyproline, whilst decreasing the urinary excretion of phosphate.

DISORDERS OF CALCIUM AND BONE METABOLISM

Hypercalcemia

Hypercalcemia is most commonly caused either by primary hyperparathyroidism or by malignancy

In practice, 90% of cases are due to either primary HPT or malignancy; a greater diagnostic challenge is presented when it becomes necessary to differentiate occult malignancy from the less common causes of hypercalcemia (Table 25.2). There is a wide individual variation in the development of symptoms and signs of hypercalcemia (Fig. 25.6).

Investigation of hypercalcemia

In the majority of cases, the cause of hypercalcemia will be identified by obtaining an accurate history, by clinical examination, and by appropriate biochemical tests. In some cases, however, additional valuable information on causation may be obtained from radiologic investigations and tissue biopsies. The development and ready availability of specific, sensitive, and reliable assays for intact PTH have enabled the clinician to discriminate primary HPT from nonparathyroid causes of hypercalcemia (particularly malignancy): an increased or inappropriately detectable intact PTH in the presence of hypercalcemia is observed in primary HPT, whereas an intact PTH below the limit of detection of the assay is usually observed in nonparathyroid causes of hypercalcemia.

Several laboratory tests may be required to differentiate the various nonparathyroid causes of hypercalcemia

In a high percentage of cases, hypercalcemia associated with malignancy is caused by tumors secreting parathyroid hormone-related protein (PTHrP) (Fig. 25.7; see also box on p. 344). Vitamin D excess or overdose may be obvious from the history, but sometimes only becomes apparent after measurement of the concentrations of vitamins D_3 (cholecalciferol), D_2 (ergocalciferol), and $1,25(OH)_2D_3$. Measurement of serum electrolytes, urea, and creatinine will confirm renal failure, and estimation of protein, albumin, and immunoglobulins may indicate the presence of myeloma (Chapter 4), which should be investigated by both serum and urine electrophoresis. Thyroid function tests (measurement of thyroid-stimulating hormone, total thyroxine, and total tri-iodothyronine) or estimation of free thyroid hormone

(see Chapter 39) enable diagnosis of thyrotoxic hypercalcemia. Rare causes of hypercalcemia may be diagnosed by estimation of lithium (toxicity or overdose), growth hormone (acromegaly), vitamin A (toxicity), and urine catecholamines (pheochromocytoma, see Chapter 42).

Primary hyperparathyroidism (HPT) is relatively common

Primary HPT is a relatively common endocrine disease, characterized by hypercalcemia associated with an increased or inappropriate concentration of intact PTH. It has an incidence ranging from 1 in 500 to 1 in 1000 of the population. In 80–85% of patients, a solitary parathyroid gland adenoma is present, and the condition is curable by successful removal of the adenoma.

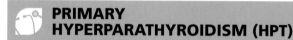

PRIMARY HYPERPARATHYROIDISM (HPT)

A 52-year-old woman presented to the accident and emergency department of her local hospital with severe right-sided flank pain. Blood was detected on stick testing of urine and radiography revealed the presence of kidney stones. The pain settled with opiate analgesia. Further questioning revealed a history of recent depression, generalized weakness, recurrent indigestion, and aches in both hands. Serum adjusted calcium was 3.20 mmol/L (12.8 mg/dL; normal range 2.2–2.6 mmol/L, 8.8–10.4 mg/dL), serum phosphate 0.65 mmol/L (2.0 mg/dL; normal range 0.7–1.4 mmol/L, 2.2–5.6 mg/dL), and PTH 16.9 pmol/L (169 pg/mL; normal range 1.1–6.9 pmol/L, 11–69 pg/mL).

Comment. Most patients with primary HPT are now identified when asymptomatic hypercalcemia is discovered on routine biochemical testing or during investigation of nonspecific symptoms. When symptomatic, primary HPT classically affects the skeleton, kidneys, and gastrointestinal tract, resulting in the well-recognized triad of complaints described as 'bones, stones, and abdominal groans'. Kidney stone disease is now the most common presenting complaint.

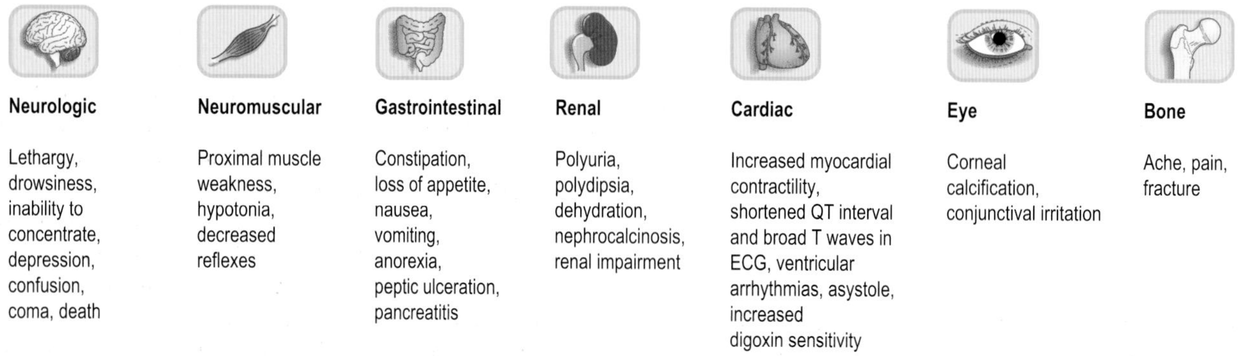

Causes of hypercalcemia	
Common causes	primary hyperparathyroidism
	malignant disease
	iatrogenic – vitamin D or vitamin D analogs
Uncommon causes	thyrotoxicosis
	multiple myeloma
	sarcoidosis
	drug-induced:
	thiazide diuretics
	lithium
	renal failure (acute and chronic)
	familial hypocalciuric hypercalcemia

Table 25.2 **Common and uncommon causes of hypercalcemia.**

Neurologic	Neuromuscular	Gastrointestinal	Renal	Cardiac	Eye	Bone
Lethargy, drowsiness, inability to concentrate, depression, confusion, coma, death	Proximal muscle weakness, hypotonia, decreased reflexes	Constipation, loss of appetite, nausea, vomiting, anorexia, peptic ulceration, pancreatitis	Polyuria, polydipsia, dehydration, nephrocalcinosis, renal impairment	Increased myocardial contractility, shortened QT interval and broad T waves in ECG, ventricular arrhythmias, asystole, increased digoxin sensitivity	Corneal calcification, conjunctival irritation	Ache, pain, fracture

Fig. 25.6 **Symptoms and signs of hypercalcemia.** Symptoms are more likely as the serum concentration of calcium increases.

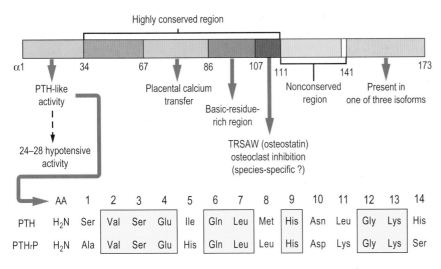

Fig. 25.7 **Parathyroid-hormone-related protein (PTHrP) synthesis, structure, and functional relationships**.

Hypercalcemia associated with malignancy (HCM)

Hypercalcemia tends to occur late in the course of malignant disease, and is usually a poor prognostic sign. Effective and relatively innocuous treatment for HCM is now available, and can markedly improve the quality of life of these patients, by relieving the symptoms of hypercalcemia.

Treatment of hypercalcemia can greatly improve the quality of life of patients

Symptomatic hypercalcemia or serum calcium concentrations exceeding 3.00 mmol/L (12 mg/dL) would merit treatment. Dehydration results from hypercalcemia-induced polyuria, reduced fluid and food intake, associated vomiting, decreased arginine-vasopressin activity (AVP, Chapter 23) at the distal tubule, and reduced renal perfusion. Fluid replacement corrects hypovolemia and provides a moderate sodium load, which will cause a concomitant increase in calcium excretion. Bisphosphonates (Fig. 25.8) have improved the management of HCM, and are the most effective drugs available for treating hypercalcemia. This group of drugs have their major effects by inhibiting osteoclast activity immediately when infused, and then exert a more prolonged effect by being incorporated into bone matrix in a position normally occupied by pyrophosphate. Calcitonin also inhibits osteoclast activity directly, and decreases renal tubular reabsorption of calcium; downregulation of calcitonin receptors subsequently occurs, and so the calcium-lowering effect lasts only 4–5 days.

Two major mechanisms of HCM are recognized

Calcium reabsorption by the kidney is often enhanced in HCM, interfering with the ability of the kidneys to limit the increased release of serum calcium that results from increased

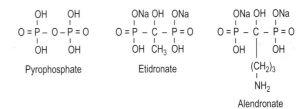

Fig. 25.8 **Structural formulae of pyrophosphate and bisphosphonates.** The P-C-P bonds of the biphosphonates can resist enzymic cleavage, and the potency of these drugs is determined by the chemical sequence attached to the carbon molecule.

osteoclast activity. There are two main sources of stimulation of the osteoclasts:

- a circulating humoral factor secreted by the tumor
- a locally active secretory factor(s) produced by the tumor or metastases in bone.

Current evidence indicates that the most common cause of HCM is the production, by tumors or their metastases, of PTHrP (see above), that can circulate in blood and exert its effects on the skeleton and kidneys. Production of PTHrP is common in breast, lung, kidney or other solid tumors, but is more rare in hematologic, gastrointestinal, and head and neck malignancies. The amino-terminal portion of PTHrP possesses PTH-like activity that results in hypercalcemia, hypophosphatemia, phosphaturia, increased renal calcium reabsorption, and osteoclast activation.

The second type of hypercalcemia is the result of increased bone resorption by osteoclasts stimulated by factors produced by the primary tumor or, more usually, by metastases, that stimulate osteoclasts by alteration of the RANKL/OPG balance. Mediators such as PTHrP, cytokines, and growth factors (e.g. IL-1, TNF-α, lymphotoxin, and TGF-α) have all

HYPOCALCEMIA IN THE NEONATE

A healthy full-term boy aged 7 days and weighing 3.5 kg was noted by the community midwife to be jittery and feeding poorly at home. On review by the pediatrician, the blood calcium was measured and found to be 1.55 mmol/L (6.2 mg/dL). The child responded to calcium supplementation and vitamin D.

Comment. Postnatal hypocalcemia is common, with most levels being above 1.75 mmol/L. In the first 36 hours of life, calcium levels fall as the relatively higher maternal levels switch the fetal parathyroid gland off. After 2 days, the concentration increases again.

Where a more profound drop in calcium is present, and particularly when it is at the end of the first week of life, other causes may be found. Here the possibilities include primary hypoparathyroidism, maternal hyperparathyroidism with hypercalcemia, and maternal vitamin D deficiency. Thus, investigations of the neonate and mother are required.

Causes of hypocalcemia		
Hypoparathyroid	**Nonparathyroid**	**PTH resistance**
postoperative	vitamin D deficiency	pseudohypoparathyroidism
idiopathic	malabsorption	hypomagnesemia
acquired hypomagnesemia	liver disease	
neck irradiation	renal disease	
anticonvulsant therapy	vitamin D resistance hypophosphatemia	

Table 25.3 **Causes of hypocalcemia.**

been shown to possess osteoclast-stimulating activity that results in significant bone resorption. Production of prostaglandins, especially those of the E series (PGE_2), has been demonstrated in several classes of tumor, particularly breast cancer. Prostaglandins stimulate osteoclastic bone resorption, and infusion of high concentrations of prostaglandins results in hypercalcemia.

Excess of vitamin D is toxic

Increasing therapeutic use of potent vitamin D analogs, hydroxylated at position 1 or at positions 1 and 25, make vitamin D toxicity the third most common cause of hypercalcemia.

Hypocalcemia

It is important to adjust serum calcium concentration for the concentration of albumin

Many acute and chronic illnesses lead to a decrease in serum albumin, which in turn decreases serum total calcium concentration. It is important that adjusted calcium is calculated in clinical situations. A serum-adjusted calcium that is below the reference range (<2.20 mmol/L; 8.8 mg/dL) may occur commonly in clinical practice. Changes in ionized calcium can result from pH changes in plasma, particularly alkalemia (Chapter 24), which increases the protein binding of calcium, causing decreased concentrations of ionized calcium.

Clinical signs of hypocalcemia are, in the main, due to neuromuscular irritability and are more obvious and severe when the onset of hypocalcemia is acute. In some cases, this irritability may be demonstrated by eliciting specific clinical

signs. Chvostek's sign is the presence of twitching of the muscles around the mouth (circumoral muscles) in response to tapping the facial nerve anterior to the ear, and Trousseau's sign is the typical contraction of the hand in response to reduced blood flow in the arm induced by inflation of a blood pressure cuff. Numbness, tingling, cramps, tetany and even seizures may be stimulated by hypocalcemia.

Hypocalcemia may be due to a low PTH concentration, secondary hyperparathyroidism or to tissue resistance to PTH

Causes of hypocalcemia can be divided into those associated with low $PTH_{(1-84)}$, those in which the decreased serum calcium results in secondary HPT, and rare cases in which there is PTH resistance (Table 25.3). Development of hypocalcemia indicates that the normal physiologic compensatory mechanisms controlled by PTH have failed and there are disturbed fluxes of calcium between bone, kidney, and intestine.

Hypoparathyroidism

The most common cause of hypoparathyroidism is as a complication of neck surgery, particularly that for pharyngeal or laryngeal tumors, thyroid disease, or parathyroid disease.

Pseudohypoparathyroidism

The group of pseudohypoparathyroidism (PHP) syndromes is characterized by hypocalcemia, hyperphosphatemia, and increased concentrations of $PTH_{(1-84)}$ (markedly increased in some patients).

The classic type of PHP is due to end-organ resistance to PTH, caused by a genetic defect resulting in an abnormal regulatory subunit of the G-protein of the adenylate cyclase complex. Confirmation of the diagnosis is made by demonstrating a lack of increase in plasma or urinary cAMP in response to the infusion of PTH.

✻ MAGNESIUM IN HYPOPARATHYROIDISM

Patients with a low plasma magnesium concentration develop a state of functional hypoparathyroidism and end-organ resistance to PTH; these patients tend not to respond to treatment with calcium supplementation alone. Secretion of PTH from the parathyroid gland requires a finite amount of magnesium to allow fusion of the secretory granules with the membrane and release of PTH (see Fig. 25.4); thus, in order to restore normal parathyroid gland function and normocalcemia, magnesium supplementation is essential.

Abnormal metabolism of vitamin D

Hypocalcemia resulting from abnormalities in vitamin D metabolism can be due to vitamin D deficiency, acquired or inherited disorders of vitamin D metabolism, and vitamin D resistance.

In addition, tissue insensitivity to $1,25(OH)_2D_3$ results in the characteristic findings of hypocalcemia, secondary HPT, and increased $11,25(OH)_2D_3$. Individually or in combination, the most common causes of vitamin D deficiency are:

- **reduced exposure to sunlight:** this is common in institutionalized elderly persons and immigrants to Western Europe from the Middle East or Indian subcontinent who wear traditional dress
- **poor dietary intake:** most Western diets contain sufficient vitamin D, but diets such as strict vegetarian or lactovegetarian have inadequate vitamin D content and, in the long term, may result in deficiency
- **malabsorption** of vitamin D may be caused by celiac disease, Crohn's disease, pancreatic insufficiency, inadequate bile salt secretion, and nontropical sprue (see Chapter 10).

Abnormalities of vitamin D metabolism are observed, among others, in patients with liver disease (deficient 25-hydroxylation, malabsorption), and renal failure (1α-hydroxylase deficiency).

METABOLIC BONE DISEASE

Osteoporosis is a common age-related disease of bone

Osteoporosis can be defined as a significant reduction of bone mineral density compared with age- and sex-matched norms, with an increased susceptibility to fractures. Osteoporosis is associated with aging and, with increasing longevity, a greater percentage of the population will become susceptible to osteoporosis and its sequelae. Bone density decreases from a peak achieved by the age of 30 years in men and women, and the rate of bone loss is accelerated in women after loss of estrogen secretion at the menopause. The progressive loss of bone that takes place with aging is a result of uncoupling of bone turnover over a prolonged period of time, with a relative increase of bone resorption or decrease in bone formation. A number of factors have been recognized as contributing to an increased risk of osteoporosis (Fig. 25.9). Seventy million people worldwide are at risk of osteoporosis.

There is much debate on the best therapeutic approach to osteoporosis, and many questions are raised about the possibility of detecting 'fast bone losers' by measuring biochemical markers of bone metabolism. Most of the available treatments decrease osteoclast activity and are therefore antiresorptive, but new therapies are available such as nightly subcutaneous injections of $PTH_{(1-34)}$ that have an anabolic action, stimulating osteoblast activity and new bone formation.

Paget's disease of bone is a disorder characterized by areas of accelerated bone turnover initiated by increased osteoclast-mediated bone resorption

Osteoclasts in Paget's disease are large, numerous, and multinucleate (up to 100 nuclei); their activity is coupled to increased osteoblast number and activity. A common biochemical abnormality in this disease is increased alkaline phosphatase, which is indicative of increased osteoblast activity. Increased collagen breakdown by osteoclasts results in a high serum and urine concentration of hydroxyproline, pyridinolines, and telopeptides. The bisphosphonates (see

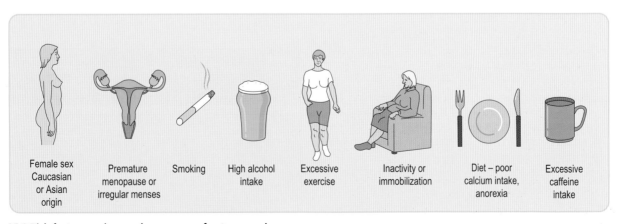

Female sex Caucasian or Asian origin   Premature menopause or irregular menses   Smoking   High alcohol intake   Excessive exercise   Inactivity or immobilization   Diet – poor calcium intake, anorexia   Excessive caffeine intake

Fig. 25.9 **Risk factors and secondary causes of osteoporosis.**

TREATMENT OF METABOLIC BONE DISEASE

Estrogen has a pivotal role in the maintenance of bone mass in women. An increased rate of osteoclast-mediated bone loss is observed immediately after the menopause, as a result of ovarian failure and the decrease in estrogen secretion. This can be prevented by hormone replacement therapy (HRT), which can be given as cyclical or continuous combined estrogen and progesterone in women with an intact uterus, or as estrogen alone in women who have had their uterus surgically removed (by hysterectomy). The Women's Health Initiative (WHI) trial established an excess of adverse events including increased breast cancer, thromboembolic disease, stroke and cardiovascular events in women receiving greater than 5 years of continuous combined HRT. Although short-term therapy is valuable for menopausal symptoms, long-term use of this type of HRT is no longer recommended as prophylaxis or treatment for osteoporosis.

Other treatments that are recommended are bisphosphonates, selective estrogen receptor modulators (SERMs), nightly injections of PTH, calcitonin and, in elderly patients, calcium with vitamin D supplementation.

OSTEOPOROSIS: A WOMAN WITH A SEVERE BACK PAIN

A 62-year-old woman was admitted to hospital because of sudden onset of severe back pain between the shoulder blades after a fall in her bathroom. Radiography detected a wedge fracture of two thoracic vertebrae with reduced bone density. A bone density scan or dual energy X-ray absorptiometry (DEXA) scan showed severely reduced density in femur and spine. She had experienced the menopause after a hysterectomy at age 41 years but had been unable to tolerate hormone replacement therapy (HRT). Biochemical investigations were all within normal limits.

Comment. Symptoms of osteoporosis develop at a late stage of the disease, and are often caused by the presence of fracture(s). Hip, vertebral, and wrist fractures are common in patients with osteoporosis, and result in significant mortality and morbidity. HRT can be used to prevent the development of bone loss in postmenopausal women but slightly increases the risk of stroke, heart attack and breast cancer.

OSTEOMALACIA: A WOMAN WITH GENERALIZED WEAKNESS AND WALKING DIFFICULTY

A 60-year-old woman who had become increasingly infirm and housebound was referred to the metabolic outpatient clinic. She had experienced a gradual onset of diffuse aches and pains throughout her skeleton but especially around the hips. She was having difficulty walking, had generalized weakness, and had recently experienced sudden severe pain in her ribs and pelvis. Radiography detected fractured ribs. Adjusted serum calcium was 2.1 mmol/L (8.4 mg/dL; normal range 2.2–2.6 mmol/L, 8.8–10.4 mg/dL), serum phosphate 0.56 mmol/L (1.7 mg/dL; normal range 0.7–1.4 mmol/L, 2.2–4.3 mg/dL), alkaline phosphatase 300 IU/L (normal range 50–260 IU/L) and PTH 12.6 pmol/L (normal range 1.1–6.9 pmol/L, 11–69 pg/mL).

Comment. In severe forms of osteomalacia, biochemical abnormalities are commonly seen, including low serum adjusted calcium, low serum phosphate, increased alkaline phosphatase and increased PTH$_{(1-84)}$. Clinically, patients may have diffuse bone pain or more specific pain related to a fracture, lateral bowing of the lower limbs, and a distinctive waddling gait. Ethnic groups with dark skin are particularly at risk in countries with low–average sunlight, as the majority of vitamin D in the body comes from synthesis by the action of UV light on 7-dehydrocholesterol. This may be exacerbated by traditional dress and a diet that is high in phytates (unleavened bread) and low in calcium and vitamin D.

Fig. 25.8) have significant antiosteoclastic activity, and are the drugs of first choice for treating Paget's disease.

Osteomalacia

The characteristic pathology in osteomalacia is the defective mineralization of osteoid in mature bone. When this occurs in the growing skeleton, there is also loss of maturation and mineralization of the cartilage cells at the growth plate; the term rickets is used to describe the clinical, radiologic, and pathologic findings seen in children. There are several diverse causes of osteomalacia, many related to abnormalities of vitamin D metabolism.

CENTRAL NERVOUS SYSTEM MAY BE INVOLVED IN THE REGULATION OF BONE METABOLISM

Recent data suggest that the central nervous system may also be involved in bone homeostasis. Leptin, an adipokine which regulates adipose tissue mass and controls appetite (see Chapter 22), has been shown to have an inhibitory effect on bone formation. Leptin-deficient animals display high bone mass. However, mutations in the signaling pathway stimulated by leptin have no effect on the bone mass, which suggest that it is a central effect, probably mediated by the sympathetic nervous system.

Summary

- Bone is a metabolically active tissue that undergoes constant remodeling.
- The major cells involved in the remodeling process are the osteoclast and osteoblast.
- Bone metabolism is closely interrelated with the metabolism of calcium which also involves the intestine and kidney.
- A calcium-sensing receptor present on the parathyroid, thyroid and kidney cells is pivotal in calcium regulation.
- The calcium balance is hormonally regulated by parathormone, vitamin D metabolites and calcitonin.

- The measurement of calcium in serum is an important test in clinical laboratories, because both hypercalcemia and hypocalcemia lead to clinical symptoms.
- Main causes of hypercalcaemia are primary hyperparathyroidism, malignancy and vitamin D excess.
- Osteoporosis, a decrease in bone density leading to bone fractures, is a major health problem.

ACTIVE LEARNING

1. Describe the RANK-RANKL signaling system in osteoclasts
2. Discuss factors that regulate osteoblast function.
3. Describe forms of calcium present in plasma. Which of them is biologically active?
4. Discuss the feedback mechanisms that maintain plasma calcium concentration.

Further reading

Boyle WJ, Simonet WS, Lacey DL. Osteoclast differentiation and activation. *Nature* 2003;**423**:337–341.

Buckley KA, Fraser WD. Receptor activator for nuclear factor kappaB ligand and osteoprotegrin: regulators of bone physiology and immune responses/potential therapeutic agents and biochemical markers. *Ann Clin Biochem* 2002;**39**:551–556.

Favus MJ (ed). *Primer on the metabolic bone disease and disorders of mineral metabolism*, 5th edn Washington, DC: American Society for Bone and Mineral Research, 2003.

Fraser WD. Paget's disease of bone. *CPD Rheumatology* 2001;**2**:8–13.

Harada S, Rodan GA. Control of osteoblast function and regulation of bone mass. *Nature* 2003;**423**:349–355.

Kronenberg HM. Developmental regulation of the growth plate. *Nature* 2003;**423**:332–336.

Richards JB, Rivadeneira F, Pastinen TM et al. Bone mineral density, osteoporosis, and osteoporotic fractures: a genome-wide association study. *Lancet* 2008;**371**:1505–1512.

Sambrook P, Cooper C. Osteoporosis. *Lancet* 2006;**367**:2010–2018.

26. Complex Carbohydrates: Glycoproteins

A D Elbein

LEARNING OBJECTIVES

After reading this chapter you should be able to:

■ Describe the general structures of oligosaccharides in various types of glycoproteins.

■ Outline the sequence of reactions involved in biosynthesis and processing of N-linked oligosaccharides to produce the various types of oligosaccharide chains.

■ Describe the role of N-linked oligosaccharides in protein folding, stability and cell–cell recognition.

■ Explain the importance of O-linked oligosaccharides in mucin function.

■ Describe how each of the monosaccharides involved in biosynthesis of N-linked and O-linked oligosaccharides is synthesized from glucose and activated for synthesis of glycoconjugates.

■ Distinguish lectins from other types of proteins and describe their role in physiology and pathology.

■ Describe several diseases that are associated with deficiencies in enzymes involved in synthesis, modification or degradation of complex carbohydrates.

INTRODUCTION

Many mammalian proteins are glycoproteins, i.e. they contain sugars covalently linked to specific amino acids in their structure. There are two major types of sugar-containing proteins that occur in animal cells, generally referred to as glycoproteins and proteoglycans. Along with glycolipids, which are presented in the next chapter, all these compounds are part of the group of sugar-containing macromolecules called glycoconjugates.

Glycoproteins (Fig. 26.1) have short glycan chains; they can have up to 20 sugars but usually contain between three and 15 sugars. These oligosaccharides are highly branched, they do not have a repeating unit, and they usually contain amino sugars (N-acetylglucosamine or N-acetylgalactosamine), neutral sugars (D-galactose, D-mannose, L-fucose) and the acidic sugar sialic acid (N-acetylneuraminic acid). Glycoproteins generally do not contain uronic acids, acidic sugars that are a major part of the proteoglycans. Glycoproteins usually contain much smaller amounts of carbohydrate than of protein, typically from just a few percent carbohydrate to 10–15% sugar by weight.

Proteoglycans (see Fig. 26.1 and Chapter 28) contain as much as 50–60% carbohydrate. In these molecules, the sugar chains are long, unbranched polymers that may contain hundreds of monosaccharides. These saccharide chains have a repeating disaccharide unit, generally made up of a uronic acid and an amino sugar.

Most proteins in cell surface membranes, that function as receptors for hormones or participate in other important membrane-associated processes such as cell–cell interactions, are glycoproteins. Many of the membrane proteins of the endoplasmic reticulum or Golgi apparatus, as well as those proteins that are secreted from cells, including serum and mucous proteins, are also glycoproteins. In fact, glycosylation is the major enzymatic modification of proteins in the body. Addition of sugars to a protein can occur either at the same time, and location, as protein synthesis is occurring in the endoplasmic reticulum, i.e. co-translationally, or following the completion of protein synthesis and after the protein has been transported to the Golgi apparatus, i.e. post-translationally. The functions of the carbohydrate chains of the resulting glycoproteins are diverse (Table 26.1).

STRUCTURES AND LINKAGES

Sugars are attached to specific amino acids in proteins

Sugars can be attached to protein in either N-glycosidic linkages or O-glycosidic linkages. N-glycosidically linked oligosaccharides are widespread in nature and are characteristic of membrane and secretory proteins. The attachment of these oligosaccharides to protein involves a glycosylamine linkage between an N-acetylglucosamine (GlcNAc) residue and the amide nitrogen of an asparagine residue (Fig. 26.2A). The asparagine that serves as an acceptor of this oligosaccharide must be in the consensus sequence Asn-X-Ser (Thr) in order to be recognized as the acceptor by the oligosaccharide transferring enzyme (see below). However, not all asparagine residues, even those in this consensus sequence, become glycosylated, indicating that other factors such as protein conformation or other properties of the protein may be involved.

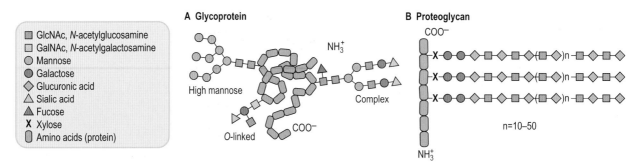

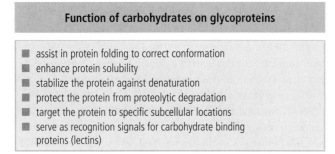

Fig. 26.1 **Generalized model of the structure of glycoproteins and proteoglycans.**

Function of carbohydrates on glycoproteins

- assist in protein folding to correct conformation
- enhance protein solubility
- stabilize the protein against denaturation
- protect the protein from proteolytic degradation
- target the protein to specific subcellular locations
- serve as recognition signals for carbohydrate binding proteins (lectins)

Table 26.1 **Function of carbohydrates on glycoproteins.**

O-linked oligosaccharides are most commonly found in proteins of mucous fluids, but also occur frequently on the same membrane and secretory proteins that contain the N-linked oligosaccharides. The *O*-linked chains typically contain three or more sugars in linear or branched chains, attached to protein by a glycosidic linkage between an N-acetylgalactosamine (GalNAc) residue and the hydroxyl group of either a serine or threonine residue on the protein (Fig. 26.2B; see Fig. 26.4). There does not appear to be a consensus sequence of amino acids for *O*-linked glycosylation, so it is not known why some serines (or threonines) become glycosylated but others do not.

A glucosyl-galactose disaccharide is frequently linked to the hydroxyl group of hydroxylysine residues in the fibrous protein, collagen (Fig. 26.2C). Hydroxylysine is an uncommon amino acid, found only in collagens and proteins with collagenous domains. Hydroxylysine is not directly incorporated into protein as such, but is produced by posttranslational hydroxylation of lysine residues. Lysine hydroxylase requires vitamin C as a cofactor, which is why vitamin C is frequently used to expedite wound healing. Collagen is first synthesized in the cell as a precursor form called procollagen. Procollagens are usually synthesized as N-linked glycoproteins, but the N-linked oligosaccharide is removed as part of that peptide that is cleaved from procollagen during its maturation to collagen. Only the *O*-linked disaccharides remain on the mature collagen molecule. The less glycosylated collagens tend to form ordered, fibrous structures, such as occur in tendons, while the more heavily glycosylated collagens are found in meshwork structures, such as basement membranes in the vascular wall and renal glomerulus (see Chapter 28).

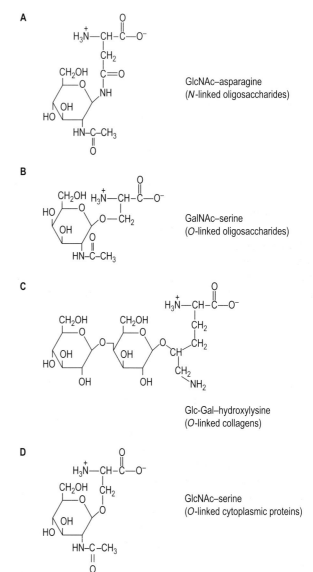

Fig. 26.2 **Various linkages of sugars to amino acids in glycoproteins.** GlcNAc, *N*-acetylglucosamine.

A single GlcNAc is found attached to the hydroxyl group of serines on a number of cytoplasmic proteins (Fig. 26.2D). The GlcNAc is linked to specific serine residues that normally become phosphorylated by protein kinases during hormonal

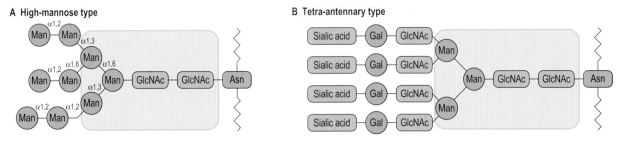

Fig. 26.3 **Typical structures of high-mannose and complex, *N*-linked oligosaccharides.** The core structure (shaded area) is common to both structures. Asn, asparagine; Gal, galactose; Man, mannose.

stimulation or other signaling events. The enzyme that adds the GlcNAc is widespread, but how it is controlled is still not clear. There is a second enzyme that removes the GlcNAc from the serines, similar to the contrasting regulatory roles of protein kinases and phosphatases. The GlcNAc addition may represent a mechanism that allows the cells to block phosphorylation of specific serine residues on selected proteins, while allowing others to still be phosphorylated. Then, the GlcNAc can be removed under appropriate conditions to allow phosphorylation.

One other amino acid that can serve as a site for glycosylation is tyrosine. The only example of this linkage is in the protein glycogenin, found at the core of glycogen (see Chapter 13). Glycogenin is a self-glucosylating protein that initially attaches a glucose to the hydroxyl group of one of its tyrosine residues. The protein then adds a number of other glucoses to the protein-linked glucose to make an oligosaccharide which serves as the acceptor for glycogen synthase.

N-linked oligosaccharides have either 'high-mannose' or 'complex' structures built on a common core

Although there are a large number of different carbohydrate structures produced by living cells, most of the oligosaccharides on glycoconjugates have many sugars and glycosidic linkages in common. All *N*-linked glycoproteins have oligosaccharide chains that are branched structures having a common core of three mannose residues and two GlcNAc residues (Fig. 26.3A and B), but differing considerably beyond the core region to give high-mannose and complex types of chains. The reason for this similarity in structure is that the high-mannose type of *N*-linked oligosaccharide is the biosynthetic precursor for all other *N*-linked oligosaccharides. As indicated below (see Fig. 26.10), the oligosaccharide is initially assembled on a carrier lipid in the endoplasmic reticulum as a high-mannose structure, then transferred to protein. It may remain as a high mannose structure, especially in lower organisms, but in animals the oligosaccharide undergoes a number of processing steps in the endoplasmic reticulum and Golgi apparatus that involve removal of some mannoses and addition of other sugars. As a result, beyond the core region, the oligosaccharides give rise to a vast array of structures that are referred to as high-mannose (Fig. 26.3A), and complex chains (Fig. 26.3B).

Complex oligosaccharides are so named because of their more complex sugar composition, including galactose, sialic acid and L-fucose. Complex chains have terminal trisaccharide sequences composed of sialic acid-galactose-GlcNAc attached to each of the branched core mannoses (Fig. 26.3A). L-Fucose may also be found attached to the core GlcNAc (see Fig. 26.1A) or in place of the sialic acids in the terminal trisaccharide sequences. In common with sialic acid, fucose is usually a terminal sugar on oligosaccharides; that is, no other sugars are attached to it. Some of the complex oligosaccharides have two trisaccharide sequences, one attached to each of the branched core mannoses, and are therefore called biantennary complex chains, whereas others have three (triantennary) or four (tetra-antennary) of the trisaccharide structures (Fig. 26.3B). More than 100 different complex oligosaccharide structures have now been identified on various cell surface proteins, providing great diversity as mediators of cellular recognition and chemical signaling events.

General structures of glycoproteins

A glycoprotein may have a single *N*-linked oligosaccharide chain or it may have several of these types of oligosaccharides. Furthermore, the *N*-linked oligosaccharides may all have identical structures or they may be quite different in structure. For example, the influenza virus coat glycoproteins, hemagglutinin and neuraminidase, are both *N*-linked glycoproteins which usually have seven *N*-linked oligosaccharide chains, of which five are biantennary complex chains and two are high-mannose structures. Thus, a range of related structures is commonly found in a single glycoprotein and, in fact, multiple different structures may also be found at a single site on a glycoprotein. Microheterogeneity of oligosaccharide structures results from incomplete processing on some chains during their biosynthesis (see Fig. 26.11). As a result, some of the oligosaccharides on a glycoprotein may be complete complex chains whereas others may be only partially processed. Oligosaccharides nearer to the amino terminus are more highly processed, perhaps because they are the earliest to be added to the protein, whereas those near the carboxy terminus are more likely to be high-mannose oligosaccharides. However, other factors such as protein conformation must also be important, since some high-mannose oligosaccharides do not undergo processing regardless of conditions.

Many N-linked glycoproteins also contain O-linked oligosaccharides of the type shown in Figure 26.4. The number of O-linked oligosaccharides varies considerably depending on the protein and its function. For example, the low-density lipoprotein (LDL) receptor is present in plasma membranes of smooth muscle cells and fibroblasts, and functions to

bind and endocytose circulating LDL, as a source of dietary cholesterol. The LDL receptor has two N-linked oligosaccharides that are located near the LDL-binding domain, and a cluster of O-linked oligosaccharides near the membrane-spanning region. As shown in Figure 26.5, this receptor has a membrane-spanning region of hydrophobic amino acids, an extended region of amino acids on the external side of the plasma membrane that contains the cluster of O-linked oligosaccharides, and a functional domain that is involved in binding LDL (see Chapter 18). Although the two N-linked chains are near the functional domain, they do not play a

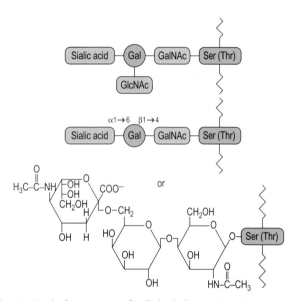

Fig. 26.4 **Typical structures of O-linked oligosaccharides.**

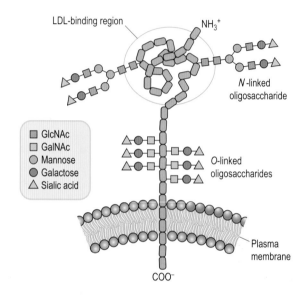

Fig. 26.5 **Model of the low-density lipoprotein (LDL) receptor.** (See also Chapter 18 and compare Fig. 18.2.)

✳ THE STRUCTURE OF N-LINKED OLIGOSACCHARIDES DEPENDS ON THE ENZYME COMPLEMENT OF THE CELL

The final structure of the N-linked oligosaccharide chain of a given glycoprotein is not coded in the genes for the proteins involved, but depends on the enzyme complement of the cell making that oligosaccharide. All cells appear to have the necessary enzymes to produce the lipid-linked saccharide precursor of the N-linked high-mannose chains, and can therefore glycosylate any membrane protein that has the appropriate asparagine in the right sequence and protein conformation. However, the glycosyl transferases and glycosidases involved in processing the oligosaccharide to its final complex structure are not so widely distributed, and a given glycosyltransferase may be present in one type of cell but not in another. For example, one cell type may have the GlcNAc transferase (GlcNAc TIII) necessary to attach a second GlcNAc on the 2-linked mannose to make a triantennary complex chain, whereas another cell may not have this GlcNAc transferase or the one to make a tetraantennary chain. Such a cell will only make biantennary chains. Enveloped viruses, such as the influenza virus or HIV, are examples of this

phenomenon, since their N-linked oligosaccharide structures reflect that of the cell in which they are grown; viruses use the cellular machinery to make all of their structures, and therefore their glycoproteins will have the same carbohydrate structures as that of the infected cell. For the virus this is beneficial since their proteins will not be recognized as foreign proteins and will escape immune surveillance. In addition, it allows the virus to attach to host cell receptors and fuse with host cell membranes by interacting with host lectins. In the biotechnology industry, this means that, although a given protein will have the identical amino acid sequence regardless of cell type, it will have different oligosaccharide structures, depending on the cell in which it is expressed. These differences in carbohydrate structure may affect the conformation and functional properties of the protein and limit its use for protein or enzyme replacement therapy. In fact, many cells used to express 'human' proteins are bioengineered to contain the complement of enzymes needed to properly glycosylate the target protein.

role in binding LDL. Instead, their function appears to be in helping the protein to fold into the proper conformation in the endoplasmic reticulum so that it can be translocated to the Golgi apparatus. The negatively charged O-linked chains, each having a sialic acid, are believed to function to keep the protein in an extended state, and to prevent it from folding back on itself.

Structure–function relationships in mucin glycoproteins

Mucins are glycoproteins that are secreted by epithelial cells lining the respiratory, gastrointestinal and genitourinary tracts. These proteins are very large in size with subunits having molecular weights of over one million daltons, and having as much as 80% of their weight as carbohydrate. Mucins are uniquely designed for their function, with about one-third of the amino acids being serines or threonines, and most of these being substituted with an O-linked oligosaccharide. Because most of these oligosaccharides carry a negatively charged sialic acid and these negative charges are in close proximity, they repel each other and prevent the protein from folding, causing it to remain in an extended state. Thus, the protein solution is highly viscous, forming a protective barrier on the epithelial surface, providing lubrication between surfaces and facilitating transport processes, such as the movement of food through the gastrointestinal system. There is a wide range of complex linear and branching oligosaccharide structures on mucins, including blood group

antigens (see Chapter 27). Some oligosaccharides participate in interaction and binding to various bacterial cell surfaces. This property may play a significant role in bacterial sequestration and elimination, limiting colonization and infection.

INTERCONVERSIONS OF DIETARY SUGARS

Normal cells can use glucose to make all the other sugars they need

Humans have a dietary requirement for some essential fatty acids and amino acids and vitamins (Chapter 11), but all the sugars that they need to make glycoconjugates can be synthesized from blood sugar, i.e. D-glucose. Figure 26.6 presents an overview of the sequence of reactions involved in interconversion of sugars in mammalian cells. All these sugar interconversion reactions involve sugar phosphates or sugar nucleotides.

Formation of galactose, mannose and fucose from glucose

Glucose is phosphorylated by hexokinase (or glucokinase in liver) as it enters the cell. Glucose-6-phosphate (Glc-6-P) can then be converted by a mutase (phosphoglucose mutase) to form Glc-1-P, which reacts with uridine 5'-triphosphate (UTP) to form UDP-Glc, catalyzed by the enzyme UDP-Glc

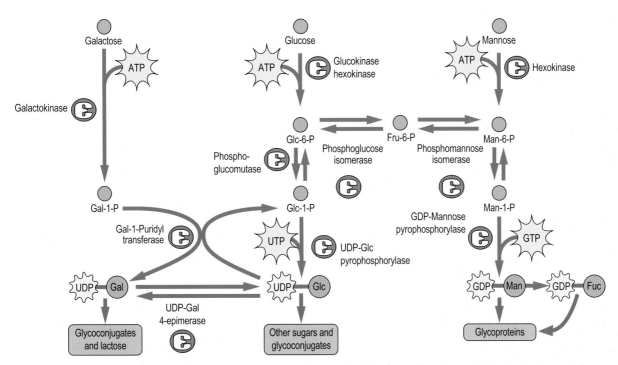

Fig. 26.6 **Interconversions of glucose, mannose, galactose, and their nucleotide sugars.** Fuc, fucose; Gal-1-P, galactose-1-phosphate; Glc-1-P, glucose-1-phosphate; Man-1-P, mannose-1-phosphate.

pyrophosphorylase. This enzyme is a pyrophosphorylase, named for the reverse reaction in which the phosphate of Glc-1-P acts to cleave the pyrophosphate bond of UTP to form UDP-Glc and pyrophosphate (PPi); cleavage of PPi by pyrophosphatase provides the driving force for the reaction. This is the same pathway used in liver and muscle for incorporation of glucose into glycogen. UDP-Glc is epimerized to UDP-galactose (UDP-Gal) by UDP-Gal 4-epimerase, providing UDP-Gal for synthesis of glycoconjugates.

Glc-6-P may also be converted to fructose-6-phosphate (Fru-6-P) by the glycolytic enzyme phosphoglucose isomerase, and Fru-6-P may be isomerized to mannose-6-phosphate (Man-6-P) by phosphomannose isomerase. The Man-6-P is then converted by a mutase (phosphomannose mutase) to Man-1-P, which condenses with GTP to form GDP-Man. GDP-Man is the form of mannose that is used in the formation of N-linked oligosaccharides and is also the precursor for the formation of activated fucose, GDP-L-fucose. Mannose is present in our diet in small amounts but it is not an essential dietary component, since it can be readily produced from glucose. However, dietary mannose can be phosphorylated by hexokinase to Man-6-P, then enter metabolism through phosphomannose isomerase.

Metabolism of galactose

Although normal animal cells can make all the galactose they need from glucose, galactose is still an important component of our diet because it is one of the sugars that make up the milk disaccharide, lactose. The pathway of galactose metabolism requires three enzymes (see Fig. 26.6). Dietary galactose is transported to the liver where it is phosphorylated

by a specific kinase, galactokinase, that attaches phosphate to the hydroxyl group on carbon 1, rather than carbon-6, to form galactose-1-phosphate (Gal-1-P). Humans lack a UDP-Gal pyrophosphorylase, so the conversion of Gal-1-P to Glc-1-P involves the participation of a sugar nucleotide, UDP-Glc. The enzyme Gal-1-P uridyltransferase catalyzes an exchange between UDP-Glc and Gal-1-P to form UDP-Gal and Glc-1-P (see Fig. 26.6). The Glc-1-P arising from galactose metabolism can by converted to Glc-6-P by phosphoglucomutase, and thus the original galactose molecule enters glycolysis.

UDP-Glc is present in only micromolar concentrations in cells so that its availability for galactose metabolism would be quickly exhausted were it not for the presence of a third enzyme, UDP-Gal-4-epimerase. This enzyme catalyzes the equilibrium between UDP-Glc and UDP-Gal, providing a constant source of UDP-Glc during galactose metabolism. The reactions catalyzed by (1) galactokinase, (2) Gal-1-P uridyltransferase, and (3) UDP-Gal 4-epimerase, are summarized below, illustrating the roundabout way by which galactose enters mainstream metabolic pathways.

(1) Gal + ATP → Gal-1-P + ADP
(2) Gal-1-P + UDP-Glc → Glc-1-P + UDP-Gal
(3) UDP-Gal UDP-Glc

Net: Gal + ATP → Glc-1-P + ADP

Metabolism of fructose

Another common sugar in the diet is fructose, which is a component of the disaccharide sucrose, or table sugar. Fructose can be metabolized by two pathways in cells as shown in Figure 26.7. Fructose can be phosphorylated by

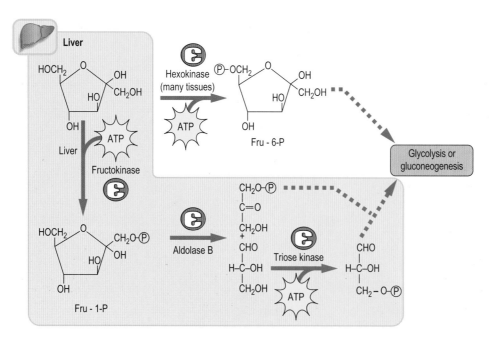

Fig. 26.7 **Metabolism of fructose by fructokinase or hexokinase.**

hexokinase, an enzyme that is present in all cells; however, hexokinase has a strong preference for glucose as a substrate, and glucose, which is present at a concentration of about 5 mmol/L in blood, is a strong competitive inhibitor of the phosphorylation of fructose. The primary pathway of fructose metabolism, which is especially important in liver after a meal, involves the enzyme fructokinase. This enzyme is a very specific kinase that phosphorylates fructose in carbon-1 (rather than the 6-position like hexokinase) to give fructose-1-phosphate (Fru-1-P). The liver aldolase is called aldolase B, and it is different in substrate specificity from the muscle aldolase A, because aldolase B can cleave both Fru-1-P and Fru-1,6-P$_2$, whereas aldolase A will only cleave Fru-1,6-P$_2$. Thus, in liver, the products of fructose cleavage are dihydroxyacetone-phosphate and glyceraldehyde

(not glyceraldehyde-3-P). The glyceraldehyde must then be phosphorylated by triose kinase in order to be metabolized in glycolysis.

It should be noted that in the liver, fructose enters glycolysis at the level of the triose phosphate intermediates, rather than as Fru-6-P as in muscle. Thus, in liver, the ingested fructose is not subject to regulation by the usual control points for regulatory enzymes, hexokinase and phosphofructokinase. By circumventing these two rate-limiting steps, fructose provides a rapid source of energy in both aerobic and anaerobic cells. This is part of the rationale behind the development of high-fructose drinks such as Gatorade®. The significance of the fructokinase, as opposed to the hexokinase, pathway of fructose metabolism is indicated by the pathology of hereditary fructose intolerance (see clinical box on p. 360).

BIOSYNTHESIS OF LACTOSE

Lactose synthase and α-lactalbumin

Lactose (galactosyl-α1,4-glucose) is synthesized from UDP-Gal and glucose in mammary glands during lactation. Lactose synthase is formed by the binding of α-lactalbumin to the galactosyl transferase that normally participates in biosynthesis of N-linked glycoproteins. α-Lactalbumin, which is expressed only in the mammary glands during lactation, converts galactosyl transferase to lactose synthase by lowering the enzyme's K_m for glucose by about three orders of magnitude, from 1 mol/L to 1 mmol/L, leading to preferential synthesis of lactose. α-Lactalbumin is the only known example of a 'specifier' protein that alters the substrate specificity of an enzyme.

GALACTOSEMIA: A BABY WHO DEVELOPED JAUNDICE AFTER BREAST FEEDING

An apparently normal newborn baby began to vomit and develop diarrhea after breast feeding. These problems, together with dehydration, continued for several days, when the child began to refuse food and developed jaundice indicative of liver damage, followed by hepatomegaly and then lens opacifications (cataracts). Measurement of glucose in the blood by a glucose oxidase assay (Chapter 3) indicated that the concentration of glucose was low, consistent with failure to absorb foods. However, glucose measured by a colorimetric method that measures total reducing sugar (i.e. any sugar that is capable of reducing copper) indicated that the concentration of sugar was quite high in both blood and urine. The reducing sugar that accumulated was eventually identified as galactose, indicating an abnormality in galactose metabolism known as galactosemia. This finding was consistent with the observation that, when milk was removed from the diet and replaced with an infant formula containing sucrose rather than

lactose, the vomiting and diarrhea stopped, and hepatic function gradually improved.

Comment. The accumulation of galactose in the blood most often is the result of a deficiency in the enzyme Gal-1-P uridyl transferase (classic form of galactosemia), which prevents the conversion of galactose to glucose and leads to the accumulation of Gal and Gal-1-P in tissues. The accumulated Gal-1-P interferes with phosphate and glucose metabolism, leading to widespread tissue damage, organ failure and mental retardation. In addition, accumulation of galactose in tissues results in galactose conversion, through the polyol pathway, to galactitol, which in the lens results in osmotic stress and development of cataracts (compare diabetic cataracts, Chapter 21). Another form of galactosemia is caused by galactokinase deficiency, but in this case Gal-1-P does not accumulate and complications are milder.

HEREDITARY FRUCTOSE INTOLERANCE: A CHILD WHO DEVELOPED HYPOGLYCEMIA AFTER EATING FRUIT

A child was brought into the emergency room suffering from nausea, vomiting and symptoms of hypoglycemia along with sweating, dizziness, and trembling. The parents indicated that these attacks occurred shortly after eating fruits (fructose) or candy (cane sugar). As a result of these symptoms, the child was developing a strong aversion to fruits so the mother was providing a large supplementation of multivitamin preparations. The child was below normal weight, but he had not exhibited any of the above unusual symptoms during the period of time when he was breast feeding, A series of clinical tests demonstrated some cirrhosis of the liver, and a normal glucose tolerance test. However, reducing substances were detected in the urine and these reducing substances did not react in the glucose oxidase test (i.e. they were not due to glucose). A fructose tolerance test was ordered using 3 g fructose/m^2 of body surface area, given intravenously in a single and rapid push. Within 30 minutes, the child displayed symptoms of hypoglycemia. Blood glucose confirmed this and revealed that the hypoglycemia was greatest after 60–90 min. Fructose concentrations reached a maximum (3.3 mmol/L) after 15 min and gradually decreased to zero by 3 h. Plasma phosphate concentration fell by 50% and tests for the enzymes alanine aminotransferase and aspartate aminotransferase indicated that they were elevated after about 90 min. The urine was also positive for fructose.

Comment. The results of a fructose tolerance test demonstrate the accumulation of fructose and its derivatives in blood and urine. The elevation of liver enzymes, alanine and aspartate aminotransferase, as well as jaundice and other symptoms indicate liver damage and suggest that Fru-1-P affects metabolism in a manner similar to that of Gal-1-P in galactosemia.

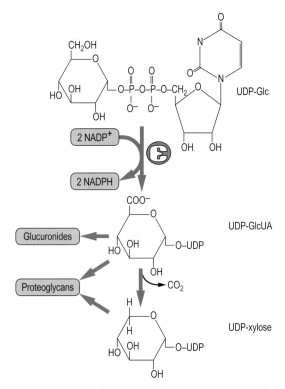

Fig. 26.8 **Conversion of UDP-Glc to UDP-glucuronic acid (UDP-GlcUA) and UDP-xylose.** Note that oxidation of UDP-Glc is a two-step reaction, from alcohol to aldehyde, then to an acid. Both reactions are catalyzed by UDP-Glc dehydrogenase.

29). UDP-GlcUA is also the precursor of UDP-xylose, a pentose sugar nucleotide. UDP-GlcUA undergoes a decarboxylation reaction that removes carbon-6 to form UDP-xylose, the activated form of xylose. Xylose is the linkage sugar between protein and glycan in proteoglycans. Xylose is also present on many plant glycoproteins, as part of their N-linked oligosaccharides, and is partly responsible for allergic reactions to peanut and nut proteins.

OTHER PATHWAYS OF SUGAR NUCLEOTIDE METABOLISM

UDP-glucose

UDP-Glc is the precursor of a number of other sugars, such as glucuronic acid, xylose and galactose, which are required for proteoglycan and/or glycoprotein synthesis. The reactions that lead to the formation of these other sugars are outlined in Figures 26.6 and 26.8. A two-step oxidation by the enzyme UDP-Glc dehydrogenase leads to the formation of the activated form of glucuronic acid (UDP-GlcUA). This sugar nucleotide is the donor of glucuronic acid, both for the formation of proteoglycans (see Chapter 28) and for the detoxification and conjugation reactions that occur in the liver to remove bilirubin, drugs and xenobiotics (see Chapter

Guanosine diphosphate-mannose (GDP-Man)

GDP-Man is the mannosyl donor for the mannose residues in the N-linked oligosaccharides. As shown in Figure 26.6, it is produced from Man-6-P and is also the precursor to GDP-L-fucose. Fucose is a 6-deoxyhexose that is an important sugar in many recognition reactions, such as inflammatory response (Fig. 26.9). The conversion of GDP-Man to GDP-fucose involves a complex series of oxidative and reductive steps, as well as epimerizations. Deficiencies in enzymes in the GDP-Man → GDP-fucose pathway are associated with a defective inflammatory response and increased susceptibility to infection. Leukocyte deficiency syndrome is caused by a defect in synthesis of the leukocyte recognition signal, sialyl Lewis-X structure (see Fig. 26.9).

CARBOHYDRATE-DEPENDENT CELL–CELL INTERACTIONS

An important example of carbohydrate-dependent cell–cell interactions occurs during inflammation. An injury, or infection, to the vascular endothelial cells elicts an inflammatory response that causes the release of cytokines (stimulatory proteins that affect cell migration) from the damaged tissue. These cytokines attract leukocytes to the site of injury or infection to remove the damaged tissue, or the invading organisms. These leukocytes must be able to stop or exit from the blood flow and attach to the injured tissue. They are able to do this because they have a carbohydrate recognition signal on their surface that is recognized by a lectin (carbohydrate-binding protein) that becomes exposed on the surface of the damaged endothelial cells. The carbohydrate signal is a tetrasaccharide called the sialyl Lewis-X antigen (Fig. 26.9), and this tetrasaccharide is a component of a glycoprotein or glycolipid on the surface of the leukocyte. The sialyl Lewis-X antigen is recognized by a lectin, E-selectin, that is located on the surface of the damaged endothelial cells. The interaction between these two enables the leukocytes to adhere to the vascular wall, even under the strong shear forces of the circulation. Figure 26.9 presents a model demonstrating the chemistry of this interaction. Selectins mediate the initial adhesive step, w hich is described as tethering, followed by rolling of leukocytes along the endothelial cell surface. In fact, leukocytes also contain a selectin, L-selectin, that probably interacts with a similar saccharide structure on the endothelial cell surface. These weak binding interactions enable leukocytes to stick to, then penetrate the interstitial layer and clean up the site of injury.

While adherence of leukocytes to endothelial cells is important in fighting infection, it can be dangerous and life threatening under other circumstances. Thus, in myocardial infarction, the leukocytes can cause blockage of arteries, leading to ischemia. Because of the significance of this interaction, several biotechnology companies are seeking to develop novel chemicals, known as glycomimetics, that mimic the structure of the sialyl Lewis-X antigen. It is hoped that administration of one of these drugs to patients who have just suffered from a heart attack will block the selectin sites and therefore prevent the binding of leukocytes to the vascular wall. Such an effect should diminish the probability of further ischemia.

Comment. This example of a protein–carbohydrate interaction is just one of many that occur in vivo. Each of these kinds of interactions involves a different lectin, each of which has a specific carbohydrate recognition site. Once the carbohydrate structure is known and the protein binding site has been mapped, it may be possible for chemists to design compounds that mimic the carbohydrate structure. These synthetic compounds should bind at the carbohydrate-binding site of the lectin and block the natural interaction. One of the difficulties with this approach is that the individual binding interactions are weak and multiple cell–cell contacts are required; these may be difficult to block by small-molecule drugs. A second problem is that synthesis of specific oligosaccharides is difficult and expensive, and that large quantities may have to be injected into the blood for effective therapy.

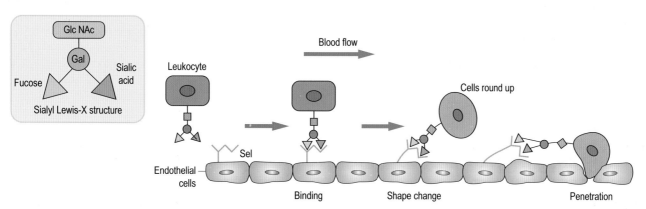

Fig. 26.9 Carbohydrate-dependent cell–cell interactions in inflammation. Sialyl Lewis-X, a tetrasaccharide antigen that forms part of the membrane structure of leukocytes, is recognized by a carbohydrate-binding protein, E-selectin (Sel), on the surface of endothelial cells. Leukocytes are first retarded by, then roll along, and eventually penetrate the endothelial monolayer. In addition, leukocytes contain ʟ-selectins, proteins that recognize saccharide structures on endothelial cells. Multiple copies of both carbohydrates and receptors participate in and strengthen these cell–cell interactions.

Amino sugars

Fru-6-P is the precursor of amino sugars

Figure 26.10 shows the pathway of formation of GlcNAc, GalNAc and sialic acid. The initial reaction involves the transfer of an amino group from the amide nitrogen of glutamine to Fru-6-Pto produce glucosamine-6-P (GlcN-6-P). An acetyl group is then transferred from acetyl-CoA to the amino group of the GlcN-6-P to form GlcNAc-6-P, which is converted to its activated form, UDP-GlcNAc, by sequential mutase and pyrophosphorylase reactions. In addition to its role as a GlcNAc donor, UDP-GlcNAc can also be epimerized to UDP-GalNAc. With few exceptions, all amino sugars in glycoconjugates are acetylated; thus they are neutral and do not contribute any ionic charge to the glycoconjugates.

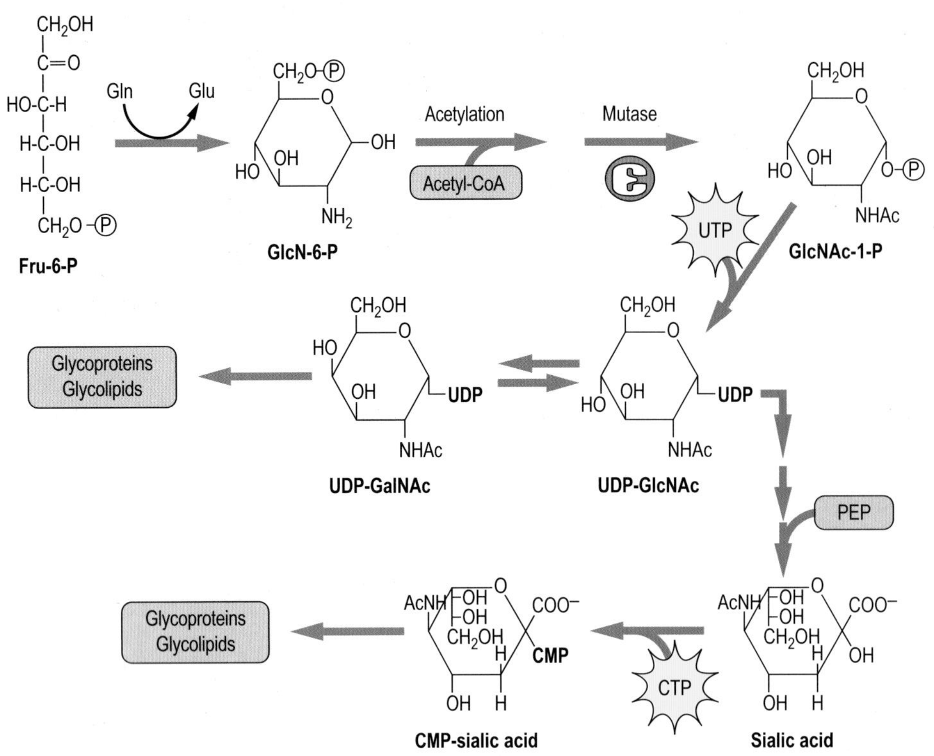

Fig. 26.10 **Synthesis of amino sugars and sialic acid.** Acetyl-CoA, acetyl coenzyme A; GlcN-6-P, glucosamine-6-phosphate; GlcNac-6P, N-acetylglucosamine-6-phosphate; GalNAc, acetylgalactosamine; HNAc, AcHN, acetamide group; PEP, phosphoenolpyruvate.

Sialic acid

UDP-GlcNAc is the precursor of *N*-acetyl-neuraminic acid (NANA), also referred to as sialic acid. Sialic acid, a 9-carbon *N*-acetylamino-ketodeoxyglyconic acid, is produced by the condensation of an amino sugar with phosphoenolpyruvate (see Fig. 26.10). Cytidine monophosphate neuraminic acid (CMP-neuraminic acid) is the activated form of sialic acid and is the sialic acid donor in biosynthetic reactions. CMP-sialic acid is the only nucleoside monophosphate sugar donor in glycoconjugate metabolism.

BIOSYNTHESIS OF OLIGOSACCHARIDES

N-linked oligosaccharides: assembly begins in the endoplasmic reticulum

The pathway of assembly of the *N*-linked oligosaccharides begins with the transfer of two GlcNAc residues to a membrane-bound lipid, called dolichyl-phosphate. Mannose and glucose residues are added to build a lipid-linked oligosaccharide intermediate, which is transferred to protein in the lumen of the endoplasmic reticulum (Fig. 26.11). Dolichols are long-chain polyisoprenol derivatives usually having about 120 carbon atoms (about 22–26 isoprene units) with a phosphate group at one end. They are synthesized in membranes using the same machinery that is used to make cholesterol, but in contrast to cholesterol, the dolichols remain as long straight chains. The length of the chain requires it to snake through the phospholipid bilayer, providing a strong anchor for the growing oligosaccharide chain.

The first sugar to be added to dolichyl-P from UDP-GlcNAc is GlcNAc-1-P to produce dolichyl-P-P-GlcNAc. A second GlcNAc is linked to the first GlcNAc followed by addition of 4–5 mannose residues from GDP-Man. Dolichyl-P-Man and dolichyl-P-Glc serve as glycosyl donors for the remaining mannoses and the three glucoses residues. Each of the sugars is transferred by a specific glycosyltransferase located in or on the endoplasmic reticulum membrane. The glucoses are not found on any of the *N*-linked oligosaccharides on glycoproteins, but are removed by glucosidases in the endoplasmic reticulum. Why are they added in the first place? They serve two very important functions. First of all, the presence of glucoses on the lipid-linked oligosaccharide has been shown to expedite the transfer of oligosaccharide from lipid to protein – the transferring enzyme (oligosaccharide transferase) has a preference for oligosaccharides that contain three glucoses and transfers those oligosaccharides to protein much faster. Secondly, the glucoses are important in directing protein folding in the endoplasmic reticulum (below).

Intermediate processing continues in the endoplasmic reticulum (ER) and Golgi apparatus

In a series of trimming or pruning reactions (Fig. 26.12), all three glucoses are removed in the ER. The oligosaccharide may then remain as a high-mannose oligosaccharide or it

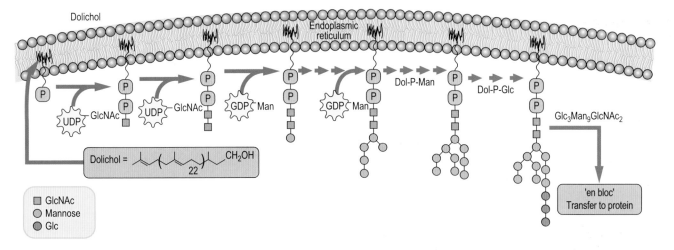

Fig. 26.11 **Synthesis of *N*-linked oligosaccharides in the endoplasmic reticulum.** GlcNAc, acetylglucosamine; Dol, dolichol; Man, mannose.

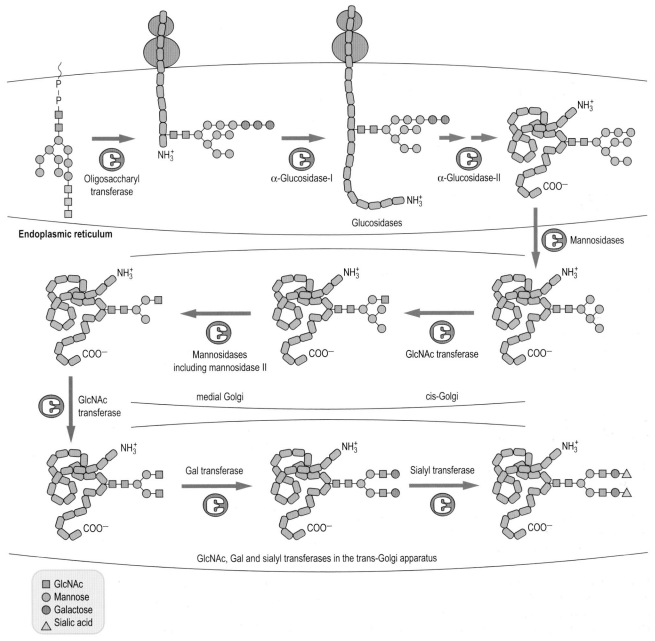

Fig. 26.12 **Processing of *N*-linked oligosaccharides from high-mannose to complex forms.** Glycoproteins are transported between the endoplasmic reticulum and Golgi compartments in vesicles. GlcNAc, *N*-acetylglucosamine.

may be further processed to a complex oligosaccharide structure. One or more mannoses may be removed in the ER, and the folded protein is then translocated to the Golgi apparatus where three or four additional mannoses may be removed to leave the core structure of three mannose and two GlcNAc residues. This core oligosaccharide is then elongated in the Golgi apparatus.

Final modifications of the N-linked oligosaccharides occur in the Golgi apparatus

After the pruning reactions in the ER and proper folding, the protein with one or more $Man_{7-8}GlcNAc_2$ oligosaccharides is transported to the Golgi apparatus where other modification reactions occur (see Fig. 26.12). Usually in the cis-Golgi, several other mannoses are removed by α-mannosidases to leave the core structure. Also in the cis-Golgi, GlcNAc residues are added to each of the mannoses. Then the protein enters the trans-Golgi fraction where the remaining sugars of the trisaccharide sequences, i.e. galactose, sialic acid and fucose, can be added to make a variety of different complex chains. The final structure of the oligosaccharide chains depends on the glycosyltransferases complement of the cell.

O-linked oligosaccharides

In contrast to the biosynthesis of *N*-linked oligosaccharides, the synthesis of the *O*-linked oligosaccharides occurs only in the Golgi apparatus by the stepwise addition of sugars from their sugar nucleotide derivatives to the protein. No lipid intermediates are involved in *O*-linked oligosaccharide formation. Figure 26.13 outlines the stepwise sequence of reactions that are involved in the assembly of an oligosaccharide chain on salivary mucin. In this sequence, GalNAc is first transferred from UDP-GalNAc to serine or threonine

residues on the protein by a GalNAc transferase in the Golgi apparatus. The resulting GalNAc-serine-protein serves as the acceptor for galactose and then sialic acid transferred from their sugar nucleotides (UDP-Gal and CMP-sialic acid) by Golgi galactosyltransferases and sialyl transferases. Other Golgi glycosyl transferases are involved in the stepwise biosynthesis of more complex mucin oligosaccharides and in the synthesis of *O*-linked oligosaccharides in proteoglycans and collagens (see Chapter 28). There are more than 100 glycosyl transferases involved in glycoconjugate synthesis in a typical cell.

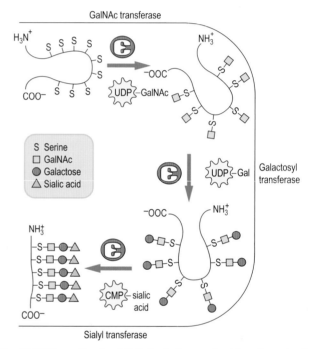

Fig. 26.13 **Biosynthesis of *O*-linked oligosaccharides of mucins in the Golgi apparatus.** GalNAc, *N*-acetylgalactosamine.

 INHIBITORS OF GLYCOPROTEIN BIOSYNTHESIS

A number of inhibitors of the biosynthesis of *N*-linked oligosaccharides have been identified and these compounds have proven to be valuable reagents for studies on the role of specific carbohydrate structures in glycoprotein function. Tunicamycin is a glycoside antibiotic that inhibits the first step in the synthesis of *N*-linked oligosaccharides, i.e. the formation of dolichyl-PP-GlcNAc (see Fig. 26.11). Tunicamycin has varied effects on glycoprotein synthesis and on cells, from benign to profound. In some cases, the protein portion of the glycoprotein is synthesized, but without its carbohydrate it is insoluble, aggregates and is degraded in the cell. Some cells will not grow in the presence of this drug, but others are not affected. A number of other inhibitors have been identified that inhibit specific steps in

the processing pathway. Many are plant alkaloids that structurally resemble the sugars glucose and mannose, and inhibit the pruning glycosidases (see Fig. 26.12). Castanospermine inhibits the ER glucosidases, whereas swainsonine and kifunensine each inhibit a different processing mannosidase. These drugs prevent the formation of complex chains and therefore are useful to evaluate structure–function relationships. Some compounds have been tested against HIV and against some cancers, and have shown positive inhibitory effects. However, they also have adverse effects on other enzymes in normal cells and are therefore not usable as viable drugs. With more specific compounds, it may be possible to manipulate glycan structures for therapeutic purposes.

FUNCTIONS OF THE OLIGOSACCHARIDE CHAINS OF GLYCOPROTEINS

N-linked oligosaccharides have an important role in protein folding

Resident proteins in the endoplasmic reticulum, known as chaperones, assist newly synthesized membrane proteins to fold into their proper conformations. Two of these chaperones, calnexin and calreticulin, bind to unfolded glycoproteins by recognition of high-mannose oligosaccharides that still contain a single glucose remaining on their structure, after the glucosidases have removed two of the three glucoses. Not all of the glycoproteins synthesized in the cell require assistance in folding but for those that do, the rate of folding is greatly accelerated by the chaperones. Incorrectly folded or unfolded proteins do not undergo normal transport to the Golgi apparatus and if they do not fold properly, they are frequently degraded in the endoplasmic reticulum or cytoplasm.

High-mannose oligosaccharides target some proteins to specific sites in the cell

Lysosomes are subcellular organelles involved in the hydrolysis and turnover of many cellular organelles and proteins. They contain a variety of hydrolytic enzymes with acidic pH optima. Most, if not all, of these lysosomal enzymes are N-linked glycoproteins that are synthesized and glycosylated in the endoplasmic reticulum and Golgi apparatus. The sorting of lysosomal enzymes occurs in the cis-Golgi. Proteins destined to be transported to the lysosomes contain a cluster of lysine residues that come together as a result of the protein folding into its proper conformation. As shown in Figure 26.14, this cluster of lysine residues serves as a docking site for an enzyme, GlcNAc-1-P transferase, that transfers a GlcNAc-1-P from UDP-GlcNAc to terminal mannose residues on the high-mannose chains of the lysosomal enzymes. A second enzyme, called an uncovering enzyme, then removes the GlcNAc, leaving the phosphate residues still attached to the mannoses on the high-mannose chains. The resulting Man-6-P residues on the high-mannose structure are now recognized by a Golgi protein called a Man-6-P receptor that somehow drags or directs the enzyme to the lysosomes. Thus, the Man-6-P residues are a targeting signal used by the cell to sort out those proteins that are destined to go to the lysosomes, and separate them from all the other proteins being synthesized in the Golgi apparatus. The Man-6-P receptor is also present on the cell surface, so that even extracellular enzymes that have this signal are endocytosed and transported to the lysosomes.

The oligosaccharide chains of glycoproteins frequently increase the solubility and stability of proteins

DEFICIENCIES IN GLYCOPROTEIN SYNTHESIS

The carbohydrate-deficient glycoprotein syndromes (CDGSs) are a recently described group of rare genetic diseases that affect the biosynthesis of glycoproteins. All patients show multisystem pathology, with severe involvement of the nervous system. Three distinct classes have been identified thus far and are characterized by a deficiency in the structure of the carbohydrate moiety of serum glycoproteins, lysosomal enzymes or membrane glycoproteins. The diagnosis of the disease is routinely made by electrophoresis of serum transferrin. In CDGS, the transferrin contains less sialic acid and therefore the protein migrates more slowly. The decrease in sialic acid results from a defect in biosynthesis of the underlying oligosaccharide structure. While a change in the migration of serum transferrin indicates that the patient is suffering from one of the CDGS, it does not identify the specific lesion. That can only be done by either characterizing the structure of the altered oligosaccharide chain(s) to determine what sugars or structures are missing, or doing a profile of key enzymes in the biosynthetic pathways, since the absence of any of these enzymes will affect the final oligosaccharide structure.

Comment. The basic defects in this group of diseases appears to be in the synthesis or processing of *N*-linked oligosaccharides. However, defects in phosphomannose isomerase and phosphomannose mutase have also been identified as causes of CDGS.

Because oligosaccharides are hydrophilic, they increase the solubility of proteins in the aqueous environment. Thus, most of the proteins that are secreted from cells are glycoproteins, including plasma proteins. These glycoproteins and enzymes generally also have high stability to heat, chemical denaturants, detergents, acids and bases. Enzymatic removal of the carbohydrate from many of these proteins greatly reduces their stability to stress. Indeed, when glycoproteins are synthesized in cells in the presence of glycosylation inhibitors, such as tunicamycin which prevents the production and therefore the attachment of the N-linked oligosaccharide chain, many of these proteins become insoluble and form inclusion bodies in the cells as a result of incorrect folding and/or decreased hydrophilicity.

Sugars are involved in chemical recognition interactions with lectins

N-linked glycoproteins on the mammalian cell surface play critical roles in cell–cell interactions and other recognition processes. One cell may contain on its cell surface a carbohydrate-recognizing protein, known as a lectin, that binds

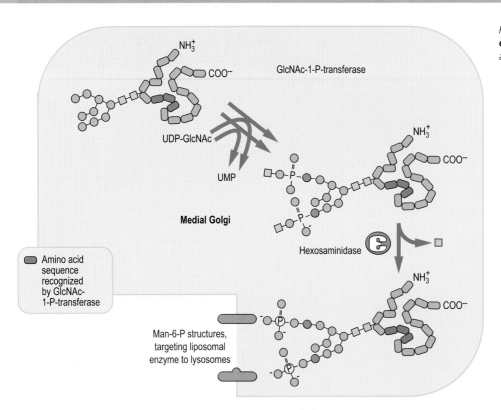

Fig. 26.14 **Targeting of lysosomal enzymes to lysosomes.** GlcNAc, *N*-acetylglucosamine; Man, mannose.

 I-CELL DISEASE

I-cell disease (mucolipidosis II) and pseudo-Hurler polydystrophy (mucolipidosis III) are rare inherited diseases that are caused by deficiencies in the machinery that targets lysosomal enzymes to the lysosomes. Clinical presentation includes severe psychomotor retardation, coarse facial features and skeletal abnormalities; death usually occurs in the first decade. In cultured fibroblasts taken from patients suffering from mucolipidosis II, newly synthesized lysosomal enzymes are secreted into the extracellular medium rather than being targeted correctly to the lysosomes. Mesenchymal cells, especially fibroblasts, contain numerous membrane-bound vacuoles in the cytoplasm containing fibrillo-granular material. These deposits are called inclusion bodies and this is the origin of the name I-cell disease.

Comment. I-cell disease results from a deficiency in synthesis of the targeting signal, Man-6-P residues on high-mannose oligosaccharides. The mutation is most commonly an absence of GlcNAc-1-P phosphotransferase, but defects in the uncovering enzyme also occur. It is likely that absence of the Man-6-P receptor protein would yield the same phenotype. In I-cell disease the lysosomes, lacking the full spectrum of hydrolase enzymes, become engorged with indigestible substances.

to a specific oligosaccharide structure on the surface of the complementary cell. The interaction between these two chemical interfaces mediates a specific chemical recognition between the cells, and such a process is a key factor

in fertilization, inflammation, infection, development and differentiation.

Carbohydrate–protein interactions are also important in nonself interactions. Many pathogens use this mechanism to recognize their target cells. *E. coli*, for example, and some other gram-negative enteric bacteria have short hair-like projections called pili on their surfaces. These pili have mannose-binding lectins at their tip that can recognize and bind to high-mannose oligosaccharides on the brush border membranes of intestinal epithelial cells. This interaction allows the bacteria to be retained in the intestine. A similar mechanism is used by some symbiotic bacteria in the intestinal tract. The influenza virus uses a hemagglutinin protein on its surface to bind to sialic acid residues on glycoproteins and glycolipids on the surfaces of target cells.

Variations in mucin structure appear to have a role in the specificity of fertilization, cell differentiation, development of the immune response, and virus infectivity. Glycoprotein ZP3, which is present on the zona pellucida of the mouse egg, functions as a receptor for sperm during fertilization. Enzymatic removal of *O*-linked oligosaccharides from ZP3 results in loss of sperm receptor activity, whereas removal of the *N*-linked oligosaccharides has no effect on sperm binding. The isolated *O*-linked oligosaccharides obtained from ZP3 also have sperm-binding activity and inhibit sperm–egg interaction and fertilization in vitro. Differences between the *O*-glycan structures of cytotoxic lymphocytes and helper cells involved in the immune response are also believed to be important in mediating cellular interactions during the immune response.

TOXICITY OF RICIN AND OTHER LECTINS

Lectins are found in a variety of foods, including beans, peanuts and dry cereals. Many plant lectins are toxic to animal cells. In edible plants, these may be less of a problem if the foods are cooked, since the lectins are denatured and therefore susceptible to intestinal proteases. On the other hand, lectins in uncooked plants are very resistant to proteases and can therefore cause serious problems. They bind to cells in the gastrointestinal tract, inhibiting enzyme activities, food digestion and nutrient absorption, and causing gastrointestinal distress and allergic reactions.

Ricin, produced by the castor bean plant, is among the most poisonous proteins known to man. These types of toxic lectins are usually composed of several subunits, one of which is the carbohydrate-recognizing or -binding site, while the other subunit is an enzyme that can catalytically inactivate ribosomes. Thus a single molecule of this catalytic subunit entering a cell can completely block protein synthesis in that cell. Other toxic lectins include modeccin, abrin and mistletoe lectin I.

CHANGES IN SUGAR COMPOSITION AND/OR STRUCTURE CAN BE DIAGNOSTIC MARKERS OF SOME TYPES OF CANCER

Changes in glycosylation of both proteins and lipids have been consistently reported on cell surface carbohydrates of various types of cancer cells, including melanomas, ovarian cancer, and hepatocellular carcinoma. While these changes are not the cause of the disease, they are being evaluated as diagnostic tools for early detection of disease. Increased levels of the enzyme GlcNAc transferase V (the transferase involved in adding a second (branching) GlcNAc residue to a mannose residue to make a triantennary complex chain) is highly expressed in some transformed cells, resulting in increased branching and production of larger N-linked oligosaccharides. Changes in O-linked oligosaccharides have also been reported, for example increased levels of sialyl Lewis-X antigen, which is thought to contribute to metastasis. Changes in the amount and sialylation of mucins are also associated with metastasis of lung and colon carcinoma cells and are being studied for their usefulness as diagnostic or prognostic biomarkers.

There is also evidence that changes in the level of fucose on some glycoproteins regulate the biologic phenotype of cancer cells, and in fact, fucosylation of the protein α-fetoprotein (AFP-L3) has been used clinically as a marker for hepatocellular carcinoma.

Comment. There is considerable evidence to indicate that the structure and composition of glycoproteins and glycolipids are altered in tumor cells, compared to normal cells. While these changes may not cause the cancer, they may have a significant effect on clinical outcome, e.g. if they limit leukocyte infiltration, assist in evading immune surveillance or facilitate metastasis. Analysis of oligosaccharide structures may be useful for early detection and diagnostic purposes and manipulation of oligosaccharide structure may prove useful in treatment of some cancers.

Summary

Glycosylation is the major posttranslational modification of tissue proteins. Glycosylation is a multicompartment activity, involving sugar interconversions and activation in the cytosolic compartment, building of complex structures on lipid intermediates in the ER, and glycosylation and pruning reactions in the ER and Golgi apparatus. The outcome is an amazingly diverse range of oligosaccharide structures on proteins. These sugars can serve a number of different functions, including:

- modification of the physical properties of the protein (solubility, stability and/or viscosity)

- aiding in the folding of the protein
- participating in the targeting of the protein to its proper location in the cell
- mediating cell–protein and cell–cell recognition during fertilization, development, inflammation and other processes.

A number of human diseases involve defects in sugar metabolism, including galactosemia and hereditary fructose intolerance, leukocyte deficiency disease, carbohydrate-deficient glycoprotein syndromes (CDGS) and lysosomal storage diseases. It is important to determine how sugars can interact in various recognition reactions and how they can provide stability and affect the physical properties of proteins and lipids since that information can provide keys to preventing or interceding in a variety of diseases.

Further reading

Asano N. Glycosidase inhibitors: update and perspectives on practical use. *Glycobiology* 2003;**13**:93R–r104R.

Boehncke WH, Schon MP. Interfering with leukocyte rolling – a promising therapeutic approach in inflammatory skin disorders? *Trends Pharmacol Sci* 2003;**24**:49–52.

Gerber-Lemaire S, Juillerat-Jeanneret L. Glycosylation pathways as drug targets for cancer: glycosidase inhibitors. *Mini Rev Med Chem* 2006;**6**:1043–1052.

Gorelik E, Galili U, Raz A. On the role of cell surface carbohydrates and their binding proteins (lectins) in tumor metastasis. *Cancer Metastasis Rev* 2001;**20**:245–277.

Kato K, Kamiya Y. Structural views of glycoprotein-fate determination in cells. *Glycobiology* 2007;**17**:1031–1044.

Marquardt T, Denecke J. Congenital disorders of glycosylation: review of their molecular bases, clinical presentations and specific therapies. *Eur J Pediatr* 2003;**162**:359–379.

Mouricout M. Interactions between the enteric pathogens and the host. An assortment of bacterial lectins and a set of glycoconjugate receptors. *Adv Exp Med Biol* 1997;**412**:109–123.

Novelli G, Reichardt JK. Molecular basis of disorders of human galactose metabolism: past, present, and future. *Mol Genet Metab* 2000;**71**:62–65.

Petri WA Jr, Haque R, Mann BJ. The bittersweet interface of parasite and host: lectin-carbohydrate interactions during human invasion by the parasite Entamoeba histolytica. *Annu Rev Microbiol* 2002;**56**:39–64.

Rubin BK. Physiology of airway mucus clearance. *Respir Care* 2002;**47**:761–768.

Websites

Carbohydrate-deficient glycoprotein syndrome: www.familyvillage.wisc.edu/lib_cdgs.htm

Galactosemia: www.galactosemia.org/

Glycoprotein biosynthesis: http://employees.csbsju.edu/hjakubowski/classes/ch331/cho/glycoproteinshtm.htm

Hereditary fructose intolerance: www.bu.edu/aldolase/HFI/

I-cell disease: www.emedicine.com/ped/topic1150.htm

Lectins: www.ansci.cornell.edu/plants/toxicagents/lectins/lectins.html

Mucopolysaccharidoses: www.mpssociety.org/

27. Complex Lipids

A D Elbein

LEARNING OBJECTIVES

After reading this chapter you should be able to:

- Describe how the various glycerol-based phospholipids are synthesized and how they are interconverted.
- Describe the multiple roles of cytidine nucleotides in activation of intermediates in phospholipid synthesis.
- Describe the various types of sphingolipids and glycolipids that occur in mammalian cells and their functions.
- Explain the etiology of lysosomal storage diseases, their pathology, and the rationale for enzyme replacement therapy for treatment of these diseases.

INTRODUCTION

Complex lipids encompass the glycerophospholipids, introduced in Chapter 3, and the sphingolipids. These molecules are found mostly in two locations, either embedded in biologic membranes or in circulating liproteins. The sphingolipids are almost exclusively in cell membranes, and primarily in the plasma membrane. They carry a wide range of carbohydrate structures which face into the exterior environment and, like glycoproteins, have a range of recognition functions. A major difference between these two classes of lipids is that glycerophospholipids are saponifiable (except plasmalogens), while sphingolipids contain no alkali-labile ester bonds. Thus, it was convenient to isolate sphingolipids from tissues by saponification, then extraction of the remaining lipids into organic solvent. Once isolated, the characterization of the glycan structure of the sphingolipids was technically challenging. Therefore, the structures were, for a long time, unknown and mysterious, leading to their name: sphinx-like or sphingolipids.

This chapter discusses the structure, biosynthesis, and function of the two major classes of polar lipids: glycerophospholipids and sphingolipids. In preparation for this chapter, it might help to review the structure of phospholipids in Chapter 3.

SYNTHESIS AND TURNOVER OF GLYCEROPHOSPHOLIPIDS

Precursors: phosphatidic acid and diacylglycerol (DAG)

All animal cells, except for erythrocytes, are able to synthesize phospholipids de novo, whereas triglyceride synthesis occurs mainly in liver, adipose tissue, and intestinal cells. As shown in Figure 27.1, phosphatidic acid and 1-2-diacylglycerol (DAG) are common intermediates in the synthesis of both triglycerides (triacylglycerols) and phospholipids. Glycerol-3-phosphate is the primary starting material for synthesis of phosphatidic acid; it is formed in most tissues by reduction of the glycolytic intermediate, dihydroxyacetone phosphate (DHAP). In liver, kidney and intestine, glycerol-3-P can also be formed directly via phosphorylation of glycerol by a specific kinase.

Glycerol-3-P is acylated by transfer of two long-chain fatty acids from fatty acyl-CoA to the hydroxyl groups at carbons 1 and 2, producing phosphatidic acid. The first fatty acid, usually a saturated fatty acid, is added to carbon-1, forming lysophosphatidic acid; the prefix 'lyso' indicates that one of the hydroxyl groups has been lysed, i.e. is not acylated. Then, a second fatty acid, usually an unsaturated fatty acid, is added to carbon-2 to form phosphatidic acid. DHAP may also be acylated by addition of a fatty acid to the 1-hydroxyl group, and this intermediate is then reduced and acylated to phosphatidic acid. Phosphatidic acid is converted to DAG by a specific cytosolic phosphatase.

Biosynthesis of phospholipids

The biosynthesis of lecithin (phosphatidylcholine) from DAG requires activation of choline to a cytidine diphosphate (CDP) nucleotide derivative. In this series of reactions, shown in Figure 27.2, the choline 'head group' is converted to phosphocholine and then activated to CDP-choline by a pyrophosphorylase reaction. The pyrophosphate bond is cleaved and phosphocholine (choline phosphate) is transferred to DAG to form lecithin. This reaction is analogous to the transfer of GlcNAc-6-P to dolichol or to the high-mannose core of lysosomal enzymes – both the sugar and a

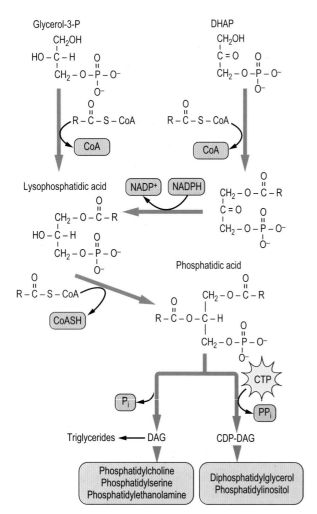

Fig. 27.1 **Pathway of formation of phosphatidic acid and its conversion to diacylglycerol (DAG) and major phospholipids.** CDP, cytidine diphosphate; CTP, cytidine triphosphate; CoASH, coenzyme A; DHAP, dihydroxyacetone phosphate; Pi, inorganic phosphate; PPi, inorganic pyrophosphate.

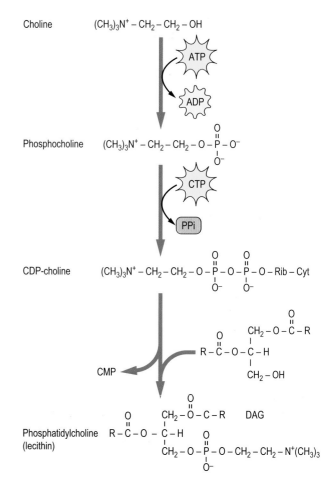

Fig. 27.2 **Formation of phosphatidylcholine by the CDP-choline pathway.** Cyt, cytosine; CDP, cytidine diphosphate, CMP, cytidine monophosphate; DAG, diacylglycerol; Rib, ribose. CTP, cytidine triphosphate.

phosphate are transferred from the nucleotide derivative. Phosphatidylethanolamine is formed by a similar pathway using cytidine triphosphate (CTP) and phosphoethanolamine, to form CDP-ethanolamine.

Both phosphatidylcholine and phosphatidylethanolamine can react with free serine by an exchange reaction to form phosphatidylserine and the free base, choline or ethanolamine (Fig. 27.3). In a secondary pathway, phosphatidylcholine can also be formed by methylation of phosphatidylethanolamine with the methyl donor, *S*-adenosylmethionine (SAM) (Fig. 27.4). The methylation pathway involves the sequential transfer of three activated methyl groups from three different molecules of SAM. Liver also has another route to phosphatidylethanolamine, involving decarboxylation of phosphatidylserine by a specific mitochondrial decarboxylase.

Phospholipids that have an alcohol as the head group, e.g. phosphatidylglycerol and phosphatidylinositol, are synthesized by an alternative pathway, which also involves

activation by cytidine nucleotides. In this case, the phosphatidic acid is activated, rather than the head group, yielding CDP-DAG (Fig. 27.5). The phosphatidic acid group is then transferred to free glycerol or inositol, to form phosphatidylglycerol or phosphatidylinositol, respectively. A second phosphatidic acid may also be added to phosphatidylglycerol to form 1,3-diphosphatidylglycerol (DPG). This lipid, known commonly as cardiolipin, is found almost exclusively in the inner mitochondrial membrane; it represents about 20% of phospholipids in heart mitochondria and is required for efficient activity of electron transport complexes III and IV and the ATP:ADP translocase.

Plasmalogens are a second major class of mitochondrial lipids, and are enriched in nerve and muscle tissue; in the heart they may account for nearly 50% of total phospholipids. The biosynthesis of plasmalogens proceeds from DHAP: it is first acylated at C-1, the acyl group exchanges with a lipid alcohol to form the ether lipid, then the ether lipid is desaturated, leading eventually to the alkenylether-phospholipid. The function of plasmalogens versus diacylphospholipids

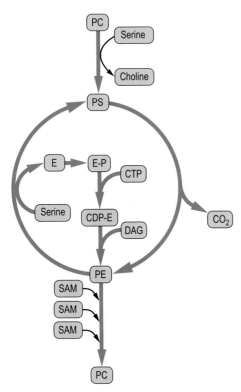

Fig. 27.3 **Pathways of interconversion of phospholipids by exchange of head groups, by methylation or by decarboxylation.** E, ethanolamine; DAG, diacylglycerol; PC, phosphatidylcholine; PS, phosphatidylserine; SAM, S-adenosylmethionine.

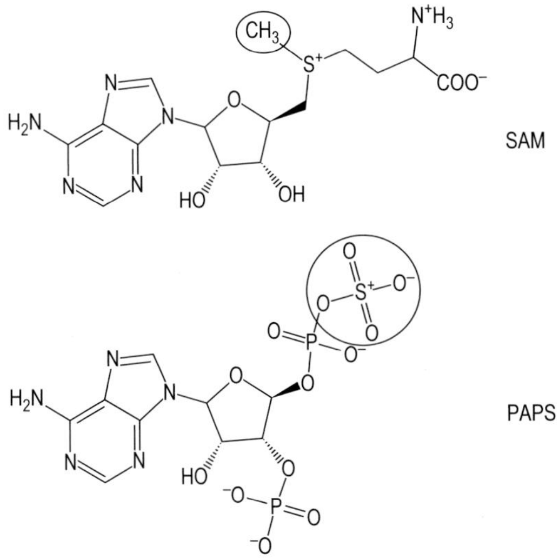

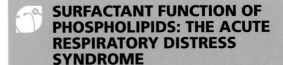

Fig. 27.4 **Structures of the methyl and sulfate donors involved in the synthesis of membrane lipids.** SAM, S-adenosylmethionine; PAPS, 3'-phosphoadenosine-5'-phosphosulfate (active sulfate).

is not clear, but there is some evidence that they are more resistant to oxidative damage, which may provide protection against oxidative stress in tissues with active aerobic metabolism (see Chapter 37).

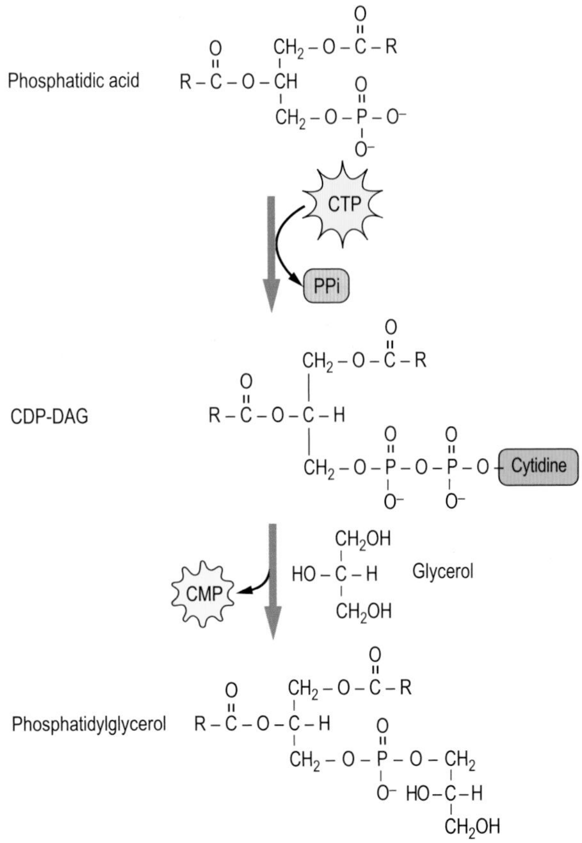

Fig. 27.5 **Formation of phosphatidylglycerol by activation of phosphatidic acid to form CDP-DAG, and transfer of DAG to glycerol.** CMP, cytidine monophosphate; CTP, cytidine triphosphate.

SURFACTANT FUNCTION OF PHOSPHOLIPIDS: THE ACUTE RESPIRATORY DISTRESS SYNDROME

Acute respiratory distress syndrome (ARDS) accounts for 15–20% of neonatal mortality in Western countries. The disease affects only premature infants and its incidence is directly related to the degree of prematurity.

Comment. Immature lungs do not have enough type II epithelial cells to synthesize sufficient amounts of the phospholipid, dipalmitoylphosphatidylcholine (DPPC). This phospholipid makes up more than 80% of the total phospholipids of the extracellular lipid layer that lines the alveoli of normal lungs. DPPC decreases the surface tension of the aqueous surface layer of the lungs, facilitating opening of the alveoli during inspiration. Lack of surfactant causes the lungs to collapse during the expiration phase of breathing, leading to ARDS. The maturity of the fetal lung can be assessed by measuring the lecithin:sphingomyelin ratio in amniotic fluid. If there is a potential problem, a mother can be treated with a glucocorticoid to accelerate maturation of the fetal lung. ARDS is also seen in adults in whom the type II epithelial cells have been destroyed as a result of the use of immunosuppressive drugs or certain chemotherapeutic agents.

Turnover of phospholipids

Phospholipids are in a continuous state of turnover in most membranes. This occurs as a result of oxidative damage, during inflammation, and through activation of lipases, particularly in response to hormonal stimuli. As shown in Figure 27.6, there are a number of phospholipases that act on specific bonds in the phospholipid structure. Phospholipases A_2 (PLA_2) and C (PLC) are particularly active during the inflammatory response and in signal transduction. Phospholipase B (not shown) is a lysophospholipase that removes the second acyl group after action of PLA_1 or PLA_2. The lysophospholipids may be degraded to phosphatidic acid or recycled (reacylated) by scavenger pathways.

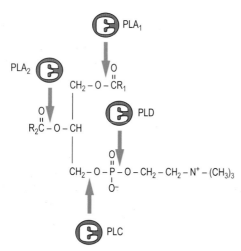

Fig. 27.6 **Sites of action of phospholipases on phosphatidylcholine.** PLA_1, PLA_2, PLC, PLD are phospholipases A_1, A_2, C, and D, respectively.

 GLYCOSYLPHOSPHATIDYLINOSITOL MEMBRANE ANCHORS

Phosphatidylinositol is an integral component of the glycosylphosphatidylinositol (GPI) structure that anchors various proteins to the plasma membrane (Fig. 27.7). In contrast to other membrane phospholipids, including most of the membrane phosphatidylinositol, GPI has a glycan chain containing glucosamine and mannose attached to the inositol. Ethanolamine connects the GPI-glycan to the carboxyl terminus of the protein. Many membrane proteins in eukaryotic cells are anchored by a GPI structure, including alkaline phosphatase and acetylcholinesterase, which have roles in bone mineralization and nerve transmission, respectively. In contrast to integral or peripheral membrane proteins, GPI-anchored proteins may be released from the cell surface by phospholipase C in response to regulatory processes.

SPHINGOLIPIDS

Structure and biosynthesis of sphingosine

Sphingolipids are a complex group of amphipathic, polar lipids. They are built on a core structure of the long-chain amino alcohol sphingosine, which is formed by oxidative decarboxylation and condensation of palmitate with serine.

 VARIABLE SURFACE ANTIGENS OF TRYPANOSOMES

The parasitic trypanosome that causes sleeping sickness, *Trypanosoma brucei*, has a protein called the variable surface antigen bound to its cell surface by a GPI anchor. This variable surface antigen elicits the formation of specific antibodies in the host, and these antibodies can attack and kill the parasite. However, some of the parasites evade immune surveillance by shedding this antigen, as if they were shedding a coat.

Comment. Trypanosomes and some other pathogens are able to shed their surface antigens because they have an enzyme, phospholipase C, that cleaves the GPI anchor at the phosphate–diacylglycerol bond, releasing the protein-glycan component into the external fluid. Surviving cells rapidly make a new coat with a different antigenic structure that will not be recognized by the antibody. Of course, this new coat will elicit the formation of new specific antibodies but the parasite can again shed this coat, and so on, in a random sequence to evade the host immune system.

DEFECTS IN GPI ANCHORING ASSOCIATED WITH GENETIC DISEASE: PAROXYSMAL NOCTURNAL HEMOGLOBINURIA

Paroxysmal nocturnal hemoglobinuria (PNH) is a complex hematologic disorder characterized by hemolytic anemia, venous thrombosis in unusual sites, and deficient hematopoiesis. The diagnosis of this disease is based on the unusual sensitivity of the red blood cells to the hemolytic action of complement (Chapter 38), because red cells from patients with PNH lack several proteins that are involved in regulating the activation of complement at the cell surface.

Comment. One of these cell surface proteins is decay accelerating factor, a GPI-anchored protein that inactivates a hemolytic complex formed during complement activation; in its absence, there is increased hemolysis. There are several genetic variants of PNH. One of these involves a defect in the GlcNAc transferase that adds *N*-acetylglucosamine to the inositol moiety of phosphatidylinositol, the first step in GPI anchor formation (see Fig. 27.7).

In all sphingolipids, the long-chain fatty acid is attached to the amino group of the sphingosine in an amide linkage (Fig. 27.8). Because of the alkaline stability of amides, compared to esters, sphingolipids are nonsaponifiable, which facilitates their separation from alkali-labile glycerophospholipids.

The synthesis of the sphingosine base of sphingolipids involves condensation of palmitoyl-CoA with serine, in which the carbon-1 of serine is lost as carbon dioxide. The product of this reaction is converted in several steps to sphingosine, which is then N-acylated to form ceramide (N-acylsphingosine). Ceramide (see Fig. 27.10) is the precursor and backbone structure of both sphingomyelin and glycosphingolipids.

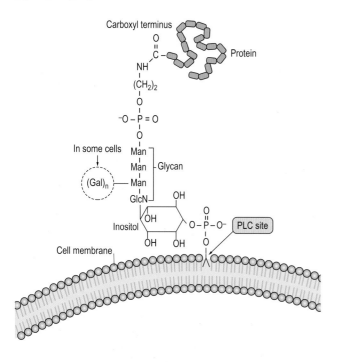

Fig. 27.7 **Structure of the glycosylphosphatidylinositol (GPI) anchor and its attachment to proteins.** Gal, galactose; GlcN, glucosamine; Man, mannose; PLC, phospholipase C.

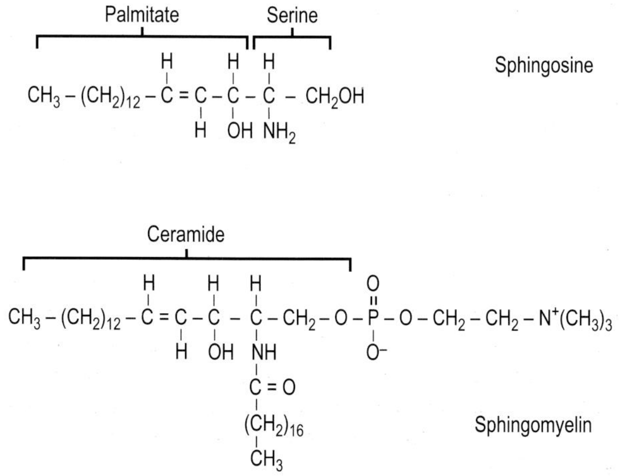

Fig. 27.8 **Structures of sphingosine and sphingomyelin**.

Sphingomyelin

Sphingomyelin (see Fig. 27.8) is found in plasma membranes, subcellular organelles, endoplasmic reticulum, and mitochondria. It comprises 5–20% of the total phospholipids in most cell types, and is mostly localized in the plasma membrane. It is the only sphingolipid that contains phosphorus, and is the major phospholipid of the myelin sheath of nerves. The phosphocholine group in sphingomyelin is transferred to the terminal hydroxyl group of sphingosine by a transesterification reaction with phosphatidylcholine. The fatty acid composition varies, but long-chain fatty acids are common, including lignoceric (24:0), cerebronic (2-hydroxylignoceric) and nervonic (24:1) acids.

Glycolipids

Sphingolipids containing covalently bound sugars are known as glycosphingolipids or glycolipids. As with glycoconjugates, in general, the structure of the oligosaccharide chains is highly variable. In addition, the glycosyltransferase distribution and glycosphingolipid content of cells varies during development and in response to regulatory processes.

Glycolipids can be classified into three main groups: cerebrosides, sulfatides and gangliosides. In all of these compounds, the polar head-group, comprising the sugars, is attached to ceramide by a glycosidic bond at the terminal hydroxyl group of sphingosine. Figure 27.9 illustrates the structure and biosynthesis of some of the simpler glycolipids. Cerebrosides are glycolipids containing only neutral and amino sugars. Gluco- and galactocerebroside (glucosyl and galactosyl ceramide) are the smallest members of this class of compounds and serve as the nucleus for elaboration of more complex structures. Sulfatides are formed by addition of sulfate from the sulfate donor, 3'-phosphoadenosine-5'-phosphosulfate (PAPS) (see Fig. 27.4), yielding, for example, galactocerebroside 3-sulfate. Finally, glycolipids containing sialic acids (N-acetyl neuraminic acid, NANA) are termed gangliosides.

Structure and nomenclature of gangliosides

The term 'ganglioside' refers to glycolipids that were originally identified in high concentrations in ganglionic cells of the central nervous system. In cells of the nervous system in general, more than 50% of the sialic acid in the cell is present in gangliosides. Gangliosides are also found in the surface membranes of cells of most extraneural tissues, but in these tissues they account for less than 10% of the total sialic acid.

The nomenclature used to identify the various gangliosides is based on the number of sialic acid residues contained in the molecule, and on the sequence of the carbohydrates (Fig. 27.10). GM refers to a ganglioside with a single (mono) sialic acid, whereas GD, GT and GQ would indicate two, three and four sialic acid residues in the molecule, respectively.

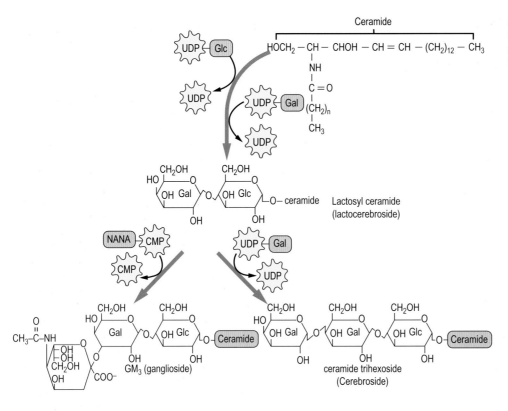

Fig. 27.9 **An outline of transferase reactions for elongation of glycolipids and formation of gangliosides.**

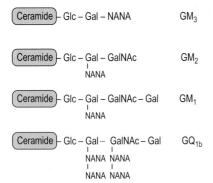

| Ceramide — Glc – Gal – NANA | GM$_3$ |

Ceramide — Glc – Gal – GalNAc GM$_2$
                         |
                       NANA

Ceramide — Glc – Gal – GalNAc – Gal GM$_1$
                         |
                       NANA

Ceramide — Glc – Gal – GalNAc – Gal GQ$_{1b}$
                    | |
                  NANA   NANA
                    | |
                  NANA   NANA

Fig. 27.10 **Generalized structures of gangliosides.** Glc, glucose; Gal, galactose; NANA, *N*-acetyl neuraminic acid; GalNAc, *N*-acetylgalactosamine.

The number after the GM, e.g. GM$_1$, refers to the structure of the oligosaccharide. These numbers were derived from the relative mobility of the glycolipids on thin layer chromatograms; the larger, GM$_1$, gangliosides migrate the most slowly.

LYSOSOMAL STORAGE DISEASES RESULTING FROM DEFECTS IN GLYCOLIPID DEGRADATION

The complex oligosaccharides on glycolipids are built up, one sugar residue at a time, in the Golgi apparatus and are degraded in a similar step-wise fashion by a series of exoglycosidases

CEREBROSIDOSES AND GANGLIOSIDOSES

Tay–Sachs disease is a gangliosidosis in which GM$_2$ accumulates as a result of an absence of hexosaminidase A (see Fig. 27.11). Individuals with this disease usually have mental retardation and blindness and die between 2 and 3 years of age. Fabry's disease is a cerebrosidosis resulting from deficiency of α-galactosidase and accumulation of ceramide trihexoside (see Fig. 27.11). The symptoms of Fabry's disease are skin rash, kidney failure, and pain in the lower extremities. Patients with this condition benefit from kidney transplants and usually live into early to mid-adulthood. Most of these lysosomal storage diseases appear in several forms (variants), resulting from different mutations in the genome. Some lysosomal storage diseases and some variants are more severe and debilitating than others. Although lysosomal storage diseases are relatively rare, they have had a major impact on our understanding of the function and importance of lysosomes.

Comment. When cells die, biomolecules, including glycosphingolipids and glycoproteins, are degraded to their individual components. Figure 27.11 presents the pathway for the degradation of a ganglioside such as GM$_1$ in the lysosomes. A number of lysosomal diseases result from the absence of an essential glycosidase (see Table 27.1). The sphingolipidoses are characterized by lysosomal accumulation of the substrate of the missing enzyme, interfering with normal lysosomal function in turnover of biomolecules.

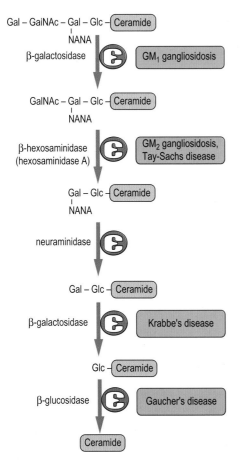

Fig. 27.11 **Lysosomal pathway for turnover (degradation) of ganglioside GM$_1$ in human cells.** Various enzymes may be missing in specific lipid storage diseases, as indicated in Table 27.1. Gal, galactose; GalNac, *N*-acetylgalactosamine; Glc, glucose; NANA, *N*-acetyl neuraminic acid.

GAUCHER'S DISEASE: A MODEL FOR ENZYME REPLACEMENT THERAPY

Gaucher's disease is a lysosomal storage disease in which afflicted individuals are missing the enzyme glucocerebrosidase. This enzyme removes the final sugar from the ceramide, allowing the lipid portion to be further degraded in the lysosomes. This disease is characterized by hepatomegaly and neurodegeneration, but there are milder variants that are amenable to treatment by enzyme replacement therapy.

For treatment of Gaucher's disease, exogenous β-glucosidase was successfully targeted to the lysosomes of macrophages using a cell surface mannose receptor. In order to do this successfully, it was necessary to produce the recombinant replacement enzyme with *N*-glycan chains containing terminal mannose residues. This was done by cleaving the glycans of the enzyme produced in mammalian cells with a combination of sialidase (neuraminidase), β-galactosidase and β-hexosaminidase to trim the complex chains down to the mannose core. An alternative recombinant glucosidase has been produced in a baculovirus-infected insect cell system. In this case, the enzyme has a high mannose oligosaccharide that is not processed to complex chains. The recombinant enzymes are administered intravenously. The success in using glucocerebrosidase for treatment of Gaucher's disease has stimulated the development of other lysosomal hydrolases for treatment of lysosomal storage diseases (see also Further reading).

Lipid storage diseases			
Disease	**Symptoms**	**Major storage product**	**Deficient enzymes**
Tay-Sachs	blindness, mental retardation, death between 2nd and 3rd year	GM$_2$ ganglioside	hexosaminidase A
Gaucher's	liver and spleen enlargement, mental retardation in infantile form	glucocerebroside	β-glucosidase
Fabry's	skin rash, kidney failure, pain in lower extremities	ceramide trihexoside	α-galactosidase
Krabbe's	liver and spleen enlargement, mental retardation	galactocerebroside	β-galactosidase

Table 27.1 **Some lipid storage diseases.**

in lysosomes (Fig. 27.11). Defects in sequential degradation of glycolipids lead to a number of lysosomal storage diseases, known as cerebrosidoses and gangliosidoses (Table 27.1). These diseases are autosomal recessive in inheritance. Heterozygotes are asymptomatic, indicating that a single copy of the gene for a functional enzyme is sufficient for apparently normal turnover of glycolipids. Like I-cell disease (see box on p. 366), the glycolipidoses are characterized by accumulation of undigested material in inclusion bodies in the cells.

FABRY'S DISEASE (INCIDENCE 1 IN 100 000)

A 30-year-old man was found to have proteinuria at an insurance medical examination. He had been seen over a number of years from around age 10 with headaches, vertigo and shooting pains in his arms and legs. No diagnosis was made and he had grown accustomed to these problems. The physician carefully examined his perineum and scrotum, identifying small, raised, red angiokeratoma.

Comment. This man was diagnosed with Fabry's disease, which often takes years before a diagnosis is confirmed by measuring

α-galactosidase A activity. His insurance was declined as proteinuria is expected to progress to renal failure within 15 years. The principal endothelial depositions of a cerebroside (ceramide trihexoside) occur in the kidney (leading to proteinuria and renal failure), the heart and brain (leading to myocardial infarction and stroke), and around blood vessels supplying nerves (leading to painful paresthesiae). Recombinant enzyme replacement therapy appears to clear the deposited cerebroside and initial studies suggest that renal function is maintained.

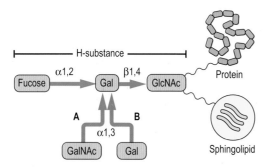

Fig. 27.12 **Relationship between the H, A, and B blood group substances.** The terminal oligosaccharide is linked through other sugars to proteins and lipids of the red cell membrane. GlcNAc, *N*-acetylglucosamine; GalNAc, *N*-acetylgalactosamine; Gal, galactose.

ABO BLOOD GROUP ANTIGENS

Blood transfusion replenishes the oxygen-carrying capacity of blood in persons who suffer from blood loss or anemia (see Chapter 5). The term 'blood transfusion' is something of a misnomer, because it involves only the infusion of washed and preserved red cells. The membranes of red blood cells contain a number of blood group antigens, of which the ABO blood group system is the best understood and most widely studied. The antigens in this group have a common precursor, called the H substance (Fig. 27.12), and an individual may have type A, type B, type AB or type O blood. Individuals with type A cells develop natural antibodies in their plasma that are directed against and will agglutinate type B and type AB red blood cells, whereas those with type B red cells develop antibodies against A substance and will agglutinate type A and type AB blood. Persons with type AB blood have neither A nor B antibodies and are called 'universal recipients', as they can be transfused with cells of either blood type. Individuals with type O blood have only H substance, not A or B substance, on their red blood cells and are 'universal donors', as their red blood cells are not agglutinated with either A or B antibodies; they may accept blood only from a type O donor.

The ABO blood group antigens are complex carbohydrates present as components of glycoproteins or glycosphingolipids of red cell membranes. The H locus codes for a fucosyltransferase. Individuals with type A blood have, in addition to the H substance, an A gene that codes for a specific GalNAc transferase that adds GalNAc α1,3 to the galactose residue of H substance, to form the A-type glycolipid. Individuals with type B blood have a B gene that codes for a galactosyl transferase that adds galactose α1,3 to the galactose residue of H substance, to form the B-type glycolipid. Individuals with type AB blood have both the GalNAc and the Gal transferases, and their red blood cells contain both the A and the B substances. Those with type O blood and only H substance on their red cell glycosphingolipids do not make either enzyme. Enzymes such as coffee bean α-galactosidase can remove the galactose from type B red cells, an approach that is being tested for increasing the supply of type O (universal donor) red cells.

The ABO antigens are present on most cells in the body but they are referred to as blood group antigens because of their association with transfusion reactions. The transfusion reaction is the result of reaction of host antibodies with transfused red cells, resulting in complement-mediated hemolysis (see Chapter 38). While the transfusion reaction demonstrates the role of carbohydrates in recognition of the foreign red cells, the physiologic function of blood group substances is unclear. Persons with an O genotype are generally as healthy as those with A or B genotype. However, there is some evidence that specific phenotypes may confer differential resistance to disease; for example, people with type A and type O blood appear to be more susceptible to smallpox and cholera, respectively.

OTHER BLOOD GROUP SUBSTANCES

The Lewis blood group antigens correspond to a set of fucosylated glycan structures. The Lewis A antigen (Lewis[a]) is synthesized by fucosyltransferase that transfers a fucose residue to a GlcNAc residue in a glycan chain (Fig. 27.13), while

Lewisᵃ   Fuc (α1 → 4)

Gal (β1 → 3) → GlcNAc-R

Fuc (α1 → 4)

Lewisᵇ   Fuc (α1 → 2)-Gal(β1 → 3) → GlcNAc-R

Fig. 27.13 **Structure of Lewis blood group antigens**.

the Lewisᵇ antigen is synthesized by the concerted action of a second fucosyltransferase which transfers fucose to a galactose residue in the same glycan chain. Note the similarity of these structures to the sialyl Lewis-X antigen in Figure 26.9 and the ABO antigens in Figure 27.12. There are 13 fucosyl transferases in the human genome. Changes in fucosylation of glycans are associated with differentiation, development, carcinogenesis and metastasis.

GLYCOLIPIDS ARE BINDING SITES FOR BACTERIA AND BACTERIAL TOXINS

Bacteria have evolved proteins called adhesins that recognize and interact with specific carbohydrate structures on glycolipids, glycoproteins and even proteoglycans. Many of the bacterial adhesins are protein subunits of pili, hair-like structures on the surfaces of the bacteria. The carbohydrate recognition domains are usually located at the tip of the pili. Most bacteria also have several different kinds of adhesins on their surfaces, each having different carbohydrate recognition sites, and these adhesins define the range of susceptible tissues that the bacteria can bind to and perhaps invade. Each individual adhesin binding is of low affinity and the binding is weak, but there are many copies of a given adhesin on the bacterial surface and they cluster together, so the total interaction is polyvalent rather than monovalent and binding becomes quite strong.

The interaction of the adhesin with its receptor can activate the signal transduction pathway and lead to events that are critical for colonization and perhaps infection. A number of bacterial adhesins target Galβ1-4Glc containing oligosaccharides. This is the disaccharide structure that is found in the animal glycolipid lactosylceramide, and this structure may be present as such or it may be capped with other sugars, as in the ABO blood group antigens. But some bacteria secrete enzymes (glycosidases) that can remove these terminal sugars to expose the lactose structure for binding to their adhesin. The epithelial cells of the large intestine express lactosylceramide, whereas the cells lining the small intestine do not express this glycolipid. As a result, *Bacterioides*, *Clostridium*, *Escherichia coli* and *Lactobacillus* only colonize the large intestine under normal conditions.

In addition to the bacterial binding, a number of toxins that are secreted from bacterial cells also bind to specific glycolipids. The best studied of these toxins is cholera toxin, i.e. the toxin produced by *Vibrio cholerae*, which binds to G-M₁ (see box). The toxin from *Shigella dysenteriae* also binds to cells of the large intestine, but it recognizes a different glycolipid, in this case the cerebroside, Galα1-4Galβceramide or Galα1-4Galβ1-4Glcβ-ceramide. These two examples show quite clearly how subtle changes in the structures of carbohydrate molecules can be recognized by different proteins, and why nature has selected carbohydrates molecules as providers of chemical recognition information. There are other toxins, such as the tetanus toxin produced by *Clostridium tetani* or botulinum toxin by *Clostridium botulinum*, which also bind to glycolipids on nerve cell membranes. These toxins recognize much more complicated glycolipids. For example, tetanus toxin binds to the glycolipid called G₁ᵦganglioside.

GANGLIOSIDE RECEPTOR FOR CHOLERA TOXIN

The galactose-containing cerebrosides and globosides in the plasma membranes of intestinal epithelial cells are binding sites for bacteria. The glycolipids appear to assist in retention of normal intestinal flora (symbionts) in the intestine but, conversely, binding of pathogenic bacteria to these and other glycolipids is believed to facilitate infection of the epithelial cells. The difference between symbiotic and parasitic bacteria depends, in part, on their ability to secrete toxins or to penetrate the host cell after the binding reaction.

Intestinal mucosal cells contain ganglioside GM₁ (see Fig. 27.10). This ganglioside serves as the receptor to which cholera toxin binds as the first step in its penetration of intestinal cells. Cholera toxin is a hexameric protein secreted by the bacterium *Vibrio cholerae*. The protein is composed of one A subunit and five B subunits. The protein binds to gangliosides by multiple interactions through the B subunits, which enables the A subunit to enter the cell and activate adenylate cyclase on the inner surface of the membrane. The cyclic AMP that is formed then stimulates intestinal cells to export chloride ions, leading to osmotic diarrhea, electrolyte imbalances, and malnutrition. Cholera remains the number one killer of children in the world today.

The P blood group antigens are glycosphingolipids on red cells and on other tissues. Again, the glycans in this blood group are synthesized by the sequential action of distinct glycosyltransferases, but so far relatively little is known about the enzymes or genes involved. The physiologic function for blood groups is unknown, but the P antigens are associated with the pathophysiology of urinary tract infections and parvovirus infections. Uropathogenic strains of *E. coli* express lectins that bind to the Galα1,4Gal moiety of the P^k and P_1 antigens. Clearly, more work is necessary to understand the genetics and biochemistry of these and other blood group antigens as well as their roles in physiology and disease.

Summary

Complex polar lipids are essential components of all cell membranes. Phospholipids are the major structural lipids of all membranes, but they also have important functional properties as surfactants, as cofactors for membrane enzymes, and as components of signal transduction systems. The primary route for de novo biosynthesis of phospholipids involves the activation of one of the components (either DAG or the head group) with CTP to form a high-energy intermediate, such as CDP-diglyceride or CDP-choline. In addition, there are exchange and modification reactions by which the animal cell interconverts various phospholipids. The other major types of membrane lipids are the sphingolipids, including sphingomyelin and various glycolipids. These lipids function as receptors for cell–cell recognition and interactions, and as binding sites for symbiotic and pathogenic bacteria and for viruses. Furthermore, various carbohydrate structures on the glycosphingolipids of red cell membranes are also the antigenic determinants responsible for the ABO and other blood types. Glycosphingolipids are degraded in the lysosomes by a complex sequence of reactions that involve a stepwise removal of sugars from the nonreducing end of the molecule, with each step involving a specific lysosomal exoglycosidase. A number of inherited lysosomal storage diseases result from defects in degradation of sphingolipids.

ACTIVE LEARNING

1. Describe the role of plasmalogens vs diacylglycerol-phospholipids in cell membrane structure and function.
2. Discuss the challenges in development of a vaccine to protect against trypanosomiasis.
3. Review current therapeutic approaches for diagnosis and treatment of acute respiratory distress syndrome (ARDS).
4. Review the mechanisms of host–pathogen interaction, focusing on the role of lectins in microbial pathogenicity.

Further reading

Allende MM, Proia RL. Lubricating cell signalling pathways with gangliosides. *Curr Opin Struct Biol* 2002;**12**:587–592.

Brady RO. Enzyme replacement for lysosomal diseases. *Annu Rev Med* 2006;**57**: 283–296.

Dowhan W. Molecular basis for membrane phospholipid diversity: why are there so many lipids? *Annu Rev Biochem* 1997;**66**:199–232.

Grabowski G. Phenotype, diagnosis, and treatment of Gaucher's disease. *Lancet* 2008; **372**:1263–1271.

Hellstrom U, Hallberg EC, Sandros J, Rydberg L, Backer AE. Carbohydrates act as receptors for the periodontitis-associated bacterium *Porphyromonas gingivalis*: a study of bacterial binding to glycolipids. *Glycobiology* 2004;**14**:511–519.

Hooper LV, Gordon JL. Glycans as legislators of host–microbial interactions: spanning the spectrum from symbiosis to pathogenicity. *Glycobiology* 2001;**11**: 1R–10R.

Lafont F, van der Goot FG. Bacterial invasion via lipid rafts. *Cell Microbiol* 2005;**7**: 613–620.

Websites

Blood groups: www.bloodbook.com/type-sys.html

Gaucher's disease: www.ninds.nih.gov/health_and_medical/disorders/gauchers_doc.htm

Paroxysmal nocturnal hemoglobinuria: www.emedicine.com/med/topic2696.htm

Tay-Sachs disease: www.ninds.nih.gov/health_and_medical/disorders/taysachs_doc.htm

28. The Extracellular Matrix

G P Kaushal, A D Elbein and W M Carver

LEARNING OBJECTIVES

After reading this chapter you should be able to:

■ Describe the composition, structure and function of the extracellular matrix (ECM) and its components, including collagens, noncollagenous proteins and proteoglycans.

■ Outline the functional roles of the ECM in tissues.

■ Outline the sequence of steps in the biosynthesis and posttranslational modification of collagens and elastin, including the structure and synthesis of crosslinks.

■ Describe the pathways of biosynthesis and turnover of proteoglycans.

■ Describe the pathology of genetic diseases resulting from errors in the synthesis or turnover of ECM components.

INTRODUCTION

The extracellular matrix (ECM) is a complex network of secreted macromolecules located in the extracellular space. Historically, the ECM has been described as simply providing a three-dimensional framework for the organization of tissues and organs; however, it has become increasingly clear that it plays a central role in regulating basic cellular processes, including proliferation, differentiation, migration and even survival. The macromolecular network of the ECM is made up of collagens, elastin, glycoproteins and proteoglycans that are secreted by a variety of cell types including fibroblasts, chondrocytes and osteoblasts. The components of the ECM are in intimate contact with their cells of origin and form a three-dimensional gelatinous bed in which the cells thrive. Proteins in the ECM are also bound to the cell surface, so that they transmit mechanical signals resulting from stretching and compression of tissues. The relative abundance, distribution, and molecular organization of ECM components vary enormously among tissues and dramatically impact the structural and functional properties of the tissue. Changes in these ECM characteristics are associated with chronic diseases, such as arthritis, atherosclerosis, cancer, and fibrosis.

COLLAGENS

Collagens are the major proteins in the ECM

The collagens are a family of proteins that comprise about 30% of total protein mass in the body. As the primary structural components of the ECM in connective tissues, collagens have an important role in tissue architecture and integrity, and in mediating a wide variety of cell–cell and cell–matrix interactions. To date, more than 25 different types of collagens have been identified. They are composed of related, but distinct, peptide chains and vary greatly in their distribution, organization, and function in tissues.

Triple-helical structure of collagens

The collagens are heterotrimeric proteins composed of three individual peptide chains. The structural hallmark of collagens is their triple-helical structure, formed by folding of the three component peptide chains. These chains vary in size, up to 1000 amino acids per chain. X-ray diffraction analysis indicates that three left-handed helical chains are wrapped around one another in a rope-like fashion, to form a superhelix structure (Fig. 28.1). The left-handed helix is more extended than the α-helix of globular proteins, having nearly twice the rise per turn and only three, rather than 3.6, amino acids per turn. Every third amino acid is glycine, because only this amino acid, with the smallest side chain, fits into the crowded central core. The characteristic, repeating sequence of collagen is Gly-X-Y, where X and Y can be any amino acid but most often X is proline and Y is hydroxyproline. Because of their restricted rotation and bulk, proline and hydroxyproline confer rigidity to the helix. The intra- and interchain helices are stabilized by hydrogen bonds, largely between peptide NH and C=O groups. The side chains of the X and Y amino acids point outward from the helix, and thus are on the surface of the protein, where they form lateral interactions with other triple helices or proteins.

Types of collagen

Some representative collagens are listed in Table 28.1. The collagen family of proteins can be divided into two main types: the fibril-forming (fibrillar) and the nonfibrillar collagens.

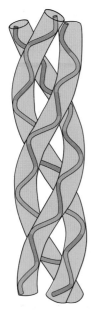

Fig. 28.1 **Three-dimensional structure of collagen**. Collagen monomer strands assume a left-handed, α-helical tertiary structure. They then associate to form a triple-stranded, right-handed superhelical quaternary structure.

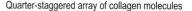

Quarter-staggered array of collagen molecules

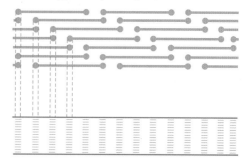

Banded appearance of fibrillar collagen

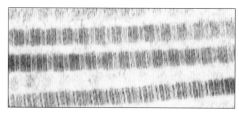

Fig. 28.2 **Formation of the quarter-staggered array of collagen molecules in a fibril**. The regular overlap of the short, nonhelical termini of the collagen chains yields a regular, banded pattern in the collagen fiber. (Electron micrograph courtesy of Dr Trevor Gray.)

Members of the collagen family		
Type	**Class**	**Distribution**
I	fibrillar	skin and tendon
II	fibrillar	cartilage, developing cornea and vitreous humor
III	fibrillar	extensible connective tissue, e.g. skin, lung and vascular system
IV	network	basement membranes, kidney, vascular wall
V	fibrillar	liver, cornea and mucosa
VI	beaded filament	most connective tissue
IX	FACIT	cartilage, vitreous humor
XI	fibril forming	cartilage, bone, placenta
XII	FACIT	embryonic tendon and skin
XIII	transmembrane domain	widely distributed
XIV	FACIT	fetal skin and tendons

FACIT, fibril-associated collagen with interrupted triple helices.

Table 28.1 **Members of the collagen family. Classification and distribution of different collagen types.**

Fibril-forming collagens

Fibril-forming collagens include types I, II, III, V, and XI (see Table 28.1). Collagen fibrils can be formed from a mixture of different fibrillar collagens. For instance, dermal collagen fibrils are hybrids of type I and type III collagen, and fibrils in corneal stroma are hybrids of type I and type IV collagen. Type I is the most abundant fibrillar collagen and occurs in a wide variety of tissues; others have a more limited tissue distribution (see Table 28.1). Type I and related fibrillar collagens form well-organized, banded fibrils and provide high-tensile strength to skin, tendons, and ligaments. As indicated above, collagens are heterotrimers composed of three α-helical peptide chains (see Fig. 28.1). The type I collagen heterotrimer is composed of two α1(I) chains and one α2(I) chain. Each of these peptide chains contains about 1000 amino acids and has a triple-helical domain structure along almost the entire length of the molecule. The collagen fibrils are formed by lateral association of triple helices in a 'quarter-staggered' alignment in which each molecule is displaced by about one-quarter of its length relative to its nearest neighbor (Fig. 28.2). The quarter-staggered array is responsible for the banded appearance of collagen fibrils in connective tissues. The fibrils are stabilized by both noncovalent forces and interchain crosslinks derived from lysine residues (see below).

Nonfibrillar collagens

Nonfibrillar collagens are a heterogeneous group containing triple-helical segments of variable length, interrupted by one or more intervening nonhelical (noncollagenous) segments. This group includes basement membrane collagens (the type IV family), fibril-associated collagens with

OSTEOGENESIS IMPERFECTA (INCIDENCE 1 IN 30 000–50 000)

A 6-year-old boy was seen in the casualty department with broken tibia and fibula occurring during a soccer game. His 6-foot-tall father explained that he had broken his legs four times while at school. The father's teeth were slightly transparent and discolored.

Comment. Osteogenesis imperfecta (OI), also called brittle bone disease, is a congenital disease caused by multiple genetic defects in the synthesis of type I collagen. It is characterized by fragile bones, thin skin, abnormal teeth and weak tendons. The majority of the individuals with this disease have mutations in genes encoding α1(I) and α2(I) collagen chains. Many of these mutations are single-base substitutions that convert glycine in the Gly-X-Y repeat to bulky amino acids, preventing the correct folding of the collagen chains into a triple helix and their assembly to form collagen fibrils. The dominance of type 1 collagen in bone explains why bones are predominantly affected. However, there is remarkable clinical variability characterized by bone fragility, osteopenia, variable degrees of short stature, and progressive skeletal deformities. The most common form of OI, with a presentation that is sometimes mistaken for child abuse, has a good prognosis, with fractures decreasing after puberty, though the general reduction in bone mass ensures lifetime risk remains high. Patients frequently develop deafness due to osteosclerosis, partly from recurrent fractures of the stapes. Bisphosphonate drugs (see Chapter 25), which inhibit osteoclast activity and thereby inhibit normal bone turnover, have reduced the incidence of fractures. Long-term follow-up studies are under way.

interrupted triple helices (FACITs), and collagens with multiple triple-helical domains with interruptions, known as multiplexins. Nonfibrillar collagens associate with the fibrillar collagens, forming microfibrils and network or mesh-like structures.

Basement membranes are relatively thin layers of ECM found on the basal aspect of epithelial cells and surrounding some other cell types including myocytes, Schwann cells and adipocytes. The basement membrane has a number of functions including anchorage of cells to surrounding connective tissue and filtration.

Type IV collagen is a major structural component of all basement membranes, where it assembles into a flexible mesh-like network. This collagen contains a long triple-helical domain interrupted by short noncollagenous sequences. These interruptions in the helical domain block continued association of two triple helices, oblige them to find another partner, and thus contribute to formation of a lattice-type structure. In the kidney, the thickened basement membrane (100–200 nm thick) on the basal aspect of the glomuerular capillary endothelial cells plays an essential role as a macromolecular filter (see Chapter 23). The meshwork of ECM proteins in the basement membrane restricts the passage of large molecules from the blood into the urine. In addition,

the inclusion of negatively charged proteoglycans (described later in this chapter) in the glomerular basement membrane restricts the passage of charged molecules. Anomalies in type IV collagen in the glomerular basement membrane result in several glomerular diseases including Goodpasture's syndrome and Alport syndrome. Goodpasture's syndrome is a rare autoimmune disease caused by the production of antibodies that specifically bind to type IV collagen of basement membranes. This condition leads to progressive worsening of basement membrane function in the kidney and sometimes in the lung. Alport syndrome results from mutations in the type IV collagen chains which cause defective collagen scaffold assembly within the basement membrane. The symptoms of both of these syndromes progress from blood in the urine (hematuria) to urine containing excessive protein (proteinuria) and eventually to kidney failure.

Synthesis and posttranslational modification of collagens

Collagen synthesis begins in the rough endoplasmic reticulum (RER)

After synthesis in the RER, the nascent collagen polypeptide undergoes extensive modification, first in the RER, then in the Golgi apparatus, and finally in the extracellular space, where it is modified to a mature extracellular collagen fibril (Fig. 28.3). A nascent polypeptide chain, preprocollagen, is synthesized initially with a hydrophobic signal sequence that facilitates binding of ribosomes to the endoplasmic reticulum (ER) and directs the growing polypeptide chain into the lumen of the ER. Posttranslational modification of the protein begins with removal of the signal peptide in the ER, yielding procollagen. Three different hydroxylases then add hydroxyl groups to proline and lysine residues, forming 3- and 4-hydroxyprolines and δ-hydroxylysine. These hydroxylases require ascorbate (vitamin C) as a cofactor (Fig. 28.3, step 1). Vitamin C deficiency leads to scurvy as a result of alterations in collagen synthesis and crosslinking (see Chapter 11).

O-linked glycosylation occurs by the addition of galactosyl residues to hydroxylysine by galactosyl transferase; a disaccharide is formed by addition of glucose to galactosyl hydroxylysine by a glucosyl transferase (Fig. 28.3, step 2). These enzymes have strict substrate specificity for hydroxylysine or galactosyl hydroxylysine, and they glycosylate only those peptide sequences that are in noncollagenous domains. N-linked glycosylation also occurs on specific asparagine residues in nonfibrillar domains. The nonfibrillar collagens, with a greater extent of nonhelical domains, are more highly glycosylated than fibrillar collagens. Thus, the extent of glycosylation may influence fibril structure, interrupting fibril formation and promoting interchain interactions required for a meshwork structure. Intra- and interchain disulfide bonds are formed in the C-terminal domains by a protein disulfide isomerase, facilitating the association and folding

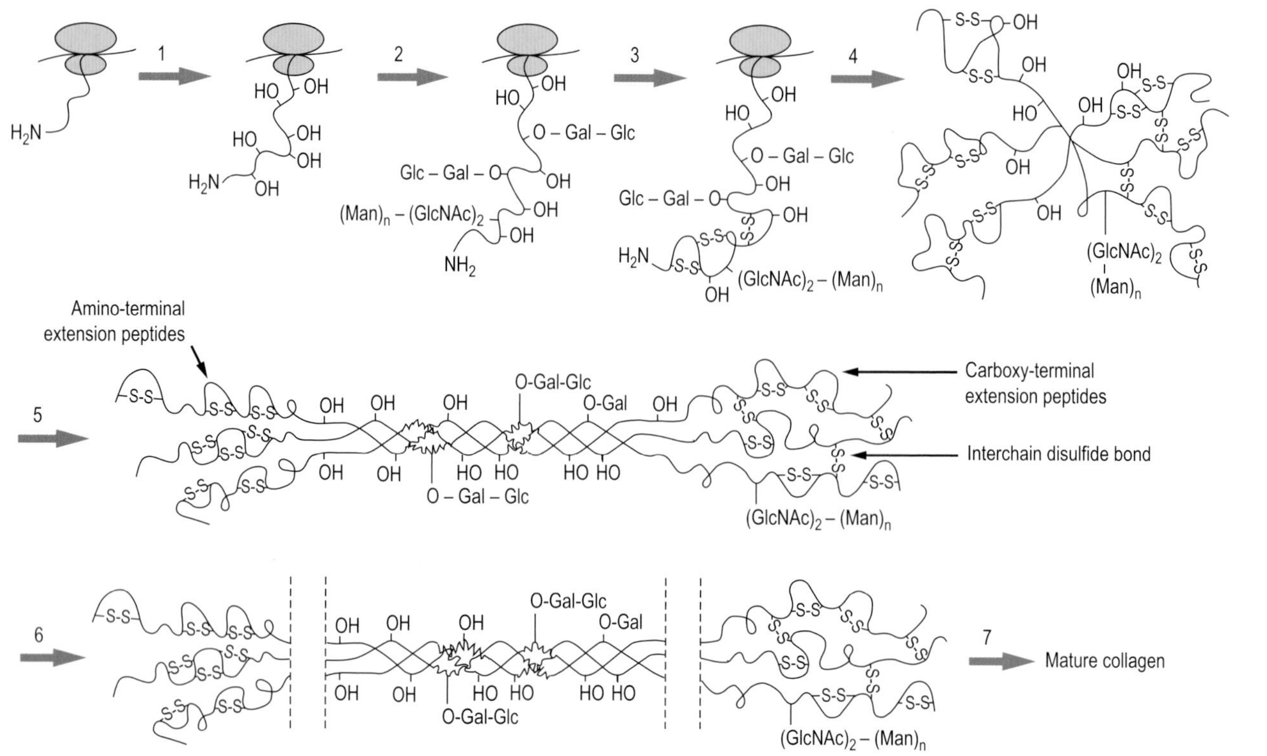

Fig. 28.3 **Biosynthesis and posttranslational processing of collagen**. Collagen is synthesized in the RER, posttranslationally modified in the Golgi apparatus, then secreted, trimmed of extension peptides, and finally assembled into fibrils in the extracellular space. (1) Hydroxylation of proline and lysine residues. (2) Addition of *O*-linked and *N*-linked oligosaccharides. (3) Formation of intrachain disulfide bonds at the *N*-terminal of the nascent polypeptide chain. (4) Formation of interchain disulfides in the *C*-terminal domains, which assist in alignment of chains. (5) Formation of triple-stranded, soluble tropocollagen, and transport to Golgi vesicles. (6) Exocytosis and removal of *N*- and *C*-terminal propeptides. (7) Final stages of processing, including lateral association of triple helices, covalent crosslinking and collagen fiber formation. Gal, galactose; Glc, glucose; GlcNAc, *N*-acetylglucosamine; Man, mannose.

of peptide chains into a triple helix (Fig. 28.3, steps 3–5). At this stage, the procollagen is still soluble and contains additional, nonhelical extensions at its *N*- and *C*-terminals.

Procollagen is finally modified to collagen in the Golgi apparatus

After assembly into the triple helix, the procollagen is transported from the RER to the Golgi apparatus, where it is packaged into cylindrical aggregates in secretory vesicles, then exported to the extracellular space by exocytosis. The nonhelical extensions of the procollagen are now removed in the extracellular space, by specific *N*- and *C*-terminal procollagen proteinases (Fig. 28.3, step 6). The 'tropocollagen' molecules then self-assemble into insoluble collagen fibrils, which are further stabilized by the formation of aldehyde-derived intermolecular crosslinks. Lysyl oxidase (not to be confused with lysyl hydroxylase involved in formation of hydroxylysine) oxidatively deaminates the amino group from the side chains of some lysine and hydroxylysine residues, producing reactive aldehyde derivatives, known as allysine and hydroxyallysine. The aldehyde groups now form aldol condensation products with neighboring aldehyde groups, generating crosslinks both within and between triple-helical molecules. They may also react with

LATHYRISM: THE RESULT OF LYSYL OXIDASE INHIBITION

Lathyrism is a diet-induced disease characterized by deformation of the spine, dislocation of joints, demineralization of bones, aortic aneurysms, and joint hemorrhages. These problems develop as a result of inhibition of lysyl oxidase, an enzyme required for the crosslinking of collagen chains. Lathyrism can be caused by chronic ingestion of the sweet pea *Lathyrus odoratus*, the seeds of which contain β-aminopropionitrile, an irreversible inhibitor of lysyl oxidase. Penicillamine, a sulfhydryl agent used for chelation therapy in heavy-metal toxicity, also causes lathyrism, because of either chelation of copper required for lysyl oxidase activity or reaction with aldehyde groups of (hydroxy)allysine, inhibiting collagen crosslinking reactions.

the amino groups of unoxidized lysine and hydroxylysine residues to form Schiff base (imine) crosslinks (Fig. 28.4). The initial products may rearrange, or be dehydrated, or reduced to form stable crosslinks, such as lysinonorleucine. Studies with

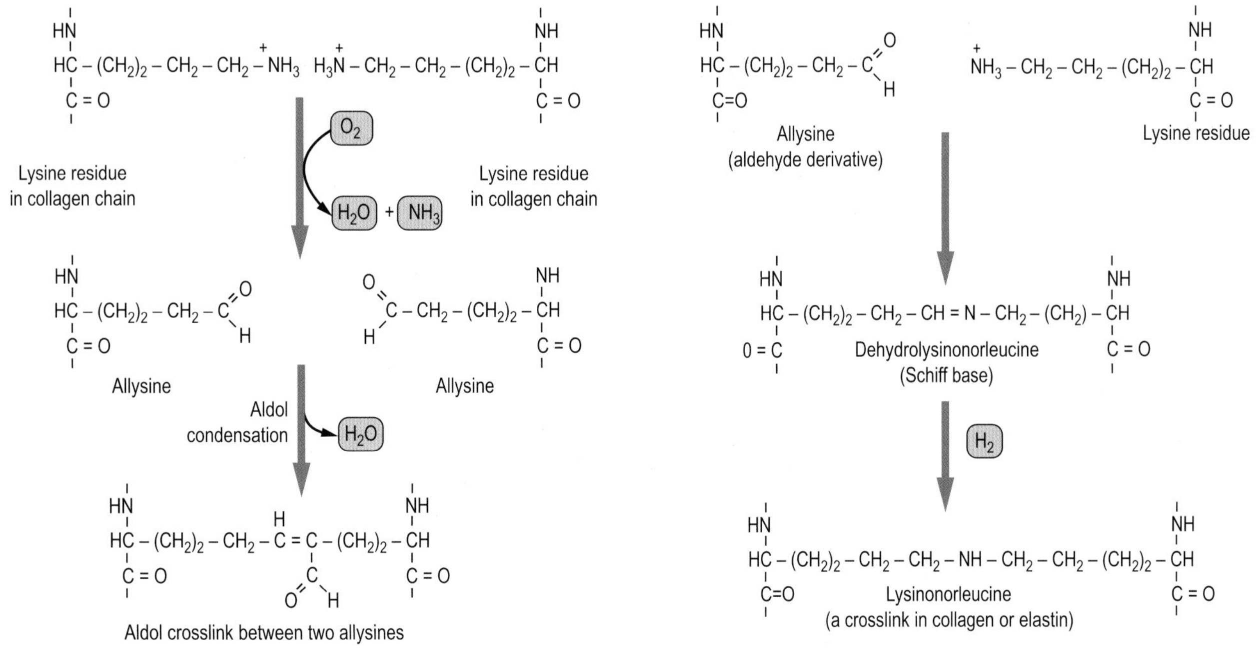

Fig. 28.4 **Collagen crosslink formation**. Allysine (and hydroxyallysine) are precursors of collagen crosslink formation by (A) aldol condensation and (B) Schiff base (imine) intermediates.

β-aminopropionitrile, which inhibits the enzyme lysyl oxidase, have illustrated that collagen crosslink formation is a major determinant of tissue mechanical properties and strength.

NONCOLLAGENOUS PROTEINS IN THE EXTRACELLULAR MATRIX

Elastin

The flexibility required for function of blood vessels, lungs, ligaments and skin is imparted by a network of elastic fibers in the ECM of these tissues. The predominant protein of elastic fibers is elastin. Unlike the multigene collagen family, there is only one gene for elastin, coding for a polypeptide about 750 amino acids long. In common with collagens, it is rich in glycine and proline residues but elastin is more hydrophobic: one in seven of its amino acids is a valine. Unlike collagens, elastin contains little hydroxyproline and no hydroxylysine or carbohydrate chains, and does not have a regular secondary structure. Its primary structure consists of alternating hydrophilic and hydrophobic, lysine and valine-rich domains. The lysines are involved in intermolecular crosslinking, while the weak interactions between valine residues in the hydrophobic domains impart elasticity to the molecule.

Elastin can stretch in two dimensions

The soluble monomeric form of elastin initially synthesized on the RER is called tropoelastin. Except for some hydroxylation

MARFAN SYNDROME: RESULT OF MUTATIONS OF THE FIBRILLIN GENE

The ultrastructure of elastic fibers reveals elastin as an insoluble, polymeric, amorphous core covered with a sheath of microfibrils that contribute to the stability of the elastic fiber. The predominant constituent of microfibrils is the glycoprotein, fibrillin. Marfan syndrome is a relatively rare genetic disease of connective tissues caused by mutations in the fibrillin gene (frequency: 1 in 10 000 births). People with this disease have typically tall stature, long arms and legs, and arachnodactyly (long, 'spidery' fingers). The disease in a mild form causes loose joints, deformed spine, floppy mitral valves (leading to cardiac regurgitation), and eye problems such as lens dislocation. In severely affected individuals, the aortic wall is prone to rupture because of defects in elastic fiber formation.

of proline, tropoelastin does not undergo posttranslational modification. During the assembly process in the extracellular space, lysyl oxidase generates allysine in specific sequences: -Lys-Ala-Ala-Lys- and -Lys-Ala-Ala-Ala-Lys-. As with collagen, the reactive aldehyde of allysine condenses with other allysines or with unmodified lysines. Allysine and dehydrolysinonorleucine on different tropoelastin chains also condense to form pyridinium crosslinks – heterocyclic structures known as desmosine or isodesmosine (Fig. 28.5). Because of the way in which elastin monomers are crosslinked in polymers, elastin can stretch in two dimensions.

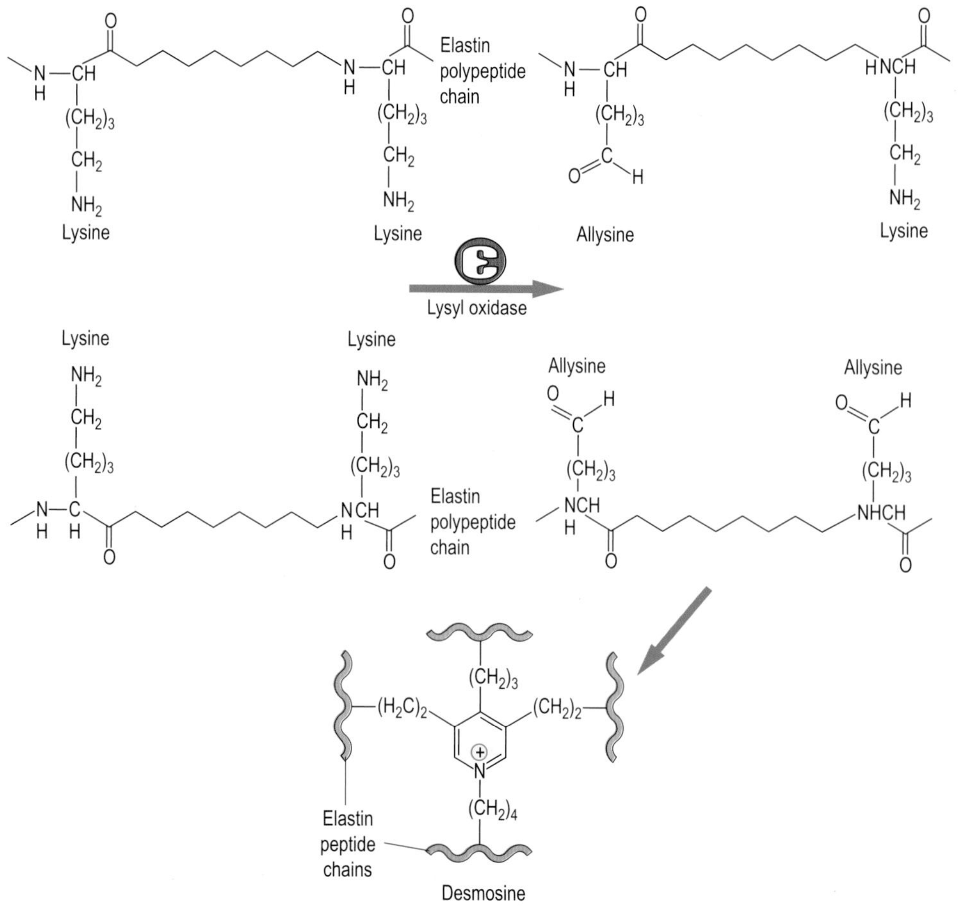

Fig. 28.5 **Desmosine – a multi-chain crosslink in elastin**. Allysine and dehydrolysinonorleucine residues in adjacent elastin chains react to form the three-dimensional elastic polymer, crosslinked by desmosine.

Fibronectin

Fibronectin is a glycoprotein present as a structural component of the ECM and also in plasma as a soluble protein. Fibronectin is a dimer of two identical subunits, each of 230 kDa, joined by a pair of disulfide bonds at their C-terminals. Each subunit is organized into domains, known as type I, II, and III domains, and each of these has several homologous repeating units or modules in its primary structure (Fig. 28.6): there are 12 type I repeats, two type II repeats, and 15–17 type III repeats. Each module is independently folded, forming a 'string of beads' type of structure. At least 20 different tissue-specific isoforms of fibronectin have been identified, all produced by alternative splicing of a single precursor messenger ribonucleic acid (mRNA). The alternative splicing is regulated not only in a tissue-specific manner but also during embryogenesis, wound healing, and oncogenesis. Plasma fibronectin, secreted mainly by liver cells, lacks two of the type III repeats that are found in cell- and matrix-associated forms of fibronectin. Because of its multidomain structure and its ability to interact with cells and with other ECM components, alterations in fibronectin expression affect cell adhesion and migration, embryonic morphogenesis, and cytoskeletal and ECM organization.

Functional domains in fibronectin have been identified by their binding affinity for other ECM components, including collagen, heparin, fibrin, and the cell surface. The type I modules interact with fibrin, heparin and collagen, type II modules have collagen-binding domains, and type III modules are involved in binding to heparin and the cell surface. The specific interactions have been further mapped to short stretches of amino acids. A short peptide containing Arg-Gly-Asp (RGD), present in the tenth type III repeat of fibronectin, binds to the integrin family of proteins present on cell surfaces; this sequence is not unique to fibronectin but is also found in other proteins in the ECM. Another sequence, Pro-X-Ser-Arg-Asn (PXSRN), present in the ninth type III repeat, is also implicated in integrin-mediated cell attachment. The integrins are a family of transmembrane proteins that bind extracellular proteins on the outside and cytoskeletal proteins, such as actin, on the inside of the cell, providing a mechanism for communication between the intracellular and extracellular environments of the cell. The loss of fibronectin from the surface of many tumor cells may contribute to their release into the circulation and penetration through the ECM, one of the first steps in tumor metastasis.

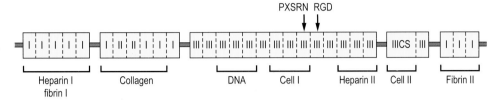

Fig. 28.6 **Structural map of fibronectin**. This shows various globular domains and domains involved in binding to various molecules in the cell and ECM. RGD, Arg-Gly-Asp; PXSRN, Pro-X-Ser-Arg-Asn.

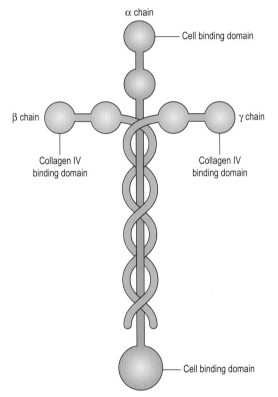

Fig. 28.7 **Structure of laminin**. This schematic illustrates the cruciform shape of a laminin heterotrimer. Labeled are some of the domains within the laminin molecule.

Laminins

Laminins are a family of noncollagenous glycoproteins found in basement membranes and expressed in variant forms in different tissues. They are large (850 kDa), heterotrimeric molecules, composed of α-, β- and γ-chains. To date, five α, four β and three γ chains have been identified which can associate to produce at least 15 different laminin variants. The three interacting chains in a heterotrimer are arranged in an asymmetric cruciform or cross-shaped molecule, held together by disulfide linkages (Fig. 28.7). Laminins undergo reversible self-assembly in the presence of calcium to form polymers, contributing to the elaborate mesh-like network in the basement membrane. Biochemical and electron microscopic studies indicate that all full-length short arms of laminin are required for self-assembly and that the polymer is formed by joining the ends of the short arms. Like fibronectin, laminins interact with cells through multiple binding sites in several domains of the molecule. The α-chains have binding sites for integrins and heparan sulfate (below). Laminin polymers are also connected to type IV collagen by a single-chain protein, nidogen/entactin, which has a binding site for collagen and, in common with fibronectin, also has an RGD sequence for integrin binding. Nidogen also binds to the core proteins of proteoglycans (below). It has a central role in formation of crosslinks between laminin and type IV collagen, generating a scaffold for anchoring of cells and ECM molecules in the basement membrane.

 MUSCULAR DYSTROPHIES

Muscular dystrophies are a heterogeneous group of genetic disorders that result in progressive decline in muscle strength and structure. To date, mutations have been identified in more than 30 genes that result in muscular dystrophies. Many of the identified gene products are components of the ECM–cell surface–cytoskeletal complex of muscle cells. In particular, one class of muscular dystrophy is caused by mutations in the α2 chain of laminin-2. These mutations prevent normal polymer formation of laminin-2 and result in abnormal basement membrane organization surrounding skeletal muscle fibers of patients with this muscular dystrophy.

 EPIDERMOLYSIS BULLOSA

Epidermolysis bullosa is a rare heritable disorder characterized by severe blistering of the skin and epithelial tissue. Three kinds are known:

- **simplex:** blistering in the epidermis, caused by defects in keratin filaments
- **junctional:** blistering in the dermal–epidermal junction, caused by defects in laminin
- **dystrophic:** blistering in the dermis, caused by mutations in the gene encoding type VII collagen.

Epidermolysis bullosa illustrates the multifactorial nature of connective tissue diseases that have similar clinical features.

PROTEOGLYCANS

Proteoglycans are gel-forming components of the ECM and comprise what has classically been called the 'ground substance'. Some proteoglycans are located on the cell surface, where they bind growth factors and other ECM components. They are composed of peptide chains containing covalently bound sugars. However, the peptide chains of proteoglycans are usually more rigid and extended than the protein portion of the glycoproteins, and the proteoglycans contain much larger amounts of carbohydrate – typically >95% carbohydrate. The sugar chains are linear, unbranched oligosaccharides that are much longer than those of the glycoproteins, and may contain more than 100 sugar residues in a chain. Furthermore, the oligosaccharide chains of proteoglycans have a repeating disaccharide unit, usually composed of a uronic acid and an amino sugar. Proteoglycan oligosaccharide chains are polyanionic because of the many negative charges of the carboxyl groups of the uronic acids, and from sulfate groups attached to some of the hydroxyl or amino groups of the sugars.

Structure of proteoglycans

The general structures of the glycosaminoglycans (GAGs), the carbohydrate part of the proteoglycans, are shown in Table 28.2. The disaccharide repeat is different for each type of GAG, but is usually composed of a hexosamine and a uronic acid residue, except in the case of keratan sulfate, in which the uronic acid is replaced by galactose. The amino sugar in GAGs is either glucosamine ($GlcNH_2$) or galactosamine ($GalNH_2$), both of which are present mostly in their N-acetylated forms (GlcNAc and GalNAc), although in some of the GAGs (heparin, heparan sulfate) the amino group is sulfated rather than acetylated. The uronic acid is usually D-glucuronic acid (GlcUA) but in some cases (dermatan sulfate, heparin) it may be L-iduronic acid (IdUA). With the exception of hyaluronic acid and keratan sulfate, all the GAGs are attached to protein by a core trisaccharide, Gal-Gal-Xyl; the xylose is linked to a serine or threonine residue of a core protein. Keratan sulfate is also attached to protein, but in that case the linkage is either through an N-linked oligosaccharide (keratan sulfate I) or an O-linked oligosaccharide (keratan sulfate II). Hyaluronic acid, which has the longest polysaccharide chains, is the only GAG that does not appear to be attached to a core protein.

Hyaluronic acid

Hyaluronic acid is composed of repeating units of GlcUA and GlcNAc. This polysaccharide chain is the longest of the GAGs, with molecular weight of 10^5–10^7 Da (250–25 000 repeating disaccharide units), and is the only nonsulfated GAG.

The chondroitin sulfates

The chondroitin sulfates are major components of cartilage. They contain GalNAc rather than GlcNAc as the amino sugar, and their polysaccharide chains are shorter: 2–5×10^5 Da. The chondroitin chains are attached to protein via the trisaccharide linkage region (Gal-Gal-Xyl), and they contain sulfate residues linked to either the 4- or 6-hydroxyl groups of GalNAc.

Dermatan sulfate

Dermatan sulfate was originally isolated from skin but is also found in blood vessels, tendon and heart valves. This GAG is similar in structure to chondroitin sulfate but has a variable amount of L-iduronic acid (IdUA), the C-5-epimer of D-GlcUA, formed in an unusual reaction by epimerization of GlcUA after it has been incorporated into the polymer. Dermatan sulfate

The proteoglycans			
Proteoglycan	**Characteristic disaccharide**	**Sulfation**	**Tissue location**
Hyaluronic acid	[4GlcUAβ1–3GlcNAcβ1]	none	joint and ocular fluids
Chondroitin sulfates	[4GlcUAβ1–3GalNAcβ1]	GalNAc	cartilage, tendons, bone
Dermatan sulfate	[4IdUAα1–3GalNAcβ1]	IdUA, GalNAc	skin, valves, blood vessels
Heparan sulfate	[4IdUAα1–4GlcNAcβ1]	GlcNAc	cell surfaces
Heparin	[4IdUAα1–4GlcNAcβ1]	$GlcNH_2$, IdUA	mast cells, liver
Keratan sulfates	[3Galβ1–4GlcNAcβ1]	GlcNAc	cartilage, cornea

GalNAc, N-acetylgalactosamine; $GlcNH_2$, glucosamine; GlcUA, D-glucuronic acid; IdUA, L-iduronic acid.

Table 28.2 **Structure and distribution of the proteoglycans.**

has a higher charge density than the chondroitin sulfates, as it contains sulfate residues on the C-2 position of some IdUA residues, and on the 4-hydroxyl groups of GalNAc.

Heparin and heparan sulfate

Heparin and heparan sulfate consist primarily of repeating disaccharide units of GlcNH$_2$ with IdUA or GlcUA, respectively. The linkage between the amino sugar and the uronic acid is uniformly 1-4, rather than the alternating 1-4/1-3 linkages seen in other GAGs. Most of the GlcNH$_2$ units of heparin are N-sulfated, whereas many of the IdUA residues are sulfated at the C-2 hydroxyl group, and the GlcNH$_2$ residues at the C-6 hydroxyl group. Heparin and heparan sulfate are the most highly charged of the GAGs. Although the structures of these two polymers are closely related, their distribution in the body and their functions are quite different: heparin is a small micro-heterogeneous molecule ($\sim$3000–30 000 Da), found intracellularly as a proteoglycan. It is released into the extracellular space as a free polysaccharide (GAG) and has strong anticoagulant activity (Chapter 7). In contrast, heparan sulfate is bound in the ECM or on the surface of cells, and has only weak anticoagulant activity.

Keratan sulfate

The final GAG structure shown in Table 28.2 is keratan sulfate (KS). This is a rather unusual GAG because it is linked to protein by either an N-linked (KS I) or an O-linked (KS II) oligosaccharide. Thus it has features common to both proteoglycans and glycoproteins. It is considered to be a proteoglycan, however, because the glycan portion has a repeating disaccharide unit and a long, linear chain. The repeating unit is composed of GlcNAc and galactose, instead of the uronic acid. Both the GlcNAc and the galactose are generally sulfated on the C-6 hydroxyl groups.

Synthesis and degradation of proteoglycans

Proteoglycans are synthesized by a series of glycosyl transferases, epimerases and sulfotransferases, beginning with the synthesis of the core oligosaccharide while the core protein is still in the RER. Synthesis of the repeating oligosaccharide and other modifications take place in the Golgi apparatus. As with the synthesis of glycoproteins and glycolipids, separate enzymes are involved in individual steps. For example, there are separate galactosyl transferases for each of the galactose units in the core, a separate GlcUA transferase for the core and repeating disaccharides, and separate sulfotransferases (see Chapter 27) for the C-4 and C-6 positions of the GalNAc residues of chondroitin sulfates. Phosphoadenosine phosphosulfate (PAPS) is the sulfate donor for the sulfotransferases. These pathways are illustrated in Figure 28.8, for chondroitin-6-sulfate.

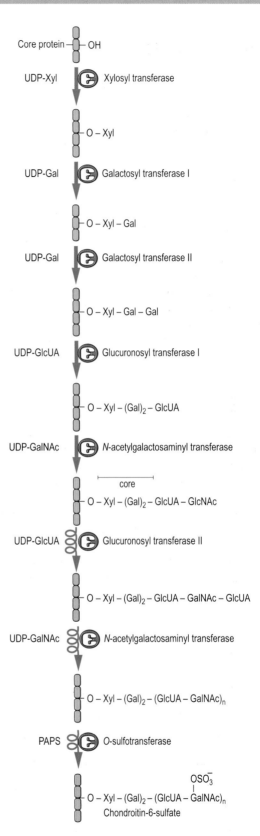

Fig. 28.8 **Synthesis of the proteoglycan, chondroitin-6-sulfate.** Several enzymes participate in this pathway. Xyl, xylose.

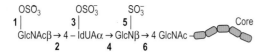

1. GlcNAc-6-sulfatase
2. Hexosaminidase
3. Iduronate sulfatase
4. Iduronidase
5. N-sulfatase
6. Glucosaminidase

Fig. 28.9 **Degradation of heparan sulfate**. This proceeds by a defined sequence of lysosomal hydrolase activities.

The mucopolysaccharidoses

Syndrome	Deficient enzyme	Product accumulated in lysosomes and secreted in urine
Hunter's	iduronate sulfatase	heparan and dermatan sulfate
Hurler's	α-iduronidase	heparan and dermatan sulfate
Morquio's A	galactose-6-sulfatase	keratan sulfate
B	β-galactosidase	keratan sulfate
Sanfilippo's A	heparan sulfamidase	heparan sulfate
B	N-acetylglucosaminidase	
C	N-acetylglucosamine-6-sulfatase	

Table 28.3 **Enzymatic defects characteristic of various mucopolysaccharidoses.**

Defects of proteoglycan degradation lead to mucopolysaccharidoses

The degradation of proteoglycans occurs in lysosomes. The protein portion is degraded by lysosomal proteases and the GAG chains are degraded by the sequential action of a number of different lysosomal acid hydrolases. The stepwise degradation of GAGs involves exoglycosidases and sulfatases, beginning from the external end of the glycan chain. This may involve the removal of sulfate by a sulfatase, then removal of the terminal sugar by a specific glycosidase, and so on. Figure 28.9 shows the steps in the degradation of dermatan sulfate. As with degradation of glycosphingolipids, if one of the enzymes involved in the stepwise pathway is missing, the entire degradation process is halted at that point and the undegraded molecules accumulate in the lysosome. The lysosomal storage diseases resulting from accumulation of GAGs are known as mucopolysaccharidoses (Table 28.3), because of the original designation of GAGs as mucopolysaccharides.

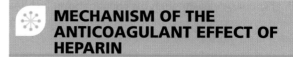

MECHANISM OF THE ANTICOAGULANT EFFECT OF HEPARIN

Heparin is a heterogeneous (3000–30 000 kDa), polyanionic oligosaccharide activator of antithrombin III (AT) (Chapter 7). AT is a slow but quantitatively important inhibitor of thrombin (factor X) and other factors (IX, XI, XII) in the blood-clotting cascade. When heparin binds to AT, it converts AT from a slow inhibitor to a rapid inhibitor of coagulating enzymes. Heparin interacts with a lysine residue in AT and induces a conformational change that promotes covalent binding of AT to the active serine centers of coagulating enzymes, inhibiting their procoagulant activity. Heparin then dissociates from the ternary complex and can be recycled for anticoagulation. The smallest, most active component of heparin is a pentasaccharide that has a K_d of ~10 μmol/L: GlcN-(N-sulfate-6-O-sulfate)-α1,4-GlcUA-β1,4-GlcN-(N-sulfate-3,6-di-O-sulfate)-α1,4-IdUA-(2-O-sulfate)-α-1,4-GlcN-(N-sulfate-6-O-sulfate). Heparin has an average half-life of 30 min in the circulation, so that it is commonly administered by infusion. Heparin does not have fibrinolytic activity; therefore, it will not lyse existing clots. In addition to its anticoagulant activity, heparin also releases several enzymes from proteoglycan binding sites on the vascular wall, including lipoprotein lipase, which is often assayed as heparin-releasable plasma lipoprotein lipase activity or postheparin lipase. Lipoprotein lipase is inducible by insulin, and decreased activity of this enzyme delays plasma clearance of chylomicrons and VLDL, contributing to hypertriglyceridemia in diabetes (Chapter 18).

There are more than a dozen such mucopolysaccharidoses, resulting from defects in degradation of GAGs. In general, these diseases can be diagnosed by the identification of specific GAG chains in the urine, followed by assay of the specific hydrolases in leukocytes or fibroblasts.

Functions of the proteoglycans

Bottlebrushes, silly putty and reinforced concrete

Proteoglycans are found in association with most tissues and cells. One of their major roles is to provide structural support to tissues, especially cartilage and connective tissue. In cartilage, large aggregates, composed of chondroitin sulfate and keratan sulfate chains linked to their core proteins, are noncovalently associated with hyaluronic acid via link proteins, forming a jelly-like matrix in which the collagen fibers are embedded. This macromolecule of macromolecules, a 'bottlebrush' structure known as aggrecan (Fig. 28.10), provides both rigidity and stability to connective tissue. Because of their negative charge, the GAGs bind large amounts of monovalent and divalent cations: a cartilage proteoglycan molecule of 2×10^6 Da would have an aggregate negative charge

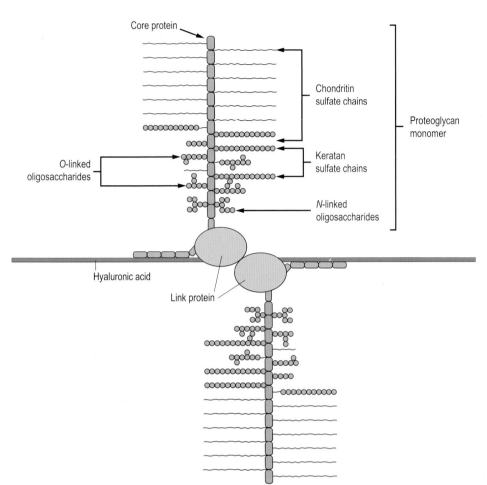

Core protein

Chondritin
sulfate chains

Proteoglycan
monomer

O-linked
oligosaccharides

Keratan
sulfate chains

N-linked
oligosaccharides

Hyaluronic acid

Link protein

Fig. 28.10 **Structure of aggrecan**. Associations between proteoglycans and hyaluronic acid form an aggrecan structure in the extracellular matrix (ECM). The extension of this structure yields a three-dimensional array of proteoglycans bound to hyaluronic acid, which creates a stiff matrix or 'bottlebrush' structure in which collagen and other ECM components are embedded.

of about 10 000. The maintenance of electrical neutrality consequently requires a high concentration of counterions. These ions draw water into the ECM, causing swelling and stiffening of the matrix, the result of tension between osmotic forces and binding interactions between proteoglycans and collagen. The structure and hydration of the ECM allow for a degree of rigidity, combined with flexibility and compressibility, enabling the tissue to withstand torsion and shock. The hyaluronic acid-proteoglycan-collagen aggregates in vertebral and articular disks have some of the viscoelastic properties of 'silly putty', bounce plus resilience, cushioning the impact between bones. These disks compress during the course of the day, expand elastically during the course of night, and deform gradually with age.

The overall structure of cartilage can be likened to that of the vertical reinforced concrete slabs poured during the construction of large buildings, in which steel rods (collagen fibers) are embedded in an amorphous layer of cement (the proteoglycan aggregates). Collagen stabilizes the network of proteoglycans in cartilage in much the same way that the reinforcing rods in the concrete provide structural strength for the cement walls. The structure of earthquake-resistant buildings, like the ECM, provides a balance between integrity and flexibility.

Although the amounts involved are low compared with those in skin and cartilage, organs such as the liver, brain, or kidney also contain a variety of proteoglycans:

- **liver:** heparan sulfate is the principal GAG; it is present both intracellularly and on the cell surface of the hepatocyte, and the attachment of hepatocytes to their substratum in cell culture is mediated, in part, by this proteoglycan
- **kidney:** changes in both the collagen and proteoglycan content of the renal basement membrane are associated with diabetic renal disease. In this case, the change in structure and charge of the proteoglycan aggregate, known as perlecan, is associated with a change in the filtration selectivity of the glomerulus (Chapter 23)
- **cornea:** two populations of proteoglycans have been identified in the cornea, one containing keratan sulfate and the other dermatan sulfate. These molecules have a much smaller hydrodynamic size than the large cartilage proteoglycans, which may be required for interaction of the corneal proteoglycans with the tightly packed and oriented collagen fibers in this transparent tissue. Corneal clouding in macular corneal dystrophy is associated with undersulfation of keratan sulfate I proteoglycan.

Other complex glycan aggregates with subtle variations in core protein structure and glycan composition are distributed in intracellular compartments, plasma membranes and in the extracellular space in a tissue-specific manner and vary with age and disease.

Some proteoglycans or GAGs, especially heparin and heparan sulfate, have important physiologic roles in binding proteins or other macromolecules:

- **mast cells** (granulated cells involved in the inflammatory response): heparin is believed to function as an intracellular binding site for proteinases in secretory granules
- **the vascular wall:** proteoglycans are involved in the binding of proteins and enzymes, such as low-density lipoprotein and lipoprotein lipase, to the vascular wall. They may also inhibit clot formation on the vascular wall by surface activation of antithrombin III (Chapter 7).

 ## EXTRACELLULAR MATRIX AND TISSUE ENGINEERING

Over the past decade, the interest in producing replacement tissues through tissue engineering has grown considerably. The ultimate goal of tissue engineering is to combine appropriate cells and biomaterials to produce tissue equivalents that favorably mimic normal tissues and organs and can replace damaged or diseased tissues. As the biologic and mechanic properties of tissues are determined in part by the heterogeneous composition and organization of the ECM, the successful generation of tissue equivalents will require the development of appropriate three-dimensional ECM scaffolds. Advances in this relatively new field will require a thorough understanding of the normal and pathologic ECM..

Summary

The ECM contains a complex array of fibrillar and network-forming collagens, elastin fibers, a stiff gelatinous matrix of proteoglycans, and a number of glycoproteins that mediate the interaction of these molecules with one another and with the cell surface. These molecules and their interactions afford structure, stability,

ACTIVE LEARNING

1. Compare the structure of heparin, its mechanism of action, its route and frequency of administration to that of other common anticoagulants, such as aspirin and coumarin derivatives.
2. Discuss factors that promote the turnover of ECM components, as part of normal growth and development and in diseases such as rheumatoid arthritis.
3. Review the consequences of genetic defects in sulfation of proteoglycans.

and elasticity to the ECM, and provide a route for communication between the intra- and extracellular environments in tissues. The heterogeneity of both the protein and the carbohydrate components of these molecules provides for great diversity in the structure and function of the ECM in various tissues.

Further reading

Bosman FT, Stamenkovic I. Functional structure and composition of the extracellular matrix. *J Pathol* 2003;**200**:423–428.
Holmbeck K, Szabova L. Aspects of extracellular matrix remodeling in development and disease. *Birth Defects Res* 2006;**78**:11–23.
Hulmes DJ. Building collagen molecules, fibrils, and suprafibrillar structures. *J Struct Biol* 2002;**137**:2–10.
Kadler KE, Baldock C, Bella J, Boot-Handford RP. Collagens at a glance. *J Cell Science* 2007;**120**:1955–1958.
Laurent GJ, Chambers RC, Hill MR, McAnulty RJ. Regulation of matrix turnover: fibroblasts, forces, factors and fibrosis. *Biochem Soc Trans* 2007;**35**:647–651.
Paez MC, Gonzalez MJ, Serrano NC, Shoenfeld Y, Anaya JM. Physiological and pathological implications of laminins: from genes to the protein. *Autoimmunity* 2007;**40**:83–94.
Parsons CJ, Takashima M, Rippe RA. Molecular mechanisms of hepatic fibrogenesis. *J Gastroenterol Hepatol* 2007;**1**:S79–84.
Stupack DG. The biology of integrins. *Oncology* 2007;**21**:6–12.

Websites

Collagen assembly: www.mc.vanderbilt.edu/cmb/collagen/index.php
Ehlers–Danlos syndrome:
- www.nlm.nih.gov/medlineplus/ehlersdanlossyndrome.html
- www.ednf.org
Heparin: www2.kumc.edu/wichita/meded/cvresource/antithrombotic/heparin/
Marfan's syndrome:
- www.marfan.org
- www.nlm.nih.gov/medlineplus/marfansyndrome.html
Mucopolysaccharidoses: www.ninds.nih.gov/health_and_medical/pubs/mps.htm

29. Role of the Liver in Metabolism

A F Jones

LEARNING OBJECTIVES

After reading this chapter you should be able to:

- Discuss the participation of the liver in carbohydrate metabolism and in particular its role in endogenous glucose production.
- Discuss the role of the liver in lipid metabolism.
- Outline changes in the hepatic protein synthesis that take place during the acute phase reaction.
- Describe ubiquitin-mediated mechanisms of proteolysis.
- Describe the pathway of heme synthesis.
- Describe the metabolism of bilirubin and the main types of jaundice.
- Comment on the mechanism of hepatotoxicity of drugs and alcohol.

XENOBIOTICS

A xenobiotic, according to the *Oxford Dictionary of Biochemistry and Molecular Biology*, is 'a substance that does not occur naturally but interferes with the metabolism of any organism'.

Hepatic function	
Function	**Markers of impairment in plasma**
Heme catabolism	↑bilirubin
Carbohydrate metabolism	↓glucose
Protein synthesis	↓albumin ↑prothrombin time
Protein catabolism	↑ammonia ↓urea
Lipid metabolism	↑cholesterol ↑triglycerides
Drug metabolism	↑drug t1/2
Bile acid metabolism	↑bile acids

t1/2 = biological half-time.

Table 29.1 **Hepatic function.** Functions of hepatic parenchymal cells and their disturbances in liver disease.

INTRODUCTION

The liver has a central role in metabolism, because of both its anatomic placement and its many biochemical functions. It receives venous blood from the intestine and thus all the products of digestion, in addition to ingested drugs and other xenobiotics, perfuse the liver before entering the systemic circulation. The hepatic parenchymal cells, the hepatocytes, have an immensely broad range of synthetic and catabolic functions, which are summarized in Table 29.1. The liver plays important roles in the regulation of carbohydrate and lipid metabolism, in amino acid metabolism, in the synthesis and breakdown of plasma proteins, and in the storage of vitamins and metals. It also has the ability to metabolize, and so detoxify, an infinitely wide range of xenobiotics. The liver also has an excretory function, in which metabolic waste products are secreted into a branching system of ducts known as the biliary tree, which in turn drains into the small intestine; the biliary constituents are then excreted in feces.

The liver has a substantial reserve metabolic capacity; mild liver disease may cause no symptoms and be detected only as biochemical changes in the blood. However, the patient with severe liver disease has a yellow pigmentation of the skin (jaundice), bruises readily, may bleed profusely, has an abdomen distended with fluid (ascites), and may be confused or unconscious (hepatic encephalopathy) (Fig. 29.1). This chapter will describe the specialized metabolic functions of the liver and the abnormalities that occur in liver disease.

STRUCTURE OF THE LIVER

The liver is the largest solid organ in the body and, in adults, weighs about 1500 g. Approximately 75% of its blood flow is supplied by the portal vein, which arises from the intestine. Blood leaving the liver enters the venous system through the hepatic vein. The biliary component of the liver comprises the gall bladder and bile ducts.

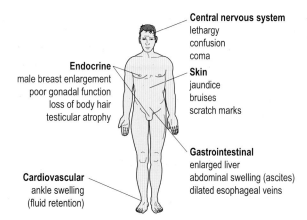

Fig. 29.1 **Clinical features of severe liver disease.**

Central nervous system
lethargy
confusion
coma

Endocrine
male breast enlargement
poor gonadal function
loss of body hair
testicular atrophy

Skin
jaundice
bruises
scratch marks

Gastrointestinal
enlarged liver
abdominal swelling (ascites)
dilated esophageal veins

Cardiovascular
ankle swelling
(fluid retention)

Structure of the liver facilitates exchange of metabolites between hepatocytes and plasma

Under the microscope, the substance of the liver is composed of a very large number of lobules, polyhedral in shape (Fig. 29.2). Blood sinusoids arise from the terminal branches of the portal vein and interconnect and interweave through these sheets of hepatocytes before joining the central lobular vein.

Sinusoids are lined by two cell types. The first are vascular endothelial cells, which are loosely connected one with another, leaving numerous gaps. There is no basement membrane between the endothelial cells and the hepatocytes. This arrangement facilitates the exchange of metabolites between hepatocyte and plasma. The second type of sinusoidal cells, known as Kupffer cells, are mononuclear phagocytes; they are generally found in the gaps between endothelial cells.

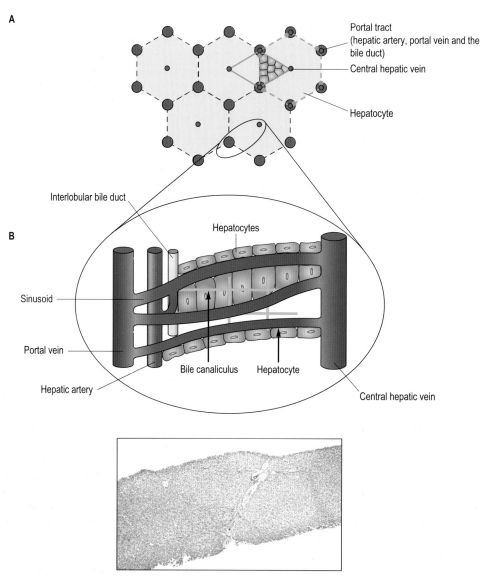

Fig. 29.2 **Structure of the liver.** (A) Outline of the structure. (B) A histologic slide of a normal liver. (Courtesy Dr J Newman, Birmingham Heartlands and Solihull NHS Trust, UK.)

LIVER AND CARBOHYDRATE METABOLISM

The liver plays a central role in glucose metabolism, specifically in maintaining the circulating concentration of glucose (Chapters 13 and 21). This function depends upon its ability both to store a supply of glucose in a polymerized form as glycogen, and to synthesize glucose from noncarbohydrate sources in the process of gluconeogenesis.

Depending on metabolic conditions, liver can either take up or produce glucose

Importantly, the liver possesses glucose-6-phosphatase which permits the release of free glucose to the blood (this process is also called 'endogenous glucose production'). Although muscle stores more glycogen than the liver, it has no glucose-6-phosphatase and hence cannot directly contribute glucose to the blood; the kidney, on the other hand, has both gluconeogenetic enzymes and glucose-6-phosphatase activities but they are quantitatively much lower than in the liver. Moreover, kidneys do not store glycogen.

The adult liver in the fasting state releases 9 g of glucose each hour to the blood to maintain the peripheral glucose concentration. The carbon substrates for the other pathway of glucose production, gluconeogenesis, are derived from lactate released by glycolysis in the peripheral tissues (the 'glucose-lactate' or 'Cori' cycle) and from hepatic deamination of amino acids generated from the proteolysis of skeletal muscle (mainly alanine, the 'glucose-alanine' cycle, see Chapter 21). Energy for gluconeogenesis comes from the β-oxidation of fatty acids. Also, the endproduct of the β-oxidation, acetyl-CoA, stimulates the activity of the pyruvate carboxylase, the first committed enzyme of gluconeogenesis.

On feeding, hepatic glucose production from gluconeogenesis is suppressed by insulin. Glucose entering the circulation after feeding enters cells by specific transporters of differing kinetic properties (see Table 8.2). The glucose transporter 1 (GLUT-1) present in the brain is not sensitive to insulin and has a low Michaelis constant (K_m), of the order of 1 mmol/L, and a low maximal velocity, around 3 mmol/L. Hence the GLUT-1 is saturated at most prevailing plasma glucose concentrations and allows the brain to extract glucose at a steady rate unlikely to be influenced by feeding or fasting. In contrast, the activity of the GLUT-2 transporter, present in both liver and pancreas, although independent of insulin, has a very high K_m (15–20 mmol/L). Thus, these tissues take up glucose at a rate which is proportional to the plasma glucose concentration. In the liver, glucose is converted to glycogen (Chapter 13). Glucose uptake by the pancreas determines β-cell insulin secretion and the GLUT-2 transporter and/or the associated hexokinase act as glucose sensors. Indeed, mutations in this pancreatic hexokinase, termed glucokinase,

are the cause of some cases of the so-called 'maturity-onset diabetes of the young' (MODY; see Chapter 21). The majority of ingested glucose, however, is disposed of by muscle and fat tissue that possess another insulin-dependent glucose transporter, GLUT-4, which, because it has a K_m similar to average plasma glucose concentration of around 5 mmol/L, becomes the most important glucose 'sink' in the fed state.

LIVER AND PROTEIN METABOLISM

The majority of plasma proteins are synthesized in the liver

Hepatocellular disease may alter protein synthesis both quantitatively and qualitatively. Albumin is the most abundant protein in blood and is synthesized exclusively by the liver (see Chapter 4). Low plasma albumin concentrations occur commonly in liver disease, but a better index of hepatocyte synthetic function is the production of the coagulation factors II, VII, IX, and X (Chapter 7), which all undergo posttranslational γ-carboxylation of specific glutamyl residues, allowing them to bind calcium. As a group, their functional concentration can be readily assessed in the laboratory by measuring the prothrombin time (PT) (see Chapter 7).

The liver also synthesizes most of the plasma α- and β-globulins. Their plasma concentrations change in hepatic disease and in systemic illness; in the latter case, these changes form part of the acute phase response to the illness (Chapter 4).

Acute phase proteins

Response to an acute insult is associated with wide-ranging changes in liver protein synthesis

The acute phase response is a term encompassing all the systemic changes which occur in response to infection or inflammation. The liver synthesizes a number of 'acute phase proteins', which have been defined as those whose plasma concentrations change by more than 25% within a week of the inflammatory or infective insult. The production of these proteins is stimulated by proinflammatory cytokines released by macrophages, and of these interleukin-1 (IL-1), IL-6 and tumor necrosis factor (TNF) have a central role. The acute phase proteins have a number of different functions. Binding proteins, opsonins, such as C-reactive protein (CRP), bind to macromolecules released by damaged tissue or infective agents and promote their phagocytosis (Chapter 4). Complement factors promote the phagocytosis of foreign molecules. Protease inhibitors, such as α1-antitrypsin and α1-antichymotrypsin, inhibit proteolytic enzymes. The latter two also promote fibroblast growth and the production of connective tissue required for the repair and resolution of the injury.

A substantial supply of amino acids is required as substrates for this increase in hepatic protein synthesis and these are derived from the proteolysis of skeletal muscle. TNF and IL-1 again are involved by stimulating the breakdown of specific intracellular proteins by the ubiquitin-proteasome system (see below).

The magnitude of the acute phase protein response is often linked to the severity of the inflammatory or infective process, such that serial measurements of the acute phase proteins in serum give useful information about the progress of the disease and response to treatment. Changes in the serum concentration of CRP are quantitatively the most marked of all the acute phase proteins This is illustrated in Figure 4.9 (see also box on p. 229). Its concentrations may increase by one or two orders of magnitude, the response is rapid and the protein has a short half-life. These properties and the relative ease with which it can be measured have led to CRP being widely used in clinical practice as a laboratory marker of infection and inflammation (see Chapters 4 and 38).

Clinical conditions associated with abnormal concentrations of liver-produced proteins in plasma

Genetic deficiency of $\alpha 1$-antitrypsin presents in infancy as liver disease or in adulthood as lung disease

Hepatic $\alpha 1$-antitrypsin belongs to the serpins, one of the family of serine protease inhibitors, and, contrary to its name, its predominant target is macrophage-derived elastase. Genetic deficiency of $\alpha 1$-antitrypsin presents in infancy as liver disease or in adulthood as lung disease caused by elastase-mediated tissue destruction; the severity of the liver disease is variable. Several isoforms of $\alpha 1$-antitrypsin exist as a result of allelic variation: the normal isoform is known as M and the two common defective isoforms as S and Z; the null allele produces no $\alpha 1$-antitrypsin.

Genetic deficiency of ceruloplasmin leads to Wilson's disease, a condition associated with liver and CNS damage

Ceruloplasmin is the major copper-containing protein of the liver and plasma, and functions as an iron oxidizing enzyme (ferroxidase): oxidation of Fe^{2+} to Fe^{3+} is necessary for the mobilization of stored iron, and nutritional copper deficiency produces anemia. Wilson's disease is a condition associated with damage to both the liver and the CNS. The liver also synthesizes proteins responsible for storage (ferritin) and transport (transferrin) of iron (see Chapters 4 and 22).

Liver cancer is associated with particularly high plasma concentrations of α-fetoprotein

α-Fetoprotein (AFP) and albumin have considerable sequence homology, and appear to have evolved by reduplication of a single ancestral gene. In the fetus, AFP appears to serve physiologic functions similar to those performed by albumin in the adult; furthermore, by the end of the first year of life, AFP in the plasma is entirely replaced by albumin. During hepatic regeneration and proliferation, AFP is again synthesized; thus high plasma concentrations of AFP are observed in liver cancer.

Protein degradation by ubiquitin-proteasome system

Ubiquitin marks intracellular proteins for proteasomal degradation

Hepatic protein turnover is highly regulated, which allows metabolic pathways to adapt to changing physiologic circumstances. Mammalian cells possess several proteolytic systems.

Plasma proteins and membrane receptors are endocytosed and then hydrolyzed by acid proteases within intracellular organelles known as lysosomes. Intracellular proteins, on the other hand, are degraded within structures known as proteasomes by the so-called ubiquitin-proteasome system (UPS) (see Chapter 33). The discoverers of protein ubiquinylation were awarded the Nobel Prize in chemistry in 2003.

Within the UPS, protein degradation occurs in two stages. First, ubiquitin, a small protein (mw 8.5 kDa), is coupled to the amino groups of protein lysyl residues, and this conjugation reaction is repeated to form chains of five or more ubiquitin molecules linked to the protein. The process involves three enzymes: an ATP-dependent ubiquitin-activating enzyme (E1), ubiquitin-conjugating enzyme (E2) and ubiquitin-protein ligase (E3). The specificity of the proteasomal degradation relies on the specificity of the enzymes responsible for the ligation of ubiquitin to protein substrate, and on the presence of particular destabilizing structures at the N-terminal end of the protein molecule, such as phosphorylated and hydroxylated residues. Incidentally, protein ubiquination is inhibited by acetylation. In the second stage, ubiquitin-bound proteins enter proteasomes, unfold and undergo proteolysis. The UPS is important in the activation of the NFκB proinflammatory pathway and the function of UPS is modified by reactive oxygen species (Chapter 37; see also Fig. 33.10).

The urea cycle and ammonia

Urea cycle is essential for the removal of nitrogen generated by amino acid metabolism

Catabolism of amino acids generates ammonia (NH_3) and ammonium ions (NH_4^+). Ammonia is toxic, particularly to the central nervous system (CNS). Most ammonia is detoxified at its site of formation, by amidation of glutamate to glutamine, which is mainly derived from muscle and used as an energy source by enterocytes. The remaining nitrogen enters the portal vein either as ammonia or as alanine, both of which are used by the liver for the synthesis of urea (Chapter 19).

Impaired clearance of ammonia causes brain damage

The urea cycle is the major route by which waste nitrogen is excreted, and is described in Chapter 19. In neonates, inherited defects of any of the enzymes of the urea cycle lead to hyperammonemia, which impairs the function of the brain, causing the condition known as encephalopathy. Such problems arise within the first 48 hours of life and inevitably are made worse by protein-rich foods such as milk (see Clinical box on p. 244).

HEME SYNTHESIS

Heme, a constituent of hemoglobin, myoglobin and cytochromes, is synthesized in most cells of the body. The liver is the main nonerythrocyte source of its synthesis. Heme is a porphyrin, a cyclic compound which contains four pyrrole

rings linked together by methenyl bridges. It is synthesized from glycine and succinyl-coenzyme A, which condense to form 5-aminolevulinate (5-ALA). This reaction is catalyzed by 5-ALA synthase, located in mitochondria, and is rate limiting in heme synthesis. Subsequently, in the cytosol, two molecules of 5-ALA condense to form a molecule containing a pyrrole ring, porphobilinogen (PBG). Then, four PBG molecules combine to form a linear tetrapyrrole compound, which cyclizes to yield uroporphyrinogen III and then coproporphyrinogen III. Final stages of the pathway occur again in the mitochondria where a series of decarboxylation and oxidation of side chains in uroporphyrinogen III yield protoporphyrin IX. At the final stage, iron (Fe^{2+}) is added by ferrochelatase to protoporphyrin IX to form heme. Heme controls the rate of its synthesis by inhibiting 5-ALA synthase (Fig. 29.3).

BILIRUBIN METABOLISM

Excess bilirubin causes jaundice

Bilirubin is the catabolic product of heme. About 75% of all bilirubin is derived from the hemoglobin of senescent red

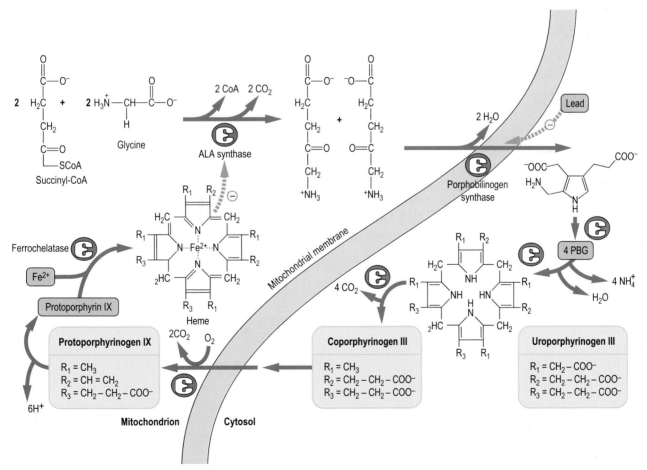

Fig. 29.3 **The pathway of heme synthesis.** Part of the pathway is located in the mitochondria and part in the cytosol. ALA, 5-aminolevulinate; PBG, porphobilinogen. Hemoglobin is discussed in Chapter 4.

PORPHYRIAS: DISEASES THAT RESULT FROM DEFECTIVE HEME SYNTHESIS

Defects in the heme synthetic pathway lead to rare disorders known as porphyrias. Different porphyrias are caused by deficiencies of different enzymes in the biosynthetic pathway, starting from 5-ALA synthase and ending with ferrochelatase. Porphyrias are classified as hepatic or erythropoietic depending on the primary organ affected.

Three porphyrias are known as acute porphyrias and can be a cause of emergency admissions with abdominal pain (which needs to be differentiated from various surgical causes). They also cause neuropsychiatric symptoms. Acute intermittent porphyria (AIC) is caused by the deficiency of hydroxymethylbilane synthase, an enzyme converting PBG to a linear tetrapyrrole; in this disorder the concentrations of 5-ALA and PBG increase in plasma and urine.

Hereditary coproporphyria is due to a defect in the conversion of coproporphyrinogen III to protoporphyrinogen III (coprooxidase). The third form of acute porphyria is the variegate porphyria, the clinical manifestations of which are very similar to AIC. Other porphyrias, such as porphyria cutanea tarda, present clinically as the sensitivity of skin to light (photosensitivity) which may cause disfiguration and scarring. Also, the pathway is inhibited by lead at the stage of porphobilinogen synthase.

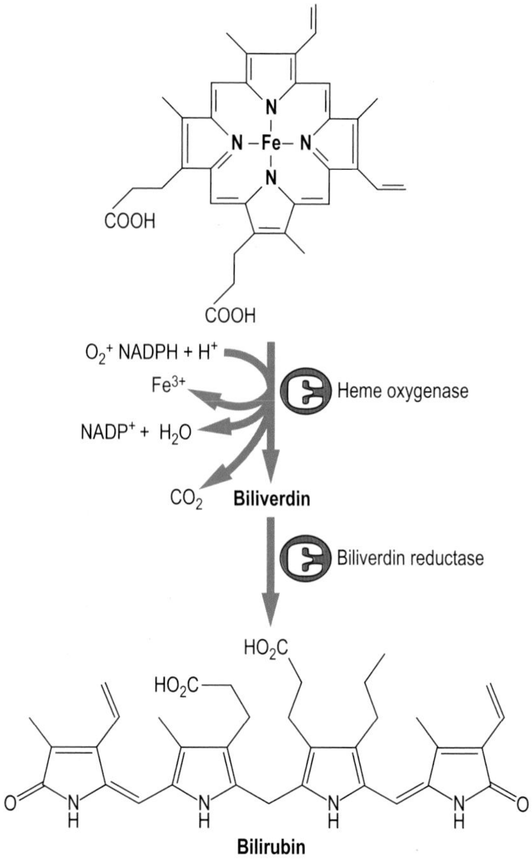

Fig. 29.4 **Degradation of heme to bilirubin.**

blood cells, which are phagocytosed by mononuclear cells of the spleen, bone marrow, and liver. In normal adults the daily load of bilirubin is 250–350 mg. The ring structure of heme is oxidatively cleaved to biliverdin by heme oxygenase, a P-450 cytochrome (see below). Biliverdin is, in turn, enzymatically reduced to bilirubin (Fig. 29.4). The normal plasma concentration of bilirubin is less than 17 μmol/L (1.0 mg/dL). Increased concentrations (more than 50 μmol/L or 3 mg/dL) are readily recognized clinically, because bilirubin imparts a yellow color to the skin (jaundice). Abnormalities in bilirubin metabolism are important pointers in the diagnosis of liver disease.

Bilirubin is metabolized by the hepatocytes and excreted in bile

Whereas biliverdin is water soluble, bilirubin, paradoxically, is not. Therefore, it must be further metabolized before excretion (Fig. 29.5). This occurs in the liver, where bilirubin is transported bound to plasma albumin; the hepatic uptake of bilirubin is mediated by a carrier and may be competitively inhibited by other organic anions. The hydrophilicity of bilirubin is increased by esterification of one or both of its carboxylic acid side chains with glucuronic acid, xylose or ribose. The glucuronide diester is the major conjugate and its formation is catalyzed by a uridine diphosphate

(UDP)-glucuronyl transferase. Conjugated bilirubin is then secreted by the hepatocyte into the biliary canaliculi.

Conjugated bilirubin in the gut is catabolized by bacteria to form stercobilinogen, also known as fecal urobilinogen, which is colorless. On oxidation, however, stercobilinogen forms stercobilin (otherwise known as fecal urobilin), which is colored; most stercobilin is responsible for the color of feces. Some stercobilin may be reabsorbed from the gut and can then be reexcreted by either the liver or the kidneys.

Bile acid and cholesterol metabolism

Bile acids are key elements in fat metabolism

Bile acids are synthesized in hepatocytes and have a detergent-like effect, solubilizing biliary lipids and emulsifying dietary fat in the gut to facilitate its digestion. Their metabolism is described in Chapters 10 and 17. Bile is also the only route of cholesterol excretion. This has been described in detail in Chapters 17 and 18.

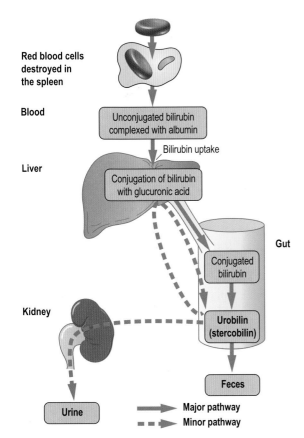

Red blood cells destroyed in the spleen

Blood

Unconjugated bilirubin complexed with albumin

Bilirubin uptake

Liver

Conjugation of bilirubin with glucuronic acid

Gut

Conjugated bilirubin

Kidney

Urobilin (stercobilin)

Feces

Urine

→ Major pathway
- - → Minor pathway

Fig. 29.5 **Normal bilirubin metabolism.**

DRUG METABOLISM

Low substrate specificity of some hepatic enzymes produces a wide-ranging capability for drug metabolism

Most drugs are metabolized by the liver. Among other effects, this hepatic metabolism usually increases the hydrophilicity of drugs and therefore their ability to be excreted. Generally, metabolites that are produced are less pharmacologically active than the substrate drug; however, some inactive prodrugs are converted to their active forms as a result of liver processing. The hepatic drug-metabolizing systems need to act on an infinite range of molecules; this is achieved by the enzymes involved having low substrate specificity. Metabolism proceeds in two phases:

- **phase I – addition of the polar group**: the polarity of the drug is increased by oxidation or hydroxylation catalyzed by a family of microsomal cytochrome P-450 oxidases
- **phase II – conjugation**: cytoplasmic enzymes conjugate the functional groups introduced in the first phase reactions, most often by glucuronidation or sulfation and also acetylation and methylation.

Three of the twelve cytochrome P-450 gene families share the responsibility for drug metabolism

The cytochrome P-450 enzymes are heme-containing proteins that colocalize with reduced nicotinamide adenine dinucleotide phosphate (NADPH):cytochrome P-450 reductase. They are present in the endoplasmic reticulum. Most metabolism associated with the cytochrome P-450 superfamily takes place in the liver but these enzymes are also present in the epithelium of the small intestine. The reaction sequence catalyzed by these enzymes is shown in Figure 29.6. There are 12 cytochrome P-450 gene families, of which three, designated *CYP1*, *CYP2* and *CYP3*, are responsible for most of the phase I drug metabolism. In fact, six enzymes, CYP1A2, CYP3A CYP2C9, CYP2C19, CYP2D6 and CYP2E1, are responsible for approximately 90% of drug metabolism. CYP3A is one of the most important cytochrome P-450 enzymes and constitutes about 50% of their activity. Each gene locus has multiple alleles.

Induction and inhibition of cytochrome P-450 enzymes is the mechanism of drug interactions

Hepatic synthesis of P-450 cytochromes is induced by certain drugs and other xenobiotic agents: this increases the rate of phase I reactions. On the other hand, drugs that form a relatively stable complex with a particular cytochrome P-450 inhibit the metabolism of other drugs that are normally substrates for that cytochrome. For instance, CYP1A2 metabolizes, among others, caffeine and theophylline. It can be inhibited by grapefruit juice, that contains a substance known as naringin, or by the antibiotic ciprofloxacin. When a person takes any of the inhibitory substances, normal substrates for CYP1A2 are metabolized more slowly and their plasma levels increase.

 ## THERAPEUTIC EXPLOITATION OF CYP3A INHIBITION

The drug ritonavir reduces the CYP3A-mediated metabolism of some of the inhibitors of human immunodeficiency virus (HIV) protease. This increases the levels of these drugs in plasma. The effect is exploited therapeutically by using combined treatment with ritonavir and protease inhibitors.

During immunosuppressive therapy the dose of the immuno-suppressant cyclosporin may need to be reduced by up to 75% if the patient also takes the antifungal drug ketoconazole (see Wilkinson in Further reading). This can precipitate adverse reactions.

The drugs that induce induction or repression of CYP3A enzymes often act through the nuclear receptor

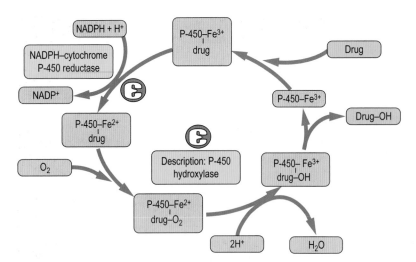

Fig. 29.6 **The role of the cytochrome P-450 system in the metabolism of drugs.**

mechanism. They combine with nuclear receptors (i.e. in case of CYP3A4, the pregnane X receptor, PXR), which then form heterodimers with retinoid X receptors (see Chapter 17). Such complexes upregulate CYP3 synthesis by binding to response elements in the gene promoter.

Cytochrome P-450 gene polymorphisms determine response to many drugs

Allelic variation that affects the catalytic activity of a cytochrome P-450 will also affect the pharmacologic activity of drugs. The best described example of such polymorphism is that of the P-450 cytochrome *CYP2D6*, which was recognized initially in the 5–10% of normal individuals who were noted to be slow to hydroxylate debrisoquine, a now little used blood pressure-lowering drug. *CYP2D6* also metabolizes a significant number of other commonly used drugs, so that 'debrisoquine polymorphism' remains clinically significant.

Genotyping of cytochromes P-450 to identify gene-relevant polymorphisms may identify an individual's capacity to metabolize a given drug. It identifies poor, intermediate, extensive and ultrarapid drug metabolizers. Such genotyping, together with measurements of therapeutic drug concentrations, is one way of preventing adverse reactions to drugs. These measures are now commonly used, for instance, in organ transplantation surgery, where the effectiveness of immunosuppressant drugs is critical to the success of a transplant.

Drug hepatotoxicity

Drugs that exert their toxic effects on the liver may do so through the hepatic production of a toxic metabolite. Drug toxicity may occur in all individuals exposed to a sufficient concentration of a particular drug. However, a drug may be toxic in some individuals at concentrations normally tolerated by most other patients. This phenomenon is known as idiosyncratic drug toxicity and may be due to a genetic or immunologic cause.

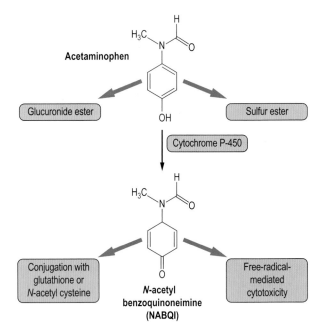

Fig. 29.7 **Metabolism of acetaminophen (paracetamol).**

The commonly prescribed drug acetaminophen (paracetamol) is hepatotoxic in excess

Acetaminophen is widely used as a painkiller. Taken in the usual therapeutic doses, it is conjugated with glucuronic acid or sulfate, which is then excreted by the kidneys. In overdose, the capacity of these conjugation pathways is overwhelmed and acetaminophen is oxidized by a liver P-450 cytochrome 3A4 to N-acetyl benzoquinoneimine (NABQI), which can cause a free radical-mediated peroxidation of membrane lipids, and consequently hepatocellular damage. NABQI may be detoxified by conjugation with glutathione but in acetaminophen overdose, glutathione stores also become exhausted, causing hepatotoxicity (Fig. 29.7). Therapeutically, a sulfhydryl compound, N-acetyl cysteine (NAC), is routinely used as an antidote to acetaminophen poisoning. It promotes detoxification of NABQI by the glutathione pathway and also scavenges

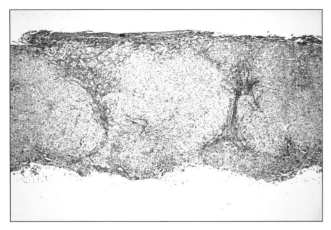

Fig. 29.8 **A histologic slide of a cirrhotic liver.** (Courtesy Dr J Newman, Birmingham Heartlands and Solihull NHS Trust, UK.)

free radicals. The risk of hepatotoxicity can be reliably predicted from measurement of the plasma concentration of acetaminophen, so that NAC can be given to those patients at risk of liver damage. Measurement of paracetamol is thus one of the emergency tests offered by clinical laboratories.

Alcohol

Alcohol excess is a major cause of liver disease

Excess intake of ethyl alcohol remains the most common cause of liver disease in the Western world (see box on p. 401). Ethanol may cause alcoholic hepatitis, steatosis due to deposition of fat or finally fibrosis (known as cirrhosis), which in turn leads to liver failure. There are over 25 000 deaths associated with liver disease in the US annually, and 40% of these are linked to alcoholic cirrhosis (see Donohue in Further reading). The microscopic features of alcoholic cirrhosis are shown in Figure 29.8.

Ethanol is oxidized in the liver, mainly by alcohol dehydrogenase, to form acetaldehyde, which is in turn oxidized by aldehyde dehydrogenase (ALDH) to acetate. Nicotinamide adenine dinucleotide (NAD^+) is the cofactor for both these oxidations, being reduced to NADH. A P-450 cytochrome, *CYP2E1*, also contributes to ethanol oxidation but is quantitatively less important than the alcohol dehydrogenase–ALDH pathway. Liver damage in patients who abuse alcohol may arise from the toxicity of acetaldehyde, which forms Schiff base adducts with other macromolecules.

Ethanol oxidation as a result of the increased ratio of NADH to NAD^+ alters the redox potential of the hepatocyte. This inhibits oxidation of lactate to pyruvate (a step that requires NAD^+ as a cofactor). This creates potential for the development of lactic acidosis and, because pyruvate is a substrate for hepatic gluconeogenesis, there is also a risk of hypoglycemia. The risk of hypoglycemia is increased in alcoholics when they fast as, because of poor nutrition, they often have low hepatic glycogen stores (see Clinical box on p. 168).

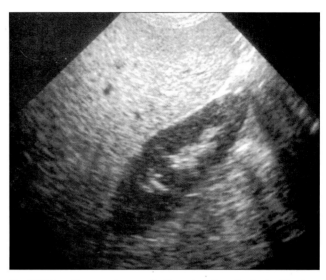

Fig. 29.9 **An ultrasound scan of a liver showing steatosis.** (Courtesy Dr A Bannerjee, Birmingham Heartlands and Solihull NHS Trust, UK.)

Also, the shift in the $NADH/NAD^+$ ratio inhibits β-oxidation of fatty acids and promotes triglyceride synthesis: their excess is deposited in the liver (hepatic steatosis) and secreted into plasma as VLDL (see Clinical box on p. 199). Hepatic steatosis can be readily diagnosed by ultrasonography of the liver when one sees a uniform increased echogenicity (Fig. 29.9). It is often associated with elevation in serum levels of the transaminase enzymes (see below) which are important laboratory markers of liver disease.

Ethanol consumption also affects the ubiquitin system of protein degradation. Chronic alcohol consumption decreases proteasome activity. This can deregulate the hepatocyte signaling system by inhibiting the Janus-signal transducer and activation of the transcription factor (JAK-STAT) pathway (see Chapter 40). The JAK-STAT pathway is involved in the acute phase response, antiviral defense and hepatic repair and inflammation and its inhibition can contribute to the development of alcoholic liver disease. Inhibition of proteasome activity may also lead to increased apoptosis (Chapter 43), a feature of alcoholic liver disease. The ethanol-induced decrease in proteasome activity prevents the degradation of CYP2E1, which is involved in peroxidation reactions; this increases oxidative stress and may be another factor contributing to alcoholic liver disease.

 BIOCHEMICAL BACKGROUND TO HEPATOMEGALY

Alcohol-induced decrease in proteasome activity may lead to the accumulation of protein in the liver, which in turn causes liver enlargement (hepatomegaly, common in alcoholic liver disease). Other ethanol-induced phenomena include increased secretion of chemokines (including IL-8 and monocyte-attractant protein-1 (MCP-1; see Chapter 18)) by hepatocytes, leading to liver infiltration by neutrophils.

ACETAMINOPHEN AND HEPATIC FAILURE

A 22-year-old woman was admitted to hospital in a semiconscious state. She had been found with a suicide note and empty acetaminophen containers. Tests revealed aspartate aminotransferase (AST) 5500 U/L, alkaline phosphatase (ALP) 125 U/L, bilirubin 70 μmol/L (4.1 mg/dL), prothrombin time 120 sec (normal value 10–15 sec), creatinine 350 μmol/L (4.0 mg/dL; normal range 20–80 μmol/L, 0.28–0.90 mg/dL), glucose 2.6 mmol/L (47 mg/dL; normal range 4.0–6.0 mmol/L, 72–109 mg/dL), and blood pH 7.1. No acetaminophen was found in her plasma.

Comment. The patient had acute hepatic failure, most probably caused by acetaminophen poisoning. Blood acetaminophen may be undetectable if the patient first comes to medical attention more than 24 h after an overdose. The hepatocellular damage worsens over the first 72 h but may improve spontaneously after that, as a result of regeneration of hepatocytes. However, in patients with a metabolic acidosis, markedly increased prothrombin times or serum creatinine >300 μmol/L (3.4 mg/dL), mortality is very high and liver transplantation may be necessary. For reference ranges see Table 29.2.

Laboratory tests in differential diagnosis of jaundice

Test	Prehepatic	Intrahepatic	Posthepatic
Conjugated bilirubin	absent	increased	increased
AST or ALT	normal	increased	normal
ALP	normal	normal	increased
Urine bilirubin	absent	present	present
Urine urobilinogen	present	present	absent

Table 29.2 **A panel of laboratory tests is essential in differential diagnosis of jaundice.** The reference ranges for liver function tests are as follows: AST (aspartate aminotransferase) 10–40 U/L, ALT (alanine aminotransferase) <50 U/L, ALP (alkaline phosphatase) 50–260 (ALP is physiologically elevated in children and adolescents), bilirubin <17 μmol/L (<1.0 mg/dL), albumin 36–52 g/L (3.6–5.2 g/dL), γ-glutamyl transpeptidase: men <90 U/L, women <50 U/L.

Symptoms of alcohol intolerance are exploited to reinforce abstinence

Both alcohol dehydrogenase and ALDH are subject to genetic polymorphisms, which have been investigated as a potential inherited basis of susceptibility to alcoholism and alcoholic liver disease. Possession of the ALDH2² allele, which encodes an enzyme with reduced catalytic activity, leads to increased plasma concentrations of acetaldehyde after the ingestion of alcohol. This causes the individual to experience unpleasant flushing and sweating, which discourages alcohol abuse.

Disulfiram, a drug that inhibits ALDH, also causes these symptoms when alcohol is taken, and may be given to reinforce abstinence from alcohol.

PHARMACOGENOMICS

The response to any particular drug will be influenced by the kinetic properties of the drug (pharmacokinetics) and its effects (pharmacodynamics). An individual's response to the drug can be influenced by genes that code for drug-metabolizing enzymes, receptors and transporters. Any variability in these genes may lead to interindividual differences in response to that drug.

The effectiveness and safety of drug therapy, particularly in elderly patients whose metabolic capacity is diminished, are currently a major problem. Approximately 3% of hospital admissions in the US are linked to drug–drug interactions and a Dutch study reported values as high as 8.4%. In the US, there are 2 million cases of adverse drug reactions annually, including 100 000 deaths. Combined with the fact that most drugs are effective in only 25–60% of patients to whom they are prescribed, this makes research into individual response to drugs absolutely essential.

Pharmacogenomics studies the effects of genetic heterogeneity on drug responsiveness

Since the liver has a central role in drug metabolism, the pharmacogenomics of some hepatic drug-metabolizing enzymes, specifically the cytochrome P-450 oxidases, is clinically very relevant. *CYP2D6* is responsible for the metabolism of more than 100 pharmaceuticals, and a polymorphism of this enzyme is responsible for the long-established variation in the metabolism of debrisoquine, mentioned above. Patients are classified as ultra-rapid, extensive, intermediate and poor metabolizers of debrisoquine. There is one *CYP2D6* genetic locus, and individuals may have two, one or no functional alleles, corresponding to extensive, intermediate and poor metabolizers respectively: gene multiplication can lead to three functional alleles and the ultra-rapid metabolizer phenotype. Seventy five *CYP2D6* alleleic variants have been identified and pharmacogenetic techniques can identify the metabolizer phenotype, thereby predicting clinical response to treatment. Although debrisoquine is now obsolete, the *CYP2D6* polymorphism is relevant for some drugs used in cardiac and psychiatric practice. For instance, poor metabolizers are more likely than other individuals to experience drug toxicity, and less likely to gain benefit from the analgesic codeine, a prodrug which is metabolized by *CYP2D6* to morphine, the active drug. A polymorphism of *CYP2C19*, again leading to extensive and poor metabolizer phenotypes, affects the metabolism of the proton pump inhibitor drugs used in gastroesophageal reflux disease and the effectiveness of treatment (Chapter 8).

ALCOHOL-RELATED LIVER DISEASE

A 45-year-old businessman had a routine medical examination, at which he was found to have a slightly enlarged liver. Tests revealed bilirubin 15 μmol/L (0.9 mg/dL), AST 434 U/L, ALT 198 U/L, ALP 300 U/L, γ-glutamyl transpeptidase (γGT) 950 U/L, and albumin 40 g/L (4 g/dL). He seemed perfectly well.

Comment. The patient has liver disease. The biochemical tests show evidence of hepatocellular damage. The increased γGT concentration is one of the most sensitive indices of excessive intake but there may also be enlarged red blood cells (macrocytosis) and an increased serum uric acid concentration. Patients may deny alcohol abuse. Needle biopsy of the liver may be necessary for diagnosis. In this patient, microscopic examination of the tissue revealed characteristic changes of alcoholic steatosis, hepatitis and central fibrosis. This may be the forerunner of cirrhosis and the patient should abstain from alcohol. Other causes, such as chronic viral infection of the liver or an autoimmune active chronic hepatitis, can be detected by blood tests. For reference ranges see Table 29.2. (Compare box on p. 168.)

GENOMICS OF LIVER DISEASE

A few hepatic diseases arise due to single gene disorders and genetic techniques can identify those with a propensity to develop a disease or confirm the diagnosis in affected individuals.

Hereditary hemochromatosis is a genetically determined disorder of iron metabolism common in northern Europeans, with a population prevalence of 1 in 200 to 1 in 300. Patients absorb excessive amounts of iron from the gut, and tissue iron overload leads to multiorgan dysfunction, including cirrhosis of the liver. A transmembrane glycoprotein, known as HFE, modulates iron uptake. Mutations in the genetic locus which encodes this protein, the HFE gene, underlie hereditary hemochromatosis. Two point mutations, *C282Y* and *H63D*, are found in the majority of those with hereditary hemochromatosis and can be identified easily by PCR-based assays. α1-Antitrypsin (AA1T) deficiency leads to early-onset lung disease and liver cirrhosis. More than 90 allelic variants of the AA1T gene, at the so-called Pi or proteinase inhibitor locus, have been described, the majority of which do not affect plasma levels or activity of AA1T. Phenotypic variants in AA1T were initially described by their relative mobility on electrophoresis, with the most common variant, M, having medium mobility. The Z and S variants are most frequently associated with AA1T deficiency, and are both due to point mutations which can also be detected by PCR assays. Wilson's disease, another hereditary cause of cirrhosis due to excess copper deposition in the liver, is also

caused by a single gene defect but multiple mutations have been found in affected patients; no routine assay is available for diagnosis. Gilbert's disease (see below) is caused by a dinucleotide polymorphism in the TATA box (see Fig. 34.1) promoter of the bilirubin UDP-glucuronyl transferase gene which impairs the hepatic uptake of unconjugated bilirubin.

BIOCHEMICAL TESTS OF LIVER FUNCTION

Clinical laboratories offer a panel of measurements on plasma or serum specimens (see Table 29.2). This group of tests is usually, and incorrectly, described as liver 'function' tests. The tests commonly include the measurements of:

- bilirubin
- albumin
- aspartate aminotransferase (AST) and alanine aminotransferase (ALT)
- alkaline phosphatase (ALP)
- γ-glutamyl transferase (γGT).

Reference ranges for these tests are given in the legend to Table 29.2.

Plasma activities of liver enzymes are markers of liver disease, and prothrombin synthesis is a good indicator of liver synthetic function.

Transaminases

Aspartate aminotransferase (AST) and alanine aminotransaminase (ALT) are involved in the interconversion of amino and ketoacids, and are required for metabolism of nitrogen and carbohydrates (Chapter 19). Both are located in the mitochondria; ALT is also found in the cytoplasm. Serum activity of ALT and AST increases in liver disease (ALT is the more sensitive measurement). In liver disease, the synthetic functions of the hepatocytes are likely to be affected, and so the patient would be expected to have a prolonged prothrombin time and low serum albumin concentration.

Alkaline phosphatase (ALP)

ALP is synthesized both by the biliary tract and by bone, but these two tissues contain different ALP isoenzymes. The origin of the ALP may be determined from the isoenzyme pattern. Alternatively, the plasma activity of another enzyme, such as γ-glutamyl transpeptidase (GGP), which also originates in the biliary tract, may be measured.

CLASSIFICATION OF LIVER DISORDERS

Hepatocellular disease

Inflammatory disease of the liver is termed hepatitis and may be of short (acute) or long (chronic) duration. Viral infections, particularly hepatitis A, B and C, are common infectious causes of acute hepatitis, whereas alcohol and acetaminophen are the most common toxicologic causes. Chronic hepatitis, defined as inflammation persisting for more than 6 months, may also be due to the hepatitis B and C viruses, alcohol, and immunologic diseases, in which the body produces antibodies against its own tissues (autoimmune diseases, Chapter 38). Cirrhosis is the result of chronic hepatitis and is characterized microscopically by fibrosis of the hepatic lobules. The term 'hepatic failure' denotes a clinical condition in which the biochemical function of the liver is severely, and potentially fatally, compromised.

Cholestatic disease

Cholestasis is the clinical term for biliary obstruction, which may occur in the small bile ducts in the liver itself or in the larger extrahepatic ducts. Biochemical tests cannot distinguish between these two possibilities, which generally have radically different causes; imaging techniques such as ultrasound are more helpful.

Jaundice

Jaundice can be pre-, post- or intrahepatic

Jaundice is clinically obvious when plasma bilirubin concentrations exceed 50 μmol/L (3 mg/dL) (see Table 29.2). Hyperbilirubinemia is the result of an imbalance between its production and excretion. The causes of jaundice (Table 29.3) are conventionally classified as:

- **prehepatic:** increased production of bilirubin (Fig. 29.10)
- **intrahepatic:** impaired hepatic uptake, conjugation or secretion of bilirubin (Fig. 29.11)
- **posthepatic:** obstruction to biliary drainage (Fig. 29.12 and box on p. 212).

Prehepatic jaundice results from excess production of bilirubin as a result of hemolysis, or a genetic abnormality in the hepatic uptake of unconjugated bilirubin. Hemolysis is commonly the result of immune disease, presence of structurally abnormal red cells or breakdown of extravasated blood. Intravascular hemolysis releases hemoglobin into

The causes of jaundice			
Type	Cause	Clinical example	Frequency
Prehepatic	hemolysis	autoimmune	uncommon
		abnormal hemoglobin	depends on region
Intrahepatic	infection	hepatitis A, B, C	common/very common
	chemical/drug	acetaminophen	common
		alcohol	common
	genetic errors:	Gilbert's syndrome	1 in 20
	bilirubin	Crigler–Najjar syndrome	very rare
	metabolism	Dubin–Johnson syndrome	very rare
		Rotor's syndrome	very rare
	genetic errors:	Wilson's disease	1 in 200 000
	specific proteins	α_1 antitrypsin	1 in 1000 with genotype
	autoimmune	chronic active hepatitis	uncommon/rare
	neonatal	physiologic	very common
Posthepatic	intrahepatic bile ducts	drugs	common
		primary bilary cirrhosis	uncommon
		cholangitis	common
	extrahepatic bile ducts	gall stones	very common
		pancreatic tumor	uncommon
		cholangiocarcinoma	rare

Table 29.3 **Causes of jaundice.**

the plasma, where it is either oxidized to methemoglobin (Chapter 5) or complexed with haptoglobin. More commonly, red cells are hemolyzed extravascularly, within phagocytes, and hemoglobin is converted to bilirubin; such bilirubin is unconjugated. Unconjugated and conjugated bilirubin can be chemically distinguished.

Intrahepatic jaundice reflects a generalized hepatocyte dysfunction. In this condition, hyperbilirubinemia is usually accompanied by other abnormalities in biochemical markers of hepatocellular function.

In neonates, transient jaundice is common, particularly in premature infants, and is due to immaturity of the enzymes

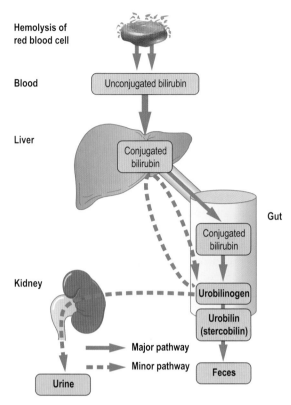

Fig. 29.10 **Prehepatic (hemolytic) jaundice.** There is an increased concentration of plasma total bilirubin due to the excess of the uncon-jugated fraction (see also Table 29.2).

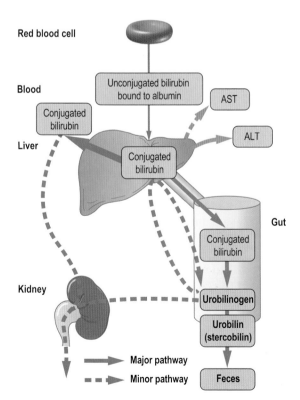

Fig. 29.11 **Intrahepatic jaundice.** Bilirubin in plasma is increased due to an increase in the conjugated fraction. Increased serum enzyme activities signify hepatocyte damage (see also Table 29.2).

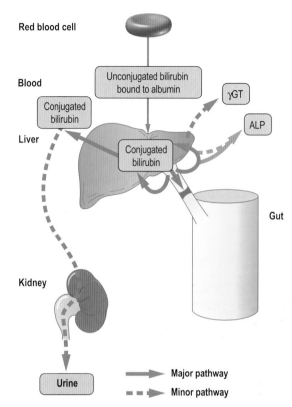

Fig. 29.12 **Posthepatic jaundice.** Plasma bilirubin is elevated due to an increase in the conjugated fraction. Obstruction of the bile duct does not allow passage of bile to the gut. Stools are characteristically pale in color. (see also Table 29.2). γGT, γ-glutamyl transpeptidase; ALP, alkaline phosphatase.

SIGNIFICANCE OF NEONATAL JAUNDICE

A normal, term baby developed jaundice on the third day of life, with a bilirubin concentration of 150 μmol/L (8.8 mg/ dL), pre-dominantly of the indirect form. The baby was otherwise well.

Comment. About 50% of normal babies become jaundiced 48 h after birth. This physiologic jaundice is caused by tem-porary inefficiency in bilirubin conjugation, and resolves in the first 10 days. The hyperbilirubinemia is unconjugated in nature; if severe, it may require phototherapy (ultraviolet light to photoisomerize bilirubin into a nontoxic form) or exchange blood transfusion to prevent damage to the brain (kernicterus). Bruising from delivery, infection or poor fluid intake may exag-gerate the hyperbilirubinemia. Jaundice in the first 24 h of life is abnormal and requires investigation to exclude hemolysis, as does physiologic jaundice severe enough to require photo-therapy. Jaundice that presents later, after 10 days, is always abnormal and is likely to indicate an inborn error of metabo-lism or structural defects of the bile ducts.

involved in bilirubin conjugation. Unconjugated bilirubin is toxic to the immature brain and causes a condition known as kernicterus. If plasma bilirubin concentrations are judged to be too high, phototherapy with blue-white light, which isomerizes bilirubin to more soluble pigments that might be excreted with bile, or exchange blood transfusion to remove the excess bilirubin is necessary to avoid kernicterus.

Posthepatic jaundice is caused by obstruction of the biliary tree. The plasma bilrubin is conjugated and other biliary metabolites, such as bile acids, accumulate in the plasma. The clinical features are pale-colored stools, caused by the absence of fecal bilirubin and urobilin, and dark urine as a result of the presence of water-soluble conjugated bilirubin. In complete obstruction, urobilinogen and urobilin are absent from urine, as there can be no intestinal conversion of bilirubin to urobilinogen/urobilin, and hence no renal excretion of reabsorbed urobilinogen/urobilin.

OBSTRUCTIVE LIVER DISEASE CAUSED BY PANCREATIC CANCER

A 65-year-old man was admitted to hospital because of jaundice. There was no abdominal pain, but he had noticed dark urine and pale stools. The gall bladder appeared palpable but not tender. Liver function tests showed bilirubin 230 μmol/L (13.5 mg/dL), AST 32 U/L, and ALP 550 U/L. Dipstick urine testing revealed the presence of bilirubin, but no urobilin.

Comment. The patient had a history typical of obstructive jaundice. The increased ALP and normal AST concentrations were consistent with this, and the absence of urobilin in the urine indicated that the biliary tract was obstructed. It was important to carry out liver imaging investigations, to find the site of the obstruction; the absence of pain suggested that gall stones were not the cause. Ultrasound showed dilatation of the bile duct and a computed tomography scan showed a mass in the head of the pancreas. During surgery, cancer of the pancreas was confirmed. For reference ranges see Table 29.2.

Genetic causes of jaundice

There are a number of genetic disorders that impair bilirubin conjugation or secretion. Gilbert's syndrome, affecting up to 5% of the population, causes a mild unconjugated hyperbilirubinemia that is harmless and asymptomatic. It is due to a modest impairment in uridine diphosphate (UDP) glucuronyl transferase activity.

Other inherited diseases of bilirubin metabolism are rare. Crigler-Najjar syndrome, which is the result of a complete absence or marked reduction in bilirubin conjugation, causes a severe unconjugated hyperbilirubinemia that presents at birth; when the enzyme is completely absent, the condition is fatal. The Dubin-Johnson and Rotor's syndromes impair the biliary secretion of conjugated bilirubin and therefore cause a conjugated hyperbilirubinemia, which is usually mild.

Summary

■ The liver plays a central role in human metabolism.
■ It is extensively involved in the synthesis and catabolism of carbohydrate, lipids and proteins.
■ It synthesizes an array of acute phase proteins in response to inflammation and infection, and laboratory measurements of such proteins are clinically useful in monitoring disease progress.
■ It is involved in the metabolism of bilirubin derived from the catabolism of heme.
■ Disease processes often cause the patient to present with jaundice due to hyperbilirubinemia.
■ The liver has a central role in the detoxification of drugs.
■ Its biochemical function is assessed in clinical practice using a panel of blood tests, called liver function tests, abnormalities of which can point to disease affecting the hepatocellular or biliary systems.

ACTIVE LEARNING

1. Discuss how the anatomic position and structure of the liver allow it to absorb and metabolize lipid, protein and carbohydrate, as well as xenobiotics from the intestine, before releasing such molecules or their derivatives to the systemic circulation.
2. Describe the function of the liver in protein synthesis and the systemic response to inflammation.
3. Outline how the liver processes bilirubin, and describe the biochemical causes of hyperbilirubinemia (jaundice) and its classification.
4. How does the liver metabolize drugs?
5. Discuss biochemical tests used by the clinical laboratory in the investigation of liver disease.

Further reading

Donohue TM, Cederbaum AI, French SW. Role of the proteasome in ethanol-induced liver pathology. *Alcohol Clin Exp Res* 2007;**31**:1446–1459.
Wijnen PAHM, Op den Buijsch RAM, Drent M et al. Review article: the prevalence and clinical relevance of cytochrome P450 polymorphisms. *Aliment Pharmacol Ther* 2007; **26**(suppl2):211–219.
Wilkinson GR. Drug metabolism and variability among patients in drug response. *N Engl J Med* 2005;**352**:2211–2221.
Zakim D, Boyer TD (eds). *Hepatology. A textbook of liver disease*, 4th edn. Philadelphia: Saunders, 2002.

Websites

www.nlm.nih.gov/medlineplus/liverdiseasesgeneral.html
www.labtestsonline.org/understanding/conditions/liver_disease.html
Cytochrome P-450: http://drnelson.utmem.edu/CytochromeP450.html
www.imm.ki.se
Pharmacogenomics: www.pharmgkb.org/index.jsp

30. Biosynthesis and Degradation of Nucleotides

A Gugliucci and R Thornburg

LEARNING OBJECTIVES

After reading this chapter you should be able to:

- Compare and contrast the structure and biosynthesis of purines and pyrimidines, highlighting differences between de novo and salvage pathways.
- Describe how cells meet their requirements for nucleotides at various stages in their cell cycle.
- Explain the biochemical rationale for using fluorouracil and methotrexate in chemotherapy.
- Describe the metabolic basis and therapy for classic disorders in nucleotide metabolism: gout, Lesch-Nyhan syndrome and SCIDS.

INTRODUCTION

Nucleotides, molecules composed of a pentose, a nitrogenous base and phosphate, are key elements in cell physiology since they are:

- precursors of deoxyribonucleic acid (DNA) and ribonucleic acid (RNA)
- components of coenzymes, e.g NAD(H), NADP(H), FMN(H$_2$), and CoA
- energy currency, driving many metabolic processes, e.g. ATP and GTP
- carriers in biosynthesis, e.g. UDP for carbohydrates and CDP for lipids
- modulators of allosteric regulation of metabolism
- second messengers, e.g. cAMP and cGMP.

We can synthesize ample amounts of purine and pyrimidine nucleotides from metabolic intermediates. In this way, although we ingest dietary nucleic acids and nucleotides, survival does not require their absorption and utilization. Because nucleotides are involved in so many levels of metabolism they are important targets for chemotherapeutic agents used in treatment of microbial and parasitic infections and cancer.

This chapter will describe the structure and metabolism of the two classes of nucleotides: purines and pyrimidines. The metabolic pathways are divided into four sections:

- de novo synthesis of nucleotides from basic metabolites, which is required in growing cells

- salvage pathways that recycle preformed bases and nucleosides and provide an adequate supply of nucleotides for cells at rest
- catabolic pathways for excretion of nucleotide degradation products, a process that is essential to limit the accumulation of toxic levels of nucleotides within cells
- biosynthetic pathways for conversion of the ribonucleotides into the deoxyribonucleotides, providing precursors for DNA.

Purines and pyrimidines

Nucleotides are formed from three components: a nitrogenous base, a five-carbon sugar, and phosphate. The nitrogenous bases found in nucleic acids belong to one of two heterocyclic groups, either purines or pyrimidines (Fig. 30.1). The major purines of both DNA and RNA are guanine and adenine.

In DNA, the major pyrimidines are thymine and cytosine, while in RNA, they are uracil and cytosine; thymine is unique to DNA and uracil is unique to RNA. When the nitrogenous bases are combined with a five-carbon sugar, they are known as nucleosides. When the nucleosides are phosphorylated, the compounds are known as nucleotides. The phosphate can be attached either at the 5′-position or the 3′-position of ribose, or both. Table 30.1 gives the names and structures of the most important purines and pyrimidines.

PURINE METABOLISM

De novo synthesis of the purine ring: synthesis of inosine monophosphate (IMP)

The demand for nucleotide biosynthesis can vary greatly. It is high during the S-phase of the cell cycle, when cells are about to divide (Chapter 43). The process is therefore very active in growing tissues, actively proliferating cells like blood cells and cancer cells, and when tissues are regenerating. Purine and pyrimidine biosynthesis are energetically expensive processes that are subject to intracellular mechanisms that sense and effectively regulate the pool sizes of intermediates and products.

The raw materials for purine synthesis are: CO$_2$, nonessential amino acids (Asp, Glu, Gly), and folic acid derivatives which act as single carbon donors. Five molecules of ATP are needed for the synthesis of IMP, the first purine

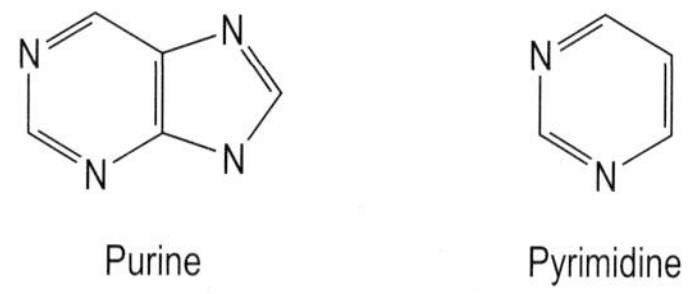

Purine   Pyrimidine

Fig. 30.1 **Classification of nucleotides.** Basic structure of purines and pyrimidines.

Names and structures of purines and pyrimidines

Structure	Free base	Nucleoside	Nucleotide
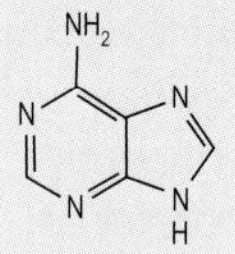	adenine	adenosine	AMP ADP ATP cAMP
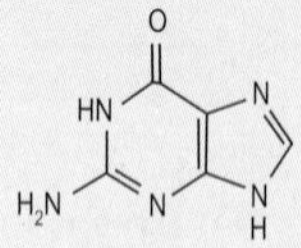	guanine	guanosine	GMP GDP GTP cGMP
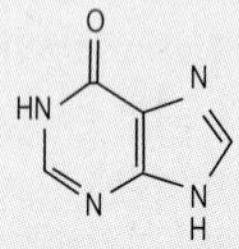	hypoxanthine	inosine	IMP
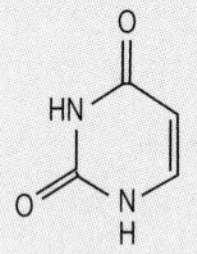	uracil	uridine	UMP UDP UTP
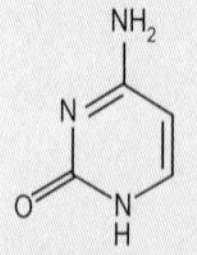	cytosine	cytidine	CMP CDP CTP
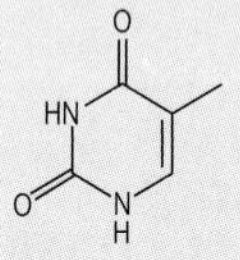	thymine	thymidine	TMP TDP TTP

Table 30.1 **Names and structures of important purines and pyrimidines.** The designation NTP refers to the ribonucleotide. The prefix d, as in dATP, is used to identify deoxyribonucleotides. dTTP is usually written as TTP, with the d-prefix implied.

product and common precursor of AMP and GMP. The starting material for synthesis of IMP is ribose 5-phosphate, a product of the pentose phosphate pathway (Chapter 12). The first step, catalyzed by ribose phosphate pyrophosphokinase (PRPP synthetase), generates the activated form of the pentose phosphate by transferring a pyrophosphate group from ATP to form 5-phosphoribosyl-pyrophosphate (PRPP) (Fig. 30.2). In a series of 10 reactions, PRPP is converted to IMP. Most of the carbons and all of the nitrogens of the purine

ring are derived from the amino acids; one carbon is derived from CO_2 and two from N^5,N^{10}-methenyl- and N^{10}-formyl-tetrahydrofolate (THF), respectively, which are derivatives of folic acid. Folate deficiency can impair purine synthesis, which can produce disease or can be exploited clinically to kill rapidly dividing cells, which have a high demand for purine biosynthesis. The endproduct of this sequence of reactions is the ribonucleotide IMP; the nucleoside is inosine and the purine base is called hypoxanthine.

Synthesis of ATP and GTP from IMP

IMP does not accumulate significantly within the cell. As shown in Figure 30.3, it is converted to both AMP and GMP. Two enzymatic reactions are required in each case (see Fig. 30.3). Distinct enzymes, adenylate kinase and guanylate kinase, use ATP to synthesize the nucleotide diphosphates from the nucleotide monophosphates. Finally, a single enzyme, termed nucleotide diphosphokinase, converts diphosphonucleotides into nucleotide triphosphates. This enzyme has activity towards all nucleotide diphosphates, including pyrimidines and purines and both ribo- and deoxyribonucleotides for synthesis of RNA and DNA, respectively.

Preformed nucleotides can be recycled by salvage pathways

In addition to de novo synthesis, cells can use preformed nucleotides obtained from the diet or from the breakdown of endogenous nucleic acids through salvage pathways. In mammals, there are two enzymes in the purine salvage pathway. Adenine phosphoribosyltransferase (APRT) converts free adenine into AMP (Fig. 30.4A). Hypoxanthine-guanine phosphoribosyltransferase (HGPRT) catalyzes a similar reaction for both hypoxanthine (the purine base in IMP) and guanine (Fig. 30.4B). Purine nucleotides are synthesized preferentially by salvage pathways, so long as the free nucleobases are available. This preference is mediated by hypoxanthine inhibition of amidophosphoribosyl transferase, step 2 of the de novo pathway. Note that step 2 is the site of inhibition of purine biosynthesis, since PRPP is also used in other biosynthetic processes including nucleotide salvage pathways.

Purine and uric acid metabolism in humans

Sources and disposal of uric acid

Uric acid is the endproduct of purine catabolism in humans; it is not metabolized and must be excreted. However, the complex renal handling of urate, described below, suggests an evolutionary advantage to having high circulating levels of urate. In fact, uric acid is one of the main circulating antioxidants. At pH 7.4, it is 98% ionized and therefore

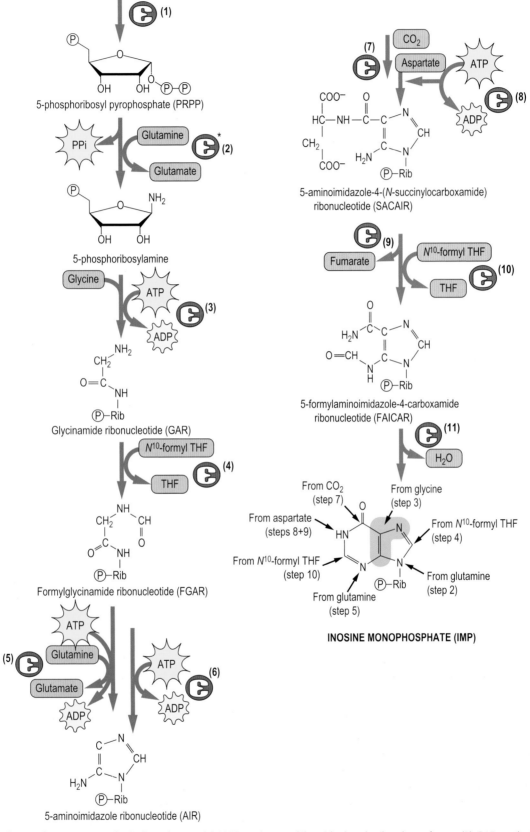

Fig. 30.2 **Synthesis of IMP.** Enzymes for indicated steps: (1) PRPP synthetase; (2) amidophosphoribosyl-transferase; (3) GAR synthetase; (4) GAR transformylase; (5) FGAM synthetase; (6) AIR synthetase; (7) AIR carboxylase; (8) SACAIR synthetase; (9) adenylosuccinate lyase; (10) AICAR transformylase; (11) IMP synthase. *The asterisk identifies the regulatory enzyme amidophosphoribosyl-transferase.

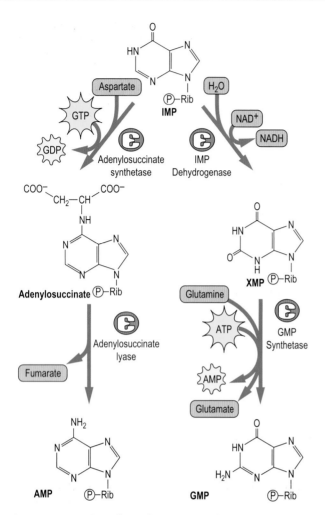

Fig. 30.3 **Conversion of IMP into AMP and GMP.** Two enzymatic reactions are needed in each branch of the pathway. XMP, xanthine monophosphate.

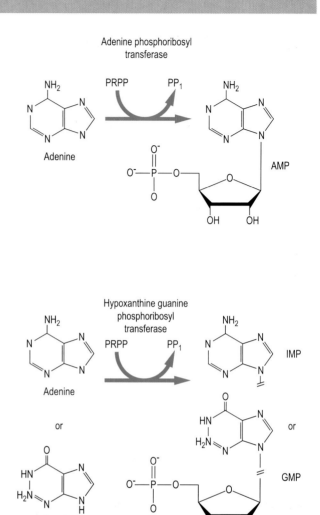

Fig. 30.4 **The purine salvage pathways.** (A) adenine phosphoribosyl transferase. (B) Hypoxanthine-guanine phosphoribosyl transferase.

circulates as monosodium urate. This salt has poor solubility, the extracellular fluid becoming saturated at urate concentrations little above the upper limit of the reference range. Therefore, there is a tendency for monosodium urate to crystallize in subjects with hyperuricemia. The most obvious clinical manifestation of this process is gout, in which crystals form in cartilage, synovium and synovial fluid. This can be accompanied by renal calculi (urate stones) and tophi (accumulation of sodium urate in soft tissues). A sudden increase in urate production, for example during chemotherapy when many cells die rapidly, can lead to widespread crystallization of urate in joints, but mainly in urine, causing an acute urate nephropathy.

There are three sources of purines in man: de novo synthesis, salvage pathways, and diet. The body urate pool (and thus plasma uric acid concentration) is governed by the relative rates of urate formation and excretion. Over half of urate is excreted by the kidney, the rest by the intestines, where bacteria dispose of it. In the kidney, urate is filtered and almost totally reabsorbed in the proximal

SALVAGE PATHWAYS ARE THE PRINCIPAL SOURCE OF NUCLEOTIDES IN LYMPHOCYTES

In humans, resting T lymphocytes, immune system cells produced in the thymus (Chapter 38), meet their routine metabolic requirements for nucleotides through the salvage pathway, but de novo synthesis is required to support growth of rapidly dividing cells. The salvage of nucleotides is especially important in HIV-infected T lymphocytes. In asymptomatic patients, resting lymphocytes show a block in de novo pyrimidine biosynthesis, and correspondingly reduced pyrimidine pool sizes. Following activation of the T lymphocyte population, these cells cannot synthesize sufficient new DNA. The activation process leads to cell death, contributing to the decline in the T lymphocyte population during the late stages of HIV infection.

The salvage pathways are especially important for many parasites as well. These organisms prey metabolically on their host, using preformed metabolites, including nucleotides. Some parasites, such as *Mycoplasma*, *Borrelia*, and *Chlamydia*, have lost the genes required for the de novo synthesis of nucleotides; they obtain these important components from their host.

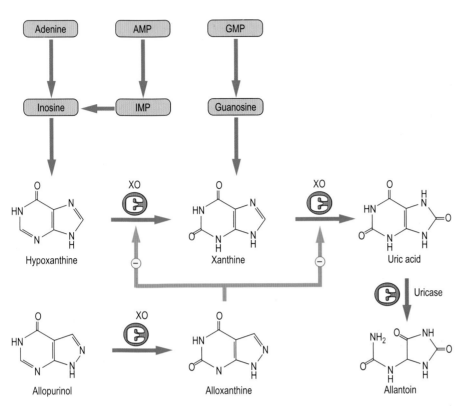

Fig. 30.5 **Degradation of purines and biochemical basis of allopurinol treatment of gout.** Inhibition of xanthine oxidase (XO) by alloxanthine is the mechanism involved in allopurinol treatment of gout. The enzyme uricase is missing in primates (including humans) but is commonly used for measurement of serum uric acid levels in humans.

 ## GOUT RESULTS FROM THE EXCESS OF URIC ACID

Diagnosis. The diagnosis of gout is primarily clinical and supported by the demonstration of hyperuricemia. About 90% of patients appear to excrete urate at an inappropriately low rate for the plasma concentration, while about 10% have excessive production. Gouty arthritis has a typically hyperacute onset (less than 24 h), with severe pain, swelling, redness and warmth in the joint(s), characteristically in the big toe. It is confirmed by the presence of tophi or sodium urate crystals in the synovial fluid. The crystals are needle-shaped, are seen inside neutrophils and have negative birefringence when viewed with polarized light.

Pathogenesis. Urate crystals in joints are phagocytized by neutrophils (leukocytes in blood and tissues). The crystals damage lysosomal and cellular membranes, causing cellular disruption and death. Release of lysosomal enzymes in the joint precipitates an acute inflammatory reaction. Several cytokines enhance and perpetuate the inflammation and other phagocytic cells, monocytes and macrophages, aggravate the inflammation.

Management. The acute attack is managed with antiinflammatory agents, including NSAIDS. Dietary changes (less meat, increased water intake, weight reduction) and changes in concurrent drug therapies, such as diuretics, may be helpful. Probenecid, a uricosuric drug, is commonly employed to reduce uricemia. Colchicine, a microtubule disruptor, may also be used during an acute attack to inhibit inflammation and phagocytosis. If the patient is already a hyperexcretor, or tophi or renal disease are present, then allopurinol is used. Allopurinol is an inhibitor of xanthine oxidase (Fig. 30.5). Allopurinol undergoes the first oxidation to yield alloxanthine, but cannot undergo the second oxidation. Alloxanthine remains bound to the enzyme, acting as a potent competitive inhibitor. This leads to reduced formation of uric acid and accumulation of xanthine and hypoxanthine, which are more soluble and are excreted in urine.

tubule. Distally, both secretion and absorption occur, so that overall urate clearance amounts to about 10% of the filtered load, i.e. 90% is retained in the body. Normally, urate excretion increases if the filtered load is increased. Because of the role of the kidney in urate metabolism, kidney diseases can lead to urate retention and urate precipitation in the kidney (stones) and urine. Dietary purines account for about 20% of excreted urate. Therefore, restricting purines in the diet (less meat) can reduce urate levels by only 10–20%.

Endogenous formation of uric acid

Each of the purine monophosphates (IMP, GMP and AMP) can be converted into their corresponding nucleosides by 5′-nucleotidase. The enzyme purine nucleoside phosphorylase then converts the nucleosides inosine or guanosine into the free purine bases hypoxanthine and guanine, respectively. Hypoxanthine is oxidized and guanine is deaminated to yield xanthine (Fig. 30.5). Two other enzymes, AMP deaminase and adenosine deaminase, convert the amino group of AMP and adenosine into IMP and inosine, respectively, which are then converted to hypoxanthine. In effect, guanine is directly converted to xanthine, while inosine and adenine are converted to hypoxanthine, then to xanthine.

Xanthine oxidase (XO), the final enzyme in this pathway, oxidizes hypoxanthine to xanthine, then xanthine to uric acid. Uric acid is the final metabolic product of purine catabolism in primates, birds, reptiles, and many insects. Other organisms, including most mammals, fish, amphibians and invertebrates, metabolize uric acid to more soluble products, such as allantoin (see Fig. 30.5).

Hyperuricemia and gout

Plasma urate concentration is, on average, higher in men than in women, tends to rise with age, and is usually elevated in obese subjects and subjects in the higher socio-economic groups. The risk of gout, a painful disease resulting from precipitation of sodium urate crystals in joints and dermis, increases with higher plasma urate concentrations (see box on p. 409). Most persons with hyperuricemia remain asymptomatic throughout life, but there is no gout without hyperuricemia. Hyperuricemia can occur due to increased formation or decreased excretion of uric acid, or both. Decreased renal excretion of urate can result from a decrease in filtration and/or secretion. Many factors (including drugs and alcohol) also affect tubular handling of urates and can cause or increase hyperuricemia.

PYRIMIDINE METABOLISM

As with the purines, the pyrimidines (uracil, cytosine and thymine) are also synthesized through a complex series of reactions using raw materials readily available in cells. One important difference is that the pyrimidine base is made first and the sugar added later. Uridine monophosphate (UMP)

is the precursor of all pyrimidine nucleotides. The de novo pathway produces UMP, which is then converted to cytidine triphosphate (CTP) and thymidine triphosphate (TTP). Salvage pathways also recover preformed pyrimidines.

De novo pathway

Pyrimidine and purine nucleoside biosynthesis share several common precursors: CO_2, amino acids (Asp, Gln), and, for thymine, N^5,N^{10}-methylene-THF. The pathway for biosynthesis of UMP is outlined in Figure 30.6. The first step, catalyzed by the enzyme carbamoyl phosphate synthetase II (CPS II), uses bicarbonate, glutamine, and 2 moles of ATP to form carbamoyl phosphate (CPS I is used in the synthesis of arginine in the urea cycle; Chapter 19). Most of the atoms required for formation of the pyrimidine ring are derived from aspartate, added in a single step by aspartate transcarbamoylase (ATCase). Carbamoyl aspartate is then cyclized to dihydroorotic acid by the action of the enzyme dihydroorotase. Dihydroorotic acid is oxidized to orotic acid by a mitochondrial enzyme, dihydroorotate dehydrogenase. Leflunomide, a specific inhibitor of this enzyme, is used for treatment of rheumatoid arthritis because blockage of this step inhibits lymphocyte activation and thereby limits inflammation. The ribosyl-5'-phosphate group from PRPP is then transferred onto orotic acid to form orotate monophosphate (OMP). Finally, OMP is decarboxylated to form UMP. UTP is synthesized in two enzymatic phosphorylation steps by the actions of UMP kinase and nucleotide diphosphokinase. CTP synthetase converts UTP into CTP by amination of UTP. This completes the synthesis of the ribonucleotides for synthesis of RNA.

Metabolic channeling by multienzymes improves efficiency

In bacteria, the six enzymes of pyrimidine (UMP) biosynthesis exist as distinct proteins. However, during the evolution of mammals the first three enzymatic activities have been fused together into CAD, a single multifunctional polypeptide encoded by a single gene. The name of the enzyme derives from its three activities: **C**arbamoyl phosphate synthetase, **A**spartate transcarbamoylase, and **D**ihydroorotase. The final two enzymatic activities of pyrimidine biosynthesis, orotate phosphoribosyl transferase and orotidylate decarboxylase, are also fused into a single enzyme, UMP synthase. As with the fatty acid synthase complex (Chaper 16), this fusion of sequential enzyme activities avoids the diffusion of the metabolic intermediates into the intracellular milieu, thereby improving the metabolic efficiency of the individual steps.

Pyrimidine salvage pathways

As with the purines, free pyrimidine bases, available from the diet or from the breakdown of nucleic acids, can be recovered

LESCH-NYHAN SYNDROME – HGPRT DEFICIENCY

The gene encoding HGPRT is located on the X-chromosome. Its deficiency results in a rare, X-linked recessive disorder, Lesch-Nyhan syndrome. The lack of HGPRT causes an overaccumulation of PRPP, which is also the substrate for the enzyme amidophosphoribosyl transferase. This stimulates purine biosynthesis by up to 200-fold. Because of increased purine synthesis, the degradation product, uric acid, also accumulates to high levels. Elevated uric acid leads to a crippling gouty arthritis and severe neuropathology resulting in mental retardation, spasticity, aggressive behavior, and a compulsion towards self-mutilation by biting and scratching.

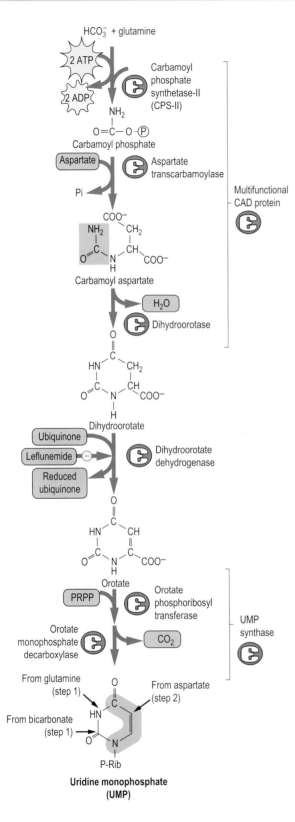

Fig. 30.6 **The metabolic pathway for synthesis of pyrimidines.** Formation of orotic acid and UMP, the first pyrimidine nucleotide.

by several salvage enzymes. Uracil phosphoribosyl transferase (UPRTase) is similar to the enzymes of the purine salvage pathways. This enzyme is required to activate some chemotherapeutic agents such as 5-fluorouracil (FU) or 5-fluorocytosine (FC). A uridine-cytidine kinase and a more specific thymidine kinase catalyze the phosphorylation of these nucleosides; nucleotide kinases and diphosphokinase complete the salvage process.

FORMATION OF DEOXYNUCLEOTIDES

Ribonucleotide reductase

Because DNA uses deoxyribonucleotides instead of the ribonucleotides found in RNA, cells require pathways to convert ribonucleotides into the deoxy forms. The adenine, guanine and uracil deoxyribonucleotides are synthesized from their corresponding ribonucleotide diphosphates by direct reduction of the 2'-hydroxyl by the enzyme ribonucleotide reductase, as shown for dUDP in Figure 30.7. The reduction of the 2'-hydroxyl of ribose uses a pair of protein-bound sulfhydryl groups (cysteine residues). The hydroxyl group is released as water, and the cysteines are oxidized to cystine during the reaction. To regenerate an active enzyme, the disulfide must be reduced back to the original sulfhydryl pair by disulfide exchange; this is accomplished by reaction with a small protein, thioredoxin. The thioredoxin, a highly conserved Fe-S protein, is in turn reduced by the flavoprotein, thioredoxin reductase.

A unique pathway to TTP

The nucleotide deoxy-TMP, abbreviated as TMP because thymine is unique to DNA, is synthesized by a special pathway involving methylation of the deoxyribose form of uridylate, dUMP (Fig. 30.8). The TMP biosynthetic pathway leads

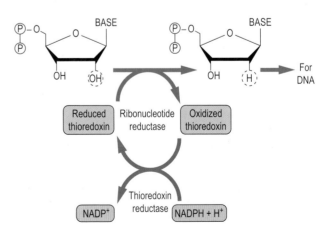

Fig. 30.7 **Formation of deoxyribonucleotides, except TTP, by ribonucleotide reductase.** Thioredoxin and NADPH (from the pentose phosphate pathway) are required for recycling of the enzyme.

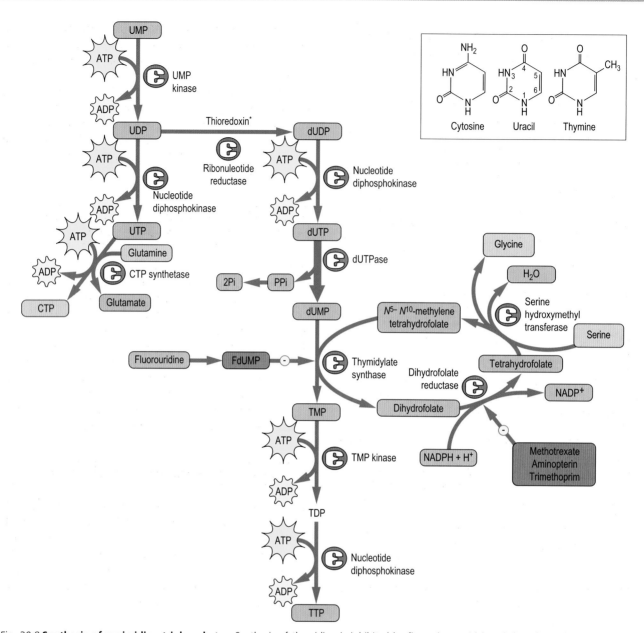

Fig. 30.8 **Synthesis of pyrimidine triphosphates.** Synthesis of thymidine is inhibited by fluorodeoxyuridylate (FdUMP), methotrexate, aminopterin and trimethoprim at the indicated sites. *Thioredoxin restores sulfhydryl residues on ribonucleotide reductase, regenerating the active enzyme (see Fig. 30.7).

from UMP to UDP, then, through ribonucleotide reductase, to dUDP. The dUDP is then phosphorylated to dUTP, which creates an unexpected biochemical problem. DNA polymerase does not effectively discriminate between the two deoxyribonucleotides, dUTP and TTP – the only difference is a methyl group at C-5. It incorporates dUTP into DNA in vitro; this reaction would lead to high rates of mutagenesis in vivo. Therefore, cells limit the concentration of dUTP by rapidly hydrolyzing dUTP to dUMP with the enzyme dUTPase. This enzyme cleaves a high-energy bond and releases pyrophosphate, which is rapidly hydrolyzed to phosphate, shifting the equilibrium ever further towards the formation of dUMP. The dUMP is converted to TMP using N^5,N^{10}-methylene-THF as

the methyl donor; the dihydrofolate product is recycled by action of the enzymes, dihydrofolate reductase and serine hydroxymethyl transferase. Two rounds of phosphorylation of TMP yield TTP for synthesis of DNA.

The synthesis of TTP is a roundabout pathway, but provides opportunities for chemotherapy through inhibition of TMP biosynthesis (see Fig. 30.8). There is only one reaction in pyrimidine synthesis that requires a THF derivative: conversion of dUMP to TMP, catalyzed by thymidylate synthase. This reaction is often rate limiting for cell division. Indeed, folate deficiency impairs cell replication, especially the replication of rapidly dividing cells. Thus, folate deficiency is a frequent cause of anemia: bone marrow cells involved in erythropoiesis

CHEMOTHERAPEUTIC TARGETS: FOLATE RECYCLING AND THYMIDYLATE SYNTHASE

Fluorodeoxyuridylate (FdUMP) is a specific, suicide inhibitor of thymidylate synthase. In FdUMP, a highly electronegative fluorine replaces the carbon-5 proton of uridine. This compound can begin the enzymatic conversion into dTMP by forming the enzyme–FdUMP covalent complex; however, the covalent intermediate cannot accept the donated methyl group from methylene THF, nor can it be broken down to release the active enzyme. The result is a suicide complex in which the substrate is covalently locked at the active site of thymidylate synthase. The drug is frequently administered as fluorouridine, and the body's normal metabolism converts the fluorouridine into FdUMP. Fluorouridine is used against breast, colorectal, gastric, and uterine cancers.

Fluorocytosine is a potent antimicrobial agent. Its mechanism of action is similar to that of FdUMP; however, it must first be converted into fluorouracil by the action of cytosine deaminase. The fluorouracil is subsequently converted into FdUMP, which blocks thymidylate synthase as above. While cytosine deaminase is present in most fungi and bacteria, it is absent in animals and plants. Therefore, in humans, fluorocytosine is not converted into fluorouracil and is nontoxic, while in the microbes, metabolism of fluorocytosine results in cell death.

Aminopterin and methotrexate are folic acid analogs that bind about 1000-fold more tightly to dihydrofolate reductase (DHFR) than does dihydrofolate. In this manner, they competitively, almost irreversibly, block the synthesis of dTMP. These compounds are also competitive inhibitors of other THF-dependent enzyme reactions used in the biosynthesis of purines, histidine, and methionine. Trimethoprim binds to DHFR, and binds more tightly to bacterial DHFRs than it does to mammalian enzymes, making it an effective antibacterial agent. Folate analogs are relatively nonspecific chemotherapeutic agents. They poison rapidly dividing cells, not just cancer cells but also hair follicles and gut endothelia, causing the loss of hair and the gastrointestinal side effects of chemotherapy.

and hematopoiesis are among the most rapidly dividing cells in the body. Inhibition of thymidylate synthase, either directly or by inhibition of THF recycling, provides a special opportunity for chemotherapy, targeting synthesis of DNA precursors in rapidly dividing cancer cells.

De novo nucleotide metabolism is highly regulated

Because nucleotides are required for mammalian cells to proliferate, the enzymes involved in de novo synthesis of both purines and pyrimidines are induced during the S-phase of cell division. Covalent and allosteric regulation also plays an important role in control of nucleotide synthesis. The multimeric protein CAD is activated by phosphorylation by protein kinases in response to growth factors, increasing its affinity for PRPP and decreasing inhibition by UTP. Both of these changes favor biosynthesis of pyrimidines for cell division.

Mole per mole, pyrimidine biosynthesis parallels purine biosynthesis, suggesting the presence of a coordinated control. Among them, one of the key points is the PRPP synthase reaction. PRPP is a precursor for all the ribo- and deoxyribonucleotides. PRPP synthase is inhibited by both pyrimidine and purine nucleotides.

Ribonucleotide reductase coordinates the biosynthesis of all four deoxynucleotides

Because a single enzyme is responsible for the conversion of all ribonucleotides into deoxyribonucleotides, this enzyme is subject to a complex network of feedback regulation. Ribonucleotide reductase contains several allosteric sites for metabolic regulation. Levels of each of the dNTPs modulate the activity of the enzyme toward the other NDPs. By regulating the enzymatic activity of deoxyribonucleotide synthesis as a function of the concentration of the different dNTPs, often described as 'cross-talk' between the pathways, the cell insures that the proper ratios of the different deoxyribonucleotides are produced for normal growth and cell division.

Catabolism of pyrimidine nucleotides

In contrast to the degradation of purines to uric acid, pyrimidines are degraded to readily soluble compounds, which are readily eliminated in urine and are not a frequent source of pathology. The pyridine nucleotides and nucleosides are converted to the free bases and the heterocyclic ring is cleaved, yielding β-aminoisobutyrate as the main excretion product, plus some ammonia and CO_2.

Summary

Nucleotides are synthesized primarily from amino acid precursors and phosphoribosylpyrophosphate by complex, metabolically expensive, multistep pathways. Not surprisingly, salvage pathways play a prominent role in nucleotide metabolism. De novo nucleotide metabolism is required for cell proliferation. Both classes of nucleotides (purines and pyrimidines) are synthesized as precursors (IMP, UMP), which are then converted into the DNA precursors (dATP, dGTP, dCTP, TTP). With the exception of TTP, ribonucleotides are converted to deoxyribonucleotides by ribonucleotide reductase. TTP is synthesized from dUMP by a special pathway involving folates. The salvage pathways have proven useful for the activation of pharmaceutical agents, while the uniqueness of the pathway for synthesis of TTP has provided a

SEVERE COMBINED IMMUNO-DEFICIENCY SYNDROMES (SCIDS) ARE CAUSED BY IMPAIRED PURINE SALVAGE PATHWAYS

SCIDS are a group of fatal disorders resulting from defects in both cellular and humoral immune function. SCIDS patients cannot efficiently produce antibodies in response to an antigenic challenge. Approximately 50% of patients with the autosomal recessive form of SCIDS have a genetic deficiency in the purine salvage enzyme, adenosine deaminase. The pathophysiology involves lymphocytes of both thymic and bone marrow origin (T and B lymphocytes), as well as 'self-destruction' of differentiated cells following antigen stimulation. The precise cause of cell death is not yet known, but may involve accumulation in lymphoid tissues of adenosine, deoxyadenosine and dATP, accompanied by ATP depletion. dATP inhibits ribonucleotide reductase and therefore impedes DNA nucleotide synthesis. The finding that deficiency of the next enzyme in the purine salvage pathway, nucleoside phosphorylase, is also associated with an immune deficiency disorder suggests that integrity of the purine salvage pathway is critical for normal differentiation and function of immunocompetent cells in man.

special target for chemotherapeutic inhibition of DNA synthesis and cell division in cancer cells. Uric acid, the final product of purine catabolism in man, produces a source of pathology: gout and kidney stones.

Further reading

Gangjee A, Jain HD, Kurup S. Recent advances in classical and non-classical antifolates as antitumor and antiopportunistic infection agents. *Anticancer Agents Med Chem* 2008;**8**:205–231.

ACTIVE LEARNING

1. Compare the roles of de novo synthesis and salvage pathways of nucleotide synthesis in various cell types, e.g. erythrocytes, lymphocytes, muscle and liver.
2. In addition to its activity as a xanthine oxidase inhibitor, what other activities of allopurinol might contribute to its efficacy for treatment of gout?
3. Discuss the use of thymidylate synthetase inhibitors and folate analogs for treatment of diseases other than cancer, e.g. arthritis, psoriasis.

Nyhan WL. The recognition of Lesch–Nyhan syndrome as an inborn error of purine metabolism. *J Inherited Metab Dis* 1997;**20**:171–178.
Sigoillot FD, Berkowski JA, Sigoillot SM, Kotsis DH, Guy HI. Cell cycle-dependent regulation of pyrimidine biosynthesis. *J Biol Chem* 2003;**278**:3403–3409.
Terkeltaub R. Gout in 2006: the perfect storm. *Bull NYU Hosp Jt Dis* 2006;**64**:82–86.
Underwood M. Diagnosis and management of gout. *BMJ* 2006;**332**:1315–1319.

Websites

Purine and pyrimidine disorders: www.amg.gda.pl/~essppmm/index.html
Gout:
- www.nlm.nih.gov/medlineplus/goutandpseudogout.html
- www.niams.nih.gov/hi/topics/gout/gout.htm; ww.nhsdirect.nhs.uk/en.asp?TopicID=221
- www.emedicine.com/neuro/topic630.htm
SCIDS: www.scid.net

31. Deoxyribonucleic Acid

R Thornburg and A Gugliucci

LEARNING OBJECTIVES

After reading this chapter you should be able to:

■ Describe the composition and structure of DNA, based on the Watson–Crick model, including the concepts of directionality and complementarity in DNA structure.
■ Describe the packaging of DNA in the nucleus.
■ Explain how replication of DNA is achieved with high fidelity.
■ Discuss the enzymes involved, the activities at replication forks, and the structures and intermediates participating in the replication process.
■ Outline the mechanism by which replication is controlled in the eukaryotic cell.
■ Describe the types of damage to DNA and the mechanisms involved in DNA repair.
■ Describe the mechanism of action of AZT for treatment of AIDS.

INTRODUCTION

Cellular nucleic acids exist in two forms, deoxyribonucleic acid (DNA) and ribonucleic acid (RNA). Approximately 90% of the nucleic acid within cells is RNA and the remainder is DNA. DNA is the repository of genetic information. This chapter deals with the structure of DNA, the manner in which it is stored in chromosomes in the nucleus, and the mechanisms involved in its biosynthesis and repair.

STRUCTURE OF DEOXYRIBONUCLEIC ACID

DNA is an antiparallel dimer of nucleic acid strands. It is composed of nucleotides containing the sugar deoxyribose. Deoxyribose is missing the hydroxyl group at the 2′-position. The chains of DNA are polymerized through a phosphodiester linkage from the 3′-hydroxyl of one subunit to the 5′-hydroxyl of the next subunit (Fig. 31.1A). Thus, DNA is a linear deoxyribose 3′,5′-phosphate chain with purine and pyrimidine bases attached to carbon-1 of the deoxyribose subunit.

Using X-ray diffraction photographs of DNA taken by Rosalind Franklin, James Watson and Francis Crick proposed a structure for DNA in 1953. This model proposed that DNA was composed of two intertwined complementary strands with hydrogen bonds holding the strands together (Fig. 31.1B). The basic simplicity of this structure led to its rapid acceptance. While some of the details of the model have been modified, its essential elements have remained unchanged since originally proposed.

Watson and Crick model of DNA

As originally presented by Watson and Crick, DNA is composed of two strands, wound around each other in a right-handed, helical structure with the base pairs in the middle and the deoxyribosyl phosphate chains on the outside. The orientation of the DNA strands is antiparallel, i.e. the strands run in opposite directions. The nucleotide bases on each strand interact with the nucleotide bases on the other strand to form base pairs (Fig. 31.2). The base pairs are planar and are oriented nearly perpendicular to the axis of the helix. Each base pair is formed by hydrogen bonding between a purine and a pyrimidine. Guanine forms three hydrogen bonds with cytosine, and adenine forms two with thymine. Because of the specificity of this interaction between purines and pyrimidines on the opposite strands, the opposing strands of DNA are said to have complementary structures. The composite strength of the numerous hydrogen bonds formed between the bases of the opposite strands and the hydrophobic interactions among the bases is responsible for the extreme stability of the DNA double helix. While the hydrogen bonds between strands are affected by temperature and ionic strength, stable complementary structures can be formed at room temperature with as few as 6–8 nucleotides.

Three-dimensional DNA

The three-dimensional structure of the DNA double helix is such that the deoxyribosyl phosphate backbones of the two strands are slightly offset from the center of the helix. Because of this, the grooves between the two strands are of different sizes. These grooves are termed the major groove and the minor groove (see Figs 31.1B and 31.2). The major groove is more open and exposes the nucleotide base pairs. The minor groove is more constricted, being partially blocked by the deoxyribosyl moieties linking the base pairs. Binding of proteins to DNA frequently occurs in the major groove and is specific for the nucleotide sequence of DNA.

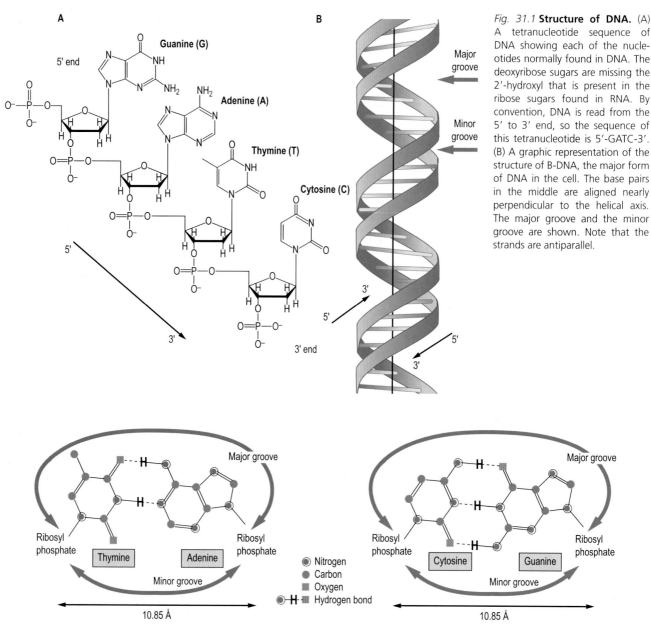

Fig. 31.1 **Structure of DNA.** (A) A tetranucleotide sequence of DNA showing each of the nucleotides normally found in DNA. The deoxyribose sugars are missing the 2'-hydroxyl that is present in the ribose sugars found in RNA. By convention, DNA is read from the 5' to 3' end, so the sequence of this tetranucleotide is 5'-GATC-3'. (B) A graphic representation of the structure of B-DNA, the major form of DNA in the cell. The base pairs in the middle are aligned nearly perpendicular to the helical axis. The major groove and the minor groove are shown. Note that the strands are antiparallel.

Fig. 31.2 **Watson–Crick base pairing of nucleotides in DNA.** The AT base pairs form two hydrogen bonds and the GC base pairs form three hydrogen bonds. Thus, GC-rich regions are more stable than AT-rich regions.

Alternative forms of DNA may help to regulate gene expression

Although the majority of DNA molecules in a cell exist in the B-form described above, alternative forms of DNA also exist. When the relative humidity of B-form DNA falls to less than 75%, the B-form undergoes a reversible transition into the A-form of DNA. In the A-form, the nucleotide base pairs are tilted 20° relative to the helical axis and the helix diameter is increased, compared to the B-form (Fig. 31.3). When the DNA strands consist of polypurine and polypyrimidine tracks, the DNA helix shows different properties. Polypurine regions are A-like, while polypyrimidine regions are B-like. These regions do not efficiently bind histones and are therefore unable to form nucleosomes (see below), resulting in nucleosome-free (exposed) regions of DNA.

Another unique form of DNA exists when the sequence of nucleotides consists of alternating purine/pyrimidine stretches. This form, termed Z-DNA, is also favored at high ionic concentrations. In Z-DNA, the base pairs flip 180° relative to the sugar nucleotide bond. This results in a novel conformation of the base pairs relative to sugar-phosphate

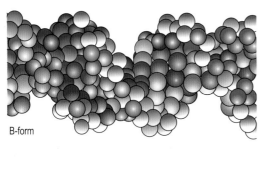

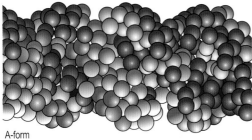

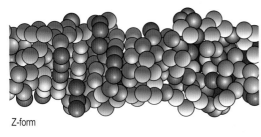

Fig. 31.3 **The structures of different forms of DNA include the B-, A- and Z-forms.** The sugar phosphate backbone of the DNA strands is colored blue. The nucleotide bases forming the internal base pairs are yellow for pyrimidines (thymine and cytosine) and red for purines (adenine and guanine).

backbones, yielding a form of DNA with a zigzag configuration (hence the name Z-DNA) along the sugar phosphate backbone. Surprisingly, this change in conformation leads to the formation of a left-handed DNA helix. While the Z-DNA form is favored at high ionic concentrations, it can also be induced at normal ionic concentrations by DNA methylation. Protein-binding interactions with these alternative forms of DNA, which are widely distributed in the genome, are involved in the regulation of gene expression.

Separated DNA strands can reassociate to form duplex DNA

Because the DNA strands are complementary and are held together only by noncovalent forces, they can be separated into individual strands. This strand separation or denaturation of DNA is commonly induced by heating the solution. The dissociation is reversible and on cooling, the interactions between the complementary nucleotide sequences reassociate

or reanneal to reform their original base pairs. This is the basis for one of the primary methods for DNA analysis, Southern hybridization (see Chapter 35). Because adenine and thymine interact through two hydrogen bonds and guanine and cytosine through three (see Fig. 31.2), AT-rich regions melt at lower temperatures than GC-rich regions in DNA. The denaturation of DNA can also be induced locally by enzymes or DNA-binding proteins. The promoter region of DNA contains a TATA sequence (the TATA box; see Fig. 34.1), an easily melted region of DNA that facilitates the unwinding of DNA during the early stages of gene expression (Chapter 34).

The human genome

The human genome contains 20 000–25 000 different protein coding genes spread over 23 chromosome pairs. These different genes represent unique DNA sequences that are present in single copies or at most only a few copies per genome. There are also several types of repeated DNA sequences within the genome. These are divided into two major classes: middle repetitive (<10 copies per genome) and highly repetitive (>10 copies per genome) sequences.

Some middle repetitive DNA consists of genes that specify transfer and ribosomal ribonucleic acids, which are involved in protein synthesis (Chapter 33), and histone proteins that are part of the nucleosome (below). Other middle repetitive DNA sequences have no known useful function but may participate in DNA strand association and chromosomal rearrangements during meiosis. The best-characterized repetitive sequence in humans is known as the Alu sequence. Between 300 000 and 500 000 Alu I repeats of about 300 base pairs are scattered throughout the human genome, comprising 3–6% of total DNA. Individual repeats of the Alu sequence may vary by 10–20% in identity. Similar sequences are found in other mammals and in lower eukaryotes.

Satellite DNA

Satellite DNA was originally identified as a subfraction of DNA with a buoyant density slightly lower than that of genomic DNA because of its higher content of AT base pairs. It consists of clusters of short, species-specific, nearly identical sequences that are tandemly repeated hundreds of thousands of times. These clusters are deficient in protein-coding genes and are found principally near the centromeres of chromosomes, suggesting that they may function to align the chromosomes during cell division to facilitate recombination. Because these repetitive sequences cover long stretches of chromosomes (100s to 1000s of kilobase pairs; kbp), determining the sequence of satellite DNA and sequencing the centromere region of DNA are major challenges to completing the sequence of eukaryotic genomes.

Mitochondrial DNA

The nucleus of eukaryotic cells contains the majority of the DNA in the cell – genomic DNA. However, DNA is also found in mitochondria and in plant chloroplasts, which is consistent with 'endosymbiont' theories for the origins of these cellular organelles; namely that they are parasites that adapted to intracellular life in symbiosis. The mitochondrial genome is small in size, circular, and encodes relatively few proteins. In humans, the mitochondrial genome encodes 22 tRNAs, two rRNAs, and 13 mitochondrial proteins that are involved in the respiratory apparatus, including subunits of NADH dehydrogenase, cytochrome b, cytochrome oxidase and ATPase.

The remainder of the proteins that are found in mitochondria (about 1000) are produced from nuclear genes, synthesized in the cytoplasm on 'free' ribosomes, then imported into the mitochondrion. This import process requires a special N-terminal 'mitochondrial-import' sequence of about 25 amino acids in length that forms an amphipathic helix which interacts with transporter and chaperone proteins in the inner and outer mitochondrial membrane and matrix. Those few proteins that are encoded by the mitochondrial genome are synthesized in the mitochondrion, using machinery similar that used in the cytoplasm for synthesis of non-mitochondrial proteins (see Chapter 33).

DNA is compacted into chromosomes

In eukaryotes, DNA is arranged in linear segments termed chromosomes. Each chromosome contains between 48 million and 240 million base pairs. The B-form of DNA has a contour length of 3.4 Å per base pair. Therefore, chromosomes have contour lengths of 1.6–8.2 cm, which is much larger than a cell. To fit within the nucleus, DNA is condensed >8000-fold into an organized structure. Interactions between DNA and mobile cations, such as Na^+, Mg^{2+}, and the polyamines such as spermidine^{3+}, play an important role in the physical properties and biologic function of DNA. Even in dilute solutions approximately three out of four DNA charges are neutralized by a cation that is in some sense 'bound'. This neutralization facilitates compaction of DNA into the densely packaged genomes of cells and deformation of DNA by proteins.

In the native chromosome, DNA is complexed with RNA and an approximately equal mass of protein. These DNA-RNA-protein complexes are termed chromatin. The majority of the proteins in chromatin are histones. Histones are a highly conserved family of proteins that are involved in the packing and folding of DNA within the nucleus. There are five classes of histones, termed H1, H2A, H2B, H3, and H4. They are all rich (>20%) in positively charged, basic amino acids (lysine and arginine). These positive charges interact with the negatively charged, acidic phosphate groups of the DNA strands to reduce electrostatic repulsion and permit tighter DNA packing.

Nucleosomes

The histone proteins associate into a complex termed a nucleosome (Fig. 31.4). Each of these complexes contains two molecules each of H2A, H2B, H3 and H4, and one molecule of H1.

The nucleosome protein complex is encircled with about 200 base pairs of DNA that form two coils around the nucleosome core. The H1 protein associates with the outside of the nucleosome core to stabilize the complex. By forming nucleosomes, the packing density of DNA is increased about sevenfold.

The nucleosome particles themselves are also organized into other, more tightly packed structures, termed 300 Å chromatin filaments. These filaments are constructed by winding the nucleosome particles into a spring-shaped solenoid structure with about six nucleosomes per turn (see Fig. 31.4). The solenoid is stabilized by head-to-tail associations of the H1 histones. Finally, the chromatin filaments are compacted into the mature chromosome, using a nuclear scaffold. The scaffold is about 400 nm in diameter and forms the core of the chromosome. The filaments are dispersed around the scaffold to form radial loops about 300 nm in length. The final diameter of a chromosome is about 1 μm.

Telomeres

The ends of the chromosomes are composed of unique DNA sequences called telomeres. These structures consist of tandem repeats of short, G-rich, species-specific oligonucleotides. In humans, the repeated sequence is TTAGGG. Telomeres can contain as many as 1000 copies of this sequence. During the synthesis of telomeres, the enzyme telomerase adds the preformed hexanucleotide repeats onto the 3'-end of the chromosome; there is no requirement for a DNA template in the elongation of telomeres. The shortening of telomeres after many cell replications has been linked to the development of cellular senescence (see advanced concept box and Chapter 44).

THE CELL CYCLE IN EUKARYOTES

Figure 31.5 shows the various phases of the growth and division of eukaryotic cells, known as the cell cycle. The G1 phase is a period of cell growth that occurs prior to DNA replication. The phase during which DNA is synthesized or replicated is termed the S-phase. A second growth phase, termed G2, occurs after DNA replication but prior to cell division. The mitosis or M-phase is the period of cell division. Following mitosis, the daughter cells either reenter the G1 phase or enter a quiescent phase termed G0, when growth and replication cease. The passage of cells through the cell cycle is tightly controlled by a variety of proteins termed cyclin-dependent kinases (see Chapter 43).

DNA is replicated by separating and copying the strands

For cells to divide, their DNA must be duplicated during the S-phase of the cell cycle. The structure of the DNA double helix and its complementarity suggested the mechanism

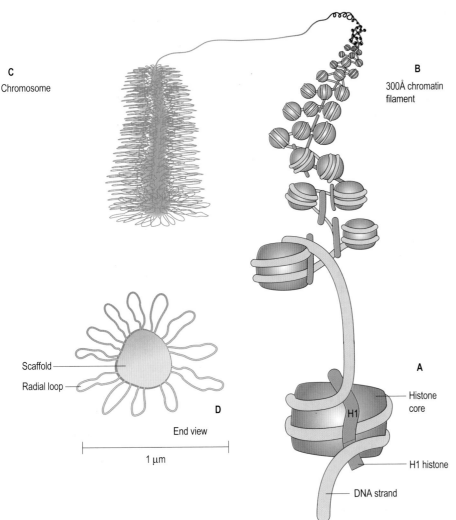

C
Chromosome

B
300Å chromatin filament

Scaffold
Radial loop

D

End view

1 μm

A

Histone core

H1

H1 histone

DNA strand

Fig. 31.4 **Structures involved in chromosome packaging.** (A) The nucleosome core is composed of two subunits each of H2A, H2B, H3, and H4. The core is twice wrapped with DNA, and the H1 histone binds to the completed complex. (B) The 300 Å chromatin filament is formed by wrapping the nucleosomes into a spring-shaped solenoid. (C) The chromosome is composed of the 300 Å filaments, which bind to a nuclear scaffold, forming large loops of chromatin material. (D) The end view of a chromosome shows the central nuclear scaffold surrounded by the radial loops of chromatin. The diameter of a chromosome is about 1 μm.

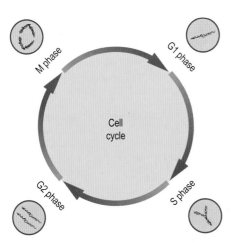

M phase

G1 phase

Cell cycle

G2 phase

S phase

Fig. 31.5 **Stages of the cell cycle.** G1 and G2 are growth phases that occur before and after DNA synthesis respectively. DNA replication occurs during the S-phase. Mitosis occurs during the M-phase, producing new daughter cells that can reenter the G1-phase (compare Fig. 43.1).

for DNA replication – strand separation followed by strand copying. The separated parent strands serve as templates for the synthesis of the new daughter strands. This method of DNA replication is described as 'semi-conservative' – each replicated duplex, daughter DNA molecule contains one parental strand and one newly synthesized strand.

DNA replication site

The site at which DNA replication is initiated is termed the 'origin of replication'. In prokaryotes, a DNA-binding protein termed DnaA binds to repeated nucleotide sequences located within the origin. Binding of 20–30 DnaA molecules to the origin of replication induces unwinding, which separates the strands in an AT-rich region adjacent to the DnaA-binding sites. Next the hexameric protein DnaB binds to the separated DNA strands. DnaB has helicase activity that catalyzes ATP-mediated unwinding of the DNA helix. DNA gyrase also participates in separation of the strands. As this complex continues unwinding the DNA strands in both directions from the origin of replication, single-stranded DNA-binding proteins coat the separated strands to inhibit their reassociation.

Once the strands are sufficiently separated, another protein, termed DNA primase, is added, resulting in the formation of a primosome complex at the replication fork. The primosome synthesizes RNA oligonucleotides complementary to each parental DNA strand. These oligonucleotides serve as primers for DNA synthesis. Once each RNA primer has been laid down, two DNA polymerase III complexes are assembled, one at each of the primed sites. Because of the unidirectional synthetic activity of the polymerase and the antiparallel nature of the two strands, the synthesis of DNA along the two strands is different (Fig. 31.6). The two daughter strands being synthesized are termed the leading strand and the lagging strand.

DNA synthesis proceeds along the leading strand in a 5′ to 3′ direction, producing a single, long, continuous strand. However, because DNA synthesis adds new nucleotides only at the 3′-end of the elongating DNA strand, DNA polymerase III cannot synthesize the lagging strand in one long continuous piece as it does for the leading strand. Instead, the lagging strand is synthesized in small fragments, 1000–5000 base pairs in length, termed Okazaki fragments (see Fig. 31.6). The primosome remains associated with the lagging strand and continues periodically to synthesize RNA primers complementary to the separated strand. As DNA polymerase III moves along the parental DNA strand, it initiates the synthesis of Okazaki fragments at the RNA primers, elongating different fragments from each primer.

When the 3′-end of the elongating Okazaki fragment reaches the 5′-end of the previously synthesized Okazaki fragment, DNA polymerase III releases the template and finds another RNA primer further back along the lagging strand, synthesizing another Okazaki fragment. Eventually, the Okazaki fragments are joined by DNA polymerase I. This enzyme, which also has a role in DNA repair, has an exonuclease activity that permits it to remove and replace a stretch of nucleotides as it proceeds along a DNA template. During DNA replication, DNA polymerase I removes the RNA primer and replaces it with DNA. Finally, DNA ligase joins the lagging-strand DNA fragments to form a continuous strand.

Eukaryotes stringently regulate DNA replication

Eukaryotic DNA synthesis is remarkably similar to prokaryotic DNA synthesis. However, eukaryotes have many more origins of replication. These are activated simultaneously during the S-phase of the cell cycle, permitting rapid replication of the entire chromosome. To insure that excess amounts of unfinished, replicating DNA do not accumulate, cells use a protein termed a licensing factor that is present in the nucleus prior to replication. Following each round of replication, this factor is inactivated or destroyed, preventing further replication until more licensing factor is synthesized later in the cell cycle.

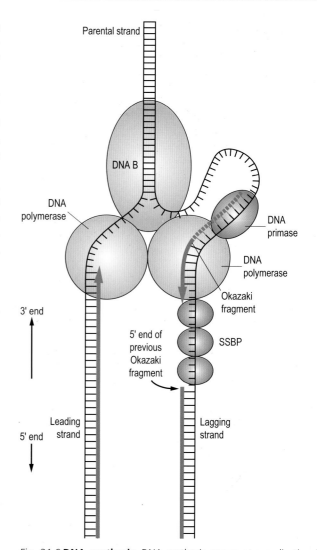

Fig. 31.6 **DNA synthesis.** DNA synthesis occurs at a replication fork producing new strands termed the leading strand and the lagging strand. The 'railroad tracks' represent double-stranded DNA. Some of the enzymes involved in DNA synthesis are shown: DNA B (helicase), DNA primase, DNA polymerase, and single-strand DNA binding protein (SSBP). The leading strand is replicated in a continuous fashion. However, for the lagging strand, RNA primers are periodically added by the DNA primase along the strand. DNA polymerase III elongates these RNA primers to form Okazaki fragments. When the Okazaki fragment is complete, the DNA polymerase III on the lagging strand will shift to the next RNA primer to initiate another Okazaki fragment. The exonuclease activity of DNA polymerase I removes the RNA primers and replaces them with DNA. DNA ligase seals the gaps in the DNA strands to complete synthesis of the lagging strand.

Licensing factor is best understood in the yeast. In yeast there is a complex called the origin recognition complex (ORC), composed of six proteins. The ORC marks the origin of replication and remains bound to the origin throughout the cell cycle. It serves as a docking site for the other components that regulate DNA replication. Early events in DNA replication include the binding of several highly unstable proteins to ORC. These proteins include CDC6/18 and CDT1,

BIOCHEMISTRY OF DNA POLYMERASES IN *ESCHERICHIA COLI*

There are several different DNA polymerases in E. *coli*. DNA polymerase III, the principal DNA replication enzyme, has the highest rate of DNA polymerization. DNA polymerase I is involved in excision repair and in the removal of RNA primers from Okazaki fragments. DNA polymerase III is a complex protein, with at least 10 distinct subunits, ranging in size from 12 kDa to 130 kDa. It requires a single-stranded template and a primer, either DNA or RNA. After binding to the template–primer complex, the enzyme first determines which nucleotide is complementary to the next available template nucleotide and allows that nucleotide to bind to the active site. The elongation reaction occurs when the 3'-hydroxyl of the previous base attacks the 5'-phosphate of the incoming deoxynucleotide triphosphate (dNTP), with release of pyrophosphate. This process results in an elongation of the DNA strand by one nucleotide. Then, in a process termed proofreading, the enzyme checks whether the newly incorporated base can form an allowed Watson–Crick base pair (i.e. AT, TA, CG or GC) with the opposing base on the template strand. If the base pair is not allowed, the enzyme removes the last added nucleotide and repeats the process. If the base pair is allowed, the enzyme advances one nucleotide along the template strand and repeats the process. The ability of DNA polymerase III to proofread DNA sequences and replace mismatched nucleotides serves to maintain the high fidelity of DNA replication.

AZT THERAPY FOR HIV INFECTION

Human immunodeficiency virus (HIV) infection results in a profound weakening of the immune system that makes the patient susceptible to a range of bacterial, fungal, protozoal and viral superinfections. Kaposi's sarcoma may also develop; it is a cancer-like disease of blood vessels caused by infection with human herpesvirus-8 (HHV-8).

Effective treatments of the HIV viral infection rely on detailed knowledge of the viral life cycle. For the AIDS virus, the viral genome is RNA. In the infected cell, it is copied into a DNA form by a viral enzyme termed reverse transcriptase. Reverse transcriptase is an error-prone enzyme that does not have the proofreading capabilities of DNA polymerase III. One therapeutic approach for treatment of AIDS takes advantage of the enzyme's promiscuity in choice of substrates. Several important antiviral drugs are nucleotide analogs that inhibit reverse transcriptase, including AZT (azido, 2',3'-dideoxy thymidine; Retrovir, Zidovudine), ddc (2',3'-dideoxycytidine; Hivid, Zalcitabine), and 3TC (2',3'-dideoxy-3'-thiacytidine; Epivir, Lamivudine). AZT, for example, is metabolized in the body into the thymine triphosphate (TTP) analog azido-TTP. The HIV reverse transcriptase misincorporates azido-TTP into the reverse-transcribed viral genome. The incorporation of azido-TTP into DNA blocks further chain elongation, because the 3'-azido group cannot form a phosphodiester bond with subsequent nucleoside triphosphates. The inability to synthesize DNA from the viral RNA template results in inhibition of viral replication (Fig. 31.7).

which facilitate binding of a group of three additional proteins: MCM2, MCM3, and MCM5. Once the MCM proteins bind, the origin exists as a prereplication complex and is 'licensed' to enter S-phase of the cell cycle. The initiation of DNA synthesis is triggered by the action of the CDC7 kinase together with other cyclin-dependent kinases. The activated MCM complex then participates in unwinding the replication origin and is thereby displaced from the origin. Following displacement, the origin forms a postinitiation complex and CDC6 is degraded, thereby preventing the reloading of the origin with additional licensing factor.

DNA REPAIR

Because DNA is the reservoir of genetic information within the cell, it is extremely important to maintain the integrity of DNA. Therefore, the cell has developed multiple, highly efficient mechanisms for the repair of modified or damaged DNA.

Types of damage to DNA: more than 10 000 modifications per cell per day

DNA can be damaged by numerous types of endogenous and exogenous agents that cause nucleotide modifications, deletions, insertions, sequence inversions and transpositions. Some of this damage is secondary to chemical modification of DNA by alkylating agents (including many carcinogens), reactive oxygen species (Chapter 37) and ionizing radiation (ultraviolet or radioactive). Both the sugar and bases of DNA are subject to modification, yielding an estimated 10 000 to 100 000 modifications of DNA per cell per day. The nature of this damage is quite variable, including modification of single bases, single or double-strand breaks, and cross-linking between bases or bases and proteins. Oxidative damage is probably the most common form of DNA damage; it is increased in inflammation, by smoking, in aging and in age-related diseases, including atherosclerosis, diabetes and neurodegenerative diseases (Chapter 44). If not repaired, the accumulated damage will lead to permanent changes in the structure of DNA, setting the stage for loss of cellular functions, cell death or cancer.

Numerous chemical and environmental agents are known that produce specific chemical modification of the nucleotides in the DNA strand, leading to mismatches during DNA synthesis. After chromosomal replication, the resulting daughter strand contains a different DNA sequence (mutation) from the parent strand. Cells use excision repair to remove alkylated

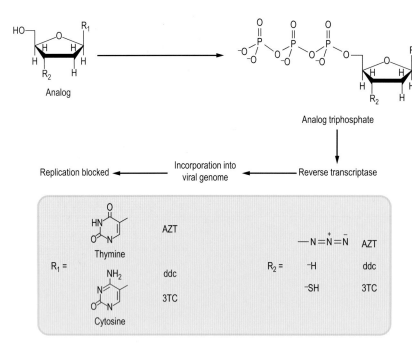

Fig. 31.7 Mechanism of action of antiretroviral chemotherapeutic agents. This class of inhibitors includes several compounds with slightly different chemical structures in the nucleobase structure and in substitution at the 3′-carbon of the sugar ring. Structures of some of the most widely used drugs are shown. These compounds are metabolized to the triphosphate form via normal cellular metabolism (see Chapter 30). The triphosphate analogs are then incorporated into the viral genome by reverse transcriptase. This blocks viral DNA synthesis because the modified 3′ end R_2 of the viral DNA molecule is not a substrate for additional rounds of DNA synthesis.

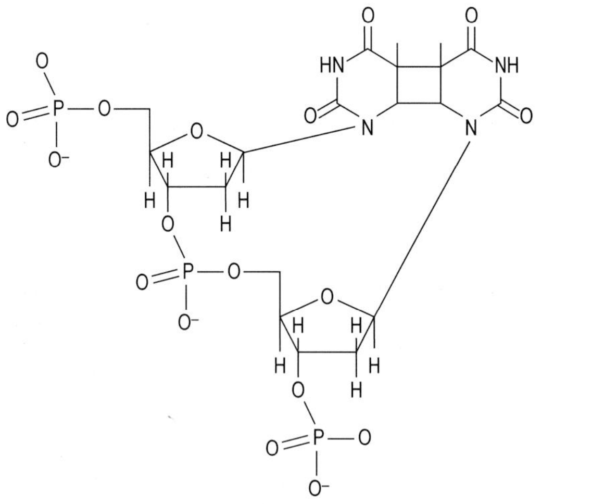

Fig. 31.8 Thymine dimer. A thymine dimer consists of a cyclobutane ring joining a pair of adjacent thymine nucleotides.

nucleotides and other unusual base analogs, thereby protecting the DNA sequence from mutations. The unmodified strand serves as the template for the repair process.

UV light produces thymine dimers: nucleotide excision repair

When short-wavelength ultraviolet (UV) light interacts with DNA, adjacent thymine bases undergo an unusual dimerization, producing a cyclobutylthymine dimer in the DNA strand (Fig. 31.8). The primary mechanism for repair of these intrastrand thymine dimers is an excision repair mechanism. An endonuclease, which appears to be specific for this type of modification, cleaves the dimer-containing

strand near the thymine dimer, and a small portion of that strand is removed. DNA polymerase I, the same enzyme that is involved in DNA biosynthesis, then recognizes and fills in the resulting gap. DNA ligase completes the repair by rejoining the DNA strands.

Deamination: excision repair

Those nucleotides that contain amines, cytosine and adenosine, may spontaneously deaminate to form uracil or hypoxanthine, respectively. When these bases are found in DNA, specific N-glycosylases remove them. This produces base pair gaps that are recognized by specific apurinic or apyrimidinic endonucleases that cleave the DNA near the site of the defect. An exonuclease then removes the stretch of the DNA strand containing the defect. A repair DNA polymerase replaces the DNA and, finally, DNA ligase rejoins the DNA strand. This repair mechanism is also referred to as excision repair.

Depurination

Single base pair alterations also include depurination. The purine-N-glycosidic bonds are especially labile, so that an estimated 3–7 purines are removed from DNA per min per cell. Specific enzymes recognize these depurinated sites, and the base is replaced without interruption of the phosphodiester backbone.

Strand breaks

Single-stranded breaks are frequently induced by ionizing radiation. These are repaired by direct ligation or by excision repair mechanisms. Double-stranded breaks are produced by ionizing radiation and some chemotherapeutic agents. Otherwise, double-stranded ends of DNA are rare in vivo; they are found at the end of chromosomes and in some

XERODERMA PIGMENTOSUM

Xeroderma pigmentosum (XP) is a group of rare, life-threatening, autosomal recessive disorders (incidence = 1/250 000) that are marked by extreme sensitivity to sunlight. Upon exposure to sunlight or ultraviolet radiation, the skin of XP patients erupts into pigmented spots, resembling freckles. Multiple carcinomas and melanomas appear early in life, exacerbated by sun exposure, and the majority of patients succumb to cancer before reaching adulthood.

XP is the result of a defect in repair of UV-induced thymine dimers in DNA. There are at least eight polypeptides (genes) involved in recognition, unwinding and excision repair of UV-induced thymine dimers. Patients with XP must avoid direct sunlight, fluorescent light, halogen light or any other source of ultraviolet light. An experimental form of protein therapy, currently undergoing clinical evaluation, involves application of a skin lotion containing the missing protein or enzyme. Ideally, this protein will enter the skin cells and stimulate the repair of UV-damaged DNA. However, protection occurs only where the lotion can be applied. For example, this treatment does not address the neurologic problems that affect about 20% of XP patients.

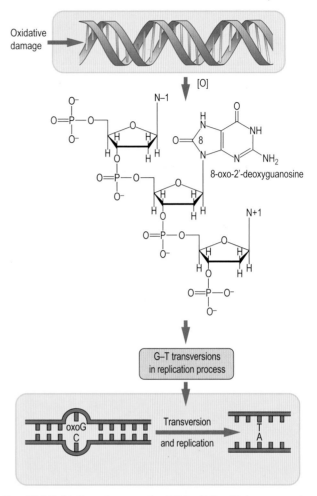

Fig. 31.9 **Oxidative damage to DNA.** 8-Oxo-2'-deoxyguanosine (oxoG) is an oxidative modification of DNA that causes mutations during replication of DNA. Replication of the strand containing oxoG frequently yields a pyrimidine A in the complementary strand which, on further replication, yields an AT base pair, instead of the original GC base pair.

specialized complexes involved in gene rearrangement. A specialized enzyme system is designed to recognize and rejoin these ends but if the ends drift away from one another, the damage is not readily repaired.

Mismatch repair

Errors that escape the proofreading activity of DNA polymerase III appear in newly synthesized DNA in the form of nucleotide mismatches. While readily repairable, the critical issue is identification of the strand to be repaired: which nucleotide strand is the daughter strand containing the error? In bacterial systems, mismatch repair is accomplished by methylation of DNA at adenine residues in specific sequences spaced along the genome; methylation does not affect base pairing. Newly synthesized strands lack methylated adenine residues, so that the mismatch repair system enzymes scan the DNA, identify the mismatch, and then repair the unmethylated strand by excision repair. A similar approach is used to correct mismatches occurring during synthesis of mammalian DNA. Defects in mismatch repair are associated with hereditary nonpolyposis colon cancer, an autosomal dominant condition in humans.

8-Oxo-2'-deoxyguanosine

About 20 different oxidative modifications of DNA have been characterized; the most studied is 8-oxo-2'-deoxyguanosine (8-oxoG) (Fig. 31.9). During the process of DNA replication, mismatches between the modified 8-oxoG nucleoside in the template strand and incoming nucleotide triphosphates

result in G-to-T transversions, thereby introducing mutations into the DNA strand. Although excision repair mechanisms are effective, 8-oxoG, like other modified bases, may be reincorporated into DNA following excision.

Recently, a mammalian protein, MTH1, was characterized that specifically degrades 8-oxo-dGTP, thereby preventing misincorporation of this altered nucleotide into DNA. Gene targeting was used to develop an MTH1 knockout mouse. Compared to the wild-type animal, the knockout showed a greater number of tumors in lung, liver, and stomach, illustrating the importance of this (and other) postrepair protection mechanisms.

In lung cells, inhalation of some particulate materials results in an increase in 8-oxoG levels. The inflammatory process may play a role in asbestos-induced formation of lung tumors. Smoking also induces oxidative damage and increases levels of DNA oxidation products in lungs, blood and urine. 8-oxoG is used as a marker of oxidative stress in many clinical studies (Chapter 44).

AMES TEST FOR MUTAGENS

Mutagens are chemical compounds that induce changes in the DNA sequence. A large number of natural and man-made chemicals are mutagenic. To evaluate the potential to mutate DNA, the American biochemist Bruce Ames developed a simple test, using special *Salmonella typhimurium* strains that cannot grow in the absence of histidine (His⁻ phenotype). These histidine auxotrophic strains contain nucleotide substitutions or deletions that prevent the production of histidine biosynthetic enzymes.

To test for mutagenesis, mutant bacteria are seeded on a culture medium lacking histidine; the suspected mutagen is added to the medium. The action of the mutagen occasionally results in the reversal of the histidine mutation, yielding a revertant strain that can now synthesize histidine and will grow in its absence. The mutagenicity of a compound is scored by counting the number of colonies that have grown, i.e. reverted to the His⁺ phenotype. There is a good correlation between results of the Ames mutagenicity test and direct tests of carcinogenic activity in animals.

Some chemicals (procarcinogens) are not mutagenic per se, but are activated to mutagenic compounds during metabolic processes, e.g. during drug detoxification in liver or kidney. Benzopyrene, for example, is not mutagenic but during its detoxification in liver, it is converted to diolepoxides which are potent mutagens and carcinogens. To provide sensitivity for detecting procarcinogens, the culture medium is supplemented with an extract of liver microsomes, a subfraction of tissue rich in smooth endoplasmic reticulum containing drug-metabolizing enzymes.

ACTIVE LEARNING

1. What are the possible functions of unusual forms of DNA?
2. Discuss the possible roles for middle repetitive and highly repetitive sequences in DNA.
3. Hereditary nonpolyposis colon cancer results from a defect in DNA mismatch repair. Why is this condition autosomal dominant?
4. What are the differences in replication and repair of nuclear vs mitochondrial DNA?

Further reading

Burhans WC, Weinberger M. DNA replication stress, genome instability and aging. *Nucleic Acids Res* 2007;**25**:2045–2056.

Cleaver JE, Crowley E. UV damage, DNA repair and skin carcinogenesis. *Front Biosci* 2002;**7**:1024–1043.

Georgakilas AG. Processing of DNA damage clusters in human cells: current status of knowledge. *Mol Biosyst* 2008;**4**:30–35.

Pavlov YI, Shcherbakova PV, Rogozin IB. Roles of DNA polymerases in replication, repair, and recombination in eukaryotes. *Int Rev Cytol* 2006;**255**:41–132.

Slijepcevic P. DNA damage response, telomere maintenance and ageing in light of the integrative model. *Mech Ageing Dev* 2008;**129**:11–16.

Spry M, Scott T, Pierce H, D'Orazio JA. DNA repair pathways and hereditary cancer susceptibility syndromes. *Front Biosci* 2007;**12**:4191–4207.

Venter JC, Adams MD, Myers EW. The sequence of the human genome. *Science* 2001;**291**:1304–1351.

Watson JD. *A passion for DNA. Genes, genomes and society.* Oxford: Oxford University Press, 2000.

Watson JD. The double helix: a personal account of the discovery of the structure of DNA. New York: WW Norton, 1980.

Summary

The human genome is composed of DNA, an antiparallel, double-stranded helical polymer of deoxyribonucleotides, stabilized by hydrogen binding between complementary bases. The DNA is packaged in the chromosome in a highly organized, condensed structure. Genetic information is replicated by a semi-conservative mechanism in which the parental strands are separated and both act as templates for daughter DNA. The replication of DNA is a complex, stringently regulated process. DNA is essentially the only polymer in the body that is repaired, rather than degraded, following chemical or biologic modification. Repair mechanisms generally involve excision of modified bases and replacement, using the unmodified strand as a template.

Websites

DNA interactive: www.dnai.org. This is the best introduction to the subject.

DNA from the beginning: www.dnaftb.org

National Human Genome Research Institute: http://www.genome.gov

DNA workshop: www.pbs.org/wgbh/aso/tryit/dna

Genetic diseases: http://www.rarediseases.org

Graphics: www.accessexcellence.org/AB/GG/structure.html

DNA repair: http://dir.niehs.nih.gov/dirlmg/DNArepair.html

DNA replication: http://dir.niehs.nih.gov/dirlmg/repl.html

Mitochondrial DNA: http://www.mitomap.org

DNA organization and nucleosomes:
- http://medweb4.bham.ac.uk/jspdf/m102pdf/DNA1.pdf
- http://medweb4.bham.ac.uk/jspdf/m102pdf/DNA2.pdf

32. Ribonucleic Acid

G A Bannon and R Thornburg

LEARNING OBJECTIVES

After reading this chapter you should be able to:

- Identify the major types of cellular RNA and the function of each.
- Describe the major steps in transcription of an RNA molecule.
- Explain the function of the different RNA polymerase enzymes.
- Describe the major differences between prokaryotic and eukaryotic mRNAs.
- Describe the different processing and splicing events that occur during synthesis of eukaryotic mRNAs.

General classes of RNA

RNA	Size and length	Percent of total cellular RNA	Function
rRNA	28S, 18S, 5.8S, 5S (26S, 16S, 5S)*	80	interact to form ribosomes
tRNA	65–110 nt	15	adapter
mRNA	0.5–6 kb	5	directs synthesis of cellular proteins

Size of rRNA in prokaryotic cells. Nt, nucleotides; Kb, kilobases; S, Svedberg units.

Table 32.1 **General classes of RNA**.

Transcription is defined as the synthesis of a ribonucleic acid (RNA) molecule using deoxyribonucleic acid (DNA) as a template. This rather simple definition describes a series of complicated enzymatic processes that result in the transfer of the genetic information stored in double-stranded DNA into a single-stranded RNA molecule that will be used by the cell to direct the synthesis of its proteins, a process known as translation. There are three general classes of RNA molecules found in prokaryotic and eukaryotic cells: ribosomal RNA (rRNA), transfer RNA (tRNA), and messenger RNA (mRNA). Each class has a distinctive size and function (Table 32.1), described by its sedimentation rate in an ultracentrifuge (S, Svedberg units) or its number of bases (nt, nucleotides, or kb, kilobases). Prokaryotes have the same three general classes of RNA as eukaryotes, but sizes and structural features differ:

- **ribosomal RNA (rRNA)** from prokaryotes consists of three different sizes of RNA, while rRNA from eukaryotes consists of four different sizes of RNA. These RNAs interact with each other, and with proteins, to form a ribosome that provides the basic machinery on which protein synthesis takes place
- **transfer RNAs (tRNAs)** consist of one size class of RNA that are 65–110 nt in length; they function as amino acid carriers and as recognition molecules that identify the mRNA nucleotide sequence and translate that sequence into the amino acid sequence of proteins
- **messenger RNAs (mRNAs)** represent the most heterogeneous class of RNAs found in cells. mRNAs generally range in size from 500 nt to ~6 kb in size (some rare but highly important mRNAs are >100 kb in size). mRNAs are carriers of genetic information, defining the sequence of all proteins in the cell; they are the 'working copy' of the genome.

In order to understand the complex series of events that lead to the production of these three classes of RNA, this chapter is divided into five parts. The first part deals with the molecular anatomy of the major types of RNA found in prokaryotic and eukaryotic cells; knowing then the chemical nature of the final products of transcription, you will be better prepared to understand the steps involved in generating these molecules. The second part describes the main enzymes involved in transcription, and their specificities. The third part describes the three steps (initiation, elongation, and termination) required to produce a protein. In the fourth section, the modifications that are made to the primary products of transcription (posttranscriptional processing) are described. This information is expanded in Chapter 34. The final section describes briefly how cells regulate gene expression at the RNA level.

MOLECULAR ANATOMY OF RIBONUCLEIC ACID MOLECULES

In general, the RNAs produced by prokaryotic and eukaryotic cells are single-stranded molecules that consist of adenine, guanine, cytosine, and uracil nucleotides joined to one another by phosphodiester linkages. The start of an RNA molecule is known as its 5′ end, and the termination of the RNA is its 3′end. Even though most RNAs are single-stranded, they exhibit extensive secondary structure, including intramolecular double-stranded regions that are important to their function. These secondary structures, one of the most common of which is called a hairpin loop (Fig. 32.1), are the product of intramolecular base-pairing that occurs between complementary nucleotides within a single RNA molecule.

rRNAs: the ribosomal RNAs

The eukaryotic rRNAs are synthesized as a single RNA transcript with a size of 45S and about 13kb long. This large primary transcript is processed into 28S, 18S, 5.8S, and 5S rRNAs (~3kb, 1.5kb, 160 and 120nt, respectively). The 28S, 5.8S, and 5S rRNAs associate with ribosomal proteins to form the large ribosomal subunit. The 18S rRNA associates with different ribosomal proteins to form the small ribosomal subunit. The large ribosomal subunit with its proteins and RNA has a characteristic size of 60S; the small ribosomal subunit has a size of 40S. These two subunits interact to form a functional 80 S ribosome (see Chapter 33). Prokaryotic rRNAs interact in a similar fashion to form these ribosomal subunits but have a slightly smaller size, reflecting the difference in prokaryotic and eukaryotic rRNA transcript size (Table 32.2).

tRNA: the molecular cloverleaf

Prokaryotic and eukaryotic tRNAs are similar in both size and structure. They exhibit extensive secondary structure

and contain several modified ribonucleotides that are derived from the normal four ribonucleotides. All tRNAs have a similar fold, with four distinct loops that have been described as a cloverleaf (Fig. 32.2). The D loop contains several modified bases, including methylated cytosine and dihydrouridine, for which the loop is named. The anticodon loop is the structure responsible for recognition of the complementary codon of an mRNA molecule: specific interaction of an anticodon of the tRNA with the appropriate codon in the mRNA is due to base pairing between these two complementary trinucleotide sequences. A variable loop, 3–21 nt in length, exists in most tRNAs but its function is unknown. Finally, there is a TψC loop, which contains a modified base, pseudouridine (ψ). Another prominent structure found in all tRNA molecules is the acceptor stem. This structure is formed by base pairing between the nucleotides at each end of the tRNA. The last three bases found at the extreme 3′ end remain unpaired, and always have the same sequence: 5′-CCA-3′. This 3′ end

rRNAs and ribosomes				
Cell type	**rRNA**	**Subunit**	**Size**	**Intact ribosome**
prokaryotic	23 S, 5 S	large	50 S	70 S
	16 S	small	30 S	
eukaryotic	28 S, 5.8 S, 5 S	large	60 S	80 S
	18 S	small	40 S	

Table 32.2 **rRNAs and ribosomes.** rRNAs interact to form ribosomes.

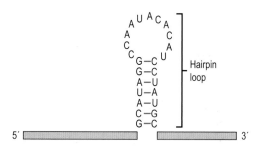

Fig. 32.1 **RNA hairpin loop.** RNA can form secondary structures called hairpin loops. These structures form when complementary bases within an individual RNA share hydrogen bonds and form base pairs. Hairpin loops are known to be important in the regulation of transcription in both eukaryotic and prokaryotic cells.

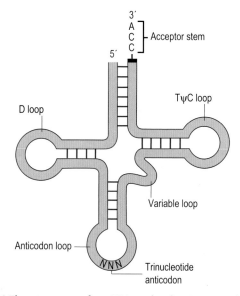

Fig. 32.2 **The structure of a tRNA molecule.** A prototypical tRNA molecule is shown and the structures important to its function are indicated. The overall structure of the molecule is due to complementary base pairing between nucleotides within a single RNA. All tRNAs have this basic structure.

of the acceptor stem is the point at which an amino acid is attached via an ester bond between the 3'-hydroxyl group of the adenosine and the carboxyl group of an amino acid in preparation for protein synthesis (see Chapter 33).

mRNA: prokaryotes and eukaryotes have dissimilar mRNAs

Prokaryotes and eukaryotes are very different kinds of organisms with dramatically different life cycles. Therefore, it is not surprising that there are differences in the structures of their genes, in their mechanisms of transcription, and in the structures of their mRNAs. In fact, we can exploit these differences with novel antibiotics that specifically target unique portions of the prokaryotic life cycle. There are a number of major differences between prokaryotic and eukaryotic mRNAs. These will be discussed in sections below. Briefly, these differences are:

- transcriptional units differ in structure: prokaryotic mRNAs are polycistronic, eukaryotic mRNAs are mono-cistronic (Fig. 32.3)
- compartmentalization of transcription and translation: prokaryotes synthesize RNA and protein in one compartment, eukaryotes separate these events in nucleus and cytoplasm
- protection at their 5' and 3' ends: ends of prokaryotic mRNAs are naked, eukaryotic mRNAs have a cap and poly(A) tail
- processing of mRNAs: prokaryotic mRNAs are not processed; eukaryotic mRNAs contain introns that are spliced out.

A major difference between prokaryotic and eukaryotic mRNAs relates to their transcriptional unit structure. In prokaryotes, transcriptional units generally contain multiple protein-coding regions (see Fig. 32.3), while in eukaryotes, each transcriptional unit generally codes for only a single protein. The polycistronic mRNAs of prokaryotes have individual start and stop codons at the beginning and end of each open reading frame, the sequence of mRNA that specifies the sequence of the polypeptide chain. Each stop codon is closely followed by another ribosome binding site and a translation start site that functions for the next open reading frame.

A second major difference between prokaryotic and eukaryotic mRNAs is the compartmentalization of the transcription and translation processes. Because prokaryotes lack a nucleus, transcription and translation are intimately coupled; prokaryotic translation is usually initiated before transcription is finished. By coupling these processes, prokaryotes increase the rate at which proteins are expressed, consistent with the relatively short life cycles of prokaryotes. In contrast, eukaryotic cells separate transcription in the nucleus from translation in the cytoplasm. Although this arrangement slows response time for protein production, it allows for much more subtle control of protein expression.

The posttranscriptional processing of mRNAs is also significantly different in prokaryotes and eukaryotes. Because of their importance, these differences will be detailed in a separate section below dealing with posttranscriptional processing of RNAs. Briefly, eukaryotes protect the 5' and 3' ends of mRNAs by addition of specific molecular structures (5' cap and polyA tail) that function to reduce mRNA

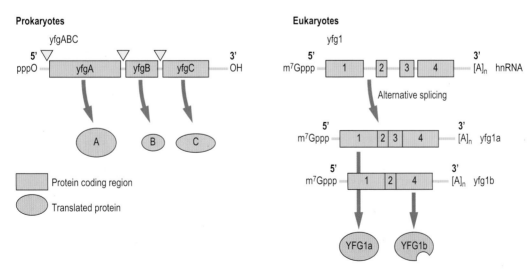

Fig. 32.3 **Prototypical structures of prokaryotic (polycistronic) and eukaryotic mRNAs.** Prokaryotic mRNAs have naked ends (triphosphate at the 5' end and hydroxyl at the 3' end). The boxes indicate those portions of the mRNA that encode a protein. Inverted triangles indicate location of ribosome-binding sites. The three genes in this cistron are translated into three different proteins. Nascent eukaryotic mRNA transcripts (heterogeneous nuclear (hnRNA)) contain both exons (blue boxes) and introns (lines). Eukaryotic mRNAs are protected by a 7-methylguanine nucleotide cap (m^7Gppp) at the 5' end and a polyA tail ($[A]_n$) at the 3' end of the mRNA. After splicing, the mature mRNAs consist only of exons plus the 5' and 3' UTRs. Alternatively spliced mRNAs are translated into different protein isoforms. *yfg:* your favorite gene; UTR: untranslated region.

turnover. Also, eukaryotic genes contain introns, untranslated sequences that are present in nascent transcripts and must be spliced out to produce mature mRNAs.

RIBONUCLEIC ACID POLYMERASES

RNA polymerases are large multimeric enzymes that transcribe defined segments of DNA into RNA with a high degree of selectivity and specificity

The enzymes responsible for the synthesis of RNA are called RNA polymerases (RNAPol). In contrast to DNA polymerases (Chapter 31), RNA polymerases do not require a primer to initiate RNA synthesis. The RNA polymerases generally consist of two high molecular-weight subunits and several smaller subunits, all of which are necessary for accurate transcription. Prokaryotes contain a single RNA polymerase that synthesizes all RNAs; however, eukaryotes contain three different RNA polymerases termed RNA polymerase I, II, and III. Each of these polymerases specializes in transcription of one class of RNA.

- RNAPol I transcribes ribosomal RNAs. The rRNAs are produced from a single transcriptional unit that is subsequently processed to produce the 18 S, 26 S, 5.8 S and 5 S rRNAs.
- RNAPol III transcribes most of the small cellular RNAs (snRNAs, below), including the tRNAs.
- RNAPol II transcribes all other genes within a eukaryotic cell, including all protein-coding genes that yield mRNA. RNAPol II is exquisitely sensitive to α-amanitin, a potent and toxic transcription inhibitor found in some poisonous mushrooms.

Yeast RNAPol II consists of a 12-subunit core. It exists in two forms. The first is an open form that is shaped like a cupped hand with a cleft that binds the DNA molecule and associated transcription factors near the start point of transcription. After melting or dissociation of the DNA strands, the complex undergoes a large structural change that closes the cleft, forming a clamp around the antisense or template strand of the DNA. Then, a specific protein (*rbp4/7*) binds to the base of the clamp, locking the clamp in the closed state. The closed form is no longer competent for transcript initiation but is capable of transcript elongation. The yeast RNAPol II structure appears to be an excellent model for the human enzyme. In addition, it is also a good model for the function of RNAPol I and III because the core subunits are either shared or are homologous between the various enzymes.

The bacterial RNA polymerase is similar to the eukaryotic enzyme complex, except the bacterial enzyme contains only four subunits ($\alpha_2\beta\beta'$) and, unlike the eukaryotic enzyme, requires only a single general transcription factor (σ-factor) to recognize the promoter and recruit the RNA polymerase to initiate transcription.

MESSENGER RIBONUCLEIC ACID: TRANSCRIPTION

Transcription is a dynamic process that involves the interaction of enzymes and DNA in specific ways to produce an RNA molecule. In order to understand this process better, it is convenient to divide it into three separate stages: initiation, elongation and termination. Transcription proceeds along the antisense or template strand, producing a complementary RNA that is identical to the sense strand of the DNA

α-AMANITIN POISONING: PICKING THE WRONG MUSHROOM

An otherwise healthy young woman presents herself to the emergency room in the early morning with severe nausea, abdominal cramping and copious diarrhea. The patient's vital signs show tachycardia and the patient's skin has poor turgor indicating dehydration. While giving her medical history, the patient explains that her symptoms began suddenly, about 6 h after she had eaten dinner. Suspecting food poisoning, the patient is asked to recall everything eaten over the past 24 h. The patient reports that she had eaten mushrooms for dinner and added that the mushrooms were picked on a recent hike through the woods. The patient is started aggressively on saline and electrolytes to replenish lost fluids and is given activated charcoal to absorb any residual or recirculating toxins in the gastrointestinal tract. The patient appears to stabilize over the next 24 h and is alert; however, she remains lethargic and the skin begins to take on a yellowish tinge. Blood work shows reduced blood glucose, elevated serum aminotransferase, and slightly elongated prothrombin time. Amylase and lipase levels are normal, indicating no pancreatic involvement, and urinalysis indicates no renal involvement. The doctor consults a gastroenterologist who advises increased monitoring of hepatorenal function and continued aggressive intravenous fluid and electrolyte treatment. After approximately 5 days, the patient recovers. What is the biochemical basis of this woman's illness?

Comment. About 95% of all mushroom fatalities in North America are associated with ingestion of the species *Amanita*. These species produce a toxin, α-amanitin, that binds to RNAPol II and inhibits its function. The first cells that encounter the toxin are those lining the digestive tract. Cells incapable of synthesizing new mRNAs die, causing acute gastrointestinal distress. Liver failure is a serious complication of α-amanitin ingestion. Jaundice and liver function tests (alkaline phosphatase, bilirubin, aminotransferase levels, and prothrombin time) indicate the level of hepatic involvement (see Chapter 29). Most accidental mushroom exposures occur in children younger than 6 years old, who because of their size absorb a larger toxin dose per kg of body weight. In an adult, the ingestion of a single *Amanita phalloides* mushroom can be fatal. Mortality rates range from 10% to 60% of all patients.

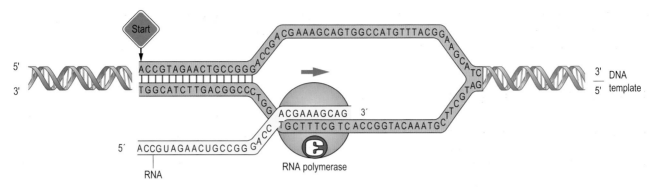

Fig. 32.4 **Transcription.** Transcription involves the synthesis of an RNA by RNA polymerase using DNA as a template. The RNA polymerase holoenzyme uses the antisense strand of DNA to direct the synthesis of an RNA molecule that is complementary to this strand.

(Fig. 32.4), except for substitution of uracil in RNA for thymine in DNA.

Initiation

Initiation involves the interaction of the RNA polymerase with DNA in a site-specific fashion. Because most genomic DNA does not encode proteins, identification of transcription start sites is crucial to obtain desired mRNAs. Special sequences termed promoters recruit the RNA polymerase to the transcription start site (Fig. 32.5). Promoters are usually located in front (upstream) of the gene that is to be transcribed. However, RNAPol polymerase III promoters are actually located within the gene.

Prokaryotic genes generally contain simple promoters. These are usually about 6–8 nt in length and are generally located immediately upstream from the start of transcription. Promoters are generally rich in adenine (A) and thymine (T). The presence of these nucleotides facilitates separation of the two DNA strands, because hydrogen bonding between A-T base pairs is weaker than between G-C base pairs. Comparisons of large numbers of prokaryotic promoters have identified two common conserved regions. These are located about 10 nucleotides and 35 nucleotides upstream (-10 and -35 sequences, respectively) from the transcription start site (see Fig. 32.5). The -10 sequence is known as the TATA box. This sequence binds the prokaryotic general transcription factor (σ-factor) that interacts and recruits the RNA polymerase to the promoter. Strong promoters tend to match the consensus sequence shown in Figure 32.5; sequences of weaker promoters differ from the consensus sequence and bind the σ-factor and the RNA polymerase less tightly.

In eukaryotic RNAPol II promoters (most genes), regulatory elements (specific small DNA sequences) termed upstream activation sequences (UASes), enhancers, repressors, CAATT and TATA box sequences are spread over several hundred to several thousand nucleotides. Individual transcription factors (activators or repressors) recognize and bind

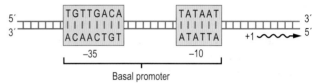

Fig. 32.5 **Prokaryotic promoters.** Promoters in prokaryotic genes are located immediately upstream of the transcription start site. Two common conserved regions have been identified that are found at -35 and -10, respectively. The consensus sequences in these regions are shown. Position $+1$ indicates the first nucleotide that will be transcribed into RNA. The TATA box is a common AT-rich promoter element.

to these UASes. The control of initiation and the regulation of gene expression are outlined in detail in Chapter 34.

Elongation

After the formation of a phosphodiester bond in the RNA complex, the RNA polymerase translocates along the template DNA strand. It is thought that the RNA polymerase accomplishes this by oscillating a small helical region of the RNA polymerase molecule between straight and bent conformations, permitting the polymerase to ratchet about 3 Å ($=1$ nucleotide step) along the antisense strand. After translocation, a new nucleotide is added. Recognition of individual ribonucleotides involves a two-step process. Initially, ribonucleotides are recognized and bind to an entry site. Binding to this site enhances the lifetime of a ribonucleotide in the active site vicinity. If the incoming ribonucleotide matches the next template base, the incoming ribonucleotide is transferred into the polymerase active site and a new phosphodiester bond is formed, thereby elongating the RNA strand and completing the cyclic process.

There are a number of protein factors that bind to and stabilize the elongation-competent RNA polymerase complex. Such factors are particularly important in viral infections.

Viruses such as adenovirus, the pox viruses, vesicular stomatitis virus (VSV), and HIV produce viral proteins that stabilize the RNA polymerase complex, either directly or by recruiting host factors that stabilize the complex. The HIV protein, TAT, is one of the better understood of these stabilization proteins. It binds elongating RNAPol II complexes that are transcribing the HIV transcript and modifies the phosphorylation state of the *C*-terminal domain of the RNA polymerase. This increases its activity, thereby enhancing viral replication.

Elongation can be a rapid process, occurring at the rate of ~40 nt per second. For elongation to occur, the double-stranded DNA must be continually unwound, so that the template strand is accessible to the RNA polymerase. DNA topoisomerases I and II, enzymes associated with the transcription complex, move along the template with the RNA polymerase, separating DNA strands so that they are accessible for RNA synthesis.

Termination

At the end of a transcriptional unit, the RNA polymerases terminate RNA synthesis at defined sites. Transcriptional termination mechanisms are much better understood in prokaryotes than in eukaryotes. In prokaryotes, termination occurs via one of two well-characterized mechanisms that both require the formation of hairpin loops in the RNA secondary structure (Fig. 32.6). In 'rho-**in**dependent' termination, a hairpin loop is formed just upstream of a sequence of 6–8 uridine (U) residues located near the 3' end of the transcript. The formation of this secondary structure dislodges the RNA polymerase from the DNA template, resulting in termination of RNA synthesis. In 'rho-dependent' termination, the *rho* protein, an ATP-dependent helicase, travels along the newly synthesized RNA, chasing the RNA polymerase. The secondary structure induced by a stable hairpin loop near the end of the transcriptional unit causes the RNA polymerase to pause, allowing the *rho* protein to catch up and then displace the RNA polymerase from the template, thereby stopping transcription.

In eukaryotes, the three RNA polymerases employ different mechanisms to terminate transcription. RNAPol I uses a specific protein, transcript termination factor 1 (TTF1), that binds to an 18 nt terminator site located about 1000 nt downstream of the rRNA coding sequence. When RNAPol I encounters the TTF1 bound to DNA, a releasing factor catalyzes the release of the polymerase from the rRNA gene. RNAPol III uses a mechanism that is similar to bacterial 'rho-independent' termination; however, the length of the uridine (U) stretch is shorter and there is no requirement for a RNA secondary structure to dislodge the RNA polymerase. The mechanism of transcription by RNAPol II, which transcribes most eukaryotic genes, is not well understood, in part because the RNAPol II products are immediately processed by removal of the nascent 3' end and addition of a polyadenosine (polyA) tail.

A STUBBORN MICROBE

POSTTRANSCRIPTIONAL PROCESSING OF RIBONUCLEIC ACIDS

The prokaryotic life strategy is to replicate as rapidly as possible when conditions support growth. Eukaryotes have a more controlled life strategy that invests more in increased regulation to achieve stable growth but limits rapid reproduction. Both strategies work well for each type of organism as evidenced by the rich diversity of life on earth; mechanisms of RNA synthesis and processing have evolved to optimize each life strategy. This is especially true for mRNAs.

Pre-rRNA and pre-tRNA

In both prokaryotes and eukaryotes, tRNAs and rRNAs are synthesized as larger precursor molecules that must be

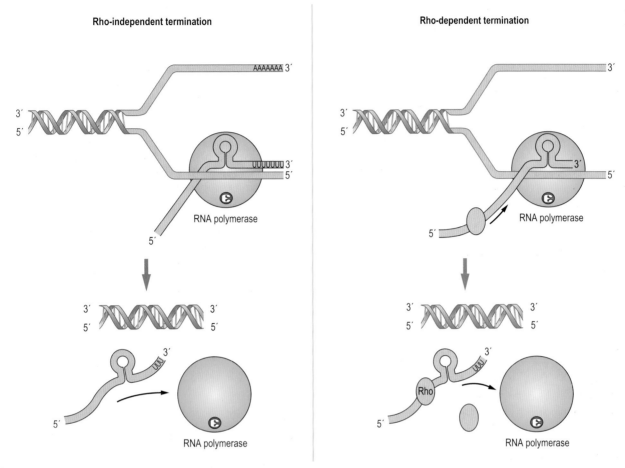

Fig. 32.6 **Transcription termination in prokaryotes.** Two mechanisms of transcription termination in bacterial cells are known. *Rho*-independent termination relies on the formation of a secondary structure in the newly transcribed RNA to dislodge the RNA polymerase from the DNA template and stop transcription. *Rho*-dependent termination requires the action of the *rho* protein. This protein moves along the newly transcribed RNA, catching up with the RNA polymerase when it pauses at the termination site, and causing the polymerase to dissociate from the DNA template.

processed to yield mature transcripts (Fig. 32.7). In prokaryotes the pre-rRNA transcript contains several features. A single 30 S rRNA transcript (~6.5 kb) contains specific leader and trailer regions located at the 5′ and 3′ ends of the transcript as well as one copy each of the 23 S, 16 S and 5 S rRNAs. The rRNA genes also contain a number of tRNAs that are embedded in the pre-rRNA transcript. The rRNA transcript must be processed to liberate the functional RNAs. Including each of the ribosomal RNAs in a single transcript is clearly advantageous to maintain the ratio of large to small ribosomal subunits.

In prokaryotes, processing of the pre-rRNA requires several RNases. Ribonuclease III (RNase III) cleaves the pre-rRNA in double-stranded regions. Such regions occur at each end of the 16 S and 23 S rRNAs and their cleavage liberates these rRNAs from the pre-rRNA transcript. The 16 S and 23 S rRNAs are further processed at the 5′ and 3′ ends; however, this trimming requires the presence of specific ribosomal proteins and occurs during ribosome assembly.

In all eukaryotes from yeast to mammals, pre-rRNA transcripts are processed in a manner similar to the prokaryotic

pre-rRNA processing. Every 35 S rRNA transcript (~9.1 kb) includes a single copy of the 18 S, 5.8 S and 25 S rRNAs. However, processing of the human rRNA is more complex. The pre-rRNA transcript must be cleaved at 11 different sites to generate the mature 18 S, 23 S, 5.8 S and 5 S rRNAs. Processing occurs on a huge ribonucleoprotein complex termed the processome. In addition to modifications by cleavage, the mature human rRNA contains 115 specific methyl group modifications (in most of these, the methyl group is added to the backbone ribosyl 2′-hydroxyl group) and 95 specific uridine to pseudouridine (ψ) conversions. These modifications are introduced into the pre-rRNA through the interaction with individual small nucleolar ribonucleolar protein complexes (snoRNPs, pronounced snorps). Each of these snoRNPs contains a unique guide RNA (~60–300 nt in length) and from one to four protein molecules. Each snoRNP is specific for a single or at most a few individual modification sites. The snoRNAs function by binding to the pre-rRNA molecules by virtue of a complementary nucleotide stretch (~10–20 nucleotides), which correctly positions a methyl transferase or a pseudouridine synthase in the

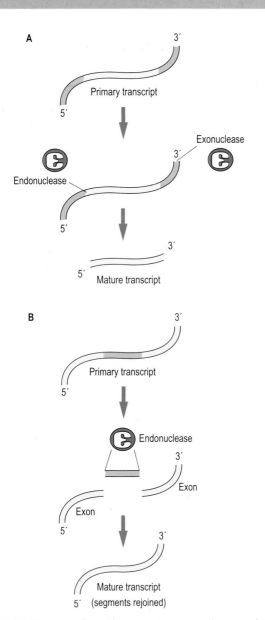

Fig. 32.7 **RNA processing.** There are two general types of RNA processing events. Processing of an RNA transcript can involve (A) the removal of excess sequences by the action of endonucleases and exonucleases as in the processing of rRNA and tRNA genes, or (B) the removal of excess sequences and the rejoining of segments of the newly transcribed RNA as in splicing of mRNAs.

RIBOZYMES: RNAs THAT ACT LIKE ENZYMES

In some instances, RNAs have a catalytic activity similar to the type of activities previously ascribed only to proteins (i.e. ribonuclease activity). These unusual catalytic molecules are known as ribozymes. The substrate specificity of a ribozyme is determined by nucleotide base pairing between complementary sequences contained within the enzyme and the RNA substrate that it cleaves. Just like proteinaceous enzymes, the ribozyme will cleave its substrate RNA at a specific site and then release it, without itself being consumed in the reaction. Some RNA viruses, especially plant viruses and virus-like particles such as hepatitis virus delta agent (HVD) that utilize a rolling-circle replicative cycle, rely on the action of ribozymes to cleave viral RNAs from the pre-RNA product.

Because sequences required for ribozyme activity have been identified, ribozymes can be designed that will cleave any RNA. Recombinant ribozymes are being considered as possible therapeutic agents for diseases that are caused by the inappropriate expression of an RNA or the expression of a mutated RNA. Theoretically, the development of a ribozyme with specificity for a particular RNA is expected to result in the selective degradation of the substrate, eliminating it from the cell and inhibiting the disease process.

finding was that the RNA portion of this complex is sufficient to cleave the RNA, i.e. the protein portion is not required for enzymatic activity. The discovery of self-splicing RNA – that is, RNA with an enzymatic activity, a ribozyme – has led to new ideas about early cellular evolution, which was originally believed to start with amino acids and proteins. It is now believed that ribonucleotides and RNA may have been the most primitive catalytic biopolymers to form on earth, providing for genetic diversity, and that DNA and proteins may have developed later. A third enzyme, RNase D, trims away the extra 3′ nucleotides from the pre-tRNAs, leaving the invariant CCA that is found at the 3′ end of every tRNA.

Pre-mRNA processing

Prokaryotes are able to rapidly alter mRNA synthesis for immediate protein production. After their immediate needs have been met, they subsequently degrade their mRNAs and reuse the ribonucleotides. A typical half-life of prokaryotic mRNA is 3 about minutes. In contrast, eukaryotes take special precautions to stably maintain their mRNAs for continued use. mRNA half-lives in eukaryotes range from a few minutes, for some highly regulated transcription factors, to as long as 30 hours for some long-lived transcripts. Prokaryotes rapidly synthesize their mRNAs and typically do not process or modify them; both the 5′ and 3′ ends of prokaryotic mRNAs are naked and unprotected.

position to modify the pre-rRNA. The processome contains >100 snoRNAs as well as more than 100 individual proteins. Studies of the processome are ongoing and a clear picture of pre-rRNA processing remains incomplete.

In addition to the rRNA genes, tRNAs are also synthesized in precursor form. As many as seven individual tRNAs can be synthesized from a single pre-tRNA gene. Processing of the tRNAs from the pre-tRNAs requires RNase P, which cleaves each tRNA from the pre-tRNA by a single cleavage at its 5′ end. RNAse P is an RNA-protein complex containing a 377 nucleotide RNA and a 20 kDa protein. A remarkable

Consequently, even newly synthesized mRNAs are rapidly degraded by normal cellular RNases. This is not a problem for these rapidly growing organisms.

Because eukaryotes maintain their transcripts for prolonged use, these organisms have evolved methods to protect each end of the mRNA. At the 5′ end, a unique structure termed a '5′ cap' is added. The cap consists of a 7-methylguanidine residue that is attached in reverse orientation to the first nucleotide of the mRNA, i.e. by a 5′ to 5′ triphosphate linkage (m^{7}Gppp). Most cellular exo-RNases do not have the ability to hydrolyze this cap from the mRNA, so the 5′ end is immune in their presence. At the 3′ end of all eukaryotic mRNAs (with the exception of histone mRNAs), a polyadenosine track is added, termed the polyA tail. The adenosine residues are not encoded by the DNA but instead are added by the action of poly(A) polymerase using ATP as a substrate. This polyA tail is frequently >250 nucleotides in length. Although it is still susceptible to the action of exo-RNases, the presence of the polyA tail significantly increases the lifetime of mRNA. The presence of the polyA tail has historically been used to isolate mRNA from eukaryotic cells.

In the more complicated posttranscriptional processing of eukaryotic mRNAs, sequences called introns (intravening sequences) are removed from the primary transcript and the remaining segments, termed exons (expressed sequences), are ligated to form a functional RNA. This process involves a large complex of proteins and auxiliary RNAs called small nuclear RNAs (snRNAs), which interact to form a spliceosome. The function of the five snRNAs (U1, U2, U4, U5, U6) in the spliceosome is to help position reacting groups within the substrate mRNA molecule, so that the introns can be removed and the appropriate exons can be spliced together precisely (Table 32.3). The snRNAs accomplish this task by binding, through base-pairing interactions, with the sites on the mRNA that represent intron/exon boundaries. Accompanying protein factors are responsible for holding the reacting components together to facilitate the reaction.

The removal of an intron and rejoining of two exons can be considered to occur in two steps (Fig. 32.8). The first step involves the breaking of the phosphodiester bond at the exon/intron boundary at the 5′ end of the intron. This is accomplished by a transesterification reaction, which occurs between the 2′-OH of an adenosine nucleotide, usually found about 30 nt from the 3′ end of the intron, and the phosphate in the phosphodiester bond of a guanosine residue located at the 5′ end of the intron. This reaction cleaves the nucleotide chain and produces a branched structure on the 3′ end in which the adenine has 2′, 3′, and 5′ phosphate groups. The intron forms a looped structure similar in appearance to that of a cowboy's lariat. The second step in the reaction involves the cleavage of the phosphodiester bond at the 3′ end of the intron, which releases the lariat structure from the complex. Splicing is completed by the joining of the 3′ end of one exon to the 5′ end of the next exon, through the formation of a regular 5′–3′ phosphodiester bond. Typically, the 3′ end of

snRNA	Size	Function
U1	165 nt	Binds the 5′ exon/intron boundary
U2	185 nt	Binds the branch site on the intron
U4	145 nt	Helps assemble the spliceosome
U5	116 nt	Binds the 3′ intron/exon boundary
U6	106 nt	Displaces U1 after first rearrangement

snRNAs and their function in splicing mRNAs

Table 32.3 **The function of small nuclear RNAs (snRNAs) in the splicing of mRNAs.**

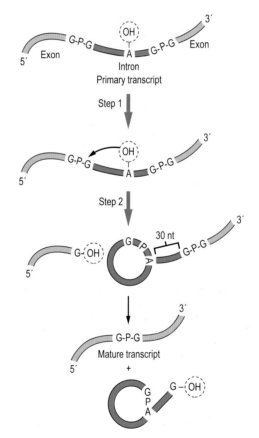

Fig. 32.8 **RNA splicing.** RNA splicing is a multistep process catalyzed by ribonucleoprotein complexes, simplified in the above diagram. In a transesterification reaction, the phosphate bond of a guanosine residue at the 5′ exon/intron boundary is broken and joined to the 2′-OH of an adenine residue located in the middle of the intron. In a later step, the phosphate bond at the 3′ intron/exon boundary is first cleaved and then the two exons are spliced together by reformation of a phosphodiester bond between the nucleotides at either end of the exons. The intron is eliminated in the form of a lariat structure, cyclized through a 2′,3′,5′-phosporylated adenosine residue.

GENOMIC IMPRINTING

snoRNAs also function in genomic imprinting. Genomic imprinting is an epigenetic (see box on p. 457) process that results in differential expression of maternal and paternal genes in a developing embryo. This process occurs in both mammals and plants. Specific genes are methylated during meiosis and thereby inactivated. This methylation occurs differentially in oocyte and spermatocyte development, thereby uniquely inactivating either the maternal or the paternal alleles during embryonic development. Genomic imprinting can affect a large number of conditions in humans including susceptibility to asthma, cancer, diabetes, obesity and a number of developmental disorders. At least 83 genes are known to be imprinted in humans, i.e. methylated and inactivated in one parent.

RNAi AS A THERAPEUTIC OPTION

Age-related macular degeneration (AMD) is the leading cause of blindness for the elderly in the developed world. AMD results from an atrophy of the macula in the retina. The result of atrophy is a loss of central vision, which can lead to the inability to read or even to recognize faces. The most severe type of AMD (the wet form) causes vision loss due to the growth of blood vessels (neovascularization) in the retinal choriocapillaries which, if untreated, leads to blood and protein leakage beneath the macula. This eventually causes scarring and irreversible damage to the photoreceptors.

One mechanism that causes neovascularization is the aberrant expression of the proangiogenic vascular endothelial growth factor (VEGF) in the retina, which results in blood vessel outgrowth. One treatment has been to use anti-VEGF antibodies (ranibizumab (Lucentis) or bevacizumab (Avastin)) injected directly into the vitreous humor of the eye. These antibodies bind to and inactivate VEGF, thereby reducing the level of angiogenesis and prolonging eyesight. The ability of a cell to downregulate specific mRNA levels coupled with the localized treatment area offered by the vitreous humor make the VEGF gene an ideal candidate for RNAi-mediated downregulation. Small RNA molecules complementary to VEGF mRNA are injected into the vitreous. When these molecules are taken into the cell, they function as siRNAs, causing degradation of VEGF mRNA and decreasing VEGF biosynthesis. Several clinical trials are under way to evaluate the use of RNAi as a therapeutic method for treatment of AMD. A similar approach might also work for treatment of diabetic retinopathy. FDA approval of AMD RNAi drugs is expected to occur in 2009. Other RNAi trials are currently under way for respiratory syncytial virus (RSV), hepatitis C, Huntington's disease, HIV and cancer.

one exon will be spliced to the 5′ end of the next closest exon, producing a transcript that exhibits all the exons in the order in which they were transcribed.

Most eukaryotic mRNAs consist of multiple introns and multiple exons. If splicing were consistent, only a single mature mRNA would result from the pre-mRNAs. However, many eukaryotic genes undergo a process called alternative splicing, in which different exons are recombined together to form multiple mature mRNAs (see Fig. 32.3). When these different mRNAs are translated, multiple protein isoforms are made. In humans, almost 60% of pre-mRNAs give rise to multiple mature mRNAs following alternative splicing. About 80% of these alternatively spliced mRNAs result in alternations in the encoded proteins (some splicing events occur in the 5′ and 3′ untranslated regions). Alternative splicing can result in insertion or deletion of amino acids in the protein sequence, shifts in reading frames, or even introduction of novel stop codons. It can also add or remove mRNA sequences that can alter regulatory elements affecting translation, mRNA stability or subcellular localization. In vertebrates (mouse, humans, and fish), the introns of many ribosomal protein genes host the sequences of the small nucleolar RNAs (snoRNAs) that function in modification of specific residues in rRNAs and tRNAs; however, many introns do not host these sequences and the function remains obscure.

Finally, in some instances, mRNAs are posttranscriptionally edited via one of several different mechanisms. These include specific C to U modifications caused by cytosine deaminases or A to I modifications caused by adenosine deaminases or deletion of single or multiple U residues to change the nucleotide sequence of the mRNA. These changes lead to codon differences that result in altered protein sequences that differ from the sequences encoded at the gene level (see Chapter 34). A large multiprotein complex termed the editosome is involved in this process. The snoRNAs that

function in rRNA and tRNA modification also function in these RNA editing processes. These snoRNAs bind to the editing sites within the mRNAs and position the editosome with either cytosine deaminase or adenosine deaminase activity at the correct position to complete the modification.

SELECTIVE DEGRADATION OR INACTIVATION OF RIBONUCLEIC ACID

RNA viruses pose a major challenge for eukaryotic cells; however, natural defense mechanisms have evolved to limit viral infection. Because RNA viruses generally form a double-strand (ds) replicative intermediate during their life cycle, this dsRNA is a unique structure that is not generally found in eukaryotic cells. It can be recognized by dsRNA binding proteins that will subsequently trigger responses to limit viral infection. One of these mechanisms involves the dsRNA-activated protein kinase (PKR). When activated by binding dsRNA, this enzyme can phosphorylate and inactivate the protein translation factor, eIF2α, thereby downregulating translation of viral RNA. Likewise, when activated by dsRNA the enzyme 2'-5' oligoadenylate synthase (2–5 A synthase) polymerizes ATP into a series of short nucleotides (2'-5' oligoadenylate, 2–5 A) that differs from the normal 5'-3' structure found in normal RNA. The most active form is a trimer, pppA-2'-p-5'-A-2'-p-5'-A. The accumulation of 2–5 A inhibits viral (and host) protein translation by activating an endoribonuclease (RNase L) that indiscriminately degrades both mRNAs and rRNAs within the cell. Both genes, PKR and 2–5 A synthase, are induced by interferon, which is itself upregulated by viral infection. This results in an efficient amplification mechanism, leading to programmed cell death (apoptosis) to limit the growth and spread of the virus.

Another important process in innate cellular immunity involves specific targeting of RNA sequences for rapid degradation. This process is termed RNA interference (RNAi) (see Chapter 34) and is sometimes called posttranscriptional gene silencing (PTGS). While this process is thought to have evolved as a defense against double-strand forms of RNA viruses, it also functions as an endogenous mechanism of gene regulation during development of many eukaryotes. PTGS begins when duplex RNA is recognized within cells by the enzyme Dicer. Dicer is an endonuclease with activity against dsRNAs. When Dicer encounters a dsRNA, it binds to the duplex RNA (the sequence is not important) and cleaves the duplex RNA into 21–25 nucleotide double-stranded fragments, termed small interfering RNAs (siRNAs). Depending on the size of the double-stranded RNA, one or many siRNAs are generated. These small fragments then encounter a multiprotein complex, termed RISC. The RISC is composed of a number of components including the enzyme Argonaut. Argonaut binds the small fragments, unwinds them, and maintains one of the strands (the guide strand) to act as an RNA targeting cofactor; the other strand is degraded. Because of the incorporated siRNA, the RISC complex is able to monitor RNAs within the cell and identify sequences complementary to its siRNA. When the RISC complex identifies a complementary RNA sequence, it will base pair with it and cleave it. Because unprotected RNA ends are readily degraded via endogenous RNases (recall the importance of a 5' cap and a 3' polyA tail in eukaryotic mRNAs), the result of this cleavage is to initiate the rapid degradation of the RNAs that are complementary to the siRNA, and thereby eliminate the viral RNA.

synthesis occurs. tRNAs function as amino acid carriers that translate the information stored in the mRNA nucleotide sequence to the amino acid sequence of proteins. In eukaryotic cells, each of these RNA classes is produced by a different, specific RNA polymerase (RNA Pol II, I or III, respectively), while in bacterial cells a single RNA polymerase synthesizes all three classes of RNA. The basic structures of rRNAs and tRNAs in eukaryotic and bacterial cells are similar. However, mRNAs from eukaryotic cells have a 5' (m^7Gppp) cap and a 3' ($[A]_n$) tail. Prokaryotic cells do not have these modifications on their 5' and 3' ends and can be polycistronic. In addition, most eukaryotic mRNAs must undergo a process called splicing to be functional, whereas prokaryotic mRNAs are functional as soon as they are synthesized. Splicing involves the removal of sequences called introns and the rejoining of exon sequences to each other to form a mature functional mRNA. The process of transcription consists of three parts: initiation, elongation, and termination. Initiation involves the recognition and binding of promoter sequences by RNA polymerase and associated transcriptional cofactors. Elongation involves the selection of the appropriate nucleotide and formation of the phosphodiester bridges between each nucleotide in an RNA molecule. Finally, termination involves the dissociation of the RNA polymerase from the DNA template. This is mediated by either RNA secondary structure or specific protein factors. Unique cellular mechanisms recognize double-stranded RNA that limit viral infection by multiple mechanisms, some that induce overall mRNA degradation and others that target specific mRNAs for degradation.

ACTIVE LEARNING

1. Which commonly used antibiotics are directed at inhibition of bacterial RNA polymerase but do not affect the mammalian complex? Why are these drugs less effective against fungal infections?

2. Review the pathogenesis of systemic lupus erythematosus, an autoimmune disease in which antibodies to ribonucleoprotein particles are implicated in the development of chronic inflammation.

3. Review the pathogenesis of the thalassemias, with emphasis on those variants in which gene mutations affect the synthesis, processing and splicing of the RNA for hemoglobin, leading to anemia.

Summary

The major products of transcription are the rRNAs, tRNAs, and the mRNAs. These RNAs perform specific functions within a cell. mRNAs carry the genetic information from nuclear DNA to ribosomes for protein synthesis. rRNAs interact with proteins to form ribosomes, the basic cellular machinery on which protein

Further reading

Akusjarvi G, Stevenin J. Remodeling of the host cell RNA splicing machinery during an adenovirus infection. *Curr Top Microbiol Immunol* 2003; **272**: 253–286.

Eisenberg I, Eran A, Nishino I et al. Distinctive patterns of microRNA expression in primary muscular disorders. *Proc Natl Acad Sci USA* 2007; **104**: 17016–17021.

Herman T, Westhof E. RNA as a drug target: chemical, modeling, and evolutionary tools. *Curr Opin Biotechnol* 1998; **9**: 66–73.

Jarad G, Simske JS, Sedor JR, Schelling JR. Nucleic acid-based techniques for post-transcriptional regulation of molecular targets. *Curr Opin Nephrol Hypertens* 2003; **12**: 415–421.

Jirtle RL, Weidman JR. Imprinted and more equal. *Am Scientist* 2007; **95**: 143–149.

Khan AU, Lal SK. Ribozymes: a modern tool in medicine. *J Biomed Sci* 2003; **10**: 457–467.

Raj SM, Liu F. Engineering of RNase P ribozyme for gene-targeting applications. *Gene* 2003; **313**: 59–69.

Sassone-Corsi P. Unique chromatin remodeling and transcriptional regulation in spermatogenesis. *Science* 2002; **296**: 2176–2178.

Wang G-S, Cooper TA. Splicing in disease: disruption of the splicing code and the decoding machinery. *Nature Rev Genet* 2007; **8**: 749–761.

Websites

RNA polymerase: www.rcsb.org/pdb/molecules/pdb40_1.html

Spliceosome:

- www.neuro.wustl.edu/neuromuscular/pathol/spliceosome.htm
- en.wikipedia.org/wiki/Spliceosome

Ribozyme: www.ribozyme.no/; highveld.com/pages/ribozyme.html

Thalassemia: www.cooleysanemia.org/; www.vgvh.org/tha//whatisit.htm

Eukaryotic transcription: nobelprize.org/nobel_prizes/chemistry/laureates/2006/chemadv06.pdf

RNAi:

- www.pbs.org/wgbh/nova/sciencenow/3210/02-cure.html
- nobelprize.org/nobel_prizes/medicine/laureates/2006/index.html

33. Protein Synthesis and Turnover

J R Patton and G A Bannon

LEARNING OBJECTIVES

After reading this chapter you should be able to:

- Describe how various RNAs involved in protein synthesis interact to produce a polypeptide.
- Outline the structure and redundancy of the genetic code.
- Explain how proteins are targeted to specific subcellular organelles.
- Describe the major steps in synthesis and degradation of a cytosolic protein.

INTRODUCTION

Protein synthesis or translation represents the culmination of the transfer of genetic information, stored as nucleotide bases in deoxyribonucleic acid (DNA), to protein molecules that are the major structural and functional components of living cells. It is during translation that this information, expressed as a specific nucleotide sequence in a ribonucleic acid (RNA) molecule, is used to direct the synthesis of a protein. The protein then folds into a three-dimensional structure that is defined, in large part, by its amino acid sequence. In order to translate an mRNA into protein, three main RNA components are necessary:

- ribosomes, containing ribosomal RNA (rRNA)
- messenger RNA (mRNA)
- transfer RNA (tRNA).

The ribosome, composed of rRNAs and a number of proteins, is a macromolecular machine on which all protein synthesis occurs. The information required to direct the synthesis of the primary sequence of the protein is contained in mRNA. The amino acids that are to be incorporated into the protein are attached to tRNAs. The ribosome interacts with the tRNA molecules and mRNA so that the correct amino acid is incorporated into the protein. The translation of mRNA begins near the 5′ end of the template and moves towards the 3′ end, and proteins are synthesized starting with their amino-terminal ends. Therefore, the 5′ end of the RNA encodes the amino-terminal end of the protein and the 3′ end of the RNA encodes the carboxyl-terminal end of the protein.

This chapter begins with an introduction to the genetic code and the components needed for protein synthesis. This is followed by presentation of the structure and function of the ribosome, detailing the process of translation by outlining the initiation, elongation, and termination of protein synthesis, and the mechanism by which proteins are targeted to specific locations in the cell. Following a discussion of posttranslational modifications of proteins, the chapter ends with description of the role of a second macromolecular complex, the proteasome, in protein turnover.

THE GENETIC CODE

The code is degenerate and not quite universal

The mRNA to be used for translation has only four nucleotides: adenosine, A; cytidine, C; guanosine, G; and uridine, U, but it will encode a protein containing as many as 20 different amino acids. So there is not a one-to-one correspondence between nucleotide and amino acid sequence; instead, a series of three nucleotides in the mRNA, known as a codon, are required to specify each amino acid. When all combinations of four nucleotides are taken into account three at a time, 64 possible codons result (Table 33.1). Three of these codons (UAA, UAG, UGA) are used as signals to stop the synthesis of a protein and do not specify an amino acid. The rest specify the 20 amino acids which illustrates a feature of the genetic code known as degeneracy: more than one codon can specify a specific amino acid. For example, codons GUU, GUC, GUA, and GUG all code for the amino acid valine. Indeed, all the amino acids, with the exception of methionine (AUG) and tryptophan (UGG), have more than one codon. The codon AUG, which specifies only methionine, encodes methionine anywhere it appears in the RNA and it also marks the starting point for protein synthesis.

The genetic code as specified by the triplet nucleotides is, for the most part, the same for bacteria and humans, and is referred to as 'universal'. However, there are exceptions and some examples are found in bacteria and mitochondria. In bacteria, if the codons GUG and UUG occur at the beginning of protein synthesis, they can be read as a methionine codon. There are also minor differences in the genetic code in mitochondria; for instance, in vertebrate mitochondria there are additional codons that can encode methionine, UGA which is normally a stop codon, encodes tryptophan, and there are additional stop codons.

1st position	2nd position				3rd position
	G	**A**	**C**	**U**	
G	Gly	Glu	Ala	Val	G
	Gly	Glu	Ala	Val	A
	Gly	Asp	Ala	Val	C
	Gly	Asp	Ala	Val	U
A	Arg	Lys	Thr	Met	G
	Arg	Lys	Thr	Ile	A
	Ser	Asn	Thr	Ile	C
	Ser	Asn	Thr	Ile	U
C	Arg	Gln	Pro	Leu	G
	Arg	Gln	Pro	Leu	A
	Arg	His	Pro	Leu	C
	Arg	His	Pro	Leu	U
U	Trp	Stop	Ser	Leu	G
	Stop	Stop	Ser	Leu	A
	Cys	Tyr	Ser	Phe	C
	Cys	Tyr	Ser	Phe	U

Table 33.1 **The genetic code.** The genetic code is degenerate, meaning more than one codon can code for an amino acid, and in many cases changing the nucleotide at the third position does not change the amino acid encoded. In order to find the sequence(s) of the codons that encode a particular amino acid, one simply finds the amino acid in the table and combines the nucleotide sequence for each position. For example, methionine (Met) is encoded by the sequence AUG. To find the amino acid that matches a codon sequence, reverse this process.

 ## SICKLE CELL ANEMIA: MUTATION OF THE GENETIC CODE

Sickle cell anemia is an example of a disease in which a single nucleotide change within the coding region of the gene for the β-chain of hemoglobin A, the major form of adult hemoglobin, yields an altered protein that has impaired function (see Chapter 5). The mutation that causes this disease is a single nucleotide change in a codon that normally specifies glutamate (GAG) and which now produces a codon that specifies valine (GUG). Under conditions of low oxygen tension, this single amino acid change causes the protein to polymerize into rod-shaped structures, resulting in deformation of red blood cells and in altered flow properties of the cells in vessels and capillaries. When hemoglobin is not bound to oxygen, the conformation of the protein exposes a hydrophobic patch, allowing the mutant proteins with valine to interact more readily and form rods. This substitution of an amino acid with an acidic side chain for an amino acid with a nonpolar, hydrophobic side chain is termed a nonconservative mutation. Conservative mutations of one amino acid by another with similar physical and chemical properties may have less severe consequences, e.g. an Arg → Lys or Asp → Glu mutation.

Another aspect of the genetic code is that once synthesis has started at an AUG codon for methionine, each successive triplet from that start point will be read in register without interruption until a termination codon is encountered. Thus the 'reading frame' of the mRNA will be dictated by the start codon. Mutations that cause the addition or deletion of even single nucleotides will cause a reading frame shift, resulting in a protein with a different (nonsense) amino acid sequence after the mutation or a protein that is prematurely terminated if a stop codon is now in frame (Table 33.2).

THE MACHINERY OF PROTEIN SYNTHESIS

Ribosomes, the molecular machines that conduct protein synthesis, consist of a small and a large subunit that, when associated with each other, possess three specific sites at which tRNAs bind. These sites are known as the aminoacyl-tRNA, or A site, the peptidyl-tRNA, or P site, and the exit site, or E

Description of change in gene sequence	mRNA sequence	Protein sequence	Result of change
Normal gene	AUG GGG AAU CUA UCA CCU GAU ...	Met-Gly-Asn-Leu-Ser-Pro-Asp-...	Normal protein
Insertion	AUG GG**C** GAA UCU AUC ACC UGA U ...	Met-Gly-Glu-Ser-Ile-Thr-Stop	Premature stop
Deletion	AUG GGG AAU CUA UC: C CUG AUC ...	Met-Gly-Asn-Leu-Ser-Leu-Ile-...	Different sequence
Deletion	AUG GGA A: UC UAA UAC CUG AUC ...	Met-Gly-Ile-Stop	Premature stop
Substitution	AUG GGG AAU CUA **CG**A CCU GAU ...	Met-Gly-Asn-Leu-Arg-Pro-Asp-...	Substitution
Substitution	AUG GGG AAU CU**G** UCA CCU GAU ...	Met-Gly-Asn-Leu-Ser-Pro-Asp-...	No change (silent)
Substitution	AUG GGG AAU CUA U**G**A CCU GAU ...	Met-Gly-Asn-Leu-Stop	Premature stop

Table 33.2 **Effect of single base mutations.** Mutations in a gene are transcribed into the mRNA and the resulting changes in the protein sequence are shown. Note that, depending on the position of the mutation, single nucleotide substitutions can result in silent changes, a change in a single amino acid (missense) or even premature termination (nonsense).

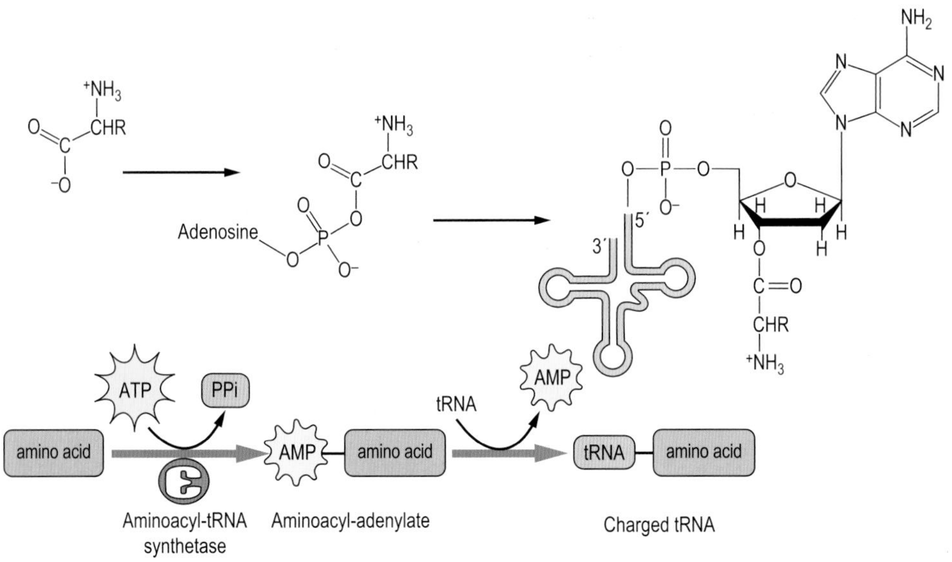

Fig. 33.1 **Activation of an amino acid and attachment to its cognate tRNA.** The amino acid must be activated by an aminoacyl-tRNA synthetase to form an aminoacyl-adenylate intermediate, before its attachment to the 3′ end of the tRNA. AMP, adenosine monophosphate; PPi, inorganic pyrophosphate.

site. The A site is where a donor tRNA molecule, carrying the appropriate amino acid on its acceptor stem, is positioned before that amino acid is incorporated into the protein. The P site is the location in the ribosome that contains a tRNA molecule with the amino-terminal polypeptide of the newly synthesized protein still attached to its acceptor stem. It is within these sites that the process of peptide bond formation takes place. This process is catalyzed by a peptidyl transferase activity, which forms the peptide bond between the amino group of the amino acid in the A site and the carboxyl terminus of the nascent peptide attached to the tRNA in the P site. The E site is where the deacylated tRNA moves once the peptide bond is formed and it will soon be exiting the ribosome. The E site, which provides a third site of interaction between tRNA and mRNA on the ribosomes, appears to be essential for maintaining the reading frame and assuring the fidelity of translation.

- A site – donor tRNA-amino acid
- P site – tRNA-growing peptide chain
- E site – site occupied by tRNA from the previous donor tRNA-amino acid.

Each amino acid has a specific synthetase that attaches it to all the tRNAs that encode it

There is a distinct tRNA molecule for most of the codons represented in Table 33.1. The amino acid is attached to the acceptor stem of the tRNA by an enzyme called aminoacyl-tRNA synthetase. This enzyme catalyzes the formation of an ester bond linking the 3′ hydroxyl group of the adenosine nucleotide of the tRNA to the carboxyl group of the amino acid (Fig. 33.1). The attachment of an amino acid to a tRNA is a two-step reaction. The carboxyl group of the amino acid is first activated by reaction with adenosine triphosphate (ATP) to form an amino-acyladenylate intermediate, which

is bound to the synthetase complex. The enzymology of activation of the carboxyl group of amino acids is similar to that for activation of fatty acids by thiokinase (Chapter 16), but, rather than transfer of the acyl group to the thiol group of coenzyme A, the aminoacyl group is transferred to the 3′-hydroxyl of the tRNA. The product is described as a charged tRNA molecule. At this point it is ready to bind to the A site of the ribosome, where it will contribute its amino acid to a growing peptide chain. There is a different synthetase specific for each of the 20 amino acids in protein. This synthetase attaches the appropriate amino acid to all the tRNAs that bind that amino acid.

✳ **FIDELITY OF TRANSLATION**

Aminoacyl-tRNA synthetases have proofreading ability

To guarantee the accuracy of protein synthesis, mechanisms have evolved to ensure selection of the correct amino acid for acylation and for proofreading of already charged tRNAs. One such mechanism is found in the enzymes responsible for attaching an amino acid to the correct tRNA. The aminoacyl-tRNA synthetases have the ability not only to discriminate between amino acids before they are attached to the appropriate tRNA, but also to remove amino acids that are attached to the wrong tRNA. In addition, these enzymes must discriminate between the multitude of tRNAs and be able to pair the correct tRNA with the appropriate amino acid. These abilities exhibited by the synthetases are accomplished by a series of hydrogen bonding interactions between the enzyme and the amino acid and between the enzyme and the tRNA. These mechanisms combine to ensure the accurate transfer of information from mRNA to protein.

Some flexibility in base pairing occurs at the 3′ base of the mRNA codon

Interaction of the charged tRNA with its cognate codon is accomplished by association of the anticodon loop in tRNA with the codon in mRNA through hydrogen bonding of complementary base pairs (Fig. 33.2). The base-pairing rules are the same as those for DNA (Chapter 31), except at the third position, or 3′ base, of the codon. At this position, nonclassic base pairs can form between this nucleotide and the first, or 5′ base, of the anticodon. The so-called wobble hypothesis of codon-anticodon pairing allows a tRNA that has an anticodon that is not perfectly complementary to the mRNA codon to recognize the sequence and allow for the incorporation of the amino acid into the growing peptide chain. Thus, if a guanine residue is at the 5′ position of the anticodon, it can form a base pair with either a cytidine or a uridine residue in the 3′ position of the codon. If the modified adenosine residue, inosine, occurs at the 5′ position of the anticodon, it can form a base pair with uridine, adenosine or even cytidine at the 3′ position of the codon (Table 33.3). This would allow a tRNA with the anticodon GAG to decode the codons CUU and CUC, both of which code for leucine. The wobble provides a mechanism for dealing efficiently with the degeneracy of the genetic code since the degeneracy occurs in the third residue of the codon.

How does the ribosome know where to begin protein synthesis?

The mRNA molecule carries the information that will be used to direct the synthesis of the protein. However, not all the information carried on the mRNA is used for this purpose. Most eukaryotic mRNAs contain regions both before and after the protein coding region, called 5′ and 3′ flanking sequences or 5′ and 3′ UTRs (untranslated regions). These sequences are involved in regulating the site and rate of protein synthesis and the stability of the mRNA. Thus, the protein coding region does not start immediately at the beginning of the mRNA which raises the question of how the ribosome knows where to start synthesis. In the case of eukaryotic cells, the ribosome first binds to the 7-methylguanine 'cap' structure (Chapter 32) at the 5′ end of the mRNA, and then moves down the molecule until it encounters the first AUG codon (Fig. 33.3). This signals the ribosome to begin synthesizing the protein, beginning with a methionine residue, and to continue until it encounters one of the termination codons. On some viral and eukaryotic mRNAs, the first AUG is not used and instead, an alternative start codon is defined by an internal ribosome entry site (IRES; see Fig. 33.3).

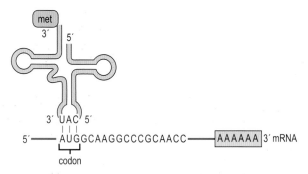

Fig. 33.2 Interaction of charged tRNA with mRNA. The interaction of a charged tRNA with an mRNA occurs by base pairing of complementary bases in the anticodon loop and the codon of the mRNA.

Prokaryotic mRNA

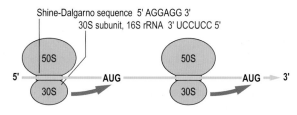

Eukaryotic mRNA

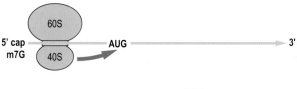

Or in some cases:

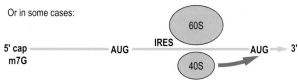

Fig. 33.3 Finding the protein-coding region. The ribosome binds to the mRNA before locating the protein-coding region. Bacterial ribosomes (a portion of 16 S rRNA) bind to complementary sequences in the mRNA that are termed Shine-Dalgarno sequences, which are a short distance from the start of the protein-coding region. Eukaryotic ribosomes bind to the 5′ cap of mRNAs and then move down the mRNA until they encounter the first AUG codon or in a few cases they bind internally at an internal ribosome entry site (IRES) and then move to the AUG.

Codon–anticodon base pairing possibilities	
Codon, third or 3′ position (mRNA)	**Anticodon, first or 5′ position (tRNA)**
G	C
U	A
A or G	U
C or U	G
A or C or U	I

Table 33.3 **Base pairing possibilities between the third position or the 3′ nucleotide of the mRNA codon and the first position or 5′ nucleotide of the tRNA anticodon.**

In the case of bacterial cells, knowing what portion of the mRNA is to be used to synthesize a protein is complicated by the fact that there can be several proteins encoded by a single mRNA, each out of register with one another, so that proteins of different sequence may be obtained from the same ribonucleotide sequence. This problem has been solved by the discovery of a sequence in the mRNA that helps to precisely position the ribosome at the beginning of each protein-coding region. This sequence, known as the Shine-Dalgarno sequence, is found in most bacterial mRNAs and is complementary to a portion of the 16 S rRNA in the small bacterial ribosomal subunit. Through the formation of hydrogen bonds the ribosome is then positioned at the start of each protein-coding region.

THE PROCESS OF PROTEIN SYNTHESIS

Translation is a dynamic process that involves the interaction of enzymes, tRNAs, ribosomes, translation factors, and mRNA in specific ways to produce a protein molecule capable of carrying out a specific cellular function. Translation is normally divided into three steps:

- initiation
- elongation
- termination.

Initiation

Initiation of protein synthesis in eukaryotes takes place when a dissociated small subunit of the ribosome forms a complex with eukaryotic initiation factors (eIF), eIF-1 A, eIF-2 and eIF-3, which binds to an eIF-2/Met-tRNA complex. This preinitiation complex is directed to the 5′ end of the mRNA by the binding of eIF-4F, and other factors, to the 5′ cap. The complex scans the mRNA until it locates the first AUG codon, using ATP to power this process. The large ribososmal subunit then binds to the small subunit/Met-tRNA/mRNA complex, and the Met-tRNA eventually is directed to the P site (Fig. 33.4), requiring eIF-5, hydrolyzing GTP and releasing initiation factors in the process. In eukaryotic cells, there are at least 12 different initiation factors. In prokaryotic cells, the process involves three initiation factors and the initiation complex first forms just 5′ to the coding region, as a result of the interaction of 16 S rRNA in small subunit with the Shine-Dalgarno sequence on the mRNA. N-Formyl methionine (fmet), encoded by AUG, is the first amino acid in all bacterial proteins, instead of methionine.

Elongation

Factors involved in the elongation stage of protein synthesis are targets of some antibiotics

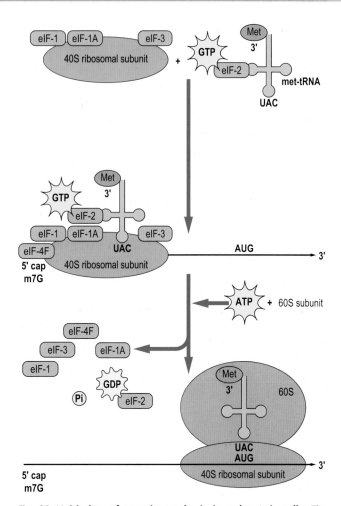

Fig. 33.4 **Initiation of protein synthesis in eukaryotic cells.** The 40S ribosomal subunit with bound initiation factors eIF-1, eIF-1A, and eIF-3, mRNA with eIF-4F bound to the 5′ cap, and met-tRNA bound to eIF-2 are brought together. Once these components are assembled, the complex translocates to the AUG (scanning and hydrolyzing ATP). The 60S ribosomal subunit completes the initiation complex and in the process the initiation factors are released. Note that, at initiation, the P site is occupied by the initiator met-tRNA. GDP, guanosine diphosphate; eIF, eukaryotic initiation factor.

After initiation is complete, the process of translating the information in mRNA into a functional protein starts. Elongation begins with the binding of a charged tRNA to the A site of the ribosome. In eukaryotic cells, the charged tRNA molecule is brought to the ribosome by the action of an elongation factor called eEF-1A (Fig. 33.5). For eEF-1A to be active, it must have a GTP molecule associated with it. If the charged tRNA is correct, one in which the anticodon of the tRNA forms base pairs with the codon on the mRNA, then GTP is hydrolyzed and eEF-1A is released. For the eEF-1A factor to bring another charged tRNA molecule to the ribosome, it must be regenerated by an elongation factor called eEF-1B which will promote the association of eEF-1A with GTP so that it may bind to another charged tRNA

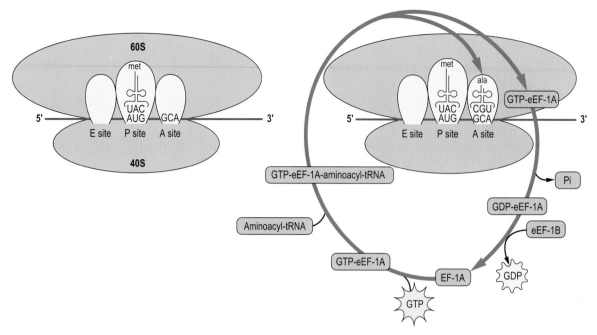

Fig. 33.5 **Recycling of elongation factor eEF-1A.** A charged tRNA molecule is brought to the A site of the initiation complex, with the aid of eEF-1A with bound GTP, to begin the process of elongation. The factor is released once GTP is hydrolyzed and the process of recycling eEF-1A is aided by the exchange factor eEF-1B. Each successive amino acid addition requires that the correctly charged tRNA molecule be brought to the A site of the ribosome. ala, alanine; Pi, inorganic phosphate.

molecule (see Fig. 33.5). Once the correct charged tRNA molecule has been delivered to the A site of the ribosome, the peptidyl transferase activity of the ribosome catalyzes the formation of a peptide bond between the amino acid in the A site and the amino acid at the end of the growing peptide chain in the P site. The tRNA-peptide chain is now transiently bound to the A site. The ribosome is then moved one codon down the mRNA (towards the 3′ end), with the help of a factor known as eEF-2, and the tRNA in the A site, with the nascent peptide chain attached, moves to the P site. The uncharged tRNA originally in the P site moves to the E site so that there is a total of nine nucleotide pairs involved in stabilization of the ribosome-mRNA-tRNA complex. The whole process recycles for addition of the next amino acid (Fig. 33.6). This complex process is identical in prokaryotic cells but the factors are different and this helps to explain the utility of antibiotics that preferentially inhibit protein synthesis in bacteria (Table 33.4).

Termination

Termination of protein synthesis in both eukaryotic and bacterial cells is accomplished when the A site of the ribosome reaches one of the stop codons of the mRNA. Protein factors called releasing factors recognize these codons, and cause the protein that is attached to the last tRNA molecule in the P site to be released (Fig. 33.7). This process is an energy-dependent reaction catalyzed by the hydrolysis of GTP, which transfers a water molecule to the end of the protein, thus

 A NONCOMPLIANT PATIENT WHO WAS PRESCRIBED AN ANTIBIOTIC

A young man you were treating for a sinus infection returns to your clinic after 1 week, still complaining of sinus headaches and stuffiness. He explains that he began to feel better about 3 days after starting to take the antibiotic tetracycline, which you had prescribed. You inquire whether he continued to take the full dose of the drug, even after he began to feel better. He reluctantly admits that, as soon as he felt better, he stopped taking the drug. How do you explain to your patient that it is important that he takes the drug for as long as you prescribed it, even if he feels better after only a few days?

Comment. As a physician, you know that tetracycline is a broad-spectrum antibiotic that inhibits the protein synthetic machinery of the bacterial cell by binding to the A site of the ribosome (Table 33.4). You also know that, if the drug is removed, protein synthesis can resume. If the drug is not taken for the entire period recommended, bacteria may begin to grow again, leading to the resurgence of the infection. Further, those bacteria that begin to grow after early termination of treatment are likely to be the most resistant to the drug. Because of the selection for more resistant mutant strains, the secondary infection is likely to be more difficult to control.

releasing it from the tRNA. After release of the newly synthesized protein, the ribosomal subunits, tRNA, and mRNA dissociate from each other, setting the stage for the translation of another mRNA (see Fig. 33.4).

PROTEIN SYNTHESIS: PEPTIDYL TRANSFERASE

Peptidyl transferase is not your typical enzyme. It is a ribozyme.

Peptidyl transferase is the activity responsible for peptide bond formation during protein synthesis. This enzyme activity catalyzes the reaction between the amino group of the aminoacyl-tRNA in the A site and the carboxyl carbon of the peptidyl-tRNA in the P site, forming a peptide bond from an ester bond. The activity is located in the ribosome, but none of the ribosomal proteins has the capacity to catalyze this reaction. Crystal structures of the bacterial 50S ribosome have shown that the peptidyl-transferase center is composed entirely of rRNA, and although the requirement for proteins or specific amino acids for positioning the tRNAs or in stabilizing rRNA structure cannot be excluded, the catalytic activity resides in the ribosomal RNA.

Antibiotics and their targets	
Antibiotic	**Target**
tetracycline	bacterial ribosome-A site
streptomycin	bacterial 30 S ribosome subunit
erythromycin	bacterial 50 S ribosome subunit
chloramphenicol	bacterial ribosome-peptidyl transferase
puromycin	causes premature termination
cycloheximide	eukaryotic 80 S ribosome

Table 33.4 **Antibiotics and their targets.** Cycloheximide is toxic to humans.

PROTEIN FOLDING

For a newly synthesized protein to become functionally active, it must be folded into a unique three-dimensional structure. Since there are too many random conformations that the newly synthesized proteins could possibly adopt, the proteins achieve their native structures with the help of a class of proteins called chaperones. Chaperones bind to exposed hydrophobic regions of unfolded proteins and prevent their interaction with each other by shielding the interactive surfaces. This restriction allows the newly synthesized protein to fold into the correct conformation without allowing the formation of nonspecific aggregates. The chaperones promote the correct folding of newly synthesized proteins by cycles of protein (substrate) binding and release regulated by an ATPase activity and by cofactor proteins. Heat shock proteins are a group of chaperone proteins that are expressed by cells in response to high temperature; they

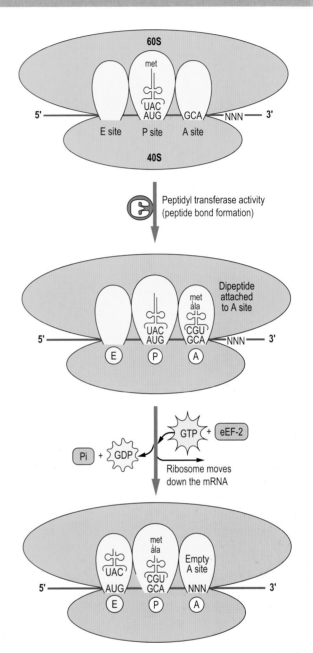

Fig. 33.6 **Peptide bond formation and translocation.** The formation of the peptide bond between each successive amino acid is catalyzed by peptidyl transferase. Once the peptide bond is formed, an elongation factor (eEF-2 in this case) will move the ribosome down one codon on the mRNA, so that the A site is vacant and ready to receive the next charged tRNA. The E-site is now occupied by the uncharged tRNA (met). NNN = codon for next amino acid.

assist in the refolding of denatured proteins, not only as a result of heat but also in response to physical and chemical stresses. The consequences of protein misfolding can be severe and there are a number of diseases that can result from faulty folding (see Chapter 2). In many cases, including some forms of cystic fibrosis (see Chapter 6) and Gaucher's disease (see Chapter 27), alterations in the amino acid sequence of a protein lead to synthesis of a misfolded protein

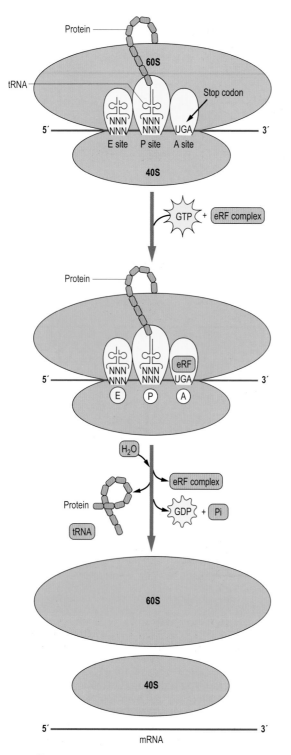

Fig. 33.7 **Termination of protein synthesis.** Termination of protein synthesis occurs when the A site is placed over a termination codon. A releasing factor complex (eRF), with eRF-1 in the A site, will cause the completed protein to be released and the ribosome, mRNA, and tRNA will dissociate from each other to begin another cycle of translation.

that is degraded in the endoplasmic reticulum or cytoplasm. Neurodegenerative disorders such as Alzheimer's have insoluble aggregates of misfolded amyloid protein in the form of plaques in the brain.

PROTEIN TARGETING AND POSTTRANSLATIONAL MODIFICATIONS

Protein targeting

An mRNA can have several bound ribosomes at one time and this is known as a polyribosome or polysome (Fig. 33.8). There are two general classes of polysomes found in cells: those that are free in the cytoplasm and those that are attached to the endoplasmic reticulum (ER). Those mRNAs encoding proteins destined for the cytoplasm or nucleus are translated primarily on polysomes free in the cytoplasm, while mRNAs encoding membrane and secreted proteins are translated on polysomes attached to the ER. Regions of the ER studded with bound ribosomes are described as the rough endoplasmic reticulum (RER).

Cellular fate of proteins is determined by their signal peptide sequences

Proteins that are destined for export, for insertion into membranes or for specific cellular organelles must in some way be distinguished from proteins that reside in the cytoplasm. The distinguishing characteristic of proteins targeted for these locations is that they contain a signal sequence usually comprising the first 20–30 amino acids on the amino-terminal end of the protein. In the case of secretory or membrane proteins, shortly after the signal sequence is synthesized, it is recognized by a ribonucleoprotein complex known as the signal recognition particle (SRP), composed of a small RNA and six proteins. The SRP binds to the signal sequence and halts translation of the remainder of the protein. This complex then binds to the SRP receptor located on the membrane of the endoplasmic reticulum. After the SRP has delivered the ribosome-bound mRNA with its nascent protein to the endoplasmic reticulum, the signal sequence is inserted through the membrane, the SRP dissociates, and translation continues with the polypeptide chain being moved, as it is synthesized, across the membrane into the interstitial space of the endoplasmic reticulum (Fig. 33.9). The protein is then transferred to the Golgi apparatus and then to its final destination.

Both mitochondrial and nucleoplasmic proteins also have signal sequences that mark them to be transported from the site of translation to their respective organelles but in contrast to secretory and membrane proteins, mitochondrial and nucleoplasmic proteins are transported after their translation is complete. In the case of proteins destined for the mitochondrion, they may have two signal sequences on their N-terminal end, depending on whether they are destined for the matrix or the intermembrane space. Mitochondrial proteins must be unfolded before they can be transported through transporters in the inner and outer membranes (TIM and TOM; see Figure 9.3). In contrast, nuclear proteins may have nuclear localization signals anywhere in the

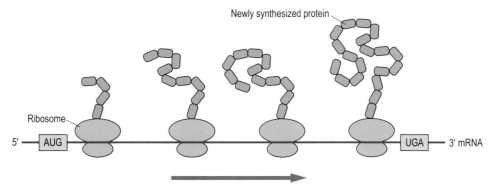

Fig. 33.8 **Protein synthesis on polysomes.** Protein can be synthesized by several ribosomes bound to the same mRNA, forming a structure known as a polysome.

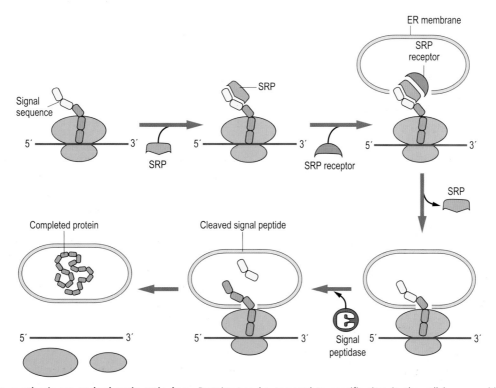

Fig. 33.9 **Protein synthesis on endoplasmic reticulum.** Proteins can be targeted to specific sites in the cell by recognition of the signal sequence by an SRP. This complex is then recognized by the SRP docking protein (SRP receptor) on the endoplasmic reticulum (ER), where the signal sequence is inserted through the membrane. A signal peptidase typically removes the signal sequence but not on every protein. Once synthesis of the protein is complete, the protein is delivered to its cellular location.

protein sequence, but exposed on the protein surface, and do not have to be unfolded before transport. Nuclear pores are very large complexes that can accommodate the recognition and transport of a protein in its native state.

Posttranslational modification

Many proteins must be altered by chemical modification of amino acids before they become biologically active; collectively, these alterations are known as posttranslational modifications. It is within the endoplasmic reticulum and

Golgi apparatus that two of the major posttranslational modifications of proteins occur. In the endoplasmic reticulum, an enzyme called signal peptidase removes the signal sequence from the amino-terminus of the protein, resulting in a mature protein that is 20–30 amino acids shorter than that encoded by the mRNA. In the endoplasmic reticulum and Golgi apparatus, carbohydrate side chains are added and modified at specific sites on the protein (Chapter 26). One of the common amino-terminal modifications of eukaryotic cells is the removal of the amino-terminal methionine residue that initiates protein synthesis. Finally, many proteins, e.g. the hormones insulin and glucagon, are synthesized as preproteins and proproteins that must be proteolytically cleaved for them to be active. The cleavage of a precursor to its biologically active form is usually accomplished by a specific protease, and is a regulated cellular event.

Proteasomes: cellular machinery for protein turnover

Protein degradation is a complex process that is critical to cellular regulation. In general, unlike DNA, damaged proteins are not repaired but degraded, and the amino acids are recycled. There are a number of reasons why a protein would need to be degraded. The protein is just worn out – it has aged passively by gradual denaturation during normal environmental stress. Proteins might also be modified by reaction with reactive intracellular compounds, such as glycolytic intermediates, or by reaction with products of lipid peroxidation during oxidative stress (Chapter 37). Other proteins might be part of cellular responses to hormones or perhaps are components of the cell cycle or are transcription factors; they need to be removed, sometimes rapidly, to attenuate the response or signal. Some of these latter proteins have characteristic amino acid sequences or N-terminal residues that promote their rapid turnover. The PEST (ProGluSerThr) sequence marks some proteins for rapid turnover, while proteins with N-terminal arginine generally have short half-lives, compared to proteins with N-terminal methionine.

Since protein degradation is a destructive process, it must be sequestered within specific cellular organelles. Lysosomes, for example, ingest and degrade damaged mitochondria and other membranous organelles. However, most soluble, cytoplasmic proteins are degraded in structures called proteasomes. The 26 S proteasome (Fig. 33.10) consists of two types of subunits: a 20 S multimeric, multicatalytic protease (MCP) and a 19 S ATPase. The proteasome is a barrel-shaped structure, formed by a stack of four rings of seven homologous monomers, α-type subunits in the outer ends and β-type subunits on the inner rings of the barrel. The proteolytic activity – three different types of threonine proteases – resides on β-subunits with active sites facing the inside of the barrel, thereby protecting cytoplasmic proteins from inappropriate degradation. The ATPase subunits are attached at either end of the barrel and act as gatekeepers, allowing only proteins destined for destruction to enter the barrel. The proteins are unfolded in a process that requires ATP and degraded by the protease activities to small peptides, 6–9 amino acids in length, that are released into the cytoplasm for further degradation.

Proteins destined for destruction are directed to the proteasome primarily by covalent modification with a very highly conserved, 76-amino acid residue protein called ubiquitin, which is found in all cells. Ubiquitin must be activated to fulfill its role (see Fig. 33.10); this is accomplished by a

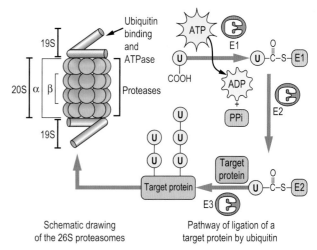

Schematic drawing of the 26S proteasomes

Pathway of ligation of a target protein by ubiquitin

Fig. 33.10 **Structure of the proteasome and the role of ubiquitin (u) in protein turnover.** The proteasome is shown at the left, a barrel-shaped structure. The 20 S multicatalytic protease in the middle rings of the barrel has protease activity on the inner face. The 19 S caps at the end of the barrel have ubiquitin binding and release and ATPase activity, and control access of proteins to the inside of the barrel for degradation. The ubiquitin cycle is involved in marking proteins for degradation by the proteasome. Ubiquitin is first activated as a thioester derivative of ubiquitin-activating enzyme E1; it is then transferred to ubiquitin-conjugating enzyme E2, then to a lysine residue on the target protein, catalyzed by ubiquitin-ligase E3. Ubiquitin is frequently copolymerized on target proteins. The more highly ubiquinated the protein, the more susceptible it is to proteasomal degradation. Note that the drawing is not to scale; the proteasome is a 26 S macromolecular complex (>2 000 000 Da); target proteins are smaller while ubiquitin molecular weight is less than 10 000 Da. (compare Chapter 29, p. 394).

✳ INHIBITING THE PROTEASOME TO TREAT CANCER

Multiple myeloma is a cancer of plasma cells (B lymphocytes), which are normally found in bone and synthesize antibodies as part of the immune system (see Chapter 2). The unchecked growth of these plasma cells results in anemia, tumors in the bones, a compromised immune response, and unfortunately usually a poor prognosis. Patients with recurring multiple myeloma have few treatment options, but a new drug that is an inhibitor of protease activity in the proteasome, bortezomib, has been added to the arsenal. It has been shown to improve the chances for survival of these patients and increase the length of time before remission, especially when combined with other therapies such as radiation or additional chemotherapy. Bortezomib appears to work by inhibiting the degradation of proteins involved in programmed cell death (apoptosis) of cancer cells, thereby enhancing the self-destruct signal in myeloma cells.

ubiquitin-activating enzyme called E1. Activation occurs when E1 is attached via a thioester bond to the C-terminus of ubiquitin by ATP-driven formation of an ubiquitin-adenylate intermediate. The activated ubiquitin is then attached to a ubiquitin carrier protein, known as E2, by a thioester linkage. A ubiquitin protein ligase known as E3 transfers the ubiquitin from E2 to a target protein, forming an isopeptide bond between the carboxyl terminus of ubiquitin and the ε-amino group of a lysine residue on a target protein. Denatured and oxidized proteins are commonly ubiquitinated by this mechanism. The 19 S subunit of the proteasome has a ubiquitin-binding site that allows proteins with a covalently attached ubiquitin protein to enter the barrel; the ubiquitin is then released by a ubiquitinase activity and recycled to the cytosol for reuse. Polymerization of ubiquitin on target proteins (poly-ubiquitination) significantly enhances the degradation of the protein.

The ubiquitin pathway leading to proteasomal degradation of proteins is complex. Although the number of E1 enzymes is typically small, there are several E2 and E3 proteins with different target specificities, and there are six different ATPase activities associated with the 19 S proteasome subunit. The ATPases are thought to be involved in denaturation of ubiquinated proteins. These variations, as well as changes during the cell cycle and in response to hormonal stimulation, provide a flexible and regulated pathway for protein turnover.

Summary

Protein synthesis is the culmination of the transfer of genetic information from DNA to proteins. In this transfer, information must be translated from the four-nucleotide language of DNA and RNA to the 20-amino acid language of proteins. The genetic code, in which three nucleotides in mRNA (codon) specify an amino acid, represents the translation dictionary of the two languages. The tRNA molecule is the bridge between these two languages. The tRNA accomplishes this task by virtue of its anticodon loop which interacts with specific codons on the mRNA and also with amino acids via its amino acid attachment site located on the 3′ end of the molecule. The process of translation consists of three parts: initiation, elongation, and termination. Initiation involves the assembly of the ribosome and charged tRNA at the initiation codon (AUG) of the mRNA. This assembly process is mediated by initiation factors and requires the expenditure of energy in the form of GTP. Elongation is a stepwise addition of the ribosome individual amino acids to a growing peptide chain by the action of the ribozyme, peptidyl transferase. The charged tRNA molecules are brought to the ribosome by elongation factors at the expense of GTP hydrolysis. Termination of protein synthesis occurs when the ribosome reaches a stop codon and releasing factors catalyze the release of a protein. After release, the newly synthesized protein must be correctly folded with the help of ancillary proteins called chaperones. Many newly synthesized proteins must also be modified, by a variety of chemical and structural changes, before they are biologically active. Once a protein is no longer needed, it is degraded intracellularly in an equally intricate, macromolecular complex called the proteasome.

ACTIVE LEARNING

1. Review the mechanism of action of various drugs that inhibit protein synthesis on the bacterial ribosome.
2. List the mechanisms that assure the fidelity of DNA and protein synthesis.
3. Describe the signal sequences that target proteins to the lysosome, the mitochondria or the nucleus.
4. Discuss the role of the N-terminal amino acid as a factor regulating the rate of turnover of a cytoplasmic protein.
5. Explain how viruses take control of the cellular protein translation machinery during viral infections to favor the synthesis of viral proteins.

Further reading

Anderson RM, Kwon M, Strobel SA. Toward ribosomal RNA catalytic activity in the absence of protein. *J Mol Evol* 2007; **64**:472–483.

Egea PF, Stroud RM, Walter P. Targeting proteins to membranes: structure of the signal recognition particle. *Curr Opin Struct Biol* 2005; **15**:213–220.

Noller H. RNA structure: reading the ribosome. *Science* 2005; **309**:1508–1514.

Ogle JM, Carter AP, Ranakrishnan V. Insights into the decoding mechanism from recent ribosome structures. *Trends Biochem Sci* 2003; **28**:259–266.

Outeiro TF, Tetzlaff J. Mechansims of disease II: cellular protein quality control. *Semin Pediatr Neurol* 2007; **14**:15–25.

Perkins ND. Post-translational modifications regulating the activity and function of the nuclear factor kappa B pathway. *Oncogene* 2006; **25**:6717–6730.

Rodnina MV, Beringer M, Wintermeyer W. How ribosomes make peptide bonds. *Trends Biochem Sci* 2006; **32**:20–26.

Websites

Genetic code: www.ncbi.nlm.nih.gov/Taxonomy/Utils/wprintgc.cgi?mode = c
tRNA database: http://lowelab.ucsc.edu/GtRNAdb/
IRES: www.iresite.org
Ribosome:
■ www.mrc-lmb.cam.ac.uk/ribo/homepage/mov_and_overview.html
■ www.weizmann.ac.il/sb/faculty_pages/Yonath/home.html
Proteasome:
■ http://users.rcn.com/jkimball.ma.ultranet/BiologyPages/P/Proteasome.html
Ubiquitin: www.rcsb.org/pdb/static.do?p = education_discussion/molecule_of_the_month/pdb60_1.html

34. Regulation of Gene Expression

J R Patton, D M Hunt and A Jamieson

LEARNING OBJECTIVES

After reading this chapter you should be able to:

■ Describe the general mechanisms of regulation of gene expression, with an emphasis on initiation of transcription.

■ Describe the many levels at which gene expression may be controlled, using steroid-induced gene expression as a model.

■ Explain how alternative mRNA splicing, alternate promoters for the start of mRNA synthesis, posttranscriptional editing of the mRNA, and the inhibition of protein synthesis by small RNAs can modulate expression of a gene.

■ Explain how the structure and packaging of chromatin can affect gene expression.

■ Explain how genomic imprinting affects gene expression, depending on whether alleles are maternally or paternally inherited.

INTRODUCTION

The study of genes and the mechanism whereby the information they hold is converted into proteins and enzymes, hormones, and intracellular signaling molecules is the realm of molecular biology. One of the most fascinating aspects of this work is the study of the mechanisms that control gene expression, both in time and in place, and the consequences if these control mechanisms are disrupted.

The goal of this chapter is to introduce the basic concepts involved in regulation of protein-coding genes and how these processes are involved in the causation of human disease. The basic mechanism of gene regulation will be described first, followed by a discussion of a specific gene regulation system to highlight various aspects of the basic mechanism. The chapter will end with a discussion of various ways in which the gene regulatory apparatus can be adapted to suit the needs of different tissues and situations.

BASIC MECHANISMS OF GENE EXPRESSION

Gene expression encompasses several different processes

The control of gene expression in humans occurs principally at the level of transcription, the synthesis of mRNA. However, transcription is just the first step in the conversion of the genetic information encoded by a gene into the final processed gene product, and it has become increasingly clear that posttranscriptional events allow for exquisite control of gene expression. The sequence of events involved in the ultimate expression of a particular gene may be summarized as:

> initiation of transcription
> →processing the transcript
> →transport to cytoplasm
> →translation of transcript into protein
> →posttranslational processing of the protein

At each of these steps conditions allow for the cell to either proceed to the next step or attenuate or halt the process. For instance, if the processing of the RNA is not correct or complete, the resulting mRNA would be useless or possibly destroyed. In addition, if the mRNA is not transported out of the nucleus, it will not be translated. Clearly, during the growth of a human embryo from a single fertilized ovum to a newborn infant, there must be numerous changes in the regulation of genes, to allow the differentiation of a single cell into many types of cells that develop tissue-specific characteristics. Similarly, at puberty there are changes in the secretion of pituitary hormones that result in the cyclic secretion of ovarian and adrenal hormones in females and the production of secondary sexual characteristics. Such programmed events are common in all cellular organisms and the production of these phenotypic changes in cells – and thus the whole organism – arises as a result of changes in the expression of key genes. The expression of genes essential for these processes varies depending on the cell type and the stage of development, but the mechanisms underlying the changes are available to basically all cells. In humans and most other eukaryotes, mechanisms that regulate gene expression are numerous; some of the requirements and options available at each stage are outlined in Table 34.1.

Regulation of gene expression		
Process	**Requirements**	**Options**
Transcription of mRNA	chromatin is relaxed (condensed chromatin is a poor template)	allele-specific transcription
	DNA in hypomethylated state (methylation of promoter inhibits transcription)	selection of alternative promoters giving different start sites
	correct trans-acting factors are present (such as transcription factors and cofactors)	
Processing of mRNA	mRNA is 5′ capped	alternative poly-A sites change the 3′ end of the mRNA
	poly-A is added to 3′ end of most messages	many transcripts are alternatively spliced, increasing coding potential
	for most mRNAs the transcript is spliced	mRNAs can be edited to change the coding sequence, changing an amino acid or creating a stop codon
		signals in the 3′ UTR of mRNAs can stabilize or mark the RNA for destruction
Translation of mRNA	mRNA must be transported to cytoplasm	mRNA can be localized in specific regions of the cytoplasm, such as the ends of axons, for local translation
	all the factors needed for protein synthesis	alternative start codons due to IRES
		translation on free ribosomes or ER
		miRNAs can inhibit translation
Turnover of proteins	unique protein half-life	structural proteins tend to turn over slowly (proteins in muscle)
		cell cycle proteins are quickly turned over to limit mitosis
		proteins that contain sequences that target them for ubiquitination

Table 34.1 **Requirements and options in the control of gene expression.**

Gene transcription requires key elements to be present in the region of the gene

The key step in the transcription of a protein-coding gene is the conversion of the information held within the DNA of the gene into messenger RNA, which can then be used as a template for synthesis of the protein product of the gene. For expression of a gene to take place, the enzyme that catalyzes the formation of mRNA, RNA polymerase II (RNAPol II), must be able to recognize the so-called startpoint for transcription of the gene. RNAPol II uses one strand of the DNA template to create a new, complementary RNA (often called the primary transcript or pre-mRNA), which is then modified in various ways, (commonly including the addition of a m^7GPPP cap at the 5′ end and the polyA tail at the 3′ end, and the removal of introns to form a mature mRNA (Chapter 32). However, RNAPol II cannot initiate transcription alone; it requires other factors to assist in the recognition of critical gene sequences and other proteins to be bound in the vicinity of the startpoint for transcription.

Promoters

Sequences that are relatively close to the start of transcription of a gene and control its expression are collectively known as the promoter. Since this is usually within a few hundred or a few thousand nucleotides of the startpoint, it is usually referred to as the proximal promoter. The promoter sequence acts as a basic recognition unit, signaling that there is a gene that can be transcribed and providing the information needed for the RNAPol II to recognize the gene and to correctly initiate RNA synthesis, both at the right place and using the correct strand of DNA as template. The promoter also plays an important role in determining that the RNA is synthesized at the right time in the right cell. Most control regions in the promoter are upstream (5′) of the transcription startpoint, and therefore are not transcribed into RNA. Occasionally, some elements of the promoter may be downstream of the startpoint for RNA synthesis, and may actually be transcribed into RNA. The

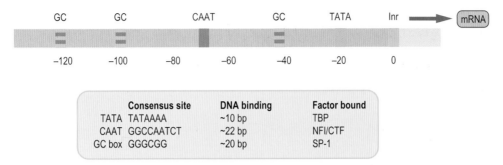

	Consensus site	DNA binding	Factor bound
TATA	TATAAAA	~10 bp	TBP
CAAT	GGCCAATCT	~22 bp	NFI/CTF
GC box	GGGCGG	~20 bp	SP-1

Fig. 34.1 **Idealized version of a promoter comprising various elements**. Each promoter element has a specific consensus sequence that binds ubiquitous transcription-activating factors. Binding of transcription factors encompasses the consensus site and a variable number of anonymous adjacent nucleotides, depending on the promoter element. CTF, a member of a protein family whose members act as transcription factors; TBP, TATA-binding protein; NFI, nuclear factor I; SP-1, ubiquitous transcription factor. Compare Figure 32.5.

structure of promoters varies from gene to gene but there are a number of key sequence elements that can be identified within the promoter. These elements may be present in different combinations, some elements being present in one gene and absent in another. Sequences further away from the transcription start site, some of which are known as enhancers, may also have a major impact on the transcription of a gene. These elements are often said to be part of the distal promoter for the gene.

The efficiency and specificity of gene expression are conferred by cis-acting elements

A promoter exerts its effect because it is on the same piece of DNA as the gene being transcribed and is referred to as a *cis*-acting sequence or element to emphasize that it affects only the neighboring gene on the same chromosome. Since the promoter is critical to gene expression, it is often regarded as being part of the gene it controls, since without it the mRNA would not be made.

The nucleotide sequence immediately surrounding the start of transcription of a gene varies from gene to gene. However, the first nucleotide in the mRNA transcript tends to be adenosine (A), usually followed by a pyrimidine-rich sequence, termed the initiator (Inr). In general, it has the nucleotide sequence Py_2CAPy_5 (Py-pyrimidine base; C-cytidine) and is found between positions -3 to $+5$ in relation to the starting point. In addition to Inr, most promoters possess a sequence known as the TATA box approximately 25 bp upstream from the start of transcription. The TATA box has an 8 bp consensus sequence that usually consists entirely of adenine-thymine (A-T) base pairs, although very rarely a guanine-cytosine (G-C) pair may be present. This sequence appears to be very important in the process of transcription, as nucleotide substitutions that disrupt the TATA box result in a marked reduction in the efficiency of transcription. The positions of Inr and the TATA box relative to the start are relatively fixed (Fig. 34.1). Having said this, it must be pointed out that there are many eukaryotic genes that do not have

an identifiable TATA box and other sequences are essential for delineating the start of transcription.

In addition to the TATA box, other commonly found *cis*-acting promoter elements have been described. For example, the CAAT box is often found upstream of the TATA box, typically about 80 bp from the start of transcription. As in the case of the TATA box, it may be more important for its ability to increase the strength of the promoter signal rather than in controlling tissue- or time-specific expression of the gene. Another commonly noted promoter element is the GC box, a GC-rich sequence; multiple copies may be found in a single promoter region.

Figure 34.1 lists some of the common *cis*-acting elements seen within promoters. These promoter elements bind protein factors (transcription factors) that recognize the DNA sequence of each particular element. Some transcription factors stimulate transcription, others suppress it; some are expressed ubiquitously, others are expressed in a tissue- or time-specific fashion. Thus the array of factors bound to a promoter region can vary from cell to cell, tissue to tissue, and be affected by the state of the organism. These factors, bound to promoter sequences, determine how actively the RNApol II copies the DNA into RNA.

Alternative promoters

Although it is clear that a promoter is essential for gene expression to occur, a single promoter may not possess the tissue specificity or developmental stage specificity to allow it to direct expression of a gene at every correct time and place. Some genes have evolved a series of promoters that confer tissue-specific expression. In addition to the use of different promoters that are physically separated, each of the alternative promoters is often associated with its own first exon and, as a result, each mRNA and subsequent protein has a tissue-specific 5′ end and amino acid sequence. A good example of the use of alternative promoters in humans is the gene for dystrophin, the muscle protein that is deficient in Duchenne muscular dystrophy (see Chapter 20). This gene uses

Identifying the function and specificity of nucleotide sequences

Consensus sequences are nucleotide sequences that contain unique core elements that identify the function and specificity of the sequence, for example the TATA box. The sequence of the element may differ by a few nucleotides in different genes but a core, or consensus, sequence is always present. In general, the differences do not influence the effectiveness of the sequence. These consensus sequences are arrived at by comparing the promoters of the same genes from different species of eukaryotes, by comparing the promoter sequences from genes that bind the same transcription factor, or by determining the actual sequence of DNA that serves as the binding element for the factor (see Fig. 34.1).

alternative promoters that give rise to brain-, muscle-, and retinal-specific proteins, all with differing N-terminal amino acid sequences.

Enhancers

Although the promoter is essential for initiation of transcription, it is not necessarily alone in influencing the strength of transcription of a particular gene. Another group of elements, known as enhancers, can regulate the level of transcription of a gene but, unlike promoters, their position may vary widely with respect to the startpoint and their orientation has no effect on their efficiency. Enhancers may lie upstream or downstream of a promoter and may be important in conferring tissue-specific transcription. For instance, a nonspecific promoter may initiate transcription only in the presence of a tissue-specific enhancer. Alternatively, a tissue-specific promoter may initiate transcription but with a greatly increased efficiency in the presence of a nearby enhancer that is not tissue specific. In some genes, for example immunoglobulin genes, enhancers may actually be present downstream of the startpoint of transcription, within an intron of the gene being actively transcribed.

Response elements

Response elements are nucleotide sequences that allow specific stimuli, such as steroid hormones (steroid response element; SRE), cyclic AMP (cyclic AMP response element; CRE) or insulin-like growth factor-1 (IGF-1, insulin response element; IRE), to stimulate or repress gene expression. Response elements are often part of promoters or enhancers where they function as binding sites for particular transcription factors. Response elements in promoters are *cis*-acting

sequences that are typically of the order of 6–12 bases in length. A single gene may possess a number of different response elements, possibly having transcription stimulated by one stimulus and inhibited by another. Multiple genes may possess the same response element, and this facilitates coinduction or corepression of groups of genes, such as in response to a hormonal stimulus.

Transcription factors

Promoters, enhancers and response elements are part of the gene; transcription factors are the proteins that recognize these structures. These sequence-specific DNA-binding proteins bind to specific nucleotide sequences and bring about differential expression of the gene during development and also within tissues of the mature organism (Fig. 34.2). Many transcription factors act positively and promote transcription, while others act negatively and promote gene silencing. The unique pattern of transcription factors present in the cell will determine in large part which portion of the genome is transcribed into RNA in any given cell. Transcription factors are sometimes referred to as '*trans*-acting' factors to emphasize that, as soluble proteins, they can diffuse within the nucleus and act on multiple different genes on different chromosomes.

There are other kinds of proteins involved in regulating transcription besides the sequence-specific transcription factors. The so-called general transcription factors, such as TFIIA, B, D, E, etc., form a complex with RNAPol II and this complex is necessary for the initiation of transcription. The general transcription factors are needed for the successful use of every promoter; they vary somewhat with the class of gene, being generally different for RNA polymerase I, II, and III. In eukaryotic cells, and mammalian cells in particular, the RNA polymerases cannot recognize promoter sequences themselves. It is the task of the gene-specific factors to create a local environment that can successfully attract the general factors, which in turn attract the polymerase itself.

In addition, other proteins can bind to the sequence-specific transcription factors and modulate their function by repressing or activating gene expression; these factors are often called coactivators or corepressors. Thus, the overall rate of RNA transcription from a gene is the result of the complex interplay of a multitude of transcription factors, coactivators and corepressors. Since there are thousands of these factors in a cell, there is an almost unimaginably large number of combinations that can occur, and thus the control of gene expression can be very specific and very subtle.

In prokaryotes, the *cis*-elements that control the start site and, in general, the initiation of transcription are placed closer to the starting point, they are fewer in number, and there is much less variety (Chapter 32). In addition, there are fewer *trans*-acting factors and the control of gene expression is much less subtle. However, understanding the limitations

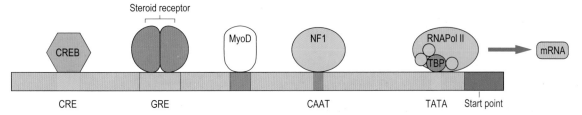

Fig. 34.2 Regulation of gene expression by specific regulatory elements. Binding of transcription factors to a steroid response element modulates the rate of transcription of the message. Different elements have varying effects on the level of transcription, some exerting greater effects than others, and may also activate tissue-specific expression. CRE, cyclic AMP response element; CREB, CRE binding protein; GRE, glucocorticoid response element; MyoD, muscle-cell-specific transcription factor; NF1, nuclear factor 1. The proteins are shown in a linear array for convenience but they interact physically with one another, both because of their size and the folding of DNA.

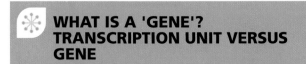

WHAT IS A 'GENE'? TRANSCRIPTION UNIT VERSUS GENE

Exactly what a 'gene' is has become increasingly difficult to define in recent years. The initial notion that a gene was a piece of DNA that gave rise to a single gene product – one gene, one protein – has been challenged. It is now clear that many functional products – different mRNA species or different protein products – may arise from a single region of transcribed DNA, as a result of differences either at the level of transcription or at the posttranscriptional level. Thus there is now a tendency to refer to such 'genes' as transcription units. The transcription unit encapsulates not only those parts of the gene such as the promoters, exons, and introns, classically regarded as the gene unit, but also the molecular elements that modify the transcription process from the initiation of transcription to the final posttranscriptional modifications. This is a shift away from the notion of a gene being one strand of DNA with exons and introns, to one of a gene being a complex structure that directs a dynamic process, giving rise to the final gene product or products at various stages of development of an organism.

of the control of gene expression in prokaryotes allows one to appreciate the flexibility of the strategies for control found in eukaryotes.

Initiation of transcription requires binding of transcription factors to DNA

For transcription to occur, transcription factors must bind to DNA. The protein known as TATA-binding protein (TBP) binds to the region of the TATA box. TBP is a general transcription factor, associated with the complex of RNAPol II and a variable number of other proteins. Binding of TBP to the TATA box directs the positioning of the transcription apparatus at a fixed distance from the startpoint of transcription and thus allows RNAPol II to be positioned exactly at the site of initiation of transcription. Once RNAPol II and a number of other transcription factors have bound to the

region of the startpoint, transcription can occur. When transcription begins, many of the transcription factors required for binding and alignment of RNAPol II are released, and the polymerase travels along the DNA, forming the pre-mRNA transcript.

Transcription factors have common structures that permit DNA binding

The binding of transcription factors to DNA involves a relatively small area of the transcription factor protein, which comes into close contact with the major and/or minor groove of the DNA double helix to be transcribed. The regions of these proteins that contact the DNA are called DNA-binding domains or motifs, and are highly conserved between species. There are a variety of DNA-binding domains, some of which occur in multiple transcription factors or multiple times in the same factor. Four common classes of DNA-binding domain are the helix-turn-helix and helix-loop-helix motifs, zinc fingers (below), and leucine zippers. Most known sequence-specific transcription factors contain at least one of these DNA-binding motifs; proteins with unknown function that contain any of these motifs are likely to be transcription factors. The average transcription factor has 20 or more sites of contact with DNA, which amplifies the strength and specificity of the contact.

In addition to a DNA-binding domain, sequence-specific transcription factors also have a transcription-regulatory domain that is required for their ability to modulate transcription. This domain may function in a variety of ways. It may interact directly with the RNA polymerase–general transcription factor complex, it may have indirect effects via coactivators or corepressor proteins, or it may be involved in remodeling the chromatin (below) and so alter the ability of the promoter to recruit other transcription factors.

One way to characterize the interaction of a transcription factor with a particular DNA sequence is to use a technique termed the electrophoretic mobility shift assay (EMSA; Fig. 34.3). This method has been used to aid in the purification of transcription factors, to identify them in complex mixtures (such as a cellular extract), to delineate the size of the binding site, and to estimate the strength of the interaction between the factor and the DNA sequence it recognizes.

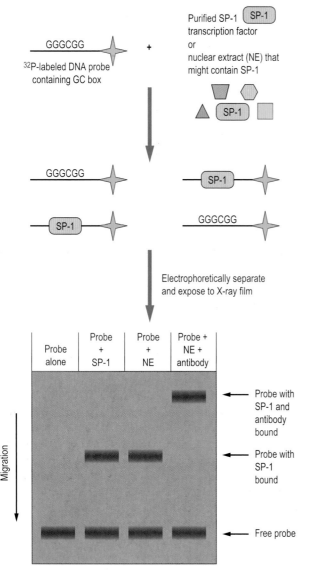

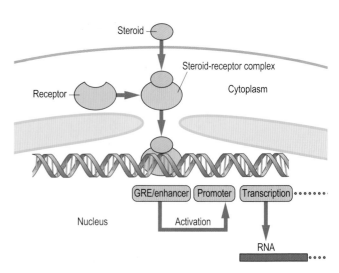

Fig. 34.4 Regulation of gene transcription by glucocorticoids. Steroids bind to receptor molecules that, in turn, bind to an enhancer, activating transcription of the gene. GRE, glucocorticoid response element.

Fig. 34.3 Electrophoretic mobility shift assay (EMSA). The basic components of the EMSA method are included in the diagram. In this example, a DNA probe that is labeled with ^{32}P is first incubated with either the purified transcription factor SP-1 or with nuclear extract (NE) that contains SP-1, and then subjected to native (nondenaturing) gel electrophoresis. If SP-1 binds to the probe it has a slower mobility in the gel than probe without protein bound (free probe). If an antibody to SP-1 is included in the reaction with NE, then the probe/SP-1 complex migrates even more slowly, confirming that the protein bound to the probe is indeed SP-1. EMSA can be used to help characterize any nucleic acid–protein interaction, including the interaction of RNA and proteins.

a common precursor, cholesterol, and thus share a similar structural backbone (Chapter 17). However, differences in hydroxylation of certain carbon atoms and aromatization of the steroid A-ring give rise to marked differences in biologic effect. Steroids bring about their biologic effects by binding to steroid-specific hormone receptors; these receptors are found in the cell cytoplasm and nucleus. For the type I (cytoplasmic) receptors, the steroid ligand induces structural changes that lead to dimerization of the receptor and exposure of a nuclear localization signal (NLS); this signal, as well as dimerization, is commonly blocked by a heat shock protein that is released on steroid binding. The ligand–receptor complex now enters the nucleus, where it binds to DNA at a specific response element, the SRE, alternatively called the hormone response element (HRE). SREs may be found many kilobases upstream or downstream of the start of transcription. The steroid–receptor complex functions as a sequence-specific transcription factor and binding of the complex to the SRE results in activation of the promoter and initiation of transcription (Fig. 34.4) or in some cases in the repression of transcription. As might be expected, because of the large number of steroids found in humans, there are correspondingly large numbers of distinct steroid receptor proteins, and each of these recognizes a consensus sequence, an SRE, in the region of a promoter.

STEROID RECEPTORS

Steroid receptors possess many characteristics of transcription factors and provide a model for the role of zinc finger proteins in DNA binding

Steroid hormones have a broad range of functions in humans and are essential to normal life. They are derived from

The zinc finger motif

Central to the recognition of the SRE in the DNA, and to the binding of the receptor to it, is the presence of the so-called zinc finger region in the DNA-binding domain of the receptor molecule. Zinc fingers consist of a peptide loop with a zinc atom at the core of the loop. In the typical zinc finger, the loop comprises two cysteine and two histidine residues

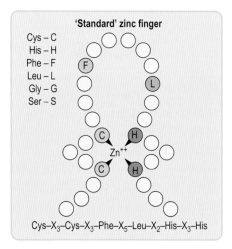
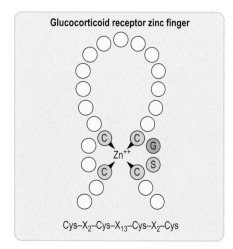

Fig. 34.5 **A 'standard' zinc finger and a steroid receptor zinc finger.** Zinc fingers are commonly occurring sequences that allow protein binding to double-stranded DNA. X, any intervening amino acid.

in highly conserved positions relative to each other, separated by a fixed number of intervening amino acids; the Cys and His residues are coordinated to the zinc ion. The zinc finger mediates the interaction between the steroid receptor molecule and the SRE in the major groove of the DNA double helix, thus enhancing the efficiency of, and conferring specificity on, the promoter. Zinc finger motifs are generally organized as a series of tandem repeat fingers; the number of repeats varies in different transcription factors. The precise structure of the steroid receptor zinc finger differs from the consensus sequence; the two are compared in Figure 34.5.

Zinc finger proteins recognize and bind to short palindromic sequences of DNA. Palindromes are DNA sequences that read the same (5′ to 3′) on the antiparallel strands, e.g. 5′-GGATCC-3′, which reads the same 5′ to 3′ sequence on the complementary strand. The dimerization of the receptor and recognition of identical sequences on opposite strands strengthen the interaction between receptor and DNA and thus enhance the specificity of SRE recognition.

Organization of the steroid receptor molecule

Steroid receptors are products of a gene family with important similarities

One central feature of all the steroid receptor proteins is the similarity in organization of their receptor molecules. Each receptor has a DNA-binding domain, a transcription-activating domain, a steroid hormone-binding domain, and a dimerization domain. There are three striking features about the structure of the steroid hormone receptors.

- The DNA-binding region always contains a highly conserved zinc finger region, which, if mutated, results in loss of function of the receptor.

- The DNA-binding regions of all the steroid hormone receptors have a high degree of homology to one another.
- The steroid-binding regions show a high degree of homology to one another.

These common features have identified the steroid receptor proteins as products of a gene family. It would appear that, during the course of evolution, diversification of organisms has resulted in the need for different steroids with varied biologic actions and, consequently, a single ancestral gene has undergone duplication and evolutionary change over millions of years, resulting in a group of related but slightly different receptors (Fig. 34.6).

STEROID RECEPTOR GENE FAMILY: THE THYROID HORMONE RECEPTORS

The steroid receptor gene family, although large, is in fact only a subset of a much larger family of so-called nuclear hormone receptors. All members of this family have the same basic structure as the steroid hormone receptors: a hypervariable *N*-terminal region, a highly conserved DNA-binding region, a variable hinge region, and a highly conserved ligand-binding domain (see Fig. 34.6). They are separated into two basic groups. Type I (cytoplasmic) receptors are a group of receptor proteins that form homodimers and bind specifically to steroid hormone response elements only in the presence of their ligand, such as the glucocorticoid receptor. Type II (nuclear) receptors form homodimers that can bind to response elements in the absence of their ligand, and may also form heterodimers with other type II receptor subunits, to form active units. The type II receptors include the thyroid hormone, vitamin D, and retinoic acid receptors.

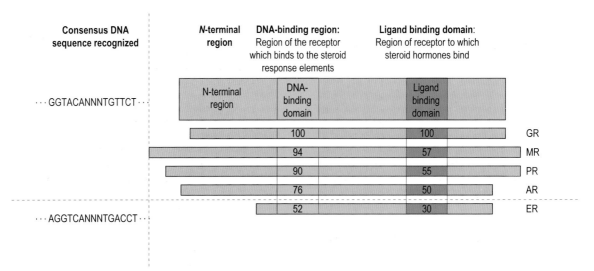

Fig. 34.6 **Similarity between different steroid receptors**. The DNA-binding and hormone-binding regions of steroid receptors share a high degree of homology. The estrogen receptor is less similar to the glucocorticoid receptor than are the others. AR, androgen receptor; ER, estrogen receptor; GR, glucocorticoid receptor; MR, mineralocorticoid receptor; PR, progesterone receptor; NNN, any three nucleotides. Numbers denote % homology to sequence in GR.

ALTERNATIVE APPROACHES TO GENE REGULATION IN HUMANS

Promoter access

DNA in the cell nucleus is packaged into nucleosomes and higher order structures in association with histones and other proteins (Chapter 31). Thus, the promoters of some genes may not be readily accessible to transcription factors, even if the transcription factors themselves are present in the nucleus. It has become evident that the degree of packaging of a promoter and the presence, absence or precise location of nucleosomes on a promoter can have major effects on the degree of access for both sequence-specific transcription factors and the RNAPol II complex associated with general transcription factors. Condensed chromatin, where the DNA is tightly associated with the nucleosomes, is usually not a good template for transcription and, in many cases, it is necessary for chromatin remodeling to occur before transcription proceeds.

Histone packaging, nucleosome stability and therefore the accessibility of DNA are controlled by reversible acetylation and deacetylation of lysine residues in the amino-terminal regions of the core histones, particularly histones H3 and H4. Histone acetyl transferases (HAT) transfer acetyl groups from acetyl-CoA to the amino group of lysines, neutralizing the charge on the lysine residue and weakening the strength of histone–DNA interactions, thereby permitting the relaxation of the nucleosome. Conversely, enzymes that remove the acetyl groups and promote the local condensation of chromosomes are known as histone deacetylases (HDAC).

Reversible acetylation and deacetylation of histones is important in controlling the activation of promoters. Indeed, some transcription factors or transcription coactivators have HAT activity themselves and can remodel chromatin. In the case of some promoters, binding of a transcription factor may result in repositioning of the nucleosomes the next time the DNA replicates, making the gene more likely to be transcribed after cell division. The dynamic interplay of chromatin structure, transcription factor and cofactor binding is important in determining whether a gene is transcribed and how efficiently the RNA polymerase synthesizes it.

Methylation of DNA regulates gene expression

Certain nucleotides, principally cytidine, can undergo enzymatic methylation without affecting Watson–Crick pairing. The methylated cytidine residues are almost always found associated with a guanosine, as the dinucleotide CG, and in double-stranded DNA the complementary cytidine is also methylated, giving rise to a palindromic sequence:

5′ mCpG 3′
3′ GpCm 5′

The presence of the methylated cytidine can be examined by susceptibility to restriction enzymes (Chapter 35) that cut DNA at sites containing CG groups only if the CG is unmethylated, compared to other restriction enzymes that cut whether or not the CG is methylated. In addition, a bisulfite sequencing technique that relies on the differential reactivity of methyl cytidine can be used to more precisely map the sites of methylation. Many genes in humans (about 50%) have what are called CpG islands (CPI) in the region of their promoters. Generally, these CPI have been found to be unmethylated

EPIGENETICS: NOVEL APPROACHES TO CHEMOTHERAPY

Methylation is one aspect of the study of epigenetics, a broad field which, in general, addresses heritable modifications of DNA and protein that do not alter the sequence of DNA, but have significant impact on gene expression. Hypermethylation of tumor suppressor genes is commonly observed in human cancers. Drugs that inhibit DNA methyl transferase activity are being tested as a means to reactivate these repressed genes for treatment of leukemias. Genes that negatively regulate cell growth are often repressed by deacetylation of histones, creating a more compact (untranscribable) form of chromatin. Inhibition of these genes supports the neoplastic phenotype of uncontrolled cell growth. Histone deacetylase (HDAC) inhibitors are being tested as therapeutic agents for treatment of rapidly growing cancers, such as lymphomas.

ALTERNATIVE SPLICING AND TISSUE-SPECIFIC EXPRESSION OF A GENE: A GIRL WITH A SWELLING ON THE NECK

A 17-year-old girl noticed a swelling on the left side of her neck. She was otherwise well, but her mother and maternal uncle have both had adrenal tumors removed. Blood was withdrawn and sent to the laboratory for measurement of calcitonin, which was greatly increased. Pathology of the excised thyroid mass confirmed the diagnosis of medullary carcinoma of the thyroid. This family has a genetic mutation causing the condition known as multiple endocrine neoplasia type 2A (MEN 2A). MEN 2A is an autosomal dominant cancer syndrome of high penetrance caused by a germline mutation in the RET protooncogene. About 5–10% of cancers result from germline mutations, but additional somatic mutations are required for cancer to develop.

Comment. Expression of the calcitonin gene provides an example of how different mechanisms may regulate gene expression and give rise to tissue-specific gene products that have very different activities. The calcitonin gene consists of five exons and uses two alternative polyadenylation signaling sites. In the thyroid gland, the medullary C cells produce calcitonin by using one polyadenylation signaling site associated with exon 4 to transcribe a pre-mRNA comprising exons 1–4. The associated introns are spliced out and the mRNA is translated to give calcitonin; elevated calcitonin is diagnostic for this condition. However, in neural tissue, a second poly-adenylation signaling site next to exon 5 is used. This results in a pre-mRNA comprising all five exons and their intervening introns. This larger pre-mRNA is then spliced and, in addition to all the introns, exon 4 is also spliced out, leaving an mRNA comprising exons 1–3 and 5, which is then translated into a potent vasodilator, calcitonin gene-related peptide (CGRP).

except in certain pathologic states and cancer. It has become clear that methylation is generally associated with regions of DNA that are less actively transcribing RNA. Demethylation of a promoter may be required for the initiation of transcription, and demethylation of a coding sequence of the gene may also be required for efficient transcription.

Alternative splicing of mRNA

In Chapter 32, the concept of the splicing of the initial transcript or pre-mRNA was introduced. Many pre-mRNAs can be spliced in alternative ways and this process, which affects an estimated 30–40% of human genes, may provide sufficient diversity to explain individual uniqueness, despite similarities in the gene complement of a species. Thus, by alternative splicing, a particular exon or exons may be spliced out on some but not all occasions. Since most genes have a number of exons (the average is about seven), some pre-mRNAs can eventually give rise to many different versions of the mRNA and likewise, the final protein. The proteins may differ by only a few amino acids or may have major differences and these often have different biologic roles. For example, whether an exon is deleted or not may affect where in the cell the protein is localized, whether a protein remains in the cell or is secreted, whether there are specific isoforms in skeletal versus cardiac muscle. Alternative splicing may also yield a truncated protein that can inhibit the function of the full-length protein. Alternative splicing is regulated, so that certain splice forms may only be seen in certain cells or tissues, at certain stages of development or under certain conditions. In the human brain, there is a family of cell surface adhesion proteins, the neurexins, which mediate the complex network of interactions between approximately 10^{12} neurones.

The neurexins are among the largest human genes, and hundreds, perhaps thousands, of neurexin isoforms are generated from only three genes by alternative promoters and splicing, providing for a diverse range of intercellular communications required for the development of sophisticated neural networks. The neurexins probably have an equally complex set of ligand isoforms, providing tremendous flexibility for reversible cellular interactions during the development of the central nervous system.

Editing of RNA at the posttranscriptional level

RNA editing involves the enzyme-mediated alteration of RNA before translation. This process may involve the insertion, deletion or conversion of nucleotides in the RNA molecule. Like alternative splicing, the substitution of one nucleotide for another can result in tissue-specific differences in transcripts. For example, *APOB*, the gene for human apolipoprotein B (apoB), a component of low-density lipoprotein, encodes a 14.1 kb mRNA transcript in the liver and a 4536-amino acid protein product, apoB100 (Chapter 18). However, in the small intestine, the mRNA is translated into a protein product, called apoB48, which is 2152 amino acids long (~48%

of 4536), those amino acids being identical to the first 2152 amino acids of apoB100. The difference in protein size occurs because, in the small intestine, nucleotide 6666 is 'edited' by the deamination of a single cytidine residue, converting it to a uridine residue. The resulting change, from a glutamine to a stop codon, causes premature termination, yielding apoB48 in the intestine (Fig. 34.7). In addition to this

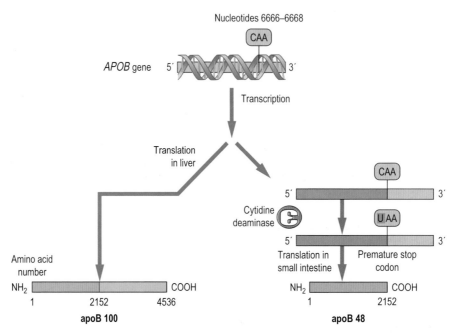

Fig. 34.7 **RNA editing of the APOB gene in man gives rise to tissue-specific transcripts.** In the small intestine, nucleotide 6666 of apoB mRNA is converted from a cytosine to uracil by the action of the enzyme cytidine deaminase. This change converts a glutamine codon in apoB100 mRNA to a premature stop codon and when the mRNA is translated the truncated product, apoB48, is produced. (See also Chapter 18.)

 IRON STATUS REGULATES TRANSLATION OF AN IRON CARRIER PROTEIN: A MAN WITH BREATHLESSNESS AND FATIGUE

A 57-year-old caucasian male presented to his family doctor with breathlessness and fatigue. He noticed that his skin had become darker. Clinical evaluation indicated cardiac failure with impaired left ventricular function as a result of dilated cardiomyopathy, a low serum concentration of testosterone and an elevated fasting concentration of glucose. Serum ferritin concentration was greatly increased, at >300 μg/L, and the diagnosis of hereditary hemochromatosis was suspected. The man was treated by regular phlebotomy until his serum ferritin was <20 μg/L, at which point the phlebotomy interval was increased to maintain the serum ferritin concentration at <50 μg/L.

Comment. In conditions of iron excess, for example in hemochromatosis, there is an increase in the synthesis of ferritin, an iron-binding and storage protein. Conversely, in conditions of iron deficiency, there is an increase in the synthesis of the transferrin receptor protein, which is involved in the uptake of iron. In both cases, the RNA molecules themselves are unchanged, and there is no change in the synthesis of the respective mRNAs. However, both the ferritin mRNA and the transferrin receptor mRNA contain a specific sequence known as the iron-response element (IRE). A specific IRE-binding protein can bind to mRNA. In iron deficiency, the IRE-binding protein binds the ferritin mRNA, prevents translation of ferritin, and binds the transferrin receptor mRNA and prevents its degradation. Thus, in iron deficiency, ferritin concentrations are low and transferrin receptor concentrations are high. In states of iron excess, the reverse process occurs and translation of ferritin mRNA increases, whereas transferrin receptor mRNA undergoes degradation, serum ferritin concentrations are high, and transferrin receptor concentrations are low (Fig. 34.8). About 10% of the US population carry the gene for hereditary hemochromatosis, but only homozygotes are affected with the disease. See also box on p.300.

cytidine deaminase, there are other enzymes that modify other mRNAs prior to translation, such as the ADARs (*adenosine deaminases acting on RNA*). ADAR2 modifies the glutamate receptor mRNA which results in the change of a single amino acid required for the function of the receptor, and although another enzyme, ADAR1, is known to be essential in mice, its substrates are unknown.

RNA interference

RNA interference (RNAi), discussed briefly in Chapter 32, is another way to control gene expression. At the heart of RNAi are very small noncoding RNAs (ncRNAs), about 20–30 nucleotides long, a group of which are called micro RNAs (miRNAs). These are involved in the attenuation or repression of translation by binding to the 3′ UTR of an mRNA and recruiting factors that inhibit protein synthesis, or by the destruction of the mRNA by an alternative pathway. It has been shown that certain pathologic states, such as cancer, change the pattern of miRNA expression in cells, thereby changing gene expression in ways that might favor proliferation. RNAi holds great promise in the treatment of human diseases where the inhibition of the expression of a gene product or the destruction of RNA would be therapeutic, such as in viral infections or cancer.

Preferential activation of one allele of a gene

The normal complement of human chromosomes comprises 22 pairs of autosomes and two sex chromosomes. In each of the pairs of autosomes the genes are present on both chromosomes: they are biallelic. Under normal circumstances, both genes are expressed without preference being given to either allele of the gene – that is, both the paternal and maternal copies of the gene can be expressed, unless there is a mutation in one allele that prevents this from occurring.

The situation with regard to sex chromosomes is slightly different. Sex chromosomes are of two types, X and Y, the X being substantially larger than the Y. Females have two X chromosomes, whereas males have one X and one Y chromosome. A region of the Y chromosome is identical to a region of the X chromosome but the X chromosome also contains genes that have no matching partner on the Y chromosome, and some genes on the Y chromosome are specific to the Y chromosome, for example SRY, a sex-determining gene. Such genes are said to be monoallelic; they offer no choice as to which allele of the gene will be expressed.

Apart from the specific cases of sex chromosomes, there would appear to be no reason why both alleles of a gene cannot be expressed. However, in humans, genes have been identified that are biallelic but only one allele – either maternal

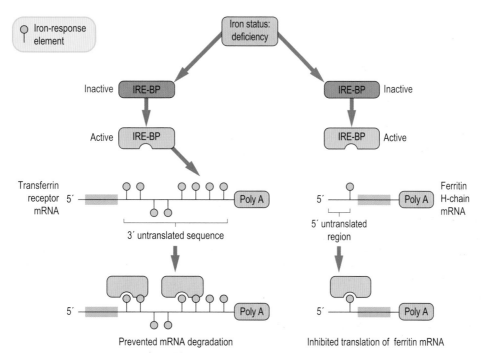

Fig. 34.8 Regulation of mRNA translation by iron status. The binding of a specific binding protein to the iron response element (IRE) of the mRNA of iron-responsive genes can alter the translation of the mRNA into functioning proteins in different ways. When iron is deficient, the iron-response element binding protein (IRE-BP) is activated and can bind to the 3′ end of the mRNA for the transferrin receptor. This prevents the degradation of the mRNA, and thus increases the amount of transferrin receptor that can be made (*left*) and thus increases the amount of iron which the receptor can deliver to the cell. However, the IRE-BP also binds to the 5′ end of the ferritin mRNA and prevents its translation (*right*). Ferritin is a protein that sequesters and stores iron in the cytoplasm, and less is needed in times of iron deficiency (compare Fig. 22.8).

Restriction of expression of biallelic genes	
Genomic imprinting	autosomal genes, imprinting may be tissue specific – monoallelic expression in some tissues, biallelic in others. Examples include insulin-like growth factor 2 (IGF-2) and Wilms' tumor susceptibility gene (WT1)
Allelic exclusion	tissue-specific production of a single allele product, for example, synthesis of a single immunoglobulin light or heavy chain in a B cell from one allele only
X chromosome inactivation	some genes on the X chromosome in females. Males exhibit only one allele of the X-linked gene but females have two, and one is inactivated by switching off nearly the entire X chromosome

Table 34.2 **Examples of types of restriction of biallelic genes in humans.** For some genes, although two alleles exist in any particular cell, only one of these alleles is active. Hence the gene behaves as if it were monoallelic although it is, in fact, biallelic.

or paternal – is preferentially expressed, despite the fact that both alleles are perfectly normal or identical. As a result, only 50% of the gene product is produced but the product is functionally active. Three different mechanisms have been identified that can restrict the expression of biallelic genes in humans (Table 34.2).

THE HUMAN GENOME PROJECT

The objectives of the International Human Genome Project included construction of a genetic map, identification of all human genes, and sequencing of the entire genome except for a few exceptionally difficult regions such as telomeres and centromeres which contain highly repetitive sequences. Working draft sequences of the human genome were presented by the International Human Genome Project collaboration and Celera Genomics in 2001. The availability of a complete reference sequence for the human genome was announced by the Human Genome Project in April 2003, just a few days prior to the 50th anniversary of the paper by Watson and Crick which first described the double helical structure of DNA. This reference sequence contains approximately 2.9 billion base pairs and represents over 90% of the approximately 3.2 billion base pairs in the human genome.

Knowledge of the human genome sequence has been important in many ways, including identification of gene changes associated with disease. It has also resulted in some surprises; for example, there appear to be fewer genes than originally anticipated. This leads to the question of why the gene number does not increase in more complex organisms by as much as might have been expected. Part of the explanation may be the frequency with which RNA transcripts undergo alternative splicing such that the same gene can give rise to different mRNAs. It has been estimated that between 30% and 40% of human genes may be able to give rise to differentially spliced mRNAs and hence to code for more than one protein per gene. In addition, complex control by hundreds of transcription factors enables cells to express huge numbers of different combinations of genes, and the subtle differences between these combinations can give rise

 X-CHROMOSOME INACTIVATION

Males have one X-chromosome whereas females have two. Thus, genes on the X-chromosome are biallelic in females but monoallelic in males. In females, however, one of the X-chromosomes in each cell is inactivated at an early stage of embryogenesis. The inactivated X may be the paternally derived or the maternally derived X-chromosome; for any particular cell, which one is inactivated is random, but the descendants of that cell will have the same X inactivated. The inactivated X-chromosome can still express a few genes, however, including XIST (inactive X–Xi-specific transcript) which codes for an RNA which plays an important role in X-chromosome inactivation. There is methylation of CpG islands on most of the genes on the inactivated chromosome and this represses transcription. The inactivated X-chromosome is reactivated during oogenesis in the female.

to enormous complexity at the cell and organism level (see Chapter 36).

Summary

The control of gene expression involves both transcriptional and posttranscriptional events that regulate the expression of a gene in both time and place and in response to numerous developmental, hormonal and stress signals. DNA sequences and DNA-binding proteins control gene expression. The DNA sequences include *cis*-acting promoters, such as the TATA box, and enhancers and response elements. The DNA-binding proteins are *trans*-acting transcription factors that bind with high specificity to these sequences, and facilitate the binding and positioning of RNAPol II for synthesis of pre-mRNA. Other factors that affect the conversion of gene to protein include access of the transcriptional apparatus to the gene, enzymatic modification of histones and nucleotides in the DNA, factors that effect alternative intron splicing, posttranscriptional editing of pre-mRNA, RNA interference, and restricted expression of biallelic genes.

ACTIVE LEARNING

1. How are steroid response elements identified in the genome? Discuss the consequences of a mutation in an SRE versus a mutation in the SRE binding protein.
2. What are the biochemical consequences of APOB gene editing in humans? Compare the effects of editing to introduce a substitution, compared to an insertion or deletion, in an mRNA molecule.
3. Some genes have promoters that have no TATA box (TATA-less genes). Without this box, what determines where the RNAPol II complex will start transcription?
4. Compare the total number of genes to the number of translated proteins that may be synthesized by the human genome. What fraction of the genes encode for transcription factors? Compare the concentration of transcription factors to the concentration of glycolytic enzymes in the cell.

Further reading

Berkhout B, Jeang KT. RISCy business: microRNAs, pathogenesis, and viruses. *J Biol Chem* 2007;**282**:26641–26645.

Brena RM, Costello JF. Genome-epigenome interactions in cancer. *Hum Mol Genet* 2007;**16**:R96–105.

Chu C-Y, Rana TM. Small RNAs: regulators and guardians of the genome. *J Cell Phys* 2007;**213**:412–419.

Collins FS, Morgan M, Patrinos A. The Human Genome Project: lessons learned from large-scale biology. *Science* 2003;**300**:286–290.

Glaser KB. HDAC inhibitors: clinical update and mechanism-based potential. *Biochem Pharmacol* 2007;**74**:659–671.

Hochheimer A, Tjian R. Diversified transcription initiation complexes expand promoter selectivity and tissue-specific gene expression. *Genes Dev* 2003;**17**:1309–1320.

International Human Genome Sequencing Consortium. Initial sequencing and analysis of the human genome. *Nature* 2001;**409**:860–921.

Li Q, Lee J-A, Black DL. Neuronal regulation of alternative pre-mRNA splicing. *Nature Rev Neurosci* 2007;**8**:819–831.

Venter JC, Adams MD, Myers EW et al. The sequence of the human genome. *Science* 2001;**291**:1304–1351.

Zhou J, Cidlowski JA. The human glucocorticoid receptor: one gene, multiple proteins and diverse responses. *Steroids* 2005;**70**:407–417.

Websites

Epigenetics: http://epigenetica.blogspot.com/
Human Genome Research Institute: www.genome.gov
Human genome resources: www.ncbi.nlm.nih.gov/genome/guide/human/
Catalog of genetic diseases: www.ncbi.nlm.nih.gov/sites/entrez?db=omim
Alternate splicing:
- http://hazelton.lbl.gov/~teplitski/alt/
- http://www.ebi.ac.uk/asd/
Non-coding RNA:
- http://biobases.ibch.poznan.pl/ncRNA/
- http://microrna.sanger.ac.uk/sequences/index.shtml
RNA editing: http://dna.kdna.ucla.edu/rna/index.aspx
RNA interference:
- www.rnaiweb.com/
- www.pbs.org/wgbh/nova/sciencenow/3210/02.html
Genomic imprinting: www.geneimprint.org/

35. Recombinant DNA Technology

W S Kistler, R G Best and A Jamieson

LEARNING OBJECTIVES

After reading this chapter you should be able to:

- Explain the chemical basis for nucleic acid hybridization, including the role of probe and target sequences in hybridization assays.
- Describe what is meant by a 'primer pair' used in the polymerase chain reaction (PCR) assay, and explain how the sequence of these primers determines the product amplified in the PCR process.
- Describe the characteristics of restriction endonucleases, including the nature of cleavage sites in DNA and the types of fragment ends produced.
- Describe the general steps used to perform a Southern blot and the type of information it provides.
- Differentiate between a cDNA and a genomic clone.
- Describe typical features of a bacterial plasmid used for cloning DNA.
- Describe the uses of hybridization and PCR technology for analysis of the human genome for forensic, genetic and diagnostic purposes.

INTRODUCTION

There are several key features to all DNA tests

Hand in hand with the development of our understanding of DNA, genes, and their functions has gone the explosion of technology for the clinical analysis of DNA and RNA. A full description of all these processes is outside the scope of this chapter, but an understanding of the basic principles of the methods and presentation of examples of some commonly used applications is essential for understanding the interpretation of DNA analysis for forensic, genetic and diagnostic services in a clinical setting. There are several key features central to all the DNA methods currently used and these will be discussed prior to outlining some of the commonly used techniques.

HYBRIDIZATION

Hybridization is based on the annealing properties of DNA

Hybridization is a fundamental feature of DNA technology. It is a process by which a piece of DNA or RNA of known nucleotide sequence, which can range in size from as little as 15 base pairs (bp) to several hundred kilobases, is used to identify a region or fragment of DNA containing complementary sequences. The first piece of DNA or RNA is called a probe. Probe DNA will form a complementary base pair with another strand of DNA, often termed the target, if the two strands are complementary and a sufficient number of hydrogen bonds is formed.

The principles of molecular hybridization

In molecular hybridization, it is essential that the probe and target are initially single-stranded

Probes can vary in both their size and their nature (Table 35.1). However, one essential feature of any hybridization reaction is that both the probe and the target must be free to base pair with one another. The process of separating the two strands of DNA is called DNA denaturation or melting. Depending on the type of hybridization reaction, probes and targets can be denatured by several different methods, for example, high temperature (80–100°C), alkaline conditions or exposure to high concentrations of urea or formamide. Once both probe and target DNA are single-stranded, mixing of the two under conditions that favor the formation of a double-stranded helix will allow complementary bases to recombine. This process is called DNA annealing or reassociation, and when a probe strand reacts with a target strand, the complex is termed a heteroduplex.

Formation of probe–target heteroduplexes is the key to the usefulness of molecular hybridization

The conditions under which DNA hybridization occurs and the reliability and specificity, or stringency, of hybridization are affected by several factors:

- **base composition:** GC pairs have three hydrogen bonds compared with the two in an AT pair. Double-stranded DNA with a high GC content is therefore more stable and has a higher meeting temperature (T_m).
- **strand length:** the longer a strand of DNA, the greater the number of hydrogen bonds between the two strands. Longer strands require higher temperatures or stronger alkali treatment to denature them; stability

Nucleic acid probes used for hybridization studies			
Probe type	**Origin**	**Probe characteristics**	**Labeling method**
DNA	cell-based DNA: cloning, polymerase chain reaction (PCR)	double-stranded cell-based: 0.1– > 100 kb PCR-based: 0.1–10 kb	random primer, nick translation
RNA	RNA transcription from phage vectors	single stranded: 1–2 kb	run-off transcription
Oligonucleotide	chemical synthesis	single-stranded: 15–50 nucleotides	end-labeling

Table 35.1 **Characteristics of some nucleic acid probes used for hybridization studies.**

varies dramatically with length for very short probes but above a few hundred base pairs, stability is relatively insensitive to length and is determined primarily by base composition.

■ **reaction conditions:** high cation concentration (typically Na^+) favors double-stranded DNA (because the negative charges on the sugar-phosphate backbone are shielded from each other), while high concentrations of urea or formamide favor single-stranded DNA (because these solutions reduce base-stacking and can compete for hydrogen bond formation). Hybridizations are said to be carried out at 'low stringency' when conditions strongly favor duplex formation, and at 'high stringency' when duplexes are only slightly more stable than single-stranded molecules.

Thus by appropriate selection of conditions (high stringency), a small 30–50 bp probe can require a perfect match to form a stable hybrid with its target. On the other hand, under low stringency a longer probe, e.g. 500 bp, might react with targets that contain multiple nucleotide mismatches (Fig. 35.1).

The stability of a nucleic acid duplex can be assessed by determining its melting temperature (T_m)

The melting temperature (T_m) is the temperature, in vitro, at which 50% of a double-stranded duplex has dissociated into single-strand form. For relatively long DNA probes, T_m is determined primarily by base composition, with AT-rich DNA melting at a lower temperature than GC-rich DNA. For humans and other mammals, the average GC content is about 40% and the melting temperature in moderate salt is about 87°C. For short oligonucleotides, such as the primers used in polymerase chain reactions (below), effects of length, composition and even the various dinucleotide sequences must be taken into consideration. This is because double-stranded DNA is stabilized by the degree of overlap by the stacked bases in successive nucleotides, and this varies depending on the specific nucleotide neighbors of a particular base. Computer programs are widely available to predict T_m values (see listing of websites at the end of the chapter).

Probes must have a label to be identified

Implicit in the use of probes to identify pieces of complementary DNA is the notion that if hybridization occurs, the heteroduplex can be specifically detected. Thus, the probe is labeled so that the probe–target duplex can be identified. There are many ways in which probes can be labeled but they fall into two categories, either isotopic, i.e. involving radioactive atoms, or nonisotopic, e.g. end-labeling probes with fluorescent tags or small ligand molecules (Table 35.2).

Many techniques involving probe hybridization and labeling still involve the use of radioisotopes such as ^{32}P, ^{35}S or ^{3}H and, as such, require a method for detecting and localizing the radioactivity. The most common method involves the process of autoradiography. Autoradiography allows information from a solid phase, e.g. a gel or fixed-tissue sample, to be detected and saved in two-dimensional form as an exposed photographic image.

Methods used for labeling nucleotide probes

Labeling of DNA or RNA probes

Both DNA and RNA can be labeled in vitro by several techniques that incorporate a labeled nucleotide (or nucleotides) into the structure of the probe. There are three general ways in which DNA can be labeled in vitro.

■ **End-labeling:** enzymatic techniques are available to add radioactive labels to the 5′ or 3′ ends of individual strands in DNA duplexes. One simple way of doing this employs polynucleotide kinase. This enzyme will transfer the terminal γ-phosphate from ATP to a free 5′ hydroxyl group at the end of a single- or double-stranded molecule. This technique, using [γ-^{32}P]dATP, is a good way to label oligonucleotides, but sensitivity is limited because only a single ^{32}P would be introduced into a long DNA strand.

■ **Polymerase-based labeling:** using a DNA polymerase, multiple labeled nucleotides are incorporated into the probe during in vitro DNA synthesis. Radioactivity

A Hybridization characteristics using a large conventional probe (>200 bases)

Match	Perfect	Single base mismatch	Multiple mismatch
Stringency	High	Intermediate	Low
Example	Human target + human probe 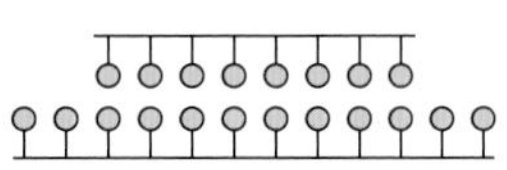	Human target + human probe with mutation 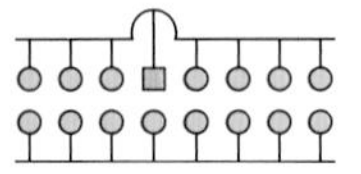	Human target + mouse probe 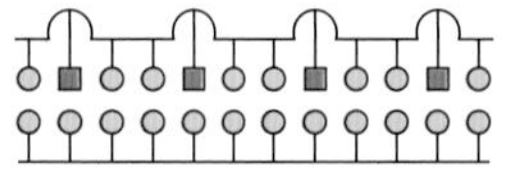
Stability	Stable	Stable	Stable

B Hybridization characteristics using a small oligonucleotide probe

Match	Perfect	Single base mismatch	
Stringency	High	High	
Example	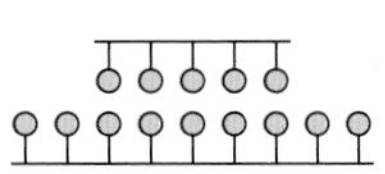	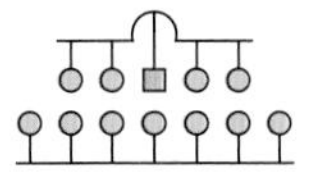	
Stability	Stable	Unstable	

Fig. 35.1 **Probe–template hybridization.** (A) Large probes, e.g. 200 bases or more, can form stable heteroduplexes with the target DNA even if there are a significant number of non-complementary bases in conditions of low stringency. (B) Oligonucleotide probes, in contrast, may discriminate between targets that differ by a single base under stringent conditions.

Labels used to prepare probes used for nucleic acid hybridization

Probe label	Characteristics	Examples
Radioactive	use radioisotopes emitting β-particles. dNTPs are incorporated into the probe DNA	^{32}P, ^{35}S
Nonradioactive	rely on the coupling of a reporter molecule to a nucleotide precursor, e.g. a dNTP. When the probe hybridizes, another protein with high affinity for the reporter group (an affinity group which has a marker group associated) binds the reporter and the bound complex can be detected	biotin and streptavidin, digoxigenin

Table 35.2 **Details of labels used to prepare probes used for nucleic acid hybridization. dNTP, deoxyribonucleoside triphosphate.**

AUTORADIOGRAPHY

For many years a commonly used imaging technique has been direct autoradiography, which involves placing the sample in immediate contact with a photographic plate, usually an X-ray film. The radioactivity of the bound probe produces a dark image on the developed film. ^{32}P is a commonly used label for nucleic acid probes because of its high specific activity. The β particle emitted is sufficiently energetic that a substantial fraction passes through ordinary film without exposing it. Therefore it is common to use the same type of intensifying screens used clinically to make film more sensitive to X-rays. Energetic β particles pass through the film but are absorbed by the intensifying screen, which then emits visible light and exposes the film.

is typically supplied as one of the four deoxynucleotide triphosphates labeled at the innermost (α) phosphate position. When a DNA fragment is heated in the presence of a mixture of oligonucleotide hexamers of random sequence, and the temperature is lowered, the hexamers will anneal at various random locations and provide starting points (primers) for elongation by a DNA polymerase. In this way, up to 25% of the nucleotides introduced will carry a radioactive tag (Fig. 35.2).

Nick translation of DNA: nick translation is an alternative technique for introducing labeled nucleotides throughout a DNA probe. In this case, a small number of single-strand breaks in the phosphodiester backbone (known as 'nicks') are introduced by an enzyme such as pancreatic DNaseI, which leaves a 3′ OH group and 5′-phosphate. If DNA polymerase I of *E. coli* is then

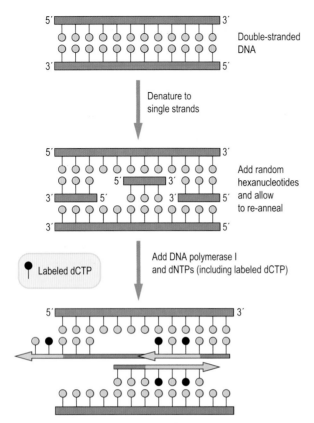

Fig. 35.2 **Random primer labeling of probe DNA.** Random hybridization of hexanucleotides to the template allows the Klenow fragment of *E. coli* DNA polymerase I to fill in the gaps, incorporating radiolabeled dCTP to create radiolabeled complementary strands of DNA.

added along with an α-^{32}P[dNTP] plus the other three unlabeled dNTPs, the enzyme will degrade the nicked DNA in the 5′ to 3′ direction, while using its polymerase activity to replace the same nucleotides in the same direction. This is possible only with DNA polymerase I because of its unique ability to both degrade double-stranded DNA in the 5′ to 3′ direction and simultaneously polymerize new nucleotides behind it in the same direction. In this manner, the original 'nick' is moved (translated) along the DNA molecule, presumably until the polymerase reaches the end of the strand.

Use of restriction enzymes to analyze genomic DNA

Southern blots are the prototype for methods that use specific hybridization probes to identify sequences in genomic DNA or in total RNA

One of the fundamental steps in the evolution of molecular biology was the discovery that DNA could be transferred from a semisolid gel onto a nitrocellulose membrane in such a way that the membrane could act as a record of the DNA information in the gel and could be used for multiple-probe experiments. The process whereby the DNA is

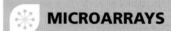 ## MICROARRAYS

Most of the methods discussed in this chapter enable one to look at one, or perhaps a few, genes at one time. However, the ability to obtain a global picture of the genes that a cell is expressing would be a major advantage. Microarray technology (Fig. 35.3) makes this possible. Depending on the intent of the study, these arrays can focus on only the expressed regions of genes (sequences that appear in mRNAs) or can include DNA targets from throughout the nonrepetitive fraction of the genome. For study of differential gene expression, thousands (or tens of thousands) of different DNAs, each corresponding to a fragment of a known gene, are spotted on a slide in an orderly array, such that the position and identity of each DNA is known. A fluorescently labeled DNA or RNA probe is then made using total RNA extracted from cells of interest. Different fluorophores can be incorporated, so that one could, for example, use a green-labeled probe derived from cancer cells and a red-labeled probe derived from normal cells from adjacent normal tissue in the same individual. The two differently colored probes are mixed together, hybridized to the DNA on the slide, and any unhybridized probe is washed away. The slide can then be scanned using an instrument that detects each probe separately at different fluorescence wavelengths. If a gene is expressed only in the tumor RNA, the spot corresponding to that gene will be green. If the gene is expressed only in the normal tissue, the spot will be red. If the gene is expressed equally in both RNAs the spot will be yellow (the sum of red and green fluorescence). The results are analyzed and the relative expression in tumor and control samples of each spot on the array can be determined. Thus, one can detect differences in the expression of a few genes (out of the thousands on the array) that correlate with a particular disease status or other condition. This is a powerful and rapid way to determine how one cell population, such as diseased cells, differs from other cells at the level of RNA expression. The same technology can be applied to analyze differences in gene expression in response to hormonal signals or environmental stresses.

Microarrays are also used to identify genomic deletions and duplications associated with developmental delays, mental retardation, structural birth defects, and contiguous gene syndromes. Genomic microarrays (which contain DNA targets distributed uniformly across chromosomes rather than only from coding regions) are useful for detecting smaller gene dosage abnormalities than can be identified with conventional karyotyping. The technique is referred to as 'molecular karyotyping' when used for this purpose. As an example, there is a remarkable amount of variation in DNA sequences between different individuals due to copy number variants (CNVs). This term describes duplications and deletions of gene-sized regions of DNA (with a median length of 100–200 kb) that have been identified in great numbers only in recent years from use of array or rapid sequencing techniques. Some of these are associated with clinically significant phenotypic effects, while others appear to be completely benign. They may account for a significant component of the genetic variation between individuals.

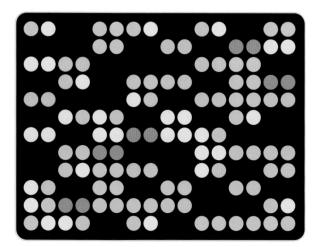

Fig. 35.3 **Microarray hybridization.** Representation of a small region of an array. The probe consisted of a mixture of green-tagged cDNA molecules derived from the mRNA of normal cells and red-tagged molecules derived from the mRNA of diseased cells. The color and brightness of the spots indicate the relative prevalence of particular mRNAs in normal as compared with diseased cells. A yellow signal indicates that a particular mRNA was equally common in both normal and diseased cells. No signal indicates genes whose expression is undetectable.

 FISHING FOR THE CAUSE OF COMPLEX PATTERNS OF BIRTH DEFECTS: THE PRADER-WILLI SYNDROME

A child is referred to her pediatrician because of poor muscle tone, developmental delay, and a nearly insatiable desire to eat (hyperphagia). The family history is negative for this unusual pattern of features. The physician orders a molecular cytogenetic test, fluorescence in situ hybridization (FISH), because of clinical suspicion of Prader-Willi syndrome (PWS), and discovers that one copy of chromosome 15 fails to hybridize to a colored probe for the small nuclear ribosomal protein N (SNRPN) gene (Chapter 31).

Comment. Microdeletions near the centromere of chromosome 15 identified in children and adults with Prader-Willi syndrome have identified the SNRPN gene to constitute a critical region for PWS. This region of chromosome 15 is imprinted (turned off) in females during gametogenesis, and therefore healthy offspring receive their only working copy from the father at conception. If the father's copy of chromosome 15 has a microdeletion that deletes SNRPN, or if both copies of chromosome are inherited from the mother, no working copy of SNRPN is expressed in the developing embryo/baby, resulting in PWS.

transferred to the membrane was first described by Ed Southern but subsequent techniques based on the transfer of RNA and proteins have also adopted the direction theme and are called Northern and Western blots, respectively (Table 35.3).

Blots used in molecular biology		
Blot	**Probe**	**Target**
Southern	Nucleotide	DNA
Northern	Nucleotide	RNA
Western	Antibody	Protein

Table 35.3 **Types of blots used in molecular biology.** Southern and Northern blots use nucleotide-based probes to hybridize to the DNA or RNA on the membrane. Western blots rely on the ability of a specific antibody to bind to a protein of interest.

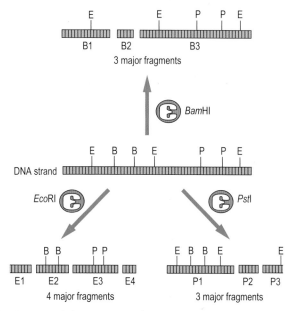

Fig. 35.4 **Restriction enzyme digestion of DNA.** Digestion of a DNA molecule by several different restriction enzymes may result in many different fragments, even though the apparent size of the fragments is similar. For example, fragments E1 and P3 are of similar size but are clearly different pieces of DNA. E, *Eco*RI site; B, *Bam*HI site; P, *Pst*I site.

Restriction enzymes are crucial in the process of performing Southern blots

Restriction endonucleases comprise a group of enzymes that cleave double-stranded DNA. These enzymes are sequence specific and each enzyme acts at a limited number of sites in DNA called 'recognition' or 'cutting' sites. Restriction endonucleases are part of the bacterial 'immune system'. Bacteria methylate their own DNA, protecting it from their own restriction enzymes, but cleave unmethylated infecting viral or bacteriophage DNAs at specific sites, thereby inactivating the virus.

If DNA is digested by a restriction enzyme, the DNA will be reduced to fragments of varying sizes depending on how many cutting sites for that restriction enzyme are present in the DNA. It is important to note that each enzyme will cut DNA into a unique set of fragments (Fig. 35.4). Many

Restriction endonucleases		
Restriction enzyme	**Restriction site**	**Ends**
*Hae*III	GG*CC CC*GG	Flush
*Msp*I	C*CGG GGC*C	Sticky
*Eco*RV	GAT*ATC CTA*TAG	Flush
*Eco*RI	G*AATTC CTTAA*G	Sticky
*Not*I	GC*GGCCGC CG CCGG*CG	Sticky

Table 35.4 **Restriction endonucleases in common use.** Enzymes can cleave DNA to produce 'flush ends' where the DNA is cut 'vertically' leaving two ends that do not have any overhanging nucleotides. However, if the DNA is cleaved 'obliquely', the DNA will have short single-stranded overhangs. Such ends are called 'sticky' because they will selectively rejoin (hybridize) to matching overhangs. The sites of cleavage of DNA by restriction enzymes are often described as *palindromic* because of their inverted repeat symmetry – they have identical sequences in opposite directions on the complementary strands.

restriction enzymes recognize sites that are typically four (e.g. *Hae*III), six (e.g. *Eco*R I) or eight nucleotides (e.g. *Not*I) in length (Table 35.4). Each enzyme recognizes its own site; variation in just one nucleotide within the recognition sequence makes a sequence completely resistant to a particular enzyme.

Southern blotting

Blotting techniques involve transfer of DNA, RNA or proteins in the semisolid phase of a gel to a solid phase that may then be used as a template for exposure to a range of molecular probes

If DNA is digested by a restriction enzyme, the resulting digest can be separated on the basis of size by gel electrophoresis. A solution of digested DNA is placed in a well in an agarose gel and an electric current applied. The rate of migration of DNA fragments depends on their size, with the smallest fragments moving furthest and the largest moving least. The size-based fractionation occurs because smaller DNA molecules can migrate more freely through the gel matrix. Medium to large DNA molecules take on random coil geometry and with increasing size have progressively greater difficulty migrating through the polysaccharide network.

Agarose gel electrophoresis is used to separate fragments ranging in size from 100 bases to approximately 20 kb

RESTRICTION ENZYME CUTTING FREQUENCY

Restriction enzymes cut DNA into fragments at sites determined by the nucleotide sequence of the DNA (Table 35.4). The frequency of the cutting sites for various different enzymes varies primarily with the length of the recognition site. Cut sites for an enzyme with a 4-base recognition site, such as *Hae*III, would occur by chance once per 256 base pair sequence. Cut sites for an enzyme with an 8-base recognition site, such as *Not*I, would occur only once in about 65 000 base pairs. Thus, frequent cutters typically generate many small fragments while rare cutters generate fewer and larger fragments. These differences can be exploited when trying to map the location of certain genes to chromosomal locations.

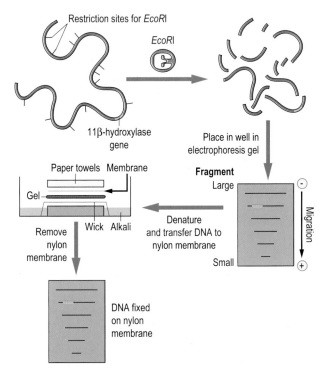

Fig. 35.5 **Southern blotting of DNA.** DNA digested with a restriction enzyme is size-fractionated by agarose electrophoresis. The agarose gel is then placed in alkali to denature the DNA. The now single-stranded DNA can pass from the gel to the nylon membrane as buffer solution flows upward by capillary action, forming a permanent record of the digested DNA.

in length (above 40 kb, resolution is minimal). Following electrophoresis, the gels are soaked in a strong alkali solution to render the DNA fragments single-stranded. These single-stranded fragments can then be transferred to a nitrocellulose or nylon membrane to which they bind readily and, if preserved properly, permanently. The process of transfer involves the passage of solute through the gel and into the

PULSED-FIELD GEL ELECTROPHORESIS

Pulsed-field gel electrophoresis (PFGE) is a technique used to separate large pieces of DNA digested by rare-cutting restriction enzymes. DNA fragments generated by rare cutters can be several hundred kilobases in size and cannot be separated by conventional agarose gel electrophoresis. Conventional gel electrophoresis uses current applied in a single dimension (see Fig. 35.5). Very large DNA fragments are thought to orient themselves so that they pass though the gel like a garden hose being drawn through a field thickly overgrown with brush. Once oriented with the voltage field, molecules of different lengths migrate at slow but similar rates. The trick to separating these large fragments is to make them change direction at regular intervals; longer DNAs take longer to orient correctly and so lag behind shorter fragments. Accordingly, in PFGE, an alternating current is applied to the gel, changing the direction of electrophoresis at intervals. The net effect of the time sequence and changes in polarity of the current is to separate large fragments by size in one dimension. Standard agarose gel electrophoresis may take 1–4h to complete, whereas PFGE often requires over 24h to complete.

filter, passively carrying the DNA and producing an image of the gel on the filter (Fig. 35.5).

DEOXYRIBONUCLEIC ACID AMPLIFICATION AND CLONING

Methods for amplification of DNA in vitro

The amplification of DNA is central to the study of molecular biology and genetics. DNA amplification makes possible an enormous increase in the number of copies of a desired DNA sequence. Two important approaches to the amplification of DNA are:

- **cell-based DNA cloning:** DNA is amplified in vivo by a cellular host such that the number of copies of the desired DNA template increases simply due to the exponential increase in number of replicating host cells
- **enzyme-based DNA cloning (cell-free):** this method is represented by the polymerase chain reaction (PCR) and involves entirely in vitro DNA amplification.

Cell-based cloning

Most cell-based cloning uses recombinant DNA in replicating bacteria; recombinant human insulin and erythropoietin are produced by this technique

Cell-based cloning is based on the ability of replicating cells, e.g. bacteria, to sustain the presence of so-called recombinant DNA within them. Recombinant DNA refers to any DNA molecule that is artificially constructed from two pieces of DNA not normally found together. One piece of DNA will be the target DNA that is to be amplified and the other will be the replicating vector or replicon, a molecule capable of initiating DNA replication in a suitable host cell.

The majority of cell-based cloning is performed using bacterial cells. In addition to the bacterial chromosome, bacteria may contain extrachromosomal double-stranded DNA that can undergo replication. One such example is the bacterial plasmid. Plasmids are circular, double-stranded DNA molecules that undergo intracellular replication and are passed vertically from the parent cell to each daughter cell. However, unlike the bacterial chromosome, plasmids used in these techniques are copied many times during each cell division. Thus, plasmids represent ideal replicons for the amplification of target DNA and methods involving the use of plasmids are widespread throughout molecular biology.

Target DNA is introduced into a replicon by using restriction enzymes to cut target and replicon DNA so that the target DNA and the linearized plasmid DNA will have complementary sticky ends (Fig. 35.6). DNA ligase then covalently joins the target to the ends of the vector to form a closed circular recombinant plasmid. Once the target DNA is incorporated into the plasmid vector, the next step is to introduce the plasmid into a host cell to allow replication to occur. The cell membrane of bacteria is selectively permeable and prevents the free passage of large molecules such as DNA in and out of the cell. However, the permeability of cells can be altered temporarily by factors such as electric currents (electroporation) and high-solute concentration (osmotic stress), so that the membrane becomes temporarily permeable and DNA can enter the cell. Such a process renders the cells competent, i.e. they can take up foreign DNA from the extracellular fluid, a process known as transformation. This process is generally inefficient, so that only a small fraction of cells may take up plasmid DNA, and often only a single plasmid per bacterium is introduced during transformation. However, it is this process of cellular uptake of plasmid DNA that forms a critical step in cell-based cloning. Individual recombinant DNAs are easily resolved from one another because they are taken up by separate cells that can be isolated simply by spreading them on an agar surface.

Following transformation, the cells are allowed to replicate, usually on a standard agar plate containing a suitable antibiotic to kill cells that do not harbor a plasmid. Colonies (clones of single cells) are then 'picked' and transferred to tubes for growth in liquid culture and a second phase of exponential increase in cell number. Thus, from a single cell and a single molecule of DNA, an extremely large number of cells containing multiple, identical recombinant plasmids can be generated in a relatively short time (Fig. 35.7). Recovery of the plasmid DNA is easy because it is a small, covalently intact circle, readily separated from the bacterial chromosomal DNA by a variety of techniques.

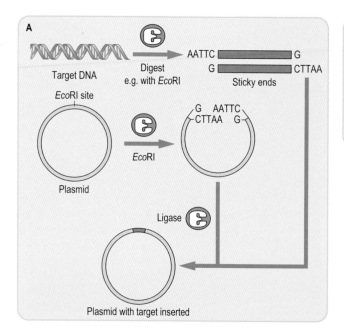
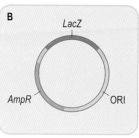

Fig. 35.6 **Formation of a plasmid containing a target gene for cloning.** (A) DNA containing the target gene is digested with a restriction enzyme that will produce 'sticky ends', e.g. *Eco*RI. The plasmid also has a restriction site for *Eco*RI, so that when digested with *Eco*RI it becomes a linear DNA strand with 'sticky ends' complementary to the target. Upon ligation, the target and vector form a recombinant molecule. (B) Structure of a typical plasmid. The plasmid contains a gene conferring resistance to the antibiotic ampicillin (AmpR), and a portion of the LacZ gene that encodes the *N*-terminal fragment of the enzyme β-galactosidase. The *E. coli* strain used for this work has a defective β-galactosidase enzyme that is complemented by the plasmid LacZ gene product to form a functional enzyme. Within the plasma LacZ gene segment is a polylinker region containing approximately 10 restriction enzyme recognition sites, which serve as sites for insertion of target DNA. The plasmid also contains ORI, the site for origin of DNA replication.

Bacterial plasmids are bio-engineered to optimize their use as vectors

Within the circular DNA of a plasmid molecule are several elements that confer specific properties on the plasmid. Naturally occurring plasmids require several modifications to convert them into efficient DNA amplification vectors:

- **a polylinker cloning site:** this is a short sequence of nucleotides that contain unique recognition sites for several common restriction enzymes
- **an antibiotic resistance gene:** the host bacterial cells used for cloning must be sensitive to an antibiotic, e.g. ampicillin or tetracycline, so that when they are transformed by the plasmid, the host cell acquires resistance to the antibiotic. This then provides a means of selecting out bacteria that contain the plasmid from those that do not. The selection step is important because of the low efficiency of introducing plasmid DNA into bacteria
- **a recombinant screening system:** it is customary for the plasmid to have an expressible gene within it that can be used to show if foreign DNA is present in the plasmid. This so-called 'marker gene' can be designed to have the polylinker sequence within its reading frame so that, if the plasmid contains the target DNA insert, the normal reading frame is disrupted and the gene becomes nonfunctioning. The most common example is the gene for β-galactosidase. Using chromogenic substrates, bacteria containing this gene can be recognized readily on

a culture plate. If there is a foreign gene insert in the plasmid, β-galactosidase is not expressed and colonies do not form the colored reaction product (see Fig. 35.7). These colonies are then selected for further study to confirm the presence of the target DNA. This selection process excludes bacteria containing plasmids that have re-cyclized, but did not incorporate the target DNA insert.

DNA cloning by the polymerase chain reaction (PCR)

The use of PCR for the amplification of DNA in vitro has revolutionized molecular biology; it is a method of copying a single template DNA molecule

PCR is a simple and quick means of generating up to 10^9 copies of a single template DNA molecule within hours. Because of its simplicity, PCR has been used for a wide range of research and clinical applications (Table 35.5). One of the most widely used clinical applications of PCR is in the identification of genetic mutations within PCR amplified DNA from 'at-risk' individuals. A standard PCR reaction requires the following:

- **DNA template:** DNA containing the sequence to be amplified
- **amplimers:** small oligonucleotide primers that will hybridize with complementary DNA sequences both

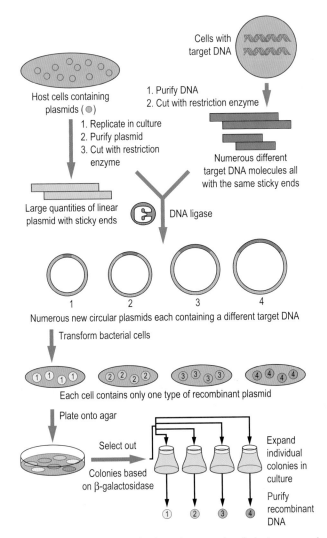

Cells with target DNA

Host cells containing plasmids (●)

1. Purify DNA
2. Cut with restriction enzyme

1. Replicate in culture
2. Purify plasmid
3. Cut with restriction enzyme

Numerous different target DNA molecules all with the same sticky ends

Large quantities of linear plasmid with sticky ends

DNA ligase

1 2 3 4

Numerous new circular plasmids each containing a different target DNA

Transform bacterial cells

Each cell contains only one type of recombinant plasmid

Plate onto agar

Select out

Colonies based on β-galactosidase

Expand individual colonies in culture

Purify recombinant DNA

Fig. 35.7 **Cell-based DNA cloning.** An example of cloning genomic DNA using bacterial cells. In general, each transformed bacterium will take up only a single plasmid molecule. Therefore individual bacterial colonies will contain many identical copies of just one particular recombinant DNA.

CELL-BASED CLONING TO PRODUCE CLINICALLY IMPORTANT PROTEINS: RECOMBINANT INSULIN

A 13-year-old girl was admitted with dehydration, vomiting and weight loss. Her blood glucose level was 19.1 mmol/L (344 mg/dL) and she had ketonuria. A diagnosis of type 1 diabetes mellitus was made. She was started on recombinant human insulin, was rehydrated, and made a prompt recovery. Compare box on page 282.

Comment. Prior to the advent of recombinant DNA technology, insulin therapy involved the use of animal insulins, most commonly pork or beef, which were chemically similar, but not identical, to human insulin. As a result of these differences, animal insulins often led to the development of antibodies, which reduced the efficacy of the insulin and could lead to treatment failures.

Insulin was the first clinically important human molecule to be produced by means of recombinant DNA technology. Following the cloning of the human insulin gene, large-scale production of pure human insulin was possible by inserting the cloned gene into a cell-based amplification system. Large amounts of insulin gene copies were produced, which were then expressed in either bacteria or yeast, and the resulting purified insulin was made available for use in treatment of diabetic patients.

One critical step in the process was the use of cDNA as a template for transcription and translation of the desired gene. Using insulin mRNA as a template, human insulin cDNA was generated by reverse transcription (formation of a complementary DNA strand using mRNA as the template). The product is a DNA molecule that contains all the coding region of the insulin gene without any introns. By this means, human recombinant insulin has almost totally replaced animal insulin in the treatment of diabetes. Other important recombinant human peptides used clinically include growth hormone, erythropoietin and parathyroid hormone.

VECTOR SYSTEMS FOR CLONING LARGE DNA FRAGMENTS

One critical factor in recombinant DNA manipulations is the size of the target DNA. Conventional bacterial plasmids, although convenient to work with, are limited in the size of insert they can accept; 1–2 kb is the common size of the insert, with an upper limit of 5–10 kb. Some modified plasmid vectors called **cosmids** can accept larger fragments up to 20 kb. Another commonly used vector that has the ability to accept larger DNA fragments is the bacteriophage **lambda** (λ). This viral particle contains a double-stranded DNA genome packaged within a protein coat. The λ-phage can infect *E. coli* cells with high efficiency and introduce its DNA into the bacterium. Infection leads to the

replication of viral DNA and the synthesis of new viral particles, which can then lyse the host cell and infect neighboring cells to repeat the process. The viral DNA is then reisolated to obtain the recombinant DNA.

Larger inserts can be cloned by using modified chromosomes from either **bacteria (bacterial artificial chromosomes, BACs)**, yeast **(yeast artificial chromosomes, YACs)** or human **(human artificial chromosomes, HACs)**. Such vectors can accommodate DNA fragments up to 1–2 Mb. BACs have been particularly important in putting together the sequence of the human genome.

Applications of PCR

Application	
Genetic marker typing	restriction site polymorphisms; microsatellite repeats
Detection of point mutations	restriction site polymorphisms; amplification refractory mutation systems
Amplification of DNA templates for DNA sequencing	double-stranded DNA; single-stranded templates
Genomic DNA cloning	PCR of gene families or genes in different species
Others	genome walking, introduction of mutations in vitro to test their effect in biologic systems

Table 35.5 **Applications of PCR.**

upstream and downstream of the desired sequence region and act as starting points for the synthesis of the newly amplified DNA strands

■ **polymerase enzyme:** typically a heat-stable polymerase, stable at temperatures required for denaturation of DNA, that will catalyze the formation of the DNA during the amplification reaction

■ **dNTPs:** these are of course essential for the synthesis of the new DNA strands by the polymerase.

PCR consists of a series of programmed temperature changes that serve to bring about a round of DNA synthesis from the primers (Fig. 35.8). The average PCR involves about 30–35 cycles of reactions, which provide as much as a billion copies of the original template ($2^{30} = 1 \times 10^9$), so that it can be visualized following electrophoresis on an agarose gel.

The cycle of the PCR comprises three steps that are repeated continuously by varying temperature in a cyclic fashion:

■ **denaturation:** heating of the reaction to approximately 95°C to ensure template and primers are single-stranded

■ **annealing:** cooling of the mixture to allow heteroduplexes of primer and template to form. The temperature for this is based on the Tm of the expected duplex (typically in the 50–65°C range)

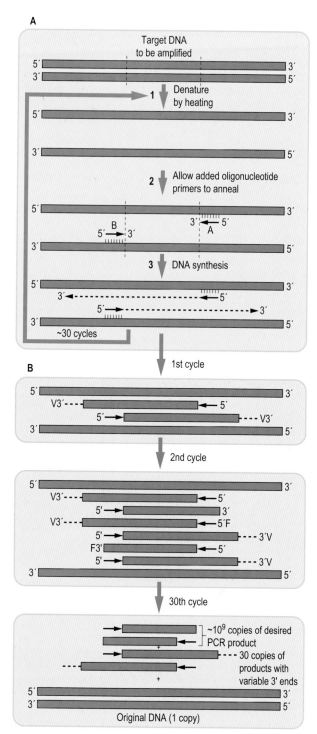

Fig. 35.8 Polymerase chain reaction (PCR) amplification of DNA. (A) Cycle 1. The target DNA is heated to 94°C to ensure complete denaturation. The mixture is then cooled to allow the oligonucleo-tide primers to hybridize to the complementary sequence in the target DNA. Specificity is provided by using two primers that anneal to sequences on opposite strands at opposite ends of the sequence to be amplified. In the presence of dNTPs, *Taq* polymerase catalyzes the elongation, beginning at the 3′ end of the primers. Two new duplex DNA molecules: one generated by each primer on its respective template. (B) Subsequent cycles. In the second cycle, products from the first cycle become templates. These templates have primers at their 5′ ends. Accordingly, the DNA made on them stops at the end of the primers used in the first cycle. From now on, molecules will accumulate during each cycle that have both ends defined by the pair of primers used. These accumulate exponentially and soon far outnumber the initial input DNA template. After 30 cycles, the original template and a trivial number of the variable-ended strands copied directly from it remain, but the number of amplified target molecules enclosed by the primers approaches 10^9. (Compare Fig. 36.4.)

- **elongation:** DNA polymerase elongates the newly synthesized DNA strand from the site of the annealed primer along the template strand (typically about 70°C).

The practical development of PCR was made possible by the discovery of heat-stable DNA polymerases that can withstand the temperature of the denaturation step and still retain enzymatic activity, e.g. *Taq* and *Pfu* polymerases. These enzymes were isolated from organisms that live and reproduce in hot springs and geysers.

The ability of PCR to amplify selectively a single template DNA relies on some prior knowledge of the nucleotide sequences in the regions flanking the target sequence

If the sequences in the regions flanking the target sequence are known, oligonucleotide primers are synthesized that are complementary to:

- the region on the sense (top) strand upstream of the target region, and
- the region on the antisense (lower) strand downstream of the target region (see Fig. 35.8).

It is essential that the sequence of the primers be unique to the target DNA being amplified. Normally a primer length of 18–20 bp is adequate for specificity, providing the primer does not lie within a region of repetitive DNA or contain simple repeats such as TGTGTGTG. Primers of a specified sequence are synthesized at low cost by many companies.

 REVERSE TRANSCRIPTASE-PCR

From whole blood or pathologic tissue, cDNA (DNA complementary to an mRNA) for a gene can be prepared by the process of reverse transcription. Reverse transcription uses a reverse transcriptase enzyme to polymerize a DNA molecule complementary to the mRNA molecule, using a single polyT primer, which binds to the mRNA at its 39 polyA tail. The reverse transcriptase proceeds along the mRNA to manufacture a complementary strand, cDNA. The resulting cDNA is then used as a template for PCR where the entire cDNA can be amplified to produce a DNA molecule containing the entire coding sequence of a gene. Clearly, in some cases, gene expression is tissue specific and one would not expect some mRNAs to be present in blood, e.g. dystrophin from muscle. However, ectopic transcription of genes occurs in white blood cells at a low frequency and allows analysis of transcripts of genes not normally expressed. This can be useful if the desired transcript is derived from a tissue that is not easily accessible or if study of the cDNA can give definitive information about the presence of a mutation. The cDNA can then be incorporated into a cell-based cloning vector for further amplification or can be introduced into a cellular expression system to produce the gene product in vitro. Such methods are used increasingly in the study of the functional aspects of mutant gene products.

Advantages and disadvantages of PCR cloning

PCR is a quick, simple and robust technique but prior sequence knowledge is needed, only a relatively small target DNA can be amplified, and DNA replication may be inaccurate

PCR has three principal advantages over cell-based cloning:

- **time:** by using PCR, a single template strand can be amplified to produce a detectable product very rapidly. Each step takes a few minutes or less, and 30 cycles of this PCR process can be completed within a few hours. Cell-based cloning is more expensive and may require days or weeks to produce a similar yield of DNA
- **sensitivity:** PCR can amplify a DNA template to usable amounts if only a single copy of the template DNA is present. Indeed, PCR protocols have been developed to allow amplification of target DNA from a single cell. This is why PCR has found such a prominent place in forensic applications and even in paleontology
- **robustness:** PCR is able to amplify DNA that is often badly degraded by time or the elements, or is present in previously inaccessible sites, e.g. formalin-fixed tissue. Only a few copies of an unmodified, relatively short sequence to be amplified need to remain intact.

Despite the apparent attraction of PCR, it is not without fault and, depending on the application, it may be an unacceptable means of amplifying DNA. The drawbacks of PCR are as follows:

- **prior sequence knowledge:** to perform PCR, flanking primers must be synthesized. For this to happen, the sequence of the target DNA, or at least its flanking regions, must be known. With the virtual completion of the human genome sequence, this issue is less important than in prior years
- **small target DNA amplification:** the size of fragments that can be amplified is limited. PCR will reliably amplify target sequences up to about 5 kb. However, larger products have been amplified recently by so-called 'long PCR' methods, allowing sequences up to 20 kb or more to be amplified
- **DNA replication may be inaccurate:** errors can be introduced during DNA polymerization by *Taq* polymerase since this enzyme lacks proofreading activity. Recently, other thermostable DNA polymerases that do carry out proofreading and have much lower error rates have become available. With suitable choice of conditions and enzymes, it is possible to obtain accurate amplification of relatively long sequences, though not the full length of typical intron-containing genes, which may exceed 50 kb.

Thus, it is safe to say that PCR provides a simple, fast and very efficient means of amplifying DNA that is partly or fully characterized, is of relatively small size and may be present in small amounts or in a poor condition. However, it is a less useful technique if the objective is to amplify gene-length DNA that is completely free of errors.

SPECIFIC METHODS USED IN THE ANALYSIS OF DEOXYRIBONUCLEIC ACID

Hybridization-based methods

There are several ways in which hybridization can be used in the study of DNA, which exploit either the stringency of the hybridization of probe to target or the utility of restriction enzymes for detecting variations in nucleotide sequences.

Restriction fragment length polymorphisms (RFLPs)

Restriction enzymes cleave DNA at specific recognition sites; if these sites are altered by mutation or polymorphism, the size of DNA fragments on a blot will differ

A single nucleotide change in the recognition site of a restriction enzyme renders the site completely resistant to cleavage. If the recognition sequence is disrupted, by either a pathogenic change in the DNA sequence resulting in a disease (a mutation) or a naturally occurring variation in the DNA sequence unaccompanied by disease (a polymorphism), the results of probing a Southern blot of DNA digested by a restriction enzyme may differ. Such differences in DNA sequence may lead to the creation of new restriction sites or the abolition of existing sites, and result in DNA fragments of novel lengths – pattern differences known as restriction fragment length polymorphisms (RFLPs) (Fig. 35.9). Historically, RFLPs have been used to identify disease-causing mutations, to study variation in noncoding DNA, and for paternity testing. Obviously, many changes in DNA would not alter a restriction site. PCR-based methods for identifying polymorphisms that do not necessarily alter restriction sites – such as short tandem repeats (STRs), single nucleotide polymorphisms (SNPs) and variable number tandem repeats (VNTRs) – have largely displaced RFLP technology.

Single nucleotide polymorphisms

Microarray technology is used to detect silent, single nucleotide differences in DNA sequences

Single nucleotide polymorphisms (SNPs) are DNA sequence variations involving single nucleotide changes that naturally occur in the population. Some of these are responsible for the changes identified as RFLPs or restriction site polymorphisms, but current techniques allow identification of these minimal variations regardless of whether or not a restriction site is present. SNPs occur in both coding and

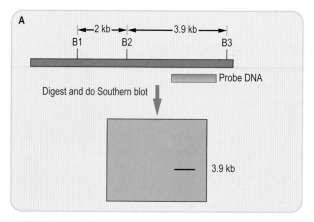

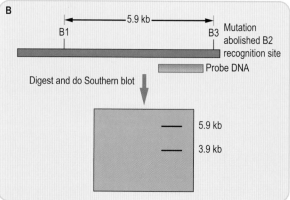

Fig. 35.9 **Restriction fragment length polymorphisms (RFLPs).** Variations in the nucleotide sequence of DNA, either due to natural variation in individuals or as a result of a DNA mutation, can abolish the recognition sites for restriction enzymes. This means that when DNA is digested with the enzyme whose site is abolished, the size of the resulting fragments is altered. Southern blotting and probe hybridization can be used to detect this change. Results are shown for (A) homozygous normal and (B) heterozygous mutant individuals. B, *Bam*HI restriction site.

noncoding regions of the genome, with an overall density of 1 per every 100–300 bp. SNPs are therefore the most densely distributed variations of all the various polymorphic markers known. SNPs that are close to one another tend to be inherited as a group. These SNP combinations or clusters, called SNPs 'haplotypes', are detected by microarray techniques to identify genes or genetic variations associated with diseases or other phenotypic traits, such as response to drug therapy. If a particular haplotype is more common in a population with diabetes, that SNP could be used to narrow in on the location and identify the gene involved in the disease. A large internationally funded project, the International HapMap Project, is designed to characterize the haplotype maps of several ethnic groups around the world to aid in discovery of genes associated with human disease. As of December 2007, approximately 4.5 million of the estimated 10–30 million SNPs in the human genome had been identified and characterized and are cataloged in a publicly accessible database.

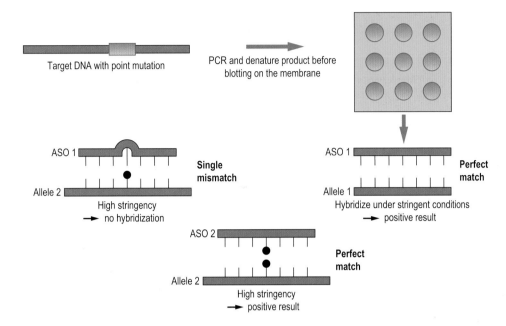

Target DNA with point mutation

PCR and denature product before blotting on the membrane

ASO 1

Allele 2

Single mismatch

High stringency
→ no hybridization

ASO 2

Allele 2

Perfect match

High stringency
→ positive result

ASO 1

Allele 1

Perfect match

Hybridize under stringent conditions
→ positive result

Fig. 35.10 **Dot-blots and allele-specific oligonucleotides.** Using a technique similar to Southern blotting, single-stranded PCR products are transferred onto a nylon membrane and fixed in situ. Allele-specific oligonucleotides (ASOs) are hybridized to the target DNA under conditions of high stringency. In this case, the ASOs are used to identify a single base substitution, with one detecting the wild type and another the mutant allele.

RFLPs CAN BE USED FOR DETECTING PATHOLOGIC MUTATIONS: A CARRIER OF THE SICKLE CELL MUTATION IN THE GLOBIN GENE

A 24-year-old Afro-Caribbean woman was referred for prenatal counseling. Her younger brother had sickle cell anemia, and she had become pregnant. Her partner was known to be a carrier of the sickle cell mutation (sickle cell trait) and she wanted to know if her child would develop sickle cell anemia. Since the patient was at risk of being a carrier, she opted to have chorionic villus sampling (CVS) performed to detect the presence or absence of the sickle cell mutation in her child. Analysis of her own DNA revealed that she was a carrier, and the CVS showed that the child was also a carrier and would not develop sickle cell anemia.

Comment. Here is a famous example in which a mutation generating the sickle allele of β-globin does alter a restriction site. One widely examined mutation is the A > T substitution at codon 6 in

the sequence for the β-globin gene. This results in a glutamine-valine (Glu-Val) mutation in the amino acid sequence of β-globin and also abolishes a recognition site for *Mst*II (CCTN(A > T)GG) in the β-globin gene. Digestion of normal human DNA with *Mst*II and probing the Southern blot with a probe specific for the promoter of the β-globin gene yields a single band of 1.2 kb as the nearest *Mst*II site is 1.2 kb upstream in the 5' region of the gene. The abolition of the codon 6 restriction site means that the fragment size seen when probing *Mst*II digested DNA is now 1.4 kb, as the next *Mst*II site is located 200 bases downstream in the intron after exon 1. Thus, patients with sickle cell anemia will show only one band, 1.4 kb, while carriers will have two bands, one 1.4 kb and another 1.2 kb, and unaffected individuals will have a single 1.2 kb band (Fig. 35.11).

Allele-specific oligonucleotides and dot-blot hybridization

This method uses a small probe to probe the blotted DNA under highly stringent conditions

The other extreme of the RFLP method is to use a small oligonucleotide probe (15–30 nucleotides) and probe the blotted DNA under conditions of high stringency. Careful choice of temperature and solvent ensures that oligonucleotides will only hybridize to complementary sequences where there is a perfect match, down to the single nucleotide level. Mutations that result from a single nucleotide change can be detected by using oligonucleotides that recognize

either the mutant or the normal allele of the gene, so-called allele-specific oligonucleotides (ASOs). ASOs can be used to screen DNA for the presence of several mutations, particularly if the template DNA is immobilized on a membrane for dot-blot analysis. Single-stranded DNA is transferred to a membrane as in the case of Southern blotting, but rather than transferring size-fractionated digested DNA, total human genomic DNA or PCR-generated fragments are blotted onto the membrane. In this way, ASOs can be hybridized to the membrane under high-stringency conditions and autoradiography performed to determine whether the DNA contains a specific allele. The process can then be repeated for other alleles (Fig. 35.10).

PCR-based methods

Detection of microsatellite repeats

This technique detects sets of tandem nucleotide repeats in mammalian genomes

Tandem microsatellite repeats are sequences that comprise a few nucleotides, typically two or three, e.g. CA or CAG, that are repeated in tandem at various locations throughout mammalian genomes, so-called microsatellite repeats. These microsatellites are small blocks of DNA that occur in noncoding regions, either intergenic or within introns of genes. The term 'satellite DNA' has been historically applied to regions of repetitive sequence in which the local base composition may differ from the overall composition of human DNA. One important feature of these microsatellite repeats is that they are highly polymorphic, i.e. the number of tandem repeats in a particular microsatellite may vary from one individual to another. This means that the two copies of a single

human microsatellite, one from each chromosome, may be of different lengths and can thus be distinguished in that individual. The number of different alleles of the microsatellite will vary depending on which microsatellite is studied, but may vary from two to 15 or more copies of the repeat per allele (Fig. 35.12). As a result of this high degree of polymorphism, microsatellite repeats are of great value in the study of genetic linkage. This is because a particular microsatellite allele may fortuitously be located in the vicinity of a pathogenic mutation. Comparison of the DNA of affected families may indicate that a particular microsatellite serves as a marker with which to trace the presence or inheritance of the mutation under study.

Mutation detection by allele-specific PCR

Only mutant DNA will be amplified using this technique

Standard PCR employs two primers to amplify both strands of the DNA and relies on the fact that each primer will reliably amplify the target strand. However, PCR can be performed using allele-specific primers, which will only amplify one allele of a target gene. For example, if a primer contains a sequence that recognizes only the mutant gene, it will only hybridize with and amplify the mutant DNA. The allele-specific primer has a sequence at its extreme 3′-nucleotides that matches the mutant gene. As the DNA polymerase requires complete hybridization of primer and template at the 3′ end of the primer, the probe will not hybridize to the normal gene. This method can be applied to the detection of specific mutations in a single gene, e.g. the gene for cystic fibrosis. It is often called an amplification refractory mutation system (ARMS) as PCR amplification will be refractory, i.e. will not occur, in the absence of the mutant allele.

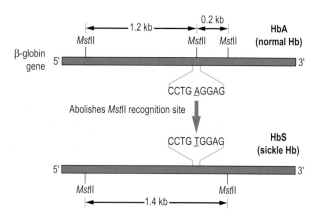

Fig. 35.11 **RFLP analysis in sickle cell anemia.** An A > T substitution at codon 6 of the β-globin gene abolishes a recognition site for the enzymes, *Mst*II, which can be used to determine the presence or absence of the mutation by studying the RFLP pattern.

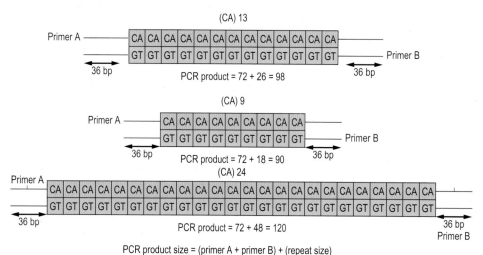

PCR product size = (primer A + primer B) + (repeat size)

Fig. 35.12 **Microsatellite repeats.** A typical microsatellite contains tandem repeats of a dinucleotide, e.g. CA. The number of repeats can vary from 2 to 20 or more. Amplification of the DNA including the microsatellite repeat is performed by PCR using a radiolabeled primer and the products are then size-fractionated on a polyacrylamide gel to aid resolution. PCR product size = 72 (primer A + primer B) + 26 (13 × 2 for each dinucleotide) = 98. In this instance, three alleles can be identified: $(CA)_{13}$, $(CA)_9$ and $(CA)_{24}$.

MICROSATELLITE REPEATS ARE IDEAL MARKERS FOR STUDY OF INHERITANCE

A 7-year-old boy was the subject of disputed paternity. His mother had identified a man as the father and maintained that he should be responsible for the child's financial well-being. All parties consented to DNA testing by means of DNA fingerprinting. Study of the DNA tests revealed that this man was the father.

Comment. It was recognized over 20 years ago that patterns of short tandem repeat (STR) microsatellites could be used for genetic fingerprinting and establishing parent–child relationships. With the development of PCR it became possible to analyze the patterns of specific microsatellite repeats rapidly. Government agencies in many countries have now agreed upon specific sets of STRs that are routinely used in law enforcement to connect crime evidence to specific individuals and in other situations where kinship is to be tested. For example, in the United States 13 loci were chosen that involve 12 different autosomes and contain variable numbers of 4-nucleotide repeats. These loci are not part of coding regions of DNA, so are relatively free of selective pressure. An additional locus is not a microsatellite but rather a sexually dimorphic region of the amelogenin gene (AMG). Taken together, these loci form the basis of the Combined DNA Index System (CODIS) used by the Federal Bureau of Investigation and US National DNA Database. The AMG locus encodes a major protein of tooth enamel and is present in active form on both the X- and Y-chromosomes, but does not cross over between the X- and Y-chromosomes during meiosis. Thus a 6 bp deletion within the AMG locus on the X-chromosome is never present on the Y, and a primer set for this region amplifies different length fragments from each sex chromosome (normal females will have only the short fragment, while normal males will have both the short and long). Interestingly, primer sets have been developed that are compatible with each other so that all 14 amplifications can be carried out simultaneously in a single tube (known as multiplex PCR). The primers are labeled with fluorescent tags, some of which are different colors. The products of the reaction are typically analyzed by capillary electrophoresis, and the differently colored primer pairs allow the products of particular STR loci to be identified in cases where fragment lengths from different loci might overlap. It is remarkable that so much information can be obtained from a single enzymatic assay.

Microsatellites have also been used to examine the linkage of a disease trait, e.g. type 1 diabetes, to certain regions of the human genome. By studying the inheritance of microsatellite markers in families or shared alleles in affected siblings, a statistical measure of the degree of coinheritance of a marker can be determined. This approach has been used successfully to identify genetic loci strongly linked to the inheritance of type 1 and type 2 diabetes, and to locate the genes causing Huntington's disease, myotonic dystrophy and other single gene disorders (Table 35.6).

Unstable trinucleotide repeats			
Disease	**Repeat**	**Normal length**	**Mutation length**
Huntington's disease	(CAG)n	9–35	37–100
Kennedy disease	(CAG)n	17–24	40–55
Spinocerebellar ataxia I (SCA I)	(CAG)n	19–36	43–81
Dentatopallidoluysian atrophy (DRPLA)	(CAG)n	7–23	49–75+
Machado–Joseph disease (SCA III)	(CAG)n	12–36	69–79+
Fragile X site A (FRAXA)	(CGG)n	6–54	200–1000+
Fragile X site E (FRAXE)	(CCG)n	6–25	>200
Fragile X site F (FRAXF)	(GCC)n	6–29	>500
Fragile 16 site A (FRA16A)	(CCG)n	16–49	1000–2000
Myotonic dystrophy	(CTG)n	5–35	50–4000
Friedreich's ataxia	(GAA)n	7–22	>200

Table 35.6 **Unstable trinucleotide repeats.** In all the cases listed, trinucleotide repeats are present in individuals without clinical disease. However, progressive increase in the number of repeats leads to the onset of clinical signs. A premutant phase has been described in some disorders, such as FRAXA, where expansions larger than normal are found but with minimal or no clinical features. These premutant states give rise to carriers – females who can subsequently pass on an expanded triplet repeat to their offspring, which may result in the disease.

Detection of deletions in genes causing disease

This is performed using primers that generate PCR products of different sizes

In patients with Duchenne muscular dystrophy, many of the disease-causing mutations are due to deletions of one of relatively few exons in dystrophin, one of the largest of human genes. Specific amplification of these exons, using primers that generate PCR products of different sizes for each exon, can be used to screen quickly for the presence of a disease-causing deletion in an affected individual or determine if the fetus of a carrier has the deletion. Such PCR is carried out by multiplex PCR in a single reaction using a single template and 5–10 different primer pairs, each generating a separate amplification product.

TRINUCLEOTIDE REPEATS IN GENES GIVE RISE TO HUMAN DISEASE

A 33-year-old woman has recently been diagnosed as having myotonic dystrophy (MD). MD is characterized by autosomal dominant inheritance, muscular weakness associated with impaired muscular relaxation, frontal balding, endocrine disorders such as diabetes, and premature ovarian failure and cataract formation. The patient has muscular problems and frontal balding, whereas her affected father, aged 60 years, has only just developed cataracts. She is concerned about the risk to her own children if she becomes pregnant.

Comment. While the majority of nucleotide repeats are noncoding and clinically silent, 11 clinical disorders have been identified where trinucleotide repeats appear directly responsible for a disease phenotype (Table 35.6), and where the repeat is said to be unstable. Unstable repeats undergo changes in the size of the repeat during meiotic division and generally undergo expansion of the size of the repeat so that with each successive meiosis, i.e. from generation to generation, the number of repeats will gradually increase. Once trinucleotide expansions reach a critical size they begin to interfere with gene function and then result in the clinical syndrome. In the case of MD, with an expansion size of 80 repeats, the patient will exhibit the signs of the disease. Owing to the instability of the triplet repeat during meiosis, offspring of this patient might expect to have a larger expansion and also display features of the disease. Similarly, successive generations may display signs of MD at a younger age. This phenomenon of progressive worsening of the clinical phenotype with successive meioses is known as *anticipation* and is the result of progressive enlargement of the trinucleotide expansions during meiosis (Fig. 35.13).

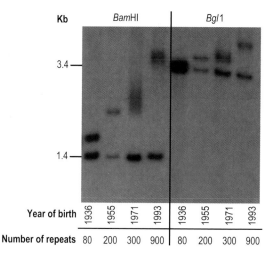

Fig. 35.13 **Molecular basis of genetic anticipation.** Myotonic dystrophy, the most common form of adult muscular dystrophy (MD), exhibits anticipation within families, i.e. the clinical features of the disease become progressively more severe and the age at onset of symptoms is younger with each successive generation. The underlying problem is the presence of an unstable trinucleotide expansion within the MD gene, which progressively expands with each meiosis. This results in the inheritance of larger mutations, which give rise to a more severe clinical picture with the tendency for the features to manifest at an earlier stage. The Southern blot illustrates the progressive increase in size of the trinucleotide expansion in successive generations of a family with MD. The normal allele size is seen at 1.4 kb for the *Bam*HI digest and 3.4 kb for the *Bgl*I digest; these enzymes have restriction sites, GGATCC and GCCNNNNNGGC respectively, yielding smaller fragments for the *Bam*HI digest. With both restriction enzymes, there is a progressive expansion in the size of the trinucleotide repeat with each generation, which is most apparent in the case of the smaller DNA fragments produced by *Bam*HI. (This is a good example of an RFLP.)

Other methods for detection of variation in DNA

Single-strand conformational polymorphism (SSCP)

SSCP is useful for analyzing PCR products of 200 bp and less and is moderately sensitive

Single-stranded DNA has a tendency to form complex structures by folding back on itself, just as tRNA molecules form hairpin structures. The mobility of single-stranded DNA in an electrophoretic gel depends not only on the length of the DNA but also on its conformation, which is determined by its DNA sequence and folding. Therefore, changes in DNA structure that do not alter the length of the target DNA, i.e. substitutions in contrast to deletions or insertions, can alter the mobility of the fragment in a nondenaturing gel, so-called single-strand conformational polymorphisms (SSCP). SSCP is performed by PCR with a radioactive primer. The reaction products are denatured to render them single-stranded and diluted to prevent intermolecular hybridization. The DNA is then electrophoresed on nondenaturing polyacrylamide gels. A control sample is also included on the gel to allow identification of the variant from the wild-type allele, based on differences in conformation and electrophoretic mobility.

Denaturant-gradient gel electrophoresis (DGGE)

DGGE uses 'melting' of double-stranded DNA

In SSCP, changes in the tertiary structure of single-stranded DNA can result in differing electrophoretic mobilities. However, this type of analysis cannot be used for double-stranded DNA. Nevertheless, if double-stranded DNA undergoes electrophoresis in a gel that contains a gradient of increasing amounts of denaturant, such as urea, double-stranded DNA will then partially denature, to form single-stranded regions and so undergo a marked change in mobility. A single nucleotide change between two alleles of a gene will affect the melting point of the alleles and thus the mobilities of amplified PCR fragments in this kind of denaturing gel.

To perform DGGE, PCR is performed using radiolabeled primers that have a GC clamp at their ends. This is a tail of guanine and cytosine residues added to the PCR primers such

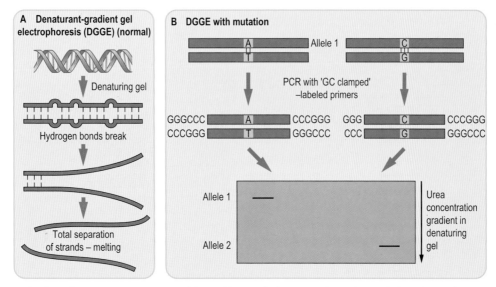

Fig. 35.14 **DGGE method to detect DNA mutations.** (A) Double-stranded DNA is electrophoresed through a gel containing a gradient of increasing concentration of denaturants, such as urea. The DNA melts at a denaturant concentration unique to that particular DNA, depending on its size and nucleotide composition. If the nucleotide sequence of a DNA is changed, e.g. by a mutation, the melting point of the DNA will be altered and thus the mobility of the DNA in the gel will be altered, allowing the change to be detected by autoradiography. (B) DGGE with mutation. In this case, a single A > C substitution has occurred. This increases the number of hydrogen bonds between the two strands and alters the mobility in the denaturant gradient. The difference in mobility through the gel only highlights the difference in the two strands' nucleotide sequence – it does not say what or where the difference is.

that the PCR product will have ends that have artificially created GC ends. These GC ends, or clamps, improve the sensitivity by preventing complete melting of double-stranded DNA. PCR products are electrophoresed in the denaturing gel and, following autoradiography, different alleles of the suspect gene are identified (Fig. 35.14). DGGE is particularly useful for rapid scanning of individually amplified exon units from a large gene with many introns.

DEOXYRIBONUCLEIC ACID SEQUENCING

At the heart of many of the foregoing techniques is the notion that at least some of the nucleotide sequence of the DNA being studied is known, particularly when PCR primers are involved. The technologies now used in the sequencing of DNA have become extremely sophisticated, and automated sequencing of large amounts of DNA is now standard practice in many centers around the world.

Chain termination (Sanger) DNA sequencing

Chain termination sequencing uses a DNA polymerase enzyme, a single-stranded template DNA, and a sequencing primer

In this method, the sequencing primer is designed to be complementary to the region flanking the sequence of interest and acts as the starting point of chain elongation. DNA

polymerization requires dNTPs to allow the strand to be elongated but, in addition, radioactive chain-terminating dideoxynucleotides (ddNTPs) are added. These are analogs of the dNTPs but differ in that they lack the 3′-hydroxyl group required for formation of a covalent bond with the 5′-phosphate group of the incoming dNTP. Therefore, during DNA polymerization, if a growing DNA chain incorporates a ddNTP, growth of the nucleotide chain is halted. A total of four reactions is carried out in parallel, each containing the primer, DNA template, polymerase and dNTPs. However, to each of the four reactions, a small amount of one radio-active ddNTP is added (ddATP, ddCTP, ddTTP, ddGTP) so that four separate reactions, the A, T, G, and C reactions, are conducted in parallel. As the chains elongate, ddNTPs, which are present at lower concentration than the natural dNTP, will be incorporated into the chain in place of the corresponding dNTP on a random basis. This means that in any one reaction mixture, there will be many chains of varying lengths which, when pooled together, represent the total collection of fragments that could terminate at that base. The DNA chains of differing lengths can be separated by electrophoresis on denaturing polyacrylamide gels. These gels allow DNA fragments that differ by only one nucleotide in length to be separated and, if the reaction involves a labeled group, either a dNTP or the primer, then electrophoresis of the four reactions in parallel, with subsequent autoradiography, will allow the sequence of the DNA to be determined (Fig. 35.15). In general, this method can produce sequence data for the 300–500 bases downstream of the sequencing primer, but some protocols permit analysis of much longer sequences.

Today, the sequencing of DNA is automated using capillary gel electrophoresis and four fluorescence-labeled ddNTPs. In

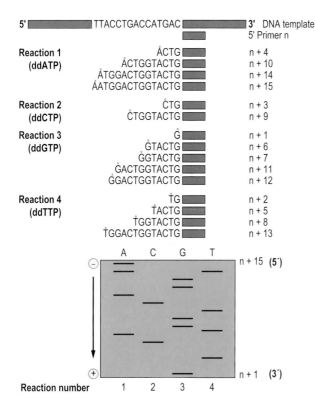

Fig. 35.15 **DNA sequencing using dideoxynucleotides**. A single reaction involving the DNA template and primer will proceed until a ddNTP is incorporated into the chain at random. This halts the reaction and that particular chain can grow no longer. Four reactions are performed in parallel; each reaction is identical with respect to the content of the four NTPs, except for the presence of tracer amounts of radiolabeled ddNTPs, either ddATP, ddCTP, ddGTP or ddTTP. Each reaction generates hundreds of different reaction products with the same 5′ end, the sequencing primer, but differing 3′ ends. The length of the 3′ end will vary from 1 to over 300 bases depending on when a ddNTP is incorporated into the chain. Once completed, the four reactions are electrophoresed in parallel on a polyacrylamide gel and the parallel ladders are read from bottom to top to yield the sequence of the DNA (see also Fig. 36.2).

this case, a single capillary gel is used but each fragment is terminated and labeled by a single fluorophore, depending on the ddNTP incorporated at the 5′ terminus. Fluorescence is recorded on a four-channel fluorimeter and the sequence of fluorophores indicates the sequence of the DNA (Fig. 35.16).

Pyrosequencing

New methods of DNA sequencing are based on different technology, but still depend on the accuracy of DNA polymerases and their absolute requirement for primers as starting points. In one of the latest techniques, individual tiny beads are prepared with many identical copies of relatively short, PCR-amplified DNA fragments. Individual beads are deposited in microwells of a plate, then DNA polymerase and a single dNTP are allowed to flow, one at a time, over the wells. When a nucleotide is added to the end of growing strands (which will happen at least once during a cycle of four dNTPs), the pyrophosphate released is used to generate a flash of light

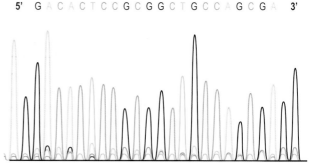

Fig. 35.16 **A portion of the DNA sequencing output generated by capillary gel electrophoresis using terminator nucleotides tagged with different dideoxy fluorophores**. As fragments elute from the end of the capillary, the fluorescence is recorded in four different channels and stored so that the entire run can be examined on a computer screen or printed. In most cases the bases are identified automatically by computer software. Depending on the specific equipment used, 500 to over 1000 nucleotides can be sequenced in a single run.

from momentary activation of luciferease. The strength of the light output from each well is proportional to the number of nucleotides added, e.g. 1, 2 or 3 intensity units for an A, AA and AAA sequence, respectively. When all four dNTPs have been cycled through multiple times, a sequence can be deduced from the pattern of light output of each well. This methodology is faster and much less expensive than previous technologies. Roughly 100 million bp of DNA sequence can be generated from a single 'massively parallel' instrument in one 7-hour run using pyrosequencing technology.

Real-time PCR (RT-PCR)

It is sometimes necessary to quantify amounts of RNA or DNA in a clinical sample. For example, in cases of human immuno-deficiency virus (HIV) infection, knowledge of the amount of viral RNA in the bloodstream can be a valuable guide to prognosis and treatment. In standard PCR reactions, one usually examines the DNA produced after 30 or more cycles, when it has been amplified a billion times or more. This is a useful qualitative test but is not good for quantification. For example, the amount of PCR products approximately doubles each cycle so small differences in efficiency at earlier cycles result in large differences at later cycles. In addition, all reactions eventually reach a plateau phase due to many reasons, including the accumulation of endproducts that inhibit the reaction, and many reactions will have reached plateau phase before 30 cycles.

To circumvent many of these problems, RT-PCR machines have been developed which measure how much product is formed at very early stages in the reaction when it is proceeding at the maximal rate. If there is more target DNA in a particular sample, fewer cycles will be needed to make a defined amount of product, so the number of cycles needed to make a defined amount of product is a measure of how much of that DNA sequence was present at the beginning of the PCR.

In RT-PCR, the formation of product is followed by using either a dye which fluoresces brightly when bound to double-stranded DNA or some form of fluorescently labeled hybridization probe. The amount of product is measured continuously at the end of every PCR cycle, e.g. by measuring fluorescence, using a probe that intercalates into double-stranded DNA and changes or increases its fluorescence on binding. Sensitive optics and powerful electronics are used so that very small amounts of product can be detected at early cycles and the process can easily be automated. This is a convenient way to quantify accurately, sensitively and quickly small amounts of DNA or RNA (which must first be transcribed to cDNA) and the technology is rapidly moving from research laboratories to clinical applications.

Summary

There are myriad DNA techniques available for the analysis of every aspect of DNA metabolism and function. However, regardless of the complexity of the methods, they all rely on the basic principles of hybridization and polymerization by appropriate enzymes. There is no doubt that the most significant recent advance in the study of DNA has been the discovery and automation of PCR. PCR is now used widely in all aspects of biomedical research, in particular in the study of human genetics. Whether in the diagnostic laboratory or in the search for new disease genes, analysis has been totally transformed by PCR. There are now many hundreds of human genetic diseases whose diagnosis can be made by a single PCR-based analysis of DNA from a single blood sample.

The virtual completion of the Human Genome Project, within just 50 years of the discovery of the three-dimensional structure of DNA, stands as one of mankind's great achievements. Of course, this vastly simplifies the study of both normal and mutant genes, since the information to design PCR primers and to predict restriction enzyme cut-sites is now available for all genes. Recombinant DNA technology has replaced complex biochemical assays as the major biologic scientific technology in most laboratories. The technology is continually evolving but at its center are several key principles that are modified to fit the application of a particular method. Understanding these principles is the key to grasping the seemingly abstract nature of some of the newer techniques.

Further reading

Cockerill FR. Application of rapid-cycle real-time polymerase chain reaction for diagnostic testing in the clinical microbiology laboratory. *Arch Pathol Lab Med* 2003;**127**:1112–1120.

Copland JA, Davies PJ, Shipley GL, Wood CG, Luxon BA, Urban RJ. The use of DNA microarrays to assess clinical samples: the transition from bedside to bench to bedside. *Recent Prog Horm Res* 2003;**58**:25–53.

Cowell JK, Hawthorn L. The application of microarray technology to the analysis of the cancer genome. *Curr Mol Med* 2007;**7**:103–120.

International HapMap Consortium, Frazer KA, Ballinger DG, Cox DR, et al. A second generation human haplotype map of over 3.1 million SNPs. *Nature* 2007;**449**:851–861.

Ivnitski D, O'Neil DJ, Gattuso A, Schlicht R, Calidonna M, Fisher R. Nucleic acid approaches for detection and identification of biological warfare and infectious disease agents. *Biotechniques* 2003;**35**:862–869.

Renwick P, Ogilvie CM. Preimplantation genetic diagnosis for monogenic diseases: overview and emerging issues. *Expert Rev Mol Diagn* 2007;**7**:33–43.

Sebat J. Major changes in our DNA lead to major changes in our thinking. *Nat Genet* 2007; **39**(7 Suppl): S3–5. (Short review on CNVs)

Sotirious C, Piccaart MJ. Taking gene-expression profiling to the clinic: when will molecular signatures become relevant to patient care? *Nat Rev Cancer* 2007; **12**:271–287.

Websites

National Center for Biotechnology Information – an entry site that leads to full genome sequences for human and mouse: www.ncbi.nlm.nih.gov

Sanger Center for Genome Analysis – an alternative presentation of data from human and other genomes: www.ensembl.org

US National Institutes of Health: a portal to health-related information. Look under 'Genetics/Birth defects': http://health.nih.gov

Institutional websites with Recombinant DNA methodology: www.genome.ou.edu/protocol_book/protocol_index.html

The International HapMap Project: www.hapmap.org/

Sanger Center website with information on copy number variants (CNVs) and their relationship to human diseases: www.sanger.ac.uk/humgen/cnv/

A description of the pyrosequencing technique: www.454.com/products-solutions/how-it-works/index.asp

Animation of Sanger sequencing: http://smcg.ccg.unam.mx/enp-unam/03-EstructuraDelGenoma/animaciones/secuencia.swf

Animation of microarray technology: www.bio.davidson.edu/courses/genomics/chip/chip.html

PCR animation: www.dnalc.org/vshockwave/pcrwhole.dcr

Plasmid cloning animation: www.sumanasinc.com/webcontent/animations/content/plasmidcloning.html

ACTIVE LEARNING

1. A 14-year-old female patient appeared to be undergoing normal sexual development, except for rather scant body hair. Her complaint was that she has never had a menstrual period. Physical examination indicated a very short vagina ending in a blind pouch. How could you use the human genome sequence to design primer pairs that would amplify exons of the androgen receptor to check for possible mutations that could account for androgen insensitivity syndrome?

2. New human pathogenic viruses appear with some regularity. If you were in charge of a large research group, how could you apply cell-based cloning techniques to establish the sequence of a new viral DNA and then suggest possible viral proteins that could be expressed to use in a recombinant vaccine? How might you make a vaccine to protect against this pathogen and several others at the same time?

3. An unsorted collection of clones derived from the DNA of an organism is called a genomic library. Similarly, an unsorted collection of clones derived from the mRNA of a particular tissue is termed a cDNA library. Why are cDNA libraries most useful if the goal is to express a specific human pituitary protein in yeast cells, but a genomic library would be required if the aim was to characterize binding sites for transcription factors in the promoter of the same gene?

36. Genomics, Proteomics and Metabolomics

A Pitt and W Kolch

LEARNING OBJECTIVES

After reading this chapter you should be able to:

- Describe what the terms genomics, transcriptomics, proteomics, and metabolomics mean.
- Discuss the differences between the -omics methods and the particular challenges.
- Give several examples of methods used in genomics.
- Describe what microarrays are and give examples of their use.
- Give examples of methods used in proteomics.
- Describe methods used in metabolomics.
- Discuss biomarkers.

INTRODUCTION

The human genome is organized into 46 chromosomes consisting of 22 pairs of autosomal chromosomes, which are shared by both sexes, and the sex-determining chromosomes, X and Y. One set of autosomal chromosomes is derived from each parent. One X chromosome is contributed by the mother and another either X or a Y from the father. The autosomal chromosomes are numbered according to their size, with 1 being the largest. Each chromosome contains genes interspersed with often large regions of nonprotein-coding DNA. Most mammalian genes consist of multiple exons, which are the parts that eventually constitute the mature mRNA, and introns, which separate the exons and are removed from the primary transcript by splicing. Surprisingly, newest estimates show that the 3 billion bases of the human genome only harbor 20 000–25 000 protein-coding genes. This is only about four times the number of genes of yeast and twice as many as the fruit fly *Drosophila melanogaster*, and less than many plants. However, mammalian cells use alternative splicing and alternative gene promoters to produce 4–6 different mRNA from a single gene, so that the number of protein-coding mRNAs, the transcriptome, may be as large as 100 000. This complexity is further augmented at the protein level by posttranslational modifications and targeted proteolysis that could generate an estimated 500 000–1 000 000 functionally different protein entities, which comprise the proteome. An estimated 10–15% of these proteins function in metabolism which collectively describes the processes used to provide energy and the basic low molecular weight building blocks of cells, such as amino acids, fatty acids and sugars. It also includes the processes that convert exogenous substances such as drugs or environmental chemicals.

A recent release of a first draft of the human metabolome lists approximately 2500 metabolites. The real size of the metabolome is unknown. It is open, as it will increase with the number of environmental substances an organism is exposed to. The relationship between the different -omes is depicted in Figure 36.1.

Studies of genome, transcriptome, proteome and metabolome pose different challenges

First, the physicochemical properties are rather uniform at the level of the genome and transcriptome, which consist entirely of DNA and RNA respectively. On the other hand, the proteome, and even more so the metabolome, consist of molecules with widely different physicochemical properties.

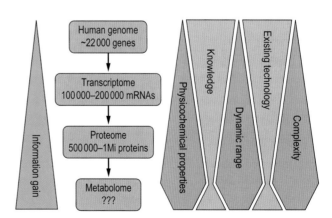

Fig. 36.1 **Relationship between the -omics.** Complexity, diversity in physicochemical properties, and dynamic range increase as we move from genes to transcripts and proteins, but may decrease again at the level of metabolites. This presents a huge technologic challenge, but also represents a rich source of information gain, especially if the different -omics disciplines can be integrated into a common view.

Due to the physicochemical homogeneity of the genome and transcriptome, methods for large-scale and multiplexed analysis are easier to establish and require a smaller range of sophisticated equipment. Furthermore, DNA and RNA can be sequenced and amplified with ease (Chapter 35). In contrast, proteins and metabolites cannot be amplified, and sequence or structure determination is much more difficult. The analysis of proteomes and metabolomes poses huge technologic challenges, mainly because of the physicochemical heterogeneity and the wide range of abundance. For instance, the concentration of proteins in human serum spans 12 orders of magnitude, while under normal conditions genes are equally abundant. Second, the complexity increases as we move from the genome to the transcriptome and proteome, while our knowledge decreases. Third, there is an increase in their dynamic nature. The genome is relatively static, whereas the transcriptome and proteome are more dynamic and can change quickly in response to internal and external cues. The most pronounced dynamic responses may manifest themselves in the metabolome as it directly reflects the interactions between organism and environment.

GENOMICS

The genome provides a way to assess the probability of a condition, but without providing information whether and when this probability will manifest itself

The 'whether and when' information can be gained from the transcriptome and proteome. The proteome is arguably the richer source due to the greater functional diversity at the protein level, which can give a detailed picture of the current state of an organism. Thus, the information provided by the -omics technologies is complementary, and their use for diagnostic purposes is increasingly available in the clinical laboratory.

Large numbers of diseases have an inheritable genetic component

Many diseases are caused by genetic aberrations and many more manifest a genetic predisposition or component. The Online Mendelian Inheritance in Man (OMIM) database currently contains 4191 entries that associate human genes with inherited diseases. Given that the number of human genes is around 22 000, this suggests that a large number of diseases have an inheritable genetic component. Thus, the genome holds a rich source of information not only about our physiology, but also about pathophysiology. Efforts to find individual disease genes were hampered by our insufficient knowledge of the genome and by the lack of high-resolution mapping methods. This situation changed with the completion of the human genome sequence in 2003 and the

 THE HUMAN GENOME PROJECT

The Human Genome Project (HGP) officially began in 1990 and culminated with the deposition of the completed sequence into public databases in 2003. However, in-depth analysis and interpretation will go on for much longer. The HGP was unique in several ways. It was the first global life science project, being coordinated by the Department of Energy and the National Institutes of Health (USA). The Wellcome Trust (UK) became a major partner in 1992, and further significant contributions were made by Japan, France, Germany, China, and other countries. More than 2800 scientists from 20 institutions around the world contributed to the paper describing the finished sequence in 2004. It also was conducted on an industrial scale with industrial-style logistics and organization. In fact, the HGP received competition from Celera Genomics, a private company founded in 1998, and the first draft sequences of the human genome were published in two parallel papers in 2001. The HGP used a 'clone-by-clone' approach where the genome was cloned first and then these large clones were divided into smaller portions and sequenced. Celera followed a fundamentally different strategy, shotgun sequencing, where the whole genome is broken up in small pieces that can be sequenced directly with the full sequence being assembled afterwards. This approach is much faster but less reliable in producing continuous sequences and much less able to mend gaps in the assembled sequence. The DNA used by the HGP was a mixture of numerous donors, whereas Celera pooled the DNA from five individuals. The 2001 draft genomes estimated the existence of 30 000–35 000 genes. The refined HGP 2003 sequence confirmed 19 599 protein-coding genes and identified another 2188 DNA predicted genes, a surprisingly low number. They are contained in 2.85 billion nucleotides covering more than 99% of the euchromatin, i.e. gene-containing DNA. The average length of continuous DNA fragments has increased from 0.8 to 38.5 million nucleotides, which greatly facilitates the mapping of disease genes. There are only 341 gaps compared to the 150 000 in the draft sequence. Moreover, the current sequence is extremely accurate, containing only one error per 100 000 base pairs. The finished sequence is accessible publicly through all major nucleotide databases.

development of novel methods for studying the genome and the transcriptome.

The genome sequencing projects were made possible by the development of high-throughput methods for DNA sequencing (Fig. 36.2) and advanced bio-informatic analysis, especially for the assembly of the sequence data. While the human genome was a major landmark, there are currently close to 3000 genome-sequencing projects ongoing worldwide with more than 600 completed. Almost 2000 are bacterial genome projects, many of them with great relevance for promoting the understanding and treatment of infectious diseases.

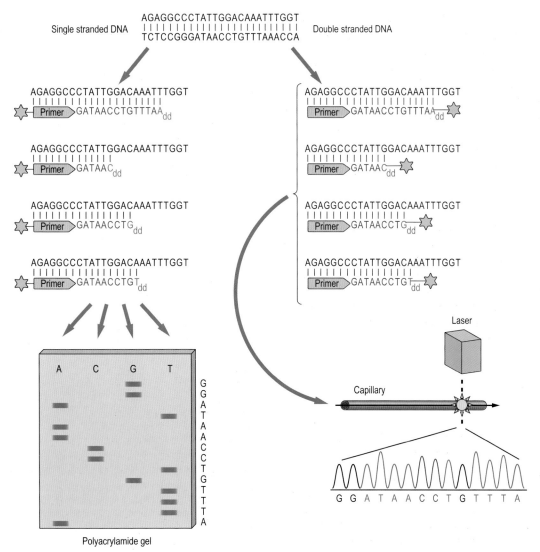

Fig. 36.2 **Principles of DNA sequence analysis by chain termination**. There are three principles of DNA sequencing: one based on chemical cleavage at specific bases (Maxam-Gilbert method); one based on measuring the extension of the complementary strand when one of the four dNTPs is added (pyrosequencing); and one based on synthesizing DNA in the presence of small amounts of chain terminating nucleotides (Sanger method). The latter is the most widely used and described in this figure. Double-stranded DNA is heat-denatured to generate single-stranded DNA. Primers (usually hexamers of random sequence) are annealed to generate random initiation sites for DNA synthesis, which is carried out in the presence of DNA polymerase, deoxynucleotides (dNTPs) and small amounts of dideoxynucleotides (ddNTPs). The ddNTPs lack the 3'-hydroxyl group which is required for DNA strand elongation. They terminate the synthesis leading to fragments of different sizes, each ending a specific nucleotide. These fragments can be separated by polyacrylamide gel electrophoresis and the sequence read from the 'ladder' of fragments on the gel. To visualize the fragments, either the DNA can be labeled by adding in radioactive or fluorescent dNTPs, or the primers can be labeled (as indicated in the figure) with a fluorescent dye. Using ddNTPs labeled with different dyes permits all four reactions being mixed together and separated by capillary electrophoresis. Online laser detection enables direct reading of the sequence. This 'capillary DNA sequencing' gives longer reads than gels, permits multiplexing, and high throughput. It was the method used for much of the human genome sequencing. (Compare Fig. 35.15.)

Karyotyping, comparative genome hybridization (CGH), chromosomal microarray analysis (CMA) and fluorescence in situ hybridization (FISH)

Karyotyping assesses the general chromosomal architecture

Amongst the early successes of exploiting genome information for the diagnosis of human disease was the discovery of trisomy 21 as the cause of Down syndrome in 1959, and the discovery of the Philadelphia chromosome as associated with chronic myelogenous leukemia (CML) in 1960. Since then karyotyping has identified a large number of chromosomal aberrations including amplifications, deletions and translocations, especially in tumors. The method is based on simple staining of chromosome spreads by Giemsa or other dyes which reveal a banding pattern characteristic for each chromosome. Thus, karyotyping assesses the characteristics of chromosomes that are visible through the light microscope.

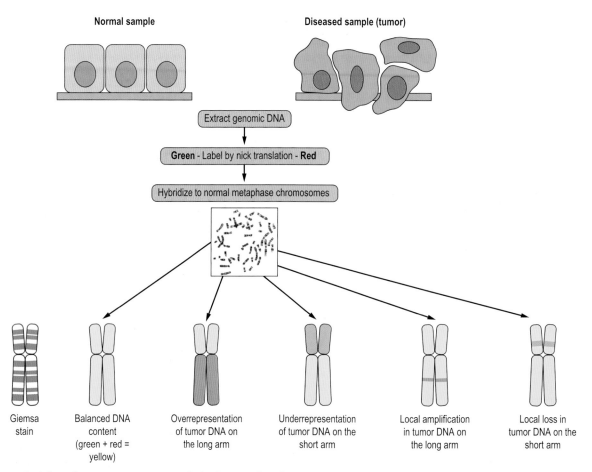

Normal sample   **Diseased sample (tumor)**

Extract genomic DNA

Green - Label by nick translation - **Red**

Hybridize to normal metaphase chromosomes

| Giemsa stain | Balanced DNA content (green + red = yellow) | Overrepresentation of tumor DNA on the long arm | Underrepresentation of tumor DNA on the short arm | Local amplification in tumor DNA on the long arm | Local loss in tumor DNA on the short arm |

Fig. 36.3 **Principles of comparative genome hybridization (CGH)**. Genomic DNA is isolated from a normal and a disease sample (here a tumor) to be compared. The DNA is labeled by nick translation with green or red fluorescent dyes, respectively, and hybridized to a normal chromosome spread. If the DNA content between samples is balanced, equal amounts of the control (green) and tumor (red) DNA will hybridize, resulting in a yellow color. Global or local amplifications or losses of genetic material will reveal themselves by a color imbalance.

Although it only reveals crude information such as number, shapes and gross alterations of general chromosomal architecture, it is still a mainstay of clinical genetic analysis.

Comparative genome hybridization compares two genomes of interest

A refinement of karyotyping is comparative genome hybridization (CGH). The principle of CGH is to compare two genomes of interest, usually a diseased against a normal control genome. The genomes that are to be compared are labeled by nick translation with two different fluorescent dyes. For nick translation, a DNAse is used to introduce breaks or 'nicks' into one DNA strand. The DNA is then incubated with DNA polymerase I, which extends the 3' end of the nick by removing nucleotides and replacing them with new nucleotides. If these carry labels such as radioisotopes or fluorescent dyes, the label becomes incorporated into the newly synthesized DNA. Due to this combination of degradation and resynthesis, the nick translates along the DNA sequence, hence the name for the method. The fluorescently labeled DNAs are then hybridized to a spread of normal chromosomes and evaluated microscopically by quantitative image analysis (Fig. 36.3). As fluorescence has a large dynamic range (i.e. the relationship between fluorescence intensity and concentration of the probe is linear over a wide range), CGH can detect regional gains or losses in chromosomes with much higher accuracy and resolution than conventional karyotyping. Losses of 5–10 megabases (Mb) are detectable by CGH, while the method is even more sensitive at picking up amplifications, which can be less than 1 Mb. Balanced changes, such as inversions or balanced translocations, escape detection as they do not change the copy number and hybridization intensity.

In chromosomal microarray analysis the labeled DNA is hybridized to an array of oligonucleotides

A further dramatic improvement in resolution is afforded by chromosomal microarray analysis (CMA; see Chapter 35). In this method, the labeled DNA is hybridized to an array of

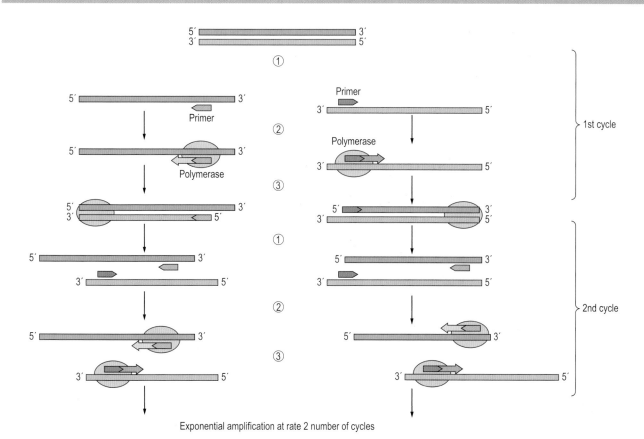

1st cycle

2nd cycle

Exponential amplification at rate 2 number of cycles

Fig. 36.4 **Polymerase chain reaction (PCR)**. This method is widely used for the amplification of DNA and RNA. The nucleic acid template is heat denatured and specific primers are annealed by lowering the temperature (step 1). The primers are extended using reverse transcriptase if the template is RNA or a DNA polymerase if the template is DNA (step 2). The result is a double-stranded product (step 3), which is heat denatured so that the cycle can start again. Typically, between 25 and 35 cycles are used. The amplification is exponential and although, because of technical reasons, the theoretical rate is not reached, PCR enables us to analyze minute amounts of DNA or RNA down to the single cell level. The use of heat-stable and high-fidelity DNA polymerases permits amplification of fragments up to several thousand base pairs long. Many variations of PCR have been developed for a wide range of applications, such as molecular cloning, site-directed mutagenesis, generation of labeled probes for hybridization experiments, quantitation of RNA expression, DNA sequencing, genotyping and many others. (Compare Fig. 35.8.)

oligonucleotides. Modern technologies for oligonucleotide synthesis and array manufacturing can produce arrays that contain several million oligonucleotides on chips the size of a microscopy slide. By choosing the oligonucleotides so that they cover the region of interest equally, a very high resolution can be achieved. The resolution obviously depends on the size of the region or genome, but is in the region of a few kilobases (kb) in the human genome. Thus copy number changes at the level of 5–10 kb can be detected. CMA is increasingly used in prenatal screening for the early detection of chromosomal defects down to the gene level. An advantage is that the probe DNA can be amplified by the polymerase chain reaction (PCR; Fig. 36.4), which allows us to work with minute amounts of starting material. However, it has to be kept in mind that the detection rates of different gene defects can vary greatly, and that these technologies must be very stringently standardized for use in clinical settings in order to minimize detection errors. Notably, neither CGH nor CMA provides information about the ploidy. As long as the DNA content is balanced and carries no further aberrations, a tetraploid genome would be indistinguishable from a diploid genome.

Fluorescence in situ hybridization can be used when the gene in question is known

If the gene of interest is already known and cloned, the recombinant DNA can be labeled and used as a probe on chromosome spreads. This method is called fluorescence in situ hybridization (FISH), and can detect gene amplifications or deletions and chromosomal translocations (see Chapter 35). Using different fluorescent labels, several genes can be stained simultaneously but the information obtained is confined to those genes under direct investigation.

Gene mutations can be studied by sequencing

The availability of cheap, fast and robust DNA sequencing has made possible the large-scale hunt for gene mutations by direct sequencing. There are many such projects on small and large scales ongoing around the world. Notable examples are the Cancer Genome Projects executed by the Wellcome

Trust Sanger Centre in the UK and the USA National Cancer Institute. The systematic sequencing of exons from cancer cell lines and human cancer samples has provided a wealth of information on gene mutations occurring in cancer. The aim of these projects is to establish a systematic map of mutations in cancer and utilize this map for risk stratification, early diagnosis and choice of the best treatment in patients.

Single nucleotide polymorphisms (SNPs) are particularly useful in identification and assessment of disease risk

Genomes in a population vary slightly by small changes, most often just concerning single nucleotides, called single nucleotide polymorphisms (SNPs; see Chapter 35). The systematic mapping of SNPs has proven extremely useful in studying genetic identity and inheritance, but most of all in the identification and risk assessment of genetic diseases. The initial draft sequences of the human genome yielded ca. 2.5 million SNPs with an estimated total number of around 10 million. The International HapMap Project tries to systematically catalog genetic variations based on large-scale SNP analysis in 270 humans of African, Chinese, Japanese and Caucasian origin.

The most common way to examine SNPs is by direct sequencing or array-based methods. For the first method, DNA is usually amplified by PCR and then sequenced. For the second method, oligonucleotide arrays containing all possible permutations of SNPs are probed with genomic DNA, so that successful hybridization only occurs when the DNA sequences match exactly.

Epigenetic changes are heritable traits not reflected in DNA sequence

Although the genome as defined by its DNA sequence is commonly viewed as the hereditary material, there are also other heritable traits that are not reflected by changes in the DNA sequence. These traits are called epigenetic changes (see box on p. 457). They are usually due to modifications that affect chromatin structure such as acetylation, methylation and the attachment of ubiquitin (ubiquitinylation). Another modification is methylation of the DNA itself, which occurs at the N5 position of cytosines, typically in the context of the sequence CpG. Methylation of CpG clusters, so-called CpG islands, in gene promoters can shut down the expression of a gene. These methylation patterns can be heritable by a poorly understood process called genomic imprinting (see Chapter 35). Aberrations in gene methylation patterns can cause diseases and are common in human tumors, often serving to silence the expression of tumor suppressor genes.

Thus, the mapping of promoter methylation patterns has become very important. The most common methods to analyze DNA methylation rely on the fact that bisulfite converts cytosine residues into uracil, but leaves 5-methylcytosine intact (Fig. 36.5). This change in the DNA sequence can be detected by several methods, including DNA sequencing of the treated versus untreated DNA, differential hybridization of oligonucleotides that specifically detect either the mutated or unchanged DNA, or array-based methods. The latter, similar to SNP analysis, also rely on differential hybridization to find bisulfite-induced changes in the DNA but due to the ability to put millions of oligonucleotide probes on an array, are able to interrogate large numbers of methylation patterns simultaneously. The main limitations are that the bisulfite modification may be incomplete, giving rise to false positives, and the severe general DNA degradation that occurs during the harsh conditions of bisulfite modification. In addition, it may be expected that the epigenome is more variable between individuals. Hence it will require a greater effort to determine systematically, but also holds more individual information that can be useful for designing personal medicine approaches.

ChIP-on-chip technique combines chromatin immunoprecipitation with microarray technology

Mapping of the occupancy of transcription factor-binding sites can reveal which genes are likely to be regulated by these factors in a given situation

The information contained in the genome is ultimately executed by the transcription of specific genes. The human genome contains many thousands of binding sites for any given transcription factor, which are short stretches of characteristic DNA sequences usually located in the promoter region of a gene. As gene array experiments (see below) show, only a few hundred of these binding sites actually seem to be used to regulate gene transcription in response to a stimulus. The challenge is to determine when, and under what conditions, a transcription factor can regulate which genes. Transcription factors need to bind to DNA directly or indirectly as part of a multiprotein complex. Thus, the systematic mapping of the occupancy of transcription factor binding sites can reveal which genes are likely to be regulated by these factors in a given situation. The technique developed for that is called ChIP-on-chip or ChIP-chip (Fig. 36.6). It combines chromatin immunoprecipitation (ChIP) with microarray technology (chip).

ChIP involves the covalent crosslinking of proteins to the DNA they are bound to in living cells, usually by formaldehyde treatment of the cells. Then, the DNA is purified and fragmented into small (0.2–1 kb) pieces by ultrasound sonication. These DNA fragments can be isolated by immunoprecipitating the crosslinked protein with a specific antibody. The DNA then is identified by PCR with specific primers that

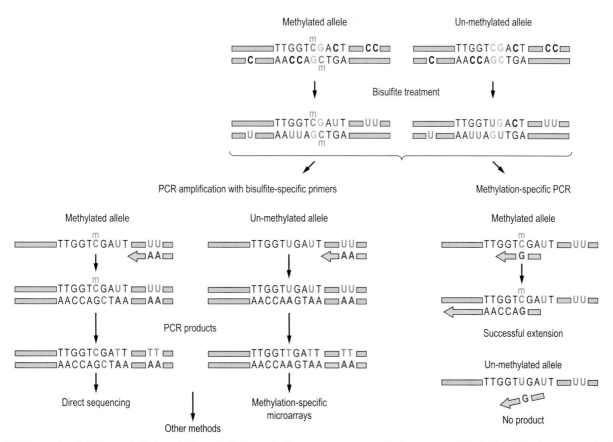

Fig. 36.5 **Analysis of DNA methylation**. DNA methylation typically occurs on cytosine in the context of 'CpG islands' (colored orange) which are enriched in the promoter regions of genes. Bisulfite converts cytosine residues to uracil, but leaves 5-methylcytosine residues unaffected. This causes changes in the DNA sequence that can be detected in various ways. Many methods use a PCR amplification step with primers that will selectively hybridize to the modified DNA (left panel). The PCR products have characteristic sequence changes where the unmodified cytosine-guanosine base pairs are replaced by thymidine-adenosine, whereas the original sequence is maintained when the cytosine was methylated. There are many methods to analyze these PCR products. The most common are direct sequencing or hybridization to a microarray that contains oligonucleotides representing all permutations of the expected changes. Another common method is methylation-specific PCR (MSP) where the primer is designed so that it can only hybridize and extend if the cytosine was methylated and hence preserved during bisulfite treatment.

amplify the DNA region one wants to examine. This method can only test one binding site at a time and therefore requires a hypothesis suggesting which site(s) should be examined. However, the availability of microarrays (chips) that represent the whole or large parts of the genome now permits the use of DNA fragments isolated as probes for the detection of all the regions where the immunoprecipitated protein is bound to in a systematic fashion and on a large scale.

ChIP-on-chip is a powerful and informative technique. An example is the combination of ChIP-on-chip with transcriptomics (see below) where the binding of transcription factors to gene promoters can be directly correlated with the transcription of these genes. However, ChIP-on-chip is not confined to investigating binding sites for transcription factors. It can be used to study any protein that interacts with DNA, and thus is increasingly used to study proteins involved in DNA replication, DNA repair and chromatin modification. Its success is critically dependent on antibodies that possess both very high affinity and specificity, as the amounts of DNA that are co-immunoprecipitated are very small, and

there is no other separation step than the specificity provided by the antibody.

Transcriptomics

Transcriptome represents the complement of RNAs that is transcribed from parts of the genome in a cell, a set of cells or an organism. Differential splicing and alternative promoter usage mean that one gene is estimated to encode an average of 4–6 transcript variants

Usually the term 'transcriptome' refers to the complement of mRNAs, i.e. transcripts that contain protein-coding sequences, but there is increasing evidence for transcription of noncoding parts of the genome which fulfill important structural or regulatory functions. The transcriptome is naturally more dynamic than the genome and may differ widely between different cell types and different conditions. Because of differential splicing and alternative promoter usage, one

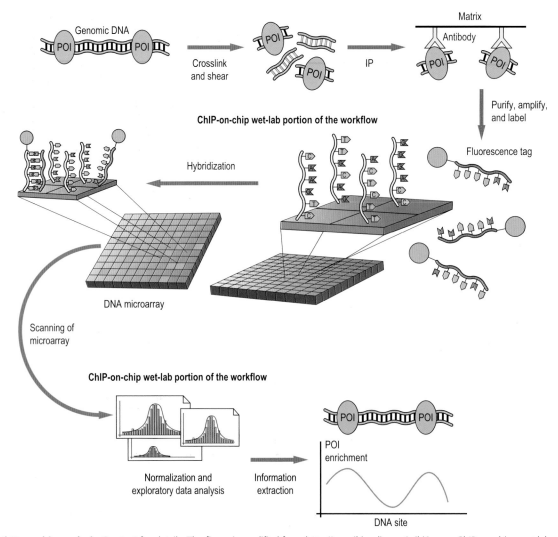

Fig. 36.6 **ChIP-on-chip analysis.** See text for details. The figure is modified from http://en.wikipedia.org/wiki/Image:ChIP-on-chip_wet-lab.png.

gene is estimated to encode an average of 4–6 variants on the transcript level. Hence, the transcriptome is also more complex than the genome. Large-scale transcriptome analysis was enabled by microarrays, and still is one of the first and most successful applications of array technology in the life sciences.

Gene (micro)arrays are tools for studying gene expression

Gene (micro)arrays contain a collection of DNA spots arranged on a solid phase slide in a defined order, with defined shape and distances, and usually at high densities, i.e. up to several millions of spots per array the size of a microscope slide (Fig. 36.7; see also Chapter 35 and box on p. 466). These spots can be cDNAs or synthetic oligonucleotides. Complementary DNA (cDNA) is made from mRNA by reverse transcriptase, an enzyme that uses RNA as a template to synthesize DNA.

As DNA is much more stable and, importantly, can be cloned into plasmids or other vectors for easy propagation and amplification in bacteria, this conversion step enables us to capture the transcribed sequences in the form of cDNA libraries. Such libraries represent a transcriptome, and whole libraries can be deposited as individual clones on a microarray slide. These were the first gene arrays.

However, cDNA arrays require that each clone is fully sequenced, propagated separately, and that each cDNA is individually isolated. Thus, they are increasingly replaced by arrays that use synthetic oligonucleotides, which can be either prefabricated and deposited on the chip or synthesized directly on the chip surface. Usually several oligonucleotide probes are used per gene. The versatility and the high quality of oligonucleotide synthesis have made oligonucleotide-based arrays standard tools in academia and industry. They are offered by several commercial vendors as part of robust assay platforms. The approaches are still evolving and currently differ mainly regarding the lengths of the oligonucleotides and the number

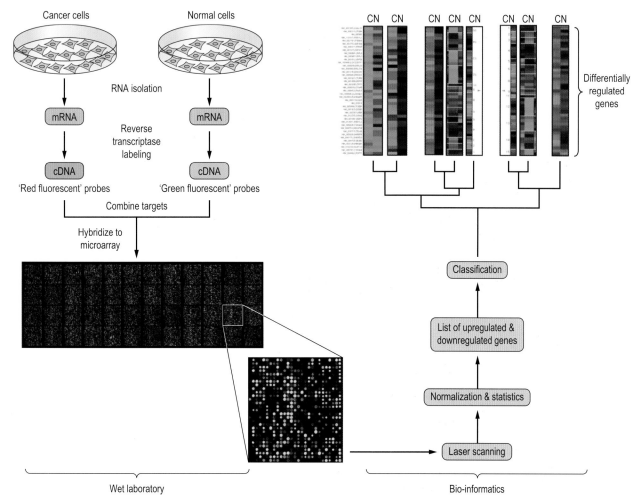

Fig. 36.7 **The workflow of a gene (micro)array experiment.** A two-color array experiment comparing normal and cancer cells is shown as an example. See text for details. A common way to display results is heatmaps, where increasing intensities of reds and greens indicate up- and downregulated genes, respectively, while black means no change. C, cancer cells; N, normal cells. The figure is modified from http://en.wikipedia.org/wiki/DNA_microarray.

per gene. Longer oligonucleotides provide better specificity and require fewer sequences per gene. Shorter oligonucleotides require more sequences per gene but are easier to manufacture and also enhance the chance of discriminating splice variants.

With enormous improvements in the density of array points, new versions of gene arrays can be designed to deliberately map exon content and splice variants. Further progress in the functional diversification of arrays is to be expected. For instance, noncoding RNAs such as siRNAs and microRNAs have recently attracted attention and are being included into arrays. This will result in a much better resolution of transcriptional changes and hopefully a better understanding of the mechanisms that cause them.

The arrays are hybridized with cDNA or cRNAs prepared from two samples that are to be compared. They are usually labeled with fluorescent dyes. For two-color detection, the samples to be compared are labeled with two different dyes, mixed and hybridized to one array. This gives information

on the relative expression of individual genes. In one-color detection, both samples are labeled with the same dye and hybridized to two copies of the same array. To facilitate comparison, the samples are often spiked with control cDNAs that allow normalization and comparison between the two arrays. This method gives absolute quantification of gene expression. It requires more chips but facilitates comparison of different arrays. For both methods, extensive bio-informatics analysis is required for normalization, i.e. reduction of errors caused by inhomogeneous hybridization across the chip and other technical variations. Additionally, there is the issue of classification of the samples identifying coregulated genes and the comparison between different experiments.

The analysis of gene array experiments is very bio-informatics intensive and also requires stringent statistical analysis. A common convention for reporting microarray experiments was introduced called minimal information for the annotation of microarray experiments (MIAME). However, the big challenge remains to go beyond classification and deduce functional information. There are many approaches but little consensus about the best method. The goal is to deduce functional information about how the changes in gene expression are generated and how they relate to biologic phenotypes. There is much more work ahead of us.

PROTEOMICS

Proteomics is the study of the protein complement of a cell, the protein equivalent of the transcriptome or genome.

The word 'proteome' was coined by Marc Wilkins in a talk in Sienna in 1994, and appeared in print for the first time in 1995. Wilkins defined the proteome as the protein complement of a cell, the protein equivalent of the transcriptome or genome. Since that time the study of the proteome, called proteomics, has evolved into a number of different themes encompassing many areas of protein science.

Proteomics is possibly the most complex of all the postgenomic sciences but is also likely to be the most informative, since proteins are the functional entities in the cell, and virtually no biologic process takes place without the intervention of a protein. Among their many roles, they are responsible for the structural organization of the cell, as they make up the cytoskeleton, the control of membrane transport (Chapter 8) and energy generation. Hence, an understanding of the proteome will be necessary to understand how biology works.

Initially, proteomics concentrated on cataloguing the proteins contained in an organelle, cell, tissue or organism, in the process validating the existence of the predicted genes in the genome. This rapidly evolved into comparative proteomics, where the protein profiles from two or more samples were compared to identify quantitative differences that could be responsible for the observed phenotype, for example from diseased versus healthy cells or looking at changes induced by drug treatment. Now proteomics also includes the study of posttranslational modifications of individual proteins, the make-up and dynamics of protein complexes, the mapping of networks of interactions between proteins, and the identification of biomarkers in disease.

Proteomics poses several challenges

It quickly became apparent that the complexity of the proteome would be a major obstacle to achieving Wilkins' initial ideal of looking at all the proteins in a cell or organism at the same time. While the number of genes in an organism is not overwhelming, the posttranslational modifications (PTMs) of proteins in eukaryotic systems, such as alternate splicing and

POSTTRANSLATIONAL MODIFICATIONS

During the process of transcription, translation and in the functioning of the cell, proteins can undergo a range of modifications. During transcription, introns are spliced out of the gene, and different splicing of the gene can result in a number of different mRNA being produced, and hence a number of proteins that differ markedly in their sequence can emerge from the same gene. After translation of the mRNA into protein, the protein can be 'decorated' with a bewildering array of additional chemical groups covalently attached to it, most of which are necessary for the activity of the protein. Some examples are given below:

- The addition of fatty acids to cysteine residues, which anchor the protein to a membrane.
- Glycosylation: the addition of complex oligosaccharides to an asparagine or serine residue, which is common in membrane proteins which have an extracellular component or are secreted. Many proteins involved in cell–cell recognition events are glycosylated, as are antibodies.
- Phosphorylation: the addition of a phosphate group to serine, threonine, tyrosine or histidine residues. This is a modification that can be added or removed, allowing the system to respond very rapidly to a changing environment. It is fundamental to signaling events in the cell. It has been estimated that one-third of all eukaryotic proteins may undergo reversible phosphorylation.
- Ubiquitination: the addition of a polyubiquitin chain that targets the protein for destruction by the proteasome. Ubiquitin is itself a small protein.
- Formation of disulfide bridges between cysteine residues in the polypeptide backbone which are close together in space once the protein is folded. These play a number of roles including adding additional structural stability, especially for exported proteins, and sense the redox balance in the cell.
- Acetylation of residues, most commonly the N-terminus of the protein or lysine. Acetylation of lysines on histones plays an important role in the gene transcription process, and drugs that target the proteins that acetylate or deacetylate histone are potential cancer therapeutics.
- Proteolytic cleavage: most proteins have the N-terminal methionine that results from the ATG initiation codon of gene translation removed. In some proteins, cleavage of the polypeptide chain occurs, such as in the activation of zymogens in the clotting cascade, or significant parts of the initial polypeptide chain are removed completely, for example in the conversion of proinsulin into insulin.

the potential addition of over 40 different covalently attached chemical groups (including the well-known examples of phosphorylation and glycosylation), mean that there may be 10 or, in extreme cases, 1000 different protein species, all fairly similar, generated from each gene, and that the predicted 22 000 genes in the human genome could give rise to 500 000 or more individual protein species in the cell. In addition, there is a wide range of protein abundance in the cell, estimated to range from less than 10 to 500 000 or more molecules per cell, and a protein's function may depend on its abundance, post-translational modifications, localization in the cell, and association with other proteins, and these may all change in fraction of a second! There is no protein equivalent of PCR that would allow for the amplification of nucleic acid sequences, so we are limited to the amount of protein that can be isolated from the sample. If the sample is small, a needle biopsy, a rare cell type, an isolated signaling complex, and ultrasensitive methods are needed to detect and analyze the proteins.

It is clear that proteomics is an extremely challenging undertaking. It is only since the introduction of new methods in mass spectrometry in the mid 1990s that an attempt could be made to analyze the proteome and new, higher-throughput and high-data content methods are being continually developed.

Proteomics in medicine

Despite the challenges, proteomics has been a vital tool in understanding fundamental biologic processes and will remain important in the armoury of scientific research. One advantage of the proteomics approach is that it is possible to discover new information about a biologic problem without having to have a clear understanding in advance of what might change. There are often more data generated from a good proteomics experiment than it is reasonable, or possible, to follow up. Proteomics has been applied successfully to the study of basic biochemical changes in many different types of biologic sample: cells, tissues, plasma, urine, CSF and even interstitial fluid collected by microdialysis. In cells isolated from cell culture, it is possible to ask complex fundamental biologic questions. Deciphering the mitogenic signaling cascades, which involve specific association of proteins in multiprotein complexes, and understanding how these can go wrong in cancer is one widely studied area. It is possible to gain information from biological fluids on the overall status of an organism because, for example, blood would have been in contact with every part of a body. Diseases at specific locations may eventually show up as changes in the protein content of the blood, as leakage from the damaged tissue occurs. This area is now often described as biomarker discovery. Tissues are a more of a challenge. The heterogeneity of many tissues makes it difficult to compare tissue biopsies which may contain differing amounts of connective tissue, vasculature, etc. Improvements in the sensitivity are overcoming this problem by allowing small amounts of material recovered from laser capture microdissection or flow cytometry to be used for the analysis. Ultimately, it would be valuable to analyze individual cells. Current approaches average out changes in the analyzed sample: thus a recorded 50% change in the level of a protein could be 50% in all the cells, or 100% in 50% of the cells in the sample.

Main methods used in proteomics

Proteomics relies fundamentally on the separation of a complex mixture of proteins or peptides, quantification of protein abundances, and identification of the proteins.

Strategies to reduce the number of proteins being analyzed while still retaining the essential information are also important, such as isolation of individual organelles or immunoprecipitation of protein complexes. A range of physicochemical properties of proteins (size, charge, hydrophobicity, etc.) adds to the complexity of the analysis, but also offers the means of separating out the complex mixtures. Separation can be achieved in many ways, but the mainstays for proteomics are polyacrylamide gel electrophoresis (PAGE), mainly two-dimensional PAGE (2DE, 2D-PAGE), and liquid chromatography, while the main method for identifying proteins is mass spectrometry. Quantification strategies depend on the techniques used, but mostly rely on staining gels with quantitative protein stains or the addition of fluorescent or isotopic tags to the proteins.

Two-dimensional gel electrophoresis (2DE)

This has been used in the study of proteins for many years but is still one of the key techniques for proteomics.

In 2DE, proteins are separated in the first dimension by differences in their isoelectric point (pI), corresponding to the pH at which a protein has no net charge. Most commonly, this is performed on strips of polyacrylamide gel mounted on a plastic backing, with a pH gradient immobilized in them. Proteins are loaded onto the strip and then a voltage is applied. Proteins at places in the pH gradient where the pH is above their pI will have a net negative charge and will move towards the cathode (the positive electrode), and those below will have a net positive charge and move towards the anode (the negative electrode). The proteins will continue to move until they reach the point in the strip where the pH is such that the positive and negative charges on the protein molecules are balanced and they have no net charge, where they will stop. The protein will over time then become concentrated at this point in the strip of gel. The strip is then placed on top of a larger slab of gel and the proteins separated in the second dimension by size, using the polyacrylamide gel as a sieve that allows smaller molecules to pass through more easily than larger ones. In order to visualize the proteins on the gel, they can be stained with a protein-specific dye, commonly Coomassie blue, or a fluorescent dye such as Sypro Ruby. Proteins show up as discrete spots on the gel, the intensity of the staining relating directly to the amount of protein present. It is usually possible to see 1500–2500 spots on a single gel. Comparison of gels from different samples run under near-identical conditions can then be used to identify the differences at the protein level (Fig. 36.8). A number of replicates is needed to differentiate general biologic variation

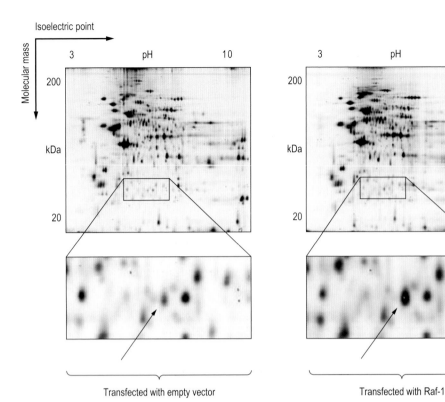

Isoelectric point

Molecular mass

Transfected with empty vector

Transfected with Raf-1

Fig. 36.8 **2D-gel electrophoresis**. Raf-1 knock-out cells were either transfected with empty vector or an expression vector for Raf-1. Cell lysates were analyzed by 2D-gel electrophoresis. The gels look very similar on first inspection, but detailed comparison shows a number of proteins that change in abundance in the cell. The spot highlighted by the arrow was cut out of the gel, the protein digested with trypsin and identified as peroxiredoxin 4 by mass spectrometry.

in the samples from real differences that are a result of the different states.

The proteins in the spots can then be identified by cutting the spots out of the gel and digesting the protein with a specific protease, usually trypsin, which cleaves at every lysine and arginine in the sequence (except where the next residue is a proline). This gives rise to a number of peptide fragments that will be unique to that protein. The molecular masses of the fragments can be measured using mass spectrometry, often referred to as the 'peptide mass fingerprint', and these experimental data compared to the data generated by taking the genome of the organism and performing an equivalent theoretical enzymatic digest. The quality of the match can be described statistically, and the probability of the identification calculated. This leads to the most likely identification of the protein (Fig. 36.9). Note that it is very difficult to identify all the proteins using this approach. The mixture of peptides can also be examined in more detail using liquid chromatography coupled to tandem mass spectrometry.

Mass spectrometry

Mass spectrometry is a technique used to determine the molecular masses of molecules in a sample. It can also be used to select an individual component from the mixture, break up its chemical structure and measure the masses of the fragments, which can then be used to determine the structure of the molecule. There are many different types of

mass spectrometers available, but the underlying principles of mass spectrometry are relatively simple. The first step in the process is to generate charged molecules, ions, from the molecules in the sample. This is relatively easily achieved for many soluble biomolecules because their polar chemistry provides groups that are easily charged. For example, the addition of a proton (H^+) to the side chain groups on the basic amino acids lysine and arginine gives a positively charged molecule. When a charged molecule is placed in an electric field, it will be repelled by an electrode of like sign and attracted by an electrode of opposite sign, accelerating the molecule towards the electrode of opposite charge. Since the force is equal for all molecules, larger molecules will accelerate less than small molecules (force = mass × acceleration), so small molecules will end up with a higher velocity. This is utilized to determine the mass. For example, after the molecules have been accelerated, the time then taken for them to travel a certain distance can be measured and related to the mass. This is called time-of-flight mass spectrometry.

A tandem mass spectrometer is effectively two mass spectrometric analyzers joined together sequentially, with an area between them, allowing molecules to be fragmented. The first analyzer is used to select one of the molecules from a mixture based on its molecular mass, which is then broken up into smaller parts, usually by collision with a small amount of gas in the intermediate region (called the collision cell). The fragments that are generated are then analyzed in the second mass spectrometer (Fig. 36.10). Fortunately, peptides tend to fragment at the peptide bond,

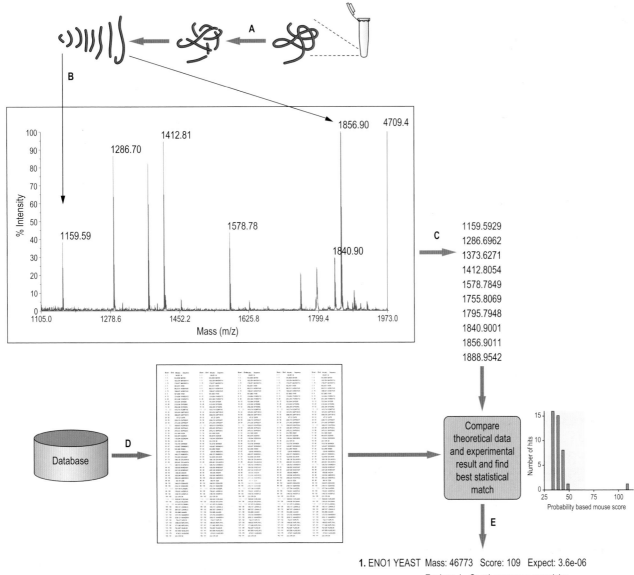

Fig. 36.9 **Protein identification by peptide mass fingerprinting (PMF)**. Shown is a typical workflow: (A) the sample is digested with a specific protease, usually trypsin, to give a set of smaller peptides which will be unique to the protein; (B) the mass of a subset of the resulting peptides is measured using mass spectrometry; (C) a list of the observed experimental masses is generated from the mass spectrum; (D) a database of protein sequences is digested theoretically in silico and a set of tables of the expected peptides generated; (E) the experimental data are compared to the theoretical digested database and a statistical score of the fit of the experimental to theoretical data is generated, giving a 'confidence' score, which indicates the likelihood of correct identification.

resulting in a spectrum that has peaks separated by the mass of the amino acid in the corresponding sequence, allowing this approach to be used to obtain sequence-related information on the peptides.

Liquid chromatography can be coupled to mass spectrometry

Liquid chromatography is an alternative method to 2DE. It separates complex mixtures on the basis of many different physicochemical properties, most commonly in proteomics the charge on the molecule and its hydrophobicity, using ion exchange chromatography or reversed phase chromatography respectively. This is achieved by having chemical groups attached to a particulate resin packed into a column and flowing a solution over this. Molecules will bind to the resin (the stationary phase) with differing affinities. Those with a high affinity will take longer to traverse the length of the column and hence will elute from the column at a later time. Molecules are therefore separated in time in the flow that

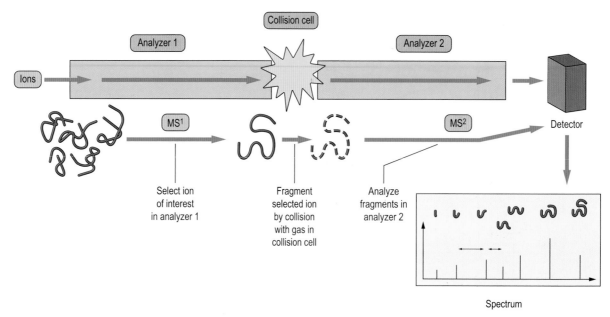

Fig. 36.10 **The basic principles of tandem mass spectrometry.** See text for details.

comes out of the column. The outlet of the chromatography system can be coupled directly to the mass spectrometer, so that the molecules eluting from the column can be monitored in real time.

Shotgun proteomics is an alternative to two-dimensional gel electrophoresis

J R Yates II developed an alternative to 2DE, which he called a multidimensional protein identification technology (MuDPIT), but methods of this type commonly go by the name of 'shotgun' analysis. In this method, the total protein content of the sample is first digested with a specific protease to break it up into peptides, and the peptides are then separated and identified by multidimensional liquid chromatography coupled to tandem mass spectrometry (Fig. 36.11). While the peptides from a protein may be spread throughout the sample, the generation of sequence data by tandem mass spectrometry allows for the identification of the proteins. The approach is made quantitative in a number of ways. If possible, samples can be grown in a selective medium that provides an essential amino acid. This can then be provided in the natural form (the 'light' form) or isotopically labeled with a stable isotope (for example, ^{13}C or ^{2}H, the 'heavy' form) that makes all of the peptides containing this amino acid appear heavier in the mass spectrometer. This is called the SILAC (stable isotope labeling with amino acids in cell culture) method. The samples are mixed together and analyzed using the shotgun approach. The ratios of 'heavy' to the equivalent 'light' peptides are used to determine the relative quantities of the protein from which they were derived.

Alternative methods include chemically reacting the proteins in the sample (using, for example, the isotope coded affinity tags, ICAT), or the peptides after digestion of the sample (e.g. in iTRAQ), with a 'light' or equivalent isotopically labeled 'heavy' chemical reagent, then mixing the samples and analyzing them as for the SILAC approach. The advantage of this methodology is that the analysis is easily automated and that approaches can be used to get information on proteins that do not work well in the 2DE approach, such as membrane proteins, small proteins and proteins with extreme pIs (e.g. histones). The disadvantage is that information on posttranslational modifications is usually lost, and digesting the sample generates a much more complex sample for the separation step.

METABOLOMICS

Metabolites are the small chemical molecules, such as sugars, amino acids, lipids and nucleotides, present in a biologic sample. The study of the metabolite complement of a sample is called metabolomics, while the quantitative measurement of the dynamic changes in the levels of metabolites as a result of a stimulus or other change is often referred to as metabonomics. The words metabolomics and metabonomics are often used interchangeably, although purists will claim that while both involve the multiparametric measurement of metabolites, metabonomics is dedicated to the analysis of dynamic changes of metabolite levels, whereas metabolomics focuses on identifying and quantifying the steady-state levels of intracellular metabolites. Metabolomics is the most commonly used generic term.

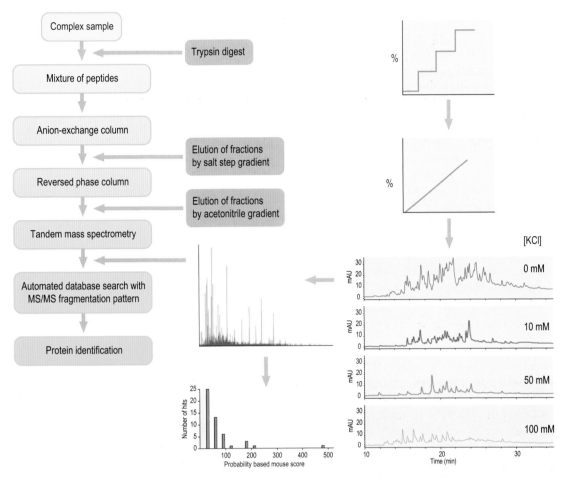

Fig. 36.11 **The 'shotgun' approach**. Illustrated is two-dimensional liquid chromatography, using a step gradient to elute individual fractions from the first dimension that are then separated in the second dimension. Direct coupling to tandem mass spectrometry allows the proteins to be identified. (Compare box on p. 16 and Fig. 2.15.)

Metabolomics gives another level of information on a biologic system. It provides information on the results of the activity of enzymes, which may not depend on the abundance of the protein alone, as this may be modulated by supply of substrates, the concentration of cofactors or products, and effect of other small molecules or proteins that modulate the activity of the enzyme (effectors). In some ways, metabolomics may be easier than proteomics. In the metabolome, there is an amplification of any changes that occur in the proteome, as the enzymes will turn over many substrate molecules for each molecule of enzyme. The methods used to look for a metabolite in each organism will be the same; as the metabolite will be identical, unlike proteins which are likely to have different sequences between organisms, the networks are more constrained, making them easier to follow, and the analysis can be done at a significantly higher throughput than proteomics. In 2007, the Human Metabolome Project released the first draft of the human metabolome consisting of 2500 metabolites, 3500 food components and 1200 drugs.

The most commonly used methods for investigating metabolites are mass spectrometry, often coupled to liquid chromatography, as used in proteomics, and nuclear magnetic resonance (NMR) spectroscopy. Identification of signals corresponding to specific metabolites can then be used to quantify these metabolites in a complex sample, and see how they change. Metabolomics can be broken down in to a number of areas.

- **Metabolic fingerprinting:** taking a 'snapshot' of the metabolome of a system, generating a set of values for the intensity of a signal from a species, without necessarily knowing what that species is. Often there is no chromatographic separation of species. It is used for biomarker discovery.
- **Metabolite profiling:** generating a set of quantitative data on a number of metabolites, usually of known identity, over a range of conditions or times. It is used for metabolomics, metabonomics and systems biology and biomarker discovery.
- **Metabolite target analysis:** the measurement of the concentration of a specific metabolite or small set of metabolites over a range of conditions or times.

Biomarkers

Biomarkers are markers that can be used in medicine for the early detection, diagnosis, staging or prognosis of disease, or for determination of the most effective therapy

A biomarker is generally defined as a marker that is specific for a particular state of a biologic system. The markers may be metabolites, peptides, proteins or any other biologic molecule, or measurements of physical properties, e.g. blood pressure. The importance of biomarkers is rapidly increasing because the trend to personalized medicine will be impossible to sustain without a detailed and objective characterization of the patients afforded by biomarkers. Biomarkers can arise from the disease process itself or from the reaction of the body to the disease. Thus, they can be found in body fluids and tissues. For ease of sample sourcing and patient compliance, most biomarker studies use urine or plasma, although saliva, interstitial fluid, nipple duct aspirates, and cerebrospinal fluid also have been used.

The most common methods for biomarker discovery have developed from those used in transcriptomics, proteomics and metabolomics, i.e. gene arrays, mass spectrometry, often coupled to chromatography, and NMR spectroscopy. Biomarker discovery is often done on small patient cohorts but, to be clinically useful, a robust statistical analysis of a large number of samples from healthy and sick individuals in well-controlled studies is required. Improvements in methods for statistical analysis coupled to detection methods that can differentiate hundreds to tens of thousands individual components in the complex sample have improved the selectivity to the level where these aims are achievable. It is usually necessary to define a number of markers that are specific for a given disease in order to achieve selectivity rather than just detecting a general systemic response such as the inflammatory response or a closely related disease. In theory, it is not necessary to actually identify what the biomarker is, although doing so may give insight into the underlying biochemistry of the disease, and many regulatory authorities demand that the markers are identified before a method can be licensed. It may also allow subsequent development of cheaper and higher throughput assays.

Some well-known examples of biomarkers are the measurement of blood glucose levels in diabetes, prostate-specific antigen for prostate cancer, and HER-2 or BRCA1/2 genes in breast cancer. Biomarker research can also elucidate disease mechanisms and further markers or potential drug targets. For example, using a 2DE approach to determine which DNA repair pathways had been lost in breast cancer led to the discovery that cancers deficient in the BRCA-1/2 genes are sensitive to the inhibition of another DNA repair protein, PARP-1. Inhibitors of PARP-1 are showing promise in clinical trials for the treatment of BRCA-1/2 deficient tumors.

Summary

- The -omics approaches hold a huge potential for the risk assessment, early detection, diagnosis, stratification and tailored treatment of human diseases.
- The -omics technologies are being introduced into clinical practice, with genomics and transcriptomics leading the way. This is mainly because DNA and RNA have defined physicochemical properties that are amenable for amplification and the design of robust assay platforms compatible with the routines of clinical laboratories. For instance, PCR is routinely used to establish paternity and in forensic medicine to determine the identity of DNA samples left at the crime scene. Genetic tests for the diagnosis of inherited diseases are in place.
- Transcriptomic-based microarray tests for breast cancer have been approved, and similar tests for other diseases will soon become available.
- Proteomics and metabolomics require specialist equipment and expertise, which are difficult to put into the routine clinical laboratory. However, their information content exceeds that of genomics and with further progress in technology, their clinical application will become reality.
- The benefits of -omics technologies are obvious, mainly in risk assessment and the design of personalized treatments. However, there are also huge ethical implications pertaining to the use of this information, and new regulatory guidelines will be needed.

NUCLEAR MAGNETIC RESONANCE SPECTROSCOPY

Nuclear magnetic resonance (NMR) spectroscopy gives useful structural information on molecules that can be used to identify them. Atomic nuclei behave like small magnets, so when they are put in a strong magnetic field they align with the field. Application of an appropriate energy (radiofrequency electromagnetic radiation) causes the nuclei to flip and align against the field. They then return to their ground state once the irradiation is turned off by flipping back, and as they do so they emit specific frequencies of radiation. These can be recorded and plotted. Each nucleus in a molecule that has a unique environment will emit a unique frequency, and nuclei bonded together or close together in space will interact with adjacent nuclei (coupling), and this can also be measured. This rich information on the molecule allows the structural elements to be determined, and the amplitude of the signals can be used to reasonably accurately quantify the amount of material. This is very useful in metabolomics. The main limitation is that the NMR spectrum quickly becomes congested with information from a complex sample, so high resolution (coming from very strong magnetic fields) is required, and the technique is relatively insensitive, having a limit of detection 3–4 orders of magnitude worse than mass spectrometry.

ACTIVE LEARNING

1. Why does the information increase when moving from studying genes to studying proteins?
2. Why do genomics and proteomics need fundamentally different technologies?
3. Why can proteomics and metabolomics use similar technologies?
4. What is a biomarker, why are biomarkers important, and what are their potential applications?

Further reading

Carrette O, Burkhard PR, Sanchez JC, Hochstrasser DF. State-of-the-art two-dimensional gel electrophoresis: a key tool of proteomics research. *Nat Protocols* 2006;**1**:812–823.

Chapman EJ, Carrington JC. Specialization and evolution of endogenous small RNA pathways. *Nat Rev Genet* 2007;**8**:884–896.

Dettmer K, Aronov PA, Hammock BD. Mass spectrometry-based metabolomics. *Mass Spectrom Rev* 2007;**26**:51–78.

Fenselau C. A review of quantitative methods for proteomic studies. *J Chromatograph B-Analyt Technol Biomed Life Sci* 2007;**855**:14–20.

Hollywood K, Brison DR, Goodacre R. Metabolomics: current technologies and future trends. *Proteomics* 2006;**6**:4716–4723.

International Human Genome Sequencing Consortium. Finishing the euchromatic sequence of the human genome. *Nature* 2004;**431**:931–945

Jordan KW, Cheng LL. NMR-based metabolomics approach to target biomarkers for human prostate cancer. *Exp Rev Proteomics* 2007;**4**:389–400.

Kolch W, Mischak H, Pitt AR. The molecular make-up of a tumour: proteomics in cancer research. *Clin Sci (Lond)* 2005;**108**:369–383.

McDonald WH, Ohi R, Miyamoto DT et al. Comparison of three directly coupled HPLC MS/MS strategies for identification of proteins from complex mixtures: single-dimension LC-MS/MS, 2-phase MudPIT, and 3-phase MudPIT. *Int J Mass Spectrom* 2002;**219**:245–251.

O'Connor M. Novel biomarkers for DNA damage response pathways: insights and applications for cancer therapy. *Proteomics* 2006; **6**(suppl2): 69–71.

Wasinger VC, Cordwell SJ, Cerpa-Poljak A et al. Progress with gene-product mapping of the Mollicutes: Mycoplasma genitalium. *Electrophoresis* 1995;**16**: 1090–1094.

Websites

Human Metabolome Project: www.metabolomics.ca/

International HapMap Project: www.hapmap.org/

Online Mendelian Inheritance in Man: www.ncbi.nlm.nih.gov/sites/entrez?db=OMIM

MIAME: www.mged.org/Workgroups/MIAME/miame.html

USA National Cancer Institute: www.cancer.gov/cancertopics/understandingcancer/CGAP

Wellcome Trust Sanger Centre (UK): www.sanger.ac.uk/genetics/CGP/Studies/

37. Oxygen and Life

J W Baynes

LEARNING OBJECTIVES

After reading this chapter you should be able to:

- Identify the major reactive oxygen species (ROS) and their sources in the cell.
- Identify targets of reactive oxygen damage and describe the effects of ROS on biomolecules.
- Identify the major antioxidant enzymes, vitamins, and biomolecules that provide protection against ROS.
- Describe the role of reactive oxygen in regulatory biology and immunologic defenses.
- Explain the role of ROS in development of chronic and inflammatory diseases.

INTRODUCTION

The element oxygen (O_2) is essential for the life of aerobic organisms (Chapter 5). Although it is highly reactive in combustion reactions at high temperature, oxygen is relatively inert at body temperature; it has a high activation energy for oxidation reactions. This is fortunate, otherwise we might spontaneously combust. About 90% of our O_2 usage is committed to oxidative phosphorylation. Enzymes that use O_2 for hydroxylation and oxygenation reactions consume another 10%, and a residual fraction, <1%, is converted to reactive oxygen species (ROS), such as superoxide and hydrogen peroxide, which are reactive forms of oxygen. ROS are important in metabolism – some enzymes use H_2O_2 as a substrate. ROS also play a role in regulation of metabolism and in immunologic defenses against infection. However, ROS are also a source of chronic damage to tissue biomolecules. One of the risks of harnessing O_2 as a substrate for energy metabolism is that we may, and do, get burned. For this reason, we have a range of antioxidant defenses that protect us against ROS.

This chapter will deal with the biochemistry of reactive oxygen, the mechanisms of formation and detoxification of ROS, and their role in human health and disease.

THE INERTNESS OF OXYGEN

In most textbooks, oxygen is shown as a diatomic molecule with two bonds between the oxygen atoms. This is an attractive presentation from the viewpoint of electron dot structures and electron pairing to form chemical bonds, but it is incorrect. In fact, at body temperature, O_2 is a biradical, a molecule with two unpaired electrons (Fig. 37.1). These electrons have parallel spins and are unpaired. Since most organic oxidation reactions, e.g. the oxidation of an alkane

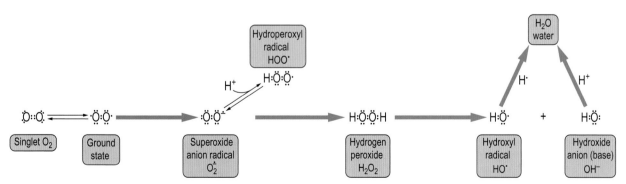

Fig. 37.1 **Structure of oxygen and reactive oxygen species (ROS).** Oxygen is shown at the far left as the incorrect double-bonded diatomic form. This form, known as singlet oxygen, exists to a significant extent only at high temperature or in response to irradiation. The diradical is the natural, ground-state form of O_2 at body temperature. ROS are partially reduced, reactive forms of oxygen. The first reduction product is the anion radical, superoxide ($O_2^{\bullet-}$), which is in equilibrium with the weak acid, hydroperoxyl radical (pKa ~4.5). Reduction of superoxide yields hydroperoxide O_2^{-2}, in the form of H_2O_2. Reduction of H_2O_2 causes a hemolytic cleavage reaction that releases hydroxyl radical (OH$^{\bullet}$) and hydroxide ion (OH^{-}). Water is the endproduct of complete reduction of O_2.

to an alcohol or an aldehyde to an acid, are two-electron oxidation reactions, O_2 is generally not very reactive in these reactions. In fact, it is completely stable, even in the presence of a strong reducing agent such as H_2. When enough heat (activation energy) is applied, one of the unpaired electrons flips to form an electron pair, which then participates in the combustion reaction. Once started, the combustion provides the heat needed to propagate the reaction, sometimes explosively.

Metabolic reactions are conducted at body temperature, far below the temperature required to activate free oxygen. In biologic redox reactions involving O_2, the oxygen is always activated by redox active metal ions, such as iron and copper; these metals also have unpaired electrons and form reactive metal-oxo complexes. All enzymes that use O_2 in vivo are metalloenzymes and, in fact, even the oxygen transport proteins, hemoglobin and myoglobin, contain iron in the form of heme (Chapter 5). These metal ions provide one electron at a time to oxygen, activating O_2 for metabolism. Because iron and copper, and sometimes manganese and other ions, activate oxygen, these redox-active metal ions are kept at very low (sub-micromolar) free concentrations in vivo. Normally, they are tightly sequestered (compartmentalized) in inactive form in storage or transport proteins, and they are locally activated at the active sites of enzymes where oxidation chemistry can be contained and focused on a specific substrate. Free redox-active metal ions are dangerous in biologic systems because, in free form, they activate O_2, and ROS cause oxidative damage to biomolecules. Damage to proteins is often site specific, occurring at sites of metal binding to proteins, suggesting that metal-oxo complexes participate in ROS-mediated damage in vivo.

REACTIVE OXYGEN SPECIES AND OXIDATIVE STRESS

ROS are reactive, strongly oxidizing forms of oxygen

Oxidative stress (OxS) is defined as a condition in which the rate of generation of ROS exceeds our ability to protect ourselves against them, resulting in an increase in oxidative damage to biomolecules (Fig. 37.2). OxS is a characteristic feature of inflammatory diseases in which cells of the immune system produce ROS in response to challenge. OxS may be localized, for instance in the joints in arthritis or in the vascular wall in atherosclerosis, or can be systemic, e.g. in systemic lupus erythematosus (SLE) or diabetes.

Among the ROS, H_2O_2 is present at highest concentration in blood and tissues, albeit at micromolar or lower concentrations. H_2O_2 is relatively stable; it can be stored in the laboratory or medicine cabinet for years but decomposes in the presence of redox-active metal ions. The hydroxyl radical (OH•) is the most reactive and damaging species; its half-life, measured in nanoseconds, is diffusion limited, i.e. determined by the time to collision with a target biomolecule. Superoxide ($O_2^{•-}$) is intermediate in stability and may actually serve as either an oxidizing or reducing agent,

IRON OVERLOAD INCREASES RISK FOR DIABETES AND CARDIOMYOPATHY

Patients with hematologic disorders such as hereditary hemochromatosis, thalassemias and sickle cell disease, or who receive frequent blood transfusions, gradually develop iron overload, a condition that increases the risk for development of cardiomyopathy and diabetes. The heart and β-cells are rich in mitochondria. The development of secondary disease in iron overload is considered the result of iron-mediated enhancement of mitochondrial ROS production in these tissues. Mutations in the mitochondrial genome may lead to progressive mitochondrial dysfunction, compromising cardiac and β-cell function. See box on page 300.

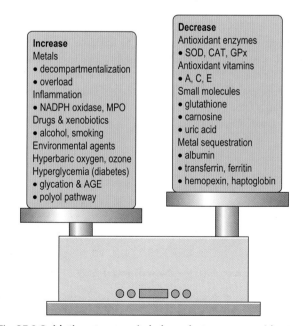

Increase
Metals
• decompartmentalization
• overload
Inflammation
• NADPH oxidase, MPO
Drugs & xenobiotics
• alcohol, smoking
Environmental agents
Hyperbaric oxygen, ozone
Hyperglycemia (diabetes)
• glycation & AGE
• polyol pathway

Decrease
Antioxidant enzymes
• SOD, CAT, GPx
Antioxidant vitamins
• A, C, E
Small molecules
• glutathione
• carnosine
• uric acid
Metal sequestration
• albumin
• transferrin, ferritin
• hemopexin, haptoglobin

Fig. 37.2 **Oxidative stress: an imbalance between prooxidant and antioxidant systems.** As described in this chapter, numerous factors contribute to the enhancement and inhibition of oxidative stress. AGE, advanced glycation endproduct; CAT, catalase; GPx, glutathione peroxidase; MPO, myeloperoxidase; SOD, superoxide dismutase.

forming H_2O_2 or O_2, respectively. At physiologic pH, the hydroperoxyl radical (HOO•, pKa ≈ 4.5), the protonated form of superoxide (see Fig. 37.1), represents only a small fraction of total O_2^{-} (about 0.1%), but this radical is intermediate in reactivity, between O_2^{-} and OH•. HOO• and H_2O_2 are small, uncharged molecules and readily diffuse through cell membranes.

ROS are formed by three major mechanisms in vivo: by reaction of oxygen with decompartmentalized metal ions (Fig. 37.3); as a side reaction of mitochondrial electron transport (Fig. 37.4); or by normal enzymatic reactions, e.g. formation of H_2O_2 by fatty acid oxidases in the peroxisome (Chapter 15). Secondary ROS are also formed by enzymatic reactions, e.g. myeloperoxidase in the macrophage catalyzes the reaction of H_2O_2 with Cl^- to produce another ROS,

hypochlorous acid (HOCl). HOCl, which is the major oxidizing species in chlorine-based bleaches, is also part of the bactericidal machinery of the macrophage (see below),

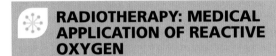

RADIOTHERAPY: MEDICAL APPLICATION OF REACTIVE OXYGEN

Radiation therapy uses a focused beam of high-energy electrons or γ-rays from an X-ray or cobalt-60 source to destroy tumor tissue. The radiation produces a flux of hydroxyl radicals (from water) and organic radicals at the site of the tumor. The localized oxidative stress causes damage to all biomolecules in the tumor cell, but the damage to DNA is critical – it prevents tumor cell replication, inhibiting tumor growth. Irradiation is also used as a method of sterilization of food, destroying viral or bacterial contaminants or insect infestations and preserving food products during long-term storage. Exposure to ionizing radiation from nuclear explosions or accidents, or breathing or ingestion of radioactive elements, such as radon gas or strontium-90, also causes oxidative damage to DNA. Cells that survive the damage may have mutations in DNA that eventually lead to development of cancers. Leukemias are particularly prominent because of the rapid division of bone marrow cells.

A Fenton reaction

$$Fe^{2+} + H_2O_2 \longrightarrow Fe^{3+} + OH• + OH^-$$

B Haber-Weiss reaction

$$O_2^{-} + H_2O_2 \longrightarrow O_2 + OH• + OH^-$$

C Metal-catalyzed Haber-Weiss reactions

Fig. 37.3 **Formation of ROS by the Fenton and Haber–Weiss reactions.** (A) Fenton first described the oxidizing power of solutions of Fe^{2+} and H_2O_2. This reaction generates the strong oxidant OH•. Cu^+ catalyzes the same reaction. (B) The Haber–Weiss reaction describes the production of OH• from O_2^{-} and H_2O_2. (C) Under physiologic conditions, the Haber–Weiss reaction is catalyzed by redox-active metal ions.

TOXICITY OF HYPEROXIA

Supplemental oxygen therapy may be used for treatment of patients with hypoxemia, respiratory distress, or following exposure to carbon monoxide. Under normobaric conditions, the fraction of oxygen in air can be increased to nearly 100% using a facial mask or nasal cannula. However, patients develop chest pain, cough and alveolar damage within a few hours of exposure to 100% oxygen. Edema gradually develops and compromises pulmonary function. The damage results from overproduction of ROS in the lung. Rats can be protected from oxygen toxicity by gradually increasing the oxygen tension over a period of several days. During this time, antioxidant enzymes, such as superoxide dismutase, are induced in the lung and provide increased protection against oxygen toxicity.

The lung is not the only tissue affected by hyperoxia. Premature infants, especially those with acute respiratory distress syndrome (Chapter 27), often require supplemental oxygen for survival. During the 1950s, it was recognized that the high oxygen tension used in incubators for premature infants increased the risk for blindness, resulting from retinopathy of prematurity (retrolental fibroplasia).

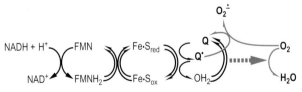

Fig. 37.4 **Formation of superoxide by mitochondria.** After the oxidation of NADH, the electron transport chain catalyzes single-electron redox reactions. The semiquinone radical, an intermediate in the reduction of Q to QH_2 by Complex I or II, is sensitive to oxidation by molecular oxygen and is considered a major source of superoxide radicals in the cell. This reaction is enhanced at high oxygen tension and also at low oxygen tension, e.g. during ischemia-reperfusion injury (see box on p. 504) when NADH is increased, the electron transport chain is saturated with electrons and the membrane potential is high.

ISCHEMIA/REPERFUSION INJURY: A PATIENT WITH MYOCARDIAL INFARCTION

A patient suffered a severe myocardial infarction, which was treated with tissue plasminogen activator, a clot-dissolving (thrombolytic) enzyme. During the days following hospitalization, the patient experienced palpitations, irregular rapid heartbeat, associated with weakness and faintness. The patient was treated with antiarrhythmic agents.

Comment. Ischemia, meaning limited blood flow, is a condition in which a tissue is deprived of oxygen and nutrients. Damage to heart tissue during a myocardial infarction occurs not during the hypoxic or ischemic phase, but during reoxygenation of the tissue. This type of damage also occurs following transplantation, and cardiovascular surgery. ROS are thought to play a major role in reperfusion injury. When cells are deprived of oxygen, they must rely on anaerobic glycolysis and glycogen stores for ATP synthesis. NADH and lactate accumulate, and all the components of the mitochondrial electron transport system are saturated with electrons (reduced), because the electrons cannot be transferred to oxygen. The mitochondrial membrane potential is increased (hyperpolarized), and when oxygen is reintroduced, great quantities of ROS are rapidly produced, overwhelming antioxidant defenses. ROS flood throughout the cell, damaging membrane lipids, DNA and other vital cellular constituents, leading to necrosis. Antioxidant supplements and drugs are being evaluated for protection of tissues prior to transplantation, during surgery and during recovery from ischemia.

REACTIVE NITROGEN SPECIES

Nitric oxide synthases (NOS) catalyze the production of the free radical, nitric oxide (NO$^{\bullet}$), from the amino acid L-arginine. There are three isoforms of NOS: nNOS in neuronal tissue, where NO$^{\bullet}$ serves a neurotransmitter function; iNOS in the immune system, where it is involved in regulation of the immune response; and eNOS in endothelial cells, where NO$^{\bullet}$, known as endothelium-derived relaxation factor (EDRF), has a role in the regulation of vascular tone.

In a side reaction, NO$^{\bullet}$ reacts with O$_2^{\bullet-}$ to form the strong oxidant, peroxynitrite (ONOO$^-$), a reactive nitrogen species (RNS) which has many of the strong oxidizing properties of OH$^{\bullet}$ but has a longer biologic half-life. ONOO$^-$ is also a potent nitrating agent; there is evidence that ONOOH degrades, in part, by homolytic cleavage to produce two reactive species, OH$^{\bullet}$ and NO$_2^{\bullet}$. Simultaneous production of NO$^{\bullet}$ and O$_2^{\bullet-}$, with the concomitant increase in ONOO$^-$ and a decrease in NO$^{\bullet}$, is thought to limit vasodilatation and cause inflammation of the vascular wall during ischemia-reperfusion injury, setting the stage for vascular disease. NO$_2^{\bullet}$, another RNS with strong oxidizing and nitrating activity, is formed by eosinophil peroxidase or myeloperoxidase catalyzed oxidation of NO$^{\bullet}$ by H$_2$O$_2$.

THE NATURE OF OXYGEN RADICAL DAMAGE

The hydroxyl radical is the most reactive and damaging ROS

The reaction of ROS with biomolecules produces characteristic products, described as biomarkers of oxidative stress. These compounds may be formed directly in the oxidation reaction with the ROS, or by secondary reactions between oxidation products and other biomolecules. The hydroxyl radical reacts with biomolecules primarily by hydrogen abstraction and addition reactions. One of the most sensitive sites of free radical damage are cell membranes, which are rich in readily oxidized polyunsaturated fatty acids (PUFA). Peroxidative damage to the plasma membrane affects the integrity and function of the membrane, compromising the cell's ability to maintain ion gradients and membrane phospholipid asymmetry. As shown in Figure 37.5, when OH$^{\bullet}$ abstracts a hydrogen atom from a PUFA, it initiates a chain of lipid peroxidation reaction, involving the secondary oxidation products, lipid peroxides and lipid peroxyl radicals. The lipid oxidation products formed in this reaction degrade to form reactive compounds, such as malondialdehyde (MDA) and hydroxynonenal (HNE). These compounds react with proteins to form adducts and crosslinks, known as advanced lipoxidation endproducts (ALE). MDA and HNE adducts to lysine residues have been measured in lipoproteins in the vascular wall in atherosclerosis and in neuronal plaque in Alzheimer's disease, implicating oxidative stress and damage in the pathogenesis of these diseases.

Hydroxyl radicals also react by addition to phenylalanine, tyrosine and nucleic acid bases to form hydroxylated derivatives and crosslinks (Fig. 37.6). Other ROS and RNS leave tell-tale tracks, such as nitro- and chlorotyrosine, formed from ONOOH and HOCl respectively, and methionine sulfoxide, formed by reaction of H$_2$O$_2$ or HOCl with methionine residues in proteins (see Fig. 37.6). Nitrotyrosine, like ALEs, is increased in atherosclerotic and Alzheimer's plaques.

ROS also react with carbohydrates to form reactive carbonyl compounds that react with protein to form crosslinks and adducts, known as glycoxidation products or advanced glycation endproducts (AGE). AGEs are increased in tissue proteins in diabetes as a result of hyperglycemia and oxidative stress, and the increase in chemical modification of proteins by AGEs and ALEs is implicated in the development of diabetic vascular, renal, and retinal complications (see Chapter 21).

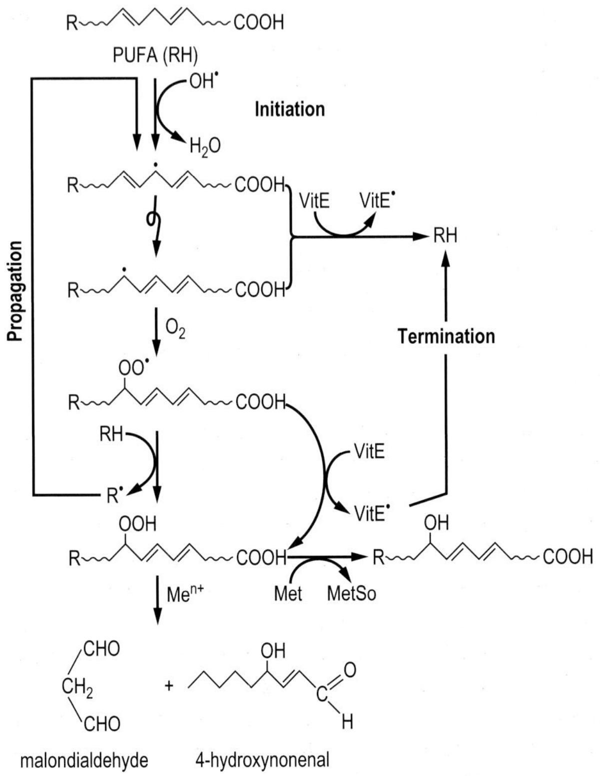

Fig. 37.5 **Pathway of lipid peroxidation.** OH• attacks PUFA, forming a carbon-centered lipid radical. The radical rearranges to form a conjugated dienyl radical. This radical reacts with ambient O_2, forming a hydroperoxyl radical, which then abstracts a hydrogen from a neighboring lipid, forming a lipid peroxide and R• which starts a chain reaction. This reaction continues until the supply of PUFA is exhausted, unless a termination reaction occurs. Vitamin E (below) is the major chain-terminating antioxidant in membranes; it reduces both the conjugated dienyl and hydroperoxyl radicals, quenching the chain or cycle of lipid peroxidation reactions. Lipid peroxides may also be reduced by methionine residues in lipoproteins, forming methionine sulfoxide and lipid alcohols. Otherwise, they decompose to form a range of 'reactive carbonyl species' such as malondialdehyde and hydroxynonenal, which react with protein to form advanced lipoxidation endproducts (ALE), which are biomarkers of oxidative stress. The reaction scheme shown here for PUFA also occurs with intact phospholipids and cholesterol esters in lipoproteins and cell membranes.

ANTIOXIDANT DEFENSES

There are several levels of protection against oxidative damage

ROS damage to lipids and proteins is repaired largely by degradation and resynthesis. Oxidized proteins, for example, are preferred targets for proteasomal degradation, and damaged DNA is repaired by a number of excision-repair mechanisms. The process is not perfect. Some proteins, such as collagens and crystallins, turn over slowly, so that damage accumulates and function may be impaired, e.g. age-dependent browning of lens proteins, crosslinking of collagen and

SENTINEL FUNCTION OF METHIONINE

Methionine (Met) residues in protein may be oxidized to methionine sulfoxide (MetSO) by H_2O_2 or HOCl. Met is generally on the surface of proteins and rarely has a role in the active site or mechanism of action of enzymes. However, there is evidence that it serves as an 'antioxidant pawn', protecting the active site of enzymes. Half of the Met residues of glutamine synthetase can be oxidized without affecting the enzyme's specific activity. These residues are physically arranged in an array that 'guards' the entrance to the active site, protecting the enzyme from inactivation by ROS. MetSO can be reduced back to methionine by the enzyme methionine sulfoxide reductase, providing a catalytic amplification of the antioxidant potential of each methionine residue.

METHIONINE OXIDATION AND EMPHYSEMA

α_1-Antitrypsin (A1AT) is a plasma protein, synthesized and secreted by liver. It is a potent inhibitor of elastase and protects tissues from damage by the neutrophil enzyme secreted during inflammation. Deficiency of this protein (about 1 in 4000 worldwide) is commonly associated with emphysema, progressive lung disease, and also hepatic damage resulting from accumulation of protein aggregates. The lung damage is attributed to failure of A1AT to inhibit elastase released by alveolar macrophages during phagocytosis of airborne particulate matter. Therapy includes replacement therapy by weekly intravenous infusion of a purified plasma concentrate or recombinant protein. Cigarette smoking and exposure to mineral dust (coal, silica) exacerbate pathology in patients with A1AT deficiency, but are also independent risk factors for emphysema and pulmonary fibrosis. Cigarette smoke and microparticulate materials activate lung macrophages, leading to release of proteolytic enzymes and increased production of ROS as a result of inflammation. The ROS cause oxidation of a specific Met residue in A1AT, irreversibly inhibiting the anti-elastase activity of this protein. Increased levels of inactive, Met(O)-containing A1AT are present in plasma of chronic smokers.

elastin, and loss of elasticity or changes in permeability of the vascular wall and renal basement membrane (see Chapter 44). The association between chronic inflammation and cancer indicates that chronic exposure to ROS causes cumulative damage to the genome in the form of nonlethal mutations in DNA.

Our first line of defense against oxidative damage is sequestration or chelation of redox-active metal ions

Endogenous chelators include a number of metal-binding proteins that sequester iron and copper in inactive form, such

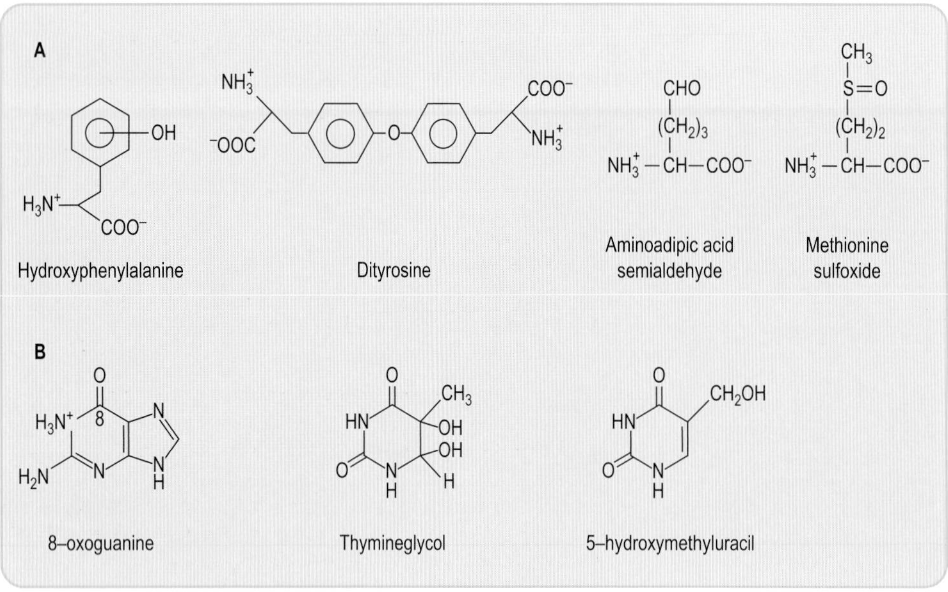

Fig. 37.6 **Products of hydroxyl radical damage to biomolecules.** (A) Amino acid oxidation products: *o-*, *m-* and *p-*tyrosine and dityrosine from phenylalanine; amino adipic acid semialdehyde from lysine; methionine sulfoxide. Other products include chlorotyrosine (from HOCl), nitrotyrosine (from ONOO⁻ and NO₂•), dihydroxyphenylalanine produced by hydroxylation of tyrosine, and aliphatic amino acid hydroperoxides, such as leucine hydroperoxide. (B) Nucleic acid oxidation products: 8-oxoguanine is the most commonly measured indicator of DNA damage.

✳ CELLULAR RESPONSE TO ROS

Cells adapt to oxidative stress by induction of antioxidant enzymes. Many of these are controlled by the antioxidant response element (ARE), also known as the electrophile response element. The central regulator of the ARE is the transcription factor Nrf2, which, on reaction with an electrophile, dissociates from its cytoplasmic inhibitor Keap1, translocates to the nucleus and activates ARE-dependent genes. Electrophilic lipid peroxidation products, such as hydroxynonenal and acrolein, are potent activators of ARE through modification of reactive thiol residues of Keap1. Keap1 also reacts with electrophilic carcinogens that alkylate DNA. ARE-dependent enzymes include catalase (CAT) and superoxide dismutase (SOD), and other enzymes that catalyze the oxidation and conjugation of carcinogens and oxidants for excretion. One of these enzymes, hepatic glutathione S-transferase, catalyzes conjugation with GSH. The conjugates are then excreted in urine as mercapturic acids, which are S-substituted *N*-acetyl-cysteine derivatives.

as transferrin and ferritin, the transport and storage forms of iron. The plasma protein haptoglobin binds to hemoglobin from ruptured red cells, and delivers the hemoglobin molecule to the liver for catabolism. Plasma hemopexin binds heme, the lipid-soluble form of iron, which catalyzes ROS formation in lipid environments; it delivers the heme to the liver for catabolism. Albumin, the major plasma protein, has a strong binding site for copper and effectively inhibits copper-catalyzed oxidation reactions in plasma. Carnosine (β-alanyl-L-histidine) and related peptides are present in muscle and brain at millimolar concentrations; they are potent copper chelators and may have a role in intracellular antioxidant protection.

Despite these manifold and potent metal chelation systems, ROS are formed continuously in the body, both by enzymes and spontaneous metal-catalyzed reactions. In these cases, there are a group of enzymes that act to detoxify ROS and their precursors. These include superoxide dismutase (SOD), catalase (CAT), and glutathione peroxidase (GPx) (Fig. 37.7). SOD converts $O_2^{\cdot-}$ to the less toxic H_2O_2. There are two classes of SOD: an MnSOD isozyme which is found in mitochondria, and CuZnSOD isozyme which is widely distributed throughout the cell. An extracellular, secreted glycoprotein isoform of CuZnSOD (EC-SOD) binds to proteoglycans in the vascular wall and is thought to protect against $O_2^{\cdot-}$ and ONOO⁻ injury. CAT, which inactivates H_2O_2, is found largely in peroxisomes, the major site of H_2O_2 generation in the cell.

GPx is widely distributed in the cytosol, in mitochondria and the nucleus. It reduces H_2O_2 and lipid hydroperoxides to water and a lipid alcohol, respectively, using reduced glutathione (GSH) as a co-substrate. GSH is a tripeptide (Chapter 2) that is present at $1-5\,mM$ concentration in all cells. The GSH is recycled by an NADPH-dependent enzyme, GSH reductase. The NADPH, provided by the pentose phosphate pathway, maintains about a 100:1 ratio of GSH:GSSG in the cell. GPx is actually a family of selenium-containing isozymes; a phospholipid hydroperoxide glutathione peroxidase will reduce lipid hydroperoxides in phospholipids in lipoproteins and membranes, while other isozymes are specific for free fatty acid or cholesterol ester hydroperoxides. There is also an isoform of GPx in intestinal epithelial cells, which is thought to have a role in detoxification of dietary hydroperoxides, e.g. in fried foods.

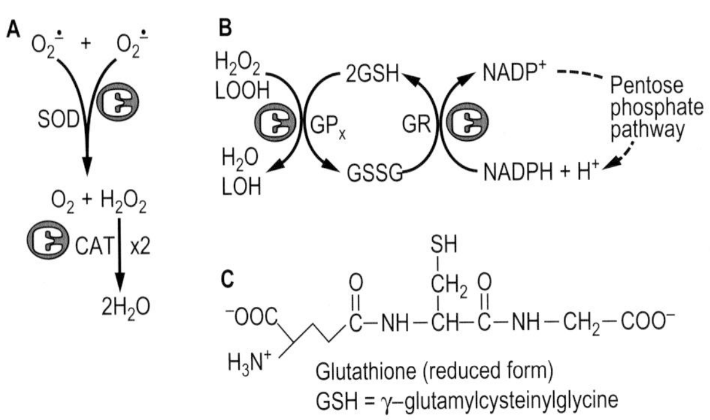

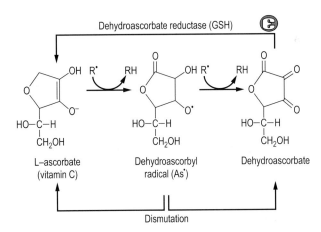

Fig. 37.7 **Enzymatic defenses against ROS.** (A) Superoxide dismutase (SOD) and catalase (CAT) are dismutases, catalyzing oxidation and reduction of separate substrate molecules; both are highly specific for their substrates, $O_2^{\bullet-}$ and H_2O_2, respectively. (B) Glutathione peroxidase (GPx) reduces H_2O_2 and lipid peroxides (LOOH), using GSH as a co-substrate. The GSH is recycled by glutathione reductase (GR) using NADPH from the pentose phosphate pathway. (C) Structure of GSH.

Fig. 37.8 **Antioxidant activity of ascorbate.** Vitamin C exists as the enolate anion at physiologic pH. The enolate anion spontaneously reduces superoxide, organic ($R^{\bullet}$) and vitamin E radicals, forming a dehydroascorbyl radical ($As^{\bullet}$). Dehydroascorbyl radical may dismutate to ascorbate and dehydroascorbate. Dehydroascorbate is recycled by dehydroascorbate reductase, a GSH-dependent enzyme present in all cells.

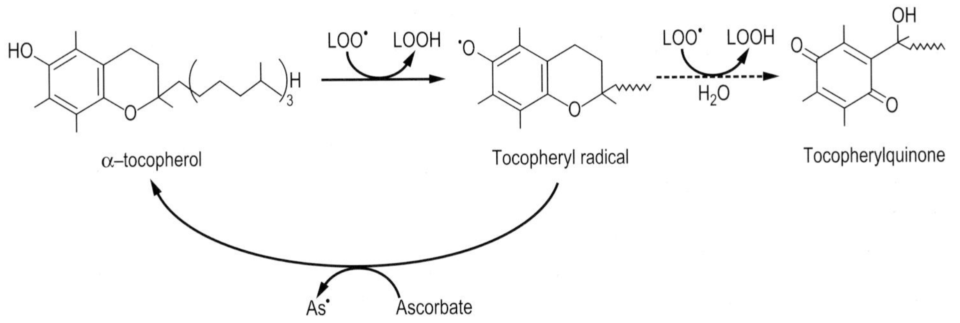

Fig. 37.9 **Antioxidant activity of vitamin E.** The term vitamin E refers to a family of related tocopherol and tocotrienol isomers with potent lipophilic antioxidant and membrane-stabilizing activity. Tocopherols reduce lipid hydroperoxyl radicals and also inactivate singlet oxygen. α-Tocopherol is the most effective form in humans and the major form of vitamin E in the diet. It consists of a chromanol ring structure with a polyisoprenoid side chain; the isoprene units are unsaturated in the tocotrienol. α, β, γ, and δ differ in the pattern of methyl groups at R_1, R_2 and R_3 (Chapter 11). The major commercial form of vitamin E is α-tocopherol acetate, which is more stable than free tocopherol during storage. The tocopheryl radical, the major product formed during antioxidant action of vitamin E, is recycled by ascorbate. Tocopheryl quinone is also formed in small quantities.

Three antioxidant vitamins, A, C and E, provide the third line of defense against oxidative damage. These vitamins, primarily vitamin C (ascorbate) (Fig. 37.8) in the aqueous phase and vitamin E (α- and γ-tocopherol; Fig. 37.9) in the lipid phase, act as chain-breaking antioxidants (see Fig. 37.5). They act as reducing agents, donating a hydrogen atom ($H^{\bullet}$) and quenching organic radicals formed by reaction of ROS with biomolecules. The vitamin C and E radicals produced in this reaction are unreactive, resonance-stabilized species; they do not propagate radical damage and are enzymatically recycled, e.g. by dehydroascorbate reductase (see Fig. 37.8). Vitamin C reduces superoxide and lipid peroxyl radicals, but also has a special role in reduction and recycling of vitamin E. In response to severe oxidative stress. vitamin C recycles vitamin E, so that vitamin E is maintained at constant concentration in the lipid phase until all the vitamin C is consumed (see Fig. 37.9). These antioxidants work together to inhibit lipid peroxidation reactions in plasma lipoproteins and membranes. Vitamin A (carotene; Chapter 11) is also a lipophilic antioxidant. Although best understood for its role in vision, it is a potent singlet oxygen scavenger and protects against damage from sunlight in the retina and skin.

THE BENEFICIAL EFFECTS OF REACTIVE OXYGEN SPECIES

While much of this chapter has focused on the dangerous aspects of reactive oxygen, it is worth closing with some recognition of the beneficial effects of ROS. Among these are the regulatory functions of NO, the role of ROS in activation

GLUTATHIONYLATION OF PROTEIN

S-glutathionylation or S-glutathiolation of proteins describes the formation of a disulfide bond between GSH and an -SH group on a target protein. S-thiolation of proteins is induced by both ROS and RNS and is thought to have a dual role in protecting cysteine against irreversible oxidation during oxidative stress and in modulating cellular metabolism (redox regulation). Target proteins include a wide range of regulatory enzymes with active site or regulatory −SH groups, such as protein kinases and transcription factors. S-thiolation also appears to protect proteins against ubiquitin-mediated proteasomal degradation during oxidative stress. It is reversed by nonenzymatic reduction by GSH or by enzymes using thiol protein cofactors (thioredoxin, glutaredoxin).

PEROXIDASE ACTIVITY FOR DETECTION OF OCCULT BLOOD

Peroxidases, such as the glutathione peroxidase (GPx), are enzymes that catalyze the oxidation of a substrate using H_2O_2. Hemoglobin and heme have a pseudoperoxidase activity in vitro. In the guaiac-based test for occult fecal blood, a stool sample is applied to a small card containing guaiac acid. Hemoglobin in a stool specimen oxidizes phenolic compounds in guaiac acid to quinones. A positive test is indicated by a blue stain along the edge of the fecal smear. Incompletely digested hemoglobin and myoglobin from animal meat and some plant peroxidases may cause false positives. Similar peroxidase-dependent assays are used to identify bloodstains at crime scenes.

of the ARE, the requirement for ROS in the bactericidal activity of macrophages, and the use of ROS as substrates for enzymes, e.g. H_2O_2 for the heme-peroxidases involved in iodination of thyroid hormone. There is also increasing

THE GLYOXALASE PATHWAY: A SPECIAL ROLE FOR GLUTATHIONE

A small fraction of triose phosphates produced during metabolism spontaneously degrades to methylglyoxal (MGO), a reactive dicarbonyl sugar. MGO is also formed during metabolism of glycine and threonine, and as a product of nonenzymatic oxidation of carbohydrates and lipids – it is a significant precursor of advanced glycation and lipoxidation endproducts (AGE/ALEs) (see Chapters 21 and 44). MGO reacts primarily with arginine residues in proteins, but also with lysine, histidine and cysteine, leading to enzyme inactivation and protein crosslinking.

MGO is inactivated by enzymes of the glyoxalase pathway, a GSH-dependent system found in all cells in the body. The glyoxalase pathway (Fig. 37.10) consists of two enzymes that catalyze an internal redox reaction in which carbon-1 of MGO is oxidized from an aldehyde to a carboxylic acid group and carbon-2 is reduced from a ketone to a secondary alcohol. The endproduct, D-lactate, does not react with proteins; D-lactate is distinct from L-lactate, the product of glycolysis, but may be converted into L-lactate, for further metabolism. Levels of MGO and D-lactate are increased in blood of diabetic patients, because levels of glucose and glycolytic intermediates, including triose phosphates, are increased intracellularly in diabetes. The glyoxalase system also inactivates glyoxal, and other dicarbonyl sugars produced during nonenzymatic oxidation of carbohydrates and lipids. Glyoxalase inhibitors are being evaluated for chemotherapy because cancer cells appear to be more sensitive to glyoxal, perhaps because of their increased reliance on glycolysis.

THE RESPIRATORY BURST IN MACROPHAGES

As outlined in Fig. 37.11, the macrophage initiates a sequence of ROS producing reactions during the burst of oxygen consumption accompanying phagocytosis. NADPH oxidase in the macrophage plasma membrane is activated to produce $O_2^{\bullet-}$ which is then converted to H_2O_2 by superoxide dismutase. The H_2O_2 is used by another macrophage enzyme, myeloperoxidase (MPO), to oxidize chloride ion, ubiquitous in body fluids, to hypochlorous acid (HOCl). H_2O_2 and HOCl mediate bactericidal activity by oxidative degradation of microbial lipids, proteins, and DNA. The macrophage has a high intracellular concentration of antioxidants, especially ascorbate, to protect itself during ROS production.

The consumption of O_2 by NADPH oxidase is responsible for the 'respiratory burst', the sharp increase in O_2 consumption for production of ROS, which accompanies phagocytosis. The endproduct of this reaction sequence, HOCl, is also the active oxidizer in chlorine-containing laundry bleaches. Intravenous infusion of dilute HOCl solutions was actually used for treatment of bacterial sepsis in battlefield hospitals during World War I, before the advent of penicillin and other antibiotics. Chronic granulomatous disease (CGD) is an inherited disease resulting from a genetic defect in NADPH oxidase. The inability to produce superoxide leads to chronic life-threatening bacterial and fungal infections.

evidence that ROS, particularly H_2O_2, are important signaling molecules involved in regulation of metabolism. The tissue concentration of H_2O_2 is estimated to be in the sub-micromolar range; estimates vary widely, from 1 to 700 nM. However, significant changes in H_2O_2 concentration occur in response to cytokines, growth factors and biomechanical stimulation. The fact that these signaling events are inhibited by peroxide scavengers or by overexpression of catalase implicates H_2O_2 in the signaling cascade. Insulin signaling, for example, appears to involve H_2O_2 as part of the mechanism for reversible inactivation of some protein tyrosine phosphatases, at the same time that protein tyrosine kinases are activated through the insulin receptor (Chapter 21). As the evidence for the signaling role of H_2O_2 has become convincing, there is increasing interest in research on the regulatory role of superoxide.

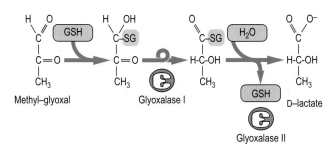

Fig. 37.10 **The glyoxalase system.** Glyoxalase I catalyzes the formation of a thiohemiacetal adduct between GSH and MGO and its rearrangement to a thioester. Glyoxalase II catalyzes the hydrolysis of the thioester forming D-lactate and regenerating GSH. Unlike GPx, this pathway does not consume GSH.

ANTIOXIDANT DEFENSES IN THE RED BLOOD CELL (RBC)

The RBC does not use oxygen for metabolism, nor is it involved in phagocytosis. However, because of the high O_2 tension in arterial blood and the heme iron content of RBCs, ROS are formed continuously in the RBC. Hb spontaneously produces superoxide ($O_2^{\bullet}$) in a minor side reaction associated with binding of O_2. The occasional reduction of O_2 to $O_2^{\bullet}$ is accompanied by oxidation of normal (ferro) Hb to methemoglobin (ferrihemoglobin), a rust-brown protein that does not bind or transport O_2. Methemoglobin may release heme, which reacts with $O_2^{\bullet}$ and H_2O_2 in Fenton-type reactions to produce hydroxyl radical (OH$^{\bullet}$) and reactive iron-oxo species. These ROS initiate lipid peroxidation reactions which can lead to loss of membrane integrity and cell death.

The RBC is well fortified with antioxidant defenses to protect itself against oxidative stress. These include catalase (CAT), superoxide dismutase (SOD) and glutathione peroxidase (GPx), as well as a methemoglobin reductase activity that reduces methemoglobin back to normal ferrohemoglobin. Normally, less than 1% of Hb is present as methemoglobin. However, persons with congenital methemoglobinemia, resulting from methemoglobin reductase deficiency, typically have a dark and cyanotic appearance. Treatment with large doses of ascorbate (vitamin C) is used to reduce their methemoglobin to functional hemoglobin.

GSH, present at ~2 mmol/L in the RBC, not only supports antioxidant defenses, but is also an important sulfhydryl buffer, maintaining —SH groups in hemoglobin and enzymes in the reduced state. Under normal circumstances, when proteins are exposed to O_2, their sulfhydryl groups gradually oxidize to form disulfides, either intramolecularly or intermolecularly with other proteins. GSH nonenzymatically reverses these reactions, leading to regeneration of the sulfhydryl group (see also Figs 12.11 and 12.12).

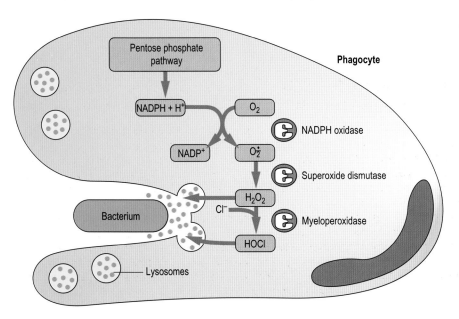

Fig. 37.11 **Generation and release of ROS during phagocytosis.** A cascade of reactions generating ROS is initiated during phagocytosis to kill invading organisms. Hydrolytic enzymes are also released from lysosomes to assist in degradation of microbial debris.

Summary

Reactive oxygen species (ROS) are the sparks produced by oxidative metabolism, and oxidative stress may be viewed as the price we pay for using oxygen for metabolism. ROS and reactive nitrogen species (RNS), such as superoxide, peroxide, hydroxyl radical, and peroxynitrite, are reactive and toxic, sometimes difficult to contain, but their production is important for regulation of metabolism, turnover of biomolecules and protection against microbial infection. ROS and RNS cause oxidative damage to all classes of biomolecules: proteins, lipids and DNA. There are a number of protective antioxidant mechanisms, including sequestration of redox-active metal ions, enzymatic inactivation of major ROS, inactivation of organic radicals by small molecules, such as GSH and vitamins, and, when all else fails, repair and/or turnover. Biomarkers of oxidative stress are readily detected in tissues in inflammation, and oxidative stress is increasingly implicated in the pathogenesis of age-related, chronic disease.

ACTIVE LEARNING

1. Review the evidence that atherosclerosis is an inflammatory disease resulting from overproduction of ROS in the vascular wall.
2. Discuss the evidence that hyperglycemia in diabetes induces a state of oxidative stress that leads to renal and vascular complications.
3. Review the data on use of antioxidants in therapy for atherosclerosis and diabetes. Based on these studies, how strong is the evidence that these diseases are the result of increased oxidative stress?
4. Discuss recent advances in the use of antioxidants for tissue protection during surgery and transplantation.

Further reading

Bonomini F, Tengattini S, Fabiano A, Bianchi R, Rezzani R. Atherosclerosis and oxidative stress. *Histol Histopathol* 2008;**23**:381–390.

Copple IM, Goldring CE, Kitteringham NR, Park BK. The Nrf2-Keap1 defence pathway: role in protection against drug-induced toxicity. *Toxicology* 2008; **246**:367–371.

Hamilton KL. Antioxidants and cardioprotection. *Med Sci Sports Exerc* 2007;**39**: 1544–1553.

Mittal A, Phillips AR, Loveday B, Windsor JA. The potential role for xanthine oxidase inhibition in major intra-abdominal surgery. *World J Surg* 2008;**32**: 288–295.

Romieu I, Castro-Giner F, Kunzli N, Sunyer J. Air pollution, oxidative stress and supplementation: a review. *Eur Respir J* 2008; **31**:179–197.

Sayre LM, Perry G, Smith MA. Oxidative stress and neurotoxicity. *Chem Res Toxicol* 2008;**21**:172–188.

Stone Jr. Yang S. Hydrogen peroxide: signaling messenger. *Antiox Redox Signal* 2006;**8**:243–270.

Wei Y, Chen K. Whaley-Connell AT, Stump CS, Ibdah JA, Sowers JR. Skeletal muscle insulin resistance: role of inflammatory cytokines and reactive oxygen species. *Am J Physiol Regul Integr Comp Physiol* 2008;**294(3)**:R673–680.

Websites

Antioxidants: www.nlm.nih.gov/medlineplus/antioxidants.html

Antioxidants and cancer: www.cancer.gov/cancertopics/factsheet/antioxidantsprevention

Antioxidants in foods: www.ific.org/publications/factsheets/antioxidantfs.cfm

Reactive oxygen species and antioxidant vitamins: http://lpi.oregonstate.edu/f-w97/reactive.html

Virtual Free Radical School: www.healthcare.uiowa.edu/research/sfrbm/virtual.html

38. The Immune Response

J A Gracie and A Farrell

INTRODUCTION

The immune system, a collection of cells, tissues and molecules, has evolved to produce a coordinated response to protect the host from, and remove, ongoing infection. Key to this is the ability to distinguish self from nonself whilst attempting to maintain the homeostasis of the body. Immunity can be categorized as being either innate (nonspecific) or adaptive (acquired/specific).

INNATE IMMUNE RESPONSE

When activated, the innate response is seen as an inflammatory response

Innate immunity is the body's first line of defense. The innate immune response protects an organism from attack, using physicochemical barriers, such as the skin and mucosal epithelia, and their associated secreted products, e.g. sweat, mucus and acid. When activated, the innate response is often seen as an inflammatory response. Inflammation is the body's response to injury or tissue damage. Its purpose is to limit, and then repair, the damage brought about by any injurious agent. It involves the interaction of the microvasculature, circulating blood cells, other cells in the tissues, and their secreted effector molecules. The cells that line blood vessels, endothelium, play a major role in the vascular effects, such as increased permeability and vasodilatation. The cellular effects involve phagocytic and secretory responses of cells that usually circulate in the blood but migrate into involved tissue, as well as of cells that are tissue resident (Table 38.1).

Inflammatory mediators contribute to the immune response

Innate immune cells synthesize and secrete a wide variety of different types of soluble chemical substances termed inflammatory mediators. The liver also produces a number of these mediators, present in the blood, including acute phase reactants such as C-reactive protein (CRP) (see Chapter 4) and components of the complement system.

The complement system

Complement is activated in a series of sequential steps

The complement system, consisting of a series of proteins, both circulating and cell membrane bound, plays an important role in antimicrobial host defense. There are

Cells involved in inflammation		
	Circulating	**Tissue based**
Polymorphonuclear leukocytes	neutrophil eosinophil basophil	
		mast cell
Mononuclear phagocytes	monocyte	macrophage
Lymphocytes		
Platelets		
Endothellal cells		

Table 38.1 **Cells involved in inflammation.**

three pathways of complement activation. As part of the innate response, and in the absence of antibody, the alternative and lectin pathways activate complement during infection by recognition of, and direct binding to, microbial surfaces. In addition, antibody produced in response to infection can bind microbial antigens and activate complement via the classic pathway. The sequential activation of the cascade by proteolytic cleavage results in an autoamplifying response producing a number of effector molecules involved in elimination of the microbial infection, as shown in Figure 38.1.

- The activation of the first component leads to the unlocking of serine protease activity.
- The activation of the next component in the sequence is achieved by it being cleaved by the first component into two unequally sized fragments.
- The larger of the resulting fragments exhibits serine protease activity and attaches to the activating surface, while the smaller fragment has distinctive biologic activities, which include the facilitation of phagocytosis (termed opsonization), the attraction of cells (chemotaxis), and the stimulating degranulation of immune cells (anaphylatoxin activity).
- This series of activation events is then repeated with further early components, thereby creating a cascade effect.
- By activating the next component, the large enzymatically active fragment of the previous component is itself inactivated.
- Instead of demonstrating enzyme activity on activation, the 'late' components of the pathway combine with each other to form a multimolecular complex that can breach the integrity of the bacterial surface by insertion into the membrane – the membrane attack complex (MAC).

Cytokines

Cytokines are soluble mediators of inflammatory and immune responses

Cytokines are soluble mediators of inflammatory and immune responses. Produced by a variety of cell types including those of the innate and adaptive immune response, these peptides or glycoproteins are active at concentrations between 10^{-9} and 10^{-15}M. In general, macrophages are often their main producers during innate responses, and T cells during adaptive responses. However, many cell types can secrete cytokines. By interacting with specific receptors on the surfaces of their target cells, the large number of cytokines now identified exhibit many effects. The majority act locally to their site of production (paracrine action) or on the cells that produced them (autocrine action). A few, however, are capable of acting on cells more distant from their site of production (endocrine). The cytokine network displays both redundancy and pleiotropy with several having

Binding and early component activation
Sequential activation of serine protease activity generates
- smaller soluble biologically active fragments and
- larger fragments that also bind to the activating surface

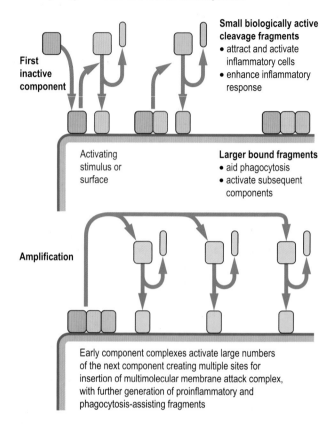

First inactive component

Small biologically active cleavage fragments
- attract and activate inflammatory cells
- enhance inflammatory response

Activating stimulus or surface

Larger bound fragments
- aid phagocytosis
- activate subsequent components

Amplification

Early component complexes activate large numbers of the next component creating multiple sites for insertion of multimolecular membrane attack complex, with further generation of proinflammatory and phagocytosis-assisting fragments

Late component activation and membrane attack complex formation

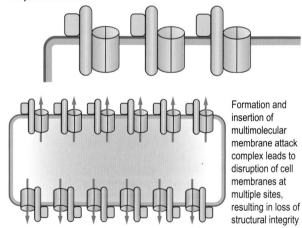

Formation and insertion of multimolecular membrane attack complex leads to disruption of cell membranes at multiple sites, resulting in loss of structural integrity

Fig. 38.1 **The complement cascade**. Activating stimuli bear surfaces that trigger complement activation, and to which the activated component can attach itself. The late components of the cascade do not show enzymatic activity. Instead, they coalesce to form a polymeric macromolecule (the membrane attack complex), which can insert itself into the activating surface (the cell wall in the case of bacteria), breach its integrity and cause osmotic lysis.

overlapping effects and an ability to act on numerous cell types. Cytokines have been grouped into smaller subfamilies, based on structure and function, as discussed briefly below. Cytokine receptors are not restricted to cells of the immune system, being found widespread on disparate cell types. For more detail on cytokine signaling, see Chapter 40.

Cytokines may be classified into families or by their principal effect

- **Colony-stimulating factors:** as the name suggests, these are involved in the development and differentiation of immune cells from bone marrow precursors.
- **Interferons (IFNs):** while IFN-α and IFN-β have a role in protection against viral replication, IFN-γ plays a significant part in regulating immune responses. Made primarily by T cells, IFN-γ activates macrophages.
- **Interleukins (ILs):** currently there are in excess of 30 interleukins recognized, participating in regulating both innate and adaptive immune responses. Made by a number of immune (and other) cell types. As the name suggests, a principal mode of action is communication between leukocytes.
- **Tumor necrosis factor (TNF) family:** a mixed collection of cytokines whose effects range from promoting inflammation (TNF-α) to stimulating osteoclasts and bone resorption (osteoprotegerin, OPG).
- **Chemokines:** these are a family of cytokines that bring about chemokinesis – movement in response to chemical stimuli. Interest has increased dramatically in the receptors for these mediators since some appear to act as coreceptors for infection, in particular HIV infection of lymphocytes.

Previously it was fashionable to describe cytokines as either pro- or antiinflammatory. It is now clear that this can be confusing given their pleiotropic effects, and comparing innate and adaptive responses or cells of origin perhaps should be considered.

- During innate responses macrophages, dendritic cells and natural killer (NK) cells are major producers of: TNF-α, IL-1, IL-6, IL-8 and many chemokines, IL-12, IL-15 and IL-18, IFN-γ (NK cells). These can all be thought of as important intercellular communicators, inducing inflammation and immune responses.
- If an adaptive or cell-mediated response develops, T cells, especially CD4⁺ T cells, become a major producer of cytokines. Their effects generally either promote or control further responses and they include: IL-2, IL-4, IL-5, IL-17, IL-10, IL-13, and TGF-β.

Cells of the innate response

Neutrophils and monocytes are normally found circulating in the bloodstream and are recruited to sites of infection by the process of extravasation. Through the interaction of receptors on the phagocyte and counterligands on vascular endothelium, cells attach, arrest and move through from the circulation to the infected tissue. Neutrophils are the most abundant leukocytes in the bloodstream, numbering 4–10 000/mm^3. Through recruitment from the bone marrow, this increases rapidly during infection and numbers often reach 20 000/mm^3. Neutrophils are generally the first cells to respond to infection, phagocytosing microbes in the circulation and moving rapidly into infected tissue. They are short-lived (normally a few hours to days) and they die rapidly after reaching the tissue.

Monocytes transform into macrophages, 'the dustbin of the immune response'

Monocytes are found in much lower numbers within the blood, 500–1000/mm^3, and by contrast with neutrophils are long-lived. Similarly to neutrophils, they can also migrate into tissue where they differentiate into macrophages. Macrophages have a number of key functions including phagocytosis of infecting microbes, antigen presentation and general removal of dying or damaged host cells. Indeed, the macrophage has often been termed the 'dustbin of the immune response'. Most organs of the body and connective tissue have resident macrophages, whose job it is to survey their environment for signs of infection.

Innate cells recognize the attacking microbes through their receptors

In order to mount an efficient response to infection, neutrophils and macrophages must realize that the body is under attack. They do so through a number of cell surface receptors. Receptors involved in microbial recognition identify structures that are shared by various microbes and which are generally not present on host cells. Such receptors are called pattern recognition receptors. Often the structures recognized by these receptors, called pathogen-associated molecular patterns (PAMPs), are required by the pathogen for survival or infectivity and are generally common to particular microbial families. The best characterized of these receptors is the Toll-like receptor (TLR) system in mammals, named after a homologous receptor system used by the *Drosophila* fruit fly for protection from infection. In man, there are at least 12 different TLRs which can form homo- or heterodimers with other family members, thus increasing the repertoire for recognition. TLRs can be either surface membrane bound or reside intracellularly. TLR4, for example, has been shown to be the receptor which recognizes lipopolysaccharide (LPS) which is found on the surface of gram-negative bacteria such as *E.coli* but is not made by mammalian cells. Other pattern recognition receptors include the more recently described nod-like receptors (NLR), which are cytoplasmic proteins which can regulate inflammatory and apoptotic responses through pathogen recognition.

A young man was brought into the emergency room in a state of shock with stridor and widespread urticaria. A companion told the admitting medic that the patient had developed difficulties in breathing shortly after eating a snack. Allergy to peanuts was suspected and a diagnosis of anaphylaxis was made. An intramuscular injection of epinephrine was given promptly and also treatment with intravenous antihistamine, corticosteroid, and cardiorespiratory support. The man recovered.

Comment. While the physiologic role of the IgE response is considered to be protection against parasite infestation, this response is seen to be subverted in those who experience atopic diseases and anaphylaxis. The major fraction of IgE is bound via receptors to mast cells in the tissues. When antigen binds and crosslinks its specific IgE on the mast cells, it triggers the degranulation of the cells and release of preformed mediators (principally histamine). When the mast cell degranulation is localized to one site it usually gives rise to only localized reactions in the form of allergic rhinitis and asthma. If the degree of sensitization with the antigen-specific IgE and/or the antigenic burden is greater, systemic degranulation can occur, with consequent anaphylactic shock. Significant vasodilatation takes place, reducing the blood pressure. This is accompanied by large increases in vessel wall permeability, leading to substantial swelling, which particularly affects the skin and other loose connective tissue such as those in the larynx. Smooth muscle spasm also occurs, leading to bronchoconstriction with consequent respiratory difficulty and wheezing. These features are accompanied by increased secretory activity of seromucous glands in the respiratory and gastrointestinal tract as well as itching of the skin.

Mannose receptors and scavenger receptors are used by neutrophils and macrophages to promote phagocytosis

Other surface receptors used by neutrophils and macrophages to promote phagocytosis and killing of microbes include mannose receptors and scavenger receptors. Microbes can be coated by soluble mediators of the immune response such as complement components or antibodies. Phagocytes in turn express a number of receptors such as complement receptors and Fc receptors which recognize these complement components and antibodies respectively. This process of coating microbial surfaces, termed opsonization, makes the phagocytic process of microbial uptake by neutrophils and macrophages more efficient.

Receptors used by the innate immune response are encoded in the germline and, unlike the receptors used by cells of the adaptive immune response (discussed below), are not produced by somatic recombination of their genes. As a result, the response elicited by such receptors is amnesic: this means that the cells will respond similarly on reinfection.

ADAPTIVE IMMUNE RESPONSE

Specificity of the response is achieved through receptors that recognize antigen

Adaptive immune responses are brought into play if our innate defenses are unsuccessful, e.g. due to the persistence of the triggering agent. The response is initiated when the lymphocytes recognize components of the infectious agent. The infectious agents are called antigens and their binding to receptors on lymphocytes triggers an adaptive response. Receptors on B cells and T cells differ and see quite different forms of antigen.

Thymic education and self-tolerance help distinguish between self and nonself

Crucial for successful adaptive responses is the requirement for such responses to distinguish between self and nonself. The immune system does this through the processes of thymic education and self-tolerance. This ensures that appropriate immune responses to infection develop. Failure of this process and inappropriate activation of the immune response by self-antigens can result in developing autoimmunity, e.g. rheumatoid arthritis or systemic lupus erythematosus.

Adaptive immune response needs time to develop

When an adaptive immune response is first initiated, relatively few components are likely to be available that could react specifically with any chosen antigenic substance. There is a delay or lag period while these components increase to a level which can ensure elimination of the antigen, or at least reduce it to a level that would be manageable by an innate immune response. This delay, however, can be disastrous for the host.

Adaptive immune response remembers specific encounters

The adaptive immune response employs a mechanism to remember a specific encounter so that if the same foreign or nonself substance is encountered again, it can be dealt with more quickly and effectively. This is called immunologic memory. Thus, in comparison to innate immunity, the adaptive response exhibits both specificity for and memory of the foreign or nonself substance.

Cells primarily responsible for adaptive response are the lymphocytes

Adaptive immunity is mediated, similarly to the innate response, by cellular and humoral elements. The cells primarily responsible are the lymphocytes. There are two major types of lymphocytes circulating in blood and present within the lymphoid tissues:

- T cells, which are responsible for a number of cellular responses
- B cells, which are responsible for humoral responses, i.e. antibody production.

In addition to the lymphocytes, professional antigen-presenting cells (APC) are required for efficient activation of the adaptive immune response.

LYMPHOCYTES

T and B lymphocytes

Distinction between T and B cells is most easily made phenotypically with reference to the cells' antigen-specific receptors

The effector cells primarily involved in the adaptive immune response are the T and B lymphocytes. In total, lymphocytes are present in the peripheral blood at $1.5–3.5 \times 10^9/L$. Of these, approximately 50–70% are T cells and 10–20% are B cells. A third population termed 'natural killer' (NK) cells, so-called because they demonstrate the ability to kill neoplastic cells without prior exposure or sensitization, are atypical lymphocytes and are generally considered to be part of the innate response. Identification of T and B cells is based on immunophenotypic or functional studies. They carry particular collections of markers that can assist in assigning their lineage. The distinction between T and B cells is most easily made with reference to their antigen receptors (Fig. 38.2).

B and T lymphocytes are activated by binding of antigen and by costimulatory molecules

The antigen recognition receptor on the B cell is a surface immunoglobulin termed 'sIg'. On binding to its antigen, it brings about the cell's activation and subsequent proliferation and differentiation. In addition to sIg, B cells express several other markers, the best characterized of which include CD19, CD20 and the major histocompatibility complex (MHC) class II molecules.

The T cell antigen receptor is termed the T cell receptor (TCR) and it is complexed with CD3. Two other CD markers whose expression appears to be mutually exclusive on T cells are the CD4 and CD8, and they are useful in further categorizing the T cell function, as discussed later.

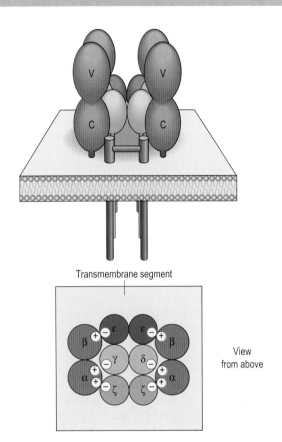

Transmembrane segment

View from above

Fig. 38.2 **Structure of the α/β, γ/δ T cell receptors.** V and C refer to the variable and constant sequence domains, respectively, of each of the α, β, γ and δ chains. Modified from Male D *et al. Immunology*, 7th edn. London: Mosby, 2006.

NK cells are currently identified by the expression of the combination of CD16 and CD56. These markers are often used in flow cytometric technology using fluorescent monoclonal antibodies to identify cell types.

Another group of surface molecules, the so-called costimulatory molecules, are also found on the surface of T and B cells. Following exposure to antigen, CD28 on T cells will bind CD80/CD86 on the APC while CD40 on B cells will bind CD40L on T cells, resulting in full activation. Without such costimulation, T and B cells will not be fully activated following exposure to antigen and could become anergic, i.e. nonresponsive.

MOLECULES INVOLVED IN ANTIGEN RECOGNITION

Antigen is recognized by specific receptors on T and B cells

The ability to recognize the enormous number of possible antigenic configurations is achieved by differences in amino acid sequence of these receptors, which gives rise to

IMMUNOGLOBULIN VARIABLE GENE RECOMBINATION EVENTS

The ability to generate molecules of variable amino acid sequence, using a basic template onto which some variation is superimposed, provides the capability to generate as many different shapes as there are sequences. This is made possible by the organization of the genes that give rise to the T and B cell antigen receptors. They both undergo similar rearrangements and recombinations to generate a vast repertoire of antigen recognition units. This is illustrated by the idealized representation of the organization of a hypothetical immunoglobulin heavy-chain gene.

One gene from each of the variable domain gene segments combines with one gene from each of the other segments (D and J) to produce a whole rearranged variable domain gene. This then associates with the gene coding for the constant domains of the particular heavy chain class being produced. In the case of a light chain, only two segments are involved in the production of a variable domain gene and this is then associated with the gene coding whichever of the light chain types is going to be produced. The whole rearranged gene can be transcribed and subsequently translated. Thus multiple gene segments contribute to the formation of each individual variable domain gene and, together with the gene encoding, the constant domains complete light- and heavy-chain genes (refer to Fig. 4.6).

differences in protein shape or conformation. The antigen and its specific receptor have a 'hand-in-glove' relationship. Both T and B cell antigen receptors show marked variability in the sequence of amino acids that come into contact with the antigen, while other parts of these molecules are relatively constant with regard to their amino acid sequences.

Unlike the antigen receptors found on innate cells which are germline encoded, the receptors found on the T and B cells are generated by random recombination of receptor genes during cell maturation. These antigen recognition receptors are clonally distributed. As a result, each clone will exhibit unique specificity for a particular antigen, thus generating the enormous pool of cells capable of responding to all antigens.

As mentioned previously, T and B cells differ in what they recognize as 'foreign'. The sIg antigen receptor found on B cells is capable of recognizing macromolecules (proteins, polysaccharides, lipids, etc.) whereas T cell receptors recognize small peptides of proteins previously processed by the APC.

Although there is a huge number of T and B cell clones each recognizing different antigens, the consequence of engagement by appropriate antigen will generally induce a similar response, i.e. signal transduction. This may lead to full cell activation: for B cells resulting in antibody production and for T cells the proliferation and promotion of the cellular adaptive immune response.

The T cell antigen receptor

T cell receptor resembles the binding portion of an immunoglobulin molecule

The TCR is a heterodimer made up of two nonidentical polypeptide chains termed α and β (see Fig. 38.2). In addition, a small unique T cell population found primarily within the gut expresses alternative TCRs, their chains being termed γ and δ. Each chain of the TCR comprises two domains – one constant and one variable amino acid sequence. The antigen-binding site of the TCR is in the cleft formed by the adjoining single N-terminal variable domains of the constituent α (Vα) or β (Vβ) chains. The effector function of the constant domain in each of the antigen receptor chains is signal transduction. The two chains come into close contact via the covalent bonds between the variable domains and noncovalent hydrophobic interactions between the opposing faces of the constant domains. Structurally, the TCR resembles the binding portion of an immunoglobulin molecule, the antigen receptor found on B cells.

MAJOR HISTOCOMPATIBILITY COMPLEX

The MHC is responsible for how T cells 'see' an antigen against a background of self

For an immune response to be initiated, antigen cannot simply bind to the nearest T cell but must be 'formally' presented to the immune system. This occurs when APC express processed antigenic peptides bound within grooves of MHC molecules on their cell surface.

The MHC complex of genes is found on the short arm of chromosome 6 and is grouped into three regions termed class I, II and III, with the same nomenclature being applied to the respective polypeptide products (Fig. 38.3). Class I and II molecules are directly involved with immune recognition and cellular interactions, whereas class III molecules are involved in the inflammatory response by coding for soluble mediators, including complement components of the innate response and TNF.

MHC class I genes are organized into several loci, the most important of which are those termed HLA-A, HLA-B and HLA-C

Alleles are transmitted and expressed in Mendelian codominant fashion. Owing to their closeness on the chromosome, they are inherited en bloc as parts of a haplotype and are expressed on the surface of all nucleated cells. The α-chains they encode have three domains, one of which is similar to those found in immunoglobulin molecules, but the other two show significant differences. The α-chains combine with β2-microglobulin to give rise to a functional class I molecule (Fig. 38.4).

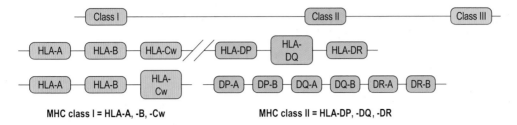

Fig. 38.3 **Genetic organization of the MHC and expressed products.** Genes of the MHC in humans are located on chromosome 6. The gene products are the human leukocyte antigens (HLA).

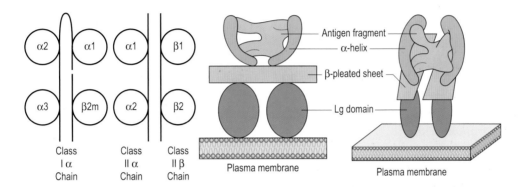

Fig. 38.4 **Class I and II MHC (HLA) structure.** On the left there are class I and class II MHC molecules. In class I molecules β2-microglobulin (β2 m) provides the fourth domain. On the right, this is related to the protein conformation in the MHC molecules.

Class II genes are HLA-DR, HLA-DQ and HLA-DP

The class II subregion genes, termed HLA-DR, HLA-DQ and HLA-DP, are organized into α- and β-loci, giving rise to α- and β-polypeptide chains, respectively. Both are of approximately the same molecular weight and combine to form a heterodimer with a tertiary structure similar to a class I molecule, with a peptide groove into which the processed antigenic fragment is inserted during antigen presentation. Unlike class I expression, class II is far more restricted, being expressed mainly on professional APCs, such as dendritic cells, as well as on macrophages and B cells.

The HLA system is intensely polymorphic

Many (currently in excess of 1000) allelic variants can be identified in each of the loci associated with antigen presentation. There are six major loci, each having between 10 and 60 functionally recognizable alleles, and as each parent passes on one set or haplotype on each chromosome, it is easy to appreciate that the likelihood of another individual in the same species having an identical set is remote.

The B cell antigen receptor

The B cell antigen receptor (BCR) is a membrane form of the immunoglobulin molecules found circulating in serum.

Immunoglobulins are Y-shaped molecules made up of four polypeptide chains (see Chapter 4, Fig. 4.6) – a pair of heavy chains each of approximate molecular weight 150 kDa and a pair of light chains each of approximate molecular weight 23 kDa. The arms interact with antigen and their structure is based on immunoglobulin domains with constant and variable sequences of amino acids in both the heavy and the light chains. It is the variably sequenced amino (NH$_2$) terminal domains of both the heavy (VH, variable heavy) and the light (VL, variable light) chains that form a pocket that constitutes the antigen-binding site; the 'fragment antigen binding' (Fab) portion sits at the end of the arms (see Fig. 4.6). The remaining relatively constant amino acid sequence domains of the chains are termed constant heavy (CH) or constant light (CL) and form the stem (Fc portion) that has a number of functions including binding complement components and binding to Fc receptors on leukocytes.

LYMPHOID TISSUES

Primary (or central) lymphoid tissues

Lymphocytes originating from common bone marrow-derived hemopoietic stem cells are initially found within primary lymphoid tissue, where they undergo early development and differentiation.

Maturation of most B cells occurs within the bone marrow

Initially, progenitor B cells rearrange their immunoglobulin genes (see below). They do so in an antigen-independent process but by interacting with stromal cells within the bone marrow. The resulting immature B cell expresses surface IgM as an antigen receptor. If they interact too strongly with environmental antigens at this stage they are removed by the process of negative selection, thus limiting the chance of autoreactivity. Following exit into the periphery, the B cells will express both surface IgM and IgD and can be activated by antigen engagement. These cells will proliferate, some becoming antibody-secreting plasma cells whilst others become long-lived memory cells.

T lymphocyte progenitors travel to the thymus where they develop into T lymphocytes

The thymus is a multilobed structure found in the midline of the body just above the heart. At the macroscopic level, there is an outer cortex and an inner medullary area within each lobule. In the thymus, T cell development progresses as the immature T cells migrate from the cortex to the medulla. The immature T cells interact with thymic epithelia and dendritic cells. These cells are thought to be responsible for the important processes of positive and negative selection that takes place as part of the 'thymic education of T cells'. During this process the T cells are assessed for their ability to interact with self MHC and receive survival signals. Cells which show excessive reactivity to self receive signals leading to their deletion whilst still within the thymus. This removes autoreactive cells which if released into the periphery could potentially induce autoimmunity. The development of both early T and B cells in the primary lymphoid tissues is independent of extrinsic antigen stimulation.

Secondary lymphoid tissues

The secondary (peripheral) lymphoid tissues comprise lymph nodes, spleen, and mucosa-associated lymphoid tissues (MALT)

These tissues are functionally organized throughout the body and have in common a degree of compartmentalization, with specific areas for T cells and B cells, and areas of overlap where they interact and respond to antigen. It is at these sites that immune reactions actually develop. For example, on exiting the thymus the naive T cells will recirculate via the bloodstream and enter the lymph nodes by appropriate upregulation of adhesion molecules and chemokine receptors, which allow them to localize in the T cell areas of the tissue.

Within the lymph node, the T cell area is the paracortex and the B cell area the follicular areas of the medulla. Here follicular structures of two types can be found: the unstimulated primary follicle, and stimulated secondary follicles, characterized by the presence of germinal centers. Lymph which drains from the tissues to the lymph nodes will carry antigens which in turn can be sampled by the APCs for presentation to the lymphocytes. On activation, the T cell will again alter chemokine receptor expression and leave the lymph node to recirculate to the site of infection where it can induce an effector response.

The spleen, an abdominal organ, contains nonlymphoid tissue (the red pulp) as well as lymphoid areas, the white pulp. Within the white pulp, follicular B cell areas are evident and the T cell areas lie between them in the interfollicular space. The spleen is used by the immune response for the presentation of blood-borne antigens.

MALT comprises the lymphoid elements adjacent to the mucosal surfaces that line internal body surfaces

They are found at the entrance to the respiratory tract and gut, and include the tonsils and adenoids. Further down the digestive tract, unencapsulated aggregates of lymphoid cells referred to as Peyer's patches are found, overlain by specialized areas of epithelium for sampling the antigenic environment. Similar to the lymph nodes and spleen, these tissues are important for initial antigen sampling and presentation, in particular for antigens which enter the body through a breach of the epithelium or via the gut.

ANTIGEN-PRESENTING CELLS

APCs are the specialized cells which display microbial antigens on their surface to allow T cell activation

Dendritic cells are the major APC and are found throughout the body. The skin and different organs have their resident population of such cells. Dendritic cells can migrate throughout the body from tissue to circulation and en route may enter the specialized secondary lymphoid organs such as lymph nodes where they may activate lymphocytes for an adaptive response. On uptake of antigen, APCs can process and reexpress it, in the context of the MHC, on the cell surface to allow presentation to the T cell. Dendritic cells are termed 'professional APC' as in addition to being able to present the antigen, they also possess a number of other cell surface molecules, e.g. CD80/86, which can provide the additional signals, so-called 'costimulation', required by a naive T cell for complete activation. Other cells which also are capable of presenting antigens and hence can be considered APCs include macrophages and B cells.

Adhesion molecules

Adhesion molecules mediate adhesion between cells

The direct cellular interactions during an immune response are dependent on the expression of the molecules and ligands that mediate adhesion between cells or between cells and the extracellular matrix. These are termed 'adhesion molecules' (see also Chapter 18). They are found on a wide variety of cell types, not only cells of the immune system, e.g. vascular endothelium. A major determinant of their expression is the prevailing cytokine environment and the surrounding connective tissue matrix. Typically, they are transmembrane glycoproteins. They deliver intracellular signals and during immune responses are primarily involved in promoting cell–cell interactions and cell migration. The latter includes the movement of innate cells from blood to tissue during infection as well as aiding lymphocytes to enter and leave lymph nodes as they circulate the body looking for activation signals as a result of antigen presentation in these peripheral organs. Adhesion molecules involved in immunity are grouped into three major families:

- **integrins**, e.g. lymphocyte function-associated antigen 1 (LFA-1), adhesion molecule 1 (MAC-1)
- **immunoglobulin supergene family adhesion molecules**, e.g. intercellular adhesion molecule 1 (ICAM-1) (CD54), platelet/cell adhesion molecule 1 (PECAM-1) (CD31)
- **selectins**, e.g. L-selectin, P-selectin.

REACTION WITH, THE RESPONSE TO AND THE ELIMINATION OF ANTIGENS

On binding to the antigen, the cell differentiates into progeny with an effector function or a memory function

On successful antigen binding, the activated lymphocyte undergoes repeated division or proliferation. Differentiation follows, which can lead to either the development of an effector function or the generation of memory.

Clonal selection creates clones of identical ells with unique antigen specificity.

The term clonal selection is given to the process whereby the immune response creates clones of identical cells, each clone having unique antigen specificity. With this clonal repertoire, the antigen determines which specific lymphocyte will be activated. The process of antigen drainage and lymphocyte recirculation to the peripheral lymphoid tissue ensures that antigen is inspected by many lymphocytes and can select for proliferation and differentiation the cell that bears a specific and reciprocal antigen receptor. Clonal selection (Fig. 38.5)

ensures not only an adequate number of effector cells to deal with the threat at the time of initial stimulation, but also a suitable number of part-primed memory cells that will be able to complete their activation more rapidly on subsequent antigen exposure.

Memory distinguishes the adaptive immune response from the innate response

How memory is generated is still the subject of research. On reexposure to the same antigen, the adaptive immune response, due to the reactivation of long-lived memory cells, mounts a more rapid and more effective response compared to the primary response. The long-lasting protection offered by vaccination is a result of immunologic memory.

Specific immune response is responsible for the elimination of antigens that are intracellular or integral to the cell surface

Adaptive immune responses are mediated by cellular and humoral elements. This response has been classically described as having cellular and humoral arms, T cells being considered responsible for cellular immunity and B cells for humoral immunity. It is now established that amongst its roles, the cellular or T cell-mediated response deals with chronic intracellular infections, mediates antitumor responses, is central to the rejection of transplanted tissue and drives contact hypersensitivity. Chronic intracellular

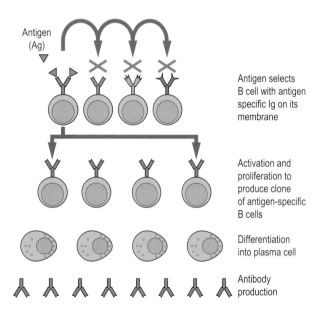

Fig. 38.5 **Clonal selection in B cells.** Antigen-specific (Ag-specific) secretory immunoglobulin (sIg) on the B cell membrane has a shape reciprocal to the antigen. Antigen-immunoglobulin binding leads to activation and proliferation to produce a clone of antigen-specific B cells. Each member of the specifically activated clone then undergoes differentiation into a plasma cell, which produces large quantities of a single homogeneous immunoglobulin with identical specificity to the sIg that triggered the response in the first instance.

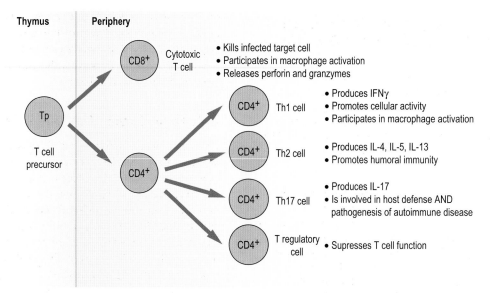

Fig. 38.6 **Functional T cell subsets.** T cell precursor cells within the thymus develop into cells with different effector functions.

infections may be bacterial (e.g. tuberculosis), viral, fungal or parasitic. In addition, T cells play key roles in the control of adaptive responses by helping or regulating other responses, e.g. helping B cells produce antibody.

T CELL RESPONSE

Distinct populations of T cells exist. All T cells, once they have left the thymus, express either CD4 or CD8 on their surface. This phenotypic distinction also has major consequences for effector function: CD4$^+$ T cells are often called T helper cells (TH), whilst CD8$^+$ cells are cytotoxic T cells (CTL). TH cells can be further subdivided. They were originally divided into TH1 and TH2 cells, but there is recent interest in a novel subset being termed TH17 due to their release of IL-17. The different subsets of T cells are shown schematically in Figure 38.6.

T cells are responsible for the regulation of the activities of the other arms of the immune response. They achieve this by direct cell–cell contact or by the secretion of soluble mediators that interact with the relevant cells, be they other T cells, B cells, cells involved in the innate immune response such as macrophages, or cells of other tissues.

Classification of T cells depends on cell surface markers

T helper cells: TH1/TH2 and TH17

This subpopulation of cells was first identified as 'helping' cellular immune responses. We have said above that T cells

need to be presented with antigen in the context of MHC on the surface of an APC. For CD4$^+$ T cells. This is done by MHC II molecules. These T cells see antigen peptides which have been processed by the APC and expressed within the binding grooves of the MHC molecule. They also receive costimulatory signals. The T cell is activated through CD28-CD80/86 ligation and will proliferate into effector cells.

The subdivision into TH1 and TH2 was originally made on the basis of their apparent function. TH1 cells appeared to function as promoting cellular responses. Once activated, they could release IFN-γ which in turn further promotes macrophage activity. In addition, they may release TNF-α which, through endothelial activation and subsequent upregulation of adhesion molecules and chemokines, would promote further leukocyte recruitment and hence perpetuate the response. TH2 cells help cellular responses in a different way. They appear to preferentially stimulate eosinophil-driven inflammation through IL-5 production. This is the major antihelminth response. By releasing IL-4 and IL-13, TH2 cells limit the TH1 activation of macrophages. Whilst all helper T cells can influence antibody production by B cells, TH2 cells, by releasing IL-4, can induce class switching and the production of an IgE response. Therefore the functions of TH cells appear to be determined by the cytokine environment they produce.

Recently, there has been much interest in another subset of TH cell which does not fit with the original TH1/TH2 paradigm. The so-called TH17 cell was originally identified in animal models of a number of autoimmune diseases including multiple sclerosis, rheumatoid arthritis and inflammatory bowel disease. Understanding the potential role of this subset, particularly in human disease, is currently a major research focus.

RECURRENT INFECTION IN AN IMMUNOCOMPROMISED CHILD

A 2-year-old child presented with a history of recurrent *Candida albicans* and chest infections. Investigations revealed a decreased number of neutrophils, IgG and IgA. Assessments of lymphocyte proliferative response showed decreased expression of CD40 on T cells. A diagnosis of X-linked hyper IgM was made and treatment with intravenous immunoglobulin was commenced.

Comment. T cell help is required for effective B cell responses. Particular interactions are required for the switch of isotype from the IgM response that is typical of a primary antibody response to the more mature IgG and or IgA isotypes seen during secondary antibody responses produced to subsequent challenges. CD40 on the T cell is required to interact with the CD40 on B cells to achieve this. In its absence, antibody production is limited to IgM and the affected individual is immunocompromised owing to the lack of the other important isotypes so critical to the integrity of the immune response. The problem of infection more typically associated with cellular problems suggests that the T cell defect has functional consequences for this arm of the immune response.

As well as restricting input, the class I and II molecules also provide a differential mechanism for processing antigens that originate from within cells, e.g. viruses, and those that arise from the extracellular environment, e.g. bacterial antigens. The different class MHC molecules also lead such antigens through different pathways to interact with the immune system, in particular with the T cells, on the basis that each will be better dealt with by differing effector systems: class I leads to CD8$^+$ T-cytotoxic responses, and class II instructs CD4$^+$ helper T to provide appropriate help to B cells for an antibody-mediated response.

T regulatory cells

Originally cells which can control a cell-mediated response were identified as 'suppressor cells'. However, the original description of a CD8$^+$ cell providing this function is no longer considered valid. The cell types now studied are the so-called T regulatory cells. This appears to be a heterogeneous group. The most studied is a CD4$^+$ T cell which appears to be able to control the action of other immune cells through a combination of soluble mediator release (IL-10 and TGF-β) and direct cell–cell contact. These cells are thought to also express the transcription factor FoxP3, which appears to be crucial for T regulatory cell development. As discussed earlier, the thymus plays an important role in deleting autoreactive T cells before they exit into the periphery by the mechanism of central tolerance. This process is not 100% efficient and it is now recognized that T regulatory cells play an important role in the process of peripheral tolerance, i.e. the holding in check cells within the circulation which if allowed would be autoreactive and cause autoimmunity. The translation to clinical applications of preventing autoimmune disease is currently under investigation. Their regulatory potential may also be applicable to induce tolerance to organ grafts.

Cytotoxic T cells (CTL) kill infected cells

The other major population of T cells based on their surface expression of CD8 is known as cytotoxic T cells. Their role is primarily to kill infected cells (e.g. virus). CD8$^+$ T cells recognize peptides of the antigen associated with MHC I on the surface of the infected cell. By doing this, they are able to limit infection. On recognition of the antigen, the CTL will become activated without the need for costimulation. It will bind tightly to the infected cell using adhesion molecules and the main method of killing infected cells is by the release of proteins such as granzymes and perforins. The result of delivery of these enzymes to the infected cell is activation of the caspase-driven apoptosis (Chapter 43). Apoptotic cells are removed by innate phagocytic cells such as macrophages.

HUMORAL SPECIFIC IMMUNE RESPONSE

Humoral immune response is characterized by the release of antibodies from fully matured plasma B lymphocytes

Humoral- or antibody-mediated specific immunity is directed at extracellular infection, especially by bacteria and their products, and also at the extracellular phase of viral infection and allogeneic cell/organ transplantation. The humoral immune response is characterized by the release of antibodies from fully matured plasma cells of the B lymphocyte lineage. As antibodies recognize many types of molecules including polysaccharides and lipids, this response is particularly efficient against extracellular pathogens. The antibody binding to structural surface components of microbes blocks the adhesion of these bacteria or viruses and prevents the harmful effects of their toxins in a process termed neutralization. However, simple antibody binding, in most situations, will not guarantee elimination of the antigen. To promote the response, the nonantigen-binding fragment of the molecule (Fc portion) is able to activate other components of the innate system, e.g. through complement activation. The diversity of effector functions is achieved by genetic recombinations of the heavy chain genes, additional to those present, to generate diversity and specificity of the antigen-binding component. Thus the original antigen specificity is preserved whilst effector functions can alter (see box on p. 516).

B cell subsets operate in the humoral immune response

Similar to the cellular response, which is mediated by a number of T cell subsets, the humoral response uses distinct B cell subsets. As noted earlier, T cells, particularly the TH cells, interact with B cells both directly and indirectly via cell surface receptors and cytokines, respectively. This happens to such a degree that effective B cell responses are often described as being T cell dependent. The B cells termed B-2 are found in the follicles of the secondary lymphoid organs. They typically respond to protein antigens and produce the high-affinity class-switched antibodies typical of humoral responses. Within the marginal zone of the spleen, there is another population of B cells which typically respond to polysaccharide antigens delivered via the bloodstream. Another population termed B-1, which express similar receptors and CD5 on their surface, is found in mucosal tissue and the peritoneum. Unlike classic follicular B cells, marginal zone and B-1 B cells predominantly make an IgM response typically to nonprotein antigens.

Antibodies illustrate the capability of the immune system for diversity

For T cell-dependent responses, reexposure to antigen will induce a secondary antibody response. The higher levels of antibody produced will have increased affinity and avidity for the particular antigen as a result of the processes of heavy chain class switching and affinity maturation. The normal human immune system is capable of producing a limitless number of highly specific antibodies with the ability of recognizing any and all nonself elements with which it comes into contact. Failure of effective immune response control can result in the production of antibodies against self-antigens, termed 'autoantibodies', and these are characteristic of a number of autoimmune diseases including systemic lupus erythematosus (SLE), rheumatoid arthritis (RA), etc.

The terms antibody, gamma globulin and immunoglobulin are synonymous

Five classes of immunoglobulin are recognized: IgG, IgA, IgM, IgD, and IgE, with subclasses being recognized for IgG (IgG1, 2, 3, and 4) and for IgA (1 and 2). When studied at the individual molecular level, no other proteins show such amino acid sequence variation between individual members of the same class or subclass. This is most evident in the NH_2-terminal domains of both heavy and light chains which are responsible for the antigen recognition portion of the molecule. Antibodies are capable of discriminating between the molecules that characterize the outer capsular coverings of differing bacterial species which may vary by a single amino acid or a monosaccharide residue. This is a consequence of the dimensions of the area recognized by the antibody molecule being 10–20 Å (10^{-10}m) and thus being significantly influenced by the alteration in three-dimensional conformation brought about by the change of a single residue.

Antibodies are good examples of how function is intimately related to structure

Antibodies (immunoglobulins) are Y-shaped molecules (see Fig. 4.6). The arms interact with antigen and the stem provides additional or effector functionality. This secondary or effector function endows the antibody with an ability to initiate immune responses which help eliminate it.

Activation of the complement system is one of the most important antibody functions

Activation of the complement system (see Fig. 38.1) is one of the most important antibody effector functions of the adaptive immune response. This is achieved by using a set of components termed the 'classic activation pathways', which comprise C1q, C1r, C1s, C4, and C-2. Sequential activation of these components leads to the activation of the pivotal and critically important C-3 component, which is an absolute requirement for full complement activation. Once this is achieved, the terminal membrane attack complex, which comprises the components C5, C6, C7, C8, and C9, is activated. This complex eventually generates the polymeric ring structure that inserts into the cell membrane of bacteria and is responsible for cell lysis. This classic pathway is triggered by C1q binding IgG or IgM that is already bound to its specific antigen (Fig. 38.7).

Two other pathways of activation exist, both constituting parts of the nonspecific immune response; they are probably older in evolutionary terms. These are the alternative pathway, which can be activated by lipopolysaccharide such as is found in gram-negative bacterial walls, and the mannose binding ligand (MBL) pathway, which can be activated by mannose and other particular carbohydrates found in the cell wall of fungi, bacteria and viruses. The effector functions of antibodies are summarized in Table 38.2.

VACCINATION

Probably the single most beneficial application developed to harness the immune response has been vaccination. The process of vaccination illustrates well the interactions of the humoral and cellular arms of the adaptive immune response and the features that characterize it best – specificity and memory. On first encounter with antigen, the immune system and antigen interact to select lymphocytes with the receptors specific for that antigen. These undergo activation, proliferation and differentiation into effector memory cells, a process that may take up to 14 days to complete (Fig. 38.8). However, the process of memory cell generation now leaves a population of cells semiprimed for that specific antigen. On subsequent exposure, the response is more rapid in view of the partly activated state of the memory cells, and more

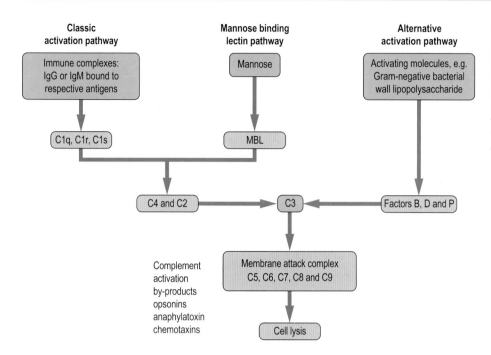

Fig. 38.7 **Complement activation pathways.** There are three possible pathways of complement activation. Only the classic pathway is triggered by the specific immune response via antibody. The mannose-binding ligand (MBL) pathway and the alternative activation pathway are triggered directly by microbes and their products independent of antibody. (Compare Fig. 38.1.)

effective as a consequence of a degree of maturation of the response, due to the differentiation of the lymphocytes that has already taken place.

With reference to antibody responses, the primary challenge elicits a predominantly IgM response. On subsequent challenge, the lymphocytes undergo further maturation and differentiation and isotype switching, and more rapidly produce a predominantly IgG response. This provides additional effector functions to that obtained with just IgM. It is this heightened and more specific response that can reduce both the severity and the duration of any damage caused by the offending antigen.

Autoimmunity is normally prevented by thymic education; a breakdown in the processes involved may lead to autoimmune disease

While the immune system's activities are mostly beneficial, there are several situations in which they can have deleterious effects. These are best considered as aberrations of the quality, quantity or direction of the response.

One particular aspect of these disorders, that of autoimmunity (self-reactivity), is avoided by the processes of central tolerance (during thymic education) and peripheral tolerance which induces clonal deletion and anergy. The self-reactive clones are eliminated or rendered impotent either through deletion within the thymus or by being controlled by T regulatory cells in the periphery. These mechanisms can be seen as a multilayered fail-safe strategy. Should these processes break down or be circumvented, the resulting state of self-reactivity and the inflammatory damage constitute autoimmune disease.

The form of disease is determined by the target antigen and the form of the immune response. At its simplest, reactions against ubiquitous antigens lead to what are termed nonorgan-specific autoimmune diseases, whereas

Type	Functions	Concentration in peripheral blood
IgG	neutralization opsonization for neutrophils and macrophages passive immunity for fetus via transplacental passage complement activation via classic pathway antibody-dependent, cell-mediated cytotoxicity natural killer – cell killing of antibody bound cells achieved by FcRs (receptors for the Fc portion) major isotype used in a secondary antibody response	6.0–16.0 g/L
IgA	defense of mucosal surfaces as the most predominant immunoglobulin produced by MALT, neutralization	0.8–4.0 g/L
IgM	neutralization most effective classic complement pathway activator predominant isotype in primary antibody responses	0.5–2.0 g/L
IgD	possible role in signal transduction and B cell maturation significance of circulating IgD is undefined	0.03 g/L
IgE	major role is defense of mucosal surfaces against multicellular microorganisms	<120 kU/L

The effector functions of antibodies

Table 38.2 **The effector functions of antibodies.**

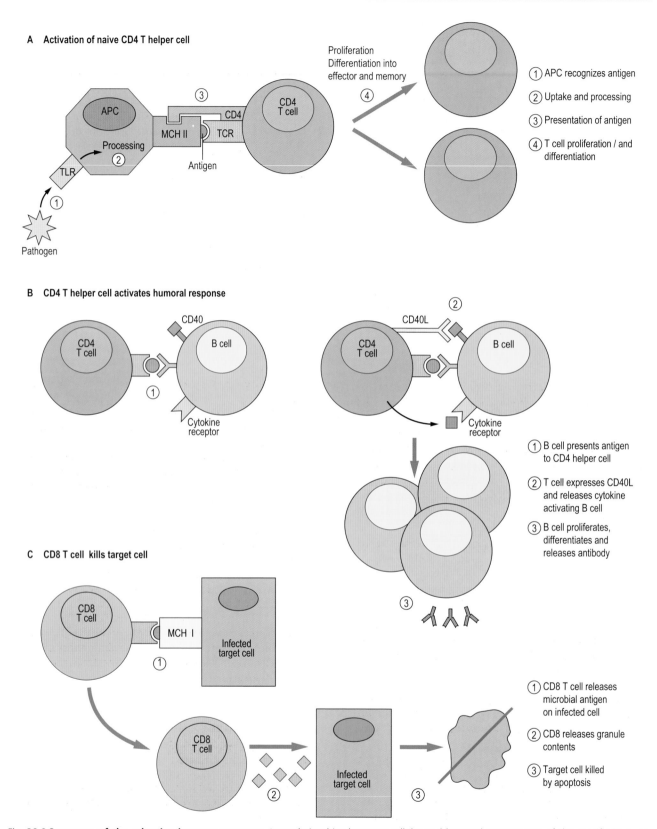

A   Activation of naive CD4 T helper cell

Proliferation
Differentiation into
effector and memory

① APC recognizes antigen

② Uptake and processing

③ Presentation of antigen

④ T cell proliferation / and
differentiation

Pathogen

B   CD4 T helper cell activates humoral response

① B cell presents antigen
to CD4 helper cell

② T cell expresses CD40L
and releases cytokine
activating B cell

③ B cell proliferates,
differentiates and
releases antibody

C   CD8 T cell kills target cell

① CD8 T cell releases
microbial antigen
on infected cell

② CD8 releases granule
contents

③ Target cell killed
by apoptosis

Fig. 38.8 **Summary of the adaptive immune response.** Interrelationships between cellular and humoral components of the specific immune response. APCs activate naive CD4 T cells which in turn can activate B cells. Cytotoxic T cells kill infected target cells.

Failure of the immune system	
Autoimmunity	inappropriate response to self antigens through the breakdown of self-tolerance can lead to autoimmune conditions.
	Examples: rheumatoid arthritis, SLE, type 1 diabetes mellitus
Hypersensitivity	inappropriate or overreaction to pathogen or antigen can often result in a response which does more harm to the body than the actual cause.
	Examples: hayfever in response to pollen, anaphylactic response to foodstuffs, e.g. peanuts
Immunodeficiency	ineffective immune response to infection can cause immunodeficiency. These can often be hereditary or induced by infection or drug treatment.
	Primary immunodeficiency is an intrinsic defect of one or more components of the immune response, e.g. antibody of impaired phagocytic function.
	Examples: X-linked agammaglobulinemia which presents as very low B cell numbers and serum immunoglobulin.
	Severe combined immunodeficiency (SCID) where thymus fails to develop and no T cells are present.
	Secondary immunodeficiency can result after infection, e.g. AIDS, where the virus infects CD4 T cells or as response to certain drugs, e.g. steroids which can impair immune cell function.

Table 38.3 **Failure of the immune system.**

reactions to unique components of individual tissues, organs or systems lead to organ-specific disease. The former are best exemplified by systemic lupus erythematosus (SLE), in which the apparent target antigens are components common to all nuclei. Damage is seen in several tissues, including the skin, joints, kidneys, and nervous system. These diseases, and the others mentioned in Table 38.3, are the focus of the discipline of clinical immunology and immunopathology. More information can be found in the books cited in the Further reading below.

Summary

- Integrated immune response to nonself or altered-self elements (antigen(s)) is made up of a number of components. Some of these show unique specificity for the particular stimulating antigen(s) and comprise the specific or adaptive immune response, whilst others recognize pathogen signatures and comprise the nonspecific or innate immune response.
- The innate response represents the first-line response and is present in all eukaryotes. The cells and soluble mediators involved are primarily those associated with the processes of inflammation and vascular activation.
- The adaptive response is more refined and usually invoked only in the face of either failure or continued stimulation of the nonspecific response. The cells responsible for the adaptive immune response are the T and B lymphocytes. The specificity they show for the inciting antigen is achieved via the use of specific antigen receptors, expressed on their cell surface.
- T cells recognize processed antigen via their receptor, interacting with antigen presented by MHC-bearing cells, leading to the secretion of additional cytokines and the generation of effector functions such as T cell help and T cell-mediated cytotoxicity

brought about by the T helper and T cytotoxic subsets respectively. Historically, T cell responses have been termed the cellular immune response. A distinct CD4$^+$ subset of T cells are termed 'T regulatory' as they function to control adaptive responses and in part prevent autoreactivity by the immune response.
- B cells recognize native antigen and secrete proteins termed antibodies which can directly bind to the antigen. Historically, B cells and their antibody products have been termed the humoral immune response.
- Both T and B cells and their products are able to recruit and utilize components of the innate response in a more effective and targeted manner, with the aim of eliminating or eradicating the antigen.
- In addition to demonstrating specificity, the adaptive immune response also demonstrates another critically important characteristic not seen with the innate response – the memory for its encounter with antigen. The benefit of this is that, on subsequent contact with the same antigen, a heightened and more efficient response will lead to a quicker removal of the causative agent, hopefully with less tissue damage than on the previous occasion.

ACTIVE LEARNING

1. Compare the function of T and B lymphocytes.
2. What are adhesion molecules and what is their role in the immune response?
3. What are the key features of the innate and adaptive immune responses?
4. What is the role of the Fc fragment of an immunoglobulin?
5. What is the role of the thymus in the immune response?

Further reading

Abbas AK, Lichtman AH. *Basic immunology*, 3rd edn Philadelphia: Saunders Elsevier, 2008.

Chapel H, Heaney M, Misbah S, Snowden N. *Essentials of clinical immunology*, 5th edn Oxford: Blackwell, 2006.

D'Cruz D, Khamashta M, Hughes GRV. Systemic lupus erythematosus. *Lancet* 2007; **369**: 587–596.

Male D, Brostoff J, Roth DB, Roitt IM. *Immunology*, 7th edn London: Mosby, 2007.

Meylan E, Tschopp J, Karin M. Intracellular patter recognition receptors in the host response. *Nature* 2006; **442**: 38–44.

Murphy K, Travers P, Walport M. *Janeway's immunobiology*, 7th edn London: Garland, 2005.

Nature Insight. Autoimmunity. *Nature* 2005; **435**: 583–627.

39. Biochemical Endocrinology

R K Semple and F F Bolander Jr

LEARNING OBJECTIVES

After reading this chapter you should be able to:

- Understand the principles governing endocrine signaling and its regulation.
- Describe the basic anatomy, organization and regulatory role of the hypothalamus and pituitary.
- Describe the regulatory processes controlling the biosynthesis, transport and mechanism of action of thyroid hormones.
- Describe the mechanisms regulating synthesis and action of glucocorticoids.
- Outline the mechanisms regulating the synthesis and activity of sex steroid hormones and their role in regulation of male and female reproduction.
- Describe the direct and indirect actions of growth hormone, including the role of IGF-I.
- Outline the role of prolactin in reproduction.
- Describe the consequences of deficiencies and excesses of hormones regulated by the hypothalamo-pituitary axis.

INTRODUCTION

As a first approximation, the human body contains 10 trillion – or 10 million million – cells, which may lie more than 2 meters apart. Coordination and regulation of the growth and multiple functions of these cells in order to meet the demands of existence in constantly fluctuating environmental conditions require precise and highly sophisticated integrative systems. The nervous system is a key part of the answer, being particularly well suited to mediating reflexes and motor actions required, for example, in 'fight or flight' situations, which may require responses in fractions of a second. The endocrine system, however, is the principal means of regulation of a wide range of less acute functions including growth, development, reproduction, many aspects of homeostasis, and the response to more chronic external stimuli and stress. Such endocrine responses occur over several seconds at their fastest, to days or weeks at their slowest. Failures in these highly elaborate, complex and often interconnected endocrine control systems are common, and lead to many very prevalent diseases.

HORMONES

The concept that organs and tissues may produce 'internal secretions' that influence the behavior of distant parts of the body probably first emerged in France in the 18th century, and by the beginning of the 20th century, adrenaline and vasopressin (ADH) had been isolated. However, it was only in 1905, shortly after isolating secretin, that Ernest Starling in London first coined the word 'hormone' to describe such internal messengers. Hormones are now understood to be chemical substances that are produced by particular glands or groups of cells, and that elicit specific responses from distant cells or organs. Classically, such hormones are blood-borne and are described as *endocrine* hormones. However, subsequently it has become clear that some hormones act locally on cells around their cell of origin – so-called *paracrine* hormones – or even on the same cell that has produced them – so-called *autocrine* hormones.

Types of hormones

Hormones have diverse chemical structures

Many different types of molecules function as hormones (Table 39.1). At the simplest level, modified amino acids, such as epinephrine (adrenaline), have hormonal activity and many such simple amines also function as neurotransmitters (Chapter 42). Other hormones are polypeptides varying in size from tripeptides (e.g. thyrotropin-releasing hormones) to complex glycoproteins (e.g. luteinizing hormone, LH). The smaller peptide hormones are synthesized as large polypeptide or protein prohormones, that are cleaved by proteolytic enzymes to release active hormone from the endocrine gland. Other hormones are derived by modification of simple lipids such as cholesterol or fatty acids.

Many glands and tissues produce hormones

Hormones are best known to be secreted from ductless glands such as the thyroid, adrenals, and pituitary which have been known to anatomists for centuries. However, many hormones are so potent that they need only circulate at tiny plasma concentrations to exert meaningful biologic effects, and may derive from small clusters of cells, or from one particular cell type scattered within a larger organ. Furthermore, it is now becoming clear that many tissues which were not

Chemical derivation of hormones

Derived from amino acids

Amino acid derivatives	catecholamines, serotonin, thyroxine
Tripeptides	TRH
Small peptides	AVP (ADH), somatostatin
Intermediate-size peptides	insulin, parathyroid hormone
Complex polypeptides and glycoproteins	gonadotropins, TSH

Derived from lipid precursors

Cholesterol derivatives	cortisol, testosterone, estradiol, vitamin D
Fatty acid derivatives	prostaglandins, leukotrienes
Phospholipid derivative	platelet-activating factor

Derived from other chemicals

Purines	adenosine
Gases	nitric oxide

AVP/ADH, arginine vasopressin or antidiuretic hormone; TRH, thyrotropin-releasing hormone; TSH, thyroid-stimulating hormone.

Table 39.1 **The chemical derivation of hormones.**

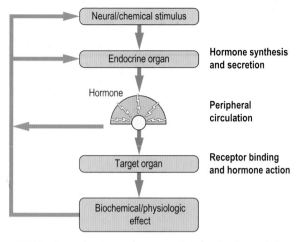

Fig. 39.1 **Basic endocrine processes.** The feedback regulation of hormone action is a classic example of self-regulation.

emphasis is on the very well-established hormonal systems which are the focus of current clinical endocrinology.

PRINCIPLES OF HORMONE ACTION

In order to function effectively to relay signals from one part of the body to others, endocrine systems must exhibit certain general properties (Fig. 39.1).

Coupling of hormone release to relevant stimuli

Some hormones function to transmit to the body important environmental cues, while others are more concerned with calibrating metabolic processes involved in maintaining homeostasis. In either situation, it is critical that there is effective translation of the magnitude of the stimulus into the amount of hormone released. How this is achieved varies depending on the stimulus. Simple homeostatic sensing mechanisms include direct coupling of parathyroid hormone release to calcium levels via a cell surface receptor which binds calcium (Chapter 25), and direct coupling of insulin secretion to plasma glucose levels via sensing of blood glucose concentration by the pancreatic β cell (Chapter 21). Many of the endocrine systems described in this chapter, in contrast, are controlled by modified neurones which secrete hormones into the bloodstream. The level of secretion of such neurones is often determined by complex synaptic inputs from many different parts of the brain as well as by the sensing of circulating metabolites and hormones. These secretory neurones thus function as important sites of integration of a variety of environmental, psychologic and physiologic cues.

NONCLASSIC ENDOCRINE ORGANS

Many tissues apart from classic ductless endocrine glands are now known to be active endocrinologically, the signals produced mediating important metabolic cross-talk between different tissues. Examples of this include production of leptin from white adipose tissue, which signals body energy stores to the brain (Chapter 22), production of fibroblast growth factor 23 (FGF23) from bone, which modulates renal phosphate handling and is ectopically produced by some tumors to produce a clinically important renal phosphate leak and osteomalacia, and production of satiety factors such as ghrelin from the small intestine. The placenta is also a highly active endocrine tissue: as well as producing βHCG, progesterone, placental growth hormone and human placental lactogen, which have well-understood roles in pregnancy, it elaborates many other hormones at high levels whose role remains to be determined.

traditionally thought to be active in endocrine terms actually secrete a wide variety of different hormones with diverse effects on other tissues. Indeed, the availability of the human genome sequence, allied to sophisticated bio-informatics and techniques such as microarray-based transcriptional profiling (Chapter 36), has led to the discovery of many new suspected hormones and hormone receptors, and understanding of the endocrine mechanisms regulating human physiology is likely to increase rapidly. Nevertheless, in this chapter the

Feedback

A major feature of most endocrine systems is negative feedback. This means that a response induced by action of a hormone feeds back to inhibit the level of hormone production. The effect of this is to damp down fluctuations in the process controlled by the hormone, thereby enhancing stability of that process and hence homeostasis. However, were negative feedback to be the only process at play, then the output of the system would remain constant. In fact, many endocrine systems, notably those controlled by the hypothalamus, display distinct rhythmicity. This is determined by the net product of the neural inputs to the relevant secretory neurones, and in this situation negative feedback serves instead to smooth out the hormonal profile and to prevent short-term instability. Furthermore, modulation of the susceptibility of the controlling neurone to feedback inhibition represents one potential mechanism of modulating the level of the output of the endocrine system.

Positive feedback refers to stimulation of hormone release by the response it provokes. This feedforward loop is inherently unstable, and leads to a rapid, exponential increase in the level of signal. This is much rarer than negative feedback in physiology, but plays an important role in some processes which require precise timing, such as the luteinizing hormone surge which precedes ovulation.

Transduction of signal at target tissues

Hormones act by binding to specific receptors, either on the cell surface or within the target cell (Chapter 40). Classically, there is a very high degree of specificity in this binding, and it is this hormone–receptor interaction that triggers and coordinates a wide range of biologic effects. Hormone receptors may be divided into different families according to their structure, and each family broadly shares signal transduction mechanisms (Chapter 40). Many amine-like hormones and peptides which cannot cross lipid bilayers act via G-protein coupled receptors, while some larger peptides such as insulin and IGF-1 act via tyrosine kinase receptors. Both of these receptor types are intrinsic plasma membrane proteins, and they each rely on cascades of sequential phosphorylation events to alter enzyme activity and gene expression. Steroid hormones, some hormones derived from fatty acids, and tri-iodothyronine, which has physicochemical properties in common with steroids (Chapter 17), enter cells before binding their receptors. These so-called nuclear hormone receptors are effectively ligand-activated transcription factors, and provide a very direct link between the exposure of a cell to hormonal ligand and alteration of patterns of gene expression (Chapter 34). Many putative receptors for unknown hormones have been identified by virtue of sequence homology among members of each of the major hormone receptor classes. It is likely that identification of the ligand for these 'orphan' receptors will significantly increase the range of endocrine hormones.

IMPRINTING IN ENDOCRINOLOGY

Gene expression may be influenced not only by the DNA sequence of genes and their promoter regions, but also by covalent modifications of DNA such as methylation of cytosine residues, which occurs particularly in promoter regions and acts to silence genes. Methylation status of some promoters depends on which parent the gene was inherited from, and because methylation patterns are preserved as cells divide, major 'parent of origin' effects can be seen, most markedly when there is a mutation in one parental allele. Several endocrine systems show significant imprinting. Best known is the IGF2-IGF2 receptor system, which acts to influence placental and fetal growth. Another important endocrine signaling gene which is imprinted is the GNAS gene, encoding a stimulatory G-protein subunit coupled to many classic endocrine peptide hormone receptors. Various different mutations have been described, and depending on which parent they are inherited from, they may produce skeletal dysplasia and resistance to various hormones, including most notably parathyroid hormone. Indeed, so-called 'pseudohypoparathyroidism' was the first reported example of end-organ resistance to a hormone. For review of the fascinating and complex biology of GNAS, readers are referred to Weinstein LS *et al*. Minireview: GNAS: normal and abnormal functions. *Endocrinology* 2004;**145**:5459–5464. (Compare p. 434 and Table 34.2.)

Turning off the signal

Levels of hormones are useful physiologic signals only if there is also an effective way of turning the signal off. Hormone inactivation usually occurs by further metabolism (e.g. proteolysis, hydroxylation, and conjugation), followed by excretion of the metabolites. Such degradation may occur in plasma, in organs such as the liver or in target tissues after receptor-mediated internalization of the hormone. The rate of clearance of different hormones varies enormously, from a few minutes (insulin), through hours (steroids) to days (thyroxine). Measurement of urinary concentrations of hormones or their metabolites can be used in some diagnostic settings, including the diagnosis of pregnancy, and in pathologies such as secretory adrenal tumors.

Many endocrine systems have additional common features.

Carrier proteins and 'free' hormones

Within the circulation, many small or hydrophobic hormones are transported bound to carrier proteins. For example, thyroxine and cortisol are transported on specific

Examples of major hormone binding proteins

Hormone	Binding protein	Approximate % bound	Notes
Thyroxine	thyroid-binding globulin (TBG)	75%	clinically significant increase in early pregnancy
	albumin	10–15%	
	transthyretin	10–15%	
Testosterone	sex hormone binding globulin (SHBG)	60–70%	levels of SHBG are strongly hormonally regulated (e.g. suppressed by insulin and increased by thyroid hormone)
Cortisol	CBG	75%	variations in cortisol BPs may be particularly misleading as it is total cortisol which is generally assayed. Thus women taking estrogens (increase CBG) may have high total but normal free cortisol, while in critical illness and malnutrition the converse is true
	albumin	15–20%	
GH	GHBP	50%	GHBP is a soluble fragment of the GH receptor. This is a common feature of many cytokine-like hormones
IGF-1	IGFBP-3	75%	there are 6 IGFBPs which modulate the paracrine activity of IGF-1, and may have signaling roles in their own right

Table 39.2 **Examples of major hormone binding proteins.**

plasma-binding globulins such as thyroid-binding globulin (TBG) and cortisol-binding globulins (CBG). This has several consequences of relevance to both physiology and clinical measurement. The transport proteins extend the biologic half-life and increase the plasma concentration of the smaller hormones, which would otherwise be eliminated rapidly in the liver or kidney. This also means that there may be large differences between the total plasma levels of hormone and the unbound or 'free' hormone in solution, which is generally the biologically active form. Thus clinical interpretation of plasma hormone levels is simplest if assays are developed to detect free hormone only, otherwise assumptions must be made about levels of binding proteins, which in turn may be significantly influenced by the nutritional and hormonal milieu. It is not only small lipophilic hormones which have plasma-binding proteins, however; both growth hormone and insulin-like growth factor 1 have plasma-binding proteins which influence bio-availability and tissue activity of the hormones in a variety of different ways (Table 39.2).

Local metabolism of hormones at target tissues

Another feature of some endocrine systems, particularly those involving steroid hormones, is local metabolism of the hormones or prohormones near their cognate receptor. This may involve conversion of an active circulating hormone to a more potent form (for example, testosterone to dihydrotestosterone by 5α-reductase in androgen-dependent hair follicles and prostate gland) or creation of an active hormone from what is effectively a circulating prohormone (e.g. thyroxine to tri-iodothyronine by de-iodinase, or synthesis of estradiol from adrenal androgens in adipose tissue). A similar mechanism is also employed to prevent mineralocorticoid receptors in the kidney being exposed to high concentrations of cortisol, with cortisol being inactivated by 11β-hydroxysteroid dehydrogenase type II, which is expressed highly near the mineralocorticoid receptors. Many other examples of such intracellular interconversion of steroid hormones have also emerged, and study of this phenomenon has sometimes been dubbed 'intracrinology' (Table 39.3).

Several hormones may control one process, or one hormone may control several processes

While it may be convenient to think of the endocrine system as being compartmentalized so that one hormone has control over one process, this is rarely the case. For example, at least four different hormones are involved in the regulation of plasma glucose concentration (see Chapter 21). Conversely, single hormones such as testosterone influence a range of metabolic processes.

All of these features of endocrine systems will be illustrated by some or all of the endocrine axes which pass through the pituitary, to be discussed later in this chapter.

Examples of hormone metabolism in target tissues

Hormone	Enzyme	Substrate	Product effect on activity
T4	deiodinase type 2	T3	generates potent T3 from nearly inactive T4 in target tissues
Testosterone	aromatase	estrogen	as well as playing an important role in the ovary in generating estrogen, aromatase is expressed in other tissues including bone, adipose tissue and hypothalamus. Even in men, this local conversion of androgens to estrogens is important in mediating effects of testosterone on bone density and central negative feedback to LH/FSH production
Testosterone	5α reductase	dihydrotestosterone	produces more potent ligand for the androgen receptor, amplifying testosterone activity locally: genetic deficiency produces pseudohermaphroditism
Cortisol	11β-hydroxysteroid dehydrogenase type II	cortisone	converts cortisol, which activates the mineralocorticoid receptor, to cortisone, which does not. The enzyme is highly expressed in mineralocorticoid-sensitive tissues such as the kidney. Genetic deficiency leads to exposure of mineralocorticoid receptors to high concentrations of active ligand, leading to severe hypertension and hypokalemia in the syndrome of apparent mineralocorticoid excess

Table 39.3 **Examples of hormone metabolism in target tissues.**

BIOCHEMICAL ASSESSMENT OF HORMONE ACTION

Laboratory testing of endocrine systems aims first to determine whether the system is functioning abnormally, and second to localize the functional defect. Most commonly, this means that levels of the hormone that elicit the relevant physiologic response at target tissues are determined, usually by immunoassay, together with measurement of one or more upstream trophic hormones, where they exist. The presence of negative feedback regulation means that the system will attempt to correct perturbations in levels of the effector hormone with compensatory changes in levels of trophic hormones. Thus assessment of at least two points in such an endocrine feedback loop is essential, and permits focusing of later diagnostic imaging on the relevant gland.

Once the hormones of most interest to the clinical problem have been chosen, care then needs to be used to ensure appropriate sampling. This should take into account whether the hormone is very unstable (for example, many small peptide hormones require blood samples to be taken into tubes on ice containing a protease inhibitor), and also whether it is produced with a circadian or other rhythm. For some hormones, such as thyroxine, which have very long half-life, timing of the sample is not critical, while for others, such as cortisol, standardized timing of the sample is essential.

A further factor to take into account in hormone testing is whether or not secretion of the hormone is pulsatile. Nearly all of the hypothalamic and pituitary hormones show some degree of pulsatility in secretion. In most cases this simply means that repeat testing in the case of mild abnormality is required, while for some hormones, such as growth hormone, which has both a short half-life and very striking secretory spikes, single measurements are often meaningless.

Because of these problems, endocrinologists commonly employ multiple testing to build up a profile of hormone levels at several points in the day. This can be an effective way of detecting subtle perturbations of the circadian rhythm, and can also lessen the impact of oscillatory secretion of the hormone. A further approach is to use provocative testing. In other words, hormone levels are measured not just in the resting state, but also after a relevant stimulus has been applied, in an attempt to assess the maximal capacity of the endocrine gland or system being tested. Frequently the stimulus is a high dose of trophic hormone (e.g. ACTH, TRH, GnRH, etc.); however, it may instead be a metabolic challenge (e.g. with an oral glucose load or severe insulin-induced hypoglycemia to mimic stress). Examples of each of these tests are given in Table 39.4.

MAJOR TYPES OF ENDOCRINE PATHOLOGY

Although each endocrine system may malfunction as a consequence of organ-specific damage or disease, for example relating to the anatomic site of the gland, there are also some general types of pathology to which endocrine cells are very susceptible. The first of these is autoimmune destruction with detectable endocrine gland-specific antibodies. This is a potential cause of loss of function of nearly all endocrine glands and, less commonly, may also cause gland hyperfunction. In fact, autoimmunity to the thyroid, adrenal and pancreatic islets accounts for more than 50% of all organ-specific autoimmune disease. This appears in part due to genetic predisposition, accounted for by both MHC and non-MHC genes, and also by poorly defined environmental factors (see Chapter 21).

Examples of commonly used provocative endocrine tests

Endocrine axis	Stimulus	Measurement	Rationale/use
H-P-Adrenal	synthetic	ACTH	cortisol tests functional integrity of adrenal glands, which rely in turn on chronic tropic actions of ACTH. This is an indirect test of pituitary/hypothalamus
H-P-Adrenal	insulin-induced hypoglycemia	cortisol	severe hypoglycemia mimics physiologic stress and robustly tests the hypothalamus, unlike the Synacthen test
H-P-Thyroid	TRH	TSH	the pattern of TSH release after TRH stimulation gives information which may be useful in diagnosing central hypothyroidism
H-P-Growth	insulin-induced hypoglycemia	GH	baseline pulsatility of GH is overcome by applying a strong stimulus to its release
H-P-Growth	oral glucose load	GH	failure of suppression of GH by glucose is used in the diagnosis of acromegaly

H-P, hypothalomo-pituitary.

Table 39.4 **Examples of commonly used provocative endocrine tests**.

 HORMONE IMMUNOASSAY

Immunoassay is the most widely applied technique for measuring hormone levels. Antibodies are produced that bind to antigenic sites on the hormone. Ideally, such antibody should possess both high specificity and affinity for the hormone of interest, e.g. the β-subunit of glycoprotein hormones.

In the first immunoassays, the antibodies were produced in the serum of animal species (e.g. rabbit or sheep) that had been immunized with human hormone preparations. Such antisera contained a range of different antibodies (polyclonal) capable of binding to different sites on the hormone antigen. However, antibody specificity and titer varied with the animal and duration of the immune response. Today most immunoassays employ monoclonal antibodies, which are produced by fusion of spleen cells from an immunized mouse with a mouse myeloma cell line. Hybridoma cells may be cloned to produce a cell line that secretes a single antibody species for an indefinite period of time.

Many commercial producers have designed proprietary methods for quantifying the hormone–antibody interaction. One of the most widely used formats is the two-site (sandwich) immunometric or ELISA assay outlined in Figure 39.2. This assay employs two antibodies binding to different epitopes on the hormone, one of which is labeled or modified to be capable of generating an optical signal. Spectrophotometric, fluorometric, luminescence and radiochemical reporter systems are in common use.

Not all immunoassays rely on labeled antibody: other approaches include nephelometry, in which appearance of light-scattering immune complexes is monitored spectrophotometrically.

 HORMONE MEASUREMENT

PROBLEM	POSSIBLE SOLUTION(S)
Short-lived or unstable hormone	Take correct sample and store on ice; consider need for protease inhibitor such as aprotinin in tube
Cyclical hormone levels	Sample only at defined time in cycle for which normal range has been established (e.g. 9 a.m.sampling for cortisol; follicular phase sampling for LH/FSH/estradiol)
Highly pulsatile pattern of secretion (e.g. GH)	Take average of multiple samples spaced out in time or use provocative stimulus before measurement (e.g. hypoglycemia)
Several possible points of dysfunction in system	Sample at two different points in the endocrine system enables anatomic localization of problem (i.e. trophic hormone plus effector hormone, e.g. TSH + T4, ACTH + cortisol)

The second major group of pathologies which present as endocrine disease is neoplasia, which may be either benign or malignant. Neoplastic cells arise as autonomous clones within endocrine glands due to somatic mutations in growth factor signaling pathways or commonly in G-protein coupled signaling pathways. They may produce disease due to either excessive and dysregulated production of biologically active hormones or damage to neighboring, normal endocrine cells, with attendant loss of hormone secretion. Very small and benign adenomas which would remain undetected in

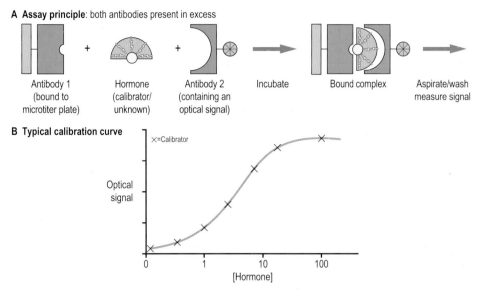

A Assay principle: both antibodies present in excess

Antibody 1 (bound to microtiter plate) + Hormone (calibrator/ unknown) + Antibody 2 (containing an optical signal) → Incubate → Bound complex → Aspirate/wash measure signal

B Typical calibration curve

×=Calibrator

Optical signal

[Hormone]

Fig. 39.2 **The sandwich design for enzyme-linked immunosorbent assay (ELISA) for the measurement of hormone concentration.** The amount of signal present on the microplate after washing of the serum/reagents is a measure of the concentration of a hormone. (Compare Fig. 40.2.)

nonendocrine tissues may produce florid disease by virtue of hormone hypersecretion coupled to the potency of hormones in eliciting biologic responses.

THE HYPOTHALAMO–PITUITARY REGULATORY SYSTEM

Hormones of the posterior pituitary gland are distinct from those of the anterior pituitary

The pituitary gland is a pea-sized, oval organ encased in a bony cavity of the skull (sella turcica) below the brain. It communicates with the hypothalamus via the pituitary stalk, which contains a complex array of axons and portal blood vessels (Fig. 39.3). The pituitary gland is divided into two lobes. The posterior pituitary (or neurohypophysis) is embryologically part of the brain, and consists largely of neurones which have cell bodies in the supraoptic and paraventricular nuclei of the hypothalamus. It is in these cell bodies that hormones are synthesized and packaged before transport on microtubules along axons to the pituitary, where they are released. The anterior lobe (adenohypophysis), accounting for approximately 80% of the gland, is embryologically derived from oral ectoderm, and has no direct anatomic continuity with the brain. Instead, it may be viewed as a target organ for endocrine hormones released from hypothalamic nuclei and transported from the median eminence by the portal circulation. Both posterior and anterior pituitary are

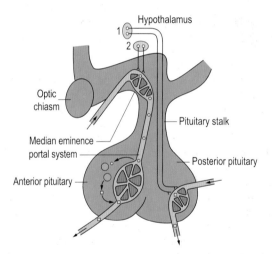

Fig. 39.3 **The hypothalamo-anterior pituitary regulatory system.** Hormones of the posterior pituitary are synthesized and packaged in the supraoptic and paraventricular nuclei of the hypothalamus (1), transported along axons and stored in the posterior pituitary prior to release into the circulation. The anterior pituitary releasing or release-inhibiting hormones are synthesized in various hypothalamic nuclei (2) and transported to the median eminence. From there they travel to the anterior pituitary via a portal venous system.

controlled largely by the hypothalamus, which is a highly connected center of the CNS, receiving synaptic inputs from vast numbers of different parts of the brain as well as sensing peripheral signals through areas of porosity in the blood–brain barrier. It thus functions as an integrative center which orchestrates a huge number of endocrine and neural processes, and entrains them to relevant external stimuli. The endocrine systems which involve the hypothalamus,

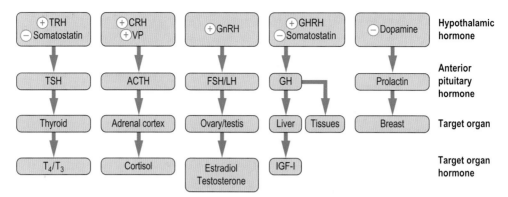

Fig. 39.4 **Hypothalamo-anterior pituitary regulatory target organ axes.** The hypothalamo-anterior pituitary regulatory system comprises five parallel endocrine axes, regulating the biosynthesis and release of: (1) thyroid hormone; (2) glucocorticoids; (3) sex steroids; (4) growth hormone; and (5) prolactin. T_4, thyroxine; T_3, tri-iodothyronine; GHRH, growth hormone-releasing hormone; GnRH, gonadotropin-releasing hormone; IGF-I, insulin growth factor-I. (+) indicates stimulatory action and (−) inhibitory action.

pituitary and downstream organs are usually termed 'axes' and are most usefully viewed as functional units for the purposes of clinical diagnosis and management (Fig. 39.4).

Hormones of the posterior pituitary gland

The posterior pituitary gland secretes two hormones into the circulation. Oxytocin is a small peptide hormone that stimulates smooth muscle contraction in the uterus and breast; it functions in parturition and lactation. Vasopressin (VP), also known as antidiuretic hormone (ADH), is a 9-amino acid cyclic peptide with functions linked to the control of water metabolism, and is described in detail in Chapter 23.

Hormones of the hypothalamo–anterior pituitary regulatory system

There are five separate endocrine axes within this system (see Fig. 39.4). Three of these are part of a complex three-level endocrine system in which the hormones of the pituitary gland (thyroid-stimulating hormone (TSH), adrenocorticotropic hormone (ACTH), follicle-stimulating hormone (FSH) and luteinizing hormone (LH)) may be regarded solely as trophic hormones for other target organs (i.e. thyroid, adrenals, gonads). In these axes, sophisticated control is exercised via a cascade in which each endocrine organ in the axis amplifies both the amount of hormone secreted and the biologic half-life of its hormone product compared with the previous organ. The fourth endocrine axis is a hybrid: growth hormone (GH) is both a trophic hormone and has actions in its own right. The fifth endocrine axis mediates the secretion of prolactin, unique in that it is not a trophic hormone. Distinct clinical syndromes are produced by either deficiency

Pituitary hormone disorders

Hormone	Deficiency	Excess
TSH	hypothyroidism	thyrotoxicosis
ACTH	hypoadrenalism	Cushing's disease
FSH/LH	hypogonadism	precocious puberty
GH	short stature	gigantism/acromegaly
Prolactin	none	galactorrhea/infertility

Table 39.5 **Clinical conditions associated with pituitary hormone disorders.**

or excess of any of the anterior pituitary hormones except prolactin, deficiency of which does not lead to clinically significant problems in humans (Table 39.5).

THE HYPOTHALAMO–PITUITARY–THYROID AXIS

Thyrotropin-releasing hormone (TRH)

TRH is manufactured in the hypothalamus and transported via the portal circulation to the pituitary where it ultimately stimulates secretion of TSH

TRH is a modified tripeptide synthesized in pulsatile fashion by peptidergic hypothalamic nuclei and transported to the anterior pituitary by the portal circulation. TRH stimulates TSH synthesis and secretion by binding to G-protein coupled receptors on the pituitary thyrotroph cell membrane that are linked to phospholipase C. The resulting increase in intracellular

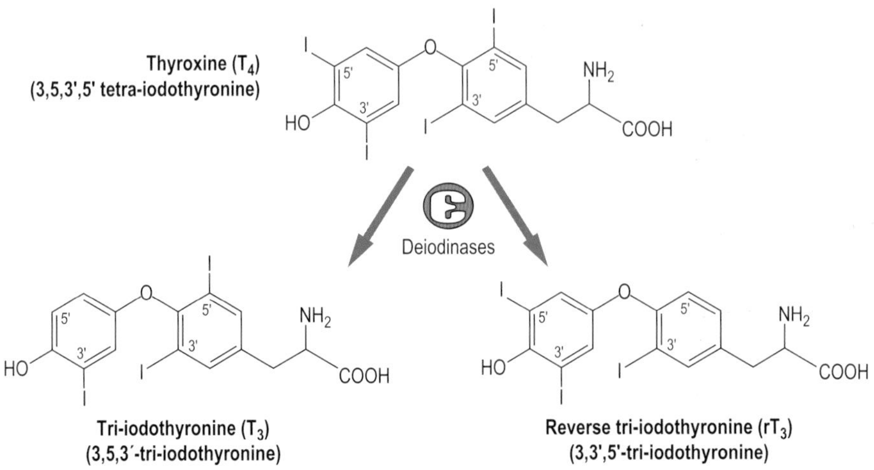

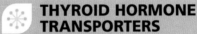

Thyroxine (T$_4$)
(3,5,3',5' tetra-iodothyronine)

Deiodinases

Tri-iodothyronine (T$_3$)
(3,5,3´-tri-iodothyronine)

Reverse tri-iodothyronine (rT$_3$)
(3,3',5'-tri-iodothyronine)

Fig. 39.5 **Structures of the thyroid hormones T$_4$, T$_3$ and rT$_3$.**

inositol trisphosphate (IP3) stimulates the release of calcium from intracellular storage sites and so leads to secretion of preformed TSH. More chronic actions of TRH include stimulation of TSH subunit biosynthesis and TSH glycosylation. The number of TRH receptors on the thyrotrophs is down-regulated both by the concentration of TRH itself and by thyroid hormones.

Thyroid-stimulating hormone

TSH, or thyrotropin, is a small glycoprotein synthesized by pituitary thyrotrophs. It consists of two noncovalently linked subunits and contains about 15% carbohydrate. The α-chain is identical to that found in other glycoprotein hormones (LH, FSH, βHCG) and so the specificity is conferred by the β-chain. The synthesis of each subunit is directed by separate messenger ribonucleic acids (mRNAs) encoded by separate genes on different chromosomes. The carbohydrate side chains are complex mixtures of unmodified, acetylated, and sulfated sugars. TSH is secreted in a pattern that is both pulsatile and circadian, and it has a plasma half-life of about 65 minutes.

TSH acts on the thyroid gland and influences virtually every aspect of thyroid hormone biosynthesis and secretion

TSH, like TRH, acts via a specific G-protein coupled receptor. However, in this case the receptor is expressed on follicular cells in the thyroid gland, and it is coupled to adenylyl cyclase and thus protein kinase A (or cAMP-dependent protein kinase). cAMP-dependent protein kinases control virtually every aspect of thyroid hormone biosynthesis and secretion, including iodide transport, iodothyronine formation, thyroglobulin proteolysis, and thyroxine de-iodination. TSH also stimulates growth of the thyroid gland. Indeed, activating somatic mutations in the TSH receptor are thought to account for many cases of multinodular goiter, a very common irregular enlargement of the thyroid gland, particularly when associated with excess secretion of thyroid hormone.

THYROID HORMONE TRANSPORTERS

Traditionally it was thought that flat, lipophilic hormones such as steroids and thyroid hormones simply diffused across lipid bilayers to reach their intracellular receptors. However, in the last few years it has been shown that the plasma membrane MCT8 protein functions as a thyroid hormone transporter, and that genetic deficiency of the protein leads to severe psychomotor retardation, and high T$_3$:T$_4$ ratios. Affected patients do not have peripheral features of hypothyroidism, however. Whether there are different thyroid hormone transporters in peripheral tissues and whether other lipophilic hormones also have similar, specific mechanisms governing cell entry remain interesting questions.

Negative feedback by thyroid hormones occurs at both hypothalamic and pituitary levels. At the pituitary level, thyroxine (T$_4$) and tri-iodothyronine (T$_3$) inhibit TSH secretion by decreasing both the biosynthesis and release of TSH through regulation of gene transcription and TSH glycosylation. T$_3$, the biologically active form of the hormone, is a more potent feedback inhibitor than T$_4$ and indeed, much of the feedback inhibition by T$_4$ requires its conversion intracellularly to T$_3$ by de-iodinase type 2.

Thyroxine and tri-iodothyronine

T$_4$ is produced exclusively in the thyroid gland and is more abundant than T$_3$, which is the biologically active form

T$_4$ (also known as tetra-iodothyronine) and T$_3$ are structurally simple molecules, being iodinated thyronines produced by the coupling of a phenyl group detached from one tyrosine to the phenyl group of a second intact tyrosine (Fig. 39.5). The biosynthesis of T$_4$ and T$_3$ occurs on the surface

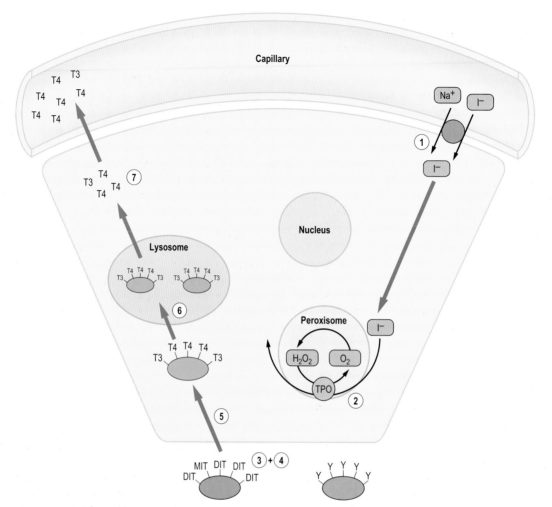

Fig. 39.6 **Mechanism of biosynthesis of thyroid hormones. 1**. Iodide is concentrated in follicular epithelial cells after entry via a sodium iodide symporter, before **2**. oxidation by thyroid peroxidase (TPO) in the peroxisome to iodine. **3**. At the plasma membrane adjacent to the follicular lumen, conversion of tyrosyl (Y) residues on the surface of thyroglobulin to either mono-iodotyrosine (MIT) or di-iodotyrosine (DIT) occurs. **4**. Coupling of iodinated tyrosines to form either T_4 (DIT + DIT) or T_3 (MIT + DIT) then occurs. **5**. Thyroglobulin is endocytosed and **6**. hydrolyzed in lysosomes to release free T_3 and free T_4. **7**. The thyroid hormones are transported to the plasma membrane and released into the bloodstream by mechanisms which are not yet clear. TSH influences virtually every step in thyroid hormone synthesis and release through the cAMP/protein kinase A pathway.

of thyroglobulin, a large tyrosine-rich glycoprotein that accounts for about 75% of the protein content of the thyroid gland. Iodination of thyroglobulin occurs after it has been secreted into the follicular lumen, and secretion of T_4 and T_3 requires enzymatic hydrolysis of thyroglobulin, which is located in the follicular colloid. During hydrolysis and subsequent de-iodination, the released iodide is conserved and reutilized (Fig. 39.6).

Thyroid hormone bioactivity is regulated by controlling the conversion of T_4 into T_3 by de-iodination; this is mediated by three de-iodinase enzymes

About 80–90% of the thyroid hormone secreted by the thyroid gland is T_4, with T_3 as the minor component. However, T_3, produced by 5′ de-iodination of T_4, is the biologically active form of the hormone, and T_4 may thus be regarded

as a prohormone. 5′ de-iodination may occur in the thyroid gland, in target tissues or in other peripheral tissues, and is accomplished by iodothyronine de-iodinases 1 and 2 (DI1 and DI2). The type 2 enzyme is particularly important in controlling nuclear T_3 levels, while the physiologic role of the kinetically inefficient type 1 de-iodinase is less clear at present. The type 3 enzyme is the major catabolic enzyme; it catalyzes the removal of an iodide from the 3 rather than 5′ position, resulting in reverse T_3, which is inactive and similarly de-iodinates and inactivates T_3. Thus, control of the de-iodination of T_4 is one method of controlling thyroid hormone bio-activity (see Fig. 39.5). About 80% of T_4 is metabolized by de-iodination with about equal amounts of T_3 and rT_3 being produced. The remaining T_4 is conjugated with sulfate or glucuronic acid and deactivated by deamidation or decarboxylation. In severe illness there is good evidence that activation of T_4 to T_3 by DI1 and DI2 is impaired, while the expression of DI3 is increased. This results in low T_3 levels, which is an early feature of the so-called 'sick euthyroid syndrome'.

The biologically active fraction of T_3 and T_4 in plasma (free T_3 or free T_4, i.e. a fraction which is not bound to protein) represents, in each case, less than 1% of the total concentration of the hormone

The daily production of T_4 is approximately 10% of the extrathyroidal pool, much of which is bound to TBG or albumin in plasma. Approximately 80% of this T_4 is converted to T_3 by extrathyroidal de-iodination. The turnover of T_3 is much greater than that of T_4. The biologically active component of T_4 and T_3 in plasma is the free fraction – that not bound to proteins. This fraction, which is a measure of thyroid hormone status, represents less than 1% of the total T_4 and T_3. Most clinical laboratories now assay free hormone levels specifically to avoid problems in interpretation of total hormone levels caused by fluctuations in binding proteins.

Biochemical actions of thyroid hormones

Thyroid hormones may be considered the accelerator pedal of metabolism

T_3 increases the metabolic rate of a wide range of tissues and thereby increases the whole-body basal metabolic rate. Most of these actions result from binding of T_3 to its nuclear receptor (see Chapter 40), and alteration in transcription rates of genes in target tissues. Among the many cellular changes which result from this altered program of gene expression, it has been shown that thyroid hormones increase ATP utilization by increasing sodium-potassium (Na^+/K^+)-dependent ATPase activity, and increase mitochondrial oxidative metabolism, in part by direct upregulation of key mitochondrial biogenesis factors. Adipose tissue lipolysis is also stimulated by cAMP-dependent activation of hormone-sensitive lipase, thus producing fatty acids that can be oxidized to generate the ATP used for thermogenesis. Increase in both glycogenolysis and gluconeogenesis occurs to balance the increased use of glucose as a fuel for thermogenesis. The rate of synthesis of many structural proteins, enzymes, and other hormones is also affected as a result of thyroid hormone action, and microarray-based transcriptomics (Chapter 36) can now be used to define the many hundreds or thousands of genes whose expression is altered by activation of the thyroid hormone receptor.

Clinical disorders of thyroid function

Thyroid disease is common, affecting almost 3% of the population; nine times as many women as men are affected

 HYPOTHYROIDISM

A 60-year-old woman comes to the clinic and complains of weight gain, intolerance of cold, and tiredness. She also says that she has recently become less alert mentally, but attributes this to aging. On questioning she admits that she has also suffered severe constipation of late. She says that two members of her family had 'thyroid trouble'. On examination, she is moderately obese, has dry, cool skin, a puffy face, and a slow heart rate of 50 beats per minute. The thyroid gland is not palpable. Her free thyroxine (T_4) was 5 pmol/L (normal range 9–25 pmol/L) and TSH was 60 mU/L (range 0.4–4 mU/L).

Comment. Symptoms of hypothyroidism at an early stage can be fairly nonspecific. The best laboratory test for the diagnosis of hypothyroidism is the plasma TSH concentration. The elevated level of TSH suggests primary thyroid disorder. Subsequently this lady's blood was shown to be positive for microsomal and antithyroglobulin antibodies. A diagnosis of lymphocytic thyroiditis (Hashimoto's thyroiditis) was made. She was treated with thyroxine.

 HYPERTHYROIDISM

A 35-year-old woman came to her physician complaining of palpitations, difficulty climbing stairs and general fatigue. She also said that she had lost 4 kg of weight recently despite a good appetite and no attempt at dieting. She also reported occasional diarrhea, and increasingly infrequent and light menstrual bleeds.

On examination, her skin was warm and moist and she had a fine tremor of outstretched hands. There was mild weakness of the thigh muscles. She had tachycardia (110/min). She also had a mild thyroid enlargement (goiter) and a bruit over the gland. Thyroid function tests show suppressed TSH level (<0.05; range 0.4–4 mU/L) and increased thyroxine (T_4 = 29; range 9–25 pmol/L) and tri-iodothyronine (T_3 = 25; range 3.5–6.5 pmol/L). Thyroid receptor antibodies were detected.

Comment. In hyperthyroidism, the TSH level is suppressed by high circulating thyroid hormones. The low TSH level and high thyroid hormone concentrations suggest hyperthyroidism. The presence of thyroid receptor antibodies confirms that the cause is Graves' disease, an autoimmune thyroid disorder.

More than 95% of thyroid disease originates in the thyroid gland and much of this is autoimmune in origin. Antibodies may arise against several components of thyroid cells, including the peroxidase-rich microsomes. Lymphocyte infiltration and progressive destruction of the thyroid gland ensue, leading to hypothyroidism, the commonest type of thyroid dysfunction. Some thyroid autoantibodies bind to the

TSH receptor. If the autoantibodies bind to but do not stimulate the gland, the thyroid hormone production falls and the patient becomes hypothyroid, with increased plasma TSH and reduced free T_4. If the autoantibodies bind and stimulate, however, they mimic the effect of TSH, breaking the normal negative feedback loop and producing thyroid oversecretion, and the patient will be hyperthyroid (thyrotoxic) with increased plasma free T_4 and suppressed TSH.

Hypothalamic and pituitary causes of hypothyroidism are often the result of impaired TSH secretion secondary to pressure from an adjacent tumor. Pituitary TSH-secreting tumors are an extremely rare cause of hyperthyroidism, and often produce abnormally high ratios of TSH α-subunit to β-subunit, and abnormal glycosylation patterns of TSH which may be useful in diagnosis.

THE HYPOTHALAMO–PITUITARY–ADRENAL AXIS

Corticotropin-releasing hormone (CRH)

CRH is a 41-amino acid peptide secreted by the paraventricular nucleus (PVN); it acts via a G-protein coupled receptor on pituitary corticotroph cells via the cAMP second messenger system to stimulate both synthesis and secretion of ACTH. A second hormone from the PVN, vasopressin (VP), potentiates the response of the pituitary to CRH, in part by increasing the amount and extent of expression of the CRH receptor. Negative feedback by cortisol inhibits both CRH and VP secretion, as well as reducing responsiveness of corticotrophs to stimulation.

Adrenocorticotropic hormone (ACTH)

ACTH is synthesized as a 241-amino acid precursor molecule, pro-opiomelanocortin (POMC). POMC is cleaved at multiple sites to release several hormonally active peptides, including the endorphins and melanocyte-stimulating hormones. In addition to the pituitary, POMC may also be produced in large quantities by certain malignancies, giving rise to ectopic ACTH syndrome.

ACTH itself is composed of 39 amino acids with the biologic activity residing in the N-terminal 24 residues. It is secreted in stress-related bursts superimposed on a marked diurnal rhythm that shows a peak at 05.00 h. It is transported unbound in plasma and has a half-life of about 10 minutes. ACTH stimulates the synthesis and release of glucocorticoid hormones by interacting with cell surface G-protein coupled receptors on the adrenal cortex that stimulate cAMP production. Acute increases in the adrenal synthesis of cortisol occur within 3 minutes, principally by stimulating the activity of cholesterol esterase. Longer-term effects of ACTH include induction of transcription of the genes that encode steroidogenic enzymes, and it is also required to maintain the zona fasciculata and zona reticularis of the gland, meaning that long-term lack of ACTH eventually abolishes the ability of the gland to respond to an acute challenge by increasing cortisol and androgen synthesis (Chapter 17).

Negative feedback by cortisol occurs within two time frames, acting at both the hypothalamic and pituitary levels. Fast feedback alters the release of hypothalamic CRH and the CRH-mediated secretion of ACTH. Slow feedback results from reduced synthesis of CRH plus suppression of POMC gene transcription, which results in reduced ACTH synthesis.

Biosynthesis of cortisol

Cortisol is the major glucocorticoid synthesized in man in the adrenal cortex and is under the direct control of pituitary ACTH

A simplified scheme of steroid biosynthesis is shown in Figure 39.7 (see also Fig. 17.11). Cholesterol is the precursor for all steroid hormones. Cleavage of the cholesterol side chain liberates the C-21 corticosteroids; further side chain cleavage yields the C-19 androgens, and aromatization of the A ring results in the C-18 estrogens. The structures of the key steroid hormones are shown in Chapter 17. Several of the steroidogenic enzymes are members of the cytochrome P-450 superfamily of oxidases (Chapter 29).

The plasma concentration of cortisol shows a pronounced diurnal rhythm, being some 10 times higher at 08.00 h than at 24.00 h. This parallels the marked diurnal rhythm of secretion of ACTH. Approximately 95% of cortisol in plasma is bound to proteins, mainly CBG. As cortisol concentration rises, the percentage of free cortisol also rises, indicating that CBG binding is saturable. Cortisol has a half-life in plasma of about 100 minutes. It is metabolized in the liver and other organs by a combination of reduction, side chain cleavage, and conjugation to produce a wide range of inactive metabolites that are excreted in urine.

Cortisol has diverse effects on metabolism and tissue growth/repair

Cortisol has wide-ranging effects on metabolism, immune function, the cardiovascular system and skeleton, mediated by alterations in expression level of thousands of genes. As the name glucocorticoid suggests, cortisol has a major influence on glucose homeostasis: it is a counterregulatory hormone, working through nuclear receptors to induce the biosynthesis of gluconeogenic enzymes, while at the same time inhibiting glucose uptake and metabolism in peripheral tissues (Chapter 21). Glycogen synthesis and deposition are increased, and lipolysis in adipose tissue is stimulated. Protein and RNA synthesis are stimulated in the liver but

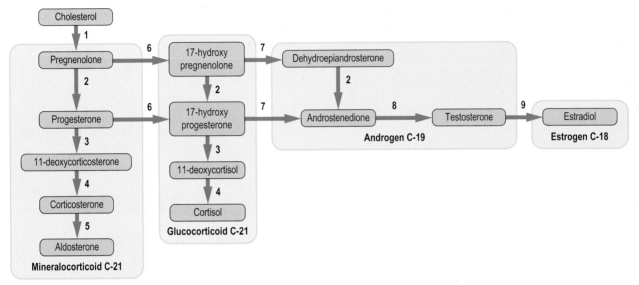

Fig. 39.7 **Summary of steroid hormone biosynthesis. 1**, cholesterol 20,22-desmolase; **2**,3β-hydroxysteroid dehydrogenaseΔα^{4,5}-oxosteroid isomerase; **3**, 21-hydroxylase; **4**, 11-hydroxylase; **5**, aldosterone synthase; **6**, 17α-hydroxylase; **7**, 17,20-lyase/desmolase; **8**, 17β-hydroxysteroid dehydrogenase; **9**, aromatase. These enzymes are part of the cytochrome P-450 dependent superfamily of NADPH-dependent monooxygenases (see also Chapter 29; compare Figs 17.10 and 17.11).

inhibited in muscle; proteolysis in muscle produces the amino acid substrates for hepatic gluconeogenesis. Cortisol works in tandem with several other hormones including insulin and GH in regulating intermediary metabolism, and these metabolic effects are best understood as part of the endocrine response to physiologic stress (Chapter 21).

Cortisol also modulates the immune system through effects on cytokine production and enhanced leukocyte apoptosis, effects which are exploited pharmacologically in the use of potent glucocorticoids to treat inflammatory conditions. It is, moreover, permissive for the effect of many vasoconstrictors such as catecholamines, has direct effects on the heart and on the kidney, where it enhances water clearance and electrolyte reabsorption, and bone, influencing turnover through a variety of mechanisms.

Clinical disorders of cortisol secretion

Hyposecretion of cortisol may occur as a result of hypothalamic, pituitary or adrenal failure

The diagnosis of the cause of cortisol hyposecretion relies on the clinical presentation, carefully timed measurement of cortisol and ACTH, and the extent of the cortisol response to synthetic ACTH (Synacthen).

Deficiencies of CRH and ACTH are often accompanied by deficiencies of other hypothalamic or pituitary hormones. Addison's disease is a primary adrenal failure in which secretion of all adrenal hormones is decreased, usually because of autoimmune disease or infection (e.g. by tuberculosis or cytomegalovirus). Biochemically, it is characterized by

hyponatremia, hyperkalemia, acidosis, and impaired cortisol response to Synacthen, together with an elevated plasma ACTH. Cortisol replacement, usually together with a mineralocorticoid, is an effective treatment for this life-threatening condition. Because glucocorticoids are also involved in normal clearance of free water, their deficiency can mask coexisting ADH deficiency, and replacement leads to dramatic diuresis. Furthermore, Addison's disease can be associated with a markedly elevated TSH which resolves with glucocorticoid therapy. This is important to recognize as erroneous diagnosis of primary hypothyroidism and treatment with thyroxine may dangerously exacerbate symptoms of hypoadrenalism.

Rarely, cortisol hyposecretion results from a genetic disorder in the steroid biosynthetic pathway: congenital adrenal hyperplasia. The most frequently affected enzyme is the steroid 21-hydroxylase (see Fig. 39.7). In nearly complete enzyme deficiency, deficiency of cortisol and aldosterone leads to salt wasting and hyponatremia in the first few days of life. Because of the loss of negative feedback by cortisol, ACTH levels rise and try to drive increased amounts of substrate through the enzymatic block at the expense of making an excess of 17-hydroxyprogesterone (17OHP) (Fig. 39.8), which is converted to androgens and may masculinize female external genitalia before birth. Partial defects in the enzyme may be compensated for by elevated ACTH levels sufficiently to maintain cortisol levels, though the build-up of metabolites proximal to the defective enzyme in the pathway still occurs. Consequently this presents in teenage girls as hirsutism and menstrual irregularity. The steroid profile of a patient with congenital adrenal hyperplasia is given in Figure 17.12.)

PRIMARY ADRENAL INSUFFICIENCY – AN ENDOCRINE EMERGENCY

A 40-year-old woman was admitted as a medical emergency following a collapse at home 2 days after contracting influenza. For 1 year she had been complaining of chronic weakness and fatigue, and lately of abdominal pain, nausea, vomiting, anorexia and confusion. She was dehydrated and hypotensive with pigmentation of the palmar creases and buccal mucosa. Biochemical analysis revealed Na^+ 115 mmol/L (135–145 mmol/L), K^+ 5.9 mmol/l (3.5–5.0 mmol/L), urea 12 mmol/L (2.5–6.5 mmol/L) and glucose 2.9 mmol/L (4.0–6.0 mmol/L). Baseline serum cortisol was 95 nmol/L rising to 110 nmol/L 30 min after administration of synthetic ACTH (Synacthen).

Comment. This is an acute presentation of Addison's disease resulting from progressive autoimmune destruction of the adrenal cortex. The nonspecific symptoms of cortisol deficiency became critical after the stress of a minor illness. The hypotension and electrolyte imbalance result from mineralocorticoid deficiency. The pigmentation is due to elevated POMC-derived peptides such as the melanocyte-stimulating hormones. The diagnosis is made by the impaired cortisol response to synthetic ACTH. Treatment is rehydration with intravenous saline, plus a bolus of intravenous hydrocortisone followed by daily maintenance therapy with hydrocortisone and a mineralocorticoid. Other autoimmune diseases commonly coexist in the patient or their family. Increased frequency of severe hypoglycemia in patients with type 1 diabetes is one presentation to watch for, because of the loss of the glucose counterregulatory effects of cortisol.

CUSHING'S SYNDROME – A DIAGNOSTIC DILEMMA

A 45-year-old woman presented with fatigue, rapid weight gain with central obesity, fullness and redness of her face (so called 'plethora'), and loss of regular menstrual periods. She was mildly hypertensive, and her family doctor had found her also to be diabetic for which she had received dietary advice. Urinary cortisol was 1000 nmol/24 h (normal <250 nmol/24 h); serum cortisol was 500 nmol/L at 24 h (normal <50 nmol/L) and her 0800 h cortisol was 550 nmol/L after 1 mg of dexamethasone (a potent synthetic glucocorticoid) (normal <50 nmol/L). Plasma ACTH was 100 ng/L (normal <80 ng/L).

Comment. This woman has hypercortisolism, known as Cushing's syndrome. The elevated urine cortisol, elevated midnight serum cortisol and failure to suppress following dexamethasone administration support the diagnosis. The ACTH result indicates that the cause is either a pituitary tumor (most likely) or ectopic ACTH secretion from an occult tumor (probably carcinoid). In this case magnetic resonance imaging (MRI) of the pituitary revealed a clear tumor of 0.5 cm diameter; diagnosis of Cushing's syndrome and localization of the problem are often not this easy! Pituitary surgery is the appropriate definitive treatment in this case.

Hypersecretion of cortisol results in Cushing's syndrome – easily the most challenging of all endocrine disorders

Exogenous glucocorticoids, commonly used to suppress the immune system in a range of inflammatory disorders, are the commonest cause of clinical Cushing's syndrome. However, Cushing's syndrome may also result from disorders of the hypothalamus, pituitary (around 80%) or adrenal gland (around 15%), or it may be the consequence of ectopic ACTH syndrome. Cortisol excess leads to remodeling of adipose tissue with deposition of fat in the face and trunk and loss of fat on the limbs, wasting of skeletal muscle, thinning of skin, and slow healing (Fig. 39.9). Cortisol excess also commonly produces diabetes and hypertension, and usually suppresses the hypothalamic gonadal axis, seen as loss of menses in women.

The diagnosis of Cushing's syndrome may be extremely demanding for several reasons.

- Because of the pronounced circadian variation in serum cortisol levels, random measurement of cortisol is of little use in the diagnosis of Cushing's syndrome. Instead, 24-hour urinary free cortisol, which provides a measurement of total production of cortisol over 1 day, is a common screening test.

- An abnormal circadian profile of cortisol secretion, with sustained levels at night when they usually almost undetectable, may produce Cushing's syndrome even if there is little, if any, increase in total daily production of cortisol. This may be detected by sampling of cortisol at 09.00 h and midnight, showing loss of normal circadian rhythm. If this test is undertaken carefully without provoking an endocrine stress response by taking blood, it can be a sensitive means of detecting hypercortisolism.

- Endogenous Cushing's syndrome usually arises from autonomously functioning secretory tumors. Some of the diagnostic challenges in Cushing's syndrome arise from the variable behavior of such tumors as they evolve. Sometimes only episodic cortisol hypersecretion is seen, with testing normal in between episodes, and sometimes aberrant receptor expression due to somatic mutations means that high levels of cortisol are secreted in response to other hormones such as gut-derived peptides.

Once these pitfalls have been overcome and cortisol excess demonstrated, the anatomic site of the problem can be investigated using a range of tests which may include ACTH measurements, dexamethasone (a synthetic glucocorticoid) suppression tests, and selective venous catheterization of the pituitary or the adrenal glands. Definitive treatment is usually surgical and should be targeted at the primary cause of the condition. However, some medical means of reducing cortisol synthesis are commonly used in preparation for surgery.

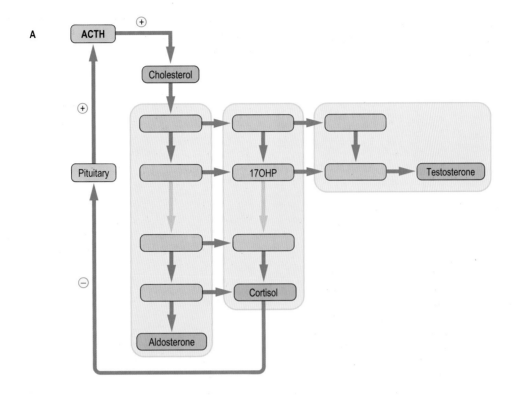

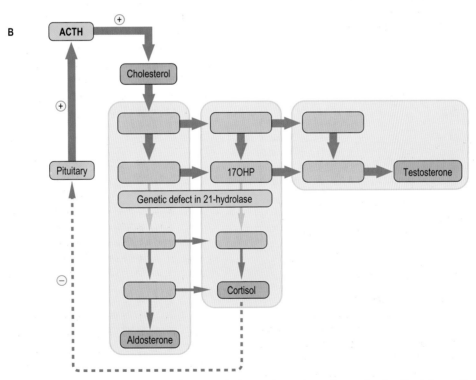

Fig. 39.8 **High levels of androgens in congenital adrenal hyperplasia are due to loss of negative feedback by cortisol.** (A) Normal negative feedback exerted by cortisol on hypothalamus and pituitary. (B) 21-Hydroxylase deficiency leads to selective loss of cortisol and aldosterone, loss of negative feedback, and ACTH hypersecretion in an attempt to correct the defect. Excess ACTH drives increased flux through all arms of the pathway before the defect, leading to clinical hyperandrogenism. 17OHP, 17-hydroxyprogesterone. Purple = mineralocorticoid pathway, pink/red = glucocorticoid pathway, blue = androgen pathway.

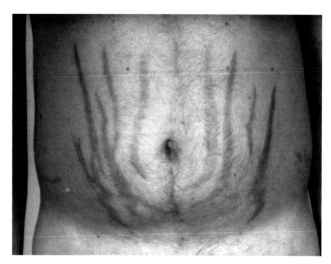

Fig. 39.9 **Cushing's syndrome due to cortisol hypersecretion.**

CUSHING'S DISEASE OF THE OMENTUM?

As described earlier, the enzyme 11β-hydroxysteroid dehydrogenase (11βHSD) type II metabolizes cortisol to inactive cortisone, thereby protecting mineralocorticoid receptors from exposure to high levels of active ligand in the kidney. A closely related second enzyme, 11βHSD type I, is widely expressed in tissues such as adipose tissue, bone and brain. Although it catalyzes the same reaction, the direction of the reaction in cells is generally the other way, leading to increases in active cortisol relative to cortisone. It has been suggested that high levels of this intracellular glucocorticoid amplifying activity in omental fat cells might contribute to central obesity and the metabolic syndrome in the absence of any circulating excess of cortisol. (Omentum is the peritoneal fold that supports stomach and viscera within the abdominal cavity.) Whether or not elevated 11βHSD I activity plays a role in the development of metabolic syndrome, its inhibition may be a useful pharmacologic strategy to improve many aspects of the condition.

GPR54: INSIGHT INTO PUBERTY FROM MICE AND MEN

For the first few months of life the hypothalamic-pituitary-gonadal axis is active before it is shut down, going into a quiescent state until it is reactivated at puberty. There are several lines of evidence suggesting that this is largely determined centrally, but the underlying cellular and molecular mechanisms have remained obscure. Recent simultaneous studies in mice and humans have, however, yielded some insight: first, deletion in mice of the gene encoding a G-protein coupled receptor of unknown function, Gpr54, produced animals which showed no evidence of sexual maturation but were otherwise normal. In parallel, human genetic studies in consanguineous (inbred) families with several members affected by hypogonadotrophic hypogonadism (i.e. low FSH, LH and sex steroids), defects in the same gene were discovered, confirming its importance also in humans. Mechanistic study suggested that GPR54 is involved in the hypothalamus in stimulating GnRH production and release. This step in defining some of the key central circuitry in controlling gonadal function has spawned considerable research activity both from those interested in teasing out the regulation of puberty and sexual function, and from those interested in exploiting this new discovery pharmacologically.

and transported to the pituitary by the portal system. It is secreted in a pulsatile fashion and induces the synthesis and secretion of both FSH and LH from the same cells. Its release is subject to negative feedback by progesterone, prolactin, and sometimes estrogen, among other hormones. GnRH acts through its cell surface receptor to increase intracellular calcium, hydrolyze phospho-inositides, and activate protein kinase C. Long-acting GnRH agonists can also cause downregulation of GnRH receptors and reduced FSH and LH secretion. Such agonists are now used to treat prostate cancer and to prepare infertile women for assisted-conception programs.

THE HYPOTHALAMO–PITUITARY–GONADAL AXIS

Gonadotropin-releasing hormone (GnRH)

GnRH is essential for the secretion of intact FSH and LH

The hypothalamus has a major role in the control of gonadal function in both males and females. Increased frequency and amplitude of hypothalamic GnRH pulses is the first measurable stage of the onset of puberty. GnRH, in turn, stimulates the secretion of pituitary FSH and LH. GnRH is a decapeptide synthesized by various hypothalamic nuclei

Follicle-stimulating hormone and luteinizing hormone

Although FSH and LH have been given their names on the basis of their function in the female, it is now clear that identical hormones are secreted and function in the male

Both FSH and LH are secreted in the male and female under the influence of GnRH, and alterations in the GnRH pulse frequency and amplitude can influence the relative amounts of FSH and LH secreted by the gonadotroph. FSH and LH are glycoproteins with an identical α-subunit (also shared with TSH) and a specific β-subunit. The gene for LH has recently

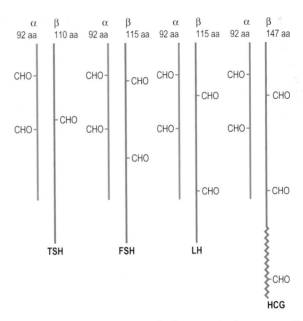

Fig. 39.10 **Relative structures of glycoprotein hormones.** The three pituitary glycoprotein hormones (TSH, FSH, LH) and the placental glycoprotein (HCG) share a common α-subunit. Hormone specificity is conveyed by the β-subunit and the resulting three-dimensional protein structure. CHO indicates the approximate location of carbohydrate side chains. HCG differs from LH solely by having an additional 32 amino acids in its β-subunit. aa, amino acids.

undergone duplication to produce HCG, a gonadotropin secreted by embryonic tissues (Fig. 39.10).

Although GnRH is essential for the secretion of intact FSH and LH, feedback from estradiol and testosterone plus gonadal peptides such as inhibin have a secondary effect. Feedback by estradiol is especially interesting because it may have either negative or positive effects on gonadotropins, depending on the stage of the menstrual cycle. An outline of the control of the hypothalamo-pituitary-gonadal axes, both for adult men and women, is shown in Figure 39.11. The half-life of LH in plasma is approximately 50 minutes; FSH has a longer half-life of about 4 hours. Both FSH and LH concentrations vary considerably depending on age and sex (Fig. 39.12).

Actions of FSH and LH on the testes

FSH and LH influence spermatogenesis

In the male, testosterone biosynthesis occurs in the Leydig cells of the testes under the primary influence of LH (see Fig. 39.11) acting through the G-protein coupled LH receptor. High intratubular testosterone levels cooperate with FSH in promoting spermatogenesis in the spermatic tubule: FSH binds to its specific receptor on the Sertoli cell of the testes and, by a mechanism similar to LH, induces increased synthesis of several proteins, including androgen-binding protein (ABP) and inhibin. ABP is secreted into the seminiferous tubular lumen where it binds testosterone (or its active form dihydrotestosterone). This ensures a high local androgen concentration that, together with FSH, brings about the meiotic divisions that are necessary for spermatogenesis. Inhibin has a role in the FSH negative feedback loop (see Fig. 39.11).

Biochemical actions of testosterone in the male

Testosterone not only influences gonadotropin regulation and spermatogenesis, but is also a natural anabolic steroid

Nearly 95% of serum testosterone comes from the testes, the remainder originating from the adrenal gland. More than 97% of this circulating testosterone is bound to protein, with equal amounts bound to albumin and to the specific sex hormone-binding globulin (SHBG), which is similar in structure to ABP. Testosterone is metabolized in target tissues to dihydrotestosterone (DHT) via 5-α reduction, more than doubling its affinity for the nuclear androgen receptor. In addition to effects on gonadotropin regulation and spermatogenesis, androgens induce the development of the reproductive tract from the Wolffian ducts during male sexual differentiation. They also have anabolic effects, stimulating protein synthesis and an increase in muscle mass (Fig. 39.13).

Clinical disorders of testosterone secretion in males

Testosterone deficiency may originate from a wide range of disorders of the hypothalamus, pituitary or testes

Endocrine failure of the testes may occur due to trauma or inflammation of the testes themselves (e.g. mumps orchitis),

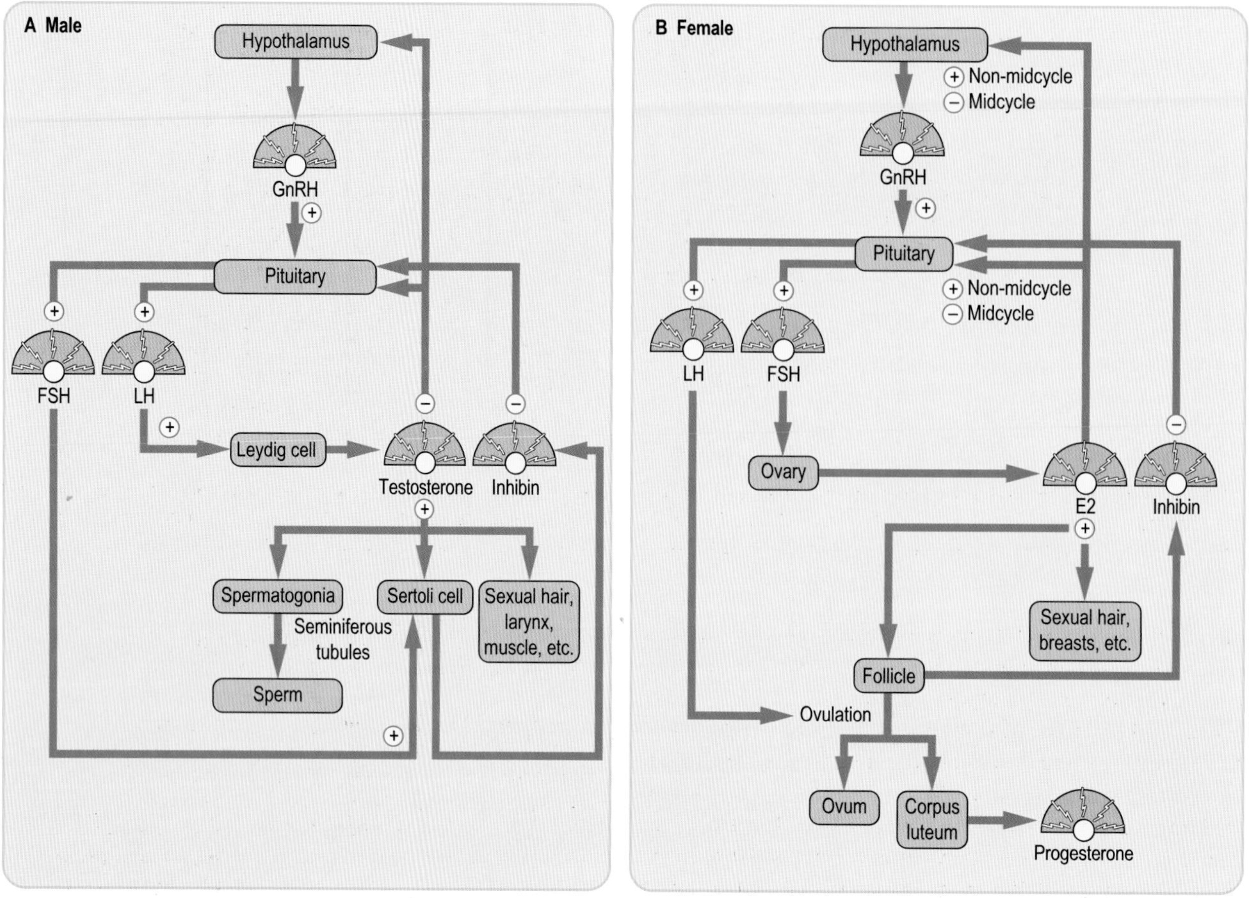

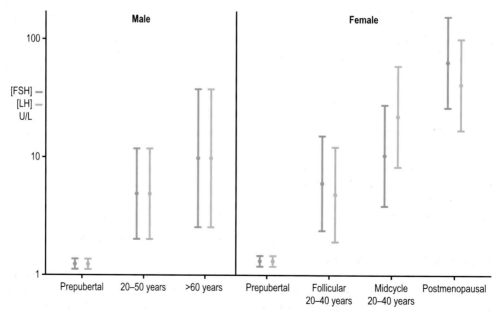

Fig. 39.11 Control of the hypothalamo-pituitary-gonadal axes. (A) In men, testosterone is produced from cholesterol in the Leydig cell under LH stimulation. Testosterone and FSH support spermatogenesis. (B) In women, estradiol (E_2) is produced by the granulosa cell and the developing follicle after feedback stimulation. E_2 feedback is mainly negative but, in midcycle, there is a positive E_2 feedback resulting in the surge of LH that causes ovulation. Progesterone (P) is secreted by the resultant corpus luteum.

Fig. 39.12 Variations in serum FSH and LH during life. Serum FSH and LH levels vary depending on age and sex.

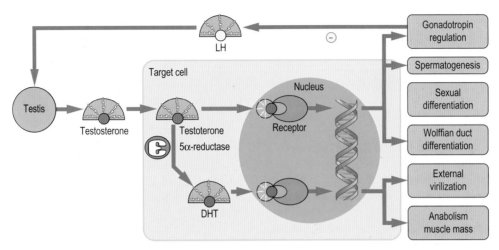

Fig. 39.13 **Mechanism of action of testosterone.** Testosterone from the testis enters a target cell and binds to the androgen receptor, either directly or after conversion to 5α-dihydrotestosterone (DHT). DHT binds more tightly than testosterone, and the DHT–receptor complex binds more efficiently to chromatin. Actions mediated by testosterone are shown by purple lines, those mediated by DHT are shown by blue lines.

or due to failure at the level of the hypothalamus or pituitary. Indeed, the gonadotrophs are among the most sensitive of the anterior pituitary cell types to pituitary damage (e.g. due to growth of an adenoma within the bony constraints of the sella turcica) and consequently gonadal failure is often the earliest manifestation of pituitary disease. There is also an interesting series of genetic disorders which manifest as gonadal failure: Klinefelter's syndrome, caused by acquisition of an additional X chromosome in males (karyotype 47XXY) presents with gynecomastia (abnormal increase in size of the male breast), eunuchoidism and varying degrees of hypogonadism, and is due to abnormal development of the testes. Serum FSH is elevated, and LH is usually elevated, but testosterone may be subnormal. Kallman's syndrome, in contrast, is a genetic hypothalamic disorder in children featuring both deficient GnRH production and commonly absent smell (anosmia) due to defective migration of GnRH and other neurones in utero; affected individuals present with delayed puberty and subnormal FSH, LH, and testosterone. Androgen deficiency may lead to muscle and fat redistribution and loss of bone mineral density, and these may be corrected, to some extent, by androgen administration (Table 39.6).

Androgen excess in males is only seen in precocious puberty

Precocious puberty is a rare condition that may result from early maturation of the normal hypothalamo-pituitary-gonadal axis, gain-of-function mutations in the LH receptor or as a result of a tumor that is secreting either androgen or HCG.

Actions of FSH and LH on the ovary

In the female, FSH promotes estradiol synthesis leading to follicular maturation, while LH leads to follicle rupture and oocyte release

| *GnRH is not easily measured clinically. | | |

Causes of hypogonadism		
Site of defect	**Biochemistry**	**Causes**
Hypothalamus	Low GnRH* Low LH, FSH Low E2/testosterone	Tumors Irradiation Genetic disorders • Kallman's syndrome • GPR54 mutations
Pituitary	High GnRH* Low LH, FSH Low E2/testosterone	Tumors Irradiation Trauma Inflammatory conditions Genetic disorders • GnRHR mutations • Mutations in pituitary transcription factors
Gonads	High GnRH* High LH, FSH Low E2/testosterone	Irradiation Physiologic (menopause) Autoimmunity Infection (e.g. mumps orchitis in men) Trauma Genetic/developmental abnormalities • Klinefelter's syndrome (47,XXY: men) • Turner's syndrome (45,XO: women)

*GnRH is not easily measured clinically.

Table 39.6 **Causes of hypogonadism.**

In the mature female, the GnRH pulse generator engages in a dynamic interplay with ovarian cells in maintaining the hormonally driven menstrual cycle (Figs 39.11 and 39.14). Primordial follicles actually begin hormone-independent growth and maturation many weeks before the start of the menstrual cycle, but only at the start of the cycle, when they have acquired the capacity to respond to FSH, are a few follicles preserved from atresia. Rising FSH concentrations stimulate estradiol synthesis in granulosa cells through induction of aromatase and other enzymes (see Fig. 39.7). As estradiol is secreted so FSH falls, and this combination plays an important role in the selection of a dominant follicle for further development, though details of the precise mechanism remain to be fully established. Follicular maturation continues under the influence of rising estradiol concentrations. Increasing estradiol, in part because of positive feedback within the dominant follicle, causes the negative central feedback of estrogen to flip into positive feedback, initiating a surge of LH. This LH binds to receptors on the dominant follicle and, in tandem with steroid hormones and other factors such as prostaglandins, induces completion of the first stage of oocyte meiosis, rupture of the follicle and release of the oocyte some 36 hours later. At this time there is a sharp fall in plasma estradiol, followed by a fall in LH. The ruptured follicle transforms into the corpus luteum, which secretes progesterone and lesser amounts of estradiol both to sustain the oocyte and to prepare the estrogen-primed uterine endometrium for implantation of a fertilized ovum and the establishment of early pregnancy. In the absence of fertilization, corpus luteum function declines, and progesterone and estradiol secretion fall. This brings about vascular changes in the endometrium leading to tissue involution and menstruation. The decline in steroid secretion stimulates FSH secretion, setting the stage for initiation of the next cycle.

Actions of steroid hormones in the female

In a woman with a normal menstrual cycle, it is the progesterone level that is of diagnostic significance

The concentrations of FSH, LH, estradiol, and progesterone vary considerably during the menstrual cycle. In a normally cycling woman, progesterone is of particular diagnostic utility: a serum concentration of more than 20 nmol/L in the luteal phase is consistent with ovulation (see Fig. 39.14). Aside from their roles in the menstrual cycle and reproduction, both estradiol and progesterone have other effects, acting via specific nuclear receptors in target cells. Estradiol, working in tandem with other hormones such as insulin-like growth factor-I (IGF-I), is responsible for linear growth, breast development and maturation of the urogenital tract and the female habitus. In adult life, both estradiol and progesterone support breast function, and estradiol has an important role in preserving bone mineral density. Progesterone is responsible for the rise in basal body temperature during the luteal phase of the menstrual cycle and decreases in progesterone secretion may contribute to premenstrual changes in mood.

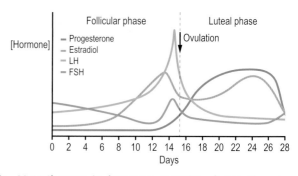

Fig. 39.14 **Changes in hormone secretion during the normal menstrual cycle.** LH, luteinizing hormone; FSH, follicle-stimulating hormone.

Disorders of steroid secretion in the female

Just as in the male, endocrine disorders of subnormal sex steroid secretion in the female may result from a wide range of disorders in the hypothalamus, pituitary or ovary

Just as for the testes, endocrine failure of the ovaries may occur due to damage or dysfunction of the ovaries themselves, or due to defects at the level of the hypothalamus or pituitary. Indeed, several pathologies, including pituitary adenomas and Kallman's syndrome, are common to men and women. However, in women the most common genetic disorder affecting the ovary is Turner's syndrome (karyotype 45X), which has characteristic somatic features including short stature, elevated plasma FSH and prepubertal estradiol, and vestigial or 'streak' ovaries. Various other endocrine causes of infertility are shown in Table 39.6, but are largely beyond the scope of this text.

Syndromes of excess ovarian steroid secretion lead to precocious puberty in children and infertility and/or hirsutism in the adult

Precocious puberty may arise from early maturation of the normal hypothalamic gonadal axis, an estradiol- or androgen-secreting cyst or tumor of the ovary or the adrenal gland, congenital adrenal hyperplasia, or severe insulin resistance. In the mature female, hypersecretion of androgen in the polycystic ovary syndrome (PCOS) may result in infertility and/or hirsutism (growth of male type and distribution of hair in women). Although the etiology of PCOS remains uncertain, it shows a strong genetic predisposition and current theories favor a key role for aberrant intraovarian androgen metabolism, in some cases strongly influenced by systemic insulin resistance. The nature of the clinically important cross-talk between insulin action and ovarian androgen production is not yet clear, however.

THE GROWTH HORMONE AXIS

Growth hormone-releasing hormone (GHRH) and somatostatin

GHRH is a 44-amino acid peptide synthesized as part of a 108-amino acid prohormone in the arcuate and ventromedial nuclei of the hypothalamus and in the median eminence. GHRH binds to its receptor on the pituitary somatotroph cell and triggers both the adenylyl cyclase and intracellular calcium-calmodulin systems (Chapter 40) to stimulate GH transcription and secretion from the anterior pituitary. Negative feedback from GH and IGF-I results in both a decrease in GHRH synthesis and secretion and an increase in somatostatin synthesis and secretion.

Somatostatin is found in two forms with 14 and 28 amino acids, both of which are produced from the same 116-amino acid gene product. Somatostatin and its receptors are found throughout the brain and also in other organs, notably the gut. Binding of somatostatin to its receptor is coupled to adenylyl cyclase by an inhibitory guanine nucleotide-binding protein, resulting in a decrease in intracellular cAMP. In the context of growth, somatostatin inhibits the secretion of GH. GHRH and somatostatin are released in separate bursts to provide a very fine level of control of GH release. Somatostatin also inhibits the production or action of many other hormones including TSH, insulin, and glucagon and gastrin. Long-acting analogs of somatostatin are thus effective in the management of GH excess as well as tumors secreting a wide range of other hormones, and as an adjunct

HORMONE REPLACEMENT THERAPY (HRT)

Women normally reach menopause at 45–55 years of age. The absence of ovarian follicles leads to an absence of estrogen and inhibin secretion resulting in a marked rise in pituitary FSH. There are vasomotor symptoms of estrogen deficiency (flushing) associated with menopause. Long-term postmenopausal estrogen deficiency is known to increase the rate of bone loss, leading to osteoporosis, and also alters lipoprotein metabolism in a way that increases the risk of cardiovascular disease. HRT with an estrogen preparation was standard practice in most developed countries both to relieve the acute symptoms and to provide prophylaxis against the long-term risks. However, recent studies have shown that HRT increases a woman's risk for breast cancer, cardiovascular disease, stroke, and pulmonary embolism. Although HRT did have a modest effect on preventing osteoporosis, there are newer drugs, the bisphosphonates, that are just as effective. The current recommendations are that HRT should only be used as short-term therapy for vasomotor symptoms that do not respond to other treatment

to pancreatic surgery to inhibit exocrine secretions from the pancreatic residue during healing.

Growth hormone

The greatest secretion of GH occurs in children and young adults, chiefly during sleep

Although GH can exist in variant forms, the major species is a 22 kDa protein. Nearly two-thirds of GH in the circulation is associated with a 29 kDa binding protein that is identical to the extracellular domain of the GH receptor. This binding protein prolongs the half-life of GH in plasma, about 20 minutes.

The normal human pituitary contains approximately 10 mg of GH; less than 5% of this is released each day. GH is released in bursts with a periodicity of 3–4 hours and greatest secretory activity occurs during sleep. At the peak of a secretory burst, the plasma GH concentration may be 100-fold greater than baseline; this means that no meaningful reference interval can be derived for this hormone, and so meaningful measurement requires either a provocative test or multiple samples over the course of a day. Secretory bursts occur most frequently in children and young adults.

Control of GH secretion

GH has a wide range of actions in regulating growth and intermediary metabolism

It is not surprising, in view of the wide range of actions of GH, that several factors other than GHRH and somatostatin can influence GH secretion. These include other hormones (estradiol) and metabolic fuels (glucose). Several pharmacologic agents are also known to influence GH secretion. These factors act at the higher centers and the hypothalamus to alter the pattern of GHRH and somatostatin secretion.

Biochemical actions of GH

Binding of GH to its receptor precipitates a complex series of intracellular events that lead to the transcription of many enzymes, hormones and growth factors, including IGF-I

The diversity of action of GH makes it difficult to understand or integrate all of its functions; thus it is convenient to think in two distinct phases (Fig. 39.15). The direct actions of GH are on lipid, carbohydrate, and protein metabolism. During hypoglycemia, GH stimulates lipolysis and induces peripheral resistance to insulin. These effects stimulate the use of

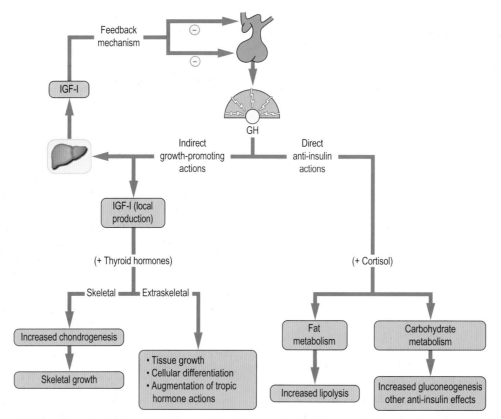

Fig. 39.15 **Biochemical functions of the growth hormone (GH).** These can be divided conveniently into direct actions on lipid and carbohydrate metabolism and indirect actions on protein synthesis and cell proliferation.

fatty acids in peripheral tissues, sparing glucose for use in the brain. Previously, GH therapy was used only for treatment of GH deficiency in children in order to stimulate growth; however, treatment is now often extended into adulthood when it can sometimes improve quality of life. This change in treatment strategy illustrates the complex effects of GH on metabolism. During growth, GH stimulates the uptake of amino acids and their incorporation into protein, especially in muscle. The indirect actions of GH are mediated by IGF-I. These actions promote the proliferation of chondrocytes and the synthesis of cartilage matrix in skeletal tissues. Although GH is most often associated with its role in stimulating linear growth, it clearly has other roles in influencing the relative amount and distribution of fat and muscle tissue. Its anabolic effects are the rationale for its current illicit use in sport.

Insulin-like growth factor I

IGF-I is the most GH-dependent of a series of growth factors

IGF-I is a 70-amino acid single-chain basic peptide, which has considerable homology with proinsulin. In response to tropic hormones like GH, IGF-I is produced in many tissues,

whose growth is then stimulated; that is, IGF-I acts as a paracrine hormone. The liver is the major source of circulating IGF-I, whose function is primarily feedback inhibition of GH secretion. In plasma and other extracellular fluids, IGF-I is complexed to a series of IGF-binding proteins (IGFBPs) of which IGFBP-3 is the most abundant. IGF-I works through the type 1 IGF receptor, which is structurally similar to the insulin receptor and linked to intracellular tyrosine kinase activity. The relative affinities of insulin and IGF-I for their respective receptors mean that, in normal physiology, there is little cross-stimulation, although in pathologic and pharmacologic situations it is possible for insulin to have some action through the IGF-I receptor, and vice versa. This has implications for states of severe insulin resistance, where local activation of the IGF1R has been suggested to underlie some clinical features such as skin overgrowth (acanthosis nigricans). Conversely, IGF-I has a limited therapeutic role in some rare conditions caused by loss of insulin receptor function.

The plasma reference interval for IGF-I in adults aged 20–60 years is fairly constant. It is much lower in young children but rises dramatically during the period of growth and progression through puberty. IGF-I concentrations fall after the sixth decade of life. Thus, IGF-I appears to be a good marker of integrated GH activity.

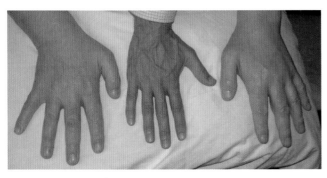

Fig. 39.16 **Acromegaly.**

Clinical disorders of GH secretion

GH deficiency in children is one of several causes of short stature, while GH excess in children leads to gigantism and, in adults, to acromegaly

The absence of a plasma reference range for GH means that GH deficiency may only be diagnosed by studying the dynamics of GH secretion, either during sleep or following a stimulation test. Basal IGF-I or IGFBP-3 measurements may serve as a preliminary screening test. Treatment is by regular injection of recombinant human GH. Adults with a definite cause of GH deficiency (hypopituitarism) are also candidates for GH replacement therapy. A rare genetic cause of short stature is Laron dwarfism in which GH levels are elevated but IGF-I levels are subnormal – a GH receptor defect is responsible.

In most cases, GH excess is caused by a pituitary tumor

GH excess is almost always due to a GH-secreting pituitary tumor, although GHRH-secreting tumors in the hypothalamus and ectopic GHRH production from pancreatic tumors have been described. In children, GH excess manifests itself as gigantism. In adults, the epiphyses of the long bones have closed and so further linear growth is not possible. Therefore, the adult form, acromegaly, is characterized by a thickening of tissues and overgrowth of the bones in the hands, feet and face (Fig. 39.16). Enlarged lips and tongue with mandibular overgrowth give rise to a classic facial appearance. Excessive sweating and joint pains are also common symptoms. Unfortunately, the progression of acromegaly is so slow that an average of 9 years elapses between the onset of symptoms and diagnosis. Classically, the diagnosis of GH excess has relied on showing inadequate GH suppression during a standard 75 g oral glucose tolerance test and on elevated IGF-I levels. However, pubescent patients may have paradoxic responses to glucose, and IGF-I levels are normally elevated during this developmental stage. Therefore MRI evidence of a pituitary tumor is critical in making the proper diagnosis. Surgery is the preferred treatment, although long-acting somatostatin is also effective. More recently, pegvisomant, a GH antagonist rationally designed based on structural features of the hormone–receptor interaction, has also proved useful in refractory cases.

THE PROLACTIN AXIS

Dopamine

Dopamine is an inhibitor of prolactin secretion

Prolactin is unique among the pituitary hormones in that it is under predominantly inhibitory control from the hypothalamus (see Fig. 36.4). Furthermore, the controlling agent is the simple molecule dopamine (Chapter 42), which is produced by tuberoinfundibular dopamine neurones. Dopamine works by stimulating the pituitary lactotroph D2 receptor to inhibit adenylyl cyclase and consequently inhibits both prolactin synthesis and secretion. Several neuropeptides, including TRH, have prolactin-releasing properties, but there is little evidence for a physiologic role.

Prolactin

Prolactin may assist breast growth and milk formation in association with other pregnancy-related hormones

Prolactin is a 23 kDa protein, which is homologous to GH. The primary role for prolactin in humans occurs during pregnancy when prolactin binds to its receptor in mammary tissue and stimulates the synthesis of several milk proteins, including lactalbumin. In other animals, prolactin also has gonadotropic, immunologic, and hematologic effects: it is required for maintenance of pregnancy in rodents, is mitogenic for some immune cells, and it ameliorates some forms of anemia. Prolactin exerts its effects on female reproductive function at multiple levels. Its actions include blocking the action of FSH on follicular estrogen secretion and enhancing progesterone levels by inhibiting steroid-metabolizing enzymes.

Clinical disorders of prolactin secretion

There are no known prolactin deficiency syndromes but hyperprolactinemia is very common

Hyperprolactinemia may result from a prolactin-secreting pituitary tumor (prolactinoma), a deficient supply of dopamine from the hypothalamus, or the use of any of a wide range of antidopaminergic drugs. In women, the presenting features of hyperprolactinemia include menstrual irregularity and galactorrhea (discharge of milk from the breast). A grossly elevated serum prolactin is usually diagnostic of a prolactinoma. For subjects with modest hyperprolactinemia, who are not taking antidopaminergic drugs, the differential diagnosis is difficult;

pituitary imaging and/or dynamic tests of prolactin secretion will assist the diagnosis of a microprolactinoma. Treatment options include long-acting dopamine agonist drugs or surgery. Prolactinomas need to be observed particularly carefully during pregnancy, when there is physiologic hyperplasia of pituitary lactotrophs in anticipation of lactation.

In men, hyperprolactinemia can cause impotence and prostatic hyperplasia. However, because other conditions more commonly produce these symptoms, the diagnosis of hyperprolactinemia is often missed until prolactinomas become very large and present as hypopituitarism with visual field defects. The latter symptoms arise when the tumor expands out of the pituitary fossa and impinges on the optic chiasm. Such tumors often shrink and fibrose with dopamine agonist therapy. For this reason it is critically important to identify which patients with large pituitary tumors have very high prolactin levels, as they may be able to avoid surgery.

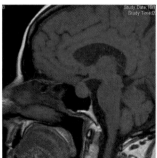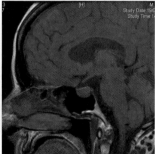

Fig. 39.17 **Effect of dopamine agonist therapy on a large prolactinoma**.

Summary

The endocrine system produces hormones, a structurally diverse group of chemical messengers that regulate and coordinate whole-body metabolism, growth, reproduction, and responses to external stimuli. The hypothalamic-anterior pituitary axis is a critical link between the brain and peripheral endocrine glands, and integrates diverse internal and external stimuli into only a few hormonal signals: it controls the synthesis and action of thyroid hormone, glucocorticoids, sex steroids, growth hormone, and prolactin. The hypothalamic-posterior pituitary axis controls the production and release of oxytocin and AVP/ADH. The action of these hormones on cells is controlled by receptors located either on cell membranes or intracellularly. Feedback mechanisms are important in controlling endocrine systems, and both overactivity and underactivity of these axes produce distinct clinical syndromes. Laboratory diagnosis of endocrine disorders relies heavily on measurement of hormones in blood; however, careful attention must often be paid to the timing of sampling, and to the nature of the sample required, before meaningful interpretation of the results is possible.

The human body contains several other endocrine systems not considered in this chapter, though they are governed by the same general principles. Some of these systems are considered in other chapters as part of the physiologic function that they control. Thus the reader is referred to Chapter 21 for carbohydrate homeostasis, Chapter 25 for calcium homeostasis and Chapter 23 for water and electrolyte homeostasis and the control of blood pressure. The intracellular signaling systems through which hormones exert their effects are described in the next chapter.

MACROPROLACTIN

Although antibody-based immunoassays are extremely powerful tools in endocrine diagnosis, they are subject to interference by endogenous antibodies in several ways. One way in which endogenous antibodies can produce confusing results is by binding and aggregating the target hormone in high molecular weight (HMW) complexes. This may be seen for several peptide hormones, but is particularly problematic for prolactin, where so-called 'macroprolactin' may account for up to 10% of cases of apparently elevated serum prolactin. This is a problem as macroprolactin is generally not biologically active, and so its detection could lead to unnecessary treatment. There are several ways around this. Most simply, as different immunoassays often have different capabilities to detect macroprolactin, use of more than one assay may provide a strong clue to its presence. Second, a common technique is to precipitate HMW complexes with polyethylene glycol (PEG) with immunoassay both before and after to establish how much signal is lost in the HMW fraction. More accurate quantification may require laborious techniques such as gel filtration.

ACTIVE LEARNING

1. Trace the two-way flow of information between hypothalamus and ovarian follicles early in the menstrual cycle.
2. How do GH, cortisol, and insulin interact to regulate lipid and carbohydrate metabolism?
3. Because dietary iodide can vary greatly, thyroid hormones need to be synthesized and stored when iodide is available but thyroid hormones are hydrophobic and cannot be contained within membrane vesicles. How does the thyroid gland solve this problem?

Further reading

Anderson MS. Autoimmune endocrine disease. *Curr Opin Immunol* 2002; **14**: 760–764.
Cooper DS. Hyperthyroidism. *Lancet* 2003; **363**: 459–468.
Dattani M, Preece M. Growth hormone deficiency and related disorders: insights into causation, diagnosis and treatment. *Lancet* 2004; **363**: 1977–1987.

Dayan CM. Interpretation of thyroid function tests. *Lancet* 2001; **357**: 619–624.

Henderson J. Ernest Starling and 'hormones': an historical commentary. *J Endocrinol* 2005; **184**: 5–10.

Melmed S. Acromegaly. *N Engl J Med* 2006; **355**: 2558–2573.

Newell Price J, Bertagna X, Grossman A, Nieman L. Cushing's syndrome. *Lancet* 2006; **367**: 1605–1617.

Roberts CGP, Ladenson PW. Hypothyroidism. *Lancet* 2004; **362**: 793–803.

Schlechte JA. Prolactinoma. *N Eng J Med* 2003; **349**: 2035–2041.

Schneider HJ, Aimaretti G, Kreitschmann-Andermahr I et al. Hypopituitarism. *Lancet* 2007; **369**: 1461–1470.

Zimmermann MB, Jooste PL, Pandav CS. Iodine-deficiency disorders. *Lancet* 2008; **372**: 1152–68

Websites

www.endo-society.org

www.endotext.org

www.thyroidmanager.org

www.pituitary.org

www.CSRF.net

www.endocrine.niddk.nih.gov/ (e.g. www.endocrine.niddk.nih.gov/pubs/cushings/cushings.htm).Hormone replacement therapy (hrt)

40. Membrane Receptors and Signal Transduction

M M Harnett and H S Goodridge

LEARNING OBJECTIVES

After reading this chapter you should be able to:

- Distinguish between steroid and polypeptide hormones, and outline their mechanisms of action.
- Describe G-protein coupled receptors.
- Outline the activation of downstream intracellular signaling cascades by heterotrimeric G-proteins.
- Discuss the generation of second messengers such as cyclic AMP, inositol trisphosphate (IP_3), diacylglycerol (DAG) and Ca^{2+}, and explain how they activate key protein kinases.
- Explain how phospholipases generate a diverse array of lipid second messengers.
- Discuss how the generation of a variety of second messengers can amplify hormone signals and lead to the generation of specific biologic responses.

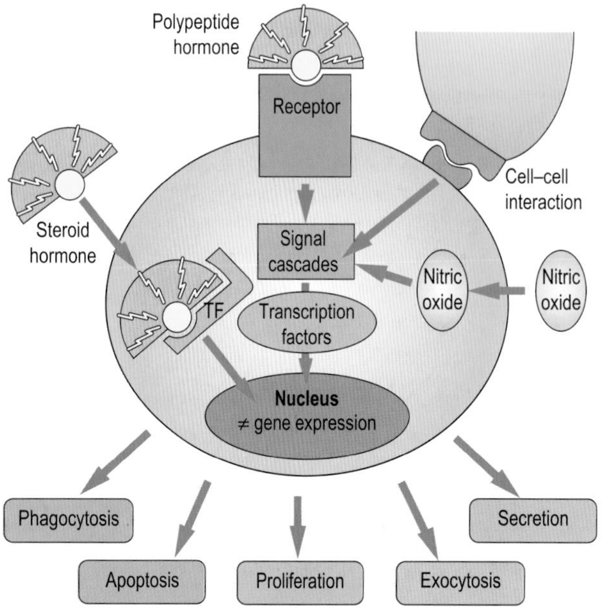

Fig. 40.1 **Mechanisms of cell signaling.** NO, nitric oxide; TF, transcription factor.

INTRODUCTION

Cells sense, respond to, and integrate a multiplicity of signals from their environment. Although some of these signals may be mediated by cell–cell contact, in multicellular organisms many signal molecules, such as hormones, originate in organs distant from their site of action and must be carried in the blood to their target effector cells. Likewise, immune cells such as phagocytes are recruited from the blood to sites of inflammation by chemoattractants. Signals generated in these ways are sensed and processed by cellular signal transduction cassettes that comprise specific cell surface membrane receptors, effector signaling elements, and regulatory proteins. These signaling cassettes serve to detect, amplify, and integrate diverse external signals to generate the appropriate cellular response (Fig. 40.1).

In this chapter, we first discuss how cell surface receptors sense and transduce their specific hormone signal by transmembrane coupling to effector enzyme systems, generating low molecular-weight molecules termed second messengers. We then discuss the diversity of these second messengers and how they influence the activity of a range of key protein kinases with distinct substrates that ultimately determine the type of obtained biologic response.

HORMONE RECEPTORS

Hormones are biochemical messengers that act to orchestrate the responses of different cells within a multicellular organism (Chapter 39). They are generally synthesized by specific tissues and secreted directly into the blood, which transports them to their target responsive organs. Hormones can broadly be subdivided into two major classes:

- steroid hormones
- polypeptide hormones.

These hormones achieve their biologic effects by interacting with specific receptors to induce intracellular signaling cascades (Table 40.1).

Intracellular receptors: steroid hormone receptors

Steroid hormones traverse cell membranes

Because of the cholesterol-based nature of their structure, steroid hormones, such as cortisol (made in the cortex of the

Classification of membrane receptors				
Receptor class	Transmembrane-spanning domains	Intrinsic catalytic activity	Accessory coupling/regulatory molecules	Examples of receptor subclasses
G-protein-coupled receptors (serpentine receptors)	multipass (seven transmembrane α-helices)	none	G-proteins	β-adrenergic α-adrenergic muscarinic chemokines (IL-8) rhodopsin (vision)
Ion-channel receptors (ligand-gated receptors)	multipass; generally form multimeric complexes	none	none	neurotransmitters ions nucleotides inositol trisphosphate (IP₃)
Intrinsic receptor tyrosine kinases	single-pass transmembrane domain, but may be multimeric (e.g. insulin receptor)	tyrosine kinase	none	epidermal growth factor (EGF) nerve growth factor (NGF) platelet-derived growth factor (PDGF) fibroblast growth factor (FGF) insulin
Tyrosine kinase-associated receptors	single-pass transmembrane domain, but generally form multimeric receptors	none	some require ITAM/ITIM-containing proteins	antigen receptors (ITAM–Src-related kinases) FcγR (ITIM–Src-related kinases) hemopoietin cytokine receptors (Janus kinases)
Intrinsic tyrosine phosphatase receptors	single-pass transmembrane domain	tyrosine phosphatase	none	CD45-phosphatase receptor
Intrinsic serine–threonine receptor kinases	single-pass transmembrane domain	serine–threonine kinase	none	tumor growth factor β (TGF-β)
Intrinsic guanylate cyclase receptors	single-pass transmembrane domain	guanylate cyclase (generates cGMP)	none	atrial natriuretic peptide (ANP) receptors
Death-domain receptors	single-pass transmembrane domain	none	death-domain accessory proteins (TRADD, FADD, RIP, TRAFs)	tumor necrosis factor (TNF-α) Fas

cGMP, cyclic guanosine monophosphate; FADD, fas-associated death domain; FcgR, Fc-g receptor (receptor for immunoglobulin G); IL, interleukin; ITAM/ITIM, immunoreceptor tyrosine activation/inhibition motif; RIP, receptor-interacting protein; Src, Src-tyrosine kinase; TRADD, TNF-receptor-associated death domain; TRAFs, TNF-receptor-associated factors.

Table 40.1 **Classification of membrane receptors**.

adrenal gland), sex hormones, and vitamin D, can traverse the plasma membrane of cells to initiate their responses via cytoplasmic located receptors called steroid hormone receptors (see Fig. 40.1). These receptors belong to a superfamily of cytoplasmic receptors called the intracellular receptor superfamily, which also transduce signals from other small hydrophobic signaling molecules such as the tyrosine-derived thyroid hormones (e.g. thyroxine) and the vitamin A-derived retinoids (e.g. retinoic acid).

Intracellular receptors for steroid and thyroid hormones and retinoids are transcription factors

The intracellular receptors for these steroid and thyroid hormones and retinoids are transcription factors; they bind to regulatory regions of the DNA of genes that are responsive to the particular steroid/thyroid hormone. Such 'ligand binding' (ligation) induces a conformational change in the transcription factor that allows it to activate or repress gene induction. Although all the target cells have specific receptors for the individual hormones, they express distinct combinations of cell type-specific regulatory proteins that cooperate with the intracellular hormone receptor to dictate the precise repertoire of genes that are induced. Hence the hormones induce distinct sets of responses in different target cells (compare Chapter 34).

Cell surface receptors: polypeptide hormone receptors

Polypeptide hormones act through membrane receptors

In contrast to the steroid hormones, polypeptide hormones cannot cross cell membranes and must initiate their effects on their target cells via specific cell surface receptors (see Fig. 40.1). As they do not themselves enter the target cell, they are termed 'first messengers' and their intracellular effects are mediated by low molecular-weight signaling molecules, such as cyclic adenosine monophosphate (cAMP) or calcium, which are called 'second messengers'. In fact, the term 'polypeptide hormones' encompasses a wide range of families of hormones, growth factors, and cytokines that use transmembrane signal transduction cassettes to elicit their biologic effects.

Receptor-independent signaling mechanisms

Some low molecular-weight signaling molecules traverse the cell membrane

Although most extracellular signals mediate their effects via receptor ligation of either cell surface or cytoplasmic receptors, some low molecular-weight signaling molecules are able to traverse the plasma membrane and directly modulate the activity of the catalytic domains of transmembrane receptors or cytoplasmic signal transducing enzymes (see Fig. 40.1). For example, nitric oxide (NO), which has been postulated to have a variety of functions including signaling the relaxation of smooth muscle cells in blood vessels, can stimulate guanylate cyclase, leading to the generation of the second messenger, cGMP. Patients with angina are treated with glyceryl trinitrate, which is converted to NO, resulting in relaxation of the blood vessels. The consequent improvement in oxygen delivery to the heart muscle eases the pain that was caused by inadequate blood flow to the heart (see box on p. 76).

RECEPTOR COUPLING TO INTRACELLULAR SIGNAL TRANSDUCTION

Some sensory systems use receptor-coupled signaling

In addition to hormone receptors, sensory systems such as vision (Chapter 41, Fig. 41.4), taste and smell use similar mechanisms of cell surface membrane receptor-coupled signal transduction (Table 40.1). Some of these receptors, for example the β-adrenergic receptors or the antigen receptors on lymphocytes, have no intrinsic catalytic activity and serve simply as specific recognition units. These receptors use a variety of mechanisms, including adaptor molecules or catalytically

active regulatory molecules such as G-proteins (guanosine triphosphatases, GTPases, which hydrolyze GTP) to couple them to their effector signaling elements, which are generally enzymes (often called signaling enzymes or signal transducers) or ion channels (Fig. 40.2). In contrast, other receptors – such as the intrinsic tyrosine kinase receptors for growth factors (e.g. platelet-derived growth factor, PDGF) or the intrinsic serine kinase receptors for molecules like transforming growth factor-β (TGF-β) – have extracellular ligand-binding domains and cytoplasmic catalytic domains. Thus, after receptor–ligand interaction (receptor ligation), these receptors can directly initiate their signaling cascades by phosphorylating and modulating the activities of target signal-transducing molecules (downstream signaling enzymes). These in turn propagate the growth factor signal by modulating the activity of further specific signal transducers or transcription factors, leading to gene induction (see Chapters 34 and 43).

G-protein coupled receptors

G-protein coupled receptors comprise a superfamily of structurally related receptors for hormones, neurotransmitters, inflammatory mediators, proteinases, taste and odorant molecules, and light photons. A classic example of this class of receptors is the β-adrenergic receptor (for which the ligand is epinephrine) as its structure–function properties have been extensively studied with respect to its activation of signal transduction cascades. G-protein coupled receptors are integral membrane proteins characterized by the seven transmembrane-spanning helices within their structure. They generally comprise an extracellular N-terminus, seven transmembrane-spanning α-helices (20–28 hydrophobic amino acids each), three extracellular and intracellular loops, and an intracellular C-terminal tail. Ligands, such as epinephrine, typically bind to the G-protein coupled receptor by sitting in a pocket formed by the seven transmembrane helices (see Fig. 13.5). G-protein coupled receptors have no intrinsic catalytic domains; they therefore recruit guanine nucleotide-binding proteins (G-proteins), via their third cytoplasmic loop, to couple to their signal transduction elements.

G-proteins

G-proteins constitute a group of regulatory molecules that are involved in the regulation of a diverse range of biologic processes, including signal transduction, protein synthesis, intracellular trafficking (targeted delivery to the plasma membrane or intracellular organelles) and exocytosis, as well as cell movement, growth, proliferation and differentiation. The G-protein superfamily predominantly comprises two major subfamilies: the small, monomeric *Ras*-like G-proteins (see Chapter 43) and the heterotrimeric G-proteins. Heterotrimeric G-proteins regulate the transduction of transmembrane signals from cell surface receptors to a

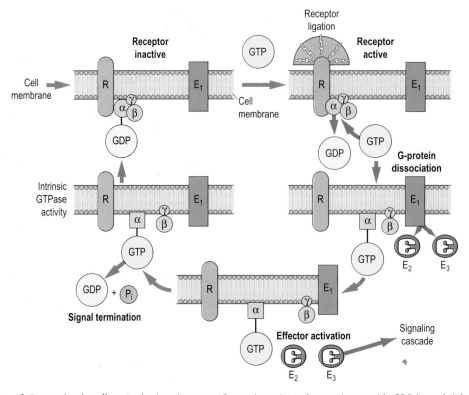

Fig. 40.2 **Mechanism of G-protein signaling.** In the inactive state, G-proteins exist as heterotrimers with GDP bound tightly to the α-subunit. None of the subunits are integral membrane proteins; however, the G-protein is anchored to the plasma membrane by lipid modification of the γ-subunits (prenylation) and some of the α-subunits (myristoylation of the $G_{i\alpha}$ family). Ligation of the receptor (R) drives exchange of GDP for GTP and induces a conformational change in Gα, which results in a decrease in its affinity both for the receptor and for the $\beta\gamma$-subunits, leading to dissociation of the receptor–G-protein complex. The activated Gα (GTP-bound) or the released $\beta\gamma$-subunits, or both, can then interact with one or more effectors, to generate intracellular second messengers that activate downstream signaling cascades. Signaling is terminated by the intrinsic GTPase activity of the α-subunit, which hydrolyzes GTP to GDP to allow reassociation of the inactive, heterotrimeric G-protein, G$\alpha\beta\gamma$. (See also Fig. 41.4.)

variety of intracellular effectors, such as adenylyl cyclase, phospholipase C (PLC), cGMP-phosphodiesterase (PDE) and ion channel effector systems (see Fig. 40.2). These G-proteins consist of three distinct classes of subunits: α (39–46 kDa), β (37 kDa), and γ (8 kDa). In general, effector specificity is conferred by the α-subunit, which contains the GTP-binding site and an intrinsic GTPase activity. However, it is now widely accepted that $\beta\gamma$ complexes can also directly regulate effectors such as phospholipase A_2 (PLA$_2$), PLC-β isoforms, adenylyl cyclase and ion channels in mammalian systems, as well as cellular responses such as mating factor receptor pathways in yeast. Four major subfamilies of α-subunit genes have been identified on the basis of their cDNA homology and function: G_s, G_i, G_q, and G_{12} (Table 40.2). Many of these Gα subunits have been shown to exhibit a rather ubiquitous pattern of expression in mammalian systems, at least at the mRNA level, but it is also clear that certain α-subunits have a tissue-restricted profile of expression. Moreover, there is evidence of differential expression of α-subunits during cellular development.

G-proteins act as molecular switches

Heterotrimeric G-proteins regulate transmembrane signals by acting as a molecular switch, linking cell surface

G-protein coupled receptors to one or more downstream signaling molecules (see Fig. 40.2).

Ligation of the receptor initiates an interaction with the inactive, GDP-bound heterotrimeric G-protein. This interaction drives exchange of GDP for GTP, inducing a conformational change in Gα, which results in a decrease in its affinity for both the receptor and the $\beta\gamma$-subunits, leading to dissociation of the receptor–G-protein complex. The activated Gα (GTP-bound) or released $\beta\gamma$-subunits, or both, can then interact with one or more effectors to generate intracellular second messengers, which activate downstream signaling cascades. Signaling is terminated by the intrinsic GTPase activity of the α-subunit, which hydrolyzes GTP to GDP to allow reassociation of the inactive heterotrimeric G-protein (G$\alpha\beta\gamma$).

SECOND MESSENGERS

Cyclic AMP (cAMP)

β-adrenergic receptors are coupled to cAMP

β-adrenergic receptors are coupled to the generation of the second messenger, cAMP. The β-adrenergic hormone epinephrine

Properties of mammalian G-proteins					
G-protein subfamily	α-subunits	Molecular mass (kDa)	Toxin substrate	Tissue distribution	Effector
G_i	G_z	41	none	brain, adrenal medulla, platelets	inhibits adenylate cyclase
	G_i	40	pertussis toxin	nearly ubiquitous	G_i α-subunits activate
	G_0	40	pertussis toxin	brain, neural systems	PLC and PLA_2 and K^+ channels, and inhibit adenylate cyclase and Ca^{2+} channels
G_s	G_t	40	pertussis/cholera toxin	retinal rods and cones	activates cGMP phosphodiesterase
	G_{gust}	40	pertussis toxin	taste buds	activates phosphodiesterase
	G_s	44–46	cholera toxin	ubiquitous	G_s activates adenylate cyclase and Ca^{2+} channels
G_{12}	G_{oll}	45	cholera toxin	olfactory neuroepithelium	activates adenylate cyclase
	G_{12}	44	none	ubiquitous	$G_{12/13}$ subunits regulate
	G_{13}	44	none	ubiquitous	Na^+/H^+ exchange, voltage-dependent Ca^{2+} channels, and eicosanoid signaling
G_q	G_q	42	none	nearly ubiquitous	PLC
	G_{11}	42	none	nearly ubiquitous	
	G_{14}	42	none	lung, kidney, liver, spleen, testis	
	G_{15}	43	none	hemopoietic cells	
	G_{16}	44	none	hemopoietic cells	

PDE, phosphodiesterase; cGMP, cyclic guanosine monophosphate; PLC, phospholipase C; PLA_2, phospholipase A_2.

Table 40.2 **Properties of the four main classes of mammalian G-protein α-subunits.** Some G-proteins can be characterized using different bacterial toxin substrates.

BACTERIAL TOXINS WHICH TARGET G-PROTEINS CAUSE A RANGE OF DISEASES

A variety of bacterial toxins exert their toxic effects by covalently modifying G-proteins and hence irreversibly modulating their function. For example, cholera toxin (choleragen) from *Vibrio cholerae* contains an enzyme (subunit A) that catalyzes the transfer of ADP-ribose from intracellular NAD to the α-subunit of G_s; this modification prevents the hydrolysis of G_s-bound GTP, resulting in a constitutively (permanently) active form of the G-protein. The resulting prolonged increase in cAMP concentrations within the intestinal epithelial cells leads to phosphokinase A-mediated phosphorylation of Cl^- channels, causing a large efflux of electrolytes and water into the gut, which is responsible for the severe diarrhea that is characteristic of cholera. Enterotoxin action is initiated by specific binding of the B (binding) subunits of choleragen (AB_5) to the oligosaccharide moiety of the monosialoganglioside, GM_1, on epithelial cells. A similar molecular mechanism has been attributed to the action of the heat-labile enterotoxin, labile toxin, secreted by several strains of *Escherichia coli* responsible for 'traveler's diarrhea'. In contrast, pertussis toxin (another AB_5 toxin) from *Bordetella pertussis*, the causative agent of whooping cough, catalyzes the ADP-ribosylation of G_i, which prevents G_i from interacting with activated receptors. Hence, the G-protein is inactivated and cannot act to inhibit adenylyl cyclase, activate PLA_2 or PLC, open K^+ channels, or open and close Ca^{2+} channels, causing a generalized uncoupling of hormone receptors from their signaling cascades.

induces the breakdown of glycogen to glucose in muscle and, to a lesser extent, in the liver. The breakdown of glycogen in the liver is predominantly stimulated by the polypeptide hormone glucagon, which is secreted by the pancreas when blood sugar is low (Chapters 13 and 21). One of the earliest signaling events after binding of these hormones to their receptors is the generation of cAMP, a small molecule that has a key role in the regulation of intracellular signal transduction, leading to the conversion of glycogen to glucose. cAMP is derived from ATP by the catalytic action of the signaling enzyme

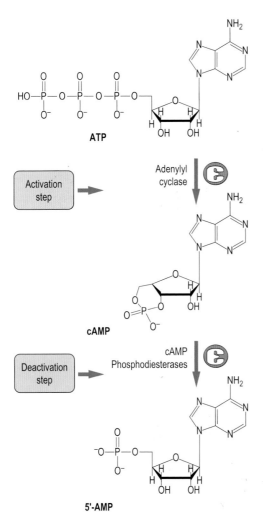

Fig. 40.3 **Metabolism of cyclic AMP.** Adenylyl cyclase catalyzes a cyclization reaction to produce the active cAMP, which is then deactivated by cAMP-phosphodiesterases. cAMP, cyclic adenosine monophosphate.

adenylyl cyclase (Fig. 40.3). This cyclization reaction involves the intramolecular attack of the 3′-OH group of the ribose unit on the α-phosphoryl group of ATP to form a phosphodiester bond; this is driven by the subsequent hydrolysis of the released pyrophosphate. The activity of cAMP is terminated by the hydrolysis of cAMP to 5′-AMP by specific cAMP-phosphodiesterases. The importance of cAMP in regulating glycogen breakdown was demonstrated by a series of experiments showing not only that hormones that activate adenylyl cyclase activity in fat cells also stimulate glycogen breakdown, but also that cell-permeant analogs of cAMP, such as dibutyryl cAMP, can mimic the effects of these hormones in inducing glycogen breakdown.

Adenylyl cyclase is activated by a G-protein

The β-adrenergic receptor is coupled to adenylyl cyclase activation by the action of the α-subunit of the stimulatory G-protein, called G_s. Because each molecule of bound hormone can stimulate many G_s α-subunits, this form of

transmembrane signaling amplifies the original hormone signal. Although hydrolysis of GTP by the intrinsic GTPase of the G_s α-subunit acts to switch off adenylyl cyclase activation, the hormone–receptor complex must also be deactivated to return the cell to its resting, unstimulated state. This receptor desensitization, which occurs after prolonged exposure to the hormone, involves phosphorylation of the C-terminal tail of the hormone-occupied β-adrenergic receptor by a kinase known as β-adrenergic receptor kinase. G-protein coupled receptors, such as α-adrenergic receptors, which act to inhibit cAMP generation, are coupled to the inhibition of adenylyl cyclase via the inhibitory, G_i-, G-protein.

Protein kinase A

Protein kinase A binds cAMP and phosphorylates other enzymes

cAMP transduces its effects on glycogen–glucose interconversion by regulating a key signaling enzyme, protein kinase A (PKA), which phosphorylates target proteins on serine and threonine residues. PKA is a multimeric enzyme comprising two regulatory (R) subunits and two catalytic (C) subunits: the R_2C_2 tetrameric form of PKA is inactive, but binding of four molecules of cAMP to the R subunits leads to the release of catalytically active C-subunits, which can then phosphorylate and modulate the activity of two key enzymes, phosphorylase kinase and glycogen synthase (Fig. 40.4), which are involved in regulation of glycogen metabolism (see Chapter 13). Involvement of such a multilayered signal transduction cascade leads to substantial amplification of the original signal at each stage of the cascade, ensuring that binding of only a few hormone molecules leads to release of a large number of sugar molecules. The amplification of a hormonal signal involving G-proteins, adenylyl cyclase, protein kinase A and phosphorylase is illustrated in Figure 40.5 (compare Fig. 13.4).

Many other cellular responses can be mediated by the cAMP-PKA signaling cassette

PKA-mediated phosphorylation can regulate the activity of a number of ion channels, such as K^+, Cl^- and Ca^{2+} channels, and that of phosphatases involved in the regulation of cell signaling. In addition, translocation of PKA into the nucleus allows modulation of the activity of transcription factors such as the cAMP-responsive-element-binding protein (CREB) or the activation transcription factor (ATF) families, leading to either the induction or the repression of expression of specific genes (see Fig. 40.4 and Chapter 34).

Phosphodiesterases

Phosphodiesterases terminate the cAMP signal

Phosphodiesterases (PDEs) terminate the cAMP signal by converting cAMP to its 5′AMP metabolite (see Fig. 40.3);

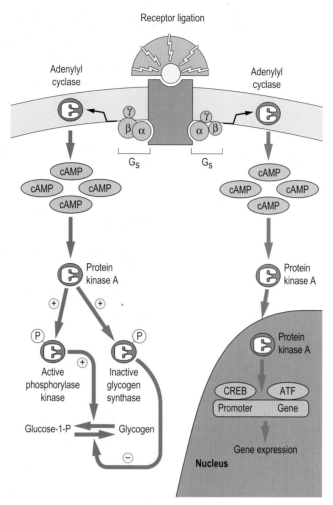

Fig. 40.4 **Protein kinase A (PKA) acts as a signaling enzyme for the second messenger, cAMP.** Binding of a stimulatory G-protein (G$_s$) to the hormone–receptor complex activates adenylyl cyclase, which catalyzes the production of cAMP. Protein kinase A is activated by binding four molecules of cAMP. Translocation of PKA into the nucleus modulates activity of transcription factors, for example CREB and ATF (see text), leading to induction or repression of gene expression. (Compare Fig. 13.6.)

thus they have the potential to play key roles in the regulation of various physiologic responses in many different cells and tissues. Indeed, they have been postulated to regulate platelet activation, vascular relaxation, cardiac muscle contraction, and inflammation, making them attractive targets for the development of selective inhibitors as potential therapeutic agents. For example, one group of compounds, the methylxanthines – which include theophylline and isobutylmethylxanthine – have been used as bronchodilators in the treatment of asthma, and are also able to exert positive inotropic responses in the heart. Moreover, drugs selective for the PDE$_3$ class of enzymes, such as milrinone, are cardiotonic and increase the force of contraction of the heart, presumably by increasing the concentrations of cAMP and stimulating PKA, leading to phosphorylation of cardiac calcium channels and a subsequent increase in intracellular calcium concentration.

Calcium ion

Calcium ion (Ca^{2+}) is a ubiquitous messenger and has an important role in the transduction of signals leading to cellular responses such as cell motility changes, egg fertilization, neurotransmission and protein secretion, as well as cell fusion, differentiation and proliferation.

Cells expend a considerable amount of energy maintaining a steep extracellular/intracellular Ca^{2+} concentration gradient; for example, the intracellular Ca^{2+} concentration in resting, unstimulated cells is of the order of 10^{-7} mol/L (100 nM), whereas the extracellular Ca^{2+} concentration is typically 10^{-3} mol/L (1 mM). This steep gradient allows for rapid, abrupt, transient changes in Ca^{2+} concentration: ligation of a wide range of hormone receptors, for example, leads to a rapid (within seconds) and transient increase in intracellular Ca^{2+}

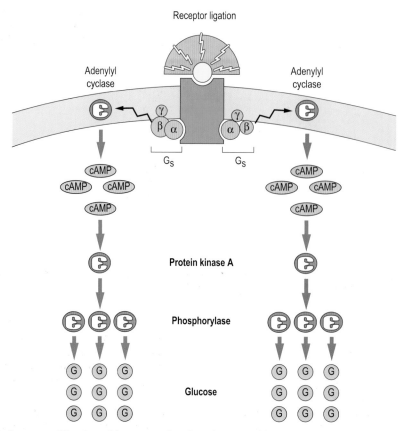

Fig. 40.5 **Signal cascade induces amplification of hormone signal.** Each activated hormone–receptor complex can stimulate multiple G_s molecules. Each adenylyl cyclase can catalyze the generation of many cAMP molecules, and each protein kinase A can activate many phosphorylase molecules, leading to the release of a large number of glucose molecules (G) as a result of glycogen degradation. (Compare Fig. 13.4.)

concentration to the micromolar range (compare Fig. 8.4). The rapid raising and lowering of Ca^{2+} concentrations is very tightly regulated and utilizes a variety of mechanisms involving cell compartmentalization. For example, intracellular Ca^{2+} concentrations can be lowered by sequestration of Ca^{2+} into the endoplasmic reticulum by Ca^{2+}-ATPases or into the mitochondria using the energy-driven electrochemical gradient. Alternatively, free Ca^{2+} can be chelated by Ca^{2+}-binding proteins such as calsequestrin.

Calmodulin

Many downstream signaling events mediated by Ca^{2+} are modulated by a Ca^{2+}-sensing and binding protein, calmodulin

Calmodulin is a 17 kDa protein found in all animal and plant cells (comprising up to 1% of cellular protein). It belongs to a family of proteins characterized by one or more copies of a Ca^{2+}-binding structural motif called an EF hand motif (Fig. 40.6). Calmodulin is composed of two similar globular domains joined by a long (6.5 nm; 65 Å) α-helix, each globular lobe having two EF hand motifs/Ca^{2+}-binding sites, 1.1 nm

(11 Å) apart. Binding of three to four calcium ions (which occurs when the intracellular calcium ion concentration is increased to about 500 nmol/L) induces a major conformational change that allows calmodulin to bind to and modify target proteins such as cAMP-PDE. Binding of several calcium ions allows cooperativity in the activation of calmodulin, such that small changes in Ca^{2+} concentration cause large changes in the concentration of an active Ca^{2+}–calmodulin (Ca^{2+}/CAM) complex, providing amplification of the original hormone signal.

Calmodulin has a wide range of target effectors, including Ca^{2+}/CAM-dependent protein kinases, which phosphorylate serine-threonine residues on proteins to regulate a variety of processes. For example, the broad-specificity kinase, Ca^{2+}/CAM-kinase II, is involved in the regulation of fuel metabolism, ion permeability, neurotransmitter biology, and myosin light-chain kinase and phosphorylase kinase activity. Interestingly, calmodulin serves as a permanent regulatory subunit of phosphorylase kinase and may also regulate non-kinase effectors such as certain adenylyl cyclase isoforms and also cAMP-PDEs, indicating 'cross-talk' between cAMP- and Ca^{2+}-dependent signaling pathways. Moreover, mice defective in the calmodulin-dependent adenylyl cyclase are deficient in

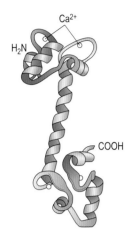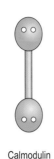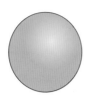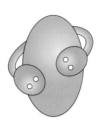

Calmodulin

Inactive
calmodulin-
dependent
kinase

Active
calmodulin-
dependent
kinase

Fig. 40.6 **Structure and function of calmodulin.** Binding of calcium induces a conformational change, allowing calmodulin to bind to and modify the activity of target signaling enzymes.

HEART FAILURE – POTENTIAL FOR TARGETING β-ADRENERGIC RECEPTOR (βAR) SIGNALING BY GENE THERAPY?

Heart disease is a major cause of death in developed countries and despite recent advances with therapies such as angiotensin-converting enzyme (ACE) inhibitors (Chapter 23), the prognosis for patients with heart failure is still relatively poor: the long-term survival (>5 years) is 50%. Normally, binding of catecholamines (epinephrine and norepinephrine) to βARs activates $G\alpha s$ to stimulate adenylyl cyclase and generate cAMP resulting in the activation of PKA and ultimately, via calcium-mediated excitation-contraction coupling, regulation of heart rate (chronotropy), contractility (inotropy) and relaxation (lusitropy). By contrast, in heart failure, myocytes exhibit characteristic changes in βAR signaling and consequent calcium mobilization, resulting in reduction of contractile function. Specifically, βAR expression is reduced and the remaining receptors appear to be desensitized due to increased levels of the negative regulator of βAR signaling, βAR kinase (βARK). Moreover, specific polymorphisms (mutations) in βARs have been identified in humans that are associated with poor prognosis following heart failure. Following on from the use of drugs targeting βAR function, such the β_2AR-specific agonist clenbuterol, much interest has focused on the therapeutic potential of modulating signaling via this pathway by cardiac gene therapy using viral vectors. For example, studies in animal models to date have suggested that there is potential therapeutic value in increasing expression of β_2AR, but not β_1AR, in terms of contractility and myocyte survival. Moreover, expression of the carboxy-terminal sequence of βARK (βARKct), which inhibits βARK-mediated desensitization of βARs, has been shown to prevent heart failure. Likewise, overexpression of downstream βAR effectors such as AC_{VI}, the major isoform of adenylyl cyclase in myocardium, has produced therapeutic effects and, indeed, clinical trials of human gene therapy using adenoviral transfer of AC_{VI} are currently progressing following preclinical studies. Finally, as βAR coupling to PKA signaling regulates the receptors and ion channels responsible for the calcium signals required for excitation-contraction coupling, downstream inotropic regulators of contractile function, such as the EF hand-type calcium sensing protein S100A1, which are also downregulated in heart failure, are also currently under study as potential therapeutic targets.

spatial memory, showing that this signal transduction system is important for learning and memory in vertebrates.

Phosphatidylinositol 4,5-bisphosphate (PIP₂)

Hydrolysis of a membrane phospholipid phosphatidylinositol 4,5-bisphosphate generates two second messengers

The major breakthrough in the search for the second messenger responsible for calcium mobilization came in the early 1980s, when it was found that stimulation of receptors that were known to increase the intracellular free Ca^{2+} concentration could activate the prior phospholipase C (PLC)-mediated hydrolysis of a minor phospholipid species, phosphatidylinositol 4,5-bisphosphate (PIP_2). PIP_2, which typically represents about 0.4% of total phospholipids in membranes, is generated from phosphatidylinositol by two kinases, phosphatidylinositol-4-kinase (PI-4-K or PI kinase) and phosphatidylinositol-5-kinase (PI-5-K or PIP kinase), both of which are found in the plasma membrane (Fig. 40.7). PIP_2 is hydrolyzed by a PIP_2-specific PLC, to generate two second messengers: inositol trisphosphate (I-1,4,5-P_3 or IP_3) and diacylglycerol (DAG). IP_3 is a water-soluble product, which is released into the cytosol and has been shown to mobilize intracellular stores of calcium. DAG is a lipid second messenger, which is anchored in the plasma membrane by virtue of

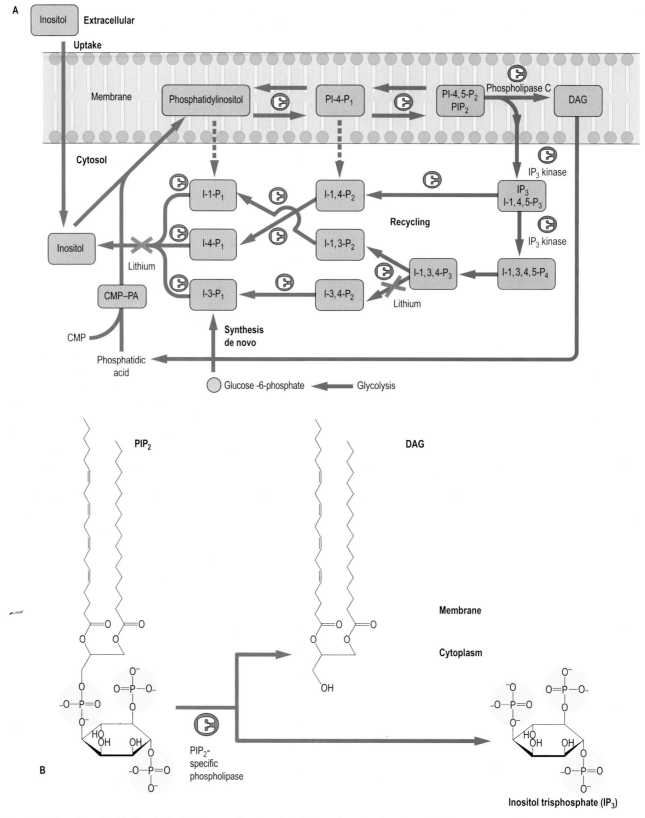

Fig. 40.7 **The phosphatidylinositol signaling cycle.** Phosphatidylinositol 4,5-bisphosphate (PIP$_2$) is generated from phosphatidylinositol by PI-4-kinase and PI-5-kinase (A). PIP$_2$ is hydrolyzed by a PIP$_2$-specific PLC, to generate two second messengers: I-1,4,5-P$_3$ (IP$_3$) and DAG (B). IP$_3$ is released into the cytosol and has been shown to mobilize intracellular stores of calcium. DAG is a lipid second messenger which is anchored in the plasma membrane and activates PKCs. IP$_3$ is degraded by (i) the sequential action of phosphatases converting I-1,4,5-P$_3$ to inositol, and (ii) an IP$_3$ kinase, which generates I-1,3,4,5-P$_4$, which is in turn sequentially degraded to inositol by inositol phosphate-specific phosphatases, some of which can be inhibited by LiCl. DAG, diacylglycerol; PA, phosphatidic acid; CMP-PA, cytosine monophosphate-phosphatidic acid (panel A).

its hydrophobic fatty acid side chains and activates a key family of signaling enzymes known as protein kinase C (PKC).

Inositol 1,4,5-trisphosphate (IP₃)

IP₃ is important in intracellular calcium mobilization

The rapid production (<1 second) and removal (t½ = 4 seconds in liver) of IP_3 that precedes an increase in intracellular Ca^{2+} concentration implied that it could be a second messenger signaling calcium mobilization. Two types of experiment confirmed that IP_3 is indeed a second messenger:

- **microinjection of IP₃ into cells**, or simply including IP_3 in incubations of cells in which detergent treatment had induced the formation of holes or pores in the plasma membrane (permeabilized cells), mobilized calcium in the absence of hormone stimulation
- **structure–function analyses** of a variety of inositol phosphate molecules suggested that calcium mobilization was dependent on specific IP_3 receptors.

IP_3 receptors that exhibit IP_3 binding and calcium release have now been cloned. These receptors are expressed on the endoplasmic reticulum of all cells as a family of related glycoproteins (molecular mass 250 kDa) comprising six transmembrane-spanning domains. The active receptor is expressed as a multimer of four IP_3 receptor molecules; this tetrameric structure gives rise to cooperativity in Ca^{2+} channel activity. It has been estimated that stimulated IP_3 (typically 2–3 mmol/L) releases 20–30 calcium ions. This calculation reveals the amplification inherent in this signaling cascade because, typically, only nanomolar concentrations of growth factor are required to elicit millimolar concentrations of this second messenger. Consistent with the transient nature of the release of intracellular calcium that is observed after hormone receptor ligation, cellular concentrations of

IP_3 are rapidly returned to resting values (0.1 mmol/L) by more than one route of degradation (see Fig. 40.7).

Diacylglycerol (DAG)

DAG activates protein kinase C

DAG fulfils its second messenger role by activating the key signaling enzyme, protein kinase C (PKC), which phosphorylates a wide range of target signal transduction proteins on serine or threonine. PKC was originally identified as a calcium- and lipid (phosphatidylserine)-dependent kinase important in the regulation of cell proliferation. However, in recent years, it has become clear that PKC is, in reality, a generic name for a superfamily of related kinases that have different tissue distribution and activation requirements (Table 40.3). Nevertheless, all these enzymes share some conserved features; most notably they comprise two major domains: an N-terminal regulatory domain and a C-terminal catalytic kinase domain. The regulatory domain contains a pseudosubstrate sequence that resembles the consensus phosphorylation site in PKC substrates. In the absence of activating cofactors (Ca^{2+}, phospholipid, DAG), this pseudosubstrate sequence interacts with the substrate-binding pocket in the catalytic domain and represses PKC activity; binding of cofactors reduces the affinity of this interaction, induces a conformational change in the PKC, and allows stimulation of PKC activity. Consistent with the fact that the activator/cofactor, DAG, is anchored in the membranes, PKC activation is generally associated with translocation from the cytosol to the plasma or nuclear membranes. Although PKC is generally considered to be a serine kinase, it can phosphorylate threonine, but never tyrosine, residues. Interestingly, PKC can phosphorylate the same protein targets as PKA but, whereas PKC generally phosphorylates the protein at serine residues, PKA usually phosphorylates threonine residues.

Protein kinase C superfamily										
	Classic PKCs				**Novel PKCs**				**Atypical PKCs**	
PKC designation	α	β1	β2	γ	δ	ε/ε′	η	θ	μ	ι/λ	ζ
Molecular mass (kDA)	82	80	80	80	78	90	80	79	115	74	72
Activators											
[Ca²⁺]	yes	yes	yes	yes	no	no	no	no		no	no
DAG	yes	yes	yes	yes	yes	yes	yes	yes		no	no
Tissue distribution	all	some	many	neural	all	neural	many	muscle, skin		ovary, testis	all
DAG, diacylglycerol.											

Table 40.3 **The protein kinase C (PKC) superfamily.** This is a multigene family, except for β1, β2 and ε/ε′, which are alternatively spliced forms of β and ε.

Phospholipases

Phospholipases hydrolyze phosphatidylcholine or phosphatidylethanolamine generating lipid second messengers

In many hormone systems, although receptor-stimulated hydrolysis of PIP$_2$ is transient and rapidly switched off (desensitized), generation of DAG is sustained. Together with the recent emergence of the multiple isoforms of PKC, some of which do not require Ca^{2+} or DAG for activation (see Table 40.3), these findings led to the discovery of additional receptor-coupled lipid signaling pathways involving hydrolysis of phosphatidylcholine or phosphatidylethanolamine (Fig. 40.8), which can give rise to DAG and other biologically active lipids (Fig. 40.9) in response to a wide range of growth factors and mitogens. Phosphatidylcholine comprises about 40% of total cellular phospholipids. It can be hydrolyzed by distinct phospholipases, generating a diversity of lipid second messengers, including arachidonic acid (generated by PLA$_2$) as well as different species of DAG (generated by PLC) and phosphatidic acid (generated by PLD). Hormone-stimulated phosphatidylethanolamine-PLD activities have also been reported.

Some hormones or growth factors can stimulate only one or other of these phospholipases, but other ligands can stimulate all these pathways after binding to their specific receptors. There is therefore the potential to generate multiple distinct species of DAG and phosphatidic acid, reflecting different fatty acid side chains (Fig. 40.10) of the PIP$_2$ (predominantly stearate/arachidonate) and phosphatidylcholine, and phosphatidylethanolamine substrates. Moreover, DAG species can be further metabolized to produce arachidonic acid via DAG lipase or, alternatively, DAG can be converted to phosphatidic acid via DAG kinase. Likewise, phosphatidic acid can be interconverted to DAG by the action of phosphatidic acid phosphohydrolase.

There is growing evidence that all these distinct lipid second messengers have different targets. For example, it has recently been suggested that the saturated/monounsaturated fatty acid-containing DAGs derived from phosphatidylcholine-specific phospholipase D (PLD) activation are unable to activate PKC isoforms, and that it is only the stearoyl-arachidonyl-phosphatidic acid species that can modulate activity of the GTPase *Ras* (see Chapter 43). Generation of these diverse but related lipid second messengers therefore provides a mechanism for initiating or terminating

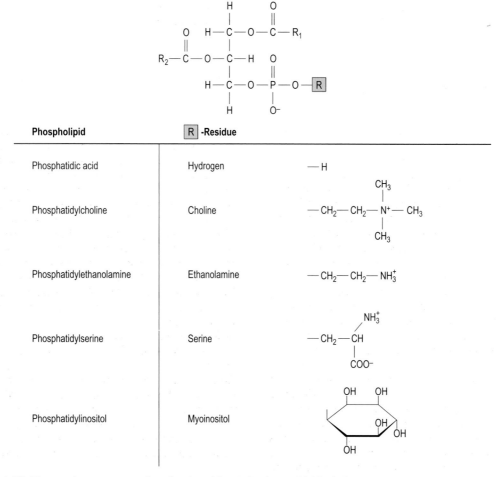

Fig. 40.8 **Potential lipid second messengers: phosphoglycerides.** R$_1$/R$_2$, fatty acid side chains.

hormone-specific responses via particular signal transducers, including differential activation of PKC isoforms.

Arachidonic acid

Arachidonic acid is a second messenger regulating phospholipases and protein kinases

Arachidonic acid is a C20 polyunsaturated fatty acid containing four double bonds (see Fig. 40.10). In addition to being implicated as a lipid second messenger involved in the regulation of signaling enzymes, such as PLC-γ, PLC-δ and PKC-α, -β and -γ isoforms, arachidonic acid is a key inflammatory intermediate. However, the arachidonic acid involved in these disparate functions appears to be generated by two distinct

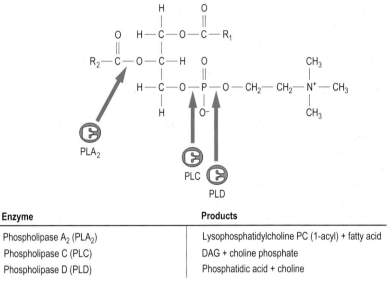

Enzyme	Products
Phospholipase A₂ (PLA₂)	Lysophosphatidylcholine PC (1-acyl) + fatty acid
Phospholipase C (PLC)	DAG + choline phosphate
Phospholipase D (PLD)	Phosphatidic acid + choline

Fig. 40.9 **Products of phosphatidylcholine breakdown.**

 ## PROTEIN KINASE C AND CANCER

Protein kinase C (PKC) was first identified as the intracellular receptor for phorbol esters, tumor-promoting chemicals used to induce skin cancer in experimental models. Since then it has become clear that PKC is the generic name for a family of serine/threonine-directed kinases involved in the regulation of normal cellular proliferation that, when dysregulated, have been implicated in promoting a range of pathologic conditions including cancer, cardiovascular disease and inflammation. The advent of transgenic and knockout mouse models has now identified distinct roles for individual PKC isoforms in all aspects (hyperproliferation, metastasis and angiogenesis) of tumorigenesis. For example, overexpression of PKCβII results in hyperproliferation of the colonic epithelium and increased susceptibility to carcinogen-induced colon cancer in mice. Consistent with this, the PKCβ-selective inhibitor enzastaurin blocks the proliferation of colon cancer cells. Interestingly, this inhibitor may have therapeutic potential in a range of other cancers as it can also inhibit the proliferation of breast cancer, glioma and T cell lymphoma cells and, indeed, is currently undergoing clinical trials in patients with advanced cancers. Similarly, overexpression of PKCα leads to hyperproliferation, tumor formation and metastasis of breast cancer cells whilst overexpression of PKCε promotes development of metastatic squamous cell carcinoma. By contrast, PKCδ generally appears to act to antagonize tumor formation as it can signal to suppress proliferation and induce apoptosis and consistent with this, overexpression of PKCδ renders mice resistant to phorbol ester-induced tumorigenesis. Signaling by various PKC isoforms is generally thought to promote metastasis by modulating both integrin-regulated adhesion and migration and also the secretion of matrix metalloproteinases required for basement membrane remodeling. Moreover, PKCs such as PKCβ are thought to transduce the VEGF and hypoxia-driven neovascularization and angiogenesis required for tumor growth and consistent with this, enzastaurin has also been shown to have antiangiogenic activity in various cancers. Fortunately, mutations in PKC isoforms resulting in human cancers are rare, although a single point mutation in PKCα (D294G) has been found in some metastatic pituitary tumors and thyroid follicular adenomas and carcinomas. Similarly, oncogenic chromosomal rearrangements involving PKC isoforms rarely occur but have been reported, for example, with respect to PKCε in thyroid cancer. Rather, expression levels are altered in many cancers and often, such changes effective in expression correlate with disease progression suggesting that they may be useful biomarkers of disease. The challenge now is to develop isoform-specific agonists and antagonists, several of which are already undergoing clinical trial, as therapies to effectively target tumors and other pathologic conditions without disrupting healthy cellular functions.

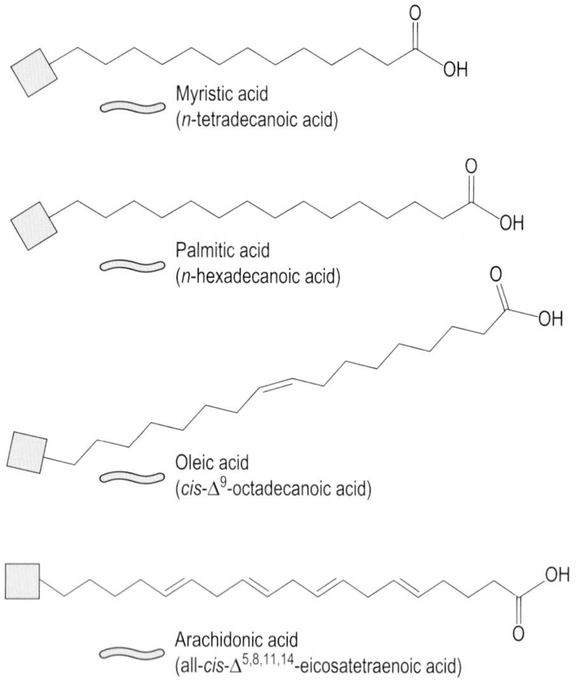

Myristic acid
(*n*-tetradecanoic acid)

Palmitic acid
(*n*-hexadecanoic acid)

Oleic acid
(*cis*-Δ^9-octadecanoic acid)

Arachidonic acid
(all-*cis*-$\Delta^{5,8,11,14}$-eicosatetraenoic acid)

Fig. 40.10 **Fatty acid side chains in phosphatidylinositol 4,5-bisphosphate (PIP$_2$) phosphatidylcholine, and phosphatidylethanolamine.**

PLA$_2$ routes. Arachidonic acid generated for signaling purposes appears to be derived by the action of a phosphatidylcholine-specific cytosolic phospholipase A$_2$ (cPLA$_2$), which has a molecular mass of 85 kDa and is regulated by phosphorylation of key serine residues. In contrast, inflammatory arachidonic acid is generated by the action of a family of low molecular-weight secretory PLA$_2$ (sPLA$_2$) proteins (14–18 kDa), which appear to be ubiquitous and are found in high concentrations in snake venom and pancreatic juices. In addition, arachidonic acid can be generated by DAG lipase.

Eicosanoids

Arachidonic acid is the precursor of eicosanoids, which encompass prostaglandins, prostacyclins, thromboxanes, and leukotrienes

As a key inflammatory mediator, arachidonic acid is the major precursor of the group of molecules termed eicosanoids, which encompass prostaglandins, prostacyclins, thromboxanes, and leukotrienes. Eicosanoids (Fig. 40.11) act like hormones and signal via G-protein coupled receptors. They have a wide variety of biologic activities, including

---

ANTI-INFLAMMATORY DRUGS TARGET PROSTAGLANDIN SYNTHESIS

Prostaglandins orchestrate myriad physiologic responses: they stimulate inflammation, regulate blood flow to organs such as the kidney, control ion transport across membranes, modulate synaptic transmission, and induce sleep. Prostaglandins are generally derived from the key inflammatory mediator, arachidonic acid, which in turn can be produced by PLA$_2$-mediated hydrolysis of various phospholipids such as phosphatidylcholine.

Nonsteroidal anti-inflammatory drugs (NSAIDs) such as aspirin and ibuprofen decrease inflammation, pain, and fever through inhibition of the synthesis of prostaglandins, by blocking the first stage whereby arachidonic acid is converted to the common prostaglandin precursor, PGG$_2$ by a cyclooxygenase enzyme. There are two forms of the enzyme. Cyclooxygenase 1 (COX-1) is mainly constitutive and found in platelets, stomach, and kidney. Cyclooxygenase 2 (COX-2) is mainly inducible and responsible for synthesis of inflammatory prostaglandins. Aspirin (acetylsalicylate) covalently modifies and irreversibly inactivates both forms of the enzyme by acetylation. Because abrogation of cyclooxygenase activity will also block production of the potent vasoconstrictor and aggregator of blood platelets, thromboxane A$_2$ (TXA$_2$, also derived from the common precursor, PGG$_2$), aspirin can also be used as a prophylactic agent, to prevent the excessive blood clotting that can lead to heart attacks and stroke. The Antiplatelet Trialists Collaboration metaanalysis of aspirin in secondary prevention showed that the reduction in risk of recurrent stroke was about 15%. The combination of aspirin with dipyridamole, which reduces platelet aggregation by increasing cAMP concentrations, may further reduce risk. Other effective antiplatelet drugs are the thienopyridines, ticlopidine and clopidogrel which block ADP-induced platelet aggregation. Selective inhibitors of COX-2 such as celecoxib are also effective treatments for inflammatory conditions such as rheumatoid arthritis and their effectiveness and tolerability are being compared with conventional NSAIDs. Moreover, the increasing evidence that COX-2 derived inflammatory mediators such as PGE$_2$ promote tumor growth and metastasis has focused interest on the use of NSAIDS as cancer therapeutics. Indeed, COX-2 expression has been shown to be elevated in colorectal cancer and the majority of adenomas and adenocarcinomas and consistent with this, population studies have shown that NSAID use is associated with reduced risk of developing colorectal cancer and familial adenomatous polyposis. This has led to clinical trials designed to assess the potential of COX-2 inhibitors, such as celecoxib, in preventing colorectal cancer either as a stand-alone drug or as a component of combination therapy. Corticosteroid hormones, such as cortisone, are also antiinflammatory drugs that target prostaglandin synthesis; in this case, however, such reagents do not affect cyclooxygenase but, rather, appear to inhibit activation of the PLA$_2$ activity that generates the key intermediate, arachidonic acid. Such drugs are therefore useful for treating inflammatory responses involving leukocyte recruitment or asthma, as targeting arachidonic acid production will, in addition to blocking synthesis of prostaglandin, also abrogate the production of leukotriene.

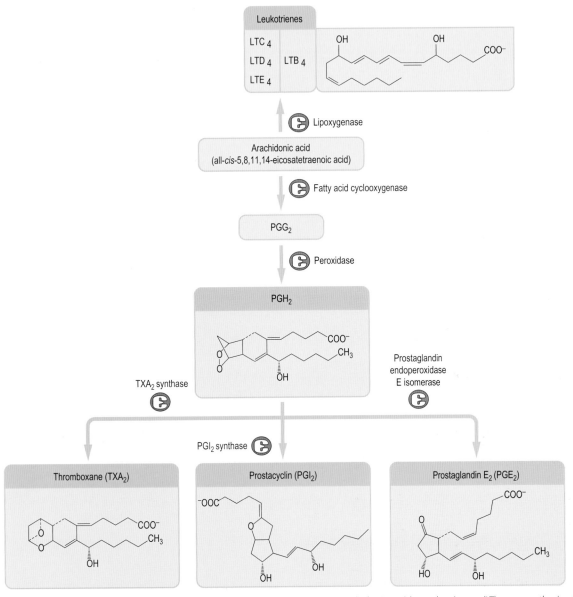

Fig. 40.11 **Synthesis of eicosanoids.** Eicosanoids are primarily derived from arachidonic acid. Leukotrienes (LT) are synthesized via a lipoxygenase-dependent pathway, whereas prostaglandins (PG), prostacyclins and thromboxanes (TX) arise from cyclooxygenase-dependent routes.

modulating smooth muscle contraction (vascular tone), platelet aggregation, gastric acid secretion, and salt and water balance, as well as mediating pain and inflammatory responses. Moreover, knockout mice defective in prostaglandin production have shown that prostaglandins have wider roles than was previously realized, being involved in the control of complex processes such as pregnancy, and tumor spread and metastasis in colon cancer (see Chapter 43).

Prostaglandins are synthesized in membranes from arachidonic acid

The first stage in the conversion of arachidonic acid to prostaglandins involves the cyclooxygenase component of prostaglandin synthase, which induces the formation of a cyclopentane ring and the introduction of four oxygen atoms to generate the intermediate, prostaglandin G_2 (PGG_2). PGG_2 is then subject to a hydroperoxidase reaction that catalyzes the two-electron reduction of the 15-hydroperoxy group to a 15-hydroxyl group and generates the highly unstable intermediate, PGH_2, which can then be converted into other prostaglandins, prostacylin and thromboxane.

Two distinct isoforms of cyclooxygenase, termed COX-1 and COX-2, have been identified. Whereas COX-1 is constitutively expressed, COX-2 is made only in response to inflammatory mediators such as cytokines. Cyclooxygenase inhibitors, the nonsteroidal antiinflammatory drugs (NSAIDs) such as aspirin and ibuprofen, act to reduce inflammation and provide pain relief by blocking this first step in the production of prostaglandins. Although the currently marketed drugs preferentially block COX-1, a number of COX-2 selective drugs are under development because it is believed that COX-2, being induced under conditions of inflammation, may have a more important role than COX-1 in mediating inflammatory responses. Moreover, the major side effects of blocking COX-1 are bleeding and the inflammation of gastric mucosa, and the use of inhibitors selective for COX-2 may make it possible to target inflammatory activity and thus avoid most of the sequelae associated with the use of COX-1 inhibitors (see box on p. 566).

McCUNE-ALBRIGHT SYNDROME (INCIDENCE 1 IN 25 000)

A 3-year-old girl was brought to hospital because her mother had been concerned about apparent breast development over the last 6 months, and a spot of blood on her pants last week. On examination, she had Tanner Stage 3 breast development. On her trunk she had three areas of brown skin pigmentation with ragged edges.

Comment. This child is suffering from McCune-Albright syndrome. She is likely to develop polyostotic fibrous dysplasia, with areas of thinning and sclerosis in her long bones which may fracture. Other endocrinopathies include thyrotoxicosis, GH hypersecretion, Cushing's syndrome (cortisol excess) and hyperparathyroidism. The cause is an activating missense mutation in the gene encoding the $G_{s\alpha}$ subunit of the G protein that stimulates cyclic AMP formation. The problem presents following a somatic cell mutation with clinical features dependent on a mosaic distribution of aberrant cells.

RADIO-IMMUNOASSAY (RIA) OF cAMP

The action of parathyroid hormone (PTH) on the renal tubule results in release of cAMP into the urine (see Chapter 25). The clinical assessment of cAMP levels is a useful indicator of parathyroid function; 90% of patients with hyperparathyroidism have increased levels of nephrogenous cAMP (urinary cAMP minus plasma cAMP filtered but not reabsorbed in the kidney). Furthermore, infusion of PTH causes a dramatic increase in urinary cAMP concentrations in patients with idiopathic hypoparathyroidism but not type I pseudohypoparathyroidism patients, who have a mutation in $G_{s\alpha}$ and thus exhibit a defective renal tubular response to PTH, resulting in reduced cAMP secretion.

cAMP levels can be analyzed by radio-immunoassay (RIA), which measures the competition for binding to an immobilized cAMP-specific antibody between ^{125}I-labeled cAMP assay reagent and unlabeled cAMP in the patient sample (Fig. 40.12). Quantitative measurement of cAMP levels can be performed using known concentrations of unlabeled cAMP assay reagent to construct a standard curve (see also Chapter 39; compare box on p. 532).

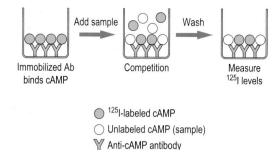

Fig. 40.12 **Measurement of cAMP by radioimmunoassay (RIA).** Unlabeled cAMP in the patient sample competes with ^{125}I-labeled cAMP assay reagent for binding to preimmobilized anti-cAMP antibody. After washing, ^{125}I levels are inversely proportional to cAMP levels in the patient sample. Quantitative analysis can be performed by constructing a standard curve. Compare the immunoradiometric sandwich assay for hormones (Fig. 39.2).

Leukotrienes

Arachidonic acid is also converted into other inflammatory and vasoactive mediators, called leukotrienes, by the action of a variety of structurally related lipoxygenases (see Fig. 40.11). For example, 5-lipoxygenase comprises both a dioxygenase activity that converts arachidonate to 5-hydroperoxyeicosatetraenoic acid (5-HPETE), and a dehydrase activity that transforms 5-HPETE to leukotriene A_4 (LTA_4). Natural deficiencies in lipoxygenases have been associated with human disease: for example, in one study, 40% of patients with myeloproliferative disorders were found to have reduced platelet lipoxygenase activity and increased synthesis of thromboxane. In addition, mice deficient in 5-lipoxygenase exhibit defects in the responses of their neutrophils to immune complexes and platelet-activating factor, supporting the idea that leukotrienes have important roles in inflammatory responses.

Summary

- Cells specifically respond to a multiplicity of signals from their environment via signal transduction cassettes, which comprise specific cell surface membrane receptors, effector signaling systems (e.g. adenylyl cyclase, phospholipases, or ion channels) and regulatory proteins (e.g. G-proteins or tyrosine kinases).

- These signal transduction cassettes serve to detect, amplify and integrate diverse external signals to generate the appropriate cellular response.

- The variety of families of cell surface receptors sense and transduce their specific hormone signal by transmembrane coupling to different effector systems to generate low molecular-weight molecules, termed second messengers, such as cAMP, IP_3, DAG, and Ca^{2+}, which mediate their signaling functions by activating key protein kinases.

- The specificity of a particular hormone response can be further heightened by the variety of available phospholipase-signaling activities (PLC, PLD and PLA$_2$). Taking into account their range of potential lipid substrates (e.g. PIP$_2$, phosphatidylcholine, and phosphatidylethanolamine) and products (e.g. DAG, phosphatidic acid and arachidonic acid), the phospholipases can generate a diverse array of lipid second messengers to influence differentially the activity of the key protein kinases. Because, for example, many of the members of the PKC family appear to have a distinct substrate repertoire of downstream signal transducers, differential activation of particular PKC isoforms can ultimately determine the specific type of biologic response obtained.

ACTIVE LEARNING

1. How are appropriate cellular responses triggered by specific hormones?
2. How do second messengers propagate intracellular signals?
3. How do NSAIDs such as aspirin and ibuprofen work?

Further reading

DeWire SM, Ahn S, Lefkowitz RJ, Shenoy SK. Beta-arrestins and cell signalling. *Ann Rev Physiol* 2007;**69**:483–510.
Lefkowitz RJ. Seven transmembrane receptors: something old, something new. *Acta Physiol (Oxf)* 2007;**190**: 9–19.
Putney JW. Recent breakthroughs in the molecular mechanism of capacitative calcium entry (with thoughts on how we got here). *Cell Calcium* 2007;**42**: 103–110.
Rozengurt E. Mitogenic signalling pathways induced by G-protein coupled receptors. *J Cell Physiol* 2007;**213**:589–602.
Scott JD. Compartmentalised cAMP signalling: a personal perspective. *Biochem Soc Trans* 2006;**34**:465–467.
Smith WL. Nutritionally essential fatty acids and biologically indispensable cyclooxygenases. *Trends Biochem Sci* 2008; **33**:27–37.

Websites

Science magazine's signal transduction knowledge environment: www.stke.org
Kimball's biology pages: www.biology-pages.info/C/CellSignaling
The Biology Project (University of Arizona): www.biology.arizona.edu/cell_bio/problem_sets/signaling
BioCarta's cell signaling pathways: www.biocarta.com/genes/CellSignaling.asp

41. Neurochemistry

E J Thompson

LEARNING OBJECTIVES

After reading this chapter you should be able to:
- Describe the cellular components of the central nervous system.
- Discuss the function of the blood–brain barrier in health and disease.
- Describe the basic principles of neuronal signaling and receptors.
- Describe adrenergic and cholinergic transmission.
- Describe the role of ion channels in nerve transmission.
- Comment on the role of sodium, potassium and calcium ions in nerve transmission.
- Discuss the process of vision as an example of a chemical process underlying neuronal function.

 GUILLAIN–BARRÉ SYNDROME

Three weeks after an acute diarrheal illness, a 65-year-old man presented with progressive ascending weakness of the limbs followed by respiratory muscle weakness requiring assisted ventilation. On examination, he was hypotonic and areflexic, with profound general weakness. Isoelectric focusing of CSF and parallel serum samples showed a similar abnormal pattern of oligoclonal bands in both.

Comment. This predominantly motor neuropathy is Guillain–Barré syndrome and the patient has antibodies developed as a result of infection with the bacterium *Campylobacter jejuni*. The organism contains the antigen ganglioside sugar GM1, which is shared with a ganglioside on peripheral nerves. Antibodies bind to peripheral motor nerves and cause the neuropathy. It is an example of molecular mimicry.

INTRODUCTION

The brain is, in many ways, a chemist's delight. This is so because it illustrates various general principles of biology applied to a highly specialized tissue that ultimately regulates all the other tissues of the body. This chapter highlights the differences between the central nervous system – that is, the brain and spinal cord – and the peripheral nervous system, which is outside the dura (the thick fibrous covering that contains the cerebrospinal fluid (CSF)).

BRAIN AND PERIPHERAL NERVE

The distinction between brain and peripheral nerve essentially reflects the division between the central nervous system (CNS) and the peripheral nervous system (PNS): a convenient dividing line being the confines of the dura, within which watertight compartment is the CSF, partially produced (about one-third of the total volume) through the action of the blood–brain barrier. Myelin insulates the axons of nerves; the chemical composition of CNS myelin is quite distinct from that of PNS myelin, not least because the two forms are produced by two different types of cells: the oligodendrocyte within the CNS and the Schwann cell within

the PNS. The distinction between the separate functions of the CNS and those of the PNS is fundamental to differential diagnosis in neurology, and many tests exist to discriminate between the two. A typical example is the difference between the demyelination of the CNS that occurs in multiple sclerosis, and the demyelination of the PNS that occurs in Guillain–Barré syndrome.

The blood–brain barrier

The term blood–brain 'barrier' is a slight misnomer, in that the barrier is not absolute but relative: its permeability depends on the size of the molecule in question

Initially, experiments based upon use of a dye (Evans' blue) bound to albumin showed that, over a period of hours, an animal progressively turned blue in all tissues, with the notable exception of the brain, which remained white. It subsequently became clear that 1 molecule in 200 of serum albumin passed normally into the CSF, which is analogous to lymph. It also became obvious that, for any given protein, the ratio of its concentrations in CSF and serum was a linear function of the molecular radius of the molecules in solution.

There are a total of six sources of the CSF which contain different 'barriers'. Under normal and pathologic conditions, proteins pass from these cellular or tissue sources into the CSF, and their degrees of filtration or rates of local synthesis, or both, vary.

The total quantity of the CSF therefore constitutes the algebraic summation of these six sources (Fig. 41.1):

- **the blood–brain barrier** (the parenchymal capillaries) gives rise to about one-third of the volume of CSF, and has been termed the interstitial fluid source
- **the blood–CSF barrier** provides the bulk of CSF (almost all of the remaining two-thirds), termed choroidal fluid, as it is principally provided by the choroid plexi (capillary tufts) situated in the lateral ventricles and, to a lesser degree, the plexi situated in the third and fourth ventricles
- **the dorsal root ganglia** contain capillaries that have a much greater degree of permeability. In the animal experiments with the Evans' blue referred to above, although the brain was otherwise white, the dorsal roots took up the blue color, reflecting their greater permeability to albumin
- **the brain parenchyma of the CNS** produces a number of brain-specific proteins. These include prostaglandin synthase (formerly called β-trace protein), which shows an 11-fold increase from the choroid plexus to the lumbar sac, and transthyretin (a protein formerly called pre-albumin which is produced locally by the choroid plexi), for which the reverse is found: it has a much greater relative concentration in ventricular than in lumbar CSF
- **CSF circulating cells**, mainly lymphocytes within the CNS, synthesize local antibodies; however, in the CNS there is strong presence of immune suppressor cells. Because of this, in brain infections such as meningitis,

steroids are given in addition to antibiotics, to suppress the potentially devastating effects, within this confined space, of inflammation associated with the intrathecal immune response
- **the meninges** represent a sixth source of CSF under pathologic conditions; they can give rise to dramatic increase in the concentrations of CSF proteins.

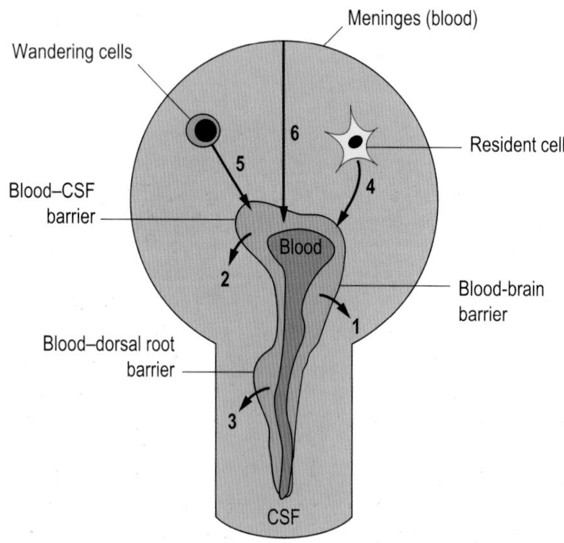

CELLS OF THE NERVOUS SYSTEM

Fewer than 10% of the cells of the nervous system are large neurones. The three major cell types in the nervous system (which each constitute about 30%) are:

- **astrocytes**, which also make up part of the blood–brain barrier
- **oligodendrocytes**, which are principally composed of fat and serve to insulate the axons
- **microglia**, which are essentially resident macrophages (scavengers).

These different cell types are associated with predominant protein molecules that are important in various brain pathologies (Table 41.1). Other minor constituents of the nervous system include the ependymal cells, which are ciliated cells secreting brain-specific proteins such as prostaglandin synthase. The brain endothelial cells also merit special comment because, unlike other tissue capillaries, these contiguous cells have tight junctions that bind them together; this feature is believed also to contribute to the blood–brain barrier,

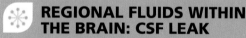

REGIONAL FLUIDS WITHIN THE BRAIN: CSF LEAK

It is essential, on clinical grounds, to distinguish CSF rhinorrhea from local nasal secretions caused by, say, influenza infection. The ENT surgeon must know whether the fluid present is CSF, as any leak must be surgically repaired lest it remain a chronic potential source of meningitis as a result of the migration of nasal flora into the subarachnoid space. One characteristic and useful marker protein in the CSF is asialotransferrin, which is transferrin lacking sialic acid. In the systemic circulation, this absence of sialic acid gives a molecular signal for the protein to be recycled, and it is thus immediately removed from the systemic circulation by all reticuloendothelial cells. The brain has no true reticuloendothelial cells along the path of CSF flow, and hence asialotransferrin is present in quite high concentrations. The aqueous humor of the anterior chamber of the eye also produces the characteristic asialotransferrin, and the same asialotransferrin can also be found in the perilymph of the semicircular canals.

Fig. 41.1 **The six main sources of cerebrospinal fluid (CSF).** The involved processes comprise passage across barriers (from the blood, i.e. 1, 2, 3) and direct sources of local production (CNS cells, i.e. 4, 5, 6).

although it is the basement membrane which is the major source of molecular sieving of the different-sized proteins.

Neurones

The significant features of neurones are their length, their many interconnections, and the fact that they do not divide postpartum

There is an archetypal notion of the electrical activity of the nervous system – in particular, of the electrical activity of neurones. However, three other biologic features of neurones are particularly worthy of note: their length, their prolific interconnections, and the fact that they do not divide postpartum. Further to the last of these features, many embryonic neurones are destined to die (through apoptosis), as

CNS cells and markers for brain pathology

Cell	Protein	Pathology
neurone	neurone-specific enolase	brain death
astrocyte	GFAP	plaque (or scar)
oligodendrocyte	myelin basic protein	de/remyelination
microglia	ferritin	stroke
choroid plexi	asialotransferrin	CSF leak (rhinorrhea)

GFAP, glial fibrillary acidic protein.

Table 41.1 **The different cells of the CNS, and their protein markers indicating brain pathologies.**

✳ IRON IN THE CNS

During normal maturation of the oligodendrocytes that form the myelin sheath, iron appears to be important, as there are increased local concentrations of this cation and of the transferrin protein that is required to bind it (including the asialo form). An apparent discrepancy between the amounts of iron and those of transferrin is readily explained by the local synthesis of the latter, particularly of the asialo form; large amounts of mRNA are found in oligodendrocytes and in the choroid plexus.

There is also local synthesis of ferritin by the normal CNS. Free iron can have a particularly toxic effect on the CNS and, by binding to it, ferritin provides a store for it. This is clearly evident in the event of cerebrovascular accidents, after which there is a further dramatic increase in the local synthesis of ferritin, to bind the iron that has been released by the destruction of red cells (compare Fig. 22.8).

they have no postembryonic target organ. The existence of cervical and lumbar swellings of the spinal cord, reflecting segmental neurones for which, respectively, the target organs were the hands and feet, is evidence for reduced diameter of the cord due to neuronal death. The capacity for memory and learning similarly indicates the importance of the plasticity of the synaptic system afforded by the extensive interconnections of and between neurones.

Because of their great length, neurones depend upon an efficient system of axonal transport

Neurones can typically be 1 m long; thus the nucleus, the source of information for the synthesis of neurotransmitters, is typically quite remote from the synaptic terminal, the site of release of those transmitters. Because of this extensive length, a crucial requirement is the neurone's ability to transport material both from the nucleus towards the synapse (anterograde transport) and from the synapse to the nucleus (retrograde transport). Neurones have evolved special characteristics to deal with this separation of their two functional sites, and to maintain electrical activity at the nodes of Ranvier (the remainder of the axon is electrically quiet during the saltatory process of electrical conduction) (Fig. 41.2).

The normal 'resting' movement within the axon is mediated by separate molecular 'motors' (motile proteins): kinesin in the case of anterograde transport and dynein in retrograde transport. The materials being transported in each direction are also rather different, and the different components of axonal structure shown in Figure 41.2 possess the capacity for different speeds of transportation (Table 41.2). During growth, a separate form of transport (toward the synapse) occurs that takes place at the rate of about 1 mm/day; this flow constitutes bulk movement of the building blocks such as the filamentous proteins.

✳ CIRCULATING CELLS IN THE CSF: 'REGIONAL' IMMUNOLOGY

As mentioned in the text, the brain is essentially an immunologically 'quiet' place. There is an almost 10-fold difference between the ratio of helper cells (CD4) to suppressor cells (CD8) in the CSF, where the ratio is 3:6, and that in the brain parenchyma, where the ratio is 0:4, reflecting a preponderance of suppressor cells within the CNS (see also Chapter 38). Approximately one-third of CNS cells are resident macrophages; within the CSF, two-thirds of the cells are lymphocytes and the remaining one-third are macrophages. There are very few lymphatic vessels within the brain itself, and CSF itself can be thought of as being analogous to lymph.

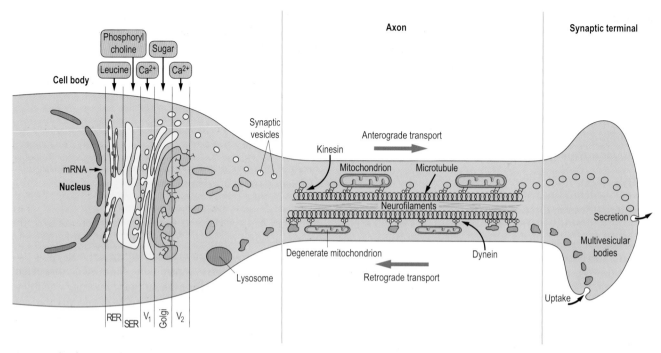

Fig. 41.2 **The functional structure of a neurone.** Within the cell body, there is specialized movement through the Golgi stack by the components required to form synaptic vesicles (V_1, V_2). In the axon, there is fast axonal transport along microtubules via the motile proteins, kinesin (in anterograde transport) or dynein (in retrograde transport). RER, rough endoplasmic reticulum; SER, smooth endoplasmic reticulum.

Differing speeds of axonal transport		
Component	**Rate (mm/day)**	**Structure and composition of transported substances**
Fast transport		
anterograde	200–400	small vesicles, neurotransmitters, membrane proteins, lipids
mitochondria	50–100	mitochondria
retrograde	200–300	lysosomal vesicles, enzymes
Slow transport		
slow component a	2–8	microfilaments, metabolic enzymes, clathrin complex
slow component b	0.2–1	neurofilaments, microtubules

Table 41.2 **Differing speeds of axonal transport.**

Neuroglial structures

Essentially, the astrocytes and the oligodendrocytes comprise the neuroglial structures

In the cortex, or gray matter, one typically finds a protoplasmic astrocyte with one set of processes surrounding the endothelial cells, thereby helping to 'filter' materials from the blood, and a separate set of processes surrounding the neurones, which are thereby being 'fed' selected substances that have been extracted from the blood for passage to the neurones. In the white matter, the astrocytes have a rather more fibrous appearance and have more of a structural role. Under pathologic conditions in which there is injury to the CNS, astrocytes can play a major part in the reaction, synthesizing large amounts of the glial fibrillary acid protein (GFAP). This is the cellular equivalent of scar tissue and is found in diseases such as multiple sclerosis, in which it is the major constituent of the characteristic plaques. Astrocytes are not found in the PNS.

The oligodendrocytes of the CNS can wrap round as many as 20 axons, forming the myelin sheath that insulates these neuronal processes from one another and stops cross-talk between neurones. There is also intense oligodendrocyte mitochondrial activity at the nodes of Ranvier, which are parallel to the sites of depolarization within the underlying axon. In the PNS, the Schwann cells form the myelin and, typically, wrap round only a single axon. As noted previously, the chemical constituents of the myelin sheath are different when produced by Schwann cells rather than by oligodendrocytes.

SYNAPTIC TRANSMISSION

One of the unique chemical characteristics of the brain is the massively high density of synapses between different neurones, at which a locally acting neurohormone is released by one axon onto many other cell bodies. On the receiving end, a given cell body will typically receive myriad cellular products via its profusely branched dendritic tree: each branch can be smothered in synapses. The first chemical messenger or 'neurotransmitter' to traverse the synaptic cleft is the neurohormone, which is released by the axon of the first cell onto the dendrite of the second cell. This action is mediated by a neurotransmitter receptor on the respondent cell. There is usually a second messenger such as a cyclic nucleotide, which may also lead to a third messenger such as a phosphorylated protein. Typically, G-proteins are found just under the neurotransmitter receptor protein spanning the cell membrane, where they act to 'couple' the first messenger (e.g. norepinephrine) to a second messenger (e.g. cyclic AMP, cAMP) (see also Chapter 40).

Neurotransmitters are normally inactivated after their postsynaptic actions on the target cell, hydrolysis being a major mechanism by which this is achieved. The best studied example is that of the enzyme acetylcholinesterase. There can also be blockade at the level of the second messenger, such as cAMP, which is broken down by the enzyme phosphodiesterase. This enzyme is inhibited by methylxanthines and caffeine, and thereby mimics many of the effects of adrenergic neurotransmission.

Synaptic transmission involves the recycling of membrane components

In addition to release of a specific neurohormone, there is also an extensive system for recycling of membrane constituents associated with this process. The synaptic vesicles contain a very high concentration of the relevant neurotransmitter, which is bounded by a membrane (see Chapter 42). During synaptic release of the transmitter, there is fusion of the synaptic vesicle membrane (containing the neurotransmitter) with the presynaptic membrane. This increase in total membrane mass is redressed by invagination of the lateral aspects of the nerve terminals, where an inward puckering movement of the membrane is effected by contractile movements of the protein clathrin. There then follows a form of pinocytosis of the excess membrane, which is transported in retrograde fashion toward the nucleus, to be digested in lysosomes.

Types of synapse

Because of the multitude of different synaptic inputs to a given neurone, the final algebraic summation results in a 'decision' at the level of the axon hillock (the site of origin of the axon from the cell body) as to whether or not to transmit an action potential down the axon as an all-or-nothing phenomenon. However, even before this decision is made, the input of a particular neurotransmitter can essentially be classified as excitatory or inhibitory.

In addition to the relatively short-term decisions concerning action potentials (Chapter 42), there is a longer-term modulation of the resting membrane potential, moving it either closer to (excitation) or further from (inhibition) the critical membrane potential, which is the level at which the resting membrane potential will finally trigger an action potential at the axon hillock. Many drugs have a longer-term effect on modulation, in addition to the short-term effect, which partially explains their addictive effect; this can be seen with alcohol or the opioid drugs. There are also long-term effects during treatment with various drugs, for example those used to treat endogenous depression, such that it may be weeks before any beneficial effects are seen.

Cholinergic transmission

Acetylcholine (ACh) is the neurotransmitter that has been best studied. As a model system, this transmitter can have two rather different effects, depending upon its site of origin

A WOMAN WITH AMYLOIDOSIS

A 75-year-old woman complained of postural dizziness, dry mouth, intermittent diarrhea, and numbness in both her feet. On examination, there was a marked decrease in blood pressure on assuming the upright posture. A chest radiogram revealed lytic lesions in the sternum. Her urine contained Bence-Jones protein. A bone marrow examination demonstrated increased numbers of plasma cells (see also Chapter 4).

Comment. Her neurologic condition was caused by amyloidosis in which the free light-chain component of myeloma globulin produced by tumor of plasma cells in the bone marrow accumulates in peripheral nerves. The light chains adopt the configuration of a β-pleated sheet, with multiple copies that are intercalated and resistant to normal proteolysis.

MULTIPLE SCLEROSIS

It is essential to make a diagnosis of a disease which relapses and remits since the patient may show no abnormalities at the time of physical examination by the clinician. Lumbar puncture therefore plays a major role with the demonstration of oligoclonal bands in CSF which are absent from the parallel serum specimen. This means that there is an intrathecal rather than a systemic immune response. The converse is seen in, e.g. neurosarcoidosis, in which the systemically synthesized immunoglobulins are transferred passively into the spinal fluid, giving rise to a so-called 'mirror' pattern, where the oligoclonal bands are the same in both CSF and serum. The test involves isoelectric focusing of CSF with a parallel serum sample. The separated immunoglobulins are exposed to anti-IgG to identify bands which are present in CSF but absent from the corresponding serum. Such patterns indicate local synthesis of IgG within the brain.

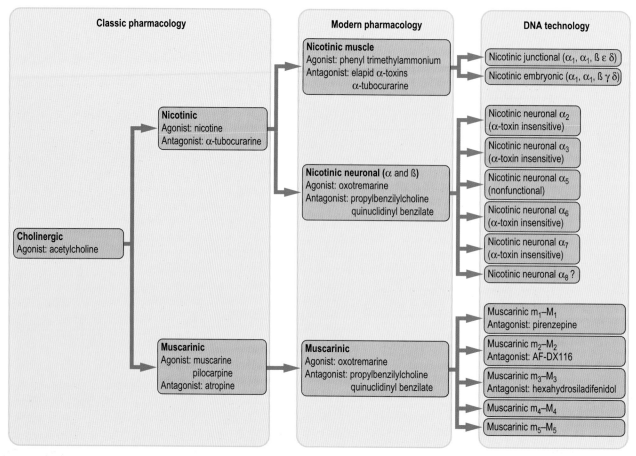

Fig. 41.3 **The history of naming: acetylcholine agonists and antagonist.** The changes in nomenclature, from early to modern terms, for the agonists and antagonists of the different central (neuronal) versus peripheral (muscle) regional actions of acetylcholine (ACh).

within the nervous system (i.e. central or peripheral): those effects originally demonstrated by experiments with nicotine are characteristic of the nicotinic receptor, whereas those demonstrated with muscarine characterize the muscarinic receptor. Modern developments in pharmacology and DNA technology have produced a complex picture of the agonists and antagonists associated with the regional actions of ACh (Fig. 41.3). The classic antagonist of the muscarinic effect is atropine and the best-studied blocker for the nicotinic receptor is the poisonous snake venom, α-bungarotoxin.

In myasthenia gravis, autoantibodies are formed against the nicotinic receptor for ACh. However, by blocking the hydrolysis of ACh, for example by means of the drug edrophonium (which inhibits the hydrolytic enzyme acetylcholinesterase), the concentration of ACh can be effectively increased (see Chapter 42).

Adrenergic transmission

After ACh, epinephrine and norepinephrine are the neurotransmitters that have received most study. Again, they have two separate receptors:

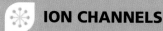

ION CHANNELS

Defects of sodium channels

Different molecular lesions at various sites of the sodium channel pores can give rise to hyperkalemic periodic paralysis. As this name suggests, the patient has intermittent muscle weakness, during which time the serum potassium concentration is increased. This is caused by an imbalance of cationic movements in which sodium enters the cell and potassium leaves it. For these patients, the abnormal flux of sodium into the muscle is not correctly regulated with its counterflux of potassium ions (see also Chapter 8).

- α-**adrenergic receptor**, blocked by phentolamine
- β-**adrenergic receptor**, blocked by propranolol.

The latter drug used to be commonly used by cardiologists (many other β-blockers are the mainstay of treatment in coronary heart disease), but neurologists also use it as part of the treatment of Parkinson's disease. This disease results from a deficiency of dopamine, the precursor of epinephrine and norepinephrine. Many adrenergic effects are promoted

CHANNELOPATHIES: AN 18-YEAR-OLD WITH MUSCLE WEAKNESS

An 18-year-old male awoke in the night with intense weakness of the proximal muscles of his arms and legs. Before retiring he had consumed a meal of pasta and cake. His brother and father had previously been similarly affected. He was taken to the emergency room of the local hospital where the weak limbs were noted to be hypotonic with depressed tendon reflexes. Serum concentration of potassium was mildly reduced at 2.9 mmol/L (normal 3.5–5.5). By the next day he had fully recovered and serum potassium had risen spontaneously to normal levels. A further attack of paralysis was induced by an infusion of intravenous glucose, thus confirming a diagnosis of familial periodic paralysis.

Comment. Hypokalemic periodic paralysis is inherited as a mendelian dominant and results from a mutation in the gene encoding the L-type calcium channel. Genetic diseases that affect ion channel function are called channelopathies (see also Chapter 8).

 BOTULISM: A WOMAN WITH BLURRED VISION AND DYSPHAGIA

Twenty-four hours after eating home-preserved vegetables, a healthy young woman experienced progressive onset of blurred vision, severe vomiting, dysphagia, and advancing limb weakness starting in the shoulders. Her doctor admitted her to hospital, and electrophysiologic studies confirmed the clinical diagnosis of botulism. Trivalent antiserum, made from inactivated toxin, was administered immediately and, with the help of assisted ventilation, the patient recovered within a few weeks.

Comment. The vegetables contained the exotoxin of the anerobe, *Clostridium botulinum*, which had not been destroyed during the preservation process. The toxin hydrolyzes the presynaptic proteins involved in the release of neurotransmitter, and thus the blockade is similar to the functional lesion in Lambert-Eaton myasthenic syndrome; however, in botulism the blockade can be lethal, especially at the level of the phrenic nerve which is essential for appropriate respiratory lung movement.

by cAMP, but other neurotransmitters have either excitatory or inhibitory effects (see Chapter 42).

Ion channels

Even at rest, the neurone is working to pump ions along ionic gradients

The 'resting' neurone is, nevertheless, continually pumping sodium out of the cell and potassium in, through ion channels. During an action potential, there is a momentary reversal of these ionic movements, such that sodium enters the cell and potassium then leaves, effectively repolarizing the resting membrane (Chapter 8). Mutations of sodium channels can occur at different sites and give rise to hyperkalemic periodic paralysis. The negative ion, chloride, moves through separate channels, which are implicated in specific pathologic states such as myotonia.

Calcium ions have an important role in the synchronization of neuronal activity

The movement of calcium ions within cells often provides a 'trigger' for the cells to synchronize an activity such as synaptic release of neurotransmitter; this synchronization of movement is also seen to have a prominent role in the sarcoplasmic reticulum of muscle (see Chapter 20). Within the central nervous system, the Lambert-Eaton syndrome is a disease that affects predominantly the P/Q subtype of calcium channels, in an example of molecular mimicry. The patient may have a primary oat cell carcinoma of the lung; the immune system responds by making antibodies against these malignant cells. However, the malignancy and the calcium channels possess a common epitope, the effect of which is that the immune response causes the release of neurotransmitter to be blocked at the presynaptic site. This is analogous to, but nevertheless can be clearly distinguished from, the condition in myasthenia gravis, in which the block is postsynaptic.

It is also worth noting that blockade of the presynaptic release of neurotransmitter may be usefully exploited by therapeutic application of botulinus toxin (a protein derived from anerobic bacteria), which contains enzymes to hydrolyze the presynaptic proteins involved in release of neurotransmitters. This toxin is used in special cases of spasticity such astorticollis, in which the patient can be relieved of the excessive contractures of the neck muscles, which turn the head chronically to one side and thus cause pain and distraction if untreated.

THE MECHANISM OF VISION

The mechanism by which the human eye can detect a single photon of light provides a marvelous example of the chemical processes underlying neuronal function. It involves both trapping of photons and the transducer effect, whereby the energy of light is converted into a chemical form, which is then ultimately transmuted into an action potential by a retinal ganglion neurone. A number of the intermediates are as yet not precisely known, but the underlying hypothesis is that the receptor protein, rhodopsin, is coupled to the G-protein. There are several sequence homologies of rhodopsin with the adrenergic β-receptor and with the muscarinic ACh receptor. The main steps take place in the following order (Fig. 41.4).

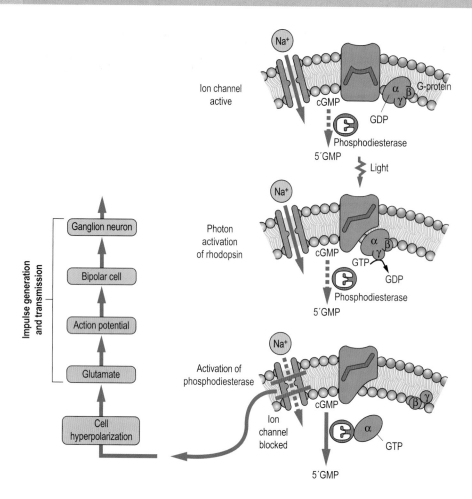

Fig. 41.4 **Neurochemistry of synaptic transmission in the mechanism of vision.** The figure shows the consequences of photon activation of rhodopsin via G-protein coupling in a rod cell. Phosphodiesterase is activated and hydrolyzes the second messenger, cGMP, thereby blocking the entry of sodium and causing hyperpolarization of the cell. Currently, the steps through which neurotransmission subsequently proceeds to produce the final ganglion neurone action potential are not known in detail. Compare G-protein coupled receptor (Fig. 40.2).

- *Cis*-retinal is converted to *trans*-retinal.
- Rhodopsin becomes activated.
- The level of cGMP decreases.
- Na^+ entry is blocked.
- The rod cell hyperpolarizes.
- There is release of glutamate (or aspartate).
- An action potential depolarizes the adjacent bipolar cell.
- This depolarizes the associated ganglion neurone, to send an action potential out of the eye.

Summary

- The nervous system contains a number of distinct cells, each of which synthesizes its own individual proteins.
- The specialized functions of the nervous system mean that these proteins are effectively compartmentalized in different loci.
- In order to facilitate communication within the brain, there are two specialized methods of moving cells, organelles and proteins: the cerebrospinal fluid and axonal transport.
- The blood–brain barrier is diverse in anatomic origin and is not absolute but relative (specifically based on molecular size).
- The synthesis of antibodies within the CSF, but not parallely in serum, is unequivocal evidence for the brain as the source of antigenic stimulation.

ACTIVE LEARNING

1. G-proteins are widely used throughout the body as 'coupling' agents between the first extracellular messenger and the second intracellular messenger. Discuss some of the different roles for which the G-protein has been adapted amongst various cell types.
2. Mitochondria play an important role in providing for the metabolic requirements of electrical activity at the nodes of Ranvier along the considerable length of the axon. Discuss the role of the two molecular motors in recycling the mitochondria required to support this function.
3. Chloride is an important anion which forms part of the complex movements with other cations such as sodium and potassium during depolarization. Discuss how congenital abnormalities in this anion transporter can give rise to abnormal activities dependent upon action potentials.
4. Discuss how the brain can produce a 'gradient' for different proteins along the rostrocaudal axis.
5. Describe the reactions in vision which illustrate how light is converted into changes in ion flux.
6. Give an example of molecular mimicry.

Further reading

Barry DM, Millecamps S, Julien JP, Garcia ML. New movements in neurofilament transport, turnover and disease. *Exp Cell Res* 2007;**313**:2110–2120.

Bos JL, Rehmann H, Wittinghofer A. GEFs and GAPs: critical elements in the control of small G proteins. *Cell* 2007;**129**:865–877.

Cannon SC. Physiologic principles underlying ion channelopathies. *Neurotherapeutics* 2007;**4**:174–183.

de Leon MJ, Mosconi L, Blennow K et al. Imaging and CSF studies in the preclinical diagnosis of Alzheimer's disease. *Ann N Y Acad Sci* 2007;**1097**:114–145.

Stein-Streilein J, Taylor AW. An eye's view of T regulatory cells. *J Leukoc Biol* 2007:**81**:593–598.

42. Neurotransmitters

S Heales

LEARNING OBJECTIVES

After reading this chapter you should be able to:

- Outline the criteria that need to be met before a molecule can be classified as a neurotransmitter.
- Identify the major neurotransmitter types and be aware that some molecules have neurotransmitter properties but cannot in the strictest sense be classified as neurotransmitters.
- Explain the generation of action potentials, appreciate how neurotransmitters can be excitatory or inhibitory and summarize the process whereby a neurotransmitter is released from the presynaptic cell.
- Describe the different neurotransmitter receptors and their general mode of action.
- Describe the major biochemical pathways for neurotransmitter synthesis and degradation.
- Identify some clinical disorders that can arise as a result of disruption of neurotransmitter metabolism.

INTRODUCTION

Neurotransmitters are molecules that act as chemical signals between nerve cells

Nerve cells communicate with each other and with target tissues by secreting chemical messengers, called neurotransmitters. This chapter describes the various classes of neurotransmitters and how they interact with their target cells. It will discuss their effects on the body, how alterations in their signaling may cause disease, and how pharmacologic manipulation of their concentrations may be used therapeutically.

DEFINITION OF A NEUROTRANSMITTER

Traditionally, for a molecule to be labeled as a neurotransmitter, a number of criteria have to be met.

- Synthesis of the molecule must occur within the neurone, i.e. all biosynthetic enzymes, substrates, cofactors, etc. are present for de novo synthesis.
- Storage of the molecule occurs within the nerve ending prior to release, e.g. in synaptic vesicles.
- Release of the molecule from the presynaptic ending occurs in response to an appropriate stimulus such as action potential.
- There is binding and recognition of the putative neurotransmitter molecule on the postsynaptic target cell.
- Mechanisms exist for the inactivation and termination of the biologic activity of the neurotransmitter.

Rigorous adherence to the above criteria means that some molecules that are involved in the cross-talk between neurones are not in the strict sense classified as neurotransmitters. Thus, nitric oxide (NO), adenosine, neurosteroids, polyamines, etc. are often termed neuromodulators rather than neurotransmitters.

CLASSIFICATION OF NEUROTRANSMITTERS

A classification of neurotransmitters based on chemical composition is shown in Table 42.1. Many are derived from simple compounds, such as amino acids (Table 42.2), but peptides are also now known to be extremely important. The principal transmitters in the peripheral nervous system are norepinephrine and acetylcholine (ACh) (Fig. 42.1; compare Fig. 41.3).

Several transmitters may be found in one nerve

An early dogma of nerve function held that one nerve contained one transmitter. However, this is now known to be an oversimplification and combinations of transmitters are the rule. The pattern of cellular transmitters may characterize a particular functional role, but details of this also remain unclear. A major low molecular-weight transmitter such as an amine is often present, along with several peptides, an amino acid, and a purine. Sometimes, there may even be more than one possible transmitter in a particular vesicle, as is believed to be the case for adenosine triphosphate (ATP) and norepinephrine in sympathetic nerves. In some cases, the intensity of stimulation may control which transmitter is released, peptides often requiring greater levels of stimulus. Furthermore, different transmitters may have a different timescale of action. Sympathetic nerves are good examples of nerves for which this is the case: it is believed that ATP causes their rapid excitation, whereas norepinephrine and

Classification of neurotransmitters

Group	Examples
amines	acetylcholine (Ach), norepinephrine, epinephrine, dopamine, 5-HT
amino acids	glutamate, GABA
purines	ATP, adenosine
gases	nitric oxide
peptides	endorphins, tachykinins, many others

5-HT, 5-hydroxytryptamine; GABA, γ-amino butyric acid.

Table 42.1 **Classification of neurotransmitters**. Neurotransmitters can be classified in several ways. The scheme shown relies on chemical similarities. All except the peptides are synthesized at the nerve ending and packaged into vesicles there; peptides are synthesized in the cell body and transported down the axon.

Neurotransmitters of low molecular weight

Compound	Source	Site of production
Amino acids		
glutamate		central nervous system (CNS)
aspartate		CNS
glycine		spinal cord
Amino acid derivatives		
GABA	glutamate	CNS
histamine	histidine	hypothalamus
norepinephrine	tyrosine	sympathetic nerves, CNS
epinephrine	tyrosine	adrenal medulla, a few CNS nerves
dopamine	tyrosine	CNS
5-HT	tryptophan	CNS, enterochromaffin gut cells, enteric nerves
Purines		
ATP		sensory, enteric, sympathetic nerves
adenosine	ATP	CNS, peripheral nerves
Gas		
nitric oxide	arginine	genitourinary tract, CNS
Miscellaneous		
ACh	choline	parasympathetic nerves, CNS

Table 42.2 **Neurotransmitters of low molecular weight**. Many neurotransmitters are of low molecular weight and are simple compounds, often derived from common amino acids.

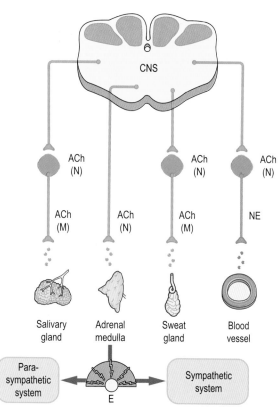

Fig. 42.1 **Transmitters in the autonomic nervous system.** Catecholamines and acetylcholine are transmitters in the sympathetic and parasympathetic nervous systems. Preganglionic nerves all release ACh, which binds to nicotinic (N) receptors. Most postganglionic sympathetic nerves release norepinephrine (NE), whereas postganglionic parasympathetic nerves release ACh, which acts at muscarinic (M) receptors. Motor neurones release ACh, which acts at distinct nicotinic receptors. E, epinephrine (see also Fig. 41.3).

the neuromodulator neuropeptide Y (NPY) cause a slower phase of action. In some tissues, NPY on its own may be able to produce a very slow excitation.

NEUROTRANSMISSION

Action potentials are caused by changes in ion flows across cell membranes

The signal carried by a nerve cell reflects an abrupt change in the voltage potential difference across the cell membrane. The normal resting potential difference is a few millivolts, with the inside of the cell being negative, and is caused by an imbalance of ions across the plasma membrane: the concentration of K^+ ion is much greater inside cells than outside, whereas the opposite is true for Na^+ ion. This difference is maintained by the action of the Na^+/K^+-ATPase (see Chapters 23 and 41). Only those ions to which the membrane is permeable can affect the potential, as they can come to an electrochemical steady state under the combined influence of concentration

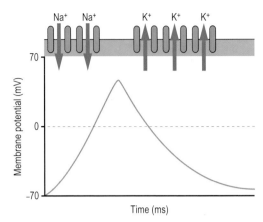

Fig. 42.2 **Generation of action potential.** Action potential is formed as follows. At the start of an action potential, the membrane is at its resting potential of about −70 mV; this is maintained by voltage-independent K⁺ channels. When an impulse is initiated by a signal from a neurotransmitter, voltage-dependent Na⁺ channels open. These allow inflow of Na⁺ ions, which alter the membrane potential to positive values. The Na⁺ channels then close and K⁺ channels, called delayed rectifier channels, open to restore the initial balance of ions and the negative membrane potential.

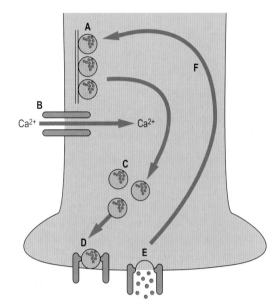

Fig. 42.3 **Release of neurotransmitters.** Neurotransmitters are released from vesicles at the synaptic membrane. (A) In the resting state, vesicles are attached to microtubules. (B) When an action potential is received, calcium channels open. (C) Vesicles move to the plasma membrane, and (D) bind to a complex of docking proteins. (E) Neurotransmitter is released, and (F) vesicles are recycled.

and voltage differences. Because the membrane in all resting cells is comparatively permeable to K⁺ as a result of the presence of voltage-independent (leakage) K⁺ channels, this ion largely controls the resting potential.

A change in voltage which tends to drive the resting potential towards zero from the normal negative voltage is known as a depolarization, whereas a process that increases the negative potential is called hyperpolarization

So far, this picture is common to all cells. However, nerve cells contain voltage-dependent sodium channels that open very rapidly when a depolarizing change in voltage is applied. When they open, they allow the inward passage of huge numbers of Na⁺ ions from the extracellular fluid (Fig. 42.2), which swamps the resting voltage and drives the membrane potential to positive values. This reversal of voltage is the action potential. Almost immediately afterwards, the sodium channels close and so-called delayed potassium channels open. These restore the normal resting balance of ions across the membrane and, after a short refractory period, the cell can conduct another action potential. Meanwhile, the action potential has spread by electrical conductance to the next segment of nerve membrane, and the entire cycle starts again.

Neurotransmitters alter the activity of various ion channels to cause changes in the membrane potential

Excitatory neurotransmitters cause a depolarizing change in voltage, in which case an action potential is more likely to occur. In contrast, inhibitory transmitters hyperpolarize the membrane and an action potential is then less likely to occur.

Neurotransmitters act at synapses

Neurotransmitters are released into the space between cells at a specialized area known as a synapse (Fig. 42.3). In the simplest case, they diffuse from the presynaptic membrane across the synaptic space or cleft, and bind to receptors at the postsynaptic membrane. However, many neurones, particularly those containing amines, have several varicosities along the axon, containing transmitter. These varicosities may not be close to any neighboring cell, so transmitter released from them has the possibility of affecting many neurones. Nerves innervating smooth muscle are commonly of this kind.

When the action potential arrives at the end of the axon, the change in voltage opens calcium channels. Calcium entry is essential for mobilization of vesicles containing transmitter, and for their eventual fusion with the synaptic membrane and release through it.

Because transmitters are released from vesicles, impulses arrive at the postsynaptic cell in individual packets, or quanta. At the neuromuscular junction between nerves and skeletal muscle cells, a large number of vesicles are discharged at a time, and a single impulse may therefore be enough to stimulate contraction of the muscle cell. The number of vesicles released at synapses between neurones, however, is much smaller; consequently, the recipient cell will be stimulated only if the total algebraic sum of the various positive and negative stimuli exceeds its threshold. As each cell in the brain receives input from a huge number of neurones, this implies that there is a far greater capability for the fine control of responses in the central nervous system (CNS) than there is at the neuromuscular junction.

Receptors

Neurotransmitters act by binding to specific receptors and opening or closing ion channels

There are several mechanisms by which receptors for excitatory neurotransmitters can cause the propagation of an action potential in a postsynaptic neurone. Directly or indirectly, they cause changes in ion flow across the membrane, until the potential reaches the critical point, or threshold, for initiation of an action potential. Receptors that directly control the opening of an ion channel are called ionotropic, whereas metabotropic receptors cause changes in second messenger systems, which in turn alter the function of channels that are separate from the receptor.

Ionotropic receptors (ion channels)

Ionotropic receptors contain an ion channel within their structure (Fig. 42.4; see also Chapter 8). Examples include the nicotinic ACh receptor and some glutamate and γ-amino butyric acid (GABA) receptors. These are transmembrane proteins, with several subunits, usually five, surrounding a pore through the membrane. Each subunit has four transmembrane regions. When the ligand binds, there is a change in the three-dimensional structure of the complex, which allows the flow of ions through it. The effect on membrane potential depends on the particular ions that are allowed to

pass: the nicotinic ACh receptor is comparatively nonspecific towards sodium and potassium and causes depolarization, whereas the $GABA_A$ receptor is a chloride channel and causes hyperpolarization.

Metabotropic receptors

All known metabotropic receptors are coupled to G-proteins

Metabotropic receptors are coupled to second messenger pathways and act more slowly than ionotropic receptors. All known metabotropic receptors are coupled to G-proteins (see Chapter 40) and, like hormone receptors, have seven transmembrane regions. Typically, they then couple either to adenylate cyclase, altering the production of cyclic adenosine monophosphate (cAMP), or to the phosphatidyl inositol pathway, which alters calcium fluxes. Ion channels that are separate from the receptor are then usually modified by phosphorylation. For instance, the β-adrenergic receptor, which responds to norepinephrine and epinephrine (see Fig. 13.5), causes an increase in cAMP, which stimulates a kinase to phosphorylate and activate a calcium channel. Some of the muscarinic class of ACh receptors have similar effects on K^+ channels.

Regulation of neurotransmitters

The action of transmitters must be halted by their removal from the synaptic cleft

When transmitters have served their function, they must be removed from the synaptic space. Simple diffusion is probably

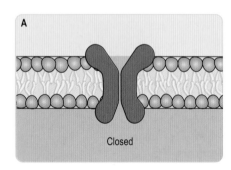

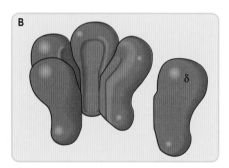

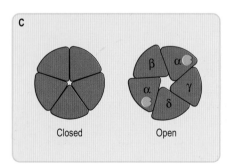

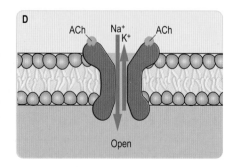

Fig. 42.4 **Mechanism of action of ionotropic receptors.** Ionotropic receptors directly open ion channels (in fact, they are themselves ion channels). The best studied example is the nicotinic ACh receptor. This is a transmembrane protein (A) consisting of five nonidentical subunits (B), each one passing right through the membrane. The subunits surround a pore (C) that selectively allows certain ions through when it is opened by a ligand (D).

the major mechanism of removal of neuropeptides. Enzymes such as acetylcholinesterase, which cleaves ACh, may destroy any remaining transmitter. Surplus transmitters may also be taken back up into the presynaptic neurone for reuse, and this is a major route of removal for catecholamines and amino acids. Interference with uptake causes an increase in the concentration of transmitter in the synaptic space; this often has useful therapeutic consequences.

Concentrations of neurotransmitters may be manipulated

The effects of neurotransmitters can be altered by changing their effective concentrations or the number of receptors. Concentrations can be altered by:

- changing the rate of synthesis
- altering the rate of release at the synapse
- blocking reuptake
- blocking degradation.

Changes in the number of receptors may be involved in long-term adaptations to the administration of drugs.

CLASSES OF NEUROTRANSMITTERS

Amino acids

It has been particularly difficult to prove that amino acids are true neurotransmitters; they are present in high concentrations because of their other metabolic roles and therefore simple measurement of their concentrations did not provide conclusive evidence. Pharmacologic studies of responses to different analogs and the cloning of specific receptors finally provided the proof.

Glutamate

Glutamate is the most important excitatory transmitter in the CNS

It acts on both ionotropic and metabotropic receptors. Clinically, the receptor characterized in vitro by N-methyl-D-aspartate (NMDA) binding is particularly important (Fig. 42.5).

The hippocampus (Fig. 42.6) is an area of the limbic system of the brain that is involved in emotion and memory. Certain synaptic pathways there become more active when chronically stimulated, a phenomenon known as long-term potentiation. This represents a possible model of how memory is laid down, and it requires activation of the NMDA receptor and the consequent influx of calcium.

Glutamate is recycled by high-affinity transporters into both neurones and glial cells. The glial cells convert it into glutamine, which then diffuses back into the neurone. Mitochondrial glutaminase in the neurone regenerates glutamate for reuse.

Glutamate and excitotoxicity

Extracellular glutamate concentration is increased after trauma and stroke, during severe convulsions, and in some

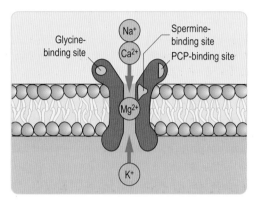

Fig. 42.5 **The NMDA glutamate receptor.** The glutamate receptor that binds N-methyl-D-aspartate (NMDA) is complex. This receptor is clinically important because it may cause damage to neurones after stroke (excitotoxicity). It contains several modulatory binding sites, so it may be possible to develop drugs that could alter its function. Glycine is an obligatory cofactor, as are polyamines such as spermine. Magnesium physiologically blocks the channel at the resting potential, so the channel can open only when the cell has been partially depolarized by a separate stimulus. It therefore causes a prolongation of the excitation. This receptor also binds phencyclidine (PCP). Because this drug of abuse can cause psychotic symptoms, it is possible that dysfunction of pathways involving NMDA receptors causes some of the symptoms of schizophrenia.

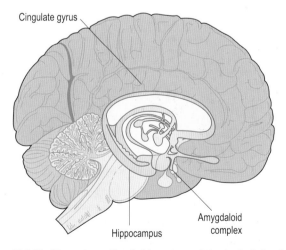

Fig. 42.6 **Limbic system.** The limbic system of the brain is involved in emotions and memory. It consists of various areas surrounding the upper brainstem, including the hippocampus, the amygdaloid body, and the cingulate gyrus. Removal of the hippocampus prevents the laying down of short-term memory, while intact amygdaloid function is required for the emotion of fear.

organic brain diseases such as Huntington's chorea, AIDS-related dementia, and Parkinson's disease. This is because of release of glutamate from damaged cells and damage to the glutamate uptake pathways.

Excess glutamate is toxic to nerve cells

The activation of NMDA receptor allows calcium entry into cells. This activates various proteases, which in turn initiate the pathway of programmed cell death or apoptosis (see also Chapter 43). There may, in addition, be changes in other ionotropic glutamate receptors that also cause aberrant calcium uptake. Uptake of sodium ions is also implicated and causes swelling of cells. Activation of NMDA receptors also increases the production of nitric oxide, which may in itself be toxic. Cell death in some models of excitotoxicity can be prevented by inhibitors of nitric oxide production, but the mechanism of toxicity is not clear.

Attempts are being made to develop drugs to inhibit NMDA activation and suppress excitotoxicity. The hope is that damage caused by stroke can be limited or even reversed. Unfortunately, many of the drugs have side effects because they bind to the phencyclidine-binding site and have unpleasant psychologic effects such as paranoia and delusions.

γ-Amino butyric acid (GABA)

GABA is synthesized from glutamate by the enzyme glutamate decarboxylase

GABA (Fig. 42.7) is the major inhibitory transmitter in the brain. There are two known GABA receptors: the $GABA_A$ receptor is ionotropic and the $GABA_B$ receptor is metabotropic. The $GABA_A$ receptor consists of five subunits that arise from several gene families, giving an enormous number of potential receptors with different binding affinities. This receptor is the target for several useful therapeutic drugs. Benzodiazepines bind to it and cause a potentiation of the response to endogenous GABA; these drugs reduce anxiety and also cause muscle relaxation. Barbiturates also bind to the GABA receptor and stimulate it directly in the absence of GABA; because of this lack of dependence on endogenous ligand, they are more likely to cause toxic side effects in overdose.

Glycine

Glycine is primarily found in inhibitory interneurones in the spinal cord, where it blocks impulses traveling down the cord in motor neurones to stimulate skeletal muscle. The glycine receptor on motor neurones is ionotropic and is blocked by

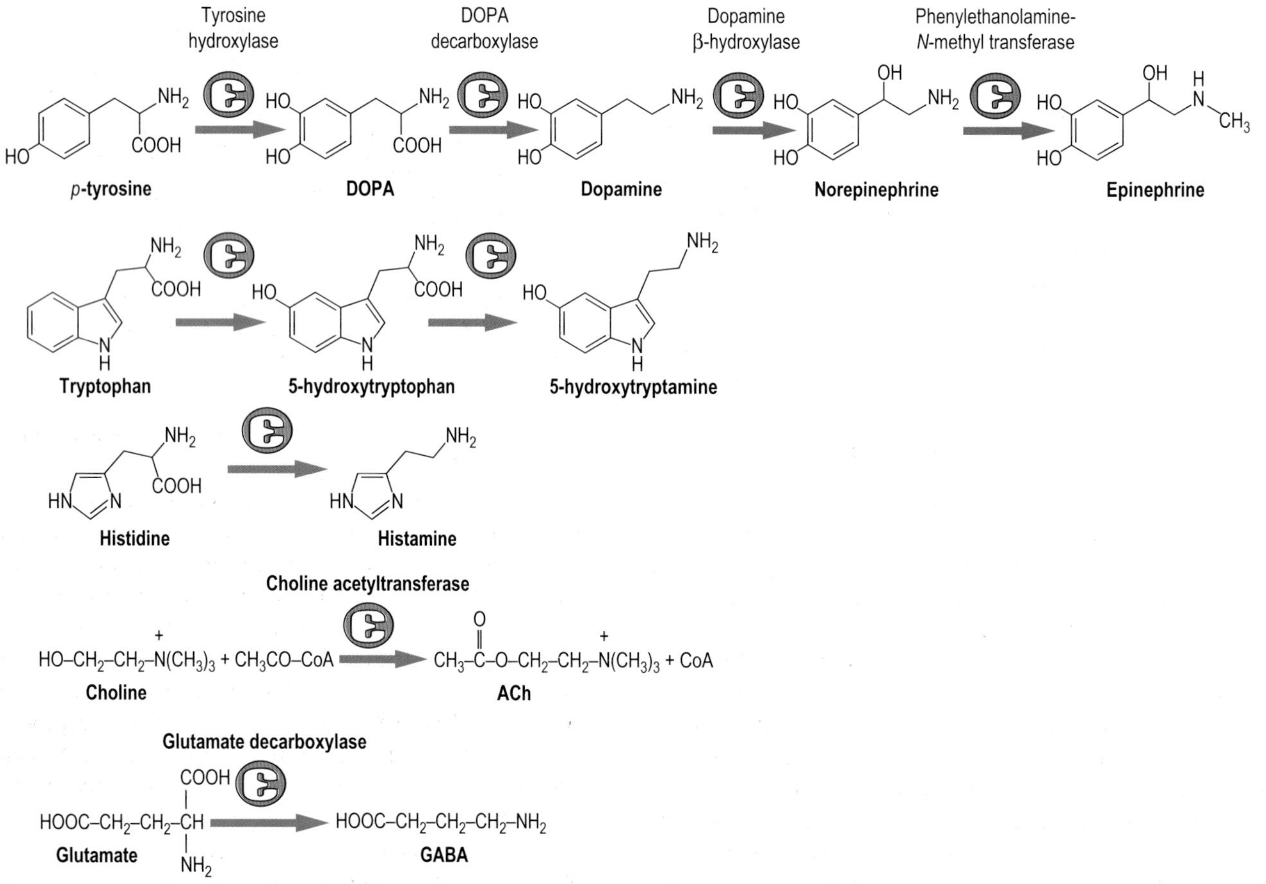

Fig. 42.7 **Synthesis of neurotransmitters.** Pathways of synthesis of neurotransmitters are simple.

DISORDERS OF NEUROTRANSMISSION: DEPRESSION AS A DISEASE OF AMINE NEUROTRANSMITTERS

Monoamine oxidase (MAO) inhibitors prevent the catabolism of catecholamines and serotonin. They therefore increase the concentrations of these compounds at the synapse and increase the action of the transmitters. Compounds with this property are antidepressants. Reserpine, an antihypertensive drug that depletes catecholamines, caused depression and is no longer in use. These findings gave rise to the 'amine theory of depression': this states that depression is caused by a relative deficiency of amine neurotransmitters at central synapses, and predicts that drugs which increase amine concentrations should improve symptoms of the condition.

In support of this theory, tricyclic antidepressants inhibit transport of both norepinephrine and serotonin into neurones, thereby increasing the concentration of amines in the synaptic cleft. Specific serotonin reuptake inhibitors (SSRIs), such as fluoxetine (Prozac), are also highly effective antidepressants. However, as the symptoms of depression do not resolve for several days after treatment is started, it is likely that long-term adaptations of concentrations of transmitters and their receptors are at least as important as acute changes in amine concentrations in the synaptic cleft.

This role of monoamines in depression is undoubtedly an oversimplification. Thus, cocaine is also an effective reuptake inhibitor but is not an antidepressant, and amphetamines both block reuptake and cause release of catecholamines from nerve terminals, but cause mania rather than relief of depression.

strychnine; motor impulses can then be passed without negative control, which accounts for the rigidity and convulsions caused by this toxin.

Catecholamines

Norepinephrine, epinephrine, and dopamine, known as catecholamines, are all derived from the amino acid tyrosine (see Fig. 42.7). In common with other compounds containing amino groups, such as serotonin, they are also known as biogenic amines. Nerves that release catecholamines have varicosities along the axon, instead of a single area of release at the end. Transmitter is released from the varicosities and diffuses through the extracellular space until it meets a receptor. This allows it to affect a wide area of tissue, and these compounds are believed to have a general modulatory effect on overall brain functions such as mood and arousal.

Norepinephrine and epinephrine

Norepinephrine (also known as noradrenaline) is a major transmitter in the sympathetic nervous system. Sympathetic nerves arise in the spinal cord and run to ganglia situated close to the cord, from which postganglionic nerves run to the target tissues. Norepinephrine is the transmitter for these postganglionic nerves, whereas the transmitter at the intermediate ganglia is ACh. Stimulation of these nerves is responsible for various features of the 'fight or flight' response, such as stimulation of the heart rate, sweating, vasoconstriction in the skin, and bronchodilation.

There are also norepinephrine-containing neurones in the CNS, largely in the brainstem (Fig. 42.8). Their axons extend in a wide network throughout the cortex and alter the overall state of alertness or attention. The stimulatory effects of

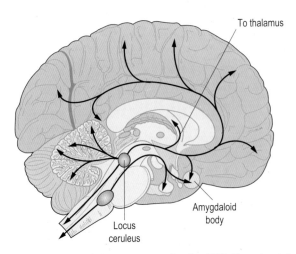

Fig. 42.8 **Norepinephrine neurones in the CNS.** Norepinephrine-containing neurones arise in the locus ceruleus in the brainstem and are distributed throughout the cortex.

amphetamines are caused by their close chemical similarity to catecholamines.

Epinephrine (also known as adrenaline) is produced by the adrenal medulla under the influence of ACh-containing nerves analogous to the sympathetic preganglionic nerves. It is more active than norepinephrine on the heart and lungs, causes redirection of blood from the skin to skeletal muscle, and has important stimulatory effects on glycogen metabolism in the liver. In response to epinephrine, a sudden extra supply of glucose is delivered to muscle, the heart and lungs work harder to pump oxygen round the circulation, and the body is then prepared to run or to defend itself (see Chapter 21). Epinephrine is not essential for life, however, as it is possible to remove the adrenal medulla without serious consequences.

The receptors for norepinephrine and epinephrine are called adrenoceptors (see Fig. 13.5). They are divided into α- and

AN UNUSUAL REACTION TO CHEESE

A 50-year-old man had been suffering from depression for some years. His condition was treated with tranylcypromine, an inhibitor of monoamine oxidase types A and B. He developed a severe, throbbing headache and his blood pressure was found to be 200/110 mmHg. The only unusual occurrence had been that he had attended a cocktail party the previous evening at which he ate cheese snacks and drank several glasses of red wine.

Comment. The patient was experiencing a hypertensive crisis caused by an interaction between the food he had eaten and the drug he was treated with – a MAO inhibitor. This drug inhibits the main enzyme that catabolizes catecholamines. Several foods, including cheese, pickled herring and red wine, contain an amine called tyramine, which is similar in structure to natural amine transmitters and is also broken down by MAO. If this enzyme is not functional, the concentrations of tyramine increase and it starts to act as a neurotransmitter. This can cause a hypertensive crisis, as it did in this patient.

PHEOCHROMOCYTOMA: A NEUROTRANSMITTER CAUSE OF HYPERTENSION

A 56-year-old woman presented with severe hypertension. She suffered from attacks of sweating, headaches, and palpitations. Her high blood pressure had not responded to treatment with an angiotensin converting enzyme inhibitor and a diuretic. A sample of urine was taken for measurement of catecholamines and metabolites. The rate of excretion of norepinephrine was 1500 nmol/24 h (253 mg/24 h) (reference range < 900 nmol/24 h, < 152 mg/24 h), that of epinephrine 620 nmol/24 h (113 mg/24 h) (reference range < 230 nmol/24 h, < 42 mg/24 h) and that of vanillylmandelic acid 60 mmol/24 h (11.9 mg/24 h) (reference range < 35.5 mmol/24 h, [<7.0 mg/24 h]) (see Fig. 42.9).

Comment. The patient had a pheochromocytoma which is a tumor of the adrenal medulla that secretes catecholamines. Both norepinephrine and epinephrine may be secreted: norepinephrine causes hypertension by activating α_1-adrenoceptors on vascular smooth muscle, and epinephrine increases heart rate by activating β_1-adrenoceptors on the heart muscle. Hypertension may be paroxysmal and severe, leading to stroke or heart failure.

Diagnosis is made by measuring catecholamines in plasma or urine, or their metabolites, such as metanephrines and vanillylmandelic acid, in urine. The tumor is usually localized by radiologic techniques such as nuclear magnetic resonance (NMR) or computed tomography (CT) scanning.

Although this is a rare cause of hypertension, comprising only about 1% of cases, it is very important to remember it, as the condition is dangerous and often amenable to surgical cure.

β-receptor classes and subclasses on the basis of their pharmacology. Epinephrine acts on all classes of the receptors but norepinephrine is more specific for α-receptors. β-Blockers, such as atenolol, are used to treat hypertension and chest pain (angina) in ischemic heart disease because they antagonize the stimulatory effects of catecholamines on the heart. Nonspecific α-blockers have limited use, although the more specific α_1-blockers, such as prazosin, and α_2-blockers, such as clonidine, can be used to treat hypertension. Certain subclasses of β-receptors are found in particular tissues; for instance, the β_2-receptor is present in lung and β_2-receptor agonists such as salbutamol are therefore used to produce bronchial dilatation in asthma without stimulating the β_1-receptor in the heart.

Norepinephrine is taken up into cells by a high-affinity transporter and catabolized by the enzyme monoamine oxidase (MAO). Further oxidation and methylation by catecholamine-O-methyl transferase (COMT) convert the products to metanephrines and vanillylmandelic acid (4-hydroxy-3-methoxymandelic acid) (Fig. 42.9), which can be measured in the urine as indices of the function of the adrenal medulla. They are particularly increased in patients who have the tumor of the adrenal medulla known as pheochromocytoma. This tumor causes hypertension because of the vasoconstrictor action of the catecholamines it produces.

Dopamine

Dopamine is both an intermediate in the synthesis of norepinephrine and a neurotransmitter. It is a major transmitter in nerves that interconnect the nuclei of the basal ganglia in the brain and control voluntary movement (Fig. 42.10). Damage to these nerves causes Parkinson's disease, which is characterized by tremor and difficulties in initiating and controlling movement. Dopamine is also found in pathways affecting the limbic systems of the brain, which are involved in emotional responses and memory. Defects in dopaminergic systems are implicated in schizophrenia, because many antipsychotic drugs used to treat this disease have been found to bind to dopamine receptors.

In the periphery, dopamine causes vasodilatation and it is therefore used clinically to stimulate renal blood flow, and is important in the treatment of renal failure (Chapter 23). The catabolism of dopamine is comparable to norepinephrine. However, the major metabolite formed is homovanillic acid (HVA).

Serotonin (5-hydroxytryptamine)

Serotonin, also called 5-hydroxytryptamine (5-HT), is derived from tryptophan (see Fig. 42.7). In addition, serotonin biosynthesis has a number of biochemical similarities to dopamine synthesis. Thus, tryptophan hydroxylase, like tyrosine hydroxylase, displays a cofactor requirement for tetrahydrobiopterin (BH_4) (see below). Furthermore, 5-hydroxytryptophan is converted to serotonin by dopa decarboxylase (also known as aromatic amino acid decarboxylase).

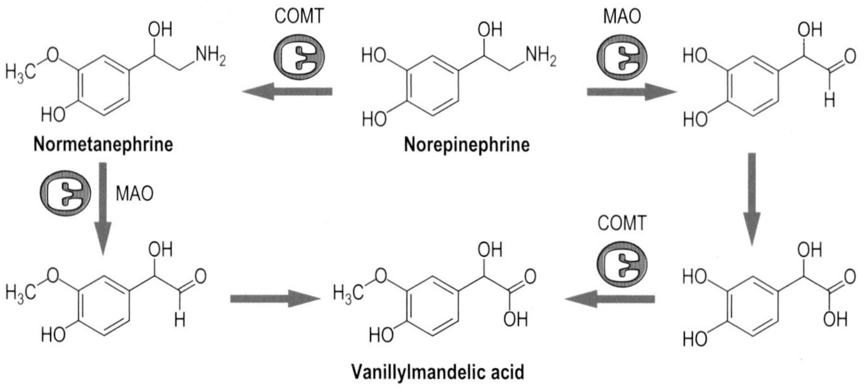

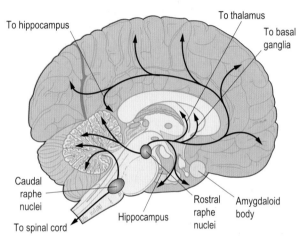

Fig. 42.9 **Catabolism of catecholamines.** Catecholamines are degraded by oxidation of the amino group by the enzyme monoamine oxidase (MAO), and by methylation by catecholamine-O-methyl transferase (COMT). The pathway shown is for norepinephrine but the pathways for epinephrine, dopamine, and 5-HT are analogous.

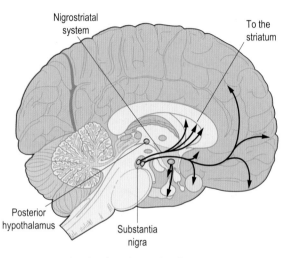

Fig. 42.10 **Dopamine in the nigrostriatal tract.** Nerves containing dopamine run in well-defined tracts. One of the most important tracts, the nigrostriatal, connects the substantia nigra in the midbrain with the basal ganglia below the cortex. Damage to this causes Parkinson's disease, with loss of fine control of movement.

Fig. 42.11 **Serotoninergic nerves in the CNS.** Serotonin-containing nerves arise in the raphe nuclei, part of the reticular formation in the upper brainstem. In common with those containing norepinephrine, they are distributed widely.

Serotoninergic neurones are concentrated in the raphe nuclei in the upper brainstem (Fig. 42.11), but project up to the cerebral cortex and down to the spinal cord. They are more active when subjects are awake than when they are asleep, and serotonin may control the degree of responsiveness of motor neurones in the spinal cord. In addition, it is implicated in so-called vegetative behaviors such as feeding, sexual behavior, and temperature control.

Acetylcholine

Acetylcholine (ACh) is the transmitter of the parasympathetic autonomic nervous system and of the sympathetic ganglia (see Fig. 41.3). Stimulation of the parasympathetic system produces effects that are broadly opposite to those of the sympathetic system, such as slowing of the heart rate, bronchoconstriction, and stimulation of intestinal smooth muscle. ACh also acts at neuromuscular junctions, where motor nerves contact skeletal muscle cells and cause them to contract. Apart from these roles, ACh may be involved in learning and memory, as neurones containing this transmitter also exist in the brain.

ACh is synthesized from choline by the enzyme choline acetyl transferase. After it is secreted into the synaptic cleft, it is largely broken down by acetylcholinesterase. The remainder is taken back up into the nerve cell by transporters similar to those for amines.

There are two main classes of ACh receptors: nicotinic and muscarinic (see Chapter 41, Fig. 41.3). Both respond to ACh but can be distinguished by their associated agonists and antagonists; they are quite different structurally and differ in their mechanisms of action.

■ **Nicotinic receptors are ionotropic**. They bind nicotine and are found on ganglia and at the neuromuscular junction. When ACh or nicotine binds, a pore opens, which

TYROSINE HYDROXYLASE AND AROMATIC AMINO ACID DECARBOXYLASE DEFICIENCIES: INHERITED CAUSES OF IMPAIRED BIOGENIC AMINE METABOLISM

Tyrosine hydroxylase is the first step in dopamine biosynthesis and inherited disorders affecting the activity of this enzyme result in brain dopamine deficiency. A number of clinical phenotypes have been described and include a progressive gait disorder and infantile parkinsonism. Treatment of tyrosine hydroxylase deficiency is by the administration of L-dopa. In order to prevent the decarboxylation of L-dopa to dopamine in the blood (by peripheral aromatic amino acid decarboxylase – AADC), an inhibitor (which does not affect the activity of the brain AADC enzyme) is given at the same time as the L-dopa. Such inhibition optimizes the transport of L-dopa across the blood–brain barrier. Within the brain, AADC can then convert the L-dopa to dopamine.

AADC catalyzes the conversion of L-dopa to dopamine and 5-hydroxytryptophan to serotonin. Consequently, an inborn error of metabolism affecting the activity of this enzyme results in a brain deficiency of both dopamine and serotonin. Patients with AADC deficiency have a clinical picture that includes a severe movement disorder, abnormal eye movements and neurologic impairment. Treatment of AADC deficiency consists of preventing the degradation of any dopamine and serotonin that may be produced by residual AADC activity, i.e. by the use of monoamine oxidase inhibitors. In addition, dopamine agonists such as pergoliode and bromocryptine are used to 'mimic' the effects of dopamine.

DEFICIENCY OF PYRIDOXAL PHOSPHATE: A CAUSE OF NEONATAL EPILEPSY

Pyridoxal phosphate (PLP), the biologically active form of vitamin B_6 (see Chapter 11), is utilized as a cofactor by more than 100 enzymes including reactions catalyzed by aromatic amino acid decarboxylase (AADC), threonine dehydratase and the glycine cleavage system. Vitamin B6 is present in the human body as a number of 'vitamers' that are precursors to PLP. A pivotal enzyme in the formation of PLP is pyridox(am)ine-5′-phosphate oxidase (PNPO). This enzyme catalyzes the conversion of the precursors pyridoxine phosphate and pyridoxamine phosphate to PLP. Deficiency of PNPO results in decreased availability of PLP and such patients, when presenting in the neonatal period, have a clinical picture that includes severe epilepsy. Biochemical analysis of CSF reveals elevated threonine, glycine and evidence of impaired AADC activity. In addition, the CSF concentration of PLP is decreased. Treatment, which can be particularly effective, is by the administration of PLP.

allows both Na^+ and K^+ to pass through. Because the action of the ligand on the channel is direct, action is rapid.

- **Muscarinic receptors, responding to the fungal toxin muscarine, are metabotropic**. They are much more widespread in the brain than are nicotinic receptors, and are also the major receptors found on smooth muscle and glands innervated by parasympathetic nerves. Atropine specifically inhibits these receptors. There are several separate muscarinic receptors, differing in their tissue distribution and signaling pathways. As yet, no clear pattern has emerged as to their specific functions.

Clinically, ACh agonists, in common with acetylcholinesterase inhibitors, are used to treat glaucoma, an eye disease characterized by high intraocular pressure, by increasing the tone of the muscles of accommodation of the eye, and to stimulate intestinal function after surgery. On the other hand, when acetylcholinesterase is inhibited by organophosphate insecticides or nerve gases, a toxic syndrome is caused by the resulting excess of ACh. There may be diarrhea, increased secretory activity of several glands, and bronchoconstriction. This syndrome can be antagonized by atropine, although longer-term treatment involves the use of drugs that can remove the insecticide from the enzyme, such as pralidoxime.

Nitric oxide gas

In autonomic and enteric nerves, nitric oxide (NO) is produced from arginine by the tetrahydrobiopterin-dependent nitric oxide synthases. NO has a number of attributed physiologic functions including relaxation of both vascular and intestinal smooth muscle and the possible regulation of mitochondrial energy production. Furthermore, within the brain, NO may have a role in memory formation. However, excessive NO formation has been implicated in the neurodegenerative process associated with Parkinson's and Alzheimer's disease. Whilst the exact mechanism whereby excessive NO causes neuronal death is not known, a growing body of evidence suggests that irreversible damage to the mitochondrial electron transport chain may be an important factor.

NO is not stored in vesicles, but released directly into the extracellular space. Consequently, NO does not, in the strictest sense, meet all the current criteria to be labeled as a neurotransmitter. NO itself diffuses comparatively easily between cells and binds directly to heme groups in the enzyme guanylate cyclase, stimulating the production of cyclic guanosine monophosphate (see also Chapter 7, and box on p. 76).

Other small molecules

ATP and other purines derived from it are now known to have transmitter functions. ATP is present in synaptic

MULTIPLE RECEPTORS FOR CATECHOLAMINES AND SEROTONIN

Dopamine and serotonin receptors

Multiple receptors have been isolated for dopamine and serotonin. Not all those that have been cloned have yet been shown to be functional, but the possible relevance in terms of drug development is obvious. In some cases, specific manipulation of particular receptors can be exploited therapeutically.

There are five known dopamine receptors, falling into two main groups (D_1-like: D_1 and D_5, and D_2-like: D_2, D_3, and D_4) that differ in their signaling pathways. D_1 receptors increase the production of cAMP, whereas D_2 receptors inhibit it. Antipsychotic drugs such as phenothiazines and haloperidol tend to inhibit D_2-like receptors, suggesting that excessive dopamine activity may be important in causing the symptoms of schizophrenia.

The D_2 receptor is a major receptor in the nerves that interconnect the basal ganglia. As it is known that destruction of these nerves causes Parkinson's disease, it is not surprising that antipsychotic drugs that inhibit the D_2 receptor tend to have the side effect of causing abnormal movements. Drugs, such as clozapine, that bind preferentially to the D_4 receptor appear to be free of such side effects, although that particular drug also binds to several other receptors.

More than a dozen serotonin (5-HT) receptors have been isolated using molecular biologic techniques. They have been divided into classes and subclasses on the basis of their pharmacologic properties and their structures. Most are metabotropic, although the 5-HT_3 receptor is ionotropic and mediates a fast signal in the enteric nervous system. The 5-HT_{1A} receptor is found on many presynaptic neurones, where it acts as an autoreceptor to inhibit the release of 5-HT.

In general, increasing the brain concentration of 5-HT appears to increase anxiety, whereas reducing its concentration is helpful in treating the condition. The antidepressant buspirone acts as an agonist at 5-HT_{1A} receptors, and presumably causes a decrease in production of 5-HT. In addition to its effects on the D_4 dopamine receptor, clozapine binds strongly to the 5-HT_{2A} receptor and it may be that a combination of a high level of 5-HT_{2A} antagonism and low D_2-binding activity is desirable for drugs that can be used to treat schizophrenia with the minimum frequency of side effects. The 5-HT_3 blocker ondansetron is an antiemetic, extensively used to prevent vomiting during chemotherapy. Migraine can be treated with sumatriptan, a 5-HT_{1D} agonist.

The central role of 5-HT in controlling brain function and the huge number of associated receptors suggest that it may possible to tailor a large number of drugs to treat specific disorders, and that pharmacologic manipulation of the function of the nervous system is probably still in its infancy.

 ANALYSIS OF CEREBROSPINAL FLUID FOR THE DETECTION OF DISORDERS OF DOPAMINE AND SEROTONIN METABOLISM

Cerebrospinal fluid (CSF) flows around the major structures of the brain and spinal cord (see also Chapter 41). During circulation, molecules reflecting cellular metabolism diffuse into the CSF. Included in this range of metabolites are the dopamine and serotonin degradation products homovanillic acid (HVA) and 5-hydroxyindoleacetic acid (5-HIAA). Furthermore, tetrahydrobiopterin (BH_4) precursors, metabolites and BH_4 itself are also released into the CSF. Thus, determination of such molecules in CSF provides a powerful indicator of the integrity of dopamine and serotonin metabolism within the central nervous system. Such analyses have identified a number of inborn errors of metabolism affecting dopamine and/or serotonin availability, e.g. disorders of BH_4 metabolism, pyridoxal phosphate metabolism, tyrosine hydroxylase deficiency and aromatic amino acid decarboxylase (dopa decarboxylase) deficiency. Quantification of the above metabolites is usually achieved by high-performance liquid chromatography (HPLC). For the above molecules, there is a concentration gradient in the CSF, known as the rostrocaudal gradient. Thus, CSF fractions taken from closer to the brain have a high concentration of these metabolites. Furthermore, for many of these metabolites, their concentration declines with age. Consequently, in view of these factors, specialist laboratories providing a diagnostic service require that the same fraction of CSF is provided for analysis. In addition, appropriate age-related reference ranges must be available for correct interpretation of the generated results.

vesicles of sympathetic nerves, along with norepinephrine, and is responsible for rapid excitatory potentials in smooth muscle. Adenosine receptors are widespread in the brain and in vascular tissue. Adenosine is largely inhibitory in the CNS, and inhibition of adenosine receptors is believed to underlie the stimulatory effects of caffeine.

Study of histamine in nerves is complicated by the large amounts that are present in mast cells. Histamine is found in a small number of neurones, mainly in the hypothalamus, although their projections are widespread throughout the brain. It has been shown to control the release of pituitary hormones, arousal, and food intake. Antihistamines designed to control allergies caused by release from mast cells act on the H_1 receptor and tend to be sedative, suggesting that other central functions also probably exist. The histamine receptor in the stomach is of the H_2 class, therefore the H_2 inhibitors, such as cimetidine and ranitidine, that are used to treat peptic ulcers have no effect on allergy.

CARCINOID SYNDROME: FLUSHING ATTACKS CAUSED BY A TUMOR

A 60-year-old man complained of attacks of flushing, associated with an increased heart rate. He also had troublesome diarrhea and abdominal pain, and had lost weight. The symptoms suggested a diagnosis of carcinoid syndrome caused by excessive secretion of serotonin and other metabolically active compounds from a tumor. To confirm this, a urine sample was taken for measurement of 5-hydroxyindoleacetic acid (5-HIAA), the major metabolite of 5-HT; the concentration was found to be 120 mmol/24 h (23 mg/24 h) (reference range 10–52 mmol/24 h, 3–14 mg/24 h).

Comment. The patient had the carcinoid syndrome, which is caused by tumors of enterochromaffin cells usually originating in the ileum which have metastasized to the liver. These cells are related to the catecholamine-producing chromaffin cells in the adrenal medulla and convert tryptophan to serotonin (5-HT). Serotonin itself is believed to cause diarrhea, but other mediators, such as histamine and bradykinin, may be more important in the flushing attacks. The urinary concentration of 5-HIAA provides a useful diagnostic test and can be used to monitor the response of the cancer to treatment.

TETRAHYDROBIOPTERIN IS AN ESSENTIAL COFACTOR FOR DOPAMINE AND SEROTONIN SYNTHESIS

Tetrahydrobiopterin (BH$_4$) is a member of the group of chemicals known as the pterins. Normally, BH$_4$ is synthesized, via a number of enzymatic steps, from the precursor guanosine triphosphate. With regard to the central nervous system, an adequate supply of BH$_4$ is essential for tyrosine and tryptophan hydroxylase activities. When acting as a cofactor, BH$_4$ is oxidized to quinonoid dihydrobiopterin (qBH$_2$). BH$_4$, under normal conditions, is regenerated from qBH$_2$ by the enzyme dihydropteridine reductase (DHPR). Several inborn errors of BH$_4$ metabolism are now known. These can arise as a result of a failure of de novo BH$_4$ synthesis or recycling by DHPR. If untreated, these patients have a number of severe neurologic problems which include mental retardation, epilepsy and a movement disorder similar to that seen in Parkinson's disease. Following diagnosis, patients are treated by L-dopa and 5-hydroxytryptophan, to bypass the metabolic block created by the BH$_4$ deficiency. Following initiation of treatment, there is usually clinical improvement, resulting from the correction of dopamine and serotonin metabolism. However, BH$_4$ is also the cofactor for all isoforms of nitric oxide synthase. There is now evidence to suggest that patients with BH$_4$ deficiency also have an impaired ability to generate NO. Thus, research is now in progress to develop means to correct this impairment of the NO signaling pathway as well, for instance by gene therapy targeting the deficient enzyme of BH$_4$ metabolism. Such an approach has the advantage of correcting the primary defect, i.e. the BH$_4$ deficiency.

MYASTHENIA GRAVIS: A DISEASE CAUSING MUSCLE WEAKNESS

A 35-year-old woman noticed that she had difficulty in keeping her eyes open. She also had periods of double vision when her voice was indistinct and nasal and she had difficulty swallowing. Her physician suspected myasthenia, a disease of nerve–muscle conduction. The serum titer of antiacetylcholine receptor antibodies was measured and found to be elevated.

Comment. The patient was suffering from myasthenia gravis. This is a disease that manifests itself as weakness of voluntary muscles and is corrected by treatment with acetylcholinesterase inhibitors. It is caused by autoantibodies directed against the nicotinic acetylcholine receptor, which circulate in serum. Because of these autoantibodies, transmission of nerve impulses to muscle is much less efficient than normal.

Drugs that inhibit acetylcholinesterase increase the concentration of acetylcholine in the synaptic space, which compensates for the reduced number of receptors. Improvement in nerve–muscle conduction in response to edrophonium can be used as a diagnostic test but requires several precautions, and long-acting acetylcholinesterase inhibitors such as pyridostigmine can be used to treat the disease but corticosteroids are often effective.

Peptides

Many peptides act as neurotransmitters

It is an open question whether all the peptides that have been described are really true neurotransmitters. Nevertheless, more than 50 small peptides have now been shown to influence neural function. All known peptide receptors are metabotropic and coupled to G-proteins (see Chapter 40), and so act comparatively slowly. There are no specific uptake pathways or degradative enzymes, and the main route of disposal is simple diffusion followed by cleavage by a number of peptidases in the extracellular fluid. This allows a peptide to affect a number of neurones before it is finally degraded.

Vasoactive intestinal peptide (VIP) is one of many peptides that affect the function of the intestine through the enteric nervous system. It was originally described as a gut hormone that affected blood flow and fluid secretion, but it is now known to be an important enteric neuropeptide, inhibiting smooth muscle contraction. It also causes vasodilatation in several secretory glands, and potentiates stimulation by ACh.

Many neuropeptides belong to multigene families

The opioid peptides (receptors) provide a good example of a multigene family. They are the endogenous ligands for opiate analgesics such as morphine and codeine. The control of pain is complex, and opioid peptides and receptors are found both in the spinal cord and in the brain itself. There are at least three genes that code for these peptides, and each contains the sequences for several active molecules:

- **proopiomelanocortin** contains β-endorphin, which binds to opiate μ-receptors, and also adrenocorticotropic hormone (ACTH) and the melanocyte-stimulating hormones (MSH), which are pituitary hormones (see Chapter 40)
- **proenkephalin A** contains the sequences for Met- and Leu-enkephalins, which bind to δ-receptors and are involved in pain regulation at local levels in the brain and spinal cord
- **prodynorphin** contains sequences for dynorphin and several other peptides, which bind to the κ class of receptors.

Opiates also affect pleasure pathways in the brain, which explains their euphoriant effects, and they also have side effects, such as respiratory depression, that limit their use. In excess, they cause contraction of the muscles of the eye, resulting in 'pinpoint' pupils. It has been shown that endorphins are released after strenuous exercise, giving the so-called 'jogger's high'. It is hoped that increased knowledge of the specific opioid receptors and neural opioid pathways will allow the development of analgesics with fewer side effects and less likelihood of abuse.

Substance P is another example of a member of a multigene family, known as the tachykinin family. It is present in afferent fibers of sensory nerves and transmits signals in response to pain. It is also involved in so-called neurogenic inflammation stimulated by nerve impulses, and is an important neurotransmitter in the intestine.

Neuropeptides can act as neuromodulators

Some peptides do act as true neurotransmitters, but they have many other actions in addition. They often alter the action of other transmitters, acting as neuromodulators but having no action of their own. For instance, VIP enhances the effect of ACh on salivary gland secretion in cat submandibular glands (glands located under the jawbone) by causing vasodilatation and potentiating the cholinergic component. NPY causes inhibition of the release of norepinephrine at autonomic nerve terminals, acting at presynaptic autoreceptors, and potentiates the action of norepinephrine in certain arteries while having only weak actions itself. Opioid peptides also are capable of modulating neurotransmitter release.

ACTIVE LEARNING

1. Does nitric oxide meet all the criteria to be defined as a true neurotransmitter?
2. Explain how a neurotransmitter such as serotonin can have so many diverse effects within the central nervous system.
3. Explain how neurotransmitters can be excitatory or inhibitory.
4. What neurotransmitter types are likely to become deficient in the brain of a patient with an inborn error affecting tyrosine hydroxylase, aromatic amino acid decarboxylase and tetrahydrobiopterin metabolism?
5. Discuss the factors that need to considered when establishing a diagnostic method for disorders of dopamine and serotonin metabolism.
6. Explain the concept of ionotropic and metabotropic receptors.

Summary

Neurones communicate at synapses by means of neurotransmitters. A large number of compounds, whether of low molecular weight, such as the biogenic amines, or larger peptides, can act as neurotransmitters. They act on specific receptors and there is normally more than one receptor for each neurotransmitter. The presence of several transmitters in the same nerves and the identification of multiple receptors suggest that there is a high degree of flexibility and complexity in the signals that can be produced in the nervous system.

Further reading

Clayton PT. B6 responsive disorders: a model of vitamin dependency. *J Inherit Metab Dis* 2006; **29**:317–326.

Hyland K. Inherited disorders affecting dopamine and serotonin: critical neurotransmitters derived from aromatic amino acids. *J Nutr* 2007;**137(6 suppl 1)**:1568S–1572S.

Lam AAJ, Hyland K, Heales SJR. Tetrahydrobiopterin availability, nitric oxide metabolism and glutathione status in the hph-1 mouse: implications for the pathogenesis and treatment of tetrahydrobiopterin deficiency states. *J Inherit Metab Dis* 2007;**30**:256–262.

Websites

www.aadcresearch.org
www.bh4.org
www.pndassoc.org

43. Cellular Homeostasis: Cell Growth, Differentiation and Cancer

M M Harnett and H S Goodridge

LEARNING OBJECTIVES

After reading this chapter you should be able to:

- Define the stages of the mammalian cell cycle.
- Describe how growth factors regulate cell proliferation.
- Outline the regulation of cell cycle progression by cyclins and cyclin-dependent kinases.
- Discuss the regulation of apoptosis by caspases and Bcl-2 family members.
- Explain how deregulation of growth control leads to the development of tumors.
- Distinguish between oncogenes and tumor suppressor genes, and describe the roles they play in tumor progression.

INTRODUCTION

In unicellular organisms such as bacteria, natural selection favors those cells that are most efficient at growing and dividing and, generally, proliferation is simply limited by the availability of nutrients. In contrast, in multicellular organisms such as human beings, there are elaborate controls on the proliferation of individual cell types to maintain the overall integrity of the organism both in terms of the number of individual cell types and also with respect to their spatial organization. Indeed, in adults, despite a plentiful supply of nutrients, the vast majority of cells are not dividing; furthermore, deregulation of growth control leads to the development of tumors and cancer. However, under certain conditions such as tissue repair and senescence, regulated growth and proliferation are promoted. Thus, as cells die, either by senescence or as a result of tissue damage, they must be replaced in a strictly regulated manner.

Cellular homeostasis maintains organ integrity through controlled cell survival, proliferation and cell death (by apoptosis) to ensure that normal cells, unlike cancerous (transformed) cells, generally stop dividing when they contact neighboring cells.

Much of what we now know about the control of normal cell growth and division has arisen from cancer research; analysis of the genetic alterations in cancer cells has revealed mutations in a large number of genes involved in the control of normal cell proliferation. These genes can be classified as proliferative or antiproliferative.

Mutated proliferative genes are called oncogenes **(cancer-causing genes)**, the normal cellular counterparts of which are called **protooncogenes.** Protooncogenes are predominantly signal transducers that act to regulate normal cell growth and division; aberrant regulation of these processes leads to cellular transformation.

In contrast, the antiproliferative genes or **tumor suppressor genes** normally act to suppress cell proliferation. Mutations that inactivate or lead to loss of expression of tumor suppressor genes therefore also lead to uncontrolled proliferation. Thus, whereas the mutant phenotype of tumor suppressor genes is usually recessive and generally requires loss or inactivation of both alleles for its expression, a mutation in only one allele of a protooncogene is required to bring about cell transformation (dominant mutant phenotype).

THE CELL CYCLE

Cells reproduce by duplicating their contents and then dividing in two; this is a closely regulated and complex process that is termed the cell cycle

In recent years, a number of key control points in the cell cycle have been elucidated. In mammals, the duration of the cell cycle varies greatly from one cell type to another, ranging from minutes to years. However, cultured immortalized mammalian cells, which are studied in experimental systems, are, typically, relatively rapidly dividing cells with a cell cycle division time of approximately 24 hours.

Traditionally, the cell cycle is divided into several phases (Fig. 43.1). Mitosis (M-phase) is the stage of cell division; in most cells this takes only about an hour. The remainder of the cell cycle, during which cell growth and deoxyribonucleic acid (DNA) synthesis occur, is known as interphase. Replication of the nuclear DNA occurs during the synthesis (S) phase of interphase. The interval between the M- and S-phases is called the G1-phase, and the interval between the S- and M-phases is called G2. The G1- and G2-phases afford time not only for cell growth but also to provide checkpoints

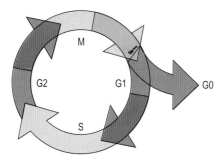

Fig. 43.1 **The phases of the cell cycle.** The mitosis (M) phase is the stage of cell division and takes about an hour in most cells. The G1, S, and G2 phases comprise the remaining interphase, during which cell growth and DNA synthesis occur. The restriction point, a point in late G1 phase, is of significance in mitogenesis (see later in text). S, the synthesis phase of interphase, during which replication of nuclear DNA occurs; G1, the interval between M- and S-phases; G2, the interval between S- and M-phases (compare Fig. 31.5).

at which the progress of the cell cycle may be controlled, and the incorporation of DNA damage prevented, before cell division. As mentioned above, individual cell cycle times vary enormously and it is during G1-phase that most of this variability occurs. This is because cells in G1-phase, which are not committed to DNA replication, can enter a specialized resting state, called G0-phase, until they receive appropriate signals allowing them to progress further through the cell cycle. In mammals, the time required for a cell to progress from the beginning of S-phase through mitosis is typically 12–24 hours irrespective of the duration of the G1-phase. Thus, almost all the variation in proliferation rates between cell types is attributable to the amount of time spent in this G0/G1 state. Furthermore, in conditions that favor cell growth, the total ribonucleic acid (RNA) and protein content of the cell increases continuously, except in M-phase, when the chromosomes are too condensed to allow transcription.

GROWTH FACTORS

Regulation of cell proliferation

Cells of a multicellular organism have to receive specific positive signals in order to grow and divide. Many of these signals are in the form of polypeptide hormones (e.g. insulin), growth factors (e.g. platelet-derived growth factor, PDGF) or cytokines (e.g. interleukins, designated IL-1 to IL-35). These growth factors bind to specific cell surface receptors and initiate intracellular signaling cascades that ultimately act to counter those negative controls in resting cells that prevent growth and block cell cycle progression. Proliferation of most cell types generally requires signaling via a specific combination of growth factors,

rather than stimulation by a single growth factor; thus a relatively small number of growth factors can selectively regulate the proliferation of many cell types. Moreover, although most factors that stimulate cell growth also stimulate cell proliferation, some factors will induce cell growth but not division. This reflects the reality that, within an organism, individual cell types vary enormously in size. Indeed, some cells, such as neurones (in the G0-phase), grow very large without ever dividing. Furthermore, although proliferating cells stop growing when they are deprived of growth factors, they continue to progress through the cell cycle until they reach the point in the G1-phase at which they can enter the G0-phase or resting state.

Growth factors bind to specific cell surface receptors, which are generally transmembrane proteins with cytoplasmic protein tyrosine kinase domains (see also Chapter 40). There are now about 50 known growth factors; PDGF was one of the first to be identified. The growth and proliferative responses to PDGF have proved to be prototypic of many other growth factors and include:

- **immediate increase in intracellular Ca^{2+}**, indicative of initiation of transmembrane signaling (see Chapter 40)
- **reorganization of actin stress fibers**, which is necessary for the anchorage dependence of cell attachment that is required for cell cycle progression
- **activation, nuclear translocation, or both, of transcription factors** (see Chapter 34) that bind to regulatory regions of the DNA of genes that are responsive to the particular growth factor. These transcription factors regulate the transcription of early response genes, which often encode additional transcription factors that are necessary for the induction of components of the cell cycle machinery such as cyclin proteins and, ultimately
- **DNA synthesis and cell division**.

Growth factors activate distinct combinations of signal transducers (see Chapter 40) and transcription factors to dictate the precise repertoire of genes that is induced, thereby enabling the initiation of characteristic differential classes of responses.

Growth factor binding generally induces receptor oligomerization and activation of the tyrosine kinase intrinsic to the receptor, causing phosphorylation of the receptor at specific sites on its cytoplasmic domains (transphosphorylation; Fig. 43.2). This tyrosine phosphorylation of the receptor creates 'docking sites' that allow protein–protein interactions, leading to recruitment and activation of signaling enzymes or 'adapter molecules', which are signal transducers that serve as enzyme modulators for signaling enzymes. Transphosphorylation of receptor cytoplasmic domains thus allows recruitment and activation of a scaffold of signal transduction elements (see Fig. 43.2) such as phospholipase C-γ (PLC-γ), GTPase-activating protein (GAP), protein tyrosine kinases (PTKs) such as *Src*, *Fyn* and *Abl*, phosphotyrosine phosphatases (PTPases) and adapter molecules such as *Shc* or *Grb2*, which we will discuss in more detail below.

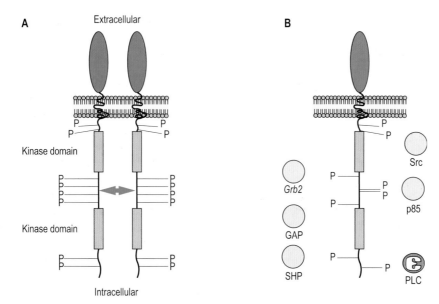

Fig. 43.2 **Recruitment of the downstream signaling element scaffold to the activated PDGF receptor.** Growth factor ligation of the receptor induces dimerization and activation of the tyrosine kinase intrinsic to the receptor cytoplasmic domains, leading to tyrosine phosphorylation (transphosphorylation, P) of the dimerized receptor at specific sites on the cytoplasmic domains (A). Docking sites thus created (B) enable protein–protein interactions that lead to recruitment and activation of downstream signaling enzymes, for example phospholipase C (PLC), GTPase-activating protein (GAP), protein tyrosine kinases (PTKs) such as *Src*, phosphotyrosine phosphatases such as SHP (SH2 domain-containing phosphatase), and adapter molecules such as Grb2 (which recruits Ras).

 ROLE OF PROTEIN TYROSINE KINASES IN SIGNAL TRANSDUCTION

Protein tyrosine kinase (PTK)-dependent interactions in cell signaling

PTKs are enzymes that transfer the γ-phosphate group of ATP to tyrosine residues on target substrate proteins. The term 'protein tyrosine kinase' is a generic term for a large superfamily of enzymes comprising both transmembrane-spanning receptors with an intrinsic tyrosine kinase activity in their cytoplasmic domains and a wide range of subfamilies of cytoplasmic tyrosine kinases such as the *Src, Abl, Syk, Tec* or Janus kinase (JAK) families. Tyrosine phosphorylation, which is a covalent modification of proteins, provides a rapid and reversible (by the action of protein tyrosine phosphatases) mechanism of modifying the enzymic activity of target proteins. In addition, it can modify their ability to act as adapter molecules to recruit other signaling molecules to the protein networks involved in transmembrane cell signaling. For example, the tyrosine phosphorylation of receptors or signaling molecules creates 'docking sites' that allow protein–protein interactions leading to recruitment of downstream signal transducers. Signal transducers are recruited to these phosphorylated tyrosines by virtue of protein–protein interaction domains, such as those called SH2 domains, contained within the sequence of many signal transducers. SH2 stands for *Src*-homology region 2, from the cytoplasmic *Src* tyrosine kinase, a signal transducing element in which this protein domain was first characterized. SH2 domains comprise approximately 100 amino acids and specifically recognize a phosphotyrosine plus the three amino acids immediately *C*-terminal to that phosphotyrosine.

 IMPORTANCE OF THE PROTEIN TYROSINE KINASES

The importance of PTKs in cell proliferation and effector function is illustrated by the defects resulting from mutations in these genes occurring in humans. For example, mutations leading to a loss of activity or expression of ZAP-70, a PTK that plays a key role in antigen-dependent T cell activation, can cause a severe combined immunodeficiency (SCID) due to severe abnormalities in T cell development. Likewise, X-linked agammaglobulinemia, an immunodeficiency characterized by lack of IgG antibody production, is due to loss of function mutations in Btk, a PTK important for B cell activation. By contrast, a chromosomal translocation, known as the Philadelphia chromosome, which involves the fusion of the breakpoint cluster region (BCR) gene from chromosome 22 (region q11) with part of the Abl gene on chromosome 9 (region q34), results in a constitutively active form of the Abl PTK that is associated with chronic myeloid leukemia (CML). The presence of this translocation is highly diagnostic of CML, since 95% of people with CML have this abnormality although it is not definitive as BCR-Abl is also found in some cases of acute lymphoblastic leukemia (ALL) and occasionally, also in acute myeloid leukemia (AML).

PDGF receptor signaling

PDGF signals through the phosphatidylinositol and Ras-MAPK cascades

Ligation of the PDGF-receptor (PDGF-R) leads to the recruitment and activation of phospholipase C-γ (PLC-γ), which catalyzes the hydrolysis of phosphatidylinositol 4,5bisphosphate (PIP$_2$) to generate the intracellular second messengers inositol 1,4,5-trisphosphate (IP$_3$) and diacylglycerol (DAG) (see Chapter 40). IP$_3$ stimulates release of Ca^{2+} from intracellular stores and DAG activates an important signal transducer family, protein kinase C (PKC). Ligation of the PDGF-R also leads to recruitment of another lipid signaling enzyme, phosphoinositide-3-kinase (PI-3-kinase). This enzyme phosphorylates PIP$_2$, yielding the lipid second messenger phosphatidylinositol 3,4,5-trisphosphate (PIP$_3$), which can also activate certain members of the PKC family. In addition, PIP$_3$ can activate another kinase called PIP$_3$-dependent kinase (see also Chapter 40).

Thirty percent of all tumors have constitutively active mutants of a signaling element called *Ras*, which acts as a molecular switch for a key signal transduction pathway in the control of growth and differentiation. *Ras* is a GTPase, which cycles between an inactive *Ras*-GDP form and an active *Ras*-GTP form (Fig. 43.3). GTP/GDP exchange is promoted by a guanine nucleotide exchange factor, called *Sos*, and the GTPase-activating protein (GAP) inactivates *Ras* by stimulating its intrinsic GTPase activity (as does the intrinsic GTPase of the α-subunit of heterotrimeric G-proteins; see Chapter 40). *Ras* is constitutively targeted to the plasma membrane by a posttranslational modification involving the addition of a lipophilic farnesyl group (Chapter 17) and is then recruited to the activated PDGF-R by interaction with an adaptor protein called *Grb2*.

One of the main effector functions of *Ras* is to regulate the mitogen-activated protein kinase (MAPK) cascade. MAPK is a serine-threonine kinase that is itself activated by phosphorylation by a dual specificity (tyrosine/threonine) MAPK kinase called MEK. MAPK has two major isoforms, extracellular regulated kinases (ERK) 1 and 2, which translocate to the nucleus and phosphorylate (on serine and threonine) key transcription factors involved in the regulation of DNA synthesis and cell division.

Cytokine receptor signaling

Cytokines are growth factors that specifically act to orchestrate the development of hemopoietic cells and the immune response

They can also have multiple effects on nonhemopoietic cell types (see Chapter 38). In common with growth factors,

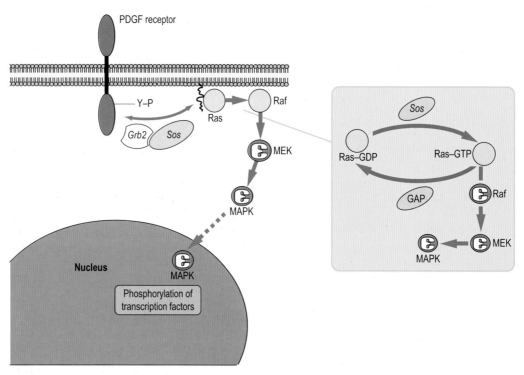

Fig. 43.3 **Recruitment and activation of Ras by the PDGF receptor.** Ras is anchored in the plasma membrane and recruited to the activated PDGF-R via interaction with the Grb2–Sos complex. Receptor-stimulated GTP/GDP exchange, and hence activation of Ras, is promoted by Sos, whereas GAP inactivates Ras by stimulating its intrinsic GTPase activity. Ras couples the PDGF-R to MAPK activation via stimulation of the intermediary kinases, Raf and MEK kinase. MAPK translocates to the nucleus and phosphorylates (on serine and threonine) key transcription factors involved in the regulation of DNA synthesis and cell division. GAP, GTP-activating protein; MAPK, mitogen-activated protein kinase.

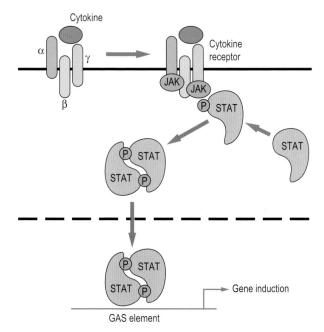

Fig. 43.4 **Cytokine receptor signaling via JAK-STAT pathways.** Following ligation by cytokine, receptors oligomerize. JAKs are recruited and phosphorylate tyrosine residues in the cytoplasmic domains of the receptor chains, enabling STAT recruitment and phosphorylation. pSTAT proteins are released from the receptor and form dimers which can rapidly translocate to the nucleus and act as transcription factors, binding to GAS elements. Different combinations of JAKs and STATs can be utilized by distinct receptors to achieve specificity. GAS, γ activation sequence; JAK, Janus kinase; STAT, signal transducer and activator of transcription.

they mediate their effects via specific cell surface receptors; although there are several major classes of receptors, many cytokine receptors belong to the superfamily called the hemopoietic receptors. These are transmembrane glycoprotein receptors characterized by their conserved extracellular domains, which contain characteristic cysteine pairs and a pentapeptide WSXWS (tryptophan-serine-any-tryptophan-serine) motif. The receptors have no intrinsic catalytic activity and many are multisubunit receptors, although not all of the chains necessarily belong to this receptor superfamily. These multisubunit receptors are generally characterized by a unique ligand-binding subunit that confers specificity, and a common signal transducer subunit that is often shared by several related cytokines and is the basis of the subdivison of the receptors into a number of distinct subfamilies. The sharing of common signal transducer subunits serves to explain the severe immunodeficiencies that result from naturally arising defects in these receptors.

As stated above, the hemopoietic receptors express no intrinsic catalytic activity; however, after ligation, these receptors stimulate tyrosine kinase activity and most cytokines, in common with the classic growth factors, can signal through PLC, PI-3-K, and *Ras*-MAPK pathways. However, a family of cytosolic protein tyrosine kinases (PTKs) has a crucial role in hemopoietic receptor signaling;

these kinases, called Janus kinases (JAKs), couple hemopoietic receptors to a novel transduction pathway that provides a direct link between receptor activation and gene transcription (Fig. 43.4). Like the *Src* kinases, the JAKs are cytosolic tyrosine kinases. They associate with the hemopoietic receptors at conserved regions near the transmembrane domain and are activated and phosphorylated after cytokine binding and oligomerization of hemopoietic receptors.

The major breakthrough in identifying the role of these kinases was obtained when the downstream targets of JAKs were identified as transcription factors called signal transducers and activators of transcription (STATs). STATs are found in a monomeric latent form in the cytoplasm of unstimulated cells. Cytokine stimulation leads to JAK-mediated phosphorylation and dimerization of STATs. STATs translocate to the nucleus, where they bind specific DNA sequences in the promoters of target genes and thus directly modulate gene inductionr (see Fig. 43.4). Recently, growth factors such as epidermal growth factor (EGF) and PDGF have also been shown to activate JAK/STAT pathways; thus this novel signaling cascade may provide a universal mechanism by which growth factors mediate gene induction and cellular responses.

REGULATION OF THE CELL CYCLE

Growth factor stimulation results in the induction of proteins involved in regulating the cell cycle, such as the cyclin-dependent kinases (CDKs) and cyclins.

Cyclins were originally defined as proteins that were specifically degraded at every mitosis

CDKs are kinases that must to bind to a cyclin in order to be active. This cyclin-dependent activation of CDKs regulates key steps in cell cycle progression (Fig. 43.5).

The activity of the cyclins is modulated by changes in their levels of expression at both the mRNA and the protein level (transcriptional and translational control). In contrast, the CDKs are expressed in relatively constant amounts and their activities are modulated by their phosphorylation status. Moreover, a further level of control has been revealed by the recent identification of CDK inhibitors (CDKIs), which bind CDKs and act as inhibitory subunits to block their catalytic activity.

Mitogenesis

Mitogenic growth factors exert their effects between the onset of G1-phase and a point in late G1-phase called the restriction point

Once the cell has passed through the restriction point, the remaining phases of the cell cycle through to M-phase are virtually unaffected by extracellular signals and are committed to progress rather than to quiesce. The retinoblastoma protein, *Rb*, controls the expression of genes that commit

X-SCID: INTERLEUKIN COMMON γ-CHAIN DEFICIENCY

X-linked severe combined immunodeficiency (X-SCID) is a disorder causing very severe immunodeficiency. It is characterized by profoundly defective cellular and humoral immunity resulting in greatly increased susceptibility to infection, and is uniformly fatal by the time the patient is 1–2 years of age unless treated by bone marrow transplantation. X-SCID males typically have profoundly defective cell-mediated and humoral immunity, with low numbers of T cells, or none at all, but normal numbers of B cells.

Comment. The gene responsible for X-SCID was initially reported to code for the γ-chain of the IL-2 receptor. It is now clear that this γ-chain is shared with the receptors for IL-4, IL-7, IL-9, IL-13, and IL-15, hence explaining the severe immunodeficiency in X-SCID as the patient is unable to respond to a number of, or all these cytokines. (See also Chapter 38.) The intracellular domain of this protein associates with the PTK, JAK3, leading to gene induction, and cell growth and proliferation. Consistent with this, mutations in JAK3 are a cause of an autosomal recessive form of SCID. Previously, transplantation of compatible bone marrow was the only effective therapy but it is now possible to repair the γ-chain defect by viral-mediated gene therapy of the patient's own bone marrow-derived B and T precursor cells as the 'repaired' cells can proliferate in response to cytokines and replace the defective cells. The finding that JAK3 mutations also resulted in SCID suggested that JAK3 may be a good therapeutic target for the development of novel immunosuppressants and indeed, JAK3 inhibitors are already undergoing preclinical and clinical trials as potential therapies not only for organ transplant rejection but also in autoimmune diseases such as psoriasis, multiple sclerosis, inflammatory bowel disease and rheumatoid arthritis. In addition, such inhibitors are likely to exhibit therapeutic potential in cancers in which aberrant JAK3 activity has been demonstrated, such as acute myeloid leukemia (AML), and colorectal and lung cancers.

MAPK SIGNALING CASCADES

The Mitogen-activated protein kinase (MAPK) cascade was originally elucidated by genetic studies in yeast, but the pathway has proved to be evolutionarily very highly conserved from yeast to mammals, allowing the mammalian elements to be identified by homology cloning. It has emerged in recent years that MAPKs are key components of an interacting network of sequential protein kinase cascades (MAPK cassettes) that serve to link early receptor-transduced signals with growth and differentiation-related transcriptional events in the nucleus. 'MAPK' is the generic name for a superfamily of signal transducing kinases that, to date, encompasses three major subfamilies, termed the extracellular regulated kinase (ERK; e.g. p44ERK1 and p42ERK2), stress activated protein kinase (SAPK) or Jun N-terminal kinase (JNK), and p38-reactivating kinase (p38RK) MAPK cassettes. These MAPK cassettes can phosphorylate transcription factors implicated in immediate early gene induction, such as AP-1 (Jun and Fos), ELK-1, and SAP1. Furthermore, whereas activation of the SAPKs and p38RKs can selectively induce apoptosis, under certain conditions, ERK1 and ERK2 generally act to promote cell survival and proliferation.

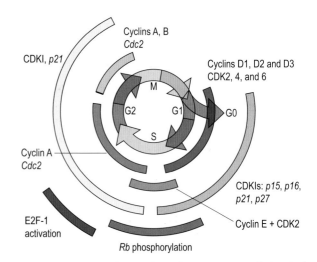

Fig. 43.5 **Regulation of the cell cycle.** Stimulation of growth factors leads to cyclin-dependent activation of the regulation of key steps in the cell cycle by CDKs and their inhibitors. The cyclins and their respective CDK partners acting at the different stages of cell cycle progression are shown. CDK, cyclin-dependent kinase; CDKI, CDK inhibitor; E2F-1, a transcription factor; *Rb*, retinoblastoma protein.

cells that are at the restriction point late in G1-phase to enter S-phase (DNA synthesis phase) of the cell cycle. Thus, in early G1-phase, hypophosphorylated *Rb* represses advance of the cell cycle by binding to, and preventing the DNA-binding activity of, a family of transcription factors, called *E2F*, which have key roles in the G1/S-phase transition. In contrast, close to the restriction point, growth factor stimulation induces the cyclin D–CDK4 and 6 complexes and then the cyclin E–CDK2 complex to hyperphosphorylate *Rb*. The resulting release of inhibition of *E2F* allows activation of genes, the products of which are important for entry into S-phase (see Fig. 43.5).

Monitoring for DNA damage

The tumor suppressor protein, *p53*, is a predominantly DNA damage-sensing protein by which the cell monitors DNA

damage throughout the cell cycle. It can halt cell cycle progression to allow DNA repair, by induction of the *p21* CDKI (WAF1), which prevents the CDK-dependent phosphorylation and inactivation of *Rb*. As WAF1 can affect a variety of cyclin–CDK complexes, it appears that growth arrest can occur at any point in the cell cycle. However, although

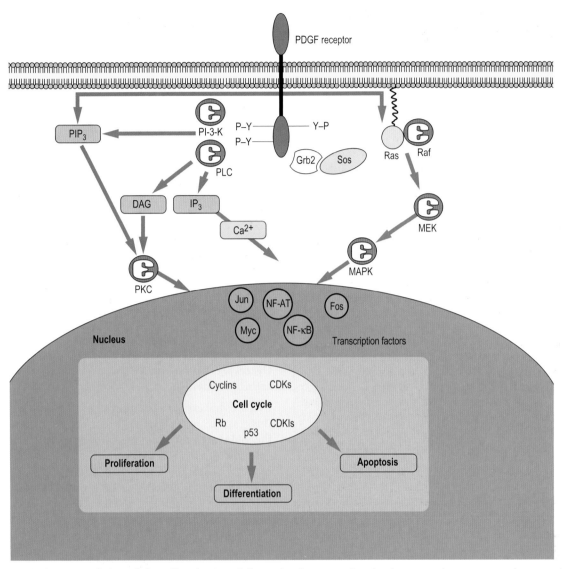

Fig. 43.6 **Growth factor regulation of the cell cycle.** Growth factor signals generated at the plasma membrane can transduce gene induction, cell cycle progression, and proliferation, differentiation or apoptosis. Growth factor receptor signaling leads to activation of transcription factors such as *Jun* and *Fos* (which dimerize to form AP-1), *Myc*, NF-AT, and NF-κB. These regulate the induction of components of the cell cycle machinery that monitor and direct cell cycle progression, cell growth arrest and cell differentiation. Induction of DNA damage that would result in the accumulation of mutations leads to cell cycle arrest and DNA repair. Alternatively if the DNA damage is too great, cell death occurs by apoptosis. DAG, diacylglycerol; IP_3, inositol-1,4,5-trisphosphate; PI-3K, phosphoinositide-3-kinase; PIP_3, inositol-3,4,5-trisphosphate; PKC, protein kinase C; PLC, phospholipidase C.

minimal repairable damage induces *p53*-mediated growth arrest to allow DNA repair and avoid accumulation of mutations by preventing replication of the damaged DNA in the S-phase, serious, irreparable damage triggers *p53*-dependent programmed cell death by apoptosis.

Growth factors and cell cycle progression

The link between growth factor receptor signaling and cell cycle progression can be seen by examining two important examples. First, the growth factor, transforming growth factor-β (TGF-β), which negatively regulates growth in many cell types, mediates many of its effects by inhibition of the

cyclin D–CDK4 and 6 complexes that promote cell cycle progression. Indeed, in some tumors, transformation appears to result from deletion or functional inactivation of TGF-β receptors or associated downstream signal-transducing elements. Second, the key signaling element, *Ras*, which has been found to be mutated to a constitutively activated form in approximately 30% of all tumors, similarly appears to exert many, if not all, of its effects ultimately by upregulating concentrations of cyclin D and, hence, by stimulating cell cycle progression. This upregulation of cyclin D expression results from stimulation of the MAPK cascade by *Ras* and the induction of the transcription factor, AP-1, which regulates induction of cyclin D expression (Fig. 43.6).

ATAXIA TELANGIECTASIA

Ataxia telangiectasia is a rare autosomal recessive disease caused by mutations in the ataxia telangiectasia-mutated (*ATM*) gene. Symptoms and signs include an unsteady gait, telangiectasia, skin pigmentation, infertility, immune deficiencies, and an increased incidence of cancer, especially lymphoreticular tumors.

Comment. ATM belongs to a protein kinase family that regulates the induction of DNA damage responses in reaction to ionizing radiation, anticancer treatment, or programmed DNA breaks during meiosis. Patients with ataxia telangiectasia show a large increase in cancer susceptibility and increased sensitivity to ionizing radiation. Ataxia telangiectasia cells show chromosomal instability, hypersensitivity to reagents that induce DNA-strand breaks, and defects in the G1/G2-phases, and altered regulation of the expression of *p53* and *p21* WAF1. *ATM* protein is constitutively expressed during the cell cycle and has been assigned a checkpoint function in monitoring DNA damage and determining whether *p53*-mediated growth arrest and DNA repair or *p53*-dependent apoptosis occurs in response to severe DNA damage. In ataxia telangiectasia, cells with mutated *ATM* fail to adequately activate *p53*, and hence to induce growth arrest or apoptosis in response to ionizing radiation. Moreover, when *p53* is also mutated, the cell cycle is deregulated and the risk of tumor formation is enhanced as a result of the accumulation of mutations.

APOPTOSIS

Apoptosis, a form of programmed cell death, occurs during normal cellular development

It is a fundamentally important biologic process that is required to maintain the integrity and homeostasis of multicellular organisms. Inappropriate apoptosis can lead to degenerative conditions, such as neurodegenerative disorders, subversion and disruption of the apoptosis machinery can result in cancer (Table 43.1) or autoimmune disease. Cells that die from damage typically swell and burst (necrosis), but apoptosis is characterized by dramatic morphologic changes in the cell, including shrinkage, chromatin condensation, cleavage, and disassembly into membrane-enclosed vesicles called apoptotic bodies that undergo rapid phagocytosis by neighboring cells. It is the accumulation of sterols in the plasma membrane and translocation of phosphatidylserine to the outer leaflet of the plasma membrane that serve to flag the apoptotic cell for elimination via phagocytosis by neighboring cells or macrophages.

Recent research has elucidated many of the biochemical signals that regulate apoptosis and has identified two key

families of proteins that appear to be central to the regulation of mammalian cell death by apoptosis. These are the family of cysteine proteases called caspases, and the B cell lymphoma protein 2 (*Bcl-2*)-related family members, which serve to modulate cell survival by regulating caspase activity.

Caspases

Caspases are involved in apoptosis

The caspases act by cleaving key target proteins, resulting in the systematic disassembly of the apoptotic cell by:

- halting cell cycle progression
- disabling homeostatic and repair mechanisms
- initiating the detachment of the cell from its surrounding tissue structures
- dismantling structural components such as the cytoskeleton
- flagging the dying cell for phagocytosis.

Overexpression of active caspases is sufficient to cause cellular apoptosis

Caspases are expressed as inactive procaspases and it is likely that caspase activation occurs in a cascade fashion, with the initial activation of a regulatory caspase serving to activate downstream effector caspases by proteolysis. Cell death receptors, such as tumor necrosis factor (TNF)-R and *Fas* (also known as CD95 or APO-1), mediate apoptotic cell death pathways in a number of cell types but particularly in cells of the immune system. They initiate apoptosis by directly recruiting procaspases, such as caspase 8, to their accessory 'death domain' transducing molecules, thereby inducing the proteolytic caspase activation cascade (Fig. 43.7). These death domain molecules include *Fas*-associated death domain protein (FADD), TNF-R associated death domain protein (TRADD), receptor interacting protein (RIP), and RIP-associated ICE-like protease with a death domain (RAIDD). The precise molecular mechanisms of effector caspase activation are as yet unknown. However, it has recently emerged that proteolysis and activation of effector caspases are facilitated by binding to cytochrome c, which is released from the mitochondria during the process of apoptosis.

The *Bcl-2* gene family

Bcl-2 is a key antiapoptotic protein

The *Bcl-2* gene family comprises structurally related proteins that form homo- or heterodimers and act to either promote or antagonize apoptosis by modulating caspase activation.

Cancer and the cell cycle

Cancer	Cell cycle element	Outcome: status of the retinoblastoma protein (Rb)

breast cancer, leukemia
testicular carcinomas
breast tumors
	cyclin expression increased as a result of gene
	  amplification or chromosomal translocation
	cyclin D1
	cyclin D2
	cyclin E
		hyperphosphorylation and inactivation of retinoblastoma
		  protein (Rb) leading to deregulated malignant cell proliferation

retinoblastomas small cell lung carcinomas osteosarcomas	mutational inactivation of Rb genes	loss of Rb control of cell cycle, leading to deregulated malignant cell proliferation
cervical carcinomas	sequestration of Rb by the human papilloma virus E7 protein	loss of Rb control of cell cycle
variety of tumor cells	deletion of CDKI genes, *p14*, *p15*	loss of inhibition of cyclin D-CDK4/6 complexes, resulting in inappropriate hyperphosphorylation and inactivation of Rb

melanomas	mutant CDK4 demonstrating resistance to CDKI gene
	  products, *p14*, *p15*
		loss of inhibition of cyclin D-CDK4/6 complexes, resulting in loss
		  of Rb control of cell cycle

Table 43.1 **Relationship between various cancers and stages of the cell cycle.** Some degree of disruption of the cell cycle machinery is likely to occur in every type of cancer cell. As most proliferative decisions are made at the restriction point in late G1-phase, the key target for cellular transformation appears to be the retinoblastoma protein, *Rb*. Indeed, it is now clear that the signal transduction events leading to *Rb* phosphorylation and functional inactivation are disrupted in many cancer cells, suggesting that *Rb* inactivation may be crucial to deregulated, malignant cell proliferation.

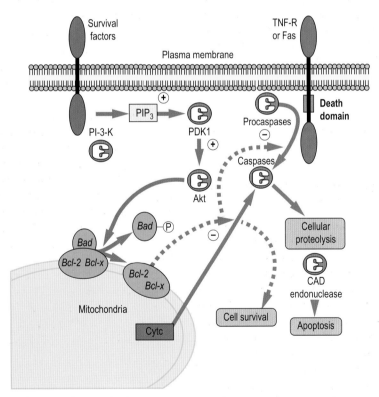

Fig. 43.7 **Regulation of apoptosis and growth factor-mediated cell rescue.** Cell death receptors, such as TNF receptor (TNF-R) or *Fas*, recruit procaspases such as caspase 8 to their 'death domain' transducing molecules (FADD, TRADD, RIP, and RAIDD), thereby inducing the proteolytic caspase activation cascade of apoptotic cell death. In contrast, the *Bcl-2* family-regulated cascade may be modulated by survival factors coupled to phosphoinositide-3-kinase (PI-3-K), leading to rescue of cells from apoptosis and promotion of cell survival. PI-3-K catalyzes the production of phosphatidylinositol 3,4,5-trisphosphate (PIP$_3$), which stimulates a PIP$_3$-dependent kinase (PDK), resulting in phosphorylation and activation of the protein kinase, *Akt*. In turn, *Akt* phosphorylates the proapoptotic *Bcl-2* family member, Bad, inducing dissociation of Bad from heterodimeric complexes with *Bcl-2* or *Bcl-x*$_L$ and allowing *Bcl-2/Bcl-x*$_L$ to antagonize cell death by preventing release of cytochrome c (Cyt c) and caspase activation. CAD, caspase-dependent endonuclase.

DEREGULATED APOPTOSIS IN TUMOR FORMATION: DISRUPTION OF THE APOPTOTIC MACHINERY IN B CELL LEUKEMIAS

During lymphopoiesis, B (75%) and T (95%) cell progenitors that fail to rearrange their antigen receptor genes in a productive, nonself manner are programmed to die by apoptosis. The finding that the cell survival gene, Bcl-2, was subject to a chromosomal translocation in human follicular lymphomas suggested that subversion of apoptotic pathways may have a key role in malignant transformation. Thus, by deregulating the key antiapoptotic protein, Bcl-2, this translocation promotes the survival of cells that would otherwise die, and which then acquire the additional mutations required for malignant transformation.

Bcl-2 has now been shown to belong to a family of proteins that, by regulating mitochondrial integrity and cytochrome C release, modulate caspase activity and hence are intimately involved in the regulation of selection of the alternative pathways of cell survival or apoptosis. Thus, whereas family members such as Bcl-2 and Bcl-x_L inhibit apoptosis, their cell survival activities can be antagonized by Bcl-x_S (a lower molecular-weight splice variant of Bcl-x_L), Bak, Bax, and Bad. The antagonistic actions of these proteins can be illustrated by studies showing that, whereas loss of Bax promotes tumor formation in mice, overexpression of Bax can suppress cellular transformation in vitro. Similarly, a number of viruses (e.g. adenovirus, Epstein–Barr virus, African swine fever virus, herpes virus Saimiri, and human herpes virus 8) enhance their replication by encoding viral homologs of Bcl-2 to promote survival of the host cell. Finally, the tumor suppressor, p53, appears to activate apoptosis, at least in part, by downregulating the expression of Bcl-2 and upregulating that of Bax; this provides an additional rationale for p53 being the most commonly mutated gene in human cancer.

ANALYSIS OF CELL CYCLE PROGRESSION AND APOPTOTIC CELLS

The DNA content of cells varies through the cell cycle, increasing during S-phase from diploid chromosomal DNA in G0/G1 to tetraploid at G2/M, before returning to diploid again after M-phase. Furthermore, subdiploid DNA content is an indicator of apoptosis as the activation of endonucleases resulting in DNA degradation is a characteristic event in apoptosis. The resulting DNA fragments, which differ in size by units of 200 base pairs, can be visualized on agarose gel electrophoresis as 'DNA ladders'. The cell cycle or apoptotic status of cells can therefore be easily assessed in the laboratory by measuring DNA content. Flow cytometry, which measures the fluorescence of individual cells, can be combined with a variety of fluorescent staining techniques to assess the proportions of cells in a population that are at the different stages of the cell cycle or undergoing apoptosis (Fig. 43.8). Similar analysis of cells or tissue can be performed by laser scanning cytometry which allows imaging and quantitative analysis of immunofluorescence in a slide-based format.

For example, staining with propidium iodide (PI), which intercalates into the DNA helix, measures the total DNA content of cells; 4'-6'-diamidino-phenylindole-2HCl (DAPI) works in a similar manner by preferentially binding to A-T base pairs. Incorporation of bromodeoxyuridine (BrdU), an analog of the DNA precursor thymidine, into the newly synthesized DNA of cells progressing through S-phase can also be detected by flow cytometry using anti-BrdU antibodies conjugated to fluorescent dyes.

Apoptosis can also be measured by the TUNEL assay in which fragments of apoptotic DNA, generated by endonuclease action, can be labeled with fluorescent dyes. Thus, the enzyme terminal deoxynucleotidyl transferase (TdT) is used to add a biotin-labeled nucleotide, such as dUTP, to the ends of the DNA fragments and then these biotin-labeled ends can be visualized by binding of the biotin ligand, streptavidin, that has been conjugated with fluorescent dyes.

Nonfluorescent carboxy-fluoresceindiacetate succinimidyl ester (CFDA SE), which is converted to fluorescent CFSE by the action of cytoplasmic esterases, is a very effective reagent for studying the division of proliferating cells. When CFSE-stained cells divide, CFSE is uniformly distributed between daughter cells; each division reduces the CFSE fluorescence intensity of daughter cells by approximately half. Flow cytometric analysis therefore reveals discrete frequency distributions of cells with progressively reduced fluorescence levels (histogram peaks), representing successive generations of cells (Fig. 43.8).

Multi-color staining using fluorescent dyes with different emission spectra can also be performed to yield extra information about cell subpopulations. For example, antibodies against cell-specific markers conjugated to other fluorescent dyes can be employed to establish whether an agent causes all cells or an individual cell type within a mixed cell population to proceed through the cell cycle, arrest in G0 phase, or undergo apoptosis.

Bcl-2 was initially discovered as a chromosomal translocation in a follicular B cell lymphoma, which was found to contribute to neoplastic growth by inhibiting normal B cell apoptosis. The molecular mechanisms underlying Bcl-2 mediated survival signals are as yet poorly defined, but it appears that Bcl-2, which is located on the outer mitochondrial membrane, may act by preventing leakage of cytochrome c from the mitochondria and, hence, activation of effector caspases (see Fig. 43.7).

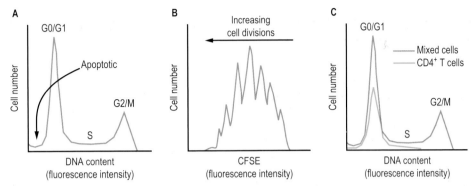

Fig. 43.8 **Analysis of cell cycle progression and apoptotic cells.** (A) Measurement of DNA content in propidium iodide (PI)- or DAPI-stained cells by flow cytometry allows assessment of the cell cycle status of individual cells in a population. Tetraploid = G2/M, diploid = G0/G1, intermediate = S-phase; subdiploid DNA content indicates cells undergoing apoptosis. (B) When CFSE-stained cells divide, CFSE is shared equally between daughter cells, reducing the fluorescence intensity of daughter cells by half with each division. Flow cytometry reveals discrete cell subpopulations representing successive generations of cells. (C) Surface staining of cells with a fluorescent antibody specific for the T helper cell marker CD4 suggests that CD4$^+$ T cells in this mixed population of cells are arrested in G0. DAPI: 4′,6′-diamidino-2-phenylindole.

CANCER

Cells that undergo mutation(s) that disrupt the regulation of cell division will divide without regard to the overall needs of the organism and become apparent as a tumor or neoplasm

As long as the neoplastic cells remain as an intact tumor, the tumor is said to be benign and can be removed surgically. However, if further mutations allow such tumor cells to invade and colonize other tissues, creating widespread secondary tumors or metastases, the tumor is described as malignant and classified as a cancer. Each cancer is derived from a single cell that has undergone some heritable mutation that allows it to outgrow its surrounding cells; by the time they are first detected, tumors typically contain a billion cells. Cancers are classified according to the tissue and cell type that they are derived from: those from epithelial cells are carcinomas, those from connective tissue or muscle cells are termed sarcomas, and those from the hemopoietic system are called leukemias. About 90% of human cancers are carcinomas, the five most common being those of the lung, stomach, breast, colon/rectum, and uterine cervix.

A single mutation is not sufficient to convert a healthy cell to a cancer cell; several rare mutations have to occur together

Mutations in DNA occur spontaneously at a rate of 10^{-6} mutations per gene per cell division (even more in the presence of mutagens). Thus, since approximately 10^{16} cell divisions occur in the human body over an average lifetime, every human gene is likely to undergo mutation on about 10^{10} occasions. Clearly then, a single mutation is not sufficient

to convert a healthy cell to a cancer cell; several rare mutations have to occur together, as demonstrated by epidemiologic studies showing that, for any given cancer, the incidence increases exponentially with age. Indeed, it has been estimated that 3–7 independent mutations are usually required, leukemias apparently needing the fewest mutations and carcinomas the most.

Tumor progression can be observed when initial minor disruptions of cell regulation escalate into a full cancer. For example, chronic myelogeneous leukemia (CML) is initially characterized by the overproduction of white blood cells, as a result of chromosomal translocation. This chronic stage of the disease remains stable for several years before transforming into the acute, rapidly progressing phase of the disease, in which the cells have accumulated several other mutations that cause them to proliferate more rapidly. Alternatively, mutations may have arisen such that committed progenitors of the cells continue to divide indefinitely, rather than terminally differentiating and dying after a strictly regulated number of cell divisions, as happens to their normal counterparts.

Mutations that block the normal development of cells towards an end-differentiated, nondividing cell, or a cell that would normally be programmed to die by apoptosis, have been shown to play an essential part in many cancers

Thus drugs that promote cell maturation may turn out to be at least as useful as those targeted to prevent cell proliferation (cytotoxic drugs). Interestingly, there is increasing evidence that aberrant signaling that has generally been associated with the development of cancer may also be associated with certain developmental disorders. For example, a number of mutations that lead to increased activation of the *Ras*-ERK MAPKinase pathway have been associated with diseases, such as neurofibromatosis 1 (defect in neurofibromin which

GENETIC MUTATIONS UNDERLYING DEVELOPMENT OF A COLORECTAL CANCER

Screening of colorectal cancer cells with DNA probes specific for known protooncogenes and tumor suppressor genes showed that 50% of these tumors had an activating point mutation in a *Ras* oncogene, and 75% of these cancers had an inactivating mutation in *p53*. Moreover, studies of familial adenomatous polyposis (FAP; see below) have shown that more than 70% of colon cancers have a mutation in the adenomatous polyposis coli (APC) gene. Indeed, it now seems clear that mutations inactivating APC may represent an early stage in the development of a colon cancer cell, because APC mutations can be detected at the same frequency in small benign polyps as in large malignant tumors. These APC mutations appear to promote the transformation of normal epithelium through a stage of hyperproliferative epithelium to early adenoma. The next stage seems to involve the activating mutation of *Ras* (rarely found in small polyps, but common in large polyps), which induces changes in cell differentiation typical of cell transformation (intermediate adenoma) and which allow the cells to grow in an anchorage-independent manner in culture. These changes are followed by a mutation in a tumor suppressor gene called 'deleted in colon carcinoma' (DCC), to generate a late adenoma that is converted to an adenocarcinoma by the subsequent loss of *p53*. Loss of the DNA-damage sensing function of *p53* allows the cells to accumulate, at a rapid rate, the further mutations required for metastasis.

Comment. Although these mutations appear to be the rate-limiting steps in a large number of colorectal cancers, it should be noted that other sequences of mutations can also generate this disease. Indeed, in about 15% of cases, patients with a hereditary syndrome called hereditary nonpolyposis colorectal cancer (HNPCC) have a mutation of the HNPCC gene that normally acts to repair mismatches in the nucleotide sequences of the DNA double helix. Thus, in such patients, the likelihood of the development of colorectal cancer is enhanced, as the HNPCC mutation decreases the fidelity of DNA replication and hence increases the tendency of the cells to undergo mutation.

THE PAPANICOLAOU OR 'PAP SMEAR' TEST OF THE UTERINE CERVIX

The epithelium of the uterine cervix resembles the epidermis of the skin, and comprises a proliferating basal layer that generates cells that differentiate into flat, keratin-rich cells that are eventually shed from the surface. Cancers of the uterine cervix are strongly associated with infection by human papilloma virus types 16 and 18 and arise from mutations in the basal epithelial cells, which are no longer then confined to the basal layer but invade the area normally occupied by the differentiated keratin-rich cells (dysplasia). These proliferating cells are shed at a less mature stage of differentiation than normal. Whereas the differentiated cells are characterized by their large size and highly condensed nuclei, the mutant cells have relatively large nuclei and little cytoplasm so that dysplasia can be identified in the Pap smear test, which simply involves microscopic examination of the morphology of a sample of cells scraped from the cervix. Dysplasia often remains stable or even spontaneously regresses. However, it may progress to a more serious lesion, called carcinoma in situ, in which the epithelium is entirely made up of undifferentiated proliferating cells with nuclei of variable size and shape. This lesion can be completely cured by surgery; however, in 20–30% of cases carcinoma in situ progresses over several years into a malignant cervical carcinoma.

Comment. Abnormal nuclear morphology is a key diagnostic tool of pathologists for identifying cancer, and correlates with the destabilization of karyotypes of cancer cells when they are cultured. These unstable karyotypes exhibit genes that become amplified or deleted, and chromosomes that are highly susceptible to loss, duplication, or translocation. These findings suggest that the cells have developed one or more mutations in the mechanisms regulating chromosomal replication, repair, recombination, or segregation, thereby facilitating the accumulation of the multiple mutations required for development of cancer.

Moreover, in order to bind to and traverse the basal lamina, the cells must express specific integrins to bind laminin, and type IV collagenase to digest the lamina.

is a *Ras* GAP) and Costello syndrome (H-*Ras*), which are characterized by craniofacial, cardiovascular and hematologic defects and impaired growth and development, including learning difficulties, as well as an increased propensity to develop a variety of tumors.

In order to metastasize, cells in a tumor must be able to escape their adhesion to neighboring cells, invade surrounding tissues, enter the blood or lymph systems and, finally, invade and colonize a new tissue. The mechanisms involved are as yet poorly understood but it appears that, in epithelia, loss of expression of the adhesion molecule, E-cadherin, has a key role in the ability of the cell to leave its parent tumor.

Oncogenes: mutant signal transducers

As mentioned above, mutations that lead to the uncontrolled proliferation of cancer cells can result either from disruption of the control of normal cell division or, alternatively, from a reduction in the normal processes of terminal differentiation or apoptosis.

This distinction is reflected by the two main groups of genes targeted for mutation: oncogenes and tumor suppressor genes (Table 43.2).

Oncogenes were first identified as viral genes that infect normal cells and transform them into tumor cells

Oncogenes, transcription factors, and tumor suppressor genes (antioncogenes)

Oncogene	Intracellular signaling role
overexpressed growth factors	*v-Sis* encodes a sequence almost identical to the active PDGF-β
	Int-2 and k-Fgf-hst are related to fibroblast growth factor (FGF)
overexpressed and/or constitutively active growth factor receptors	v-ErbB is analogous to the activated cytoplasmic domain of EGF-receptor (EGF-R)
	v-Fms is related to macrophage colony stimulating factor receptor (M-CSF-R)
	v-kit is related to PDGF-R
	Mas is related to the G-protein-coupled angiotensin receptor also, overexpression of normal receptors can lead to transformation
G-proteins	mutated Gs (*gsp*) in pituitary/thyroid tumors mutated Gi (*gip2*) in adrenocortical/ovarian tumors
	Ras: mutated in 30% of human tumors
kinases	Src, Abl: protein tyrosine kinases
	Raf: serine-threonine kinase
oncomodulin	calcium-binding protein similar to calmodulin, found only in cancer cells
growth regulation genes	*Jun* and *Fos*: transcription factors
	Myc: a transcription factor regulating Cdc25 protein tyrosine phosphatase
	Myb and *Mos*: regulate Gi/S-phase transition
	Cdc2: regulation of S/M-phase transition
	Bcl-2 family: cell survival
tumor suppressor genes	*p53*: most frequently mutated gene in human cancer; cell cycle and apoptosis regulator
	Rb gene; cell cycle regulator
	neurofibromatosis gene – analogous to *Ras* GTP-ase activating protein (GAP)

Table 43.2 **Factors involved in the uncontrolled proliferation of cancer cells.**

For example, the Rous sarcoma virus, which is a retrovirus that causes connective tissue tumors in chickens, will infect and transform fibroblast cells grown in cell culture. The transformed cells outgrow the normal cells and exhibit a number of growth abnormalities, such as a loss of cell contact-mediated inhibition of growth and loss of anchorage dependence of growth. In addition, the cells have a rounded appearance and can proliferate in the absence of growth factors. Moreover, the cells are immortal, do not senesce, and can induce tumor formation when injected into a suitable animal host.

The key to understanding cell transformation lies in the mutation of a normal cellular gene that controls cell growth. The use of mutant Rous sarcoma viruses that, despite multiplying normally, have lost the ability to transform host cells showed that it was the *Src* gene that was responsible for such cell transformation. The breakthrough in our understanding of how this single gene could transform cells in culture came when it became apparent that the viral oncogene was a mutated homolog of a normal cellular gene. This gene is now called the *c-Src* protooncogene and has been identified as a protein tyrosine kinase signal transducer involved in the normal control of cell growth. As expression of this gene is not essential to the survival of the retrovirus, it is likely that *Src* was accidentally incorporated by the virus from a previous host genome and was somehow mutated in the process. In the case of the Rous sarcoma virus, the introns normally present in c-*Src* are spliced out and, in addition, there are a number of mutations causing amino acid substitutions, resulting in a constitutively active enzyme.

Cell transformation can, however, also result from oncogenes that are not constitutively activated but rather, are overexpressed in an abnormally high number of copies, as a consequence of the gene being under the control of powerful promoters or enhancers in the viral genome. Alternatively, for retroviruses, DNA copies of the viral RNA inserted into the host genome at or near sites of protooncogenes (insertional mutation) can cause abnormal activation of these protooncogenes. In this situation, the altered genome is inherited by all progeny of the original host cell.

Most human tumors are nonviral in origin and arise from spontaneous or induced mutations. Approximately 85% of human tumors arise as a result of point or deletion mutations, rather than through viral involvement. These mutations may be spontaneous or induced by carcinogens or radiation, resulting in overexpression or hyperactivity of the protooncogenes. In addition, karyotyping of tumor cells has shown, for example, that the conversion of the *Abl* (tyrosine kinase) protooncogene into an oncogene in CML results from a chromosomal translocation between chromosomes 9 and 22, with breakpoints in the *Abl* and *Bcr* genes, respectively, leading to the generation of a chromosome called the Philadelphia chromosome. This translocation results in the generation of a fusion protein comprising the N-terminus of *Bcr* and the C-terminus of *Abl*. The *Abl* kinase domain of this fusion protein is hyperactive and drives the abnormal proliferation of a clone of hemopoietic progenitors in the bone marrow. In other cases, the translocation brings the oncogene under the control of an inappropriate promoter. For example, in Burkitt's lymphoma, overexpression of the *Myc* gene occurs through its translocation into the vicinity of one of the Ig loci. Because *Myc* normally acts as a nuclear proliferative signal, overexpression of *Myc* induces the cell

Selected inherited cancer syndromes		
Syndrome	**Cancer**	**Gene product**
Familial retinoblastoma	retinoblastoma osteosarcoma	Rb 1: cell cycle and transcriptional regulation
Li-Fraumeni	sarcomas, adrenocortical carcinomas carcinomas of breast, lung, larynx, and colon brain tumors leukemia	p53: transcription factor DNA damage and stress
Familial adenomatous polyposis (FAP)	colorectal cancer: colorectal adenomas, duodenal and gastric tumors, jaw osteomas, and desmoid tumors (Gardner syndrome), medulloblastoma (Turcot syndrome)	APC: regulation of β-catenin, microtubule binding
Wiedmann–Beckwith syndrome	Wilms' tumor, organomegaly, hemihypertrophy, hepatoblastoma, adrenocortical cancer	p57/KIP2: cell cycle regulator
Neurofibromatosis type 1 (NF1)	neurofibrosarcoma AML brain tumors	GTP-ase activating protein (GAP) for *p21*Ras
Hereditary papillary renal cancer	renal cancer	Met HGF-receptor
Familial melanoma	melanoma pancreatic cancer dysplastic nevi atypical moles	*p16* (CDK): inhibitor of cyclin-dependent kinase (CDK4/6) cyclin-dependent kinase (CDK4)

Table 43.3 **Selected inherited cancer syndromes.** AML, acute myeloid leukemia; HGF, hepatocyte growth factor; KIP2, 57 kDa inhibitor of cyclin-CDK complexes.

to divide, even under conditions that would normally dictate growth arrest.

Oncogene actions are dominant and mutation in only one allele is therefore sufficient to transform culture cells

Studies in transgenic mice overexpressing mutiple oncogenes have illustrated the point, made above, that human cancers are usually generated after the accumulation of mutations over several years. For example, transgenic mice overexpressing either the *Myc* or *Ras* oncogenes typically exhibit some tissues that are abnormally large. Occasionally, with age, some of these mice develop a few tumors, in a manner that is consistent with the expression of an inherited oncogene that increases the risk of accumulating further mutations and, hence, of initiating cancers. However, the vast majority of these transgenic cells do not develop any cancers. In contrast, double transgenic mice overexpressing both the *Myc* and the *Ras* oncogenes develop cancers at a much greater rate – a phenomenon known as oncogene collaboration. An example of such synergistic action in human cancers is provided by B cell lymphoma, which relies on cooperation between overexpressed *Myc* (to drive inappropriate cell division) and *Bcl-2* (to inhibit apoptosis and promote B cell survival).

Tumor suppressor genes

Subversion of the cell cycle

Mutations in tumor suppressor genes are recessive and, thus, mutations in both copies of the gene are usually required for transformation. As it is very difficult to identify the loss of function of a single gene in a cell, much of the initial information relating to tumor suppressor genes was obtained by studying a range of inherited cancer syndromes (Table 43.3).

The retinoblastoma (Rb) gene

The rare human cancer retinoblastoma affords a good example of a cancer syndrome that has been an important source of information on tumor suppressor genes. In this cancer, neural progenitor cells in the immature retina are transformed by an unusually low number of mutations. Retinoblastoma occurs in childhood, with an incidence of about 1 in 20000. In the hereditary form of the disease, multiple tumors occur, affecting both eyes, whereas in the (very rare) nonhereditary form, only one eye is affected by a single tumor. Sufferers of both forms of the disease were found to

FAMILIAL ADENOMATOUS POLYPOSIS (FAP) AND COLON CANCER

Investigation of inherited cancer genes has advanced our understanding of somatic mutations in sporadic cancers and the function of these signaling elements in the normal regulation of cell growth. FAP, a rare condition affecting 1 in 7000 in the USA, is characterized by inactivating germline mutations in the APC gene. Although germline mutations in APC are infrequent, somatic mutations in APC are present in more than 70% of adenomatous polyps and carcinomas of the colon and rectum. APC acts to promote degradation of the protein, β-catenin, in normal cells; β-catenin, through its interactions with transcription factors, drives transcriptional activation. Thus, in APC-mutated cells, β-catenin accumulates and binds and activates transcription factors, resulting in deregulated growth control and cancer. Additional evidence for a key role for β-catenin signaling in cancer development has been provided by cancer cells bearing β-catenin mutations that render β-catenin insensitive to APC-mediated degradation and repression of transcriptional activation.

Comment. Studies of the use of aspirin in humans have suggested that inhibitors of cyclooxygenase (COX: enzymes that have a key role in the conversion of the inflammatory mediator, arachidonic acid, to various prostaglandins; see Chapter 40) can alter the natural history of colon cancer. A randomized, double-blind trial showed that aspirin prevented adenomas from arising in patients with previous colorectal cancer. Indeed, not only does the risk of the disease appear to be reduced in regular users of aspirin, but also the risk of fatal or metastatic colon cancer appears to be reduced by up to 50% in chronic users of the drug. This effect of aspirin appears to result from inhibition of COX-2, which is expressed at high levels in most colon tumors, and reflects the important roles that prostaglandins have in the pathogenesis of cancer as a result of their modulation of a wide range of cellular responses such as mitogenesis, cellular adhesion, immune surveillance, and apoptosis.

have a deletion of a specific band on chromosome 13; analysis of this genetic defect in individual patients showed that patients with the hereditary disease had a deletion or loss-of-function mutation of the Rb gene in every cell. This mutation predisposed these cells to become cancerous, because a single somatic mutation to knock out the remaining copy of Rb gene was sufficient to initiate a cancer. In fact, in approximately 70% of cases, the second Rb gene and its flanking regions on the chromosome are either completely deleted or replaced with the corresponding regions of the defective chromosome by a process of mitotic recombination (loss of heterozygosity). In contrast, although patients with the nonhereditary disease show no mutations in either copy of their Rb genes in noncancerous cells, both copies are defective in their cancer cells. This explains the rarity of the nonhereditary disease, because somatic mutations in both copies of Rb in a single retinal cell are required for transformation. Given the key role of the retinoblastoma protein, Rb, in the negative regulation of cell cycle progression (see above), it is perhaps not surprising that loss of Rb function plays such a major part in tumor progression. Thus, although retinoblastoma is a rare disease, mutations of Rb are not and occur in many of the most common cancers such as lung, breast, and bladder carcinomas.

Tumor suppressor protein *p53*

p53 is a cell cycle regulator that has a key role not only in regulating G1/S-phase cell cycle progression but also in monitoring DNA damage

Individuals with only one functional copy of the *p53* gene are predisposed to develop a wide range of tumors, including sarcomas, carcinomas of the lung, breast, larynx and colon, brain tumors and leukemias. In common with retinoblastoma, this syndrome, called Li-Fraumeni syndrome, is rare and tumor cells in affected patients have defects in both copies of *p53*. Again like retinoblastoma, although the Li-Fraumeni syndrome is rare, the incidence of *p53* mutations in common cancers is extremely high. Deletion of *p53*, in addition to allowing uncontrolled cell cycle progression, also permits replication of damaged DNA, leading to further carcinogenic mutations or gene amplification; it is perhaps not surprising, therefore, that the most common genetic lesion in cancer is found in *p53*.

Summary

- Most protooncogenes and tumor suppressor genes that have been identified function in signal transduction to mimic the effects of persistent mitogenic stimulation, thereby uncoupling cells from normal external controls.

- These signaling pathways converge on the machinery that controls passage of the cell through the G1-phase and prevent cell cycle exit.

- In addition, other genes, many of which are targeted by cancer-specific chromosomal translocations, lead to aberrant lineage-specific differentiation and developmental decisions that would normally induce apoptosis. The two tumor suppressor proteins, p53 and Rb, which have key roles in determining cell cycle progression and apoptosis, and the genes coding for these proteins, are most frequently disrupted in cancer cells.

Further reading

Bensaad K, Vousden KH. p53: new roles in metabolism. *Trends Cell Biol* 2007;**17**: 286–291.

Branzei D, Foiani M. Regulation of DNA repair throughout the cell cycle. *Nat Rev Mol Cell Biol* 2008;**9**:297–308.

Meier P, Vousden KH. Lucifer's labyrinth – ten years of path finding in cell death. *Mol Cell* 2007;**28**:746–754.

Rozengurt E. Mitogenic signalling pathways induced by G-protein coupled receptors. *J Cell Physiol* 2007;**213**:589–602.

Youle R, Strasser A. The BCL-2 protein family: opposing activities that mediate cell death. *Nat Rev Mol Cell Biol* 2008;**9**:47–59.

Websites

Virtual Library of Cell Biology (cell cycle, apoptosis, etc.): www.vlib.org/Science/Cell_Biology

Kimball's biology pages: www.biology-pages.info

Nature's Encyclopedia of Life Sciences: www.els.net

Genetics of Cancer Resource Center: www.intouchlive.com/cancergenetics

44. Aging

J W Baynes

LEARNING OBJECTIVES

After reading this chapter you should be able to:

- Describe the relationship between aging and disease.
- Explain the Gompertz plot and how it describes the rate of aging of different species.
- Differentiate between biologic and chemical theories of aging.
- Explain the precepts of the free radical theory of aging, including identification of characteristic oxidation products that accumulate in long-lived proteins with age.
- Outline the evidence that the rate of mutation of DNA is an important determinant of the rate of aging.
- Outline the evidence in support of the mitochondrial theory of aging and describe how this theory interfaces with the free radical theory of aging.
- Describe the etiology and pathology characteristic of several diseases of accelerated aging.
- Describe the effects of caloric restriction on the rate of aging of rodents.

INTRODUCTION

Aging may be defined as the time-dependent deterioration in function of an organism. While it has broad-based physiologic effects, aging is fundamentally the result of changes in cellular structure and function, biochemistry and metabolism (Table 44.1). The result of aging, even healthy aging, is increased susceptibility to disease and increased probability of death – the endpoint of aging. However, aging is not a disease. Diseases affect a fraction of the population; aging affects all of us, whether it is programmed or stochastic.

With the aging of the population, gerontology and geriatric medicine are becoming increasingly important. This chapter presents an overview on biochemical and physiologic changes associated with aging, in general, and with the aging of specific organ systems. It includes a review of current theories on aging (there are several theories and, in general, the more theories there are, the less we really understand about something) and concludes with a discussion of the relationship between cancer and aging and an update on approaches to lifespan extension.

Aging of complex systems

Excluding genetic defects, childhood disease and accidents, humans survive until about age 50 with limited maintenance requirements or risk of death; then we become increasingly frail and our death rate increases with time, reaching a maximum at about age 76. Our lifespan is affected by our genetics and our environmental exposure, and our death is usually attributable to failure of a critical organ system (cardiovascular, renal, pulmonary, etc.). The capacity of these interdependent physiologic systems usually declines as a linear function of age, leading to an exponential increase in our age-specific death rate (Fig. 44.1). Historically, improvements in health care and environment have resulted in 'rectangularization' of the survival curve – our mean lifespan has increased but without a significant effect on our maximum lifespan (see Fig. 44.1A).

The Hayflick limit – replicative senescence

Differentiated cells from animals undergo only a limited number of cell divisions (population doublings) in tissue

Changes in biochemistry and physiology during aging	
Biochemical	**Physiologic**
Basal metabolic rate	Lung expansion volume
Protein turnover	Renal filtration capacity (glomerular)
Glucose tolerance	Renal concentration capacity (tubular)
Reproductive capacity	Cardiovascular performance
Telomere shortening	Musculoskeletal system
Oxidative phosphorylation	Nerve conduction velocity Endocrine and exocrine systems Immunological defenses Sensory systems (vision, audition)

Table 44.1 **Decline in biochemical and physiologic systems with age.**

culture, unless they become transformed to cancer cells by mutation or infection with certain viruses. The number of potential cell divisions is greater in longer-lived animals, suggesting a relationship between cell division potential and longevity. Human neonatal fibroblasts will divide about 60 times, then enter a non-dividing state, while fibroblasts from mice and rats, which have shorter lifespans, undergo fewer cell divisions in vitro. Cells from younger donors have greater replicative capacity and a greater number of cell divisions in cell culture, but the number of dividing cells decreases with age. This limited doubling capacity, described by Dr Leonard Hayflick, is known as the Hayflick limit. The relevance of the Hayflick limit to human aging is still debated – certainly human cells retain some replicative capacity, even at advanced age, and major tissues, such as muscle and nerve, are largely postmitotic, i.e. not actively dividing. However, changes in the metabolism of senescent cells, including decreased responsiveness to hormones and the decline in their synthetic and degradative capacities, e.g. in the immunologic and reticuloendothelial systems, may affect our adaptability and susceptibility to stress and age-related diseases, placing limits on our lifespan.

Mathematical models of aging

In the early 19th century, Gompertz observed that the age-specific death rate of humans increased exponentially after 35 years of age, and that human survival curves could be modeled by what is now known as the Gompertz equation (Fig. 44.2):

$$m_t = Ae^{\alpha t}$$

The term m_t is the age-specific death rate at age t; α is the slope, the effect of time on the death rate; and A, the y-axis intercept, is the death rate at birth. The Gompertz–Makeham equation:

$$m(t) = Ae^{\alpha t} + B$$

adds a constant, B, to correct for the age-independent death rate, e.g. as a result of infant mortality or accidents, and provides a better fit to actuarial data.

The Gompertz plots in Figure 44.2 illustrate the time-dependent changes in death rate for three different species of vertebrates and for flies raised at different temperatures. Shorter-lived mammals have a greater age-adjusted rate of death (α), while the death rate for poikilotherms varies with ambient temperature – flies live longer when grown at lower temperatures. This observation has been interpreted as evidence for 'rate of living' or 'wear and tear' theories of aging. Flies, being more active at higher temperature, consume more energy and die more rapidly. Flies that are restrained, e.g. in a matchbox, rather than a large carboy, also live longer; wingless flies live longer; and male flies, segregated from females, also live longer. In each case, in small enclosures, without

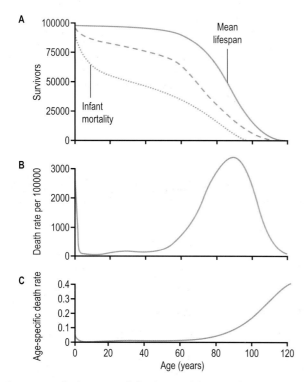

Fig. 44.1 **Survival curve and death rate.** (A) Mean lifespan is defined as the age at which 50% of a population survives (or has died). The negative slope of the survival curve reaches a maximum at the mean lifespan of a species. The dashed line describes a survival curve in the Third World where infant mortality and disease significantly decrease mean lifespan. The dotted line describes the survival curve for the United States in the early part of the 20th century. The solid line applies to 21st-century Europe. (B) The death rate reaches a maximum at the mean lifespan. (C) The age-specific death rate, defined as the number of deaths per time at a given age, e.g. deaths per 100 000 persons of a specific age per year, increases exponentially with age. The lifespan or maximum lifespan potential (MLSP) is defined as the maximum age attainable by a member of the population, which is about 120 years for humans.

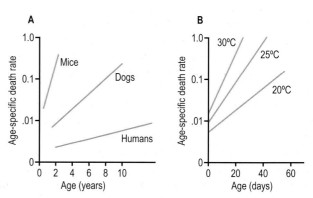

Fig. 44.2 **Gompertz plots for humans and other species.** (A) Humans and other vertebrates. (B) Flies raised at various temperatures (adapted from the work of Prof RS Sohal).

wings, and in the absence of the opposite sex, male flies are less active, have lower basal metabolic rates, and have longer mean and maximum lifespans. None of these strategies for lifespan extension is applicable to humans.

THEORIES OF AGING

Theories of aging can be divided into two general categories: biologic and chemical

Biologic theories treat aging as a genetically controlled event, determined by the programmed expression or repression of genetic information. Aging and death are seen as the orchestrated endstage of birth, growth, maturation and reproduction. Apoptosis (programmed cell death) and thymic involution are examples of genetically programmed events at the level of cells and organs, and the decline in the immunologic, neuroendocrine and reproductive systems may be seen, in a broader context, as evidence for action of a biologic clock affecting the integrated functions of an organism. Biologic theories attribute differences in lifespan to interspecies differences in genetics but also provide an explanation for the observation that there is a genetic component to longevity within a species, e.g. in families with a history of longevity. Differences in lifespan among species are also closely correlated with the efficiency of DNA repair mechanisms. Longer-lived species have more efficient DNA repair processes (Fig. 44.3). Numerous diseases of accelerated aging (progeria) also illustrate the importance of genetics and maintenance of the integrity of the genome during aging.

Chemical theories of aging treat it as a somatic process resulting from cumulative damage to biomolecules. At one extreme, the error-catastrophe theory proposes that aging is the result of cumulative errors in the machinery for replication, repair, transcription, and translation of genetic information. Eventually, errors in critical enzymes, such as DNA and RNA polymerases or enzymes involved in the synthesis and turnover of proteins, gradually affect the fidelity of expression of genetic information and permit the accumulation of altered proteins. The propagation of errors and resultant accumulation of dysfunctional macromolecules lead eventually to the collapse of the system. Consistent with this theory, increasing amounts of immunologically detectable, but denatured or modified, functionally inactive enzymes accumulate in cells as a function of age.

More general chemical theories treat aging as the result of chronic, cumulative chemical (nonenzymatic) modification, insults or damage to all biomolecules (Table 44.2). Like rust or corrosion, the accumulation of damage with age gradually affects function. This damage is most apparent in long-lived tissue proteins, such as lens crystallins and extracellular collagens, which accumulate chemical modifications with age. These proteins gradually brown with age as a result of formation of a wide range of conjugated

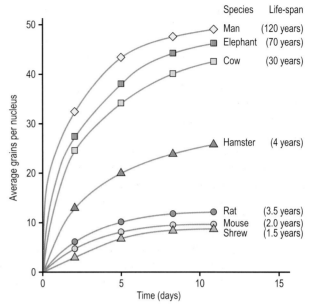

Fig. 44.3 **Relationship between DNA repair activity and longevity.** Fibroblasts from various species were irradiated briefly, forming thymine dimers and thymine glycol (Chapter 31). The oxidized bases are removed and replaced by excision repair. DNA repair was assessed by the rate of incorporation of a [³H]thymidine tracer into DNA by autoradiography (adapted from Hart RW, Setlow RB. Correlation between deoxyribonucleic acid excision-repair and life-span in a number of mammalian species. *Proc Natl Acad Sci USA* 1974;**71**:2169–2173).

Chemistry and aging		
Protein modification	**DNA modification and mutation**	**Other**
crosslinking	oxidation	lipofuscin
oxidation	depurination	inactive enzymes
deamidation	substitutions	
D-aspartate	insertions and deletions	
protein carbonyls	inversions and transpositions	
glycoxidation		
lipoxidation		

Table 44.2 **Age-dependent chemical changes in biomolecules.** Long-lived proteins, such as lens crystallins and tissue collagens, accumulate damage with age. Modification and crosslinking of proteins occurs as a result of nonoxidative (deamidation, racemization) or oxidative (protein carbonyls) mechanisms or by reactions of proteins with products of carbohydrate or lipid peroxidation (glycoxidation, lipoxidation). Damage to DNA is often silent, i.e. modified forms of nucleotides may not accumulate, but the damage increases in the form of mutations resulting from errors in repair.

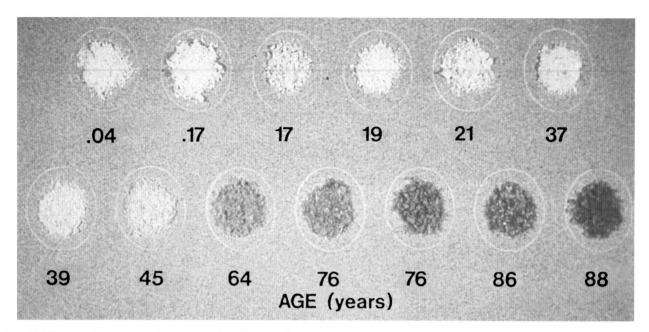

Fig. 44.4 **Changes in lens protein and costal cartilage with age.** Browning is a characteristic feature of the aging of proteins, not just in the lens, which is exposed to sunlight, but also in tissue collagens throughout the body. Crosslinking of proteins also increases with browning. Crosslinking contributes to the gradual insolubilization of lens protein with age. Aggregates of lens protein disperse light, contributing to the development of 'senile' cataracts. Crosslinking of articular and vascular collagens decreases the resilience of vertebral disks and compliance of the vascular wall with age. These changes in extracellular proteins, shown here for costal collagen, are similar to changes induced by reaction of carbohydrates and lipids with protein during the cooking of foods, a process known as the Maillard or browning reaction. At one level, humans have been described as low-temperature ovens, operating at 37°C, with long cooking cycles (~75 years). Many of the Maillard reaction products detected in the crust of bread and pretzels have been identified in human crystallins and collagens, and increase with age. (See also discussion of diabetic complications in Chapter 21.)

compounds with absorbance in the yellow-red region of the spectrum (Fig. 44.4). Chemical damage to the integrity of the genome also occurs, but is more difficult to quantify because of the efficiency of repair processes that excise and repair modified nucleotides. As noted in Table 44.2, there are a number of silent consequences of DNA damage. This damage is primarily endogenous but is enhanced by xenobiotic and environmental agents.

Organ system theories of aging incorporate various aspects of the above theories. These theories attribute aging to the failure of integrative systems, such as the immunologic, neurologic, endocrine or circulatory system. While they do not assign a specific cause, these theories integrate biologic and chemical theories, acknowledging both genetic and environmental contributions to aging.

The free radical theory of aging

The most widely accepted chemical theory of aging is the free radical theory of aging (FRTA). This treats aging as the result of cumulative oxidative damage to biomolecules: DNA, RNA, protein, lipids, and glycoconjugates. From the viewpoint of the FRTA, longer-lived organisms have lower rates of production of reactive oxygen species (ROS; Chapter 37), better antioxidant defenses, and more efficient repair or turnover processes. While it is a chemical theory, the FRTA does not ignore the importance of genetics and biology in limiting the production of ROS, and in antioxidant and repair mechanisms. It also interfaces with other theories of aging, such as the rate of living theory because the rate of generation of ROS is a function of the overall rate and/or extent of oxygen consumption, and the crosslinkage theory because some products of ROS damage crosslink protein. Finally, as a chemical hypothesis, the FRTA does not exclude cumulative chemical damage, independent of ROS, such as racemization and deamidation of amino acids, but focuses on ROS as the primary source of damage and the fundamental cause of aging.

The FRTA is supported by the inverse correlation between basal metabolic rate (rate of oxygen consumption per unit weight) and maximum lifespan of mammals, and by evidence of increased oxidative damage to proteins with age. Protein carbonyl groups, such as glutamic and aminoadipic acid semialdehyde, formed by oxidative deamination of arginine and lysine, respectively, are formed in proteins exposed to ROS. The steady-state level of protein carbonyls in intracellular proteins increases logarithmically with age and at a rate inversely proportional to the lifespan of species.

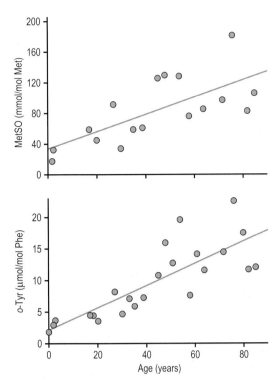

Fig. 44.5 **Accumulation of amino acid oxidation products in human skin collagen with age.** Methionine is oxidized to methionine sulfoxide (MetSO) by HOCl or H_2O_2; *ortho*-tyrosine is a product of hydroxyl radical addition to phenylalanine. Despite a 100-fold difference in their rate of accumulation in collagen, levels of MetSO and *o*-tyrosine correlate strongly with one another, indicating that multiple ROS contribute to oxidative damage to proteins (adapted from Wells-Knecht MC *et al.* Age-dependent accumulation of *ortho*-tyrosine and methionine sulfoxide in human skin collagen is not increased in diabetes: evidence against a generalized increase in oxidative stress in diabetes. *J Clin Invest* 1997;**100**:839–846).

Protein carbonyls are also much higher in fibroblasts from patients with progeria (accelerated aging), e.g. Werner's or Hutchinson-Gilford syndromes, compared to age-matched subjects. Similar concentrations of protein carbonyls are also present in tissues of old rats and elderly humans, arguing that similar changes occur at old age in a range of organisms, regardless of the difference in their lifespans.

Figure 44.5 illustrates the accumulation of two relatively stable amino acid oxidation products in human skin collagen: methionine sulfoxide and *ortho*-tyrosine. These compounds are formed by different mechanisms involving different ROS (Chapter 37) and are present at significantly different concentrations in skin collagen, but increase in concert with age. Other amino acid modifications that accumulate in skin collagen with age include advanced glycoxidation and lipoxidation endproducts (AGE/ALEs), such as carboxymethyllysine and pentosidine (Fig. 44.6 and see Fig. 21.16), and D-aspartate.

D-aspartate is a nonoxidative modification of protein that is formed by spontaneous, age-dependent racemization of L-aspartate, the natural form of the amino acid in protein.

PROGERIAS: ACCELERATED AGING RESULTING FROM DEFECTS IN DNA REPAIR

Certain genetic diseases are considered models of accelerated aging (progeria). These monogenic diseases display many, but never all, of the features of normal aging; few progeric patients develop dementia or age-related pathologies, such as Alzheimer's disease. The progerias are sometimes described as caricatures of aging, but are useful models for understanding the aging process. Werner's and Bloom's syndromes are autosomal recessive diseases caused by mutation of distinct DNA helicase genes which have a role in repair of damaged DNA. Patients with Werner's syndrome appear normal during childhood, but stop growing in their teens. They gradually show many symptoms of premature aging, including graying and loss of hair, thinning of skin, development of early cataracts, impaired glucose tolerance and diabetes, atherosclerosis and osteoporosis, and increased rates of cancer. Death usually occurs in their mid-40s from cardiovascular disease. Fibroblasts from Werner's patients divide only about 20 times in cell culture and have higher levels of protein-bound carbonyl groups, an indicator of increased oxidative stress.

Bloom's syndrome is characterized by increased frequency of chromosomal breaks, dwarfism, photosensitivity and increased frequency of cancer and leukemia; death occurs typically in the mid-20s. Ataxia-telangiectasia, or fragile chromosome syndrome, is associated with increased loss of telomeres with cell division and deficiency in repair of double-strand DNA breaks. It is caused by a defect in a protein kinase involved in signal transduction, cell cycle control and DNA repair. Hutchinson-Gilford syndrome is a severe, pediatric form of progeria. Patients have many of the symptoms of Werner's syndrome, but the symptoms appear at an earlier age and death usually occurs by the mid-20s. This syndrome is caused by a defect in a gene for lamin, a component of the nuclear envelope. Hutchinson-Gilford is one of several distinct syndromes associated with lamin mutations, which cause an increase in nuclear fragility and aberrant mRNA splicing; as in Werner's syndrome, cultured fibroblasts become prematurely senescent. These progeric diseases suggest that efficient repair of DNA is essential for normal aging.

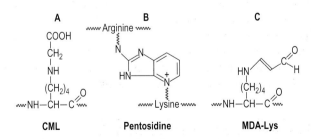

Fig. 44.6 **Structure of major advanced glycoxidation and lipoxidation endproducts (AGE/ALEs).** (A) The AGE/ALE, $N^{\varepsilon-}$(carboxymethyl)lysine (CML), which is formed during both carbohydrate and lipid peroxidation reactions. (B) The AGE pentosidine, a fluorescent crosslink in proteins. (C) The ALE, malondialdehyde-lysine (MDA-Lys), a reactive ALE that may proceed to form aminoenimine (RNHCH=CHCH=NR) crosslinks in proteins (see also Fig. 21.16).

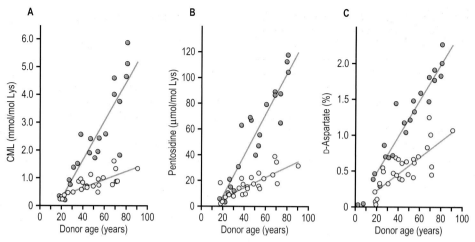

Fig. 44.7 **Accumulation of advanced glycoxidation and lipoxidation endproducts (AGE/ALEs) and D-aspartate in collagens with age.** N$^{\varepsilon-}$(carboxymethyl)lysine (CML) is formed by oxidative mechanisms from glycated proteins or reaction of glucose, ascorbate or lipid peroxidation products with protein. The fluorescent crosslink pentosidine is formed by oxidative reaction of glucose or ascorbate with proteins. D-Aspartate is formed nonoxidatively by racemization of L-aspartate residues in protein. Differences in rate of accumulation of both oxidative and nonoxidative biomarkers are attributable to differences in rates of turnover of collagens (adapted from Verzijl N et al. Effect of collagen turnover on the accumulation of advanced glycation endproducts. *J Biol Chem* 2000;**275**:39027–39031).

The more rapid turnover of skin, compared to articular, collagen yields a lower rate of accumulation of D-aspartate in skin collagen with age and also explains the difference in rates of accumulation of AGE/ALEs in skin versus articular collagen. AGE/ALEs are even higher in lens crystallins, which have the slowest rate of turnover among proteins in the body. Deamidation of asparagine and glutamine is another nonoxidative chemical modification that increases with age in proteins; it has been described primarily in intracellular proteins.

The rate of accumulation of these modifications depends on the rate of turnover of the collagens (Fig. 44.7) and is accelerated by hyperglycemia and hyperlipidemia in diabetes and atherosclerosis. The increase in AGE/ALEs and oxidative crosslinking of collagen is thought to impair the turnover and contribute to the thickening of basement membranes with age. Increased age-adjusted levels of AGE/ALEs in collagen are implicated in the pathogenesis of complications of diabetes and atherosclerosis. These products are also increased together in the brain in various neurodegenerative diseases, including Alzheimer's and Parkinson's disease and Creutzfeld-Jakob (prion) disease.

The age pigment lipofuscin is a less well-characterized but characteristic biomarker of aging. It accumulates in the form of fluorescent granules, derived from lysosomes, in the cytoplasm of postmitotic cells at a rate that is inversely related to species lifespan. It is considered the accumulated, indigestible debris of reactions between lipid peroxides and proteins. Lipofuscin may account for 10–15% of the volume of cardiac muscle and neuronal cells at advanced age, and its rate of deposition in cardiac myocytes in cell culture is accelerated by growth under hyperoxic conditions. In flies, the rate of accumulation of lipofuscin varies directly with ambient

temperature and activity, and inversely with lifespan, consistent with the effects of these variables on lifespan (see Fig. 44.2B).

In summary, there is a wide range of chemical modifications, both oxidative and nonoxidative, that accumulate in proteins with age. While attention is often focused on modification of protein, the real damage from free radicals and oxidative stress is at the level of the genome; if the DNA is not repaired correctly, the cell will die, its capacity may be impaired or the damage will be propagated. Damage to DNA accumulates not in the form of modified nucleic acids but as chemically 'silent' errors in repair – insertions, deletions, substitutions, transpositions and inversions of DNA sequences – that affect the expression and structure of proteins. Because repair is fairly efficient in humans compared to other animals, and the composition of DNA does not change on repair, mutations in DNA are not detectable in tissues by conventional analytic techniques. However, the presence of oxidized pyrimidines and purines in urine provides evidence of chronic oxidative damage to the genome.

Mitochondrial theories of aging

Mitochondrial theories of aging are a blend of biologic and chemical theories, treating aging as the result of chemical damage to mitochondrial DNA (mtDNA). Mitochondria contain proteins specified by both nuclear and mitochondrial DNA but only 13 mitochondrial proteins are encoded by mitochondrial DNA. While this may seem trivial, these include essential subunits of the three proton pumps and ATP synthase. MtDNA is especially sensitive to mutations: mitochondria are the major site of ROS production in the

BIOMARKERS OF OXIDATIVE STRESS AND AGING

Advanced glycoxidation and lipoxidation endproducts (AGE/ALEs) are carbohydrate- and lipid-derived chemical (nonenzymatic) modifications and crosslinks in protein. They are formed by reaction of proteins with products of oxidation of carbohydrates and lipids (see Fig. 44.6). Some compounds, such as N^ε-(carboxymethyl)lysine (CML), may be formed from either carbohydrates or lipids; others, such as pentosidine, are formed only from carbohydrates, and others, such as the malondialdehyde adduct to lysine, are formed exclusively from lipids. Carbohydrate sources of AGEs include glucose, ascorbate, and glycolytic intermediates; ALEs are derived from oxidation of polyunsaturated fatty acids in phospholipids. Lysine, histidine and cysteine residues are the major sites of AGE/ALE formation in protein. Over 30 different AGE/ALEs have been detected in tissue proteins, and many of these are known to increase with age. AGE/ALEs are useful biomarkers of the aging of proteins and their exposure to oxidative stress.

ALZHEIMER'S DISEASE: OXIDATIVE STRESS IN NEURODEGENERATIVE DISEASE

Alzheimer's disease (AD) is the most common form of progressive cognitive deterioration in the elderly. It is characterized microscopically by the appearance of neurofibrillary tangles and senile plaques in cortical regions of the brain. The tangles are localized inside neurones, and are rich in τ (tau) protein, which is derived from microtubules; it is hyperphosphorylated and polyubiquitinated. Plaques are extracellular aggregates, localized around amyloid deposits, formed from insoluble peptides derived from a family of amyloid precursor proteins. AD affects primarily cholinergic neurones, and drugs that inhibit the degradation of acetylcholine within synapses are a mainstay of therapy. A similar approach is used for preservation of dopamine in dopaminergic neurones in Parkinson's disease, i.e. by inhibiting the degradative enzyme, monoamine oxidase. Several studies have shown that both AGEs and ALEs are increased in tangles and plaques in brain of AD patients, compared with age-matched controls. Other indicators of generalized oxidative stress in the AD brain include increased levels of protein carbonyls, nitrotyrosine and 8-OH-deoxyguanosine, all detected by immunohistochemical methods. The amyloid protein is toxic to neurones in cell culture and appears to provoke oxidative stress and inflammatory responses in glial cells. Significant quantities of decompartmentalized, redox-active iron are also detectable histologically in the AD brain and can be removed reversibly (in vitro) by treatment with chelators, such as desferrioxamine. Based on these data, oxidative stress is strongly implicated in the development and/or progression of AD, and chelators are being evaluated clinically for treatment of AD. Epidemiologic studies also indicate that long-term treatment with nonsteroidal antiinflammatory drugs, such as ibuprofen and Tylenol, may reduce the risk of AD and delay its onset or slow its progression.

AGING OF THE CIRCULATORY SYSTEM

The extracellular matrix of the aorta and major arteries becomes thicker and more highly crosslinked with age, contributing to both the decrease in elasticity and the capacity of the endothelium to dilate blood vessels in response to physical and chemical stimuli. These changes occur naturally with age, independent of pathology, but may account for the increase in cardiovascular risk in the elderly. AGEs and ALEs are implicated in the crosslinking of the vascular extracellular matrix, explaining the age-adjusted increase in arterial crosslinking in diabetes and dyslipidemia. A new class of drugs, known as AGE-breakers, is being evaluated clinically for reversal of increased vascular stiffness in aging and disease.

cell (see Fig. 37.4), mtDNA is not protected by a sheath of histones, and mitochondria have limited capacity for DNA repair.

Mitochondrial diseases commonly involve defects of energy metabolism, including the pyruvate dehydrogenase complex, pyruvate carboxylase, electron transport complexes, ATP synthase, and enzymes of ubiquinone biosynthesis. These defects can be caused by mutations in both nuclear and mitochondrial DNA, but mtDNA suffers many more mutations than nuclear DNA. Such defects often result in the accumulation of lactic acid because of impaired oxidative phosphorylation, and may cause cell death, especially in skeletal (myopathies) and cardiac muscles (cardiomyopathies) and nerve (encephalopathies), all of which are heavily dependent on oxidative metabolism. The number of mitochondria and multiple copies of the mitochondrial genome in the cell may provide some protection against mitochondrial dysfunction as a result of mutation, but loss of fully functional mitochondria, and sometimes the number of mitochondria, is a characteristic feature of aging.

GENETIC MODELS OF INCREASED LIFESPAN

The effect of genetics on longevity is readily apparent in animal models. Different strains of mice, for example, vary by more than twofold in lifespan, and there are also significant differences in the lifespan of male and female mice of the same strain raised under identical conditions. Deficiencies in some hormones or defects in their receptors or postreceptor signaling pathways have a significant effect on mouse lifespan. The most profound effects are observed in Ames and Snell dwarf mice. These mice have different pituitary defects, both resulting in negligible secretion of growth hormone

TELOMERES: A CLOCK OF AGING

Telomeres are the repetitive sequences at the ends of chromosomal DNA, typically thousands of copies of short, highly redundant, repetitive DNA, TTAGGG in humans (Chapter 31). DNA polymerase requires a double-stranded template for replication; RNA primers at the 5' end of the template serve to initiate DNA synthesis. However, at the extreme ends of the chromosomes, DNA synthesis is restricted, because there are no sequences further upstream for DNA primase engagement. Therefore, each round of chromosome replication results in chromosome shortening. The enzyme telomerase is a reverse transcriptase containing an RNA with a sequence complementary to the telomere DNA. It functions to maintain the length of telomeres at the 3'-end of chromosomes. Telomerase is found in fetal tissues, adult germ cells and in tumor cells. but the somatic cells of multicellular organisms lack telomerase activity. This has led to the hypothesis that shortening of the telomere may contribute to the Hayflick limit and is involved in aging of multicellular organisms. Increased expression of telomerase in human cells results in elongated telomeres and an increase in the longevity of those cells by at least 20 cell doublings. Cells from individuals with premature aging diseases (progeria) also have short telomeres. In contrast, cancer cells, which are immortal, express an active telomerase activity. All of these observations suggest that the decrease in telomere length is associated with cellular senescence and aging. Knockout mice, in which the telomerase gene has been deleted, have chromosomes lacking detectable telomeres. These mice have high frequencies of aneuploidy and chromosomal abnormalities. The disease, autosomal dyskeratosis congenita, features a mutation in the telomerase locus, with inability of somatic cells to reconstitute their telomeres, and hence loss of epidermis and hematopoietic marrow. This disease has many of the characteristics of accelerated aging.

AGING OF MUSCLE: DAMAGE TO MITOCHONDRIAL DNA

Old age is characterized by a general decrease in skeletal muscle mass (sarcopenia) and strength, as a result of a decrease in both the number of motoneurones and the number and size of myofibers. The fiber loss is accompanied by an increase in interstitial, fibrous connective tissue, and a reduction in capillary density, which limits the blood supply. The decrease in muscle mass and strength contributes to frailty and increased risk of mortality. The loss in skeletal muscle mass may also contribute to glucose intolerance in the elderly as a result of the decreasing mass of tissue available to take up glucose from blood.

One of the major changes in muscle biochemistry with age is an increase in the number of muscle cells with mitochondria deficient in cytochrome oxidase, which limits the muscle's ability to do work. As mitochondria become less efficient in oxidizing NADH, they become more reduced, and the accumulation of partially reduced ubiquinone (semiquinone) promotes the reduction of molecular oxygen, leading to increased superoxide production in older mitochondria (see Chapter 37). Under these conditions, when oxidative phosphorylation is impaired, cells appear to generate ATP primarily by glycolysis. NADH is also oxidized extramitochondrially, primarily by NADH oxidases in the plasma membrane, which produce hydrogen peroxide, but no ATP.

$$\text{NADH oxidase: } NADH + H^+ + O_2 \rightarrow NAD^+ + H_2O_2$$

These changes are observed in both cardiac and skeletal muscle and appear to result from major, random deletions in mitochondrial DNA (25–75% of total mtDNA), which are then amplified by clonal expansion, leading to fiber atrophy and breakage. The muscle fiber is only as strong as its weakest link, so that small regions of fiber loss affect overall muscle capacity. Fortunately, sarcopenia can be delayed and partially reversed by resistance exercise, thus the emphasis on regular exercise among the elderly.

(GH; stimulates IGF-1 secretion by liver), thyroid-stimulating hormone and prolactin (see Chapter 39). Their body weights are decreased as young adults by about 35% and their maximum lifespan increased by about 45% compared to littermates, but oddly they become obese with age. Similar effects on weight and lifespan are observed in mice with defects in GH or IGF-1 receptors or signal transduction. Many of these strains are fragile: Ames and Snell dwarfs are hypothyroid, hypoglycemic and hypoinsulinemic, and have low body temperature; they have impaired reproductive capacity, are more susceptible to infection, and require special housing conditions to maintain body temperature. Treatment of hypothyroidism in Snell dwarfs resulted in a restoration of a near normal lifespan, while hypophysectomy of young rats increases their maximum lifespan by 15–20%. Thus, three hormones that have a profound effect on metabolism and growth (growth hormone, IGF-1 (and insulin) and thyroxine) also have profound effects on lifespan.

In humans, the most significant genetic determinant of lifespan is sex: women live longer than men. Genetics accounts for an estimated 20–50% of the remaining variance in lifespan, the other 50–80% being attributed to environment and random developmental variations. It is estimated (in 2008) that there are at least 30 genes that have a significant effect on human lifespan. The cross-breeding of human populations and the many allelic combinations of these genes may obscure effects seen in inbred strains of worms or rodents. However, there is a recent report that Ashkenazi Jews who live past age 95 have a higher frequency of mutations in the gene for the IGF-1 receptor (IGF-1R). There are other genes or gene products that are associated with increased longevity in humans, e.g. variants in ApoE, ApoC3 and CETP. However, these genes seem to increase mean lifespan, probably by modulating the cardiovascular effects of dietary cholesterol, rather than cause an increase in maximum lifespan.

ANTI-AGING INTERVENTIONS – WHAT WORKS AND WHAT DOESN'T

Antioxidant supplements

Based on the FRTA, it seems reasonable to speculate that antioxidant supplementation should have an effect on longevity. In fact, however, there is no rigorous, reproducible experimental evidence that antioxidant supplements have any effect on maximum lifespan of humans or other vertebrates. At the same time, antioxidant supplements, most of which include vitamins, may improve health, particularly in those subjects with vitamin deficiencies. Thus, effects of antioxidant therapy on mean (and healthy) lifespan are not unexpected. Failure to affect maximum lifespan may result from the fact that there are so many mechanisms for production and control of free radicals and inhibiting or reversing damage to biomolecules. Many of these processes depend on the activity of enzymes that detoxify ROS or regenerate endogenous antioxidants. These enzymes, such as superoxide dismutase and glutathione peroxidase (Chapter 37), are induced in response to oxidative stress and may also be repressed during times of low oxidative stress. Thus, the body may respond to maintain a homeostatic balance between prooxidant and antioxidant forces (see Fig. 37.2), countering efforts to enhance antioxidant defenses. This response may be essential, for example, to maintain effective bactericidal activity during the respiratory burst accompanying phagocytosis.

Calorie restriction

Calorie restriction (CR) is the only intervention that consistently extends maximum lifespan in a variety of species, including mammals, fish, flies, worms, and yeast. Reduction in total caloric intake is the essential feature of this intervention, i.e. the beneficial, life-extending effects are observed whenever CR is applied and regardless of dietary composition, although early and prolonged intervention has more impressive effects. As shown in Figure 44.8, CR leads to a significant increase in both the mean and maximum lifespan of laboratory rats, equivalent to extending human lifespan to about 180 years. Calorie-restricted rats have fewer muscle fibers lacking in cytochrome oxidase and decreased levels of deletions in muscle mitochondrial DNA. CR mice also have lower levels of inducible genes for hepatic detoxification, DNA repair and response to oxidative stress (heat shock proteins), suggesting a lower rate of oxidative stress and damage to proteins and DNA.

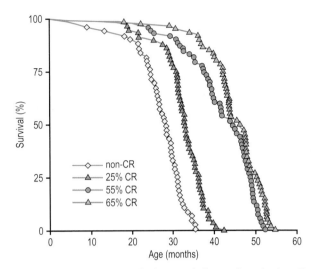

Fig. 44.8 **Calorie restriction (CR) extends longevity of mice.** The non-CR group received food *ad libitum*. Other groups were restricted by 25%, 55% and 65% of the *ad lib* diet, starting at 1 month of age (adapted from Weindruch R *et al.* Retardation of aging in mice by dietary restriction. *J Nutr* 1986;**116**:651–654).

CR also delays the onset of a wide range of age-related diseases, including cancer (Fig. 44.9), and is, in fact, the most potent, broad-acting cancer prevention regimen in rodents. It is argued that the extension of maximum lifespan by CR is achieved by delaying the onset of cancer. Long-lived animals are more efficient in protecting their genome and thereby delaying the onset of cancer, but CR may limit damage even more, preserving the integrity of the genome and thereby leading to a longer lifespan. While CR has not been tested in humans, obesity is a risk factor for cancer in humans.

In CR experiments, it has been difficult to differentiate between the effects of dietary restriction on energy expenditure (rate of living) versus the reduction in body weight that accompanies dietary restriction. FIRKO (adipose tissue (fat) insulin receptor knockout) mice have a 15–25% decrease in body mass, largely because of a 50% decrease in fat mass. However, these mice consume identical amounts of food per day as control littermates, actually more than the control animals when normalized to their body weight. They also have an ~20% increase in lifespan, suggesting that the decrease in body or fat mass is more important than caloric intake in determining maximum lifespan potential. In another study, overexpression of the gluconeogenic enzyme PEPCK in skeletal muscle produced a leaner mouse, with 50% of body weight and 10% of fat mass, compared to controls. These mice were seven times as active and ate 60% more than control mice, but lived longer and had longer reproductive life. Overall, the decrease in body weight or adiposity during CR, rather than the decrease in food consumption, appears to have the greater effect on lifespan extension. One general outcome from these dietary and genetic experiments is that mitochondrial efficiency, measured as lower

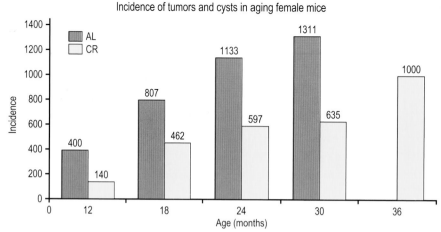

Fig. 44.9 Effect of calorie restriction (CR) on development of tumors in mice. Over 1000 mice, 50:50 male and female, from four different genotypes were divided into two groups, one fed *ad libitum* (AL), the other receiving 60% of the caloric intake of the control group (CR), but with comparable intake of vitamins, minerals and micronutrients. Cohorts of animals were sacrificed at specified times and total lesions (tumors plus cysts) were measured. At 24 months, 51% AL and 13% CR mice had tumors. Note the absence of tumors in control mice at 36 months – all of the control mice are dead! CR extended the mean and maximum lifespan of the mice and also delayed the onset of cancer (adapted from Bronson RT, Lipman RD. Reduction in rate of occurrence of age related lesions in dietary restricted laboratory mice. *Growth Dev Aging* 1991;**55**:169–184).

rates of ROS/ATP production, appears to be an important determinant of longevity.

Studies on CR in longer-lived, primate species have been under way since the late 1980s and there is clear evidence of cardiovascular and overall health benefits of CR in primates, although effects on maximum lifespan are not yet available. Even if CR can be shown to extend human lifespan, it is unlikely that humans will be able to adopt the strict dietary control required for this regimen. There are also some risks associated with caloric restriction, e.g. sterility and possibly increased susceptibility to environmental stress and microbial infection. However, understanding the biologic mechanisms of the effects of CR may lead to alternative strategies that mimic CR and extend lifespan.

Summary

Aging is characterized by a gradual decline in the capacity of physiologic systems, leading eventually to failure of a critical system, then death. At the biochemical level, aging is considered the result of chronic chemical modification of all classes of biomolecules. According to the free radical theory of aging, ROS are the primary culprits, causing alterations in the sequence of DNA (mutations) and structure of proteins. Longevity is achieved by developing efficient systems to limit and/or repair chemical damage. Caloric restriction is, at present, the only widely applicable mechanism for delaying aging and extending the mean, healthy, and maximum lifespan of species. CR appears to work, in part, by inhibiting the production of ROS and limiting damage to biomolecules, delaying many of the characteristic features of aging, including cancer.

ACTIVE LEARNING

1. Discuss the nature of protein carbonyls and lipofuscin and their relevance to aging.
2. Discuss the relative importance of chemical damage to protein and DNA during aging.
3. Review recent literature on mouse genetic models of mammalian aging and discuss the relationship between growth rate, obesity, calorie restriction and aging in the mouse.
4. Nearly a dozen genes have been identified that, when mutated, extend the lifespan of animals. Why are the wild type genes preserved in the gene pool?
5. Discuss the evidence that caloric restriction increases the mean, healthy and maximum lifespan of primates.

Further reading

Capri M, Salvioli S, Sevini F et al. The genetics of human longevity. *Ann NY Acad Sci* 2006;**1067**:252–263.

Chomyn A, Attardi G. MtDNA mutations in aging and apoptosis. *Biochem Biophys Res Commun* 2003;**304**:519–529.

Finch CF. *The biology of human longevity: inflammation, nutrition, and aging in the evolution of lifespans.* Amsterdam: Academic (Elsevier), 2007.

Harper ME, Bevilacqua L, Hagopian K, Weindruch R, Ramsey JJ. Ageing, oxidative stress, and mitochondrial coupling. *Acta Physiol Scand* 2004;**182**:321–331.

Hayflick L. Biological aging is no longer an unsolved problem. *Ann NY Acad Sci* 2007;**1100**:1–13.

Rincon M, Rudin E, Barzilai N. Insulin/IGF-1 signaling in mammals and its relevance to human longevity. *Exp Gerontol* 2005; **40**:873–877.

Terzioglu M, Larsson NG. Mitochondrial dysfunction in mammalian ageing. *Novartis Foundation Symp* 2007;**287**:197–213.

Tosato M, Zamboni V, Ferrini A, Cesari M. The aging process and potential interventions to extend life expectancy. *Clin Interv Aging* 2007;**2**:401–412.

Ungvari Z, Parrado-Fernandez C, Csiszar A, de Cabo R. Mechanisms underlying caloric restriction and lifespan regulation: implications for vascular aging. *Circ Res* 2008; **102**:519–528.

Websites

Caloric restriction: www.calorierestriction.org
Lecture notes on gerontology:
- www.pathguy.com/lectures/aging.htm
- www.benbest.com/lifeext/aging.html
Progeria: www.progeriaresearch.org/index.html
Telomeres: www.telomeres.net/

Selected clinical laboratory reference ranges

Yee Ping Teoh and M H Dominiczak

Reference ranges are values of a given substance (analyte) obtained in a reference population, which is usually a group of healthy individuals. These reference values represent the physiologic quantities of a substance (concentrations, activities or counts) to be expected in healthy persons. The term 'reference range' is preferred over 'normal range' because the reference population can be clearly defined whereas no clear definition exists for what is 'normal' in a clinical sense. Deviation above or below the reference range may be associated with a disease process, and the severity of the disease process may be associated with the magnitude of the deviation.

When data from a large cohort of healthy subjects fit a Gaussian distribution, the reference limits is defined as two standard deviations above and below the mean. This would constitute the central 95% interval of the distribution. Most analyte distributions are, however, non-Gaussian and these values are usually mathematically transformed (e.g. logarithmic, reciprocal, exponential transformation) to produce a Gaussian distribution.

The interpretation of results from laboratory tests is based on comparing them with reference values. If the value falls outside the reference interval, it signifies that the result varies from that seen in the reference population. Note that it is not necessarily abnormal: by definition, 5% of individuals in a reference population will have results outside the reference range (1 in 20 subjects). However, the further the result is from the reference range, the greater is the probability that it is associated with a pathology.

In some cases (such as with glucose, lipids or cardiac troponin measurements), instead of reference values, we use clinical decision limits; these are usually derived from epidemiologic studies linking the levels of a particular analyte with either the presence or the risk of a particular disease.

The reference values given here are either those used in North Glasgow University Hospitals, Glasgow, UK, or are quoted from publications listed in Further Reading below. Throughout the tables, intervals are given in SI and conventional units, together wherever possible with the factor for converting from SI to conventional units.

These values are given for guidance only and the reader should always check their local laboratory ranges before interpreting laboratory tests. Remember also that laboratory tests must always be interpreted in the context of clinical data derived from other sources, including medical history and physical examination.

To convert from an SI unit to a conventional unit, multiply by the conversion factor.

To convert from a conventional unit to an SI unit, divide by the conversion factor.

Unless indicated, the ranges given are for serum/plasma concentrations.

Blood gases	SI units	Conversion factor (SI to conventional units)	Conventional units
Arterial pH	7.37–7.44		
H^+ ion activity	36–43 nmol/L		
Arterial oxygen partial pressure (PaO_2)	10.5–13.5 kPa	×7.5	79–101 mmHg
Mixed venous oxygen partial pressure (PaO_2)	5.5–6.8 kPa	×7.5	41–51 mmHg
Arterial carbon dioxide partial pressure ($PaCO_2$)	4.6–6.0 kPa	×7.5	34–45 mmHg
Arterial bicarbonate	19–24 mmol/l	×1.0	19–24 mEq/L
Base excess	±2 mmol/l	×1.0	±2 mEq/L
Anion gap ($Na^+ + K^+$) – ($HCO_3^- + Cl^-$)	12–16 mmol/l	×1.0	12–16 mEq/L
Carboxyhemoglobin	0.005–0.01%		
Methemoglobin	<1.5%		

Serum electrolytes and markers of renal function	SI units	Conversion factor (SI to conventional units)	Conventional units
Sodium	135–145 mmol/L	×1.0	135–145 mEq/L
Potassium	3.5–5.0 mmol/L	×1.0	3.5–5.0 mEq/L
Chloride	95–108 mmol/L	×1.0	95–108 mEq/L
Bicarbonate	20–25 mmol/L	×1.0	20–25 mEq/L
Urea	2.5–6.5 mmol/L	×6.02	16.2–39 mg/dL
Creatinine	20–80 umol/L	×0.0113	0.23–0.90 mg/dL
Magnesium	0.7–1.0 mmol/L	×2.43	1.7–2.4 mg/dL
Osmolality	285–295 mmol/kg	×1.0	285–295 mOsm/kg

Serum proteins, bone and markers of liver function	SI units	Conversion factor (SI to conventional units)	Conventional units
Total protein	60–80 g/L	×0.1	6–8 g/dL
Albumin	36–52 g/L	×0.1	3.6–5.2 g/dL
Globulins	19–33 g/L Calculated value = (total protein − albumin)	×0.1	1.9–3.3 g/dL
Immunoglobulins:			
IgG	6–16 g/L		
IgA	0.8–4.0 g/L		
IgM	0.5–2.0 g/L		
C-reactive protein (CRP)	<95 nmol/L	×0.105	<10 mg/L
Haptoglobin	0.2–2 g/L	×100	20–200 mg/dL
Ferritin	31–450 pmol/L	×0.445	14–200 μg/L
Fibrinogen	5.8–11.8 umol/L	×0.345	2–4 g/L
$\beta 2$-microglobulin	1.2–2.4 mg/L		
Calcium:			
total calcium	2.20–2.60 mmol/L	×4.0	8.8–10.4 mg/dL
ionized calcium	1.1–1.3 mmol/L		4.4–5.2 mg/dL
Phosphate	0.7–1.4 mmol/L	×3.1	2.2–4.3 mg/dL
Bilirubin	<17 μmol/L	×0.058	<1 mg/dL
Alkaline phosphatase adults	50–260 U/L		
Alanine aminotransferase (ALT)	<50 U/L		
Aspartate aminotransferase (AST)	10–40 U/L		
γ-glutamyl transferase (GGT):			
men	<90 U/L		
women	<50 U/L		

Selected hormones	SI units	Conversion factor (SI to conventional units)	Conventional units
Thyroid stimulating hormone (TSH)	0.4–4.0 mU/L		
Free T4	9–25 pmol/L	×0.08	0.7–2.0 ng/dL
Total T4	55–144 nmol/L	×0.08	4.4–12 μg/dL
Free T3	3.5–6.5 pmol/l	×65	228–422 pg/dL
Total T3	0.9–2.8 nmol/L	×0.65	0.6–1.8 ng/mL
Cortisol (plasma):			
at 08:00h	190–690 nmol/L	×0.036	7–15 μg/dL
at 24:00h	<50 nmol/L		<2 μg/dL
urinary free cortisol	<250 nmol/24h		<9 μg/dL
Short Synacthen test:			
basal cortisol	>225 nmol/L	×0.036	8 ug/dL
increment	>200 nmol/L		7 ug/dL
30 min cortisol	>500 nmol/L		18 ug/dL
Adrenocorticotropin (ACTH)	<17.6 pmol/l	×4.55	<80 ng/L
Aldosterone:			
supine	83–271 pmol/L	×0.03	3–10 ng/dL
upright	139–832 pmol/L		5–30 ng/dL
Plasma renin activity:			
supine	0.51–2.64 ng/ml/h		
upright	0.98–4.18 ng/ml/h		
Follicle stimulating hormone (FSH):			
follicular phase	3–13 U/L	×1.0	3–13 mIU/mL
midcycle phase	9–18 U/L		9–18 mIU/mL
luteal phase	1–10 U/L		1–10 mIU/mL
postmenopausal	18–150 U/L		18–150 mIU/mL
Luteinizing hormone:			
follicular phase	2–15 U/L	×1.0	2–15 mIU/mL
midcycle phase	22–90 U/L		22– mIU/mL
luteal phase	1–19 U/L		1–19 mIU/mL
postmenopausal	16–64 U/L		16–64 mIU/mL
Prolactin:			
men	<400 mU/L		
women	<630 mU/L		
Progesterone (midluteal phase)	>20 nmol/L	×0.33	>6.4 ng/mL
17-hydroxyprogesterone	<50 nmol/L	×0.32	<16 pg/L
Human chorionic gonadotrophin (hCG)	<5 U/L Varies with gestational age		
Testosterone:			
men (<50 years)	10–36 nmol/L	×28.8	288–1038 ng/dL
women (<50 years)	1.0–3.2 nmol/L		29–92 ng/dL
Sex hormone binding globulin:			
men (<50 years)	6–45 nmol/L	×0.112	0.7–3.1 μg/mL
women (<50 years)	30–120 nmol/L		3.4–13.5 μg/mL
Insulin	<13 mU/L undetectable in hypoglycemia	×6.9	<90 pmol/L

(continued)

Selected hormones	SI units	Conversion factor (SI to conventional units)	Conventional units
C-peptide	0.36–1.12 nmol/L	×3	1.1–3.4 ng/mL
Parathyroid hormone	1.1–6.9 pmol/L	×9.16	11–69 pg/mL
Brain natriuretic peptide (BNP):			
NT-proBNP (<75 years)	<125 pg/mL		
BNP	<100 pg/mL		

Trace elements, metal-binding proteins and vitamins	SI units	Conversion factor (SI to conventional units)	Conventional units
Ceruloplasmin	200–450 mg/L	×100	20–45 mg/dL
Copper	10–22 µmol/L	×6.54	65.4–144 µg/L
Zinc	9–20 µmol/L	×6.5	78–118 µg/dL
Selenium	0.8–2.0 µmol/L	×79	6–16 mg/dL
Iron	10–30 µmol/L	×5.59	56–167 µg/dL
Transferrin	2.2–4.0 µmol/L	×0.8	1.8–3.2 g/L
Ferritin			30–280 mg/L
Vitamin A	1.05–2.8 µmol/L	×28.6	30–80 µg/dL
Vitamin B_1 (as erythrocyte thiamine diphosphate)	275–675 ng/g Hb		
Vitamin B_2 (flavin adenine nucloetide)	220–410 nmol/L	×0.038	8.4–15.6 µg/dL
Vitamin B_6 (pyridoxal phosphate)	20–140 nmol/L	×0.247	4.9–34.6 ng/mL
Vitamin C (ascorbic acid)	15–90 µmol/L	×0.176	2.6–15.8 mg/L
25-hydroxy vitamin D	25–170 nmol/L	×0.4	10–68 µg/L
Vitamin E (tocopherol)	15–45 µmol/L	×0.43	6.5–19.4 µg/mL
Vitamin B_{12}	138–780 nmol/l	×1.36	187–1060 ng/L
Folate	12–33 µmol/L	×0.442	5.3–14.6 µg/L

Therapeutic drug monitoring	SI units	Conversion factor (SI to conventional units)	Conventional units
Carbamazepine	1.0–2.8 μmol/L	×4.2	4.0–12.0 mg/L
Digoxin	1.0–2.6 nmol/L	×0.78	0.5–2.0 μg/L
Gentamicin:		×0.48	
trough	<4 μmol/L		<2 mg/L
1 hour post dose	10.4–21 μmol/L		5–10 mg/L
Lithium	0.6–1.0 mmol/L	×1.0	0.6–1.0 mEg/L
Phenytoin:		×0.25	
adults	40–80 μmol/L		10–20 mg/L
neonates	25–40 μmol/L		6.25–10 mg/L
Phenobarbitone:		×0.23	
adults	60–180 μmol/L		14–41 mg/L
neonates	60–120 μmol/L		14–28 mg/L
Theophylline:		×0.18	
adult	55–110 μmol/L		10–20 mg/L
neonates	28–55 μmol/L		5–10 mg/L
Sodium valproate	350–700 μmol/L	×0.14	50–100 mg/L
Vancomycin:	<7.0 μmol/L	×1.44	<10 mg/L
2 h end infusion trough	12.5–18 μmol/L		18–26 mg/L

Analytes where clinical decision limits are used	SI units	Conversion factor (SI to conventional units)	Conventional units
Total cholesterol (desirable)	≤4.0 mmol/L	×38.6	≤155 mg/dL
LDL-cholesterol (optimal) (Calculated LDL = Chol − HDL-C − 0.46 × TG)	≤2.0 mmol/L	×38.6	≤77 mg/dL
HDL-cholesterol (desirable)	≥1.0 mmol/L (men) ≥1.2 mmol/l (women)	×38.6	40 mg/dL 46 mg/dL
Triglycerides (desirable)	≤1.7 mmol/L	×88.4	<150 mg/dL
Glucose:		×18	
normal range (plasma)	4.0–6.0 mmol/L		72–109 mg/dL
fasting	<6.1 mmol/L		<110 mg/dL
impaired fasting glucose	≥6.1 mmol/L but <7.0 mmol/L		≥110 mg/dL but <126 mg/dL
diabetes	≥7.0 mmol/L		≥126 mg/dL
Glycated hemoglobin (DCCT calibrated) acceptable glycemic control	<7% (varies with type of patient)		
Cardiac troponin:			
Troponin–I	<0.1 μg/L	×1.0	<0.1 ng/mL
Troponin–T	<0.1 μg/L	×1.0	<0.1 ng/mL

For more details on lipid values and goals of treatment see http://www.nhlbi.nih.gov/guidelines/cholesterol/atp3xsum.pdf (US recommendations) and http://www.bcs.com/download/651/JBS2final.pdf (British recommendations)

Neurotransmitters and their metabolites	SI units	Conversion factor (SI to conventional units)	Conventional units
Norepinephrine: plasma urine	1094–1625 pmol/L <900 nmol/24h	0.169	185–275 ng/L <152 mg/24h
Epinephrine: plasma urine	164–464 pmol/L <230 nmol/24h	0.182	30–85 ng/L <42 mg/24h
Urine vanillylmandelic acid	<35.5 mmol/24h	0.198	<7.0 mg/24h
Urine 5-hydroxy indoleacetic acid (5-HIAA)	10–52 mmol/24h	0.191	3–14 mg/24h

Miscellaneous	SI units	Conversion factor (SI to conventional units)	Conventional units
Creatine kinase	210 U/L		
Amylase	0–100 U/L		
Urate: male female	0.2–0.5 mmol/L 0.1–0.4 mmol/L	×16.8	5.0–8.0 mg/dL 2.5–6.2 mg/dL
Ammonia	15–88 µmol/L	×1.7	25–150 µg/dL
Lactate	0.7–1.8 mmol/L	×9.0	6–16 mg/dL
Urine porphobilinogen	<9 µmol/24h	0.226	<2 mg/24h

Cerebrospinal fluid (CSF)	SI units	Conversion factor (SI to conventional units)	Conventional units
Protein	<0.45 g/L		
Glucose	3.3–4.4 mmol/L (normal >65% of plasma glucose)	×18.0	59–79 mg/dL
Lactate	<2.2 mmol/L	×9.0	<20 mg/dL

Urine	SI units	Conversion factor (SI to conventional units)	Conventional units
Microalbumin			
Albumin/creatinine ratio: men women	<20 mg/L ACR <2.5 mg/mmol creat ACR <3.5 mg/mmol creat		
Albumin excretion rate	AER <20 μg/min		
Sodium	75–300 mmol/24h	×1.0	75–300 mEq/24h
Potassium	40–100 mmol/24h	×1.0	40–100 mEq/24 hour
Chloride	100–250 mmol/24hours	×1.0	150–250 mEq/24h
Urea	420–720 mmol/24h	×0.028	11.8–20.2 g/24h
Calcium	2.5–7.5 mmol/24h	×40	100–300 mg/24h
Magnesium	2.5–8.0 mmol/24hours	×24.3	61–194 mg/24h
Phosphate	10–40 mmol/24h	×0.03	0.31–1.24 g/24h
Copper	0.2–0.6 μmol/24h	×6.54	1.3–3.9 μg/24h
Creatinine	9–18 mmol/24h	×0.11	1.0–2.0 g/24h
Osmolality	50–1200 mmol/kg	×1.0	50–1200 mOsm/kg

Reference intervals for hematology tests	SI units	Conventional units
Hemoglobin: men women newborns children	8.1–11.2 mmol/L 7.4–9.9 mmol/L 10.2–12.1 mmol/L 7.0–10.2 mmol/L	13.0–18.0 g/dL 12.0–16.0 g/dL 16.5–19.5 g/dL 11.2–16.5 g/dL
Hematocrit	41–46%	41–46 mL/dL
Mean corpuscular hemoglobin (MCH)	26–34 pg/cell	26–34 pg/cell
Mean corpuscular volume (MCV)	80–96 fL	80–96 μm^3
Mean corpuscular hemoglobin concentration (MCHC)	320–360 g/L	32–36 g/dL
Erythrocyte cell count: men women	4.4–5.9 × 10^6/mL 3.8–5.2 × 10^6/mL	4.6–6.2 million/mm^3 3.8–5.2 million/mm^3
Leukocytes, total	4.0–11.0 × 10^9/L	4000–11 000/mm^3
Leukocytes, differential count: neutrophil lymphocytes monocytes eosinophil basophil	2–7.5 × 10^9/L 1.3–4 × 10^9/L 0.2–0.8 × 10^9/L 0.04–0.4 × 10^9/L 0.01–0.1 × 10^9/L	45–74% 16–45% 4.0–10% 0.0–7.0% 0.0–2.0%
Platelets	150–400 × 10^9/L	150 000–400 000/mm^3
Reticulocytes	25–75 × 10^9/L	0.5–1.5% of erythrocytes

(continued)

Reference intervals for hematology tests	SI units	Conventional units
Erythrocyte sedimentation rate (ESR)	2–10 mm/h	
Activated partial thromboplastin time (APTT)	30–50 sec	
Prothrombin time (PT)	10–15 sec	
INR Therapeutic range (differs according to underlying condition)	0.9–1.2 2.0–4.0	
Thrombin clotting time (TCT)	11–18 sec	
Fibrinogen	2.0–4.0 g	200–400 mg/dL
Bleeding time (template)	2.0–10.0 min	2.0–10 min
d-Dimer	<0.25 g/L	

Further reading

Bakerman S. *Bakerman's ABC of interpretive laboratory data*. 4th edn Scottsdale, AZ: Interpretive Laboratory Data, 2002; Comment: p.580.

Burtis C, Ashwood ER. *Tietz textbook of clinical chemistry*, 3rd edn Philadelphia: Saunders, 1999; Comment: p.1917.

Dominiczak MH (ed). *Seminars in clinical biochemistry*. Glasgow: University of Glasgow, 1997; Comment: p.415.

Jakob M. *Normal values pocket book*. Hermosa Beach, CA: Borm Bruckmeier, 2002; Comment: p.220.

Index

Please note that page references relating to non-textual content such as Figures or Tables are in *italic* print